MW00845431

5TH EDITION

MANUAL FOR
Radiation Oncology Nursing Practice and Education

Edited by

Maurene McQuestion, RN, BA, BScN, MSc, CON(C)

Lorraine C. Drapek, DNP, FNP-BC, AOCNP®

Mary Ellyn Witt, MS, RN, AOCN®

Oncology Nursing Society
Pittsburgh, Pennsylvania

ONS Publications Department

Publisher and Director of Publications: William A. Tony, BA, CQIA
Senior Editorial Manager: Lisa M. George, MPH, BA, CHES
Acquisitions Editor: John Zaphyr, BA, MEd
Staff Editor: Andrew Petyak, BA
Associate Staff Editor: Casey S. Kennedy, BA
Design and Production Administrator: Dany Sjoen
Editorial Assistant: Rachel Geffrey, BFA

First printing, May 2021; second printing, March 2024

Library of Congress Cataloging-in-Publication Data

Names: McQuestion, Maurene, editor. | Drapek, Lorraine C., editor. | Witt,
  Mary Ellyn, editor. | Oncology Nursing Society, issuing body.
Title: Manual for radiation oncology nursing practice and education /
  edited by Maurene McQuestion, Lorraine C. Drapek, Mary Ellyn Witt.
Other titles: Radiation oncology nursing practice and education
Description: 5th edition. | Pittsburgh, Pennsylvania : Oncology Nursing
  Society, [2021] | Includes bibliographical references and index.
Identifiers: LCCN 2021001111 (print) | LCCN 2021001112 (ebook) | ISBN
  9781635930436 (paperback) | ISBN 9781635930443 (ebook)
Subjects: MESH: Oncology Nursing--education | Radiation Oncology--education
  | Outline
Classification: LCC RC266 (print) | LCC RC266 (ebook) | NLM WY 18.2 |
  DDC 616.99/40231--dc23
LC record available at https://lccn.loc.gov/2021001111
LC ebook record available at https://lccn.loc.gov/2021001112

Publisher's Note

Printed in the United States of America

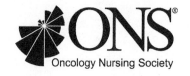

Oncology Nursing Society

Innovation   •   Excellence   •   Advocacy   •   Inclusivity

Contributors

Editors

Maurene McQuestion, RN, BA, BScN, MSc, CON(C)
Clinical Nurse Specialist, Radiation Medicine Programme
Co-Lead, Head and Neck Cancer Survivorship Programme
Princess Margaret Cancer Centre
University Health Network
Toronto, Ontario, Canada

Lorraine C. Drapek, DNP, FNP-BC, AOCNP®
Nurse Practitioner, Radiation Oncology, Gastrointestinal Service
Massachusetts General Hospital
Boston, Massachusetts

Mary Ellyn Witt, MS, RN, AOCN®
Survivorship Care Coordinator
University of Chicago Cancer Center at Silver Cross Hospital
New Lenox, Illinois

Authors

Brittany Adams, FNP-C
Advanced Practice Nurse
Provision Center for Proton Therapy
Knoxville, Tennessee
IV.G. Treatment of patients who are pregnant; VIII.G. Proton beam therapy

Deborah Hutchinson Allen, PhD, RN, CNS, FNP-BC, AOCNP®
Nurse Scientist, Director of Nursing Research and Evidence-Based Practice
Duke University Health System
Durham, North Carolina
V.A. Brain and central nervous system

Karen J. Allen, MSN, ANP-BC, RN, OCN®
Nurse Practitioner, Department of Radiation Oncology
Duke Cancer Institute
Duke University Health System
Durham, North Carolina
V.A. Brain and central nervous system

Shaylene Baumgartner, MSN, RN
Nursing Instructor
Clarkson College
Omaha, Nebraska
IV.A. Fatigue

Susan Weiss Behrend, RN, MSN, AOCN®
Clinical Nurse Specialist, Department of Nursing
Fox Chase Cancer Center
Philadelphia, Pennsylvania
VI.C. Benign conditions and benign tumors

Sarah Belcher, PhD, RN, OCN®
Assistant Professor, Health and Community Systems
University of Pittsburgh School of Nursing
Pittsburgh, Pennsylvania
IV.E. Sexual function and dysfunction

Renata Benc, RN, BA, MSc(A), CON(C)
Clinical Nurse Consultant, Division of Oncology
Jewish General Hospital
Integrated Health and Social Services University Network for West-Central Montréal
Montréal, Québec, Canada
IV.B. Skin reactions

Theresa S. Brown, PharmD, BCOP, CPP
Clinical Oncology Pharmacist
Duke Cancer Center
Duke University Health System
Durham, North Carolina
X.A. Radiosensitizers and concurrent chemotherapy and biotherapy

Deborah W. Bruner, PhD, RN
Senior Vice President for Research
Emory University
Atlanta, Georgia
IV.E. Sexual function and dysfunction

Sarah Buchanan, RD
Registered Dietitian
Princess Margaret Cancer Centre
University Health Network
Toronto, Ontario, Canada
IV.H. Nutritional issues

Angela Cashell, MRTT, MSc
Clinical Educator, Radiation Medicine Program
Princess Margaret Cancer Centre
University Health Network
Toronto, Ontario, Canada
VIII.A. External beam radiation therapy (teletherapy)

Emilie Cecil, MS, CRNP
Nurse Practitioner
Radiation Oncology, Head and Neck Cancer
Johns Hopkins Hospital
Baltimore, Maryland
V.B. Head and neck

Rustica Cerillo, BSN, RN, OCN®
Clinical Nurse IV
Duke Cancer Institute
Duke University Health System
Durham, North Carolina
V.E. Gastrointestinal tract and abdomen

Barbara Clendinning, RN, BSN, OCN®
Registered Nurse
Duke Cancer Institute
Duke University Health System
Durham, North Carolina
V.G. Male pelvis and prostate

Rachel W. Conklin, MMS, PA-C
Physician Assistant, Radiation Oncology Survivorship and Telemedicine
Vanderbilt University Medical Center
Nashville, Tennessee
IV.K. Cardiac toxicities and cardiac implantable electronic devices

Kimberly DeBaun, RN, BSN, CNML
Nurse Manager, Radiation Oncology
Duke Cancer Center
Duke University Health System
Durham, North Carolina
*VIII.B. Low-dose-rate and high-dose-rate
   brachytherapy*

**Susan A. DiStasio, DNP, ANP-C, APRN,
AOCNP®**
Nurse Practitioner, Radiation Oncology
Norris Cotton Cancer Center
Dartmouth Hitchcock Medical Center
Lebanon, New Hampshire
IV.C. Pain

Kathryn Ericson, RN, BSN, PCCN
Clinical Nurse III, Radiation Oncology
Duke Cancer Center
Duke University Health System
Durham, North Carolina
*VIII.B. Low-dose-rate and high-dose-rate
   brachytherapy*

Marsha Fair, BSN, RN
Radiation Oncology Nurse
Johns Hopkins Hospital
Baltimore, Maryland
V.B. Head and neck

Lisa Feldsien, BSN, BSN, OCN®
Staff Nurse, Radiation Oncology
Baptist Health Paducah
Paducah, Kentucky
IX.D. Patients with special needs

**Maria B. Fenton-Kerimian, APRN-BC, MA,
RN, BSN, OCN®**
Nurse Practitioner
Weill Cornell Medicine
New York, New York
V.C. Breast

Marcia Flynn-Post, RN, BA, MHST, CON(C)
Nurse Manager, Clinical Trials
Princess Margaret Cancer Centre
University Health Network
Toronto, Ontario, Canada
XI.C. Cancer clinical trials

Olivia Franek, BSN, RN, OCN®
Clinical Nurse IV
Duke Cancer Center
Duke University Health System
Durham, North Carolina
V.E. Gastrointestinal tract and abdomen

Sarah Hales, MD, PhD, FRCPC
Psychiatrist and Assistant Professor
Princess Margaret Cancer Centre
University Health Network
Toronto, Ontario, Canada
IX.F. Patients with mental illness

Tina Q. Harris, MS, NP-C, AOCNP®
Executive Managing Director
Chattanooga Tumor Clinic
Chattanooga, Tennessee
*X.B. Radioimmunotherapy and
   radiopharmaceuticals*

Hilda Haynes-Lewis, PhD, ANP-BC, AOCNP®
Nurse Practitioner
Montefiore Medical Center
New York, New York
IV.J. Late effects of treatment

John Vernon Hillson, BA, RN, BSN, OCN®
Clinical Nurse III, Radiation Oncology
Duke Cancer Center
Duke University Health System
Durham, North Carolina
*X.A. Radiosensitizers and concurrent
   chemotherapy and biotherapy*

**Karol J. Huenerberg, MSN, FNP-BC,
APNP, AOCNP®**
Nurse Practitioner, Radiation Oncology
University of Wisconsin Hospitals and Clinics
Madison, Wisconsin
IV.I. Neutropenia

Melissa James, BSN, RN, BMTCN, OCN®
Nurse Educator
Barbara Ann Karmanos Cancer Center
Detroit, Michigan
*VIII.D. Total body irradiation and
   hematopoietic stem cell transplantation*

Rana Jin, RN, BSN, MSN, CON(C)
Clinical Nurse Specialist, Geriatric
   Oncology
Princess Margaret Cancer Centre
University Health Network
Toronto, Ontario, Canada
*IX.E. Patients with cognitive changes and
   dementia*

Anet Julius, RN, BScN, MN, CON(C)
Director of Professional Practice
Princess Margaret Cancer Centre
University Health Network
Toronto, Ontario, Canada
V.H. Female pelvis

Marcelle Kaplan, RN, MS, CNS
Oncology Nursing Consultant
Merrick, New York
*VII. Oncologic Emergencies, Spinal Cord
   Compression and Superior Vena Cava
   Syndrome*

Melissa A. Kerr, BSN, RN, OCN®
Certified Registered Nurse
Sentara Radiation Oncology
Virginia Beach, Virginia
IX.D. Patients with special needs

Amber Killam, RN, MScN, CON(C)
Nurse Educator, Medical Oncology
   Department
The Ottawa Hospital
Ottawa, Ontario, Canada
IV.B. Skin reactions

Pam Laszewski, BSN, RN, OCN®
Clinical Leader
Barbara Ann Karmanos Cancer Center
Detroit, Michigan
*VIII.D. Total body irradiation and
   hematopoietic stem cell transplantation*

Jennifer Li, BSc, CCRP
Clinical Research Manager
Princess Margaret Cancer Centre
University Health Network
Toronto, Ontario, Canada
XI.C. Cancer clinical trials

**Rachel Lopez, MSN, APRN, FNP-C,
AOCNP®**
Nurse Practitioner, Multi-Specialty Surgery
Albany Medical Center
Albany, New York
VI.A. Sarcomas

Allison Loucks, APN
Clinical Nurse Specialist, Geriatric
   Oncology
Princess Margaret Cancer Centre
University Health Network
Toronto, Ontario, Canada
*IX.E. Patients with cognitive changes and
   dementia*

Laura Mitchell, RN, MN, CON(C)
Interim Senior Professional Practice
   Leader
Princess Margaret Cancer Centre
University Health Network
Toronto, Ontario, Canada
*IV.F. Fertility; IX.B. Adolescent and young
   adult radiation oncology*

**Tayreez Mushani, RN, BScN, MSH,
CON(C), CHPCN(C)**
Advanced Practice Nurse Educator
University Health Network
Toronto, Ontario, Canada
VIII.H. Cobalt therapy

Shannon Nixon, MN, NP
Nurse Practitioner, Malignant Hematology
Princess Margaret Cancer Centre
University Health Network
Toronto, Ontario, Canada
VI.B. Lymphomas

Eugenia Perevalova, DMP, DABR
Medical Physicist
University of Chicago Comprehensive
   Cancer Center at Silver Cross Hospital
New Lenox, Illinois
II. Practice of Radiation Oncology

Dorothy Pierce, DNP, NP-C, CRN
Advanced Practice Nurse
Rutgers Cancer Institute of New Jersey
New Brunswick, New Jersey
*III. Radiation Protection and Safety; VIII.C.
   Stereotactic radiosurgery; VIII.E. Total
   skin irradiation*

Joanne Pun, BSc, RD, CNSC
Registered Dietitian
Princess Margaret Cancer Centre
University Health Network
Toronto, Ontario, Canada
IV.H. Nutritional issues

Martine Puts, RN, PhD
Canada Research Chair in the Care of Frail
  Older Adults
Associate Professor
Lawrence. S. Bloomberg Faculty of Nursing
University of Toronto
Toronto, Ontario, Canada
*IX.E. Patients with cognitive changes and
  dementia*

Annette Quinn, RN, MSN
Clinical Nurse Specialist
UPMC
Pittsburgh, Pennsylvania
X.C. Immunotherapy

Lindy Romanovsky, MD, BCH, BAO
Staff Geriatrician
Sinai Health System
Clinical Associate
University Health Network
Toronto, Ontario, Canada
*IX.E. Patients with cognitive changes and
  dementia*

**Susan "Kate" Sandstrom, RN, MSN,
APRN-CNP, AOCN®**
Certified Nurse Practitioner, Radiation
  Oncology
Seidman Cancer Center
University Hospital
Cleveland, Ohio
XII. Patient, Caregiver, and Family Education

**Jennifer Schmid, MSN, BS, RN, FNP-C,
OCN®, EMT-P**
Nurse Practitioner, Radiation Oncology
Henry Ford Allegiance Health
Jackson, Michigan
XI.A. Survivorship

Rickinder Sethi, MD, FRCPC
Clinical Psychiatry Fellow
Princess Margaret Cancer Centre
University Health Network
Toronto, Ontario, Canada
IX.F. Patients with mental illness

Brenda L. Silvia, ANP-C
Nurse Practitioner
Massachusetts General Hospital
Boston, Massachusetts
V.F. Bladder

Fay Strohschein, RN, PhD
Senior Clinical Research Coordinator
Oncology and Aging Program
Jewish General Hospital
Montréal, Québec, Canada
IX.C. Older adult radiation oncology

Nannette Thomas, DNP, CNP
Nurse Practitioner
Sarcoma and Connective Tissue Oncology
  Service
Department of Radiation Oncology
Massachusetts General Hospital
Boston, Massachusetts
*I. Scope of Practice for the Registered
  Nurse*

Keri Wagner, RN, FNP-C, OCN®
Nurse Leader, Nurse Practitioner
Memorial Sloan Kettering Cancer Center
  Commack
Commack, New York
V.D. Thorax

Ann Walsh, RN, MSN, OCN®
Radiation Oncology Nurse Navigator
Baptist MD Anderson
Jacksonville, Florida
IV.D. Distress and coping

Nicole Marie Wilson, BSN, RN, OCN®
Registered Nurse
Duke Cancer Center
Duke University Health System
Durham, North Carolina
IX.B. Pediatric radiation oncology

Shiby Wilson, DNP, MSN, RN, FNP-C
Advanced Practice Registered Nurse, CNS
  and Pediatric Services
Department of Radiation Oncology
University of Texas MD Anderson Cancer
  Center
Houston, Texas
VIII.F. Total lymphoid irradiation

Christine Zywine, RN(EC), MSN, CON(C)
Nurse Practitioner, Palliative Radiation
  Oncology Program
Princess Margaret Cancer Centre
University Health Network
Toronto, Ontario, Canada
IV.L Bone metastasis; XI.B. Palliative care

Disclosure

Editors and authors of books and guidelines provided by the Oncology Nursing Society are expected to disclose to the readers any significant financial interest or other relationships with the manufacturer(s) of any commercial products.

A vested interest may be considered to exist if a contributor is affiliated with or has a financial interest in commercial organizations that may have a direct or indirect interest in the subject matter. A "financial interest" may include, but is not limited to, being a shareholder in the organization; being an employee of the commercial organization; serving on an organization's speakers bureau; or receiving research funding from the organization. An "affiliation" may be holding a position on an advisory board or some other role of benefit to the commercial organization. Vested interest statements appear in the front matter for each publication.

Contributors are expected to disclose any unlabeled or investigational use of products discussed in their content. This information is acknowledged solely for the information of the readers.

The contributors provided the following disclosure and vested interest information:

Maurene McQuestion, RN, BA, BScN, MSc, CON(C): Canadian Association of Nurses in Oncology, employment or leadership position

Lorraine C. Drapek, DNP, FNP-BC, AOCNP®: QED Therapeutics, honoraria

Deborah Hutchinson Allen, PhD, RN, CNS, FNP-BC, AOCNP®: Nursing and Patient Care Innovations LLC, consultant or advisory role

Sarah Belcher, PhD, RN, OCN®: Oncology Nursing Society Metro Atlanta chapter, honoraria; National Institute of Nursing Research, Sigma Theta Tau International Alpha Epsilon chapter, research funding

Deborah W. Bruner, PhD, RN: City of Hope, honoraria

Emilie Cecil, MS, CRNP: Unitech Medical, other remuneration

Tina Q. Harris, MS, NP-C, AOCNP®: Advanced Practitioner Society for Hematology and Oncology, Chattanooga Area Nurses in Advanced Practice, Health Disparities Task Force for Hamilton County, Tennessee, employment or leadership position; Oncology Nursing Foundation, other remuneration

Marcelle Kaplan, RN, MS, CNS: Western Schools, employment or leadership position

Pam Laszewski, BSN, RN, OCN®: Oncology Nursing Society Metro Detroit chapter, honoraria

Shannon Nixon, MN, NP: AbbVie, AstraZeneca, Celgene, consultant or advisory role

Licensing Opportunities

The Oncology Nursing Society (ONS) produces some of the most highly respected educational resources in the field of oncology nursing, including ONS's award-winning journals, books, online courses, evidence-based resources, core competencies, videos, and information available on the ONS website at www.ons.org. ONS welcomes opportunities to license reuse of these intellectual properties to other organizations.

Licensing opportunities include the following:

- **Reprints**—Purchase high-quality reprints of ONS journal articles, book chapters, and other content directly from ONS, or obtain permission to produce your own reprints.
- **Translations**—Translate and then resell or share ONS resources internationally.
- **Integration**—Purchase a license to incorporate ONS's oncology-specific telephone triage protocols or other resources into your institution's EMR or EHR system.
- **Cobranding**—Display your company's logo on ONS resources for distribution to your organization's employees or customers.
- **Educational reuse**—Supplement your staff or student educational programs using ONS resources.
- **Customization**—Customize ONS intellectual property for inclusion in your own products or services.
- **Bulk purchases**—Buy ONS books and online courses in high quantities to receive great savings compared to regular pricing.

As you read through the pages of this book, think about whether any of these opportunities are the right fit for you as you consider reusing ONS content—and the contents of this book—for your organization.

Contact licensing@ons.org with your licensing questions or requests.

Table of Contents

Introduction

Advances in technology, research, and evidence-based practice have led to improvements in the care of patients receiving radiation therapy. The knowledge and expertise required by nurses must focus on the needs of patients who come into their care at any point across the trajectory of the cancer journey. These patients may be currently receiving specialized radiation therapy or have received it previously. Nurses may work in tertiary or quaternary care hospital settings and large academic medical centers and provide care to patients undergoing multimodal therapies or clinical trial protocols, both of which can include radiation. Others may work in stand-alone radiation therapy settings, local urgent care locations, and remote community settings. Regardless of the geographic location and range of specialty practices, nurses may have varying levels of knowledge and skill when caring for patients receiving radiation therapy as part of overall cancer care. Across settings, nurses provide care for patients who are dealing with symptoms and acute side effects of radiation therapy, as well as late effects occurring months or years after treatment.

The Oncology Nursing Society has published the fifth edition of *Manual for Radiation Oncology Nursing Practice and Education* to support nurses nationally and internationally who work in diverse settings caring for patients who will receive, are receiving, or have received radiation therapy. This manual is an excellent resource for individual nurses new to working in a radiation therapy setting, regardless of their years in oncology nursing, as well as to nurses wanting to advance their knowledge in radiation biology and protection, diverse radiation therapy modalities, combination treatments, site- or disease-specific considerations, symptom management, special populations, and care during transition points. Additionally, this manual can be a resource to advanced practice clinicians, educators, and administrators, with a focus on support for nursing staff seeking the education and skills required to care for patients receiving radiation therapy and their families.

The fifth edition has had significant updates and changes to the content. Many sections that had been updated in past editions now required a new focus or a complete rewrite as a result of the advances in technology, treatment options, and symptom management. New sections have been added based on input from radiation oncology nurses or because of changes in treatment options, the needs of specific patient populations, and observations from clinical practice. New topics include patients with cognitive changes and dementia; general distress and coping; patients with mental illness; special populations, such as women who are pregnant and adolescents and young adults; special needs related to late effects of treatment and cardiac toxicities; and treatment modalities, including cobalt therapy and immunotherapy.

Comprehensive literature reviews were completed by authors for updates, revisions, and new information, along with extensive review by the editors and external peer review. References to articles, texts, guidelines, and respected websites for medical, nursing, or professional associations are provided within each section. Readers are encouraged to seek mentors and supplement their knowledge as they seek out strategies to apply their learning to practice. Participation in research or quality improvement projects will continue to identify new knowledge and advance the integration of research, education, and practice.

We hope that this manual will be helpful to readers' knowledge, skill development, and evidence-based practice, and we hope it will be used to support excellent quality care for patients receiving radiation therapy and their families.

Maurene McQuestion, RN, BA, BScN, MSc, CON(C)
Lorraine C. Drapek, DNP, FNP-BC, AOCNP®
Mary Ellyn Witt, MS, RN, AOCN®

ACOG—American College of Obstetricians and Gynecologists

ACoS CoC—American College of Surgeons Commission on Cancer

ACR—American College of Radiology

ADLs—activities of daily living

AJCC—American Joint Committee on Cancer

ALARA—as low as reasonably achievable

ALTENS—acupuncture-like transcutaneous electrical nerve stimulation

ANA—American Nurses Association

ANC—absolute neutrophil count

APA—American Psychiatric Association

ASCO—American Society of Clinical Oncology

ASD—acute stress disorder

ASTRO—American Society for Radiation Oncology

ATP—adenosine triphosphate

AVM—arteriovenous malformation

AYA—adolescent and young adult

Bq—becquerel

BCG—bacillus Calmette-Guérin

CAM—complementary and alternative medicine

CD—cluster of differentiation

CDC—Centers for Disease Control and Prevention

CDT—complete decongestive therapy

CGA—comprehensive geriatric assessment

cGy—centigray

Ci—curie

CIED—cardiac implantable electronic device

CINV—chemotherapy-induced nausea and vomiting

CNS—central nervous system

CPR—cardiopulmonary resuscitation

CRF—cancer-related fatigue

CSF—cerebrospinal fluid

CT—computed tomography

CTCAE—Common Terminology Criteria for Adverse Events

CTEP—Cancer Therapy Evaluation Program

CTLA-4—cytotoxic T-lymphocyte antigen 4

CTV—clinical target volume

CYP450—cytochrome P450

DCIS—ductal carcinoma in situ

DLBCL—diffuse large B-cell lymphoma

dps—disintegration per second

DSM-5—*Diagnostic and Statistical Manual of Mental Disorders* (5th edition)

DVHs—dose-volume histograms

EBRT—external beam radiation therapy

EORTC—European Organization for Research and Treatment of Cancer

EPA—U.S. Environmental Protection Agency

ESAS— Edmonton Symptom Assessment System

ESCC—epidural spinal cord compression

FDA—U.S. Food and Drug Administration

FITT—frequency, intensity, time, and type

FLAIR—fluid-attenuated inversion recovery

FTD—frontotemporal dementia

G₂—gap 2 phase

G8—Geriatric 8 tool

GnRH—gonadotropin-releasing hormone

GTV—gross target volume

GVHD—graft-versus-host disease

Gy—gray

HDR—high-dose-rate

HPA—hypothalamic–pituitary–adrenal

HPV—human papillomavirus

HSCT—hematopoietic stem cell transplantation

HSOS—hepatic sinusoidal obstruction syndrome

ICRP—International Commission on Radiological Protection

ICRU—International Commission on Radiation Units and Measurements

IGRT—image-guided radiation therapy

IMRT—intensity-modulated radiation therapy

ITV—internal target volume

LDR—low-dose-rate

LENT-SOMA—Late Effects of Normal Tissue–Somatic, Objective, Management, Analytic

LET—linear energy transfer

LGBTQ—lesbian, gay, bisexual, transgender, queer or questioning

MAO—monoamine oxidase

mCi—millicurie

MeV—megaelectron volt

MHC—major histocompatibility complex

mrem—millirem

MRI—magnetic resonance imaging

mSv—millisievert

mTOR—mechanistic target of rapamycin

MV—megavolt

NCCN—National Comprehensive Cancer Network

NCI—National Cancer Institute

NCRP—National Council on Radiation Protection and Measurements

NRC—U.S. Nuclear Regulatory Commission

NSAIDs—nonsteroidal anti-inflammatory drugs

NSCLC—non-small cell lung cancer

OARs—organs at risk

OCTN—oncology clinical trial nurse

ONS—Oncology Nursing Society

PCP—primary care provider

PDE5—phosphodiesterase type 5

PD-L1—programmed cell death-ligand 1

PD-1—programmed cell death protein 1

PET—positron emission tomography

PRBCs—packed red blood cells

PSA—prostate-specific antigen

PTSD—post-traumatic stress disorder

PTV—planning target volume

rad—radiation absorbed dose

RD—registered dietitian

RDN—registered dietitian nutritionist

RINV—radiation-induced nausea and vomiting

RION—radiation-induced optic neuropathy

RSO—radiation safety officer

RT—radiation therapy

RTOG—Radiation Therapy Oncology Group

SBRT—stereotactic body radiation therapy

SCLC—small cell lung cancer

SCP—survivorship care plan

SEER—Surveillance, Epidemiology, and End Results

SI—International System

SINS—Spinal Instability Neoplastic Score

SNHL—sensorineural hearing loss

SNRI—serotonin–norepinephrine reuptake inhibitor

SPMI—serious and persistent mental illness

SRS—stereotactic radiosurgery

SSRI—selective serotonin reuptake inhibitor

Sv—sievert

SVC—superior vena cava

SVCS—superior vena cava syndrome

TBI—total body irradiation

3DCRT—three-dimensional conformal radiation therapy

TLI—total lymphoid irradiation

TMJ—temporomandibular joint

TNF-α—tumor necrosis factor-alpha

TNM—tumor-node-metastasis

UNEP—United Nations Environment Programme

VES-13—Vulnerable Elders Survey-13

VEGF—vascular endothelial growth factor

VMAT—volumetric modulated arc therapy

WBC—white blood cell

I. Scope of Practice for the Registered Nurse

A. Professional nursing practice
1. Professional nursing practice is defined and regulated at four levels (American Nurses Association [ANA], 2015).
   a) Practice is defined nationally through the scopes and standards of practice, codes of ethics, and specialty certifications.
   b) States regulate practice through boards of nursing and nurse practice acts.
   c) Institutions outline policies and procedures.
   d) Nurses are individually licensed and, consequently, are responsible for their individual decisions and actions.
2. The third edition of *Nursing: Scope and Standards of Practice* (ANA, 2015) refined the definition of *nursing* and maintained existing language referring to "protection, promotion, and optimization of health and abilities," as well as the nurse's role in prevention, facilitation of healing, alleviation of suffering, and advocacy for patients and families (Bowe et al., 2017).
3. The concepts in the ANA definition are foundations of basic nursing practice and generalizable to all areas of practice. Completion of an approved nursing education program may be in a diploma, associate degree (United States), or baccalaureate curriculum. Licensure to practice after successful testing grants legal sanction to practice to the new nurse.

B. Radiation nursing specialty
1. The radiation oncology nurse is a professional RN who functions independently and interdependently with the radiation oncology team to provide quality patient care (Altman, Butler, & Shern, 2016).
   a) Nurses provide clinical care, education, psychosocial support, and consultation.
   b) Radiation oncology nurses may participate in the leadership roles of clinician, educator, administrative manager, consultant, or researcher.
   c) Radiation oncology nurses provide evidence-based practice throughout the trajectory of care with assessments, symptom management, outcome identification, planning, implementation, and evaluation.
   d) Nurses also provide support to patients and families during new patient visits, active radiation therapy (RT), and weekly review clinics, in nurse-led radiation support clinics, and through long-term follow-up.
2. Radiation oncology nursing is a complex specialty requiring an overall, basic understanding of the pathophysiology of cancer and its treatment.
   a) Radiation oncology specialty education provides an understanding of RT as a local cancer treatment. Providing informed and competent holistic care to patients with cancer and their families requires an interest and commitment to lifelong learning.
   b) Radiation oncology nursing practice is based on philosophic tenets identified by the Oncology Nursing Society (ONS) in *Oncology Nursing: Scope and Standards of Practice* (Lubejko & Wilson, 2019).
   c) Specialty nursing practice in oncology, specifically radiation oncology nursing, requires specialized knowledge and critical thinking skills to make independent patient care decisions within a nurse's scope of practice beyond basic nursing education (prelicensure programs).
   d) Specialized training and education provided by the employing institution during a designated orientation period and supporting attendance at continuing professional educational programs provide opportunities to develop new knowledge and advanced critical thinking skills. ONS provides diverse levels of educational opportunities to learn about radiation oncology, ranging from basic science and novice clinical skills to advanced concepts of complex concurrent systemic therapy during RT.
   e) As professional nurses gain experience over time, novice skills develop into expert practice skills. Additionally, interprofessional oncology workforce training for team-based cancer care and education, as well as oncology certification, is desirable to provide competent quality care for the radiation oncology patient population (Ferrell, McCabe, & Levit, 2013; ONS, 2016).
3. Standards of care refer to professional nursing activities that radiation oncology nurses demonstrate through the use of the nursing process.
   a) The nursing process is the foundation of clinical decision-making and encompasses all significant action taken by nurses within the scope of practice of their licensure, providing care to patients and families (Lubejko & Wilson, 2019).
   b) The Canadian Association of Nurses in Oncology (2018) developed *Radiation Oncology Nursing Practice Standards and Competencies* based on the vision that all patients, regardless of geography, receiving radiation care and treatment should receive that care from oncology nurses who meet a standard of practice through a comprehensive education program to ensure competency.

C. Advanced practice nursing: Nurse practitioner and clinical nurse specialist
1. General
   a) A master's degree is the minimum education required for entry into the advanced practice nursing roles of nurse practitioner or clinical nurse specialist.
   b) The four advanced practice roles recognized in the United States are the certified registered nurse anes-

thetist, certified nurse midwife, nurse practitioner, and clinical nurse specialist.
2. ONS framework: ONS's *Oncology Nursing: Scope and Standards of Practice* provides the framework from which advanced practice nursing roles can be delineated (Lubejko & Wilson, 2019).
3. Cancer Care Ontario guidelines
   a) Cancer Care Ontario (2018) has developed guidelines and advice on clarifying the roles of clinical nurse specialists and nurse practitioners in the delivery of cancer care.
   b) The organization has also published guidelines on the effective use of advanced practice nurses in the delivery of adult cancer services (Bryant-Lukosius et al., 2015).
   c) In January 2018, Cancer Care Ontario published additions to the guidelines that included expert recommendations on clinical nurse specialist and nurse practitioner roles, providing unpublished emerging practice evidence to fill in the gaps of previous guidelines (Nowell et al., 2018).
4. Advanced practice nursing in radiation oncology
   a) Advanced practice nursing in radiation oncology spans the continuum of cancer care from screening and cancer risk reduction to diagnosis and treatment, survivorship, palliative care, and the end of life.
   b) Nurse practitioners and clinical nurse specialists may participate in institutional review boards and quality outcome and indicator monitoring, function as administrators or nurse leaders, and be involved in strategic planning and restructuring of the healthcare and cancer care system.
5. Nurse practitioner role in radiation oncology
   a) In the United States, certification through successful postgraduate testing by a national nursing organization (e.g., American Association of Nurse Practitioners) is required to apply for advanced practice licensure.
      (1) State licensure, in addition to employer credentialing, is required to enter into a general advanced practice role.
      (2) The role in radiation oncology requires specialized education not offered in a general prelicensure nurse practitioner program.
      (3) The education and role of nurse practitioners as direct clinical care providers qualifies them to diagnose, treat, and manage acute and chronic illness within the scope of practice and to directly bill for services provided (American Association of Nurse Practitioners, 2019a).
      (4) Clinical care may be provided to patients independently or in collaboration with a physician.
      (5) Nurse practitioners have prescriptive authority for pharmacologic treatment of medical conditions. Prescribing pain medication (controlled substances) requires federal and state registration. Radiation oncology nurse practitioners have a significant role in pain and symptom management.
      (6) The nurse practitioner role in research may include investigator-initiated studies or participation in collaborative group protocols with an interprofessional team (American Association of Nurse Practitioners, 2019b).
   b) Currently, nurse practitioners working in the United States require two state licenses to practice: RN and advanced practice RN (American Association of Nurse Practitioners, 2019c).
      (1) License to practice and scope of practice of nurse practitioners are granted by an individual state's nurse practice act.
      (2) Scope-of-practice authority varies by state and may be full practice, reduced practice, or restrictive (supervisory) authority.
      (3) The practice authority of each state is determined by state legislation and the nurse practice act.
6. Clinical nurse specialist role in radiation oncology
   a) A clinical nurse specialist is an expert clinician whose role includes components of patient care, leadership, education of patients and staff, academic appointments, consultation, and research (Cancer Care Ontario, 2018; ONS, 2008).
   b) The role may be further defined by the employing institution or job description.
   c) Clinical nurse specialists provide complex health interventions and affect outcomes for high-risk patient populations; collaborate on health issues with patients, families, and interprofessional teams; and influence administrators and policy makers within and beyond various institutions, facilitating system change and advancing the profession of nursing.

References

Altman, S.H., Butler, A.S., & Shern, L. (Eds.). (2016). *Assessing progress on the Institute of Medicine report The Future of Nursing*. National Academies Press. https://doi.org/10.17226/21838

American Association of Nurse Practitioners. (2019a). Scope of practice for nurse practitioners. https://www.aanp.org/advocacy/advocacy-resource/position-statements/scope-of-practice-for-nurse-practitioners

American Association of Nurse Practitioners. (2019b). Standards of practice for nurse practitioners. https://www.aanp.org/advocacy/advocacy-resource/position-statements/standards-of-practice-for-nurse-practitioners

American Association of Nurse Practitioners. (2019c). State practice environment. https://www.aanp.org/advocacy/state/state-practice-environment

American Nurses Association. (2015). *Nursing: Scope and standards of practice*. Author.

Bowe, P., Culver, D., Gecsedi, R., Henker, R., Koyama, K., Lee, C.A.B., ... McNail, S. (2017). *American Nurses Association recognition of a nursing specialty, approval of a specialty nursing scope of practice statement, acknowledg-*

ment of specialty nursing standards of practice, and affirmation of focused practice competencies. American Nurses Association. https://www.nursingworld.org/~4989de/globalassets/practiceandpolicy/scope-of-practice/3sc-booklet-final-2017-08-17.pdf

Bryant-Lukosius, D., Cosby, R., Bakker, D., Earle, C., Fitzgerald, B., & Burkoski, V. (2015). *Effective use of advanced practice nurses in the delivery of adult cancer services in Ontario.* Cancer Care Ontario. https://www.cancercareontario.ca/en/guidelines-advice/types-of-cancer/2166

Canadian Association of Nurses in Oncology. (2018). *Radiation oncology nursing practice standards and competencies.* https://cdn.ymaws.com/www.cano-acio.ca/resource/resmgr/standards/ronp_s&c_web(2).pdf

Cancer Care Ontario. (2018). *Clarifying the role of the clinical nurse specialist and nurse practitioners in delivery of cancer care in Ontario.* https://www.cancercareontario.ca/sites/ccocancercare/files/guidelines/full/APN%20Role%20Clarity_Final.pdf

Ferrell, B., McCabe, M.S., & Levit, L. (2013). The Institute of Medicine report on high-quality cancer care: Implications for oncology nursing. *Oncology Nursing Forum, 40,* 603–609. https://doi.org/10.1188/13.ONF.603-609

Lubejko, B.G., & Wilson, B.J. (2019). *Oncology nursing: Scope and standards of practice.* Oncology Nursing Society.

Nowell, A., Campbell, C., Kiteley, C., Giroux, J., Moody, L., Martelli, L., ... Jain, P. (2018). *Expert recommendation report on clinical nurse specialist and nurse practitioner roles in the delivery of adult cancer services in Ontario.* Cancer Care Ontario. https://www.cancercareontario.ca/en/guidelines-advice/types-of-cancer/52201

Oncology Nursing Society. (2008). *Oncology clinical nurse specialist competencies.* https://www.ons.org/oncology-clinical-nurse-specialist-competencies

Oncology Nursing Society. (2016). The impact of nursing workforce issues on quality cancer care [Position statement]. *Oncology Nursing Forum, 43,* 16–17. https://doi.org/10.1188/16.ONF.16-17

II. Practice of Radiation Oncology

A. Principles of radiation therapy
1. Definition of RT
   a) RT is the use of high-energy x-rays or other radiation particles to treat malignant and some benign conditions.
   b) Radiation with sufficient energy to disrupt atomic structures by ejecting orbital electrons is known as *ionizing radiation* (Gibbons, 2020).
2. Types of ionizing radiation commonly used in treatment (Gibbons, 2020; see Figure 1)
   a) Electromagnetic radiation: X-rays and gamma rays have the same characteristics but differ in origin.
      (1) X-rays: photons (i.e., "packets" of energy generated from an electrical machine, such as a linear accelerator) emitted from electrons transitioning to a lower atomic orbital or when striking a target
      (2) Gamma rays: photons emitted from the nucleus of a radioactive source (e.g., cobalt-60, cesium-137, iridium-192)
   b) Particulate radiation: Alpha particles, protons, neutrons, electrons, and beta particles are types of particulate radiation.
      (1) Alpha particles: large, positively charged particles with poor penetrating ability; emitted during disintegration (i.e., decay) of some radioactive sources (e.g., radium); have a mass approximately 8,000 times that of an electron
      (2) Protons: large, positively charged particles that may be generated by a cyclotron or a linear accelerator; have a mass approximately 2,000 times that of an electron
      (3) Neutrons: large, uncharged particles that may be generated by a cyclotron or a linear accelerator; have the same mass as protons
      (4) Electrons: small, negatively charged particles accelerated to high energies by a linear accelerator
      (5) Beta particles: electrons emitted during disintegration of radioactive sources
3. Sources of radiation for treatment (Gibbons, 2020; see Figure 1)
   a) Megavoltage machines: Megavoltage machines are used in external beam RT (EBRT).
      (1) Linear accelerator
         (a) A linear accelerator generates ionizing radiation from electricity.
         (b) Commercially available machines produce x-rays and electrons with an energy range 4–25 megaelectron volt (MeV). The energy of therapeutic x-rays is expressed in megavolts (MV) because the x-ray beam is made up of a spectrum of energies. The energy of therapeutic electrons is expressed in terms of MeV because the electron beam is almost monoenergetic before incidence on the patient surface.
         (c) Linear accelerators may have multiple energies of both x-rays and electrons so that various depths of treatment may be selected.
         (d) The high-energy electron beam can treat superficial tumors and give high skin doses, and x-rays can treat intermediate to deep-seated tumors and give low to moderate skin doses.
      (2) Cobalt-60 machine: A radioactive source (cobalt-60) emits gamma rays; treatment depth is comparable to a 4 MV x-ray beam (intermediate penetration).
      (3) Cyclotron: A cyclotron is a large, electrically powered machine that produces neutrons or protons.

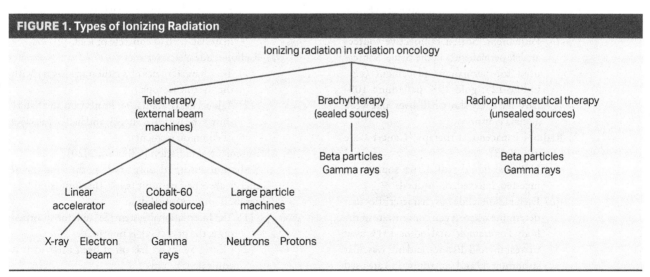

FIGURE 1. Types of Ionizing Radiation

Note. Based on information from Gibbons, 2020; Van Dyk, 1999.

b) Radionuclides: Radionuclides are radioactive sources that emit radiation in the form of alpha particles, beta particles, gamma rays, or a combination. Each radionuclide emits particles or rays with energies that are characteristic of that specific radionuclide (Gibbons, 2020).

(1) Brachytherapy (internal radiation): Brachytherapy is a technique that uses sealed radioactive sources placed directly into (interstitial) or adjacent to (intracavitary, intraluminal, surface) tumors. Therapy can be done alone or combined with EBRT. Radioactive particles or rays penetrate the sealed container to give a high radiation dose to the tumor with rapid dose falloff in the surrounding normal tissue.

(a) Temporary

 i. Sealed radioactive sources (e.g., iridium-192, cesium-137) are removed after the prescribed dose is reached in the calculated time period.

 ii. High-dose-rate (HDR) treatment: One or several doses are administered and separated by at least six hours. Each dose is administered over a few minutes. Iridium-192 is commonly used for HDR.

 iii. Low-dose-rate (LDR) treatment: Continuous LDR treatment is administered over several days in a protected, lead-shielded room. Cesium-137 tubes have been popular for intracavitary LDR, but their use in the United States has greatly diminished over the past decade because of limited availability from manufacturers and excellent results using low-energy brachytherapy sources, which greatly restrict a patient's radiation exposure (Khan, Gibbons, & Sperduto, 2016).

(b) Permanent: Sealed radioactive sources are left permanently in the tissue. Sources used for permanent placement (e.g., iodine-125, gold-198, palladium-103) have relatively short half-lives and weak gamma emissions.

(2) Radiopharmaceutical therapy (Cancer Care Ontario, 2015)

(a) Unsealed liquid radioactive sources are ingested, injected, or instilled.

(b) Each radionuclide has characteristics that determine where it can concentrate in the body. For example, oral iodine-131 is used to treat thyroid diseases, and intravascular strontium-89 and samarium-153 are used to treat multiple bone metastases.

4. Radioactivity (Gibbons, 2020)

a) Isotope

(1) An isotope is a variant of a chemical element, with a different number of neutrons.

(2) The nucleus contains protons and neutrons. The number of protons determines the element, and the number of neutrons determines the isotope.

(3) An element may have both stable and radioactive isotopes.

b) Nuclei

(1) Nuclei of radioactive elements have excess energy.

(2) Radioactive materials (also known as *radionuclides*, *radioactive sources*, or *isotopes*) decay and emit radiation in the form of alpha particles, beta particles, and gamma rays until they become stable.

(3) Radioactivity, or radioactive decay, is the spontaneous emission (disintegration) of highly energetic particles or rays from the nucleus of an element.

(4) Radioactivity is measured in disintegration per second (dps).

c) Half-life

(1) Half-life is the period of time required for a radioactive substance to lose half of its radioactivity through nuclear decay.

(2) The spontaneous decay or expulsion of particles and rays from a radionuclide occurs at a characteristic rate for each element.

d) Radioactivity

(1) A radioactive element radiates energy that is characteristic of that element.

(2) Some radioactive sources emit more penetrating radiation than others and, therefore, require more shielding to absorb the radiation.

(3) Half of the radioactivity from a source is absorbed by one half-value layer of a shielding material, such as concrete or lead.

e) Radionuclide characteristics

(1) The characteristics of a radionuclide vary with the specific isotope.

(2) Table 3 in III. Radiation Protection and Safety shows the half-life, energy, and half-value layer of common elements.

5. Measurement of radiation (Gibbons, 2020)

a) Radiation-absorbed dose (rad) is the amount of energy absorbed per unit mass. This unit is no longer used for prescribed dose.

(1) The International System (SI) unit for absorbed dose, the gray (Gy), is now used.

(2) Centigray (cGy) has often been used, as it is equivalent to rad.

(3) 1 Gy = 100 rad = 100 cGy.

b) Dose equivalent is used in radiation protection.
  (1) Badge readings have been reported in milli-rem (mrem).
  (2) Sievert (Sv) is the SI unit for dose equivalent.
  (3) 1 Sv = 100 rem.
c) Activity of radioactive sources has been measured in curies (Ci) and millicuries (mCi), as well as becquerel (Bq), the SI unit.
  (1) Ci and Bq are measured as dps.
  (2) $1 \text{ Ci} = 3.7 \times 10^{10}$ dps.
  (3) $1 \text{ Bq} = 1 \text{ dps} = 2.7 \times 10^{-11}$ Ci.

B. Radiobiology

1. Radiobiology is the study of events that occur after ionizing radiation is absorbed by a living organism.
   a) Ionizing radiation can result in breaking of chemical bonds and, eventually, in biologic change (Hall & Giaccia, 2018; see Figure 2).
   b) The nature and severity of effects and the time in which they appear depend on the amount and type of radiation absorbed and the rate at which it is administered. Early- and late-responding tissues are affected differently by these factors. Interaction of radiation in cells is random and has no selectivity for any structure or site (Hall & Giaccia, 2018).
2. If critical sites are damaged by radiation, the probability of cell death is higher than if noncritical sites are damaged.
   a) DNA is considered to be the critical target for radiation damage.
   b) Cells can successfully repair much of the damage caused by ionizing radiation (Hall & Giaccia, 2018).
3. Damage to DNA may lead to cell alteration or death. All living cells, whether healthy or cancerous, are susceptible to the effects of radiation and may be injured or destroyed by RT. Injury generally is expressed at the time of cell division (reproductive death).
   a) Physical stage: excitation and ionization of atoms or molecules
   b) Radiochemical stage: formation of free radicals, which are highly reactive
   c) Biologic stage: damage to critical target (DNA, which is composed of two strands that form a double helix)
     (1) Single chromosomal strand breaks: These generally are repaired readily and have little biologic consequence (Hall & Giaccia, 2018). Misrepair (incorrect repair) may result in mutation.
     (2) Double chromosomal strand breaks: Double chromosomal strand breaks are thought to be the most significant damage produced in chromosomes by radiation and may result in cell death, mutation, or carcinogenesis. Double chromosomal strand breaks may activate an oncogene or inactivate a tumor suppressor gene (Hall & Cox, 2010).
4. In an irradiated volume of tissue, there are several potential effects to a single cell (Halperin, Wazer, Perez, & Brady, 2019; see Figure 3).
   a) No effect or no cell injury occurs in critical target.
   b) Radiation damage to critical target is repaired, and the cell continues to function and divide.
   c) Radiation damage to critical target is misrepaired, and mutation occurs.
   d) Cell death occurs.
5. Radiation-induced chromosome aberration effects also occur (Hall & Cox, 2010).
   a) Cell death induced by radiation
     (1) Chromosome damage may cause reproductive failure (death at the time of cell division).
     (2) Apoptosis (programmed cell death), the process that occurs during normal development of organs and tissues, is enhanced by toxic treatments, such as RT (Pinar et al., 2010).
   b) Mutation (germ cells): heritable change in genes expressed in later generations (a large variation in mutation types exists)
   c) Carcinogenesis (somatic cells): chromosome aberration that may cause oncogene activation or suppressor gene loss (Hall & Giaccia, 2018)
6. Radiosensitivity is the innate sensitivity of cells, tissues, or tumors to radiation.
   a) Healthy and cancer cells are affected by radiation. Cells vary in their expressed sensitivity to radiation.
     (1) Generally, rapidly dividing cells (e.g., mucosa) are most sensitive and are referred to as *radiosensitive*.
     (2) Nondividing or slowly dividing cells (e.g., muscle cells, neurons) generally are less radiosensitive or are radioresistant.
     (3) Exceptions include small lymphocytes and salivary gland cells, which are nondividing but very radiosensitive. These may experience an interphase death (death prior to mitosis) (Hall & Giaccia, 2018).

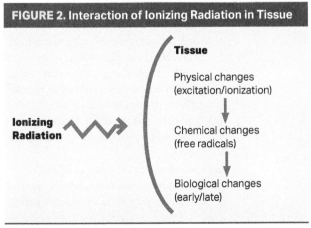

FIGURE 2. Interaction of Ionizing Radiation in Tissue

Ionizing Radiation

Tissue

Physical changes (excitation/ionization)

↓

Chemical changes (free radicals)

↓

Biological changes (early/late)

Note. Based on information from Fritz-Niggli, 1995; Hall & Giaccia, 2018.

FIGURE 3. Possible Response of a Cell in Irradiated Volume of Tissue

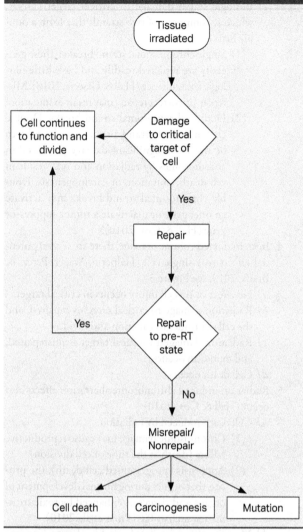

Note. Based on information from Fritz-Niggli, 1995; Hall & Cox, 2010; Halperin et al., 2019.

b) Manifestations of radiation effects occur at different times for different tissues (Hall & Cox, 2010).
   (1) Acutely responding tissues demonstrate effects in hours to days after RT and include the bone marrow, ovaries, testes, lymph nodes, salivary glands, oral mucosa, stomach, small bowel, colon, larynx, esophagus, arterioles, skin, bladder, capillaries, and vagina.
   (2) Subacutely responding tissues demonstrate effects in weeks to several months after RT and include the lungs, liver, kidneys, heart, spinal cord, and brain.
   (3) Late-responding tissues, including the lymph vessels, thyroid, pituitary gland, breasts, bones, cartilage, pancreas (endocrine), uterus, and bile ducts, rarely show acute effects and demonstrate effects months to years after RT.

c) Multiple factors influence radiation sensitivity (Hall & Cox, 2010).
   (1) Cell cycle phase
       (a) Cells in the late gap 2 (G_2) and mitosis (M) phases are more sensitive.
       (b) Cells in the late synthesis (S) phase are most resistant to radiation.
   (2) Oxygen
       (a) The presence of oxygen enhances radiation damage.
       (b) When oxygen is not present, chemical damage in DNA may be repaired.
       (c) Reoxygenation occurs as the tumor shrinks during RT, and previously hypoxic cells become better oxygenated.
       (d) Hypoxia may contribute to radioresistance.
   (3) Differentiation
       (a) Poorly differentiated tumors generally are more sensitive. Far more radiation is required to destroy the function of a differentiated cell than to destroy a dividing cell (Hall & Giaccia, 2018).
       (b) However, poor differentiation of a tumor is associated with a poor disease-free survival rate, perhaps because of a more aggressive natural history (Halperin et al., 2019).
   (4) Proliferative capacity
       (a) Rapidly dividing cells generally are more sensitive to the effects of radiation.
       (b) Nondividing or slowly dividing cells generally are radioresistant.
   (5) Repair of radiation damage
       (a) A greater repair capability of the healthy tissue correlates to greater effectiveness of the treatment. Most repairs are thought to occur within six hours after a treatment.
       (b) DNA damage can be repaired to its original state or misrepaired with errors (mutations).
   (6) Tumor size
       (a) Tumor size is a major factor in dose-response outcomes of RT.
       (b) Larger tumors generally are more difficult to control than small tumors of the same type. Control of large tumors may require a radiation dose that would result in unacceptable damage to healthy tissue.
       (c) Often, the tumor bulk indicates a poorly oxygenated mass that is less radiosensitive.
   (7) Fractionation
       (a) Overview (Hall & Giaccia, 2018)
           i. Fractionation is the division of a total prescribed dose into smaller daily doses, or fractions. Daily fractions generally are 1.8–2 Gy.

ii. Fraction size is the dominant factor in determining late effects on tissue, with large fractions causing an increase in late effects.

iii. Fractionation varies depending on goal of therapy.

(b) Hyperfractionation

i. Multiple daily fractions (e.g., 1.5 Gy twice a day) are delivered, generally separated by at least six hours to allow for repair of damage to the normal tissues from the first dose before administration of the second dose.

ii. The intent is to decrease late effects while achieving equal or improved tumor control and equal or only slightly increased early effects.

iii. A higher total physical dose is administered.

(c) Hypofractionation

i. The total dose of radiation is divided into large doses, and treatments may be given less than once a day.

ii. A lower total physical dose is administered, but a higher biologically equivalent dose is expected because of the larger fractional doses.

iii. Hypofractionation may have high potential for therapeutic gain, as well as economic and logistic advantages for some tumors. For example, per American Society for Radiation Oncology (ASTRO) guidelines, RT for selective patients with prostate cancer can be hypofractionated to 2.4–3.4 Gy per fraction treated daily for fewer total fractions (Morgan et al., 2018).

(8) Quality of radiation

(a) Energy of various types of radiation is distributed differently in tissues. Heavy particles (e.g., neutrons, alpha particles) ionize densely and quickly; light particles (e.g., electrons) ionize sparsely in tissues (Gibbons, 2020).

(b) Linear energy transfer (LET) is the distribution of energy along the ionization track in irradiated material.

i. High LET radiation is densely ionizing and is influenced to a lesser degree by the cell cycle phase and the presence of oxygen (i.e., more effective on hypoxic cells than low LET radiation).

ii. Less repair occurs with high LET radiation. Low LET radiation is sparsely ionizing.

(c) Relative biologic effectiveness of a radiation type is dependent on LET. High LET radiation is more biologically damaging than low LET radiation.

(9) Chemotherapy (Hall & Giaccia, 2018; Halperin et al., 2019)

(a) Mutations in molecular pathways that govern DNA repair, cell cycle, and cell death can also be activated by chemotherapy agents.

(b) A given dose kills a constant fraction of cells that divide soon after exposure to the drug.

(c) The goals of combining chemotherapy agents with RT are to improve locoregional tumor control, to decrease or eliminate distant metastases, or both, while preserving organ and tissue integrity and function.

(d) Specifically, such agents reduce the number of cells in tumors undergoing RT by their independent cytotoxic action and render tumor cells more susceptible to killing by ionizing radiation.

(e) Improvements in treatment outcome have been achieved with traditional chemotherapy agents, such as cisplatin and 5-fluorouracil, but selection of the most effective drug or the optimal treatment approach remains a significant challenge.

7. Radiation effects on healthy cells and cancer cells differ (Hall & Cox, 2010).

a) Although healthy cells and cancer cells are affected by radiation and respond similarly to RT, only cancer cells are believed to undergo reoxygenation.

b) Malignant tumors differ greatly in radiosensitivity because of innate sensitivity, mitotic activity, hypoxic component, and blood supply.

c) Dividing a dose into multiple daily fractions spares normal tissues because of damage repair between fractions and repopulation of cells if overall time is sufficient. Dose fractionation increases damage to cancer cells because of reoxygenation of the tumor and reassortment of cancer cells into more sensitive phases of the cell cycle.

d) Side effects are the result of radiation damage to healthy cells.

8. A biomarker, or biologic marker, is a substance used as an indicator of a biologic state, such as normal biologic processes, pathogenic processes, or radiobiologic responses to RT treatments.

a) Better markers identifying the undesirable cells, such as cancer stem cells, and better tools to image them must be developed.

b) Newer biologic techniques are rapidly changing the landscape for biomarker identification, validation, and clinical trial design in order to move radiation oncology from precision medicine to precise, personalized medicine (Story & Wang, 2018).

C. Dose prescription, treatment planning, and simulation
  1. Specification of dose and volume
      a) The method of writing and interpreting a prescription is essential to the success of treatment.
      b) The International Commission on Radiation Units and Measurements (ICRU, 1993) definition of treatment volume is separated into three distinct boundaries: visible tumor, a region to account for uncertainties in microscopic tumor spread, and a region to account for positional uncertainties. These boundaries create the following volumes (Khan et al., 2016; see Figure 4).
          (1) Gross target volume (GTV) is the gross extent of the malignant growth as determined by palpation or an imaging study.
          (2) Clinical target volume (CTV) is the tissue volume that contains the GTV and subclinical microscopic malignant disease.
          (3) Internal target volume (ITV) is defined by considering variations in size, shape, and position of the CTV within the patient (e.g., filling of stomach or bladder, movements due to respira-

tion). This internal margin is difficult or impossible to control and is considered an optional tool in helping to delineate the planning target volume (PTV) (ICRU, 1999).
          (4) PTV is defined by specifying the internal margins that must be added around the CTV to compensate for physiologic variations of CTV and by the setup margin related to variations in patient position and beam position, both intrafractionally and interfractionally (ICRU, 1999).
      c) ICRU (1999) also defined two other dose volumes.
          (1) Treated volume is enclosed by an isodose surface that is selected and specified by the radiation oncologist as being appropriate to achieve the purpose of treatment (e.g., 95% isodose surface).
          (2) Irradiated volume is the volume that receives a significant dose in relation to normal tissue tolerance (e.g., 50% isodose surface).
      d) Organs at risk (OARs) are defined as healthy tissues whose radiation sensitivity may significantly influence treatment planning or prescribed dose (e.g., rectum and bladder for prostate treatment). OARs are classified as *serial, parallel,* or *serial-parallel* (ICRU, 1999).
          (1) The spinal cord is classified as a serial organ, indicating that a dose above the tolerance limit, even to a small volume, can totally impair the function of the organ (e.g., myelitis).
          (2) The lung is classified as a parallel organ, meaning that the main parameter for impairing pulmonary function is the proportion of the organ that receives a dose above the tolerance level.
          (3) The heart can be considered as having a combined serial (coronary arteries) and parallel (myocardium) structure.
      e) A planning OAR volume is defined by an OAR with an added margin to compensate for organ movements and changes in shape and size, as well as the setup uncertainties, to avoid serious complications (e.g., 3 mm margin for spinal cord for head and neck treatment) (ICRU, 1999, 2010).
      f) In Report 62, ICRU (1999) defined a series of doses including the minimum, maximum, and mean dose for dose reporting purposes.
          (1) Additionally, an ICRU reference dose is defined at the ICRU reference point.
          (2) The ICRU reference point is chosen based on the following criteria: it must be clinically relevant, be defined in an unambiguous way, and be located where the dose can be accurately determined (not in a region with steep dose gradients).
          (3) In general, this point should be in the central part of the PTV.

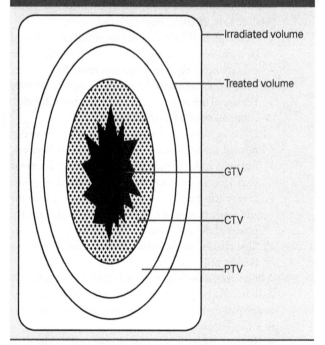

FIGURE 4. Schematic Illustration of the Boundaries of Tumor Volumes[a]

Irradiated volume

Treated volume

GTV

CTV

PTV

[a] As defined by International Commission on Radiation Units and Measurements (1993) Report 50

CTV—clinical target volume; GTV—gross tumor volume; PTV—planning target volume

Note. Based on information from Khan et al., 2016.

g) Dose-volume histograms (DVHs) play an essential role in evaluating and reporting three-dimensional dose distributions (ICRU, 2010).

    (1) A cumulative DVH plots the fraction of a structure receiving at least a given dose.

    (2) A differential DVH plots the fraction of a structure receiving a dose within a specified dose interval.

2. Treatment planning: As a multistage process, RT requires comprehensive treatment planning, entailing interactions among medical physicists, dosimetrists, radiation oncologists, resident physicians (if available on the team), and radiation therapists, as well as the use of various computer programs and hardware devices for dosimetric planning and quality assurance. The following are the steps in the treatment planning process (Gibbons, 2020; Klein et al., 2009).

a) Computed tomography (CT) simulation using a dedicated CT scanner (e.g., flat table, laser lights for patient positioning, reproducible immobilization, and external markings to ensure a consistent position during the course of imaging and treatment)

b) Patient data acquisition (CT, magnetic resonance imaging [MRI], positron-emission tomography [PET])

c) Data transfer to treatment planning system

d) Image registration, or fusion of images from different studies into one dataset (i.e., mapping of structures seen in MRI onto the CT images)

e) Image segmentation (slice-by-slice delineation of target volumes, and OARs)

f) Treatment design (modality, beam arrangements, beam aperture design, modifiers)

g) Computation of dose distributions

h) Plan optimization and evaluation (review of isodose distributions to find optimal dose to the tumor and spare healthy tissue, DVHs, or other physical or biologic dosimetric parameters)

i) Plan implementation (data transfer to record and verify system, preparation of plan documents)

j) Patient-specific quality assurance (review of the plan, independent check of monitor units or minutes based on the prescribed dose, additional measurements to verify the dose)

3. Verification simulation: Verification simulation is the process of aiming and defining the radiation beams to meet the goals of the prescribed therapy. The process is mainly concerned with geometric aspects of a treatment, such as the orientation of beams, beam sizes, and placement of marks on the patient to allow for reliable reproduction of treatment geometry from day to day. Unforeseeable problems with a patient setup or treatment technique also can be solved during simulation.

a) Treatment simulator

    (1) A treatment simulator is an apparatus that uses a diagnostic x-ray tube but duplicates a radia-

tion treatment unit in terms of its geometric, mechanical, and optical properties.

    (2) These units were commonly used until the early to mid-2000s, but modern verification simulation is performed mostly at the medical linear accelerator.

b) Image-guided RT (IGRT)

    (1) IGRT is an advanced imaging system that uses image guidance for target localization before and during treatment.

    (2) IGRT systems use imaging technology to identify and correct problems arising from inter- and intrafractional variations in patient setup and anatomy, such as shapes and volumes of treatment target and OARs.

    (3) As the PTVs are made increasingly conformal, the accuracy requirements of PTV localization and its dosimetric coverage during each treatment become increasingly stringent, so IGRT systems allow for frequent two- or three-dimensional imaging to correlate the actual tumor position with the radiation treatment plan to ensure accurate target dose delivery (Bissonnette et al., 2012).

c) On-board imagers

    (1) On-board imagers are accelerator-mounted imaging systems.

    (2) Many modern linear accelerators are equipped with two kinds of imaging systems: kilovoltage x-ray imager, in which a conventional x-ray tube is mounted on the accelerator with an opposing flat-panel image detector, and megavoltage electronic portal imaging device with its own flat-panel image detector.

    (3) The kilovoltage imager can be used in both the radiographic and fluoroscopy mode to check patient setup or track the movement of fiducial markers due to respiratory motion.

    (4) The megavoltage imager can provide portal verification before each treatment, as well as monitoring of target position during treatment delivery (Gibbons, 2020).

4. Three-dimensional conformal RT (3DCRT)

a) The goal of 3DCRT is to conform the dose distribution as closely as possible to the target volume and minimize the dose to the surrounding healthy tissue (Khan et al., 2016).

b) 3DCRT requires the availability of three-dimensional anatomic information and a computer-based treatment planning system that can calculate the optimal dose distribution in accordance with the clinical objectives.

    (1) Computer graphics are used to design fields and beam arrangement, allowing for a beam's-eye-view visualization of the delineated targets and other structures.

(2) The term *beam's-eye-view* denotes display of the segmented target and normal structures in a plane perpendicular to the central axis of the beam, which is used to set field margins for each field (Khan et al., 2016).

   c) 3DCRT is commonly delivered with photon and electron beams using multileaf collimators or custom-designed blocks (cutouts) to shape uniform open fields (to match the beam's-eye-view projection of the PTV) or using wedges to account for the effect of surface irregularities and internal heterogeneities (to achieve uniform dose at a selected treatment depth, usually through the middle of the target volume).

5. Intensity-modulated RT (IMRT)

   a) IMRT is an advanced form of 3DCRT in which the fluence distribution in the plane perpendicular to the incident beam is modulated in order to customize optimal dose distributions (Khan et al., 2016).

   b) Because of the conformal dose distributions and steep dose gradients that can be achieved with IMRT, requirements for patient immobilization, target and structure delineation, treatment planning, beam delivery, and dose verification are more stringent (Gibbons, 2020; Halperin et al., 2019; Khan et al., 2016).

   c) A treatment-planning computer system is needed to divide each beam into small subdivisions (i.e., beamlets, field segments) and determine optimum setting of their fluences or weights.

      (1) The optimization process involves inverse planning in which beamlet weights or intensities are adjusted to satisfy predefined dose distribution criteria for the composite plan (Gibbons, 2020).

      (2) Inverse or forward planning allows for superior target coverage and healthy tissue sparing based on the specified dose requirements for the treatment volumes and dose constraints on the OARs.

   d) A hardware system must be capable of delivering the intensity-modulated beams. The generated fluence files are electronically transmitted to the linear accelerator, which is computer controlled. IMRT fields are commonly delivered using computer-controlled multileaf collimators. However, beam intensity modulation also can be achieved using complex physical compensators (Gibbons, 2020).

   e) IMRT is time and resource intensive. Adequate time to perform reviews and quality checks is essential. Therefore, as noted by Moran et al. (2011), "Team members need to acknowledge that initiation of treatment may need to be delayed to allow time for necessary [quality assurance] checks and subsequent investigations of problems" (p. 195).

6. Stereotactic radiosurgery (SRS)

   a) SRS is a single-fraction RT for treating intracranial lesions using head immobilization and delivery of radiation through multiple noncoplanar beams or arcs.

   b) The same procedure when used for delivering multiple dose fractions is called *stereotactic RT*.

   c) Both techniques involve three-dimensional imaging to localize the lesion and deliver a high degree of dose conformity while sparing as much as possible of the healthy brain.

   d) The requirements in terms of accurate beam calibration, treatment planning, accuracy of delivery, and quality assurance are more stringent than in other areas of RT. The active collaboration among all professionals in the stereotactic RT program is critical for treatment quality and patient safety (ICRU, 2017).

7. Stereotactic body RT (SBRT) (Benedict et al., 2010; Khan et al., 2016)

   a) SBRT has been established as a highly effective local therapy for a variety of tumors in the spine, lung, liver, pancreas, kidney, and prostate.

   b) It requires accurate targeting, effective immobilization, and tumor motion management to deliver a large dose in a few fractions (typically fewer than five), which results in a high biologic effective dose.

   c) Conformation of high doses to the target and rapid falloff doses away from the target is critical.

   d) In order to reduce healthy tissue toxicity, two approaches are used to account for tumor motion: minimization of target motion via immobilization (e.g., abdominal compression or breath-hold techniques), or, alternatively, to account for physiologic tumor motion via tracking or gating.

D. Purpose of radiation therapy

1. RT is used to treat local or regional disease and, rarely, systemic disease. The aim is to destroy malignant cells in the treated volume of tissue while minimizing damage to healthy tissues.

2. RT can be selected for various purposes (Gosselin, 2018; Ma, 2012).

   a) Definitive treatment: RT is prescribed as the primary treatment modality, with or without chemotherapy, for the treatment of cancer. Examples can include cancers of the head and neck, lung, prostate, and bladder, as well as Hodgkin lymphoma.

   b) Neoadjuvant treatment: RT is prescribed prior to definitive treatment, usually surgery, to improve the chance of successful resection. Examples include esophageal or colon cancers.

   c) Adjuvant treatment: RT is given after definitive treatment (surgery or chemotherapy) to improve local control. Examples include breast, lung, or high-risk rectal cancers.

   d) Prophylactic treatment: RT is delivered to asymptomatic, high-risk areas to prevent growth of cancer.

(1) Examples are prophylactic cranial irradiation in lung cancer or central nervous system (CNS) cancers to prevent relapse of certain forms of leukemia.

(2) In addition, RT can be given prophylactically to treat several benign conditions, such as keloids and heterotopic bone (single fraction of 7 Gy to prevent abnormal bone formation in joints) (Cadieux, DesRosiers, & McMullen, 2016).

e) Palliation: RT is given to manage symptoms of bleeding, pain, airway obstruction, or neurologic compromise to alleviate life-threatening problems in incurable illness or to improve a patient's quality of life. Examples may include relieving spinal cord compression or superior vena cava syndrome (SVCS), opening airways in patients with pneumonia, or relieving pain from bone metastases.

E. Tissue tolerance dose

1. Tissue tolerance dose is the radiation dose to which healthy tissue can be irradiated and continue to function. Great progress has been made in the field of healthy tissue tolerance based on work by Emami (2013) and the extensive review by QUANTEC (Quantitative Analyses of Normal Tissue Effects in the Clinic) (Bentzen et al., 2010; see Table 1).

2. Organs vary in their ability to tolerate radiation injury. The tolerance to radiation of healthy tissue depends on the ability of the dividing cells to produce enough mature cells to maintain function of the organ. The tolerance dose is the dose of radiation that results in an acceptable probability of a treatment complication (Hall & Giaccia, 2018).

3. The dose prescribed to eradicate a cancer ultimately is dependent on the healthy tissue's tolerance to the dose.

F. Factors related to radiation-induced injury of healthy tissue (Halperin et al., 2019)

1. Patient-related factors

a) Age

(1) Children: growth-related factors (e.g., growth retardation, endocrine changes)

(2) Adults: limited available data

b) Hemoglobin level

(1) Low hemoglobin has been found to decrease local control probability in cancers such as squamous cell carcinoma of the head and neck (Hoff, 2012), carcinoma of the cervix (Barkati et al., 2013; Gangopadhyay, Das, Nath, & Biswas, 2014), and transitional carcinoma of the bladder (Schubert et al., 2016).

TABLE 1. Normal Tissue Tolerance for Standard Fractionation

Organ	Endpoint	Rate (%)	Dose-Volume Parameter	D_{max} (Gy)	D_{mean} (Gy)
Brain	Symptomatic necrosis	< 3		< 60	
		< 5		< 65	
Brainstem	Necrosis or cranial neuropathy	< 5	D100 < 54 Gy		
		< 5	D1–10 cc ≤ 59 Gy	< 64 Point	
Spinal cord	Grade ≥ 2 myelopathy	≤ 1		50	
Optic nerve and chiasm	Optic neuropathy	< 3		< 55	< 50
		3–7		55–60	
Retina	Blindness	< 1		< 50	
Cochlea	Hearing loss	< 15			≤ 45
Parotid 1	Grade 4 xerostomia	< 20			< 20
Parotid 2		< 20			< 25
Mandible	ORN	< 5		< 70 Point	
Pharyngeal constrictors	PEG tube dependent	< 5			< 50
	Aspiration	< 5			< 60
Larynx	Grade ≥ 2 edema	< 20	V50 < 27%		< 44
Brachial plexus	Clinically apparent nerve damage	< 5		< 60	

(Continued on next page)

TABLE 1. Normal Tissue Tolerance for Standard Fractionation *(Continued)*

Organ	Endpoint	Rate (%)	Dose-Volume Parameter	D_{max} (Gy)	D_{mean} (Gy)
Lung	Symptomatic pneumonitis	5	V5 < 42%, V20 < 22%		7
		10	V20 < 31%		13
		20	V20 < 40%		20
		30			24
		40			27
Esophagus	Grade ≥ 2 esophagitis	< 30	V35 < 50%	< 74 point	
			V50 < 40%		
			V70 < 20%		
	Grade ≥ 3 esophagitis	≤ 10	V60 < 30		< 34
Heart	Pericarditis	< 15	V30 < 46%		< 26
	Long-term cardiac mortality	< 1	V25 < 10%		
Liver	RILD, normal liver	< 5			≤ 30
	RILD, liver disease	< 5			≤ 28
Kidney 1	Renal dysfunction	< 5	Equivalent of 1 kidney < 18 Gy		
Kidney 2	Renal dysfunction	< 5			< 18
Stomach	Ulceration		D100 < 50 Gy		
Small bowel	Acute grade ≥ 3 toxicity	< 10	V15 < 120 cc		
	Late obstruction/perforation	< 5	V50 < 5%		
Rectum	Grade ≥ 2/≥ 3 late toxicity	< 10/< 15	V50 < 50%		
	Grade ≥ 2/≥ 3 late toxicity	< 10/< 15	V60 < 35%		
	Grade ≥ 2/≥ 3 late toxicity	< 10/< 15	V65 < 25%		
	Grade ≥ 2/≥ 3 late toxicity	< 10/< 15	V70 < 20%		
	Grade ≥ 2/≥ 3 late toxicity	< 10/< 15	V75 < 15%		
Bladder	Grade ≥ 3 late toxicity	< 6	D100 < 65 Gy		
		?	V65 ≤ 50%		
			V70 ≤ 35%		
			V75 ≤ 25%		
			V80 ≤ 15%		
Penile bulb	Severe erectile dysfunction	< 35			< 50
Femoral head	Necrosis	< 5	D100 < 52 Gy		

Parotid 1, sparing single parotid gland; Parotid 2, combined parotid glands; Kidney 1, bilateral partial kidney RT; Kidney 2, bilateral whole kidneys; Vx, volume of the organ receiving ≥ x Gy; Dx, minimum dose received by x% of the organ; D_{max}, maximum radiation dose; D_{mean}, mean radiation dose

ORN—osteoradionecrosis; PEG—percutaneous endoscopic gastrostomy; RILD—radiation-induced liver disease; RT—radiation therapy

Note. From "Tolerance of Normal Tissue to Therapeutic Radiation," by B. Emami, 2013, *Reports of Radiotherapy and Oncology, 1*, p. 39 (http://radioncology.com/articles/2782.html). Copyright 2013 by Kowsar. Reprinted with permission.

(2) Little information is available concerning hemoglobin level related to healthy tissue reactions.

c) Smoking can enhance some early and late side effects (Hoff, 2012).

d) Tumor invasion may interfere with healthy tissue reactions.

e) Infections may increase healthy tissue injury, especially when the immune system is compromised.

2. Intrinsic radiosensitivity (Halperin et al., 2019)

a) Genetic syndromes: some associated with increased sensitivity to RT (e.g., ataxia telangiectasia)

b) Autoimmune diseases (e.g., systemic lupus erythematosus)

G. Considerations for radiation therapy

1. Diagnosis and staging: tumor histology and extent of disease

2. General condition of the patient and comorbid conditions

3. Tumor site: whether healthy tissues are included in treatment fields

4. Combination therapy (e.g., chemotherapy, surgery, immunotherapy, hyperthermia): goal of improving the therapeutic ratio relative to the use of a single modality (Brodsky, 2019; Hall & Cox, 2010)

5. Available treatment facilities

H. Radioresponsiveness of healthy tissue (see Figure 5)

1. Expression of healthy tissue injury varies greatly from patient to patient.

2. Response of a tissue or organ primarily depends on the radiosensitivity of the cells and the kinetics of the population in which the cells are functioning.

3. Treatment characteristics include total dose, dose per fraction or dose rate, and overall treatment time.

4. With combined modality therapy (e.g., sequential or concomitant chemotherapy), interactions may substantially influence side effects of RT.

I. Side effects

1. Early side effects (Hall & Giaccia, 2018)

a) Early side effects occur during or immediately after RT in tissues with a rapid rate of turnover (e.g., epidermal layer of the skin, gastrointestinal epithelium, hematopoietic system).

b) Extent of effects depends on total dose, dose per fraction, and overall treatment time (Hall & Giaccia, 2018).

c) Injury can repair rapidly and may be completely reversible.

2. Late side effects

a) Late side effects occur more than three months after irradiation in predominantly slowly proliferating tissues (e.g., heart, kidney, lung, liver, CNS).

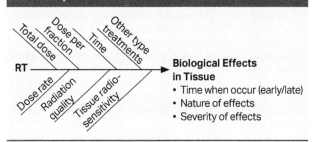

FIGURE 5. Factors Affecting Tissue Radioresponsiveness

Note. Based on information from Hall & Giaccia, 2018.

b) Extent of effects depends highly on dose per fraction. High dose per fraction results in more severe late effects (Hall & Giaccia, 2018).

c) Late damage may improve but is never completely repaired.

d) The time from RT to a specific late effect is the latent period.

e) Late injury expression is time dependent. The severity and percentage of patients expressing the injury increase over time (Hall & Giaccia, 2018). Some lesions, such as those associated with atherosclerosis and heart disease, may occur decades after RT and are an increasing problem as patients live longer (Halperin et al., 2019).

References

Barkati, M., Fortin, I., Mileshkin, L., Bernshaw, D., Carrier, J.-F., & Narayan, K. (2013). Hemoglobin level in cervical cancer: A surrogate for an infiltrative phenotype. *International Journal of Gynecological Cancer, 23,* 724–729. https://doi.org/10.1097/igc.0b013e31828a0623

Benedict, S.H., Yenice, K.M., Followill, D., Galvin, J.M., Hinson, W., Kavanagh, B., ... Yin, F-F. (2010). Stereotactic body radiation therapy: The report of AAPM Task Group 101. *Medical Physics, 37,* 4078–4101. https://doi.org/10.1118/1.3438081

Bentzen, S.M., Constine, L.S., Deasy, J.O., Eisbruch, A., Jackson, A., Marks, L.B., ... Yorke, E.D. (2010). Quantitative Analyses of Normal Tissue Effects in the Clinic (QUANTEC): An introduction to the scientific issues. *International Journal of Radiation Oncology Biology Physics, 76*(3 Suppl.), S3–S9. https://doi.org/10.1016/j.ijrobp.2009.09.040

Bissonnette, J.-P., Balter, P.A., Dong, L., Langen, K.M., Lovelock, D.M., Miften, M., ... Yoo, S. (2012). Quality assurance for image-guided radiation therapy utilizing CT-based technologies: A report of the AAPM TG-179 *Medical Physics, 39,* 1946–1963. https://doi.org/10.1118/1.3690466

Brodsky, A.N. (2019). *Cancer immunotherapy and you: Patient education webinar series.* https://www.cancerresearch.org/blog/january-2019/cancer-immunotherapy-2018-review-2019-predict

Cadieux, C.L., DesRosiers, C., & McMullen, K. (2016). Risks of secondary malignancies with heterotopic bone radiation therapy for patients younger than 40 years. *Medical Dosimetry, 41,* 212–215. https://doi.org/10.1016/j.meddos.2016.02.001

Cancer Care Ontario. (2015). *Radiopharmaceuticals for the palliation of painful bone metastases: Program in Evidence-Based Care practice guideline report 14-1.* https://www.cancercareontario.ca/en/content/radiopharmaceuticals-palliation-painful-bone-metastases

Emami, B. (2013). Tolerance of normal tissue to therapeutic radiation. *Reports of Radiotherapy and Oncology, 1,* 35–48. http://radioncology.com/articles/2782.html

Fritz-Niggli, H. (1995). 100 years of radiobiology: Implications for biomedicine and future perspectives. *Cellular and Molecular Life Sciences, 51,* 652–664. https://doi.org/10.1007/bf01941263

Gangopadhyay, A., Das, J., Nath, P., & Biswas, J. (2014). Haemoglobin levels may predict toxicities in patients on pelvic chemoradiation for carcinoma of the cervix—Experience of a regional cancer centre. *Ecancermedicalscience, 8,* 431. https://doi.org/10.3332/ecancer.2014.431

Gibbons, J.P. (Ed.). (2020). *Khan's the physics of radiation therapy* (6th ed.). Wolters Kluwer Health.

Gosselin, T.K. (2018). Principles of radiation therapy. In C.H. Yarbro, D. Wujcik, & B.H. Gobel (Eds.), *Cancer nursing: Principles and practice* (8th ed., pp. 267–284). Jones and Bartlett Learning.

Hall, E.J., & Cox, J.D. (2010). Physical and biologic basis of radiation therapy. In J.D. Cox (Ed.), *Radiation oncology: Rationale, technique, results* (9th ed., pp. 3–49). Elsevier Mosby.

Hall, E.J., & Giaccia, A.J. (2018). *Radiobiology for the radiologist* (8th ed.). Wolters Kluwer.

Halperin, E.C., Wazer, D.E., Perez, C.A., & Brady, L.W. (Eds.). (2019). *Perez and Brady's principles and practice of radiation oncology* (7th ed). Wolters Kluwer.

Hoff, C.M. (2012). Importance of hemoglobin concentration and its modification for the outcome of head and neck cancer patients treated with radiotherapy. *Acta Oncologica, 51,* 419–432, https://doi.org/10.3109/0284186x.2011.653438

International Commission on Radiation Units and Measurements. (1993). *Prescribing, recording, and reporting photon beam therapy* (ICRU Report 50). Author.

International Commission on Radiation Units and Measurements. (1999). *Prescribing, recording, and reporting photon beam therapy (Supplement to ICRU Report 50)* [ICRU Report 62]. Author.

International Commission on Radiation Units and Measurements. (2010). *Prescribing, recording, and reporting photon-beam intensity-modulated radiation therapy (IMRT)* [ICRU Report 83]. Oxford University Press.

International Commission on Radiation Units and Measurements. (2017). *Prescribing, recording, and reporting of stereotactic treatments with small photon beams* [ICRU Report 91]. Oxford University Press.

Khan, F.M., Gibbons, J.P., & Sperduto, P.W. (Eds.). (2016). *Khan's treatment planning in radiation therapy* (4th ed.). Wolters Kluwer.

Klein, E.E., Hanley, J., Bayouth, J., Yin, F.-F., Simon, W., Dresser, S., ... Holmes, T. (2009). American Association of Physicists in Medicine Radiation Therapy Committee Task Group 142 report: Quality assurance of medical accelerators. *Medical Physics, 36,* 4197–4212. https://doi.org/10.1118/1.3190392

Ma, C.-M.C. (2012). The practice of radiation oncology. In R.R. Iwamoto, M.L. Haas, & T.K. Gosselin (Eds.), *Manual for radiation oncology nursing practice and education* (4th ed., pp. 17–27). Oncology Nursing Society.

Moran, J.M., Dempsey, M., Eisbruch, A., Fraass, B.A., Galvin, J.M., Ibbott, G.S., & Marks, L.B. (2011). Safety considerations for IMRT: Executive summary. *Practical Radiation Oncology, 1,* 190–195. https://doi.org/10.1016/j.prro.2011.04.008

Morgan, S.C., Hoffman, K., Loblaw, D.A., Buyyounouski, M.K., Patton, C., Barocas, D., ... Sandler, H. (2018). Hypofractionated radiation therapy for localized prostate cancer: An ASTRO, ASCO, and AUA evidence-based guideline. *Practical Radiation Oncology, 8,* 354–360. https://doi.org/10.1016/j.prro.2018.08.002

Pinar, B., Herníquez-Hernández, L.A., Lara, P.C., Bordon, E., Rodriguez-Gallego, C., Lloret, M., ... De Almodovar, M.R. (2010). Radiation-induced apoptosis and initial DNA damage are inversely related in locally advanced breast cancer patients. *Radiation Oncology, 5,* 85. https://doi.org/10.1186/1748-717x-5-85

Schubert, T., Todenhöfer, T., Mischinger, J., Schwentner, C., Renninger, M., Stenzl, A., & Gakis, G. (2016). The prognostic role of pre-cystectomy hemoglobin levels in patients with invasive bladder cancer. *World Journal of Urology, 34,* 829–834. https://doi.org/10.1007/s00345-015-1693-2

Story, M.D., & Wang, J. (2018). Developing predictive or prognostic biomarkers for charged particle radiotherapy. *International Journal of Particle Therapy, 5,* 94–102. https://doi.org/10.14338/ijpt-18-00027.1

Van Dyk, J. (Ed.). (1999). *The modern technology of radiation oncology: A compendium for medical physicists and radiation oncologists.* Medical Physics Publishing.

III. Radiation Protection and Safety

A. Nursing implications: Precedence of knowing specific information regarding radiation protection regulations, principles, and practices allows nurses to do the following.

1. Avoid unnecessary radiation exposure (Wilson-Stewart, Shanahan, Fontanarosa, & Davidson, 2018)
2. Focus on the needs of patients receiving radionuclides versus possibly providing hasty care and minimal interaction (Badawy, Mong, Lykhum, & Deb, 2016)
3. Adapt radiation safety practices to new therapeutic radionuclide procedures and treatments (Alavi, Dabbagh, Abbasi, & Mehrdad, 2017)
4. Teach patients, families, and others in healthcare settings about radiation protection practices (Jones & Mathieson, 2016; O. Kim et al., 2018)
5. Alleviate possible fears and misconceptions regarding radiation exposure (Fencl, 2015; Jones & Mathieson, 2016)
6. Put radiation exposure risks into perspective with other health risks (Morishima et al., 2016)

B. Purpose of radiation protection regulations (Kase et al., 2018)

1. To prevent clinically significant radiation-induced deterministic effects by keeping exposed healthcare professionals and the public at a certain threshold dose
   a) Deterministic effects are likely detrimental health problems that occur in someone exposed to ionizing radiation (Petrinec, Šoštarić, & Babić, 2019).
   b) Effects usually are associated with a threshold dose (Petrinec et al., 2019).
   c) The severity of effect increases as dose increases (Kamiya et al., 2015; Kazzi, Buzzell, Bertelli, & Christensen, 2015).
   d) Effects are predictable and based on acute, large-dose exposures as seen in historical studies of atomic bomb survivors, Chernobyl nuclear power plant workers, and individuals treated with RT for benign diseases decades ago (Bouville & Kryuchkov, 2014; Kamiya et al., 2015; Song, 2018).
   e) A small group of deterministic effects appears beyond the acute period, such as radiation-induced cataracts in occupational exposure and total body irradiation (TBI).
      (1) Coppeta et al. (2019) highlighted that the absence of radiologic protection devices leads to an exceedance of the current threshold for deterministic effects on the crystalline lens after several years of work.
      (2) Coppeta et al. (2019) stated that published data determined radiation dose to the lens to be 0.05–0.66 millisieverts (mSv) per procedure.
      (3) The International Commission on Radiological Protection (ICRP) set the dose limit for the crystalline lens to be 20 mSv per year, or 100 mSv in five years, provided that the value for a single year does not exceed 50 mSv (Coppeta et al., 2019).
   f) Acute, large-dose effects are rare in occupational exposure but can occur with major mishandling of radionuclide source, equipment problems, or nuclear power plant disasters (Held & Woloschak, 2016; Song, 2018).

2. To limit the risk of stochastic effects to a reasonable level concerning societal needs, values, and economic factors (Kase et al., 2018)
   a) Stochastic effects are detrimental health effects that can occur from low-level, long-term exposure to ionizing radiation (Kazzi et al., 2015).
   b) Effects occur regardless of total dose or threshold dose (Kamiya et al., 2015; Schroderus-Salo et al., 2019).
   c) Risk of effects is based on the linear no-threshold model, a statistical model suggesting that any increase in radiation exposure dose leads to an incremental increase in risk. Although the acceptance of this model has been heavily debated in the radiation protection scientific community, most recent reviews by the National Council on Radiation Protection and Measurements (NCRP) and other scientific consensus panels hold this model to be true (S.Y. Chen et al., 2014; Domenech, 2017; Kamiya et al., 2015; Kase et al., 2018).
   d) In the future, the main effect of low-dose radiation exposure from medical imaging may be up to 2% of cancers (Hobbs et al., 2018)
   e) Leukemia and solid cancers have been linked with ionizing radiation because the incidence or mortality ascertained from the Life Span Study of atomic bomb survivors serves as a primary input for ICRP in defining dose limits, dose constraints, and reference levels for protection of workers and the public in planned, accidental, and existing exposure situations (Rühm et al., 2016).
      (1) J. Chen and Xie (2019) mentioned that most types of leukemia other than chronic lymphocytic leukemia could be induced by ionizing radiation with a minimum latency of approximately two years.
      (2) Moreover, acute forms of leukemia tend to predominate and occur more rapidly after exposure than chronic granulocytic leukemia (J. Chen & Xie, 2019; Kase et al., 2018).
   f) Offspring of exposed individuals can have genetic effects also, and Anderson (2019) reported that biologic effect is influenced by LET.
      (1) Kyriakopoulou et al. (2018) were unable to rule out the plausibility that cumulative parental exposure may have an etiologic role in the development of acute leukemia in the offspring (Bouville et al., 2018).

(2) Consequently, according to the United Nations Environment Programme (UNEP, 2016), if radiation damage occurs in reproductive cells (sperm or ovum), this can lead to heritable effects in descendants.

(3) Furthermore, radiation can directly damage an embryo or fetus already developing within the womb (Brent et al., 2013; UNEP, 2016).

g) Several factors can influence cancer induction, including age, genetic heritage, gender, and an individual's immune susceptibility (Kutanzi, Lumen, Koturbash, & Miousse, 2016).

3. To keep radiation exposure to individuals or groups at a dose limit that is *as low as reasonably achievable* (ALARA)

a) The ALARA concept has been present for more than 30 years in radiation protection regulations (Badawy, Deb, Chan, & Farouque, 2016; S.Y. Chen et al., 2014; Domenech, 2017).

b) Regulations aim to keep the public and workers safe from harmful radiation exposure (Fencl, 2015; Haygood, 2013).

4. To apply individual dose limits to ensure that radiation exposure does not result in individuals or groups of individuals exceeding levels of acceptable risk (S.Y. Chen et al., 2014; Simon & Linet, 2014)

C. Sources of radiation exposure: Since the 1980s, a dramatic shift and increase has occurred in the amounts of ionizing radiation the average person receives from various sources. The expected average radiation exposure in the United States in the 1980s was 3.6 mSv (360 mrem), and this increased to 6.2 mSv (620 mrem) in 2006 (Bolus, 2013; Haygood, 2013).

1. Natural background radiation

a) Radon, a naturally occurring gas in soil and other sources, is the leading source of natural radiation (American Cancer Society, 2015; Government of Canada, 2020b; Lecomte et al., 2014; Worrell, Gibson, & Allen, 2016). In the 1980s, an individual's exposure to natural background radiation represented 83% of exposure, but decreased to 50% in 2006 (Bolus, 2013). For example, background radiation (radon in the home), accounted for roughly 68% of exposure in 1980 and decreased to 37% in 2006 (Bolus, 2013).

b) Cosmic radiation exposure depends on the altitude of a geographic area. Because air is thinner at higher altitudes, less cosmic radiation is filtered from outer space, thus increasing exposure. Cosmic rays account for 11% of background radiation exposure (American Cancer Society, 2015; Bolus, 2013; Yamamoto, 2013).

c) Other natural sources include minimal amounts of radionuclides found in humans from ingesting food and water containing radionuclides, such as potassium-40 (Abojassim, Dahir, Alaboodi, & Abonasria, 2016; Bolus, 2013; Inoue et al., 2017).

2. Occupational exposure: Occupational exposure from the nuclear power industry and other industries using ionizing radiation represented 0.1% of public exposure in 2006 versus 0.3% in 1980 (Bolus, 2013; Bouville et al., 2018; Yamamoto, 2013).

3. Consumer products: Consumer products, such as televisions and microwave ovens, represented 4% of public radiation exposure in 2006 versus 2% in 1980 (Batool, Bibi, Frezza, & Mangini, 2019; Bolus, 2013; Duarte, de Figueiredo Silva Hafner, & Malvestiti, 2015).

4. Medical sources

a) Exposure from medical sources

(1) The use of medical radiation sources has increased sevenfold in the United States since the early 1980s to 2006.

(2) Medical sources constituted 15% of ionizing radiation exposure in the 1980s.

(3) By 2006, medical source radiation increased to 48% (Bolus, 2013; Kase et al., 2018).

(a) The increase in exposure is mostly the result of interventional fluoroscopy, nuclear medicine procedures, CT, and PET-CT (Hobbs et al., 2018).

(b) Hobbs et al. (2018) researched imaging utilization from 1996 to 2010 and found that the mean per capita radiation exposure from CT examinations doubled and the number of patients receiving high (20–50 mSv) and very high (> 50 mSv) annual radiation doses also doubled.

i. Because of the dramatic increase in medical radiation exposure, radiation protection organizations and regulators are now focusing on reducing unnecessary radiation exposure.

ii. Steps taken to reduce excess medical imaging include advising consumers to keep track of medical imaging procedures and to question the need for these examinations (Ria et al., 2017; Saeed et al., 2018).

b) Types of medical exposure

(1) Diagnostic x-rays from external radiograph studies (general x-rays), including portable x-ray units, fluoroscopy, dental x-rays, CT scans, and mammograms, are common sources (Tomà, Cannatà, Genovese, Magistrelli, & Granata, 2017). In RT, this includes CT localization scans used in IGRT (Nabavizadeh et al., 2016).

(a) Fluoroscopy for diagnostic imaging represents the largest source of occupational exposure in medicine because the operator must be present in the examination room and the x-ray tube used may be energized for considerable periods (Nabaviza-deh et al., 2016).

(b) General radiography poses little exposure if the operator is protected behind the shielded barrier (Nabavizadeh et al., 2016).

(c) Radionuclides are used in nuclear medicine studies, which include a bone scan, thyroid scan, heart scan, PET scan, radionuclide angiography, lymphoscintigraphy, and sentinel lymph node localization (Nabavizadeh et al., 2016).

(d) Radionuclides are used in laboratory departments, for in vitro studies on blood, urine, or cells, as well as radioimmunoassay and other laboratory research studies (Boice, 2014; Qaim, 2017).

(2) Therapeutic sources of radiation

(a) EBRT and teletherapy, which emit x-rays, gamma rays, electrons, protons, and neutrons, are common therapeutic sources (Gross, Frank, Hsu, Diaz, & Gitelis, 2015).

(b) Because personnel are not permitted inside the treatment room for EBRT, this source represents little exposure risk unless lower-energy contact therapy orthovoltage sources are used and operated by personnel or if inadequate shielding is used for external beam equipment (Gross et al., 2015).

(c) The patient receiving EBRT is not radioactive and poses no exposure risk to personnel, the public, or family (Gross et al., 2015).

(3) Radionuclide sources used in internal RT

(a) Sealed sources (brachytherapy) may include iodine-125, iridium-192, and cesium-137. Seeds or ribbons are placed directly into tissues (interstitial brachytherapy) or applicators in body cavities (intracavitary brachytherapy). Table 2 lists sealed radionuclides and their physical properties (Domenech, 2017; Flynn et al., 2019; Mostafa, Rachid, & Ahmed, 2016; Thomadsen, 2018).

(b) Remote afterloading brachytherapy involves radioactive sources (iridium-192) with a highly specific activity that deliver HDR radiation in a short period.

   i. The radioactive source is housed in a shielded unit and poses no exposure risk to staff when inserted remotely into patients (Domenech, 2017).

   ii. It is crucial that proper safeguards and procedures are used to ensure that the radioactive source is returned to the machine.

   iii. In the past 20 years, use of remote afterloading brachytherapy has increased, especially in the treatment of gynecologic malignancies, sarcomas, and other solid tumors. This has led to a dramatic decrease in radiation exposure to healthcare professionals (Domenech, 2017; Erickson, Bittner, Chadha, Mourtada, & Demanes, 2017; Mostafa et al., 2016; Thomadsen, 2018).

(c) Unsealed sources are given as oral, IV, and colloidal radiopharmaceutical therapy (e.g., iodine-131, strontium-89, samarium-153, yttrium-90, phosphorus-32). Table 3 lists therapeutic radiopharmaceuticals and their physical properties (Hashempour, Ghorbani, Amato, & Knaup, 2019).

D. Radiation protection organizations: Several organizations are involved in radiation protection guidelines and standards, delineate practice, and enact general criteria to determine compliance (Wernli, 2016).

1. NCRP

   a) NCRP is a nongovernmental, nonprofit organization first chartered by the U.S. Congress in 1964 (NCRP, 2014, 2015).

   b) The organization collects, analyzes, develops, and disseminates information to the public regarding protection against radiation and radiation measurements, quantities, and units, specifically related to radiation protection.

   c) NCRP provides a means for cooperation among organizations concerned with radiation and radiation protection so that they may effectively utilize resources progress in scientific work.

   d) NCRP develops concepts related to radiation quantities, units, and measurements; the application of these concepts; and radiation protection.

   e) NCRP cooperates with ICRU and other national and international organizations (government and private) concerned with radiation and radiation protection.

   f) The organization publishes guidelines on all aspects of radiation protection for ionizing and nonionizing radiation exposure (Kase et al., 2018; NCRP, 2014; St. Germain, Silberstein, Vetter, Williamson, & Zanzonico, 2006).

   g) Table 4 lists the current NCRP limits of ionizing radiation exposure for radiation workers and the public (de Jong, 2017).

   h) Regulatory agencies in the United States usually adhere to the NCRP guidelines.

2. ICRP (n.d.)

TABLE 2. Physical Properties of Brachytherapy Radionuclides

Radionuclide	Half-Life	Photon Energy (MeV)	Half-Life Layer (mm Pb)	Exposure-Rate Constant[a] Γδ (R cm² mCi¹ h¹)	Physical Form
$^{226}Ra^b$	1,600 y	0.83 (mean)	12	8.25[c]	Tubes, needles
$^{222}Rn^b$	3.83 d	0.83 (mean)	12	8.25[c]	Seeds
^{60}Co	5.25 y	1.25 (mean)	12	13	Plaques, needles
^{137}Cs	30 y	0.662	6.5	3.2	Tubes, needles
^{192}Ir	74.02 d	0.397(β max)	3	4.59	Seeds in ribbons, wires, source on cable
^{125}I	60.14 d	0.028	0.025	1.45	Seeds
^{103}Pd	17 d	0.020	0.008	0.86	Seeds
^{198}Au	2.7 d	0.412	3.3	2.35	Seeds
$^{90}Sr/^{90}Y$	28.2 y	2.24 (β max)	N/A[d]	N/A[d]	Plaques
^{241}Am	432 y	0.60	0.12	3.14	Tubes
^{169}Yb	32 d	0.093 (mean)	0.48	3.27	Seeds
^{131}Cs	9.69 d	0.030	0.030	1.24	Seeds
^{145}Sm	340 d	0.043	0.060	0.885	Seeds

[a] This subscript notation δ in Γδ is used to denote that the calculated value does not include the contributions of radiations removed (i.e., attenuated by the presence of encapsulating materials).
[b] Listed for historical significance only
[c] 0.5 mm platinum-iridium filtration
[d] N/A = not applicable

Am—americium; Au—gold; Co—cobalt; Cs—cesium; I—iodine; Ir—iridium; Pb—lead; Pd—palladium; Ra—radium; Rn—radon; Sm—samarium; Sr—strontium; Y—yttrium; Yb—ytterbium

Note. From *Management of Radionuclide Therapy Patients* (NCRP Report No. 155, p. 43), by J. St. Germain, E.B. Silberstein, R.J. Vetter, J.F. Williamson, and P.D. Zanzonico, 2006, National Council on Radiation Protection and Measurements. Copyright 2006 by National Council on Radiation Protection and Measurements. Reprinted with permission of the National Council on Radiation Protection and Measurements, http://NCRPonline.org.

a) ICRP is an independent, registered nonprofit charity established in the United Kingdom to advance the science of radiation protection for the public benefit.

b) ICRP is involved with guidance on all aspects of radiation protection.

c) ICRP offers recommendations intended to help management and professional staff with responsibilities for radiologic protection to regulatory and advisory agencies.

d) Radiation protection legislation in most countries adheres to ICRP recommendations.

E. U.S. and Canadian regulatory agencies

1. U.S. Nuclear Regulatory Commission (NRC)

a) NRC provides direct regulatory authority over the medical use of reactor-produced radionuclides, including those for therapeutic and diagnostic purposes (U.S. NRC, 2019).

b) NRC regulates the use of by-product materials and materials made radioactive in a reactor (Medical Use of Byproduct Material, 2013).

c) NRC regulates the use of radioactive materials used in medicine per the Code of Federal Regulations, including the following requirements (Standards for Protection Against Radiation, 1991; U.S. NRC, 2003).

(1) Establishing dose limits for radiation workers and the public

(2) Monitoring and labeling of radioactive materials

(3) Posting specific warning signs in places using radiation sources

(4) Reporting theft or loss of radioactive materials

(5) Enforcing penalties for noncompliance with NRC regulations

(6) Publishing tables of individual radionuclide exposure limits

d) NRC (2003) issues full medical licenses to individuals using radionuclides for medical use in hospital and outpatient settings.

e) NRC specifies what instructions should be given to nursing staff who care for brachytherapy patients

(Basran, Baxter, & Beckham, 2015; Medical Use of Byproduct Material, 2013).

    (1) Size and appearance of the brachytherapy sources

    (2) Safe handling and shielding instructions in case of dislodgment

    (3) Procedures for visitor control

    (4) Procedures for the patient or human research control

    (5) Procedures for notifying the radiation safety officer (RSO) if the patient has a medical emergency or dies

  f) All NRC regulations are now available online at www.nrc.gov.

2. U.S. Food and Drug Administration (U.S. FDA, 2018)

  a) FDA regulates the design and manufacture of radiation devices and equipment.

  b) FDA regulates the development of radiopharmaceuticals.

3. State radiation commissions and agencies

  a) States can be licensed by the NRC or can be classified as agreement states. Agreement states, per state law, assign all responsibility for radiation protection to a state agency. Agreement states may require radiation protection practices in addition to the NRC guidelines. Figure 6 shows the current agreement and nonagreement states (Pryor, 2016; U.S. NRC, 2019).

  b) Individual states have radiation protection agencies that are responsible for setting state guidelines and enforcing the national standards and guidelines. States also regulate radiation-producing equipment (e.g., linear accelerators). Nurses are encouraged to become familiar with their individual state's radiation regulation programs (O. Kim et al., 2018).

4. Canadian Nuclear Safety Commission (2014)

  a) The Nuclear Safety Commission regulates nuclear substances and radiation devices to protect the health and safety of Canadians and the environment.

  b) The Nuclear Safety Commission safeguards against loss of nuclear materials.

  c) The Nuclear Safety Commission regulates and grants licenses to medical facilities that use radionuclides.

  d) The Nuclear Safety Commission establishes exposure dose limits for the public and occupational workers.

5. Canadian Radiation Protection Bureau (Government of Canada, 2020a)

  a) The Radiation Protection Bureau manages the National Dose Registry, which contains the occupa-

TABLE 3. Physical Properties of Photon- and Beta-Emitting Radionuclides Commonly Used in Therapeutic Radiopharmaceuticals

Radionuclide	Physical Half-Life	Specific Gamma-Ray Constant[a][b] (R cm² mCi¹ h¹)	Maximum Beta-Ray Energy (MeV)	Specific Bremsstrahlung Constant[a][b] (R cm² mCi¹ h¹)	
Photon- and Beta-Emitters				Soft Tissue Zeff = 7.9	Bone (calcium) Zeff = 21
¹³¹I	8.04 d	2.23	0.81	0.000768	0.00204
¹⁷⁷Lu	6.7 d	0.222		0.000385	0.00102
¹⁵³Sm	47 h	0.712	0.497, 0.44	0.000597	0.0.00159
¹⁸⁶Re	89 h	0.143	0.8	0.00121	0.00322
¹⁸⁸Re	17 h	0.320	1.07	0.00154	0.00409
Beta-Emitters					
³²P	14.3 d	-	1.71	0.00405	0.0108
³³P	25.4 d	-	0.25	0.000658	0.00175
⁸⁹Sr[c]	50.5 h	-	1.49	0.00314	0.00843
⁹⁰Y	64.1 h	-	2.28	0.00564	0.015

[a] Values for constants from NUREG-1556, Vol. 9 (U.S. NRC, 2005), and for ¹⁷⁷Lu only (Unger & Trubey, 1982).

[b] The specific gamma-ray constant is a physical quantity that is expressed in conventional units of R cm² mCi¹ h¹. The specific gamma-ray constant and the analogous specific bremsstrahlung are therefore expressed in these conventional units.

[c] Although ⁸⁹Sr emits a gamma ray, it is grouped with the beta emitters because the frequency of its gamma-ray emissions, < 0.01% per decay, is negligibly low.

I—iodine; Lu—lutetium; P—phosphorus; Re—rhenium; Sm—samarium; Sr—strontium; Y—yttrium

Note. From *Management of Radionuclide Therapy Patients* (NCRP Report No. 155, p. 75), by J. St. Germain, E.B. Silberstein, R.J. Vetter, J.F. Williamson, and P.D. Zanzonico, 2006, National Council on Radiation Protection and Measurements. Copyright 2006 by National Council on Radiation Protection and Measurements. Reprinted with permission of the National Council on Radiation Protection and Measurements, http://NCRPonline.org.

TABLE 4. Recommended Dose Limits

Population	Annual Effective Dose Limit (mSv)
Adult workers	50
Adult worker who declares her pregnancy	0.5 mSv month^{-1}
Members of the public	1
Family member of patient	5
Pregnant women and children	1
Trained and monitored family member of patient	50
Adult lifetime	Age × 10 mSv

Note. From *Management of Radionuclide Therapy Patients* (NCRP Report No. 155, p. 17), by J. St. Germain, E.B. Silberstein, R.J. Vetter, J.F. Williamson, and P.D. Zanzonico, 2006, National Council on Radiation Protection and Measurements. Copyright 2006 by National Council on Radiation Protection and Measurements. Reprinted with permission of the National Council on Radiation Protection and Measurements, http://NCRPonline.org.

tional radiation dose records of all radiation-monitored workers in Canada.
   b) The Radiation Protection Bureau researches exposure trends for radiation workers and the health outcomes of occupational exposures to radiation.
   c) The Radiation Protection Bureau provides advice to federal departments and agencies, other levels of government, industry, universities, hospitals, workers, and the public on health issues related to radiation exposure.
6. Institutional committees and individuals responsible for radiation protection
   a) Institutional radiation safety programs and radiation safety committees
      (1) These groups are designated by hospital or institution administration and are authorized by the state and NRC to oversee and monitor the radiation protection program of an institution.
      (2) Groups must meet quarterly to review the hospital or institution's radiation protection program and should have a nursing representative (O. Kim et al., 2018).
   b) RSO or delegated trained personnel responsibilities
      (1) RSO implements and monitors the institution's radiation protection program (Domenech, 2017; Haygood, 2013; Spruce, 2017).
      (2) RSO trains personnel, including nurses, in radiation protection practices, as well as educates patients and families on discharge precautions with certain radionuclide procedures (Domenech, 2017; Haygood, 2013; Spruce, 2017).
      (3) RSO serves as the primary resource person regarding institutional radiation protection

practices and issues (Domenech, 2017; Haygood, 2013; Spruce, 2017).
      (4) RSO monitors radiation doses received by occupationally exposed individuals and the public in and around the medical facility (Domenech, 2017; Spruce, 2017).
      (5) RSO monitors radiation exposure from patients who are receiving internal RT in inpatient and outpatient settings (Domenech, 2017; Haygood, 2013; Spruce, 2017).
      (6) RSO determines when patients treated with radionuclides can be discharged from radiation isolation (Domenech, 2017; Spruce, 2017).
      (7) RSO is responsible for inventory and receipt of radioactive sources (Haygood, 2013).
      (8) RSO is responsible for the removal of radioactive waste or contamination (Boice, Cohen, Mumma, & Ellis, 2019).

F. Radionuclide factors determining the type and amount of radiation protection practices
   1. Type and energy of radiation emission from radionuclide: Radionuclides can give off one or mixed emission spectra depending on the specific radionuclide (Domenech, 2017; Elgqvist, Timmermand, Larsson, & Strand, 2016).
   a) Alpha particles
      (1) Alpha particles are composed of two protons and two neutrons that travel at high speed but have poor penetrating capability because of their large size (Domenech, 2017; Elgqvist et al., 2016; U.S. Environmental Protection Agency [EPA], n.d.-b).
      (2) Alpha particles have energies ranging 5–9 MeV and travel in straight lines (Domenech, 2017; Elgqvist et al., 2016).
      (3) Maximum distance particles can travel is less than 5 cm in the air (Domenech, 2017; Elgqvist et al., 2016).
      (4) A sheet of paper, clothes, or a range of greater than 5 cm is adequate to shield a person from external alpha particle radiation (Domenech, 2017; Elgqvist et al., 2016).
      (5) High quantities of alpha particle sources (e.g., radon) when inhaled or swallowed can pose an inherent hazard inside the body. Alpha particles transfer relatively large amounts of ionizing energy to living cells (high LET and relative biologic effectiveness) (Bouville et al., 2018; Domenech, 2017; Elgqvist et al., 2016).
      (6) Alpha particles have a high dose equivalent and are more dangerous compared to other types of radiation, given that ionizations from alpha particles are very close together, resulting in more damage to DNA and the cells (NCRP, 2014; U.S. EPA, n.d.-b).

(a) Dose equivalent is a quantity used in radiation protection to place all radiation on a standard scale for calculating tissue damage.

(b) Dose equivalent is the absorbed dose multiplied by a quality factor.

(c) The quality factor accounts for the differences in radiation effects caused by different types of ionizing radiation. Alpha particles produce a more significant amount of damage per unit of an absorbed dose than other radiation, as the weighted quality factor is 20 times that of beta or gamma radiation (Elgqvist et al., 2016; Haygood, 2013; Sgouros, Hobbs, & Josefsson, 2018; U.S. EPA, n.d.-b; U.S. FDA, 2018).

(7) Because of their poor penetrating range in tissues, alpha particles can only discharge their energy in a small number of cells and can be blocked, for example, by skin or a sheet of paper (Bouville et al., 2018; Dauer et al., 2018).

(a) Pure alpha emitters were not traditionally used in RT until the emergence of radiolabeled antibodies. Experimental monoclonal antibodies labeled with pure alpha particle emitters, such as bismuth-213, can be more cytotoxic than beta-radiolabeled antibodies, as alpha emitters have greater biologic effectiveness because of their high LET.

(b) Some evidence has also shown that alpha-radiolabeled antibodies may kill tumor cells that are in hypoxic environments.

b) Beta particles

(1) Beta particles are negatively charged electrons emitted from the nucleus of a decaying radioactive particle. They have deeper penetration than alpha particles and travel approximately ½ inch inside human tissue. They can be shielded by something as thin as a pad of paper.

(2) Examples of pure beta particle radionuclides used in therapy are phosphorus-32, yttrium-90, strontium-98, and samarium-153 (Elgqvist et al., 2016; Haygood, 2013; Mancini-Terracciano et al., 2017; U.S. EPA, n.d.-b).

(3) Once a pure beta particle radionuclide is instilled or injected into a patient's body, the body will supply adequate shielding (Conti & Eriksson, 2016; Elgqvist et al., 2016; Haygood, 2013; Mancini-Terracciano et al., 2017; U.S. EPA, n.d.-b).

(4) If a specific dose of some beta emitters is used systemically, a patient's body fluids may be tem-

FIGURE 6. U.S. Nuclear Regulatory Commission Agreement and Non-Agreements States

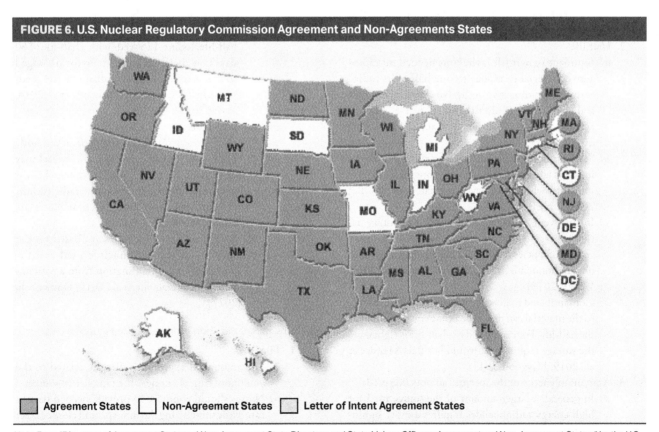

☐ Agreement States ☐ Non-Agreement States ☐ Letter of Intent Agreement States

Note. From "Directory of Agreement State and Non-Agreement State Directors and State Liaison Officers: Agreement and Non-Agreement States," by the U.S. Nuclear Regulatory Commission, 2020 (https://scp.nrc.gov/asdirectory.html). In the public domain.

porarily radioactive (Elgqvist et al., 2016; Haygood, 2013; Mancini-Terracciano et al., 2017; U.S. EPA, n.d.-b).

(5) Beta particles can pose an internal radiation hazard if inhaled or ingested (Elgqvist et al., 2016; Haygood, 2013; Mancini-Terracciano et al., 2017; U.S. EPA, n.d.-b).

c) Gamma rays

(1) High-energy electromagnetic radiation is given off by specific radionuclides when their nuclei transition from a higher to a lower energy state (U.S. EPA, n.d.-b).

(2) Gamma rays have a wide range of energies and penetrating capabilities. Higher power requires thicker material for gamma radiation shielding (Elgqvist et al., 2016; Haygood, 2013; U.S. EPA, n.d.-b).

(3) High-energy gamma-emitting radionuclides require both specified distances and shielding to reduce a person's exposure (Elgqvist et al., 2016; Haygood, 2013; U.S. EPA, n.d.-b).

(4) Patients receiving high-energy gamma radionuclides (e.g., cesium-137, iridium-192) may need to be in radiation isolation and behind lead shields (Elgqvist et al., 2016; Haygood, 2013; Smith & Kearfott, 2018).

(5) Low-energy gamma emitters, such as iodine-125 and palladium-103, do not require radiation isolation and lead shielding (S.Y. Chen et al., 2014).

2. Half-life

a) Radioactive half-life is the time needed for radioactive material to reduce to one-half of its radioactivity by radioactive decay. No chemical or physical operation can alter the decay rate of a radioactive substance (S.Y. Chen et al., 2014; UNEP, 2016).

b) Sealed radionuclides are chosen for either permanent implants (short half-life, low emissions) or temporary implants, which may have long half-lives (NCRP, 2014; UNEP, 2016).

c) In the event of dislodgment, spill, or contamination, storage of the radioactive source is a primary concern. Policies related to these incidents are based on a radionuclide's half-life (S.Y. Chen et al., 2014; UNEP, 2016).

d) Contaminated radioactive waste may require storage so the material can decay for a time equal to 10 times the half-life. For example, if the half-life is eight days, the storage requirement would be 80 days (Boice et al., 2019; Haygood, 2013).

3. Amount of energy of the specific radionuclide used

a) In general, a larger amount of the source used for high-energy radionuclides requires a more significant amount of radiation safety protection measures (NCRP, 2014).

b) The amount of energy that requires radiation isolation is determined by regulatory agencies, such as NRC, from guidelines established by NCRP (2014).

4. Radionuclide form: The two basic types of radionuclides are used. Sealed sources include rods, ribbons, needles, and seeds, all of which are surgically implanted into tumor tissues or in special applicators placed in body cavities. Unsealed sources include liquids, capsules, and colloids, all of which can be ingested, injected, or instilled into the body (Domenech, 2017).

a) Sealed sources

(1) With sealed sources, the source, not the patient, is radioactive.

(a) The radioactive material is encapsulated, and safety measures are based on the source itself and the likelihood of dislodgment.

(b) The patient and body fluids are not radioactive.

(c) For temporary implants, once the source has been removed and returned to the safe storage and the area has been surveyed and checked for any dislodged sources, no further radiation protection measures are required (S.Y. Chen et al., 2014; Domenech, 2017).

(2) With permanent implants, precautions for dislodged sources may be in place for a specified time based on the energy of the source and the half-life. Iodine-125 seeds with a half-life of 60 days may dictate a longer time for dislodged source precautions than palladium-103 seeds with a half-life of 17 days (Lecomte et al., 2014; Pryor, 2015).

b) Unsealed sources

(1) With unsealed sources, the patient and body fluids (blood, urine, feces, saliva, sweat) may be radioactive for a specified time, which is determined by the energy of the radionuclide, amount used, and half-life (Bouville et al., 2018; Domenech, 2017).

(2) Radiation safety measures are based on the specifics of the radionuclide used and the possibility of contamination from a patient's body fluids (Bouville et al., 2018; Domenech, 2017).

G. Principles of radiation protection (see Figure 7)

1. Time

a) The amount of exposure is directly related to the amount of time spent near the radioactive source.

b) Nurses should continue to provide needed patient care while minimizing the time spent in close contact with a gamma radionuclide source inside a patient, which poses a radiation exposure risk.

FIGURE 7. Cardinal Principles of Time, Distance, and Shielding

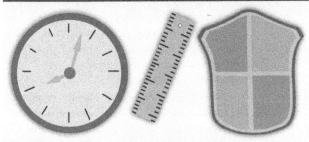

Time: To decrease exposure to penetrating beta and gamma ionizing radiation, decrease the time of exposure.

Distance: To decrease the amount of radiation exposure, increase the distance from the source. The intensity of the radiation is inversely proportional to the square of the distance from the source. For example, doubling the distance from the source will reduce the intensity of radiation by a factor of 4.

Shielding: Shielding is useful for absorbing radiation exposure. Select the right shielding to stop the type of radiation being used.

Note. From "RadTown Radiation Protection: Teacher Information" by U.S. Environmental Protection Agency, 2019 (https://www.epa.gov/radtown/radtown-radiation-protection-teacher-information). In the public domain.

c) If a time limit for direct patient contact per nursing shift has been established (determined by the RSO), this should be posted on a patient's hospital room door.

d) The time limit for a patient's visitors also should be displayed. Strategies to minimize time include the following (Fencl, 2015; Haygood, 2013).

  (1) Provide necessary patient education before the procedure (Haygood, 2013).

  (2) Teach, observe, and document the patient's ability to perform self-care measures before the procedure (Haygood, 2013).

  (3) Evaluate the patient's understanding of the procedure. Discuss the reasoning for limiting staff and family exposure. This explanation will help prevent the patient from feeling alienated (Haygood, 2013).

  (4) Provide the maximum amount of direct nursing care before the radioactive source is placed or administered (Haygood, 2013).

  (5) Assemble all necessary equipment and supplies in the patient's room before the procedure to avoid unnecessary trips, and ensure that equipment (e.g., telephone, television) in the patient's room works appropriately before the radioactive source is administered (Haygood, 2013).

  (6) Check on the patient frequently via intercom or telephone, anticipate the patient's needs, and encourage the patient to communicate any problems or concerns to the staff via intercom or telephone (Haygood, 2013).

  (7) Use time efficiently when in contact with the patient and organize care. Nurses caring for patients who have undergone specific radioactive procedures may want to practice routine care activities (e.g., logrolling the patient from side to side, visually checking the position of the gynecologic applicator, emptying a Foley catheter bag) (Haygood, 2013).

  (8) Rotate the nursing and ancillary staff caring for the patient receiving radioactive implants and reassure the family that care is a priority and the patient will not be neglected (Bibbo, Benger, Sigalas, & Kirkwood, 2018; Haygood, 2013).

2. Distance
  a) The amount of radiation exposure a person receives is inversely related to the distance from the radioactive source or radioactive patient (inverse square law) (U.S. EPA, n.d.-a).

    (1) By doubling the distance from the source, exposure is decreased by a factor of 4 (2^2).

    (2) For example, an exposure rate of 40 mrem/hour at 1 meter would reduce to an exposure rate of 10 mrem/hour at a distance of 2 meters.

  b) The following are examples of nursing care measures that maximize distance from a radioactive source (Haygood, 2013; U.S. EPA, n.d.-a).

    (1) With direct patient contact, nurses should stand as far away from the sealed radioactive source as possible. For example, nurses can stand at the head of the bed to take vital signs when in the room with a patient who has a gynecologic implant. Nurses should talk to patients from the doorway rather than inside the room (U.S. EPA, n.d.-a).

    (2) Nurses should assist patients with needed tasks (e.g., unwrapping food items) from a distance (U.S. EPA, n.d.-a).

    (3) Nurses should reinforce the teaching of self-care activities while standing at a distance from a patient (Haygood, 2013).

3. Shielding
  a) The amount of radiation exposure received from a specified radioactive source can be decreased by the use of absorbing material (shield) placed between the source and the person receiving the exposure (S.Y. Chen et al., 2014; Domenech, 2017; U.S. EPA, n.d.-b).

  b) Figure 8 shows the type of shielding that can stop different forms of ionizing radiation (S.Y. Chen et al., 2014; Domenech, 2017; U.S. EPA, n.d.-b).

  c) The amount of exposure decreased by shielding will vary with the energy of the source and the thickness of the shielding material.

  d) *Half-value layer* refers to the thickness of a material required to reduce radiation exposure to half of its original exposure amount. For example, the

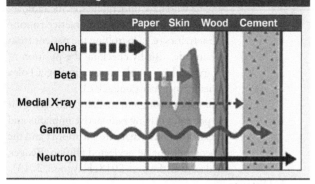

Note. From "Radiation Basics," by U.S. Nuclear Regulatory Commission, 2017 (https://www.nrc.gov/about-nrc/radiation/health-effects/radiation-basics .html). In the public domain.

half-value layer of cesium-137 is 6 mm of lead or 10 cm of concrete.

  e) The following are common suggestions for shielding to reduce exposure when shielding is appropriate (Baalamurugan et al., 2019; Domenech, 2017; Hinrichsen, Finck, Östlund, Rääf, & Andersson, 2018; Sabet, Cryer, & Waterhouse, 2016; Semmler et al., 2019; U.S. EPA, n.d.-a).

   (1) Keep the shielding between the source and the person exposed. Build shields into the walls and floors of designated treatment rooms that are used for radioactive procedures that use high-energy gamma sources (Domenech, 2017; U.S. EPA, n.d.-a).

   (2) Continue to apply principles of time and distance, even with shields, to further reduce radiation exposure (Domenech, 2017; U.S. EPA, n.d.-a).

   (3) Consider that maneuvering the shield may require increased nursing time in the room, making some uses of shields unwarranted (Domenech, 2017; U.S. EPA, n.d.-a).

   (4) Select the correct material for shielding based on the type of emitters (e.g., lead for high-energy gamma sources, plastic for pure beta sources) (Domenech, 2017; U.S. EPA, n.d.-a).

   (5) Use more shielding in institutions that perform large numbers of gamma-emitting radioactive procedures (Domenech, 2017; Haygood, 2013; Ortiz López et al., 2018).

H. Radiation monitoring devices (see Figure 9)
  1. Overview
   a) Although ionizing radiation cannot be detected by human senses, detection devices (personal monitoring device or survey monitor) can measure the amounts of radiation exposure received by an individual (Garcia-Sanchez, Angosto, Riquelme, Berna, & Ramos-Amores, 2018).

   b) Monitoring devices do not offer any radiation exposure protection. They only physically measure levels or amounts of exposure (Bouville et al., 2018; Domenech, 2017).
  2. Types of personal dosimetry monitors
   a) Personal monitoring devices
    (1) Personal monitoring devices are recommended for individuals who need constant radiation exposure monitoring in the occupational setting. Monitors are recommended for all occupationally exposed individuals who, in the judgment of the RSO, have the potential to receive significantly more than 10% of the annual effective dose limit during the ordinary course of their duties, as well as individuals who enter radiation areas (Basran et al., 2015; Haygood, 2013).

    (2) Electronic personal dosimeters should be worn consistently at work during times of potential and actual exposure and should not be worn outside of work (Basran et al., 2015; Haygood, 2013).

    (3) The dosimeter is not to be shared or exchanged with other staff (Basran et al., 2015; Haygood, 2013).

    (4) The dosimeter should not be exposed to excessive heat or moisture (Basran et al., 2015; Haygood, 2013).

    (5) The dosimeter should not remain on the lab coat or placed in a room with radiation sources when it is not being worn (Basran et al., 2015; Haygood, 2013; König, Etzel, Thomas, & Mahnken, 2019).

    (6) The dosimeter should be worn on the area of the body that the highest deep, shallow, and eye-dose equivalent is expected to be received. In general, this is on the front of the body between the waist and collar. For specialized work in which the highest dose is at the head level, such as fluoroscopy, the dosimeter should be worn at the collar (Domenech, 2017; König et al., 2019; Yoder et al., 2019).

    (7) The dosimeter should be read according to the institutional schedule, and the cumulative record of personal monitor readings should be kept on file at the institution (Alkhorayef et al., 2018; Haygood, 2013).
   b) Ring dosimeter (Domenech, 2017)
    (1) A ring dosimeter is an individual monitoring device similar to a personal dosimeter but is worn on the finger and is used by personnel who are handling radioactive material.

    (2) Guidelines are similar to those of a personal dosimeter.

FIGURE 9. Example of Radiation Monitoring Devices

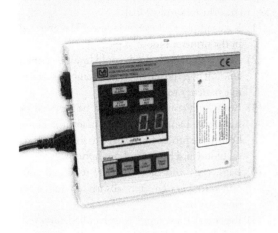
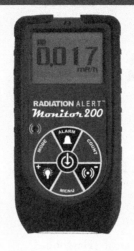
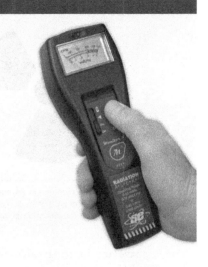

Digital area monitor, monitor 4 survey meter, and ranger survey meter

Note. Images courtesy of Biodex Medical Systems Inc. Used with permission.

c) Pocket ion chamber dosimeter
  (1) A pocket ion chamber dosimeter is a light-weight radiation measurement instrument that gives the same readouts of radiation exposure as a personal dosimeter but is used by individuals who do not need continual radiation exposure monitoring but rather periodic monitoring for scheduled radioactive procedures.
  (2) Unlike an individual monitor, different personnel can share pocket dosimeters.
  (3) The amount of radiation exposure received is known immediately for each person who wears the monitoring device.
  (4) Pocket dosimeters are especially useful for nursing and healthcare staff and family members who are in contact with people being cared for in inpatient or outpatient units that infrequently use diagnostic or therapeutic radioactive materials (Domenech, 2017; Haygood, 2013; König et al., 2019).
  (5) Use of pocket ion chamber dosimeters should adhere to the following.
    (a) Dosimeters should be left at the nurses' station or outside a patient's room with the exposure dose record sheet that keeps track of individual exposure amounts. These devices should not be kept near a radioactive source (Garcia-Sanchez et al., 2018).
    (b) Pocket dosimeters should be worn in the same place as a personal dosimeter—where the highest dose may be received (Yoder et al., 2019).
    (c) Dosimeters should be read before entering a patient's room and again after leaving a patient's room.

    i. The readings should be recorded on the dose record sheet.
    ii. Information to record includes the name of the person exposed, date, time, dosimeter readouts, time spent in the room, and readings before entering and after leaving the room (Basran et al., 2015).
  (d) Dosimeters should be handled gently. If dropped, tapped, or knocked, pocket ion chamber dosimeters can show inaccurate readings and may need to be recalibrated by the radiation safety staff or radiation oncology dosimetry staff (Domenech, 2017).
  (e) Dosimeters should be read by holding them up toward the light in a horizontal position and reading the point at which the hairline crosses the numbered scale (Haygood, 2013).
  (f) Dosimeters should have their records kept on file and monitored by the RSO and radiation safety staff (Basran et al., 2015; Haygood, 2013).

I. Recognition of radiation-restricted areas: Federal and state laws require the posting of appropriate radiation protection warning signs in areas containing potential and real radiation exposure (Haygood, 2013).

  1. Radiation caution sign (see Figure 10)
    a) Caution signs have a yellow background with magenta lettering and should specify the specific radionuclide source and radiation precautions (Haygood, 2013).
    b) Caution signs should be placed on the door of the rooms, both inpatient and outpatient, that

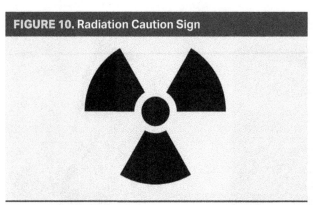

FIGURE 10. Radiation Caution Sign

Note. From "Radtown Radiation Protection: Teacher Information," by U.S. Environmental Protection Agency, 2019 (https://www.epa.gov/radtown/radtown-radiation-protection-teacher-information). In the public domain.

have any ionizing radiation present (Haygood, 2013).

   c) For rooms of patients treated with sealed radioactive sources, the caution sign needs to specify any restrictions for staff and visitors. The sign needs to remain in place until the source is removed and the room surveyed for possible source dislodgment or until exposure risk is no longer present (Bibbo et al., 2018; Haygood, 2013).

   d) For rooms of patients treated with unsealed radioactive sources, the caution sign needs to specify restrictions for staff and visitors and remain in place until the room is surveyed and all contaminated articles are removed (Bibbo et al., 2018).

2. Therapeutic radionuclide information sheets (Haygood, 2013)

   a) Information sheets should be placed in a patient's inpatient or outpatient chart (Bibbo et al., 2018).

   b) Document radionuclide information should include the name of the radionuclide, dose, specific activity, administration method, and date of administration (Bibbo et al., 2018; Haygood, 2013).

J. Special radiation protection considerations and issues related to discharge of patients treated with radiopharmaceuticals or permanent implants (Bibbo et al., 2018)

1. Pure beta emitters (yttrium-90, strontium-89, samarium-153)

   a) The administration of yttrium-90 (radiolabeled antibody) is safely performed on an outpatient basis. Some patients need to be treated as inpatients for medical reasons, not because of radiation protection hazard. Samarium-153 and strontium-89 can be given as an outpatient injection (Bobin, Thiam, & Chauvenet, 2017; Conti & Eriksson, 2016; Fons-Castells, Tent-Petrus, & Llauradó, 2017; Haygood, 2013).

   b) There is no external radiation exposure risk to patients' family members and healthcare professionals in contact with the patient (Haygood, 2013).

   c) Possible internal exposure risk from unintentionally ingested beta particles can prompt an internal hazard to healthcare professionals.

     (1) For example, radioactive iodine-131 is excreted in the urine or blood.

     (2) Excretion in body fluids could result in a small amount of radioactivity to be extant on surfaces in a patient's room.

     (3) Body fluid contamination can be ingested by surface to hand to mouth contact; therefore, healthcare professionals need to follow universal blood and body fluid precautions.

     (4) Bags, vials, and tubes that are used and contain pure beta emitters absorb any radiation that may be present.

     (5) In general, these supplies are handled, surveyed, and discarded by designated radiation safety personnel (Haygood, 2013; S.-T. Kim, Yoo, & Park, 2018; Sgouros et al., 2018).

   d) Patients receiving pure beta emitters can be discharged immediately after treatment without any activity limits, and no dose-rate limit measurements need to be taken (Haygood, 2013).

   e) The person administering pure beta radiopharmaceuticals should wear gloves, use a plastic syringe cover over the medication, and be careful not to spray or drip the medication (Domenech, 2017; Sgouros et al., 2018).

   f) Patients should be encouraged to use regular toilet facilities, avoid urine leakage, and double-flush toilets. Anyone handling a patient's urine, especially in the first 24 hours after the injection, should wear gloves (Haygood, 2013; Nasser, Cohen, Dauer, & Zelefsky, 2016; Yoder et al., 2019).

   g) After LDR prostate brachytherapy, precaution recommended to a patient and partner is the use of condoms for sexual relations for one week after injection. It is theoretically possible for a seed to be expelled in the semen (Nasser et al., 2016; Yoder et al., 2019; Zain, 2018).

   h) After discharge, patients should clean up any spilled urine and dispose of any urine- or blood-contaminated material (e.g., flush it down the toilet; place it in a plastic bag in household trash) to prevent it from being handled by others (Haygood, 2013; Yoder et al., 2019).

2. Radioactive iodine-131 for thyroid cancer or hyperthyroidism

   a) In 1997, NRC revised its patient release regulations, allowing for larger activities of radioactive iodine-131 to be given as an outpatient administration. Previously, NRC required any individual receiving 30 mCi or greater of radioactive iodine-131 to be an inpatient setting in radiation isolation and discharged after an exposure rate of less than 5 milliroentgen/hour at 1 meter was obtained. The newer regulation allows patients to be released if the total effective dose equivalent to any other individual is not likely to exceed 5 mSv (Bibbo et al., 2018; U.S. NRC, 1997).

b) With systemic gamma-emitting radionuclides, such as iodine-131, a patient's body fluids (blood, urine, saliva, feces, semen) pose a temporary radiation hazard, as well as the patient being an external hazard to individuals in close contact with the patient (Bibbo et al., 2018; Haygood, 2013; Pae, 2018).

c) Studies have shown that the amounts of radiation exposure received by household members of patients discharged after receiving iodine-131 have been below the limit of 1 mSv/year (Bibbo et al., 2018; Harrison et al., 2016).

d) Discharge instructions are based on not only the amount of iodine-131 given, but on several other factors, such as where a patient will be discharged to and who will be in the home, including children, the sex and age of each household member, and sleeping partner information.

   (1) The medical facility or occupational settings should provide radiation risk precautions to protect pregnant women or minors.

   (2) Patients should be provided discharge instructions regarding transportation to and from the medical facility and the home; physical challenges; and incontinence or ostomy care. Ability to comprehend instructions is paramount.

   (3) Figure 11 provides an example of discharge instructions given to a patient who has received radioactive iodine therapy (Bibbo et al., 2018; Domenech, 2017; Idota et al., 2017; Long, Frank, & Ehrlich, 2017).

   (4) Discharge instructions for unsealed sources, such as radioactive iodine, can be determined by a computer program specific to the particulars of outpatient radioactive iodine therapy. A copy of these instructions should be given to the patient and family and placed in the patient's record (Domenech, 2017; Idota et al., 2017).

3. Iodine-125 and palladium-103 prostate seed implants

   a) Prostate implants can be inserted as an outpatient procedure. Once the seeds are in place, there is little radiation exposure risk to others (Hanada, Yorozu, Kikumura, Ohashi, & Shigematsu, 2014; Inada et al., 2018).

   b) NRC guidelines allow discharge of patients if the exposure rate at 1 meter is at or below 0.01 mSv/hour for iodine-125 and 0.03 mSv/hour for palladium-103 (S.Y. Chen et al., 2014; Sheetz & Steiner, 2018; Stish et al., 2018).

   c) Hanada et al. (2014) conducted a study involving direct radiation exposure measurement to family members of patients with prostate cancer who received iodine-125 seeds. Results showed that radiation exposure to family members was low.

   (1) Based on two study periods, the mean estimated lifetime exposure doses were 7.61 mSv (range 0.45–20.21 mSv) and 6.84 mSv (range 0.41–19.20 mSv) for patients and 0.19 mSv (range 0.02–0.54 mSv) and 0.25 mSv (range 0.04–1 mSv) for family members (Hanada et al., 2014).

   (2) In reference to palladium-103, according to Nasser et al. (2016) in their study of 20 patients treated with iodine-125 and 82 patients with palladium-103, results showed that in the weeks immediately after prostate seed implantation, the estimated intrarectal dose rates are higher for palladium-103 than iodine-125, noting that palladium-103 decays at a faster rate.

   (3) Moreover, radiation exposure from palladium-103 is lower than iodine-125. Therefore, anal intercourse time should be kept as low as possible approximately two to six months after LDR prostate brachytherapy with iodine-125 and palladium-103 (Nasser et al., 2016).

   (4) Conversely, postimplantation radiation exposures to spouses and other family members, as assessed by worn dosimeter monitoring studies, have been calculated at 0.07–0.1 mSv following either iodine-125 or palladium-103 prostate brachytherapy (Stish et al., 2018).

   (5) Prospectively, the amount of exposure is less than the amount of cosmic radiation experienced annually by a person living at sea level (Stish et al., 2018).

   (6) Research has shown that an individual who received prostate brachytherapy could hold a child on his lap for at least 30 minutes every day immediately following an iodine-125 implant, and the child would not exceed a 0.5 mSv exposure threshold (Stish et al., 2018).

   (7) Prospectively, a person flying from New York to Tokyo receives 0.0055 mSv, and someone flying from New York to Seattle receives 0.005 mSv (Federal Aviation Administration, 2016).

d) Discharge instructions to patients who received iodine-125 or palladium-103 vary per institution but should contain the following information (S.Y. Chen et al., 2014).

   (1) Instructions should name and describe the radioactive sources (e.g., "small metallic seeds, about ⅓ to ½ inch long") (Stish et al., 2018).

   (2) Instructions should recommend lengths of activites to minimize exposure to others, including holding or cuddling children, closeness to pregnant women, sleeping restrictions with a partner, and sexual intercourse (Nasser et al., 2016).

FIGURE 11. Example Instruction Sheet

**Radiation Safety Precautions for
Radiopharmaceutical Therapy Patients**

Note: Please carefully read and follow the instructions in this document.

If you or your healthcare provider have any questions or concerns regarding the radionuclide therapy you have received, please contact:

Dr. J. Smith

Nuclear Medicine Attending Physician

at _____(111) 222-3333_____ or _____0000_____

      Telephone number   Emergency or pager telephone number

Patient **John Q. Patient**, Medical Record Number **1111-11-111**, received a therapeutic dose of **6.475 MBq (175 mCi)** of **Iodine-131 Sodium Iodide** at **General Hospital** on **January 1, 2004**, at **9:00 am** and should observe the following radiation safety precautions at home as follows.

- Avoid close contact [less than 1 meter (3 feet) away from] with pregnant women and children until **1 day** after the administration of the radionuclide therapy.
- Do not hold or embrace children for more than 10 minutes a day until **21 days** after the day your radionuclide therapy was administered. *This requires that you avoid contact with these children altogether during your* **first day** *after the day your radionuclide therapy was administered.*
- Unless you work alone (for example, driving a truck), do not return to work until **1 day** after the day your radionuclide therapy was administered.
- Do not sleep in the same bed with your sleeping partner until **7 days** after the day your radionuclide therapy was administered.
- However, if your sleeping partner is pregnant, do not sleep in the same bed with your sleeping partner until **24 days** after the day your radionuclide therapy was administered. This requires that you avoid contact with your pregnant sleeping partner *altogether* during the **first day** after the day your radionuclide therapy was administered.

Patient: **Patient, John Q.**
MRN: **1111-11-111**

In addition, the following precautions should be observed until 1 day after the administration of your radiopharmaceutical therapy.

- To the extent that is reasonable, generally try to remain as far away from individuals around you as possible.
- After using the toilet, flush twice and, as usual, wash your hands. If possible, use paper towels to dry your hands and dispose of the paper toweling in the trash.
- You should otherwise observe good personal hygiene and may shower, bathe, shave, etc., as you normally would, rinsing the shower stall, tub, or sink thoroughly after use.
- Wipe up any spills of urine, saliva, or mucus with tissues or a small amount of disposable (i.e., flushable) paper toweling, and dispose of the tissue or toweling down the toilet.
- Use nondisposable plates, bowls, spoons, knives, forks, and cups. If possible, you should use a separate sponge or washcloth from that used by the rest of your household to wash plates, bowls, spoons, knives, forks, and cups that you have used. Rinse the sink thoroughly after use, wipe the fixtures with paper towels, and dispose of the paper toweling in the trash.
- If you use a dishwasher, wash your plates, bowls, spoons, knives, forks, and cups separately from those of the rest of your household.
- Use the same set of plates, bowls, spoons, knives, and forks for 1 day after your radionuclide therapy.
- Store and launder your soiled/used clothing and bed linens separately from those of the rest of your household, running the rinse cycle two times at the completion of the machine laundering.
- Do not share food or drinks with anyone.
- After using the telephone, wipe the receiver (especially the mouthpiece) with paper towels, and dispose the paper towels in the trash.

Signature Section (example release form)

**I have read this form and all of my questions have been answered.
By signing below, I acknowledge that I have read and accept all of the information above.**

_____   _____

Signature of patient or patient representative   Print name of patient or representative

_____

Date

_____

Relation of personal representative to patient

Note. From *Management of Radionuclide Therapy Patients* (NCRP Report No. 155, pp. 166–168), by J. St. Germain, E.B. Silberstein, R.J. Vetter, J.F. Williamson, and P.D. Zanzonico, 2006, National Council on Radiation Protection and Measurements. Copyright 2006 by National Council on Radiation Protection and Measurements. Reprinted with permission of the National Council on Radiation Protection and Measurements, http://NCRPonline.org.

(3) Prostate brachytherapy patients are counseled on the use of public transportation and avoidance of prolonged close contact with the general public, especially pregnant women and children, to ensure any unnecessary risk is avoided (Stish et al., 2018).

(4) Instructions should include precautions regarding possible dislodged seeds.

(a) Instructions should include use of condoms and how long to use them; straining their urine (to collect any dislodged seeds) for at least seven days after implantation; and actions to be taken if a dislodged seed or pellet is found.

(b) If a dislodged pellet is found, it should not be touched with bare hands; it should be picked up with tweezers or a spoon.

(c) Dislodged seeds should be placed in a container with a tight lid and kept in a location away from people. The patient should notify the person in the treatment facility who placed the seeds (Bibbo et al., 2018; Haygood, 2013; Miller, 2017).

4. Patient information card or letter concerning radiopharmaceutical or radionuclide procedure

a) Patients discharged with radiopharmaceuticals or radionuclides in the body should have a letter or wallet identification card from the physician or medical facility specifying radionuclide therapy (Kaniuka-Jakubowska et al., 2012).

b) Patients may set off very sensitive alarms that detect radioactivity, such as those found in airports, train stations, government buildings, tunnels, and border crossings (Kaniuka-Jakubowska et al., 2012).

c) Patients treated with iodine-131 have activated security alarm detectors after radioiodine administration (Kaniuka-Jakubowska et al., 2012). Iodine-131 has a half-life of eight days; thus, it will remain active for 80–90 days (Alkhorayef et al., 2018; Barrett, Stiles, & Patterson, 2012).

5. Special radiation protection considerations (Kawthalkar, Sequeira, Arya, & Baheti, 2019)

a) In a freestanding facility not associated with a hospital, it is recommended that the local fire, emergency medical services, and police departments are aware of radiation hazards.

b) All freestanding facilities also are regulated by NRC and state radiation control organizations.

6. Special populations: radiation exposure of pregnant employees (Brent et al., 2013)

a) Embryos and fetuses are the most radiosensitive living tissues (Brent et al., 2013; Maquilan et al., 2018).

b) The first trimester is the most radiosensitive period of a fetus (Brent et al., 2013; Maquilan et al., 2018).

c) Because of the radiosensitivity of an embryo, a pregnant woman has a dose limit of 5 mSv (0.5 rem) during pregnancy, per NCRP guidelines (Brent et al., 2013; Ghatan, Fassiotto, Jacobsen, Sze, & Kothary, 2016; Maquilan et al., 2018).

d) Many institutions recommend that pregnant women do not provide care to patients who are receiving radionuclide therapy. However, by law, pregnant women cannot be restricted from providing this care, as long as NCRP guidelines for exposure limits are followed (Maquilan et al., 2018; NCRP, 2014).

e) A pregnant woman assumes all responsibility for the exposure of the fetus until the pregnancy is officially declared.

(1) Once a pregnancy is declared, the supervisors and RSO are responsible for ensuring that the woman's monitored radiation exposure does not exceed the 5 mSv (0.5 rem) dose limit.

(2) The RSO also is required to evaluate the work area and recommend further procedures to reduce exposure (Brent et al., 2013; Ghatan et al., 2016; Haygood, 2013; Marx, 2018).

7. Emergency procedures: General guidelines for emergency procedures, including radioactive spills and loss or rupture of a sealed radioactive source, can be found in S.Y. Chen et al. (2014) and Domenech (2017).

a) Dislodged source guidelines

(1) Notify the radiation oncologist and RSO regarding any dislodged source as soon as it is discovered (Domenech, 2017; Haygood, 2013).

(2) Have a lead storage container available to store any displaced source and have long-handled forceps available to pick up the source. Only individuals with training in handling radioactive sources should be permitted to handle dislodged sources. Bare hands should never be used to pick up a radioactive source (Domenech, 2017; Haygood, 2013).

(3) The patient also should be instructed never to pick up a dislodged radioactive source and to contact the staff if a dislodgment is suspected immediately (Basran et al., 2015; Domenech, 2017; Haygood, 2013).

(4) The time the source became dislodged should be recorded and communicated to the radiation oncology team to determine the therapeutic radiation dose that the patient received (Bibbo et al., 2018).

(5) Radiation safety staff should survey all applicators, dressings, and linens that may contain a dislodged source before removing them from the room (Domenech, 2017; Haygood, 2013; Zain, 2018).

b) Cardiopulmonary resuscitation (CPR) of patients who have received radionuclide therapy (Kazzi et al., 2015; Zain, 2018)

(1) CPR in patients with sealed radionuclides

(a) Begin CPR immediately per guidelines.

(b) Immediately notify personnel who can properly remove the sealed source and place it in a lead container (Haygood, 2013; Kazzi et al., 2015; Zain, 2018).

(c) Once the source is removed and properly stored, and the area is surveyed, no additional risk of exposure is present (Kazzi et al., 2015).

(2) CPR in patients with unsealed sources (e.g., iodine-131) (Henkin et al., 2011)

(a) Begin CPR immediately in the usual manner as recommended.

(b) Notify radiation safety personnel and radiation oncologist (Haygood, 2013; Zain, 2018).

(c) The priority is the patient, and staff exposure is likely to be minimal. Thirty minutes of resuscitation of a patient with 100 mCi of iodine-131 would result in approximately 100 mrem exposure at one foot, a 200 mrem/hour exposure absorbed dose rate (Kaiser Permanente, 2002).

(d) People performing CPR should wear gloves, a gown, and shoe covers (Kazzi et al., 2015; Zain, 2018).

(e) All equipment used for CPR should be surveyed for radiation contamination before removal from the room (Kazzi et al., 2015).

(f) All personnel involved in CPR should remain in the immediate location of the patient's room and be cleared to leave the area by radiation safety personnel (Kazzi et al., 2015; Zain, 2018).

8. Other situations

a) Information on handling other situations involving patients with radionuclides, such as dialysis, emergency surgery, death, autopsy, cremation, and organ donation, can also be found in St. Germain et al. (2006).

b) Al Aamri, Ravichandran, and Al Balushi (2019) noted that radioactive iodine treatment for thyroid cancer has activity at 1.85–7 GBq.

c) Idota et al. (2017) described a case involving a patient with prostate cancer who died within one year of implantation of iodine-125, noting that the prostate and all radioactive implants should have been removed before the body was cremated.

d) Calais (2017) reported a cremation of a patient who suffered a fatal cardiac arrest after administration of 7,200 MBq of sodium-131 iodides.

(1) The family needed the authorization to arrange for the body cremation after three weeks by which time the whole-body activity had decayed to approximately 1,000 MBq (Calais, 2017).

(2) Calais (2017) mentioned that removal of the thyroid or remnants before cremation is warranted to reduce exposure during handling or viewing of the body and to reduce contamination and emissions from the crematorium.

K. Nursing education in radiation protection

1. Nurses caring for patients treated with radionuclides should receive specific training in radiation protection and periodic review in radiation protection practices per institutional guidelines (Clarijs, Coeck, Van Bladel, & Fremout, 2015; Fencl, 2015; Morishima et al., 2016).

2. Education is effective in increasing nurses' knowledge about radiation safety practices (Fencl, 2015; O. Kim et al., 2018).

3. NRC regulations require instruction in radiation protection measures for nurses caring for patients receiving radionuclides (Demeter, Applegate, & Perez, 2016; Fencl, 2015; Miller, 2017).

L. Related websites

1. American College of Radiology (ACR): www.acr.org
2. American Association of Physicists in Medicine: www.aapm.org
3. Canadian Nuclear Safety Commission: www.cnsc.gc.ca
4. FDA: www.fda.gov
5. Health Physics Society (Ask the Experts): www.hps.org
6. ICRP: www.icrp.org
7. NCRP: www.ncrponline.org
8. NRC: www.nrc.gov
9. Radiological Society of North America: www.rsna.org

References

Abojassim, A.A., Dahir, D.M., Alaboodi, A.S., & Abonasria, A.H. (2016). Annual effective dose of gamma emitters in adults and children of some types of rice consumed in Iraq. *Journal of Food Protection, 79,* 2174–2178. https://doi.org/10.4315/0362-028x.jfp-16-242

Al Aamri, M., Ravichandran, R., & Al Balushi, N. (2019). Radioactive iodine (I-131) therapy isolation rooms: Introduction of lead glass window on the wall for patient comfort and better ambience. *World Journal of Nuclear Medicine, 18,* 42–44. https://doi.org/10.4103/wjnm.wjnm_18_18

Alavi, S.S., Dabbagh, S.T., Abbasi, M., & Mehrdad, R. (2017). Medical radiation workers' knowledge, attitude, and practice to protect themselves against ionizing radiation in Tehran Province, Iran. *Journal of Education and Health Promotion, 6,* 58. https://doi.org/10.5812/ircmj.29394

Alkhorayef, M., Sulieman, A., Mohamed-Ahmed, M., Al-Mohammed, H.I., Alkhomashi, N., Sam, A.K., & Bradley, D.A. (2018). Staff and ambient radiation dose resulting from therapeutic nuclear medicine procedures. *Applied Radiation and Isotopes, 141,* 270–274. https://doi.org/10.1016/j.apradiso.2018.07.014

American Cancer Society. (2015). Natural background radiation. http://www.cancer.org/cancer/cancer-causes/radiation-exposure/x-rays-gamma-rays/natural-background-radiation.html

Anderson, RM. (2019). Cytogenetic biomarkers of radiation exposure. *Clinical Oncology, 31,* 311–318. https://doi.org/10.1016/j.clon.2019.02.009

Baalamurugan, J., Ganesh Kumar, V., Chandrasekaran, S., Balasundar, S., Venkatraman, B., Padmapriya, R., & Bupesh Raja, V.K. (2019). Utilization of induction furnace steel slag in concrete as coarse aggregate for gamma radiation shielding. *Journal of Hazardous Materials, 369,* 561–568. https://doi.org/10.1016/j.jhazmat.2019.02.064

Badawy, M.K., Deb, P., Chan, R., & Farouque, O. (2016). A review of radiation protection solutions for the staff in the cardiac catheterisation laboratory. *Heart, Lung and Circulation, 25,* 961–967. https://doi.org/10.1016/j.hlc.2016.02.021

Badawy, M.K., Mong, K.S., Lykhun, U.P., & Deb, P. (2016). An assessment of nursing staffs' knowledge of radiation protection and practice. *Journal of Radiological Protection, 36,* 178–183. https://doi.org/10.1088/0952-4746/36/1/178

Barrett, B., Stiles, M., & Patterson, J. (2012). Radiation risks: Critical analysis and commentary. *Preventive Medicine, 54,* 280–282. https://doi.org/10.1016/j.ypmed.2011.12.017

Basran, P.S., Baxter, P., & Beckham, W.A. (2015). Reducing radiation risks for patients with permanently implanted radioactive sources requiring unrelated surgery. *Journal of Applied Clinical Medical Physics, 16,* 159–166. https://doi.org/10.1120/jacmp.v16i5.5372

Batool, S., Bibi, A., Frezza, F., & Mangini, F. (2019). Benefits and hazards of electromagnetic waves, telecommunication, physical and biomedical: A review. *European Review for Medical and Pharmacological Sciences, 23,* 3121–3128. https://doi.org/10.26355/eurrev_201904_17596

Bibbo, G., Benger, T., Sigalas, V., & Kirkwood, I. (2018). Radioiodine (^{131}I) therapies performed in a paediatric hospital: Facilities and procedures. *Australasian Physical and Engineering Sciences in Medicine, 41,* 747–756. https://doi.org/10.1007/s13246-018-0658-3

Bobin, C., Thiam, C., & Chauvenet, B. (2017). A radionuclide calibrator based on Cherenkov counting for activity measurements of high-energy pure β⁻-emitters. *Applied Radiation and Isotopes, 119,* 60–65. https://doi.org/10.1016/j.apradiso.2016.10.018

Boice, J.D., Jr. (2014). Implications of radiation dose and exposed populations on radiation protection in the 21st century. *Health Physics, 106,* 313–328. https://doi.org/10.1097/hp.0000000000000024

Boice, J.D., Jr., Cohen, S.S., Mumma, M.T., & Ellis, E.D. (2019). The Million Person Study, whence it came and why. *International Journal of Radiation Biology.* Advance online publication. https://doi.org/10.1080/09553002.2019.1589015

Bolus, N.E. (2013). NCRP report 160 and what it means for medical imaging and nuclear medicine. *Journal of Nuclear Medicine Technology, 41,* 255–260. https://doi.org/10.2967/jnmt.113.128728

Bouville, A., & Kryuchkov, V. (2014). Increased occupational radiation doses: Nuclear fuel cycle. *Health Physics, 106,* 259–271. https://doi.org/10.1097/hp.0000000000000066

Bouville, A., Toohey, R.E., Beck, H.L., Dauer, L.T., Eckerman, K.F., Hagermeyer, D., ... Zeitlin, C.J. (2018). *Deriving organ doses and their uncertainty for epidemiologic studies (with a focus on the One Million U.S. Workers and Veterans Study of Low-Dose Radiation on Health Effects)* [NCRP Report No. 178]. National Council on Radiation Protection and Measurements. https://ncrponline.org/shop/reports/report-no-178-deriving-organ-doses-and-their-uncertainity-for-epidemiologic-studies

Brent, R.L., Frush, D.P., Gorson, R.O., Harms, R.W., Kroger, L.A., Linet, M.A., ... Woo, S.Y. (2013). *Preconception and prenatal radiation exposure: Health effects and protective guidance* (NCRP Report No. 174). National Council on Radiation Protection and Measurements. https://ncrponline.org/shop/reports/report-no-174-preconception-and-prenatal-radiation-exposure-health-effects-and-protective-guidance-2013

Calais, P.J. (2017). Gaussian plume atmospheric modelling and radiation exposure calculations following the cremation of a deceased thyroid cancer patient treated with iodine-131. *Journal of Radiological Protection, 37,* 247–265. https://doi.org/10.1088/1361-6498/aa51e2

Canadian Nuclear Safety Commission. (2014). Our mission. http://www.cnsc.gc.ca/eng/about-us/our-mission.cfm

Chen, J., & Xie, L. (2019). Domestic radon exposure and childhood leukaemia and lymphoma: A population-based study in Canada. *Radiation Protection Dosimetry, 184,* 486–492. https://doi.org/10.1093/rpd/ncz068

Chen, S.Y., Barnett, D.J., Buddemeier, B.R., Covello, V.T., Kiel, K.A., Lipoti, J.A., ... Wallo, A. (2014). *Decision making for late-phase recov-ery from major nuclear or radiological incidents* (NCRP Report No. 175). National Council on Radiation Protection and Measurements. https://ncrponline.org/shop/reports/report-no-175-decision-making-for-late-phase-recovery-from-major-nuclear-or-radiological-incidents-2014

Clarijs, T., Coeck, M., Van Bladel, L., & Fremout, A. (2015). Basic radiation protection training for nurses and paramedical personnel: Belgian experience and future perspectives. *Radiation Protection Dosimetry, 165,* 506–509. https://doi.org/10.1093/rpd/ncv070

Conti, M., & Eriksson, L. (2016). Physics of pure and non-pure positron emitters for PET: A review and a discussion. *EJNMMI Physics, 3,* 8. https://doi.org/10.1186/s40658-016-0144-5

Coppeta, L., Pietroiusti, A., Neri, A., Spataro, A., DeAngelis, E., Perrone, S., & Magrini, A. (2019). Risk of radiation-induced lens opacities among surgeons and interventional medical staff. *Radiological Physics and Technology, 12,* 26–29. https://doi.org/10.1007/s12194-018-0487-9

Dauer, L.T., Bouville, A., Toohey, R.E., Boice, J.D., Jr., Beck, H.L., Eckerman, K.F., ... Zeitlin, C. (2018). Dosimetry and uncertainty approaches for the million person study of low-dose radiation health effects: Overview of the recommendations in NCRP report No. 178. *International Journal of Radiation Biology.* Advance online publication. https://doi.org/10.1080/09553002.2018.1536299

de Jong, J.R. (2017). Personnel and public people. In A.W.J.M. Glaudemans, J. Medema, A.K. van Zanten, R.A.J.O. Dierckx, & C.T.B. Ahaus (Eds.), *Quality in nuclear medicine* (pp. 117–130). Springer. https://doi.org/10.1007/978-3-319-33531-5_7

Demeter, S., Applegate, K.E., & Perez, M. (2016). Internet-based ICRP resource for healthcare providers on the risk and benefits of medical imaging that uses ionising radiation. *Annals of the ICRP, 45*(Suppl. 1), 148–155. https://doi.org/10.1177/0146645316637786

Domenech, H. (2017). *Radiation safety: Management and programs.* Springer. https://doi.org/10.1007/978-3-319-42671-6

Duarte, I.A.G., de Figueiredo Silva Hafner, M., & Malvestiti, A.A. (2015). Ultraviolet radiation emitted by lamps, TVs, tablets, and computers: Are there risks for the population? *Anais Brasileiros De Dermatologia, 90,* 595–597. https://doi.org/10.1590/abd1806-4841.20153616

Elgqvist, J., Timmermand, O.V., Larsson, E., & Strand, S.-E. (2016). Radiosensitivity of prostate cancer cell lines for irradiation from beta particle-emitting radionuclide ^{177}Lu compared to alpha particles and gamma rays. *Anticancer Research, 36,* 103–110. http://ar.iiarjournals.org/content/36/1/103.long

Erickson, B.A., Bittner, N.H.J., Chadha, M., Mourtada, F., & Demanes, D.J. (2017). The American College of Radiology and the American Brachytherapy Society practice parameter for the performance of radionuclide-based high-dose-rate brachytherapy. *Brachytherapy, 16,* 75–84. https://doi.org/10.1016/j.brachy.2016.05.006

Federal Aviation Administration. (2016). What aircrews should know about their occupational exposure to ionizing radiation. https://www.faa.gov/data_research/research/med_humanfacs/oamtechreports/2000s/media/0316.pdf

Fencl, J.L. (2015). Guideline implementation: Radiation safety. *AORN Journal, 102,* 629–639. https://doi.org/10.1016/j.aorn.2015.10.010

Flynn, R.T., Adams, Q.E., Hopfensperger, K.M., Wu, X., Xu, W., & Kim, Y. (2019). Efficient ^{169}Yb high-dose-rate brachytherapy source production using reactivation. *Medical Physics, 46,* 2935–2943. https://doi.org/10.1002/mp.13563

Fons-Castells, J., Tent-Petrus, J., & Llauradó, M. (2017). Simultaneous determination of specific alpha and beta emitters by LSC-PLS in water samples. *Journal of Environmental Radioactivity, 166,* 195–201. https://doi.org/10.1016/j.jenvrad.2016.04.035

Garcia-Sanchez, A.-J., Angosto, E.A., Riquelme, P.A.M., Berna, A.S., & Ramos-Amores, D. (2018). Ionizing radiation measurement solution in a hospital environment. *Sensors, 18,* 510. https://doi.org/10.3390/s18020510

Ghatan, C.E., Fassiotto, M., Jacobsen, J.P., Sze, D.Y., & Kothary, N. (2016). Occupational radiation exposure during pregnancy: A survey of attitudes and practices among interventional radiologists. *Journal of Vascular Interventional Radiology, 27,* 1013–1020.e3. https://doi.org/10.1016/j.jvir.2016.03.040

Government of Canada. (2020a, January 16). Radiation Protection Bureau. https://www.canada.ca/en/health-canada/corporate/about-health-canada/branches-agencies/healthy-environments-consumer-safety-branch/environmental-radiation-health-sciences-directorate/radiation-protection-bureau.html

Government of Canada. (2020b, February 21). Radon. https://www.canada.ca/en/health-Canada/services/radon.html

Gross, C.E., Frank, R.M., Hsu, A.R., Diaz, A., & Gitelis, S. (2015). External beam radiation therapy for orthopedic pathology. *Journal of American Academy of Orthopaedic Surgeons, 23,* 243–252. https://doi.org/10.5435/jaaos-d-14-00022

Hanada, T., Yorozu, A., Kikumura, R., Ohashi, T., & Shigematsu, N. (2014). Assessing protection against radiation exposure after prostate ^{125}I brachytherapy. *Brachytherapy, 13,* 311–318. https://doi.org/10.1016/j.brachy.2013.12.001

Harrison, J.D., Balonov, M., Martin, C.J., Ortiz Lopez, P., Menzel, H.-G., Simmonds, J.R., ... Wakeford, R. (2016). Use of effective dose. *Annals of the ICRP, 45*(Suppl. 1), 215–224. https://doi.org/10.1177/0146645316634566

Hashempour, M., Ghorbani, M., Amato, E., & Knaup, C. (2019). Effect of beta particles spectrum on absorbed fraction in internal radiotherapy. *Asia Oceania Journal of Nuclear Medicine and Biology, 7,* 71–83. https://doi.org/10.22038/AOJNMB.2018.11610

Haygood, J. (2013). *Radiation safety procedures and training for the radiation safety officer: Guidance for preparing a radiation safety program.* iUniverse.

Held, K.D., & Woloschak, G.E. (2016). NCRP program area committee 1: Basic criteria, epidemiology, radiobiology and risk. *Health Physics, 110,* 98–100. https://doi.org/10.1097/hp.0000000000000402

Henkin, R.E., Del Rowe, J.D., Grigsby, P.W., Hartford, A.C., Jadvar, H., Macklis, R.M., ... Rosenthal, S.A. (2011). ACR–ASTRO practice guideline for the performance of therapy with unsealed radiopharmaceutical sources. *Clinical Nuclear Medicine, 36,* e72–e80. https://doi.org/10.1097/RLU.0b013e318224b814

Hinrichsen, Y., Finck, R., Östlund, K., Rääf, C., & Andersson, K.G. (2018). Comparison of experimental and calculated shielding factors for modular buildings in a radioactive fallout scenario. *Journal of Environmental Radioactivity, 189,* 146–155. https://doi.org/10.1016/j.jenvrad.2018.04.005

Hobbs, J.B., Goldstein, N., Lind, K.E., Elder, D., Dodd, G.D., III, & Borgstede, J.P. (2018). Physician knowledge of radiation exposure and risk in medical imaging. *Journal of the American College of Radiology, 15,* 34–43. https://doi.org/10.1016/j.jacr.2017.08.034

Idota, N., Nakamura, M., Masui, K., Kakiuchi, Y., Yamada, K., & Ikegaya, H. (2017). Lessons learned from autopsying an unidentified body with iodine-125 seeds implanted for prostate brachytherapy. *Journal of Forensic Sciences, 62,* 536–540. https://doi.org/10.1111/1556-4029.13296

Inada, M., Monzen, H., Matsumoto, K., Tamura, M., Minami, T., Nakamatsu, K., & Nishimura, Y. (2018). A novel radiation-shielding undergarment using tungsten functional paper for patients with permanent prostate brachytherapy. *Journal of Radiation Research, 59,* 333–337. https://doi.org/10.1093/jrr/rry030

Inoue, M., Yamashita, S., Fujimoto, K., Kofuji, H., Miki, S., & Nagao, S. (2017). Simple ^{40}K removal by acidified water leaching for estimating low level of radiocesium in fishery products following Fukushima Dai-ichi nuclear power plant accident. *Applied Radiation and Isotopes, 120,* 17–21. https://doi.org/10.1016/j.apradiso.2016.11.008

International Commission on Radiological Protection. (n.d.). Governance. http://www.icrp.org/page.asp?id=3

Jones, E., & Mathieson, K. (2016). Radiation safety among workers in health services. *Health Physics, 110*(Suppl. 2), s52–s58. https://doi.org/10.1097/hp.0000000000000485

Kaiser Permanente. (2002). *Radiation safety for nurses.* https://kpnursing.org/_SCAL/professionaldevelopment/orientation/LAMC/rs_nurse.pdf

Kamiya, K., Ozasa, K., Akiba, S., Niwa, O., Kodama, K., Takamura, N., ... Wakeford, R. (2015). Long-term effects of radiation exposure on health. *Lancet, 386,* 469–478. https://doi.org/10.1016/s0140-6736(15)61167-9

Kaniuka-Jakubowska, S., Lewczuk, A., Mizan-Gross, K., Obołończyk, Ł., Lass, P., & Sworczak, K. (2012). Giving radioiodine? Think about airport security alarms. *Revista Española de Medicina Nuclear e Imagen Molecular, 31,* 148–150. https://doi.org/10.1016/j.remn.2011.10.012

Kase, K.R., Cool, D.A., Ansari, A., Boice, J.D., Jr., Bushberg, J.T., Dauer, L.T., ... Woloschak, G.E. (2018). *Management of exposure to ionizing radiation: Radiation protection guidance for the United States (2018)* [NCRP Report No. 180]. National Council on Radiation Protection and Measurements. https://ncrponline.org/shop/reports/report-no-180-management-of-exposure-to-ionizing-radiation-radiation-protection-guidance-for-the-united-states-2018-2018

Kawthalkar, A.S., Sequeira, R.A., Arya, S., & Baheti, A.D. (2019). Non-radiation occupational hazards and health issues faced by radiologists—A cross-sectional study of Indian radiologists. *Indian Journal of Radiology and Imaging, 29,* 61–66. https://doi.org/10.4103/ijri.ijri_403_18

Kazzi, Z., Buzzell, J., Bertelli, L., & Christensen, D. (2015). Emergency department management of patients internally contaminated with radioactive material. *Emergency Medicine Clinics of North America, 33,* 179–196. https://doi.org/10.1016/j.emc.2014.09.008

Kim, O., Kim, M.S., Jang, H.J., Lee, H., Kang, Y., Pang, Y., & Jung, H. (2018). Radiation safety education and compliance with safety procedure—The Korea nurses' health study. *Journal of Clinical Nursing, 27,* 1–28. https://doi.org/10.1111/jocn.14338

Kim, S.-T., Yoo, J.-R., & Park, J.M. (2018). An investigation into internal exposure management needs for nuclear medicine practitioners and temporary visitors through I-131 internal dose assessment: Focusing on large hospitals in South Korea. *PLOS ONE, 13,* e0209244. https://doi.org/10.1371/journal.pone.0209244

König, A.M., Etzel, R., Thomas, R.P., & Mahnken, A.H. (2019). Personal radiation protection and corresponding dosimetry in interventional radiology: An overview and future development. *Fortschritte auf dem Gebiet der Röntgenstrahlen, 191,* 512–521. https://doi.org/10.1055/a-0800-0113

Kutanzi, K.R., Lumen, A., Koturbash, I., & Miousse, I.R. (2016). Pediatric exposures to ionizing radiation: Carcinogenic considerations. *International Journal of Environmental Research and Public Health, 13,* 1057. https://doi.org/10.3390/ijerph13111057

Kyriakopoulou, A., Meimeti, E., Moisoglou, L., Psarrou, A., Provatopoulou, X., & Dounias, G. (2018). Parental occupational exposures and risk of childhood acute leukemia. *Materia Socio-Medica, 30,* 209–214. https://doi.org/10.5455/msm.2018.30.209-214

Lecomte, J.-F., Solomon, S., Takala, J., Jung, T., Strand, P., Murith, C., ... Janssens, A. (2014). ICRP publication 126: Radiological protection against radon exposure. *Annals of the ICRP, 43,* 5–73. https://doi.org/10.1177/0146645314542212

Long, B.W., Frank, E.D., & Ehrlich, R.A. (2017). *Radiography essentials for limited practice* (5th ed.). Elsevier.

Mancini-Terracciano, C., Donnarumma, R., Bencivenga, G., Bocci, V., Cartoni, A., Collamati, F., ... Faccini, R. (2017). Feasibility of beta-particle radioguided surgery for a variety of "nuclear medicine" radionuclides. *Physica Medica, 43,* 127–133. https://doi.org/10.1016/j.ejmp.2017.10.012

Maquilan, G., Bussière, M.R., McCormack, J., Medich, T., Niemierko, A., & Shih, H.A. (2018). Radiation safety for pregnant workers at proton facility. *International Journal of Radiation Oncology, Biology, Physics, 100,* 560–564. https://doi.org/10.1016/j.ijrobp.2017.11.016

Marx, M.V. (2018). Baby on board: Managing occupational radiation exposure during pregnancy. *Techniques in Vascular and Interventional Radiology, 21,* 32–36. https://doi.org/10.1053/j.tvir.2017.12.007

Medical use of byproduct material, 10 C.F.R. § 35 (2013). https://www.nrc.gov/reading-rm/doc-collections/cfr/part035/

Miller, D.L. (2017). Make radiation protection a habit. *Techniques in Vascular and Interventional Radiology, 21,* 37–42. https://doi.org/10.1053/j.tvir.2017.12.008

Morishima, Y., Chida, K., Katahira, Y., Seto, H., Chiba, H., & Tabayashi, K. (2016). Need for radiation safety education for interventional cardiology staff, especially nurses. *Acta Cardiologica, 71,* 151–155. https://doi.org/10.1080/ac.71.2.3141844

Mostafa, L., Rachid, K., & Ahmed, S.M. (2016). Comparison between beta radiation dose distribution due to LDR and HDR ocular brachytherapy applicators using GATE Monte Carlo platform. *Physica Medica, 32,* 1007–1018. https://doi.org/10.1016/j.ejmp.2016.07.636

Nabavizadeh, N., Elliott, D.A., Chen, Y., Kusano, A.S., Mitin, T., Thomas, C.R., Jr., & Holland, J.M. (2016). Image guided radiation therapy (IGRT) practice patterns and IGRT's impact on workflow and treatment planning: Results from a national survey of American Society for Radiation Oncology members. *International Journal of Radiation Oncology, Biology, Physics, 94,* 850–857. https://doi.org/10.1016/j.ijrobp.2015.09.035

Nasser, N.J., Cohen, G.N., Dauer, L.T., & Zelefsky, M.J. (2016). Radiation safety of receptive anal intercourse with prostate cancer patients treated with low-dose-rate brachytherapy. *Brachytherapy, 15,* 420–425. https://doi.org/10.1016/j.brachy.2016.03.012

National Council on Radiation Protection and Measurements. (2014). *NCRP: Achievements of the past 50 years and addressing the needs of the future* (50th annual meeting program). Author. https://ncrponline.org/wp-content/uploads/2018/08/Annual/pp50.pdf

National Council on Radiation Protection and Measurements. (2015). Mission. https://ncrponline.org/about/mission

Ortiz López, P., Dauer, L.T., Loose, R., Martin, C.J., Miller, D.L., Vañó, E., ... Yoder, C. (2018). ICRP publication 139: Occupational radiological protection in interventional procedures. *Annals of the ICRP, 47*(2), 1–118. https://doi.org/10.1177/0146645317750356

Pae, J.S. (2018). CBRNE—Radiation emergencies. https://emedicine.medscape.com/article/834015-overview

Petrinec, B., Šoštarić, M., & Babić, D. (2019). The role of physics in radioecology and radiotoxicology. *Archives of Industrial Hygiene and Toxicology, 70,* 3–13. https://doi.org/10.2478/aiht-2019-70-3225

Pryor, K.H. (2015). Radiation safety of sealed radioactive sources. *Health Physics, 108,* 172–177. https://doi.org/10.1097/hp.0000000000000225

Pryor, K.H. (2016). End of life decisions for sealed radioactive sources. *Health Physics, 110,* 168–174. https://doi.org/10.1097/hp.0000000000000398

Qaim, S.M. (2017). Nuclear medicine data for production and medical application of radionuclides: Present status and future needs. *Nuclear Medicine and Biology, 44,* 31–49. https://doi.org/10.1016/j.nucmedbio.2016.08.016

Ria, F., Bergantin, A., Vai, A., Bonfanti, P., Martinotti, A.S., Redaelli, I., ... Samei, E. (2017). Awareness of medical radiation exposure among patients: A patient survey as the first step for effective communication of ionizing radiation risks. *Physica Medica, 43,* 57–62. https://doi.org/10.1016/j.ejmp.2017.10.014

Rühm, W., Azizova, T.V., Bouffler, S.D., Little, M.P., Shore, R.E., Walsh, L., & Woloschak, G.E. (2016). Dose-rate effects in radiation biology and radiation protection. *Annals of the ICRP, 45*(Suppl. 1), 262–279. https://doi.org/10.1177/0146645316629336

Sabet, M., Cryer, D., & Waterhouse, D. (2016). Shielding design for Cs-137 rod-type standard point source for well chamber constancy checks. *Australasian Physical and Engineering Sciences in Medicine, 39,* 951–956. https://doi.org/10.1007/s13246-016-0481-7

Saeed, M.K., Al-shaari, H., Almarzooq, M.M.S., Alsareii, S.A., Aljerdah, S.A., & AL-ayed, M.S. (2018). Radiation awareness among physicians about the hazards of radiologic examinations on the health of workers and their patients in Saudi Arabia. *Journal of Radiation Research and Applied Sciences, 11,* 299–304. https://doi.org/10.1016/j.jrras.2018.04.001

Schroderus-Salo, T., Hirvonen, L., Henner, A., Ahonen, S., Kääriäinen, M., Miettunen, J., & Mikkonen, K. (2019). Development and validation of a psychometric scale for assessing healthcare professionals' knowledge in radiation protection. *Radiography, 25,* 136–142. https://doi.org/10.1016/j.radi.2018.12.010

Semmler, J., Kuang, W., Volchek, K., Toor, A., Snaglewski, A., Khan, Z., & Azmi, P. (2019). Large area decontamination after radiological incident. *Journal of Environmental Radioactivity, 199–200,* 66–74. https://doi.org/10.1016/j.jenvrad.2019.01.009

Sgouros, G., Hobbs, R., & Josefsson, A. (2018). Dosimetry and radiobiology of alpha-particle emitting radionuclides. *Current Radiopharmaceuticals, 11,* 209–214. https://doi.org/10.2174/1874471011666180426130058

Sheetz, M., & Steiner, C. (2018). Compliance with the U.S. Nuclear Regulatory Commission revised licensing guidance for radioactive seed local-

ization. *Health Physics, 115,* 402–408. https://doi.org/10.1097/hp.0000000000000889

Simon, S.L., & Linet, M.S. (2014). Radiation-exposed populations: Who, why, and how to study. *Health Physics, 106,* 182–195. https://doi.org/10.1097/hp.0000000000000006

Smith, T., & Kearfott, K.J. (2018). Practical considerations for gamma-ray spectroscopy with NaI (Tl): A tutorial. *Health Physics, 114,* 94–106. https://doi.org/10.1097/hp.0000000000000804

Song, J.H. (2018). An assessment of the environmental contamination caused by the Fukushima accident. *Journal of Environmental Management, 206,* 846–852. https://doi.org/10.1016/j.jenvman.2017.11.068

Spruce, L. (2017). Back to basics: Radiation safety. *AORN Journal, 106,* 42–49. https://doi.org/10.1016/j.aorn.2017.05.001

Standards for protection against radiation, 10 C.F.R. § 20 (1991). https://www.nrc.gov/reading-rm/doc-collections/cfr/part020

St. Germain, J., Silberstein, E.B., Vetter, R.J., Williamson, J.F., & Zanzonico, P.D. (2006). *Management of radionuclide therapy patients* (NCRP Report No. 155). National Council on Radiation Protection and Measurements. https://ncrponline.org/shop/reports/report-no-155-management-of-radionuclide-therapy-patients-2006

Stish, B.J., Davis, B.J., Mynderse, L.A., McLaren, R.H., Deufel, C.L., & Choo, R. (2018). Low dose rate prostate brachytherapy. *Translational Andrology and Urology, 7,* 341–356. https://doi.org/10.21037/tau.2017.12.15

Thomadsen, B. (2018). Radiation protection responsibility in brachytherapy. *Health Physics, 116,* 189–204. https://doi.org/10.1097/hp.0000000000001005

Tomà, P., Cannatà, V., Genovese, E., Magistrelli, A., & Granata, A. (2017). Radiation exposure in diagnostic imaging: Wisdom and prudence, but still a lot to understand. *La Radiologia Medica, 122,* 215–220. https://doi.org/10.1007/s11547-016-0709-3

Unger, L.M., & Trubey, D.K. (1982). *Specific gamma-ray dose constants for nuclides important to dosimetry and radiological assessment.* Oak Ridge National Laboratory.

United Nations Environment Programme. (2016). *Radiation effects and sources.* Author. http://hdl.handle.net/20.500.11822/7790

U.S. Environmental Protection Agency. (n.d.-a). Protecting yourself from radiation. https://www.epa.gov/radiation/protecting-yourself-radiation

U.S. Environmental Protection Agency. (n.d.-b). Radiation basics. http://www.epa.gov/radiation/radiation-basics

U.S. Food and Drug Administration. (2018, March 27). Labeling requirements for radiation emitting devices and products. https://www.fda.gov/medical-devices/device-labeling/labeling-requirements-radiation-emitting-devices-and-products

U.S. Nuclear Regulatory Commission. (1997). *Release of patients administered radioactive materials.* https://www.nrc.gov/docs/ML0833/ML083300045.pdf

U.S. Nuclear Regulatory Commission. (2003). *Dose standards and methods for protection against radiation and contamination.* https://www.nrc.gov/reading-rm/basic-ref/students/for-educators/08.pdf

U.S. Nuclear Regulatory Commission. (2005). *Consolidated guidance about materials licenses: Program-specific guidance about medical use licenses—Final report* (NUREG-1556, Vol. 9). Author. https://www.nrc.gov/docs/ML1925/ML19256C219.pdf

U.S. Nuclear Regulatory Commission. (2019). *The NRC: Who we are and what we do.* https://www.nrc.gov/docs/ML2000/ML20003E672.pdf

Wernli, C. (2016). A short history and critical review of individual monitoring. *Radiation Protection Dosimetry, 170,* 4–7. https://doi.org/10.1093/rpd/ncw025

Wilson-Stewart, K., Shanahan, M., Fontanarosa, D., & Davidson, R. (2018). Occupational radiation exposure to nursing staff during cardiovascular fluoroscopic procedures: A review of literature. *Journal of Applied Clinical Medical Physics, 19,* 282–297. https://doi.org/10.1002/acm2.12461

Worrell, J., Gibson, P., & Allen, D.H. (2016). Radon exposure: Using the spectrum of prevention framework to increase healthcare provider awareness. *Clinical Journal of Oncology Nursing, 20,* 664–666. https://doi.org/10.1188/16.cjon.664-666

Yamamoto, L.G. (2013). Risks and management of radiation exposure. *Pediatric Emergency Care, 29,* 1016–1029. https://doi.org/10.1097/pec .0b013e3182a380b8

Yoder, R.C., Dauer, L.T., Balter, S., Boice, J.D., Jr., Gorgan, H.A., Mumma, M.T., ... Vetter, R.J. (2019). Dosimetry for the study of medical radiation workers with a focus on the mean absorbed dose to the lung, brain and other organs. *International Journal of Radiation Biology.* Advance online publication. https:// doi.org/10.1080/09553002.2018.1549756

Zain, A.M. (2018, September). *Radioactive patient collapsed: To flee or to resus* [Presentation slides]. Lecture presented at the Inaugural Malaysian Nuclear Medicine Conference, Kuala Lumpur, Malaysia. http://storage.unitedwebnetwork .com/files/362/80119d91716ab390388546e41e5c715b.pdf

IV. Symptom Management

A. Fatigue

1. Pathophysiology
    a) The underlying etiology of cancer-related fatigue (CRF) in patients receiving RT is multifactorial, which includes cognitive, emotional, psychosocial, and somatic factors (O'Higgins, Brady, O'Connor, Walsh, & Reilly, 2018).
    b) Although the cause is unknown, up to 80% of patients receiving chemotherapy or RT will experience CRF (National Comprehensive Cancer Network [NCCN], 2020a).
    c) Poirier (2011) stated that fatigue from RT usually occurs during the second week of treatment and gradually increases during treatment. Fatigue is usually the most severe when a patient completes RT. The following effects of RT are possible causes of fatigue.
        (1) Serotonin dysregulation (O'Higgins et al., 2018)
            (a) Cancer or its treatment may disrupt serotonin (5-hydroxytryptamine) levels and upregulation of serotonin receptors.
            (b) The influence of serotonin on appetite, sleep, memory, learning, temperature regulation, mood, behavior, cardiovascular function, muscle contraction, endocrine regulation, and depression suggests that serotonin may have an effect on central fatigue.
            (c) Central fatigue comes from the CNS, which controls voluntary movement, and may result from the failure to transmit CNS neuronal impulses.
            (d) Central fatigue can be described as inability to complete physical or mental tasks that require internal cues. Proinflammatory cytokines, such as tumor necrosis factor-alpha (TNF-α) may dysregulate the feedback loop, causing an increase of serotonin release.
        (2) Hypothalamic–pituitary–adrenal (HPA) axis dysfunction (O'Higgins et al., 2018)
            (a) Cancer or its treatment may change the pattern of cortisol release by the HPA axis, which is the central regulatory system of cortisol.
            (b) Cortisol plays a role in the cardiovascular system, immune system function, and metabolism.
            (c) Suppression of the HPA axis can lead to lower energy levels. Serum cortisol varies, with the most concentration observed after waking and tapering during the day.
        (3) Circadian rhythm disruption (O'Higgins et al., 2018).
            (a) Changes in cortisol secretion rhythm and rest–activity pattern have been associated with increased fatigue in patients with cancer.
            (b) A flatter diurnal cortisol slope, which causes disruptions in an individual's arousal or sleep patterns, was observed in those with greater fatigue.
            (c) Circadian rhythm dysregulation caused by cancer is complex. It may be related to genetic factors or psychosocial, environmental, and behavioral components, as well as host response to the malignancy.
            (d) Patients with cancer have a higher incidence of altered sleep patterns, more wakefulness during normal sleep times, and more fatigue during normal activity times.
        (4) Muscle metabolism and adenosine triphosphate (ATP) dysregulation (O'Higgins et al., 2018)
            (a) ATP is the basis for energy needed for skeletal muscle functioning, and cancer or its treatment may compromise regeneration of ATP in skeletal muscle.
            (b) This dysregulation results in an increase of metabolic byproducts and can lead to a decrease in physical capabilities.
            (c) Also referred to as *peripheral fatigue*, it is still unclear if ATP dysregulation is a cause of CRF.
        (5) Vagal afferent nerve activation (O'Higgins et al., 2018)
            (a) The vagal nerve primarily contains fibers that control visceral autonomic, motor, and sensory functions to the brain stem.
            (b) The vagal afferent nerve hypothesis suggests that somatic muscle activity inhibition and occurrence of "sickness behavior" results from cancer or treatment stimulating vagal afferent nerves. This may contribute to loss of skeletal muscle tone, general weakness, fatigue, and decreased ability to concentrate.
        (6) Cytokine dysregulation (O'Higgins et al., 2018).
            (a) Increases in plasma levels of proinflammatory cytokines resulting from tumor by-products or treatment are associated with increased fatigue.
            (b) Patients with cancer and survivors experiencing fatigue show markedly elevated serum levels of proinflammatory cytokines compared to nonfatigued survivors and healthy controls.

d) Risk factors: CRF severity varies between patients and has not been directly associated with a certain disease or treatment (Bower, 2014).

  (1) Anemia

    (a) Defined as a hemoglobin level of 11 g/dl or less, anemia may be the result of cancer or its treatment (NCCN, 2020b).

    (b) Cancer-related anemia is attributable to a number of factors, including bleeding, hemolysis, bone marrow infiltration, and suboptimal nutrition.

    (c) Anemia can result from cancer treatment, such as hormone therapy used to treat different types of cancer (e.g., prostate cancer, breast cancer) (Feng et al., 2015).

    (d) Decreased oxygenation of vital organs is a likely cause of fatigue.

  (2) Nutritional deficits (NCCN, 2020a)

    (a) Nutritional deficits occur because of a loss in appetite, difficulty swallowing, diarrhea, or constipation.

    (b) Bowel obstructions can occur because of cancer or treatment.

    (c) Fatigue can be a result of decreased caloric intake and electrolyte imbalances.

  (3) Nutritional disturbances

    (a) Nutritional intake may be affected with those diagnosed with cancer or by cancer treatment.

    (b) Patients will frequently experience nausea, vomiting, decreased or poor appetite, mucositis, diarrhea, or constipation (NCCN, 2020a).

    (c) Cachexia is frequently seen in patients with cancer and leads to CRF.

    (d) Those with anorexia or cachexia have a disruption in muscle protein metabolism, which leads to a decrease in muscle mass. This has the potential to reduce ATP regeneration (O'Higgins et al., 2018).

  (4) Emotional distress

    (a) Patients with cancer frequently experience depression, which is strongly associated with fatigue.

    (b) The relationship between depression and fatigue is unclear.

    (c) Fatigue is typically a symptom of depression. However, depression can stem from the fatigue that causes interferences with social and occupational activities (Bower, 2014).

    (d) Greater mental fatigue has been correlated with anxiety for individuals with brain tumors (Purcell et al., 2010).

  (5) Sleep disorders

    (a) Sleep disorders have shown to be correlated with CRF (Bower, 2014).

    (b) Symptoms include difficulty falling asleep, waking throughout the night, or difficulty staying asleep.

    (c) Poor sleep reduces quality of life, immune function, and ability to function throughout the day (Mahtani, 2017).

  (6) Cancer therapies

    (a) Treatments received prior to RT may influence the level of fatigue at the initiation of treatment (Purcell et al., 2010).

    (b) Treatment with chemotherapy followed by RT may result in greater fatigue than RT alone (Dhruva et al., 2010).

    (c) Fatigue was found to be worse on treatment days, with decrease in severity of symptoms on days off of treatment.

  (7) Comorbidities: Comorbidities that may contribute to increased fatigue include cardiopulmonary, hepatic, and renal dysfunction (Mitchell, 2014).

  (8) Site of RT

    (a) Patients receiving RT for head and neck cancer, for example, are more likely to experience fatigue from treatment. This is likely caused by inflammation (Xiao et al., 2016).

    (b) When RT is combined with chemotherapy, fatigue can be worse for patients with head and neck cancer (Ferris et al., 2018).

2. Incidence and prevalence

  a) Fatigue affects patients' quality of life, as well as survival rates (Xiao et al., 2016). The absence of a standard definition of fatigue is a challenge in assessing the prevalence of CRF (Mitchell, 2014).

  b) Three prevalent studies examining CRF showed that the prevalence of fatigue varied depending on the patients studied, the timing of measurement, and the definition or measure of fatigue. Based on these studies, strong evidence supports that fatigue is a significant problem during and after cancer treatment.

    (1) Jones et al. (2016) studied CRF through a self-administered questionnaire.

      (a) The study used the Functional Assessment of Cancer Therapy–Fatigue.

      (b) The participants were survivors of stage I–III breast, prostate, and colorectal cancer.

      (c) The study used three cohorts: 6–18 months after treatment, 2–3 years after treatment, and 5–6 years after treatment.

      (d) A total of 1,294 questionnaires were completed. The results demonstrated that approximately one-third of cancer survivors showed clinically significant levels of fatigue up to six years after primary treatment.

(2) Roila et al. (2019) conducted a cross-sectional study on all patients with cancer in any phase of treatment or disease who attended any of the 24 participating centers on two nonconsecutive days.

    (a) Participants completed the Brief Fatigue Inventory questionnaire and reported any pharmacologic or nonpharmacologic treatment for fatigue.

    (b) A total of 1,394 participants were included, and 866 reported fatigue.

    (c) Fatigue lasted longer than four months in 50.9% of participants. Strong predictors of fatigue were reduced physical activity, anxiety, pain, insomnia, anemia, and depression.

(3) Poirier (2011) conducted a secondary data analysis of a convenience sample of 77 patients from a previous study that investigated the correlation between fatigue and employment patterns in patients who had received RT.

    (a) Approximately 44% of patients were receiving treatment to the breast and the remainder to the chest, abdomen, pelvis, head and neck, and prostate.

    (b) Fatigue had a statistical difference between baseline and end of treatment in three roles studies: primary roles (activities of daily living [ADLs]), secondary roles (work or school activities), and tertiary roles (leisure activities).

    (c) Participants who received RT to the lung, pelvis, or head and neck showed more disruption in their roles.

    (d) CRF affected those who lived alone more than those who did not.

3. Assessment

  a) NCCN (2020a) recommends that all patients with cancer be screened for fatigue at their initial oncology visit, at regular intervals during treatment, and after treatment has been completed.

  b) Fatigue can best be assessed by a self-report because it is a subjective experience and a symptom perceived by the patient (NCCN, 2020a). Those who are assessed to have fatigue should have a comprehensive evaluation. It has been determined that a patient's report of fatigue is superior to a physician's assessments (Ferris et al., 2018).

  c) The first step is to screen for the presence or absence of fatigue using a question such as, "Are you experiencing fatigue?"

    (1) If fatigue is present, a 0–10 numeric rating scale can be used to rate the severity of fatigue. A score of 0–3 indicates mild fatigue; 4–6 indicates moderate fatigue; and 7–10 indicates severe fatigue.

    (2) NCCN (2020a) recommends that a score of 4 or greater should trigger a more comprehensive evaluation of fatigue.

    (3) Some patients may be unable to numerically rate their fatigue. These patients can rate their fatigue as mild, moderate, or severe (NCCN, 2020a).

  d) Comprehensive evaluation should include the following assessments.

    (1) Focused history

      (a) Disease and treatment status: Disease progression or recurrence is frequently a reason why patients will seek evaluation for CRF. Evaluation should include ruling out recurrence or progression and obtaining information on current medications, nonprescription drugs or supplements, chemotherapy, RT, and date of most recent treatment (NCCN, 2020a).

      (b) Laboratory values: Assessment for anemia, hypothyroidism, dehydration, and infection evaluates reversible causes of CRF (Polek, 2017).

      (c) In-depth fatigue history (onset, pattern, duration, change over time, associated or alleviating factors, interference with function): Fatigue levels for patients with cancer can vary depending on the time of day (Dhruva et al., 2010).

      (d) Medications, side effects, and drug interactions

      (e) Review of systems

    (2) Assessment of treatable contributing factors (NCCN, 2020a)

      (a) Pain

      (b) Emotional distress (e.g., anxiety, depression)

      (c) Anemia

      (d) Sleep disturbance

      (e) Nutritional status (e.g., weight, intake, fluid and electrolyte balance)

      (f) Activity level (decreased activity or fitness)

      (g) Medication side effects

      (h) Alcohol or substance abuse

      (i) Comorbid conditions (e.g., infection, cardiac, pulmonary, renal, hepatic, neurologic, or endocrine)

  e) Few valid and reliable fatigue assessment tools are available that are appropriate for use in clinical practice. Desirable characteristics of a clinical practice tool include brevity, ease of completion and scoring, and information to guide interpretation of scores.

    (1) The NCCN fatigue screening tool is a 0–10 scale, with 0 indicating no fatigue and 10 indi-

cating extreme fatigue. Based on consensus within the NCCN fatigue guidelines panel, a score of 4 or greater (defined as moderate fatigue) should be further evaluated with a focused health history and physical examination (NCCN, 2020a).

(2) The fatigue criterion of the Common Terminology Criteria for Adverse Events (CTCAE) is measured as grades 1–3 (grade 1: fatigue is relieved by rest; grade 2: fatigue is not relieved by rest and limits instrumental ADLs; grade 3: fatigue is not relieved by rest and limits self-care ADLs) (National Cancer Institute [NCI] Cancer Therapy Evaluation Program [CTEP], 2017). No empirically based cut score is available.

(3) The Multidimensional Fatigue Inventory is a 20-item, self-report instrument that addresses five areas of fatigue: general, physical, mental, reduced motivation, and reduced activity.

   (a) Each area includes four items to rate on a 1–5 scale.

   (b) Total scores range 20–100, with a higher score indicating greater fatigue.

   (c) The Multidimensional Fatigue Inventory has well-established validity and reliability for use with patients receiving RT (Lin et al., 2009; Smets, Garrsen, Bonke, & DeHaes, 1995).

(4) Numerous multi-item questionnaires have been evaluated as valid and reliable measures of fatigue, including the NCCN Problem List, Piper Fatigue Score-12, and Functional Assessment of Cancer Therapy–Fatigue. NCCN (2020a) outlines each tool based on the length and ease of use, number and type of dimensions, and for which types of patients the tool has been validated.

f) Follow-up assessment is used to track fatigue over time and evaluate the effectiveness of fatigue management strategies.

(1) Fatigue assessment should be conducted at regular intervals during treatment and after treatment completion (NCCN, 2020a).

(2) Fatigue may be a distressing symptom during and after cancer treatment; therefore, ongoing assessment is necessary (Mitchell et al., 2014).

4. Management
  a) Pharmacologic management
    (1) Anemia
      (a) NCCN (2020a) recommends using the guidelines for hematopoietic growth factors in evaluating and managing anemia as a treatable cause of fatigue.

      (b) Treatments for anemia may include iron replacement for iron-deficiency anemia and transfusion of packed red blood cells (PRBCs).

      (c) Erythropoietin-stimulating agents can also be effective treatment for anemic patients.

        i. The use of erythropoietin-stimulating agents has shown to decrease the need for PRBC transfusions in patients undergoing chemotherapy.

        ii. In a study of 2,192 patients who received erythropoietin-stimulating agent therapy, 65% of patients had an increase in hemoglobin of 1 g/dl or more.

        iii. However, increase in hemoglobin takes longer with erythropoietin-stimulating agents than PRBC transfusion (NCCN, 2020b).

    (2) Pain
      (a) NCCN (2019) has established guidelines for adult cancer pain for evaluation and management of pain. A 0–10 scale and faces pain scale are acceptable methods for assessing pain.

      (b) Acetaminophen or nonsteroidal anti-inflammatory drugs (NSAIDs) are recommended for mild cancer pain.

      (c) For moderate, weak, or episodic pain, short-acting opioids are recommended.

      (d) Severe or intractable pain requires stronger, long-acting opioid medication.

      (e) Pain control should target the root cause of pain, with additional analgesics or other therapies, including antidepressants, anticonvulsants, and corticosteroids.

    (3) Depression
      (a) Literature supporting pharmacologic management of depression indicates that major depression affects approximately 16% of patients with cancer. Pharmacologic interventions combined with psychosocial interventions can be beneficial in the treatment of depression (Li et al., 2016).

      (b) Selective serotonin reuptake inhibitors (SSRIs) and serotonin–norepinephrine reuptake inhibitors (SNRIs) are used to treat depression and anxiety.

        i. SSRIs, such as fluoxetine, sertraline, paroxetine, citalopram, and escitalopram, can be used to treat depression.

        ii. SSRIs and SNRIs have been found to be effective and can also be prescribed for anxiety and hot flashes.

        iii. SNRIs have the ability to improve nausea, increase appetite, and improve sleep (Li et al., 2016).

(c) Tricyclic antidepressants include nortriptyline, desipramine, and imipramine.
  i. Side effects include constipation, dry mouth, orthostatic hypotension, weight gain, and sedation.
  ii. They should be used with caution in patients with cancer because of potentially dangerous interactions with other medications (Grassi, Nanni, Rodin, Li, & Caruso, 2018).

(d) Monoamine oxidase (MAO) inhibitors prevent monoamine oxidase from breaking down neurotransmitters.
  i. Examples include imipramine, phenelzine, isocarboxazid, and tranylcypromine.
  ii. MAO inhibitors are usually the third or fourth line of treatment for depression.
  iii. Patients should be provided with education on the specific food and drug interactions and side effects associated with these medications (Wimbiscus, Kostenko, & Malone, 2010).

(4) Sleep disturbance
  (a) Patients with cancer may have altered sleep patterns related to a variety of factors, such as pain, stress, or medications. Benzodiazepines and nonbenzodiazepine hypnotics have shown effectiveness in alleviating insomnia in this group.
  (b) Benzodiazepines (e.g., lorazepam, temazepam, diazepam, clonazepam) are a widely used class of drugs to treat insomnia. These drugs may cause daytime sleepiness, issues with sleep maintenance, rebound insomnia, and memory issues. They also have potential drug–drug interactions (NCCN, 2020a).
  (c) Nonbenzodiazepine hypnotics (e.g., eszopiclone, zolpidem, zaleplon) are useful in decreasing sleep latency, increasing total sleep time, and providing greater continuity of sleep (Joffe et al., 2010).
  (d) Mirtazapine is a noradrenergic and specific serotonergic antidepressant. The medication works quickly, can improve sleep, and has other therapeutic benefits in addition to treating depression (Alam, Voronovich, & Carley, 2013).

(5) Comorbid conditions
  (a) NCCN (2020a) recommends evaluation and optimal management of noncancer comorbidities throughout the course of treatment.
  (b) Treatment may necessitate new medications, adjustment of current medications, or both.

(6) General pharmacologic strategies for management of fatigue
  (a) Once treatable causes have been assessed and ruled out, pharmacologic interventions should be considered.
  (b) Methylphenidate has been evaluated for its effectiveness when treating CRF. Studies have shown it reduces fatigue compared to the placebo. However, patients have experienced side effects, such as headache and nausea (NCCN, 2020a).
  (c) Dexamethasone treatment showed significant improvement in CRF in a study of patients with advanced stage cancer who reported moderate to severe CRF. It also improved quality of life (Yennurajalingam et al., 2013).

b) Nonpharmacologic management: Strong evidence supports use of a variety of nonpharmacologic interventions to reduce fatigue.
  (1) Exercise: Physical exercise can greatly reduce the effects of CRF, as well as improve quality of life and physical functioning (Schmitz et al., 2010).
    (a) Patients frequently try to sleep to reduce fatigue, but this can worsen CRF symptoms (Jones et al., 2016).
    (b) The suggested exercise prescription for patients undergoing chemotherapy or RT can vary. The American Cancer Society (2019) recommends 150 minutes of moderate-intensity or 75 minutes of vigorous-intensity exercise, ideally spread throughout the week.
    (c) Moderate activity involves effort comparable to that of brisk walk.
    (d) Vigorous activity results in increased heart rate and respiratory rate compared to moderate activity (American Cancer Society, 2019).
    (e) Strength training is suggested two to three times per week and should include large muscle groups.
    (f) Stretching and flexibility exercises should be done on days with other types of physical activity (Schmitz et al., 2010).
    (g) Exercise has the strongest evidence to support its benefits in managing CRF during and after treatment (NCCN, 2020a).
      i. The exercise prescription should include the type of exercise; initial intensity, duration, and frequency;

and rate of progression to higher levels.

ii. Currently, there is insufficient evidence to recommend a specific amount of physical activity (NCCN, 2020a).

iii. For individuals who are just beginning physical exercise, amounts less than those recommended are still beneficial.

iv. Amount of physical activity can be increased over time. However, men older than 40 years, women older than 50 years, and those with chronic conditions (heart problems) should discuss it with their physician first (American Cancer Society, 2019).

v. A professional with appropriate expertise should prescribe exercise.

vi. For deconditioned individuals and those with bone metastases, referral to a rehabilitation program may be appropriate.

vii. Patients should avoid exercising one to two days after receiving chemotherapy or during periods of neutropenia, low platelets, anemia, or fever.

viii. If patients experience dyspnea, chest pain, dizziness, pain, or nausea and vomiting during activity, they should discontinue exercise and seek medical attention (NCCN, 2020a).

(2) Psychosocial interventions: A strong correlation exists between emotional distress and fatigue; however, the relationship is not clear. Patients frequently experience anxiety and depression during cancer (NCCN, 2020a).

(a) Education: Education about fatigue should be given to all patients with cancer, especially when they are beginning treatments that may cause fatigue (e.g., chemotherapy, RT, biotherapy).

i. Patients should understand that CRF might be a consequence of treatment, and their fatigue does not necessarily mean that the disease is progressing or that the treatment is not working.

ii. Reassuring patients that CRF is common is helpful because fear of progression can lead to patients underreporting CRF (NCCN, 2020a).

(b) Energy conservation: Teaching energy conservation and activity management strategies has been shown to reduce CRF during cancer treatment.

i. The goal is to plan out daily activities to ensure the patient can set realistic expectations and participate in specific or special events.

ii. Patients can delegate certain tasks and plan for times to rest (NCCN, 2020a).

(c) Behavior interventions: Behavioral interventions to optimize sleep include the following (Mitchell et al., 2014).

i. Stimulus control
 • Preparing a bedtime routine
 • Going to bed when sleepy
 • Avoiding caffeine or alcohol near bedtime
 • Maintaining regular arising time
 • Getting out of bed when unable to sleep
 • Using the bed for only sleep and sexual activities
 • Avoiding long naps in the afternoon

ii. Sleep restriction: limiting amount of time in bed to closely approximate time asleep

iii. Cognitive therapy
 • Reducing or eliminating unrealistic sleep expectations and misconceptions about the cause of insomnia
 • Emphasizing the consequences of sleeplessness and anxiety resulting from failed attempts to control sleep

(d) Relaxation training: Progressive muscle relaxation and relaxation breathing have been shown to reduce fatigue (Mitchell et al., 2014).

i. This type of training includes flexing and relaxing each body part in succession, guided imagery (imagining a restful scene with all senses), diaphragmatic breathing (taking slow deep breaths that expand the whole diaphragm and push out the abdomen), body scan (focusing attention on each body part while in a relaxing position), and meditation (focusing on a word, sound, or object while clearing other thoughts from the mind).

ii. Related interventions that have some evidence of effectiveness include massage and healing touch (Mitchell et al., 2014).

iii. Activities such as journaling, yoga, meditation, or listening to quiet music can also help promote sleep (NCCN, 2020a).

    (3) Nutrition: Cancer and its treatment can cause changes in nutritional status.

        (a) Patients usually decrease the amount of oral nutrient intake because of nausea or vomiting.

        (b) Fatigue can be mitigated when patients have balanced fluid and electrolytes (NCCN, 2020a).

    (4) Other recommendations: NCCN (2020a) suggests nutrition consultation, physically based therapies (e.g., massage), psychosocial interventions (e.g., supportive expressive therapies), cognitive behavioral therapy for sleep, and bright white light therapy.

5. Documentation: Documentation of fatigue assessment at regular intervals can include the following.

  a) NCCN (2020a) fatigue assessment

  b) CTCAE scale (NCI CTEP, 2017)

  c) Additional documentation

    (1) Treatable factors that contribute to fatigue

    (2) Impact of fatigue on daily activities

    (3) Recommended interventions for fatigue

    (4) Outcomes of intervention

6. Nursing implications

  a) RT will affect the lives of patients while on treatment and after treatment is completed.

    (1) Radiation oncology nurses have the opportunity to assist patients through different challenges by knowing what to expect.

    (2) Social and financial changes can affect patients.

    (3) Working-age patients may not have accumulated much paid time off, presenting an added stress to those patients experiencing the side effects of radiation. In fact, not all patients will have paid sick leave or be able to take time off from work, even if they do not get paid (Poirier, 2011).

    (4) Younger adult patients may have children, thus affecting the level of fatigue they experience (Banthia, Malcarne, Ko, Varni, & Sadler, 2009).

  b) Current research is not consistent about whether a patient's age influences the risk of CRF.

    (1) Hamre et al. (2013) and Butt et al. (2010) stated that older patients are more prone to fatigue.

    (2) Banthia et al. (2009) noted that younger patients are more at risk for fatigue.

    (3) Fagundes et al. (2011) and Luctkar-Flude, Groll, Woodend, and Tranmer (2009) reported no correlation between patient age and CRF.

    (4) This contradicting information emphasizes the importance of frequent assessment of fatigue.

7. Patient, caregiver, and family education

  a) Desirable patient, caregiver, and family education outcomes include the following.

    (1) Adequate knowledge of fatigue and strategies for managing fatigue

    (2) Demonstration of fatigue management skills (e.g., energy conservation, relaxation strategies)

    (3) Self-report of decreased fatigue

    (4) Ability to maintain important activities despite fatigue

    (5) Family support for modification of patient activities

  b) The following teaching tools can be utilized.

    (1) The Patient-Reported Outcomes CTCAE (PRO-CTCAE) is a questionnaire developed by NCI with common activities drawn from CTCAE (NCI Division of Cancer Control and Population Sciences, 2019).

        (a) The goal of the PRO-CTCAE is to improve the quality of adverse event reporting in clinical trials, identify the patient prospective, and improve detection of potential serious adverse events.

        (b) The following questions refer to fatigue. Response options include none, mild, moderate, severe, and very severe.

            i. What was the severity of your fatigue, tiredness, or lack of energy at its worst?

            ii. How much did fatigue, tiredness, or lack of energy at its worst interfere with your usual or daily activities?

    (2) The webpage "What is Fatigue or Weakness?" (American Cancer Society, 2020) provides information about how long fatigue will last, potential causes, and additional resources for management of fatigue.

    (3) *Walking . . . A Step in the Right Direction* is an educational brochure adapted by ONS (2016) from materials produced by the National Institute of Diabetes and Digestive and Kidney Diseases, National Institutes of Health.

    (4) Websites: Many health-related sites contain accurate updated information about fatigue.

        (a) "Getting Help for Fatigue" (American Cancer Society): www.cancer.org/content/dam/cancer-org/cancer-control/en/booklets-flyers/getting-help-for-fatigue.pdf

        (b) "Life With Cancer": www.nccn.org/patients/resources/life_with_cancer/default.aspx

        (c) American Society of Clinical Oncology (ASCO) Cancer.Net: www.cancer.net

        (d) NCI information on fatigue: www.cancer.gov/about-cancer/treatment/side-effects/fatigue

c) If pain is an issue, patients should be involved in developing a pain management plan and set realistic expectations.

  (1) Pain can be treated with scheduled analgesics.

  (2) Breakthrough pain can be managed using short-acting analgesics (NCCN, 2019).

d) Patients are frequently ready to make lifestyle changes when they are diagnosed with cancer.

  (1) Providers should discuss an exercise plan with patients to help prevent fatigue.

  (2) Physicians and nurses may encourage "physical activity," rather than "exercise," to encourage patients to have a less sedentary lifestyle. This may be just as effective for patients as educating on more formal exercise recommendations (Nyrop et al., 2016).

e) Nurses can use the FITT principle to help patients set goals for physical activity.

  (1) The FITT principle includes the frequency, intensity, time, and type of physical activity (Lee, 2017).

  (2) Nurses may also assist patients in finding activities they enjoy, encouraging patients to find an exercise partner, setting realistic goals, and providing rewards for staying active (Tasillo, 2017).

f) The internet is readily available to help patients stay connected to others and can be especially helpful for patients who are experiencing depression or are too tired to participate in social activities. Nurses are in the position to provide individual patient-centered care plans that are unique to patient needs (Poirier, 2011).

References

Alam, A., Voronovich, Z., & Carley, J.A. (2013). A review of therapeutic uses of mirtazapine in psychiatric and medical conditions. *Primary Care Companion for CNS disorders, 15,* PCC.13r01525. https://doi.org/10.4088/PCC.13r01525

American Cancer Society. (2019). ACS guidelines for nutrition and physical activity. https://www.cancer.org/healthy/eat-healthy-get-active/acs-guidelines-nutrition-physical-activity-cancer-prevention/guidelines.html

American Cancer Society. (2020). What is fatigue or weakness? https://www.cancer.org/treatment/treatments-and-side-effects/physical-side-effects/fatigue/what-is-cancer-related-fatigue.html

Banthia, R., Malcarne, V.L., Ko, C.M., Varni, J.W., & Sadler, G.R. (2009). Fatigued breast cancer survivors: The role of sleep quality, depressed mood, stage and age. *Psychology and Health, 24,* 965–980. https://doi.org/10.1080/08870440802110831

Bower, J.E. (2014). Cancer-related fatigue—Mechanisms, risk factors, and treatments. *Nature Reviews Clinical Oncology, 11,* 597–609. https://doi.org/10.1038/nrclinonc.2014.127

Butt, Z., Rao, A.V., Lai, J.-S., Abernethy, A.P., Rosenbloom, S.K., & Cella, D. (2010). Age-associated differences in fatigue among patients with cancer.

Journal of Pain and Symptom Management, 40, 217–223. https://doi.org/10.1016/j.jpainsymman.2009.12.016

Dhruva, A., Dodd, M., Paul, S.M., Cooper, B.A., Lee, K., West, C., ... Miaskowski, C. (2010). Trajectories of fatigue in patients with breast cancer before, during, and after radiation therapy. *Cancer Nursing, 33,* 201–212. https://doi.org/10.1097/NCC.0b013e3181c75f2a

Fagundes, C.P., Murray, D.M., Hwang., B.S., Gouin, J.-P., Thayer, J.F., Sollers, J.J., III, ... Kiecolt-Glaser, J.K. (2011). Sympathetic and parasympathetic activity in cancer-related fatigue: More evidence for a physiological substrate in cancer survivors. *Psychoneuroendocrinology, 36,* 1137–1147. https://doi.org/10.1016/j.psyneuen.2011.02.005

Feng, L.R., Chen, M.-K., Lukkahatai, N., Hsiao, C.-P., Kaushal, A., Sechrest, L., & Saligan, L.N. (2015). Clinical predictors of fatigue in men with non-metastatic prostate cancer receiving external beam radiation therapy. *Clinical Journal of Oncology Nursing, 19,* 744–750. https://doi.org/10.1188/15.CJON.744-750

Ferris, M.J., Zhong, J., Switchenko, J.M., Higgins, K.A., Cassidy, R.J., III, McDonald, M.W., ... Beitler, J.J. (2018). Brainstem dose is associated with patient-reported acute fatigue in head and neck cancer radiation therapy. *Radiotherapy and Oncology, 126,* 100–106. https://doi.org/10.1016/j.radonc.2017.08.008

Grassi, L., Nanni, M.G., Rodin, G., Li, M., & Caruso, R. (2018). The use of antidepressants in oncology: A review and practical tips for oncologists. *Annals of Oncology, 29,* 101–111. https://doi.org/10.1093/annonc/mdx526

Hamre, H., Zeller, B., Kanellopoulous, A., Ruud, E., Fosså, S.D., Loge, J., ... Kiserud, C.E. (2013). Serum cytokines and chronic fatigue in adults surviving after childhood leukemia and lymphoma. *Brain, Behavior, and Immunity, 30,* 80–87. https://doi.org/10.1016/j.bbi.2013.01.006

Joffe, H., Petrillo, L., Viguera, A., Koukopoulos, A., Silver-Heilman, K., Farrell, A., ... Cohen, L.S. (2010). Eszopiclone improves insomnia and depressive and anxious symptoms in perimenopausal and postmenopausal women with hot flashes: A randomized, double-blinded, placebo-controlled crossover trial. *American Journal of Obstetrics and Gynecology, 202,* 171.e1–171.e11. https://doi.org/10.1016/j.ajog.2009.10.868

Jones, J.M., Olson, K., Catton, P., Catton, C.N., Fleshner, N.E., Krzyzanowska, M.K., ... Howell, D. (2016). Cancer-related fatigue and associated disability in post-treatment cancer survivors. *Journal of Cancer Survivorship, 10,* 51–61. https://doi.org/10.1007/s11764-015-0450-2

Lee, J.Q. (2017). FITT principle for physical activity. In L.M. Bernardo & B.J. Becker (Eds.), *Integrating physical activity in cancer care: An evidence-based approach* (pp. 39–62). Oncology Nursing Society.

Li, M., Kennedy, E.B., Byrne, N., Gérin-Lajoie, C., Katz, M.R., Keshavarz, H., ... Green, E. (2016). Management of depression in patients with cancer: A clinical practice guideline. *Journal of Oncology Practice, 12,* 747–756. https://doi.org/10.1200/JOP.2016.011072

Lin, J.-M.S., Brimmer, D.J., Maloney, E.M., Nyarko, E., BeLue, R., & Reeves, W.C. (2009). Further validation of the Multidimensional Fatigue Inventory in a US adult population sample. *Population Health Metrics, 7,* 18. https://doi.org/10.1186/1478-7954-7-18

Luctkar-Flude, M., Groll, D., Woodend, K., & Tranmer, J. (2009). Fatigue and physical activity in older patients with cancer: A six-month follow-up study. *Oncology Nursing Forum, 36,* 194–202. https://doi.org/10.1188/09.ONF.194-202

Mahtani, R.L. (2017). Insomnia in the cancer patient: A complex problem. *Breast Journal, 23,* 385–386. https://doi.org/10.1111/tbj.12761

Mitchell, S.A. (2014). Cancer-related fatigue. In C.H. Yarbro, D. Wujcik, & B.H. Gobel (Eds.), *Cancer Symptom Management* (4th ed., pp. 27–44). Jones and Bartlett Learning.

Mitchell, S.A., Hoffman, A.J., Clark, J.C., DeGennaro, R.M., Poirier, P., Robinson, C.B., & Weisbrod, B.L. (2014). Putting Evidence Into Practice: An update of evidence-based interventions for cancer-related fatigue during and following treatment. *Clinical Journal of Oncology Nursing, 18*(Suppl. 6), 38–58. https://doi.org/10.1188/14.CJON.S3.38-58

National Cancer Institute Cancer Therapy Evaluation Program. (2017). *Common terminology criteria for adverse events* [v.5.0]. https://ctep.cancer.gov/protocoldevelopment/electronic_applications/ctc.htm#ctc_50

National Cancer Institute Division of Cancer Control and Population Sciences. (2019). What is PRO-CTCAE? https://healthcaredelivery.cancer.gov/pro-ctcae/overview.html

National Comprehensive Cancer Network. (2019). *NCCN Clinical Practice Guidelines in Oncology (NCCN Guidelines®): Adult cancer pain.* [v.3.2019]. https://www.nccn.org/professionals/physician_gls/pdf/pain.pdf

National Comprehensive Cancer Network. (2020a). *NCCN Clinical Practice Guidelines in Oncology (NCCN Guidelines®): Cancer-related fatigue* [v.1.2020]. https://www.nccn.org/professionals/physician_gls/pdf/fatigue.pdf

National Comprehensive Cancer Network. (2020b). *NCCN Clinical Practice Guidelines in Oncology (NCCN Guidelines®): Hematopoietic growth factors* [v.2.2020]. https://www.nccn.org/professionals/physician_gls/pdf/growthfactors.pdf

Nyrop, K.A., Deal, A.M., Williams, G.R., Guerard, E.J., Pergolotti, M., & Muss, H.B. (2016). Physical activity communication between oncology providers and patients with early-stage breast, colon, or prostate cancer. *Cancer, 122,* 470–476. https://doi.org/10.1002/cncr.29786

O'Higgins, C.M., Brady, B., O'Connor, B., Walsh, D., & Reilly, R.B. (2018). The pathophysiology of cancer-related fatigue: Current controversies. *Supportive Care in Cancer, 26,* 3353–3364. https://doi.org/10.1007/s00520-018-4318-7

Oncology Nursing Society. (2016). *Walking ... A step in the right direction* [Brochure]. https://www.ons.org/sites/default/files/2019-01/Patient%20Education%20Brochure_012919.pdf

Poirier, P. (2011). The impact of fatigue on role functioning during radiation therapy. *Oncology Nursing Forum, 38,* 457–465. https://doi.org/10.1188/11.ONF.457-465

Polek, C. (2017). Cancer. In S.L. Lewis, L. Bucher, M.M. Heitkemper, & M.M. Harding (Eds.), *Medical-surgical nursing: Assessment and management of clinical problems* (10th ed., pp. 234–269). Elsevier.

Purcell, A., Fleming, J., Bennett, S., McGuane, K., Burmeister, B., & Haines, T. (2010). A multidimensional examination of correlates of fatigue during radiotherapy. *Cancer, 116,* 529–537. https://doi.org/10.1002/cncr.24731

Roila, F., Fumi, G., Ruggeri, B., Antonuzzo, A., Ripamonti, C., Fatigoni, S., ... Ballatori, E. (2019). Prevalence, characteristics, and treatment of fatigue in oncological cancer patients in Italy: A cross-sectional study of the Italian Network for Supportive Care in Cancer (NICSO). *Supportive Care in Cancer, 27,* 1041–1047. https://doi.org/10.1007/s00520-018-4393-9

Schmitz, K.H., Courneya, K.S., Matthews, C., Demark-Wahnefried, W., Galvão, D.A., Pinto, B.M., ... Schwartz, A.L. (2010). American College of Sports Medicine roundtable of exercise guidelines for cancer survivors. *Medicine and Science in Sports and Exercise, 42,* 1409–1426. https://doi.org/10.1249/MSS.0b013e3181e0c112

Smets, E.M.A., Garssen, B., Bonke, B., & De Haes, J.C.J.M. (1995). The multidimensional fatigue inventory (MFI) psychometric quantities of an instrument to assess fatigue. *Journal of Psychometric Research, 39,* 315–325. https://doi.org/10.1016/0022-3999(94)00125-O

Tasillo, K.E. (2017). Overview. In L.M. Bernardo & B.J. Becker (Eds.), *Integrating physical activity in cancer care: An evidence-based approach* (pp. 1–12). Oncology Nursing Society.

Wimbiscus, M., Kostenko, O., & Malone, D. (2010). MAO inhibitors: Risks, benefits, and lore. *Cleveland Clinic Journal of Medicine, 77,* 859–882. https://doi.org/10.3949/ccjm.77a.09103

Xiao, C., Beitler, J.J., Higgins, K.A., Conneely, K., Dwivedi, B., Felger, J., ... Miller, A.H. (2016). Fatigue is associated with inflammation in patients with head and neck cancer before and after intensity-modulated radiation therapy. *Brain, Behavior, and Immunity, 52,* 145–153. https://doi.org/10.1016/j.bbi.2015.10.016

Yennurajalingam, S., Frisbee-Hume, S., Palmer, J.L., Delgado-Guay, M.O., Bull, J., Phan, A.T., ... Bruera, E. (2013). Reduction in cancer-related fatigue with dexamethasone: A double blind, randomized, placebo-controlled trial in patients with advanced cancer. *Journal of Clinical Oncology, 31,* 3076–3082. https://doi.org/10.1200/JCO.2012.44.4661

B. Skin reactions
  1. Pathophysiology
    a) Skin is composed of two main layers—epidermis and dermis—and serves as a protective barrier (see Figure 12).
      (1) Epidermis (superficial layer)
        (a) During normal skin regeneration, superficial cells are shed through normal desquamation.
        (b) New cells form in the basal layer of the epidermis, migrate to the superficial layer, and continuously replace those that are shed.
        (c) The basal layer of the epidermis proliferates rapidly; therefore, it is particularly sensitive to RT.
      (2) Dermis (deep layer containing blood vessels, glands, nerves, and hair follicles): The dermis layer provides the supportive structure required for the epidermis to renew.
    b) Radiation-induced skin reactions or skin toxicity
      (1) Radiation-induced skin reactions or skin toxicity is also referred to as *radiation dermatitis*, *radiodermatitis*, or *radiation skin injury*.
      (2) Skin changes caused by ionizing radiation have been documented since the beginning

FIGURE 12. Layers of the Skin

Note. Image courtesy of National Cancer Institute. Illustration created by Don Bliss (https://visualsonline.cancer.gov/details.cfm?imageid=4366). In the public domain.

of the 20th century (Feight, Baney, Bruce, & McQuestion, 2011).

(3) Although the histologic effects of radiation-induced skin damage have long been described in the literature, the pathogenesis driving these changes is understood to a lesser degree, and treatments for radiation-induced skin reactions are underdeveloped (Borrelli et al., 2019).

(a) Ionizing radiation damages the mitotic ability of stem cells within the basal layer, thus preventing the process of repopulation and weakening the integrity of the skin.

(b) Repeated radiation exposure impairs cell division within the basal layer, and a skin reaction develops (Archambeau, Pezner, & Wasserman, 1995).

(c) The high proliferative capacity and oxygenation requirements of basal epidermal cells make them very radiosensitive (Evans, Schrlau, Chalian, Zhang, & Koch., 2006).

(d) In addition to causing direct DNA damage, ionizing radiation generates reactive oxygen and nitrogen species that lead to localized inflammation.

(e) This inflammatory process ultimately develops into a fibrotic one characterized by increased collagen deposition, poor vascularity, and scarring.

(f) Transforming growth factor-beta serves as the primary mediator in this response, along with a host of other proinflammatory cytokines and growth factors (Straub et al., 2015).

(4) Novel technological advancements, such as high-precision IMRT, and the development of new treatment schedules have been successful in partly ameliorating, but not eliminating, radiation-induced skin reactions. IMRT has been associated with a significantly lower incidence of acute skin toxicity and a more prominent skin-sparing effect compared to 3DCRT (Ghosh, Tallari, & Malviya, 2016; Jo, Kim, & Son, 2017).

(5) Temporary and partial hair loss occurs at 30 Gy, and permanent hair loss can occur at 55 Gy (Chao, Perez, & Wang, 2018).

(6) Various types of skin reactions occur at different dosages (approximate) (Feight et al., 2011).

(a) Epilation: 20 Gy
(b) Erythema: 20–40 Gy
(c) Dry desquamation and pruritus: greater than 30 Gy
(d) Moist desquamation: greater than 40 Gy

(e) Hypopigmentation: 45 Gy
(f) Hyperpigmentation: 45 Gy

(7) Radiation-induced skin reactions result in myriad of complications, including delays in treatment, diminished aesthetic appeal, and reduced quality of life (Singh, Alavi, Wong, & Akita, 2016).

(a) Chronic soft tissue fibrosis can alter tissue form and function, causing significant cosmetic and functional disturbances, which can significantly affect quality of life (Borrelli et al., 2019).

(b) Acute reactions usually occur within 90 days of radiation exposure (Bray, Simmons, Wolfson, & Nouri, 2016).

(c) A variety of cellular mediators are involved in the healing process (Cohen, Jorizzo, & Kircik, 2007).

(d) In the acute phase, radiation increases the permeability of blood vessels, leading to tissue edema and intravascular thrombosis and fibrosis (Archambeau et al., 1995).

(e) The early symptoms of radiation-induced skin damage include pigment alterations, erythema, edema, desquamation, ulceration, and loss of skin elasticity (Borrelli et al., 2019).

c) Risk factors: Several factors can increase the risk of a skin reaction.

(1) Treatment related (Chao et al., 2018; Porock, Kristjanson, Nikoletti, Cameron, & Pedler, 1998)

(a) Type of energy (electrons vs. photons)
(b) Use of tangential fields (higher doses received within thinner areas)
(c) Use of parallel opposed fields (two skin proximal surfaces)
(d) Skin bolus (gel-like sheets applied over the skin to ensure higher dose)
(e) Skin types (higher tolerance in the scalp than the trunk or groin)
(f) More oxygenated cells than hypoxic cells
(g) Size of treatment field
(h) RT dose, use of a radiosensitizer, or previous radiation exposure

(2) Nontreatment related (Chao et al., 2018; Porock et al., 1998).

(a) General skin condition
(b) Moist areas of the body causing friction (e.g., axilla, inframammary areas, groin, perineum)
(c) Skin folds and bony prominences
(d) Age, nutrition, and hydration status
(e) Prior exposure to chemotherapy agents associated with radiation recall (e.g., doxo-

rubicin) and underlying medical conditions (e.g., scleroderma, lupus, diabetes)

   (f) Conditions associated with delayed wound healing (e.g., hypertension, smoking)

   d) Healing

   (1) Healing typically does not start until one to two weeks after the end of treatment.

   (2) The healing process is considered a continuous process of three to four overlapping phases (Broughton, Janis, & Attinger, 2006) regulated by a complex network of cytokines, growth factors, and their cellular receptors (Haubner, Ohmann, Pohl, Strutz, & Gassner, 2012).

   (a) Hemostasis (may or may not be considered one of the steps)

   (b) Clotting and inflammation

   (c) Cell migration and proliferation

   (d) Skin remodeling and maturation

   (3) Repetitive radiation injury disrupts the inflammatory and proliferative phases of wound healing, resulting in repetitive inflammatory responses and ongoing cellular regeneration (Dormand, Banwell, & Goodacre, 2005; Haubner et al., 2012).

   (4) Radiation induces other changes in healing, including an upregulation and cascade of inflammatory cytokines leading to changes to the extracellular matrix and collagen formation (Borrelli et al., 2019).

   (5) Changes in the healing process can result in post-radiation fibrosis, a late effect of treatment.

   (a) The fibrotic pathways activated in the acute phase result in progressive deposition of collagen and substantial dermal induration even years after the initial radiation exposure (Borrelli et al., 2019).

   (b) Chronic radiodermatitis is marked by significant induration of the dermis and subcutaneous tissue, telangectasia, and hyalinization of collagen of the reticular dermis.

   (c) The epidermis may be hyperplastic or become atrophic, ulcerated, and necrotic.

   (d) Reduced perfusion in irradiation skin impairs its wound healing potential and complicates reconstructive strategies (Borrelli et al., 2019; Bray et al., 2016).

   e) Radiation recall (Bray et al., 2016; Burris & Hurtig, 2010)

   (1) Radiation recall is an acute inflammatory reaction confined to an area previously exposed to radiation in response to a systemic drug, occurring weeks to months after RT and within days to weeks following treatment with a triggering agent (e.g., doxorubicin, docetaxel, pacli-

taxel, gemcitabine, capecitabine, methotrexate, hydroxyurea, tamoxifen, cetuximab).

   (2) Incidence has been reported in up to 6% of patients undergoing RT (Burris & Hurtig, 2010).

   (3) Radiation recall manifests with maculopapular eruptions, dry desquamation, pruritus, swelling, and ulcerations.

   (4) Certain drugs appear to be associated with this phenomenon, but the cause and incidence are unknown.

2. Incidence and prevalence

   a) Up to 95% of patients with cancer receiving RT will develop some form of radiation-induced skin reaction, including erythema, dry desquamation, and moist desquamation (McQuestion, 2011; Ryan, 2012).

   b) To date, the most effective chemoradiation strategies for locally advanced cancers integrate nontargeted cytotoxic chemotherapies (e.g., cisplatin, 5-fluorouracil, taxanes) that increase healthy tissue toxicities.

   (1) To mitigate treatment-related side effects and allow for more potent radiosensitizing chemotherapy agents, molecularly targeted approaches are required to sensitize tumors and protect healthy tissues.

   (2) Antibody-drug conjugates are emerging as a tumor-targeted delivery strategy to restrict localization of drugs to tumors while sparing healthy tissue (Sievers & Senter, 2013).

   c) The incidence rate of radiation-induced skin reactions is difficult to predict and monitor, as the severity and occurrence are not well documented.

   (1) Radiation dermatitis is among the most common side effects experienced by patients receiving RT for sarcoma and breast, anal, vulva, and head and neck cancers (McQuestion, 2011; Salvo et al., 2010). The proximity of the treatment target to the skin in these cancers makes it difficult to spare the skin from higher doses of radiation.

   (2) The skin is vulnerable to damage during treatment of cancer in which skin-sparing techniques for delivering RT are not yet possible, such as with breast, head and neck, and anal cancers (Borrelli et al., 2019).

3. Assessment

   a) Radiation-induced skin reactions occur on a continuum ranging from erythema to moist desquamation (Feight et al., 2011; Glover & Harmer, 2014; Singh et al., 2016).

   (1) Erythema

   (a) Erythema can appear as redness around the treatment field and may be edematous and feel warm.

(b) This is a result of the release of histamine-like substances with basal keratinocyte destruction.

(2) Dry desquamation

   (a) Dry desquamation results in dry, flaky skin, as well as pruritis.

   (b) This is caused by compensatory mitosis to replace damaged cells where new cells are produced faster than damaged cells are removed.

(3) Moist desquamation

   (a) Moist desquamation occurs typically around regions of friction.

   (b) Skin may blister and become moist and edematous, and exudate may be present because of stem cell apoptosis and sloughing of the epidermis.

   (c) Loss of hair follicles, nails, skin appendages, and sebaceous glands in the treatment field can occur, as well as textural changes (e.g., scales).

b) Skin assessment

(1) A skin assessment should be completed at baseline, prior to initiation of treatment, and reassessments should occur minimally at weekly appointments throughout treatment, as well as at post-treatment follow-up appointments.

(2) Assessment should include objective evaluation of physical changes (e.g., changes in color, appearance of erythema, patchy dry desquamation, patchy or confluent moist desquamation, drainage, odor, possible infection), as well as patient symptoms (e.g., sensations of dryness, pruritus, or pain).

(3) The distress and impact associated with radiation dermatitis on quality of life, daily living, self-care ability, and financial impact of caring for the skin reaction also are important areas of assessment (Feight et al., 2011; Gosselin et al., 2017).

(4) Assessment should always include visual inspection of skin included in the treatment fields and exit sites.

c) Grading or scoring tools

(1) Several commonly used practitioner grading or scoring tools are available for assessment and documentation of radiation dermatitis.

(2) Each assessment tool can be used to identify grades or ranges of skin reactions from erythema to dry and moist desquamation, but most do not capture patient symptoms or impact of skin reactions (Feight et al., 2011; see Table 5).

   (a) The Radiation Therapy Oncology Group (RTOG) Acute Radiation Morbidity Scoring Criteria assesses intensity or severity of reaction (Cox, Stetz, & Pajak, 1995).

   (b) The RTOG and European Organization for Research and Treatment of Cancer (EORTC) toxicity criteria assess late complications including fibrosis, induration, skin contracture, and necrosis. It is a toxicity tool used in clinical trials but is also routinely used in clinical practice (Cox et al., 1995).

   (c) CTCAE is an adverse event reporting tool that uses a severity scale for grades of desquamation (NCI CTEP, 2017).

   (d) The Skin Toxicity Assessment Tool is composed of three areas of assessment: patient and treatment factors, objective scoring of grades of desquamation, and patient symptoms (Berthelet et al., 2004).

   (e) The Radiation-Induced Skin Reaction Assessment Scale uses weighted categories (e.g., moist desquamation weighted higher than dry desquamation) for an overall score that incorporates the effect on the patient (symptom scale) (Noble-Adams, 1999a, 1999b).

4. Management

  a) Overview

(1) The goal of skin care management is to enhance patient comfort, maintain skin integrity, promote healing, and prevent infection if the skin breaks down (McQuestion, 2011).

(2) More research is needed for well-designed studies to confirm some of the current recommendations (Leventhal & Young, 2017).

(3) Few randomized studies support specific products for the management of skin breakdown due to RT.

  b) General interventions

(1) All surgical wounds should be healed before initiating RT.

(2) It is vital to maintain skin integrity throughout RT.

   (a) Several studies demonstrate how basic hygiene and self-care improve a patient's sense of well-being, as well as demonstrating the importance of hygiene, to reduce the overgrowth of *Staphylococcus aureus*, and hydration as self-care strategies (see Table 6) (Bensadoun et al., 2013; Bolderston, Lloyd, Wong, Holden, & Robb-Blenderman, 2006; Bostock & Bryan, 2016; Brown & Pinnix, 2018; Glover & Harmer, 2014; Leventhal & Young, 2017; McQuestion, 2006; Morley, Cashell, Sperduti, McQuestion, & Chow, 2014; Wong et al., 2013; Yee et al., 2018).

TABLE 5. Primary Scoring Systems for Assessment of Acute Radiation Dermatitis

Grade	Radiation Therapy Oncology Group	Common Terminology Criteria for Adverse Events
0	No change	No change
1	Faint erythema, dry desquamation, epilation, decreased sweating	Faint erythema or dry desquamation
2	Tender or bright erythema, moderate edema, patchy moist desquamation	Moderate to brisk erythema, mostly confined to skin folds and creases, moderate edema
3	Moist desquamation in areas other than skin folds, pitting edema	Moist desquamation in areas other than skin folds and creases, bleeding induced by minor trauma or abrasion
4	Ulceration, hemorrhage, necrosis	Life-threatening consequences, skin necrosis or ulceration of full thickness dermis, spontaneous bleeding from involved site; skin graft indicated
5	Death	Death

Note. Based on information from Cox et al., 1995; National Cancer Institute Cancer Therapy Evaluation Program, 2017.

(b) In general, studies support basic hygiene to maintain skin integrity.
  i. Hygiene includes washing the affected area daily with mild perfume-free soap and patting dry to avoid friction to the area.
  ii. Patients can apply water-based moisturizer daily to hydrate affected areas, from the start of treatment, with no restrictions to timing of application prior to each fraction.
  iii. Studies have refuted the long-held practice myth that lotions, creams, or ointments applied to skin prior to RT would have a bolus effect on the skin.
  iv. Tse et al. (2016) assessed 17 topical agents and dressings and reported that no cream, gel, or dry dressing increased the skin dose with typical clinical application of a topical agent. More than twice the typical application of a product would be needed to create a clinically meaningful dose increase (Morley et al., 2014).
  v. Patients no longer need to restrict product application for any period of time prior to their treatment (Baumann et al., 2018; Bieck & Phillips, 2010; Brown & Pinnix, 2018; Fackrell, Kirby, Sanghera, & Hartley, 2015; Iyama et al., 2018; Tse et al., 2016).
(3) Patients should avoid perfumes, aftershave, alcohol-based products, cornstarch, baby powder, extreme temperatures of heat or cold (e.g., ice packs, hot water bottles), and sun exposure to the affected area.

(4) Patients should use electric razors only, and avoid use of shaving cream, aftershave creams, shaving lotions, or any alcohol-containing products on the treatment area.
(5) Patients can use deodorant or antiperspirant if the skin is intact. Studies have demonstrated no difference in dermatitis as it relates to deodorants or antiperspirants containing aluminum or those without it (Bolderston et al., 2018; Lewis et al., 2014; Morley et al., 2014; Salvo et al., 2010; Wong et al., 2013; Yee et al., 2018).
(6) To reduce friction, patients should avoid wearing tight-fitting clothes, shirts with collars for treatment to the head and neck, or underwire bras for treatment to the breast. Providers should advise patients to wear cotton if possible.
(7) Providers can support patients in reducing factors that interfere with skin healing by encouraging them to maintain good nutrition (e.g., adequate intake of protein) and to quit smoking.
c) Measures to delay the onset and reduce the severity of skin reactions
  (1) Hydrating products
    (a) Few studies have demonstrated that the use of nonsteroidal hydrating products results in less dermatitis, compared to no treatment (Sekiguchi et al., 2018; Yee et al., 2018).
    (b) Creams, lotions, and moisturizers should only be applied to intact skin (Bauer, 2016; Haruna, Lipsett, & Marignol, 2017; Hindley et al., 2014; Lucas, Lacouture, Thompson, & Schneider, 2018; Sekiguchi et al., 2018; Sio et al., 2016; Wong et al., 2013; Yee et al., 2018).

TABLE 6. Management of Radiation Dermatitis and Minimizing Skin Reactions

Radiation Therapy Oncology Group Grade	Interventions or Self-Care Measures	Rationale	Expected Outcome	Product Examples
All grades	Hygiene: Gently wash skin using lukewarm water in bath or shower; avoid extremes of temperature. Use only a mild soap with thorough rinsing. Use baby shampoo on scalp if area is treated, and sitz bath in peri-anal areas. Pat dry with a soft, clean towel; avoid rubbing.	Washing is subjectively associated with being important for patients' well-being. It reduces overgrowth of *staphylococcus aureus* (i.e., normal skin bacteria).	Delays the onset of dry or moist desquamation (same outcome for subsequent interventions).	Dove®, Neutrogena®, Pears®, baby soaps
	Do not use cosmetic products on irradiated skin (perfume, make-up, aftershave). Avoid use of lanolin-based products (potential allergen) and products with SPF.	Lanolin is a known sensitizer and can cause increased risk of sensitivity (contact dermatitis).		–
	Antiperspirant and deodorant are safe to use on intact skin.	No bolus effect is demonstrated with use of antiperspirant and deodorant or metallic-based products (e.g., zinc, aluminum).		–
	Wear loose clothing. Wear cotton or soft fabrics next to the skin in the treatment area. If treatment to breast area, wear cotton sports bras; do not wear underwire bras.	Prevent skin-to-skin friction.		–
	Do not use cornstarch or baby powder, especially in areas of skin folds, such as the, perineum, breast, or underarm.	These products create an environment for fungal and bacterial infections. They dry skin and can create unwanted aerosol particles.		–
	Shaving: Use an electric razor only. Do not use shaving cream, aftershave, or any alcohol-based products.	Electric razors minimize friction and prevent cuts or open areas. This avoids use of products that are drying and/ or irritating.		–
	Do not apply adhesive tape on treatment area.	This prevents skin shearing and tears.		–
	Do not place restrictions on timing of application of lotions or creams before or after each fraction.	This reduces friction and improves patient comfort, without bolus effects with treatment.		–
	Avoid using anything hot or cold on the area (e.g., heating pads, ice packs).	This prevents thermal injury.		–
Grade 0 • Intact skin • Use only one; do not use these products concurrently.	Moisturizing: Apply hydrophilic (water-based), lanolin-free, simple lubricant or moisturizing cream. There are no time restrictions.	Moisturizing keeps the skin hydrated and supple and maintains skin integrity. Moisturizing reduces trauma and friction and provides protection.	Delays the onset of dry or moist desquamation	Glaxal Base™ cream, Lubriderm® unscented lotion, Vaseline® Intensive Care™, Aveeno®

(Continued on next page)

Radiation Therapy Oncology Group Grade	Interventions or Self-Care Measures	Rationale	Expected Outcome	Product Examples
Grade 0 *(cont.)*	Barrier creams: Use from first day of treatment until 2 weeks post or as long as skin intact.	Barrier cream reduces friction and protects skin from water loss. Patients can shower.	Delays the onset of dermatitis and minimize moist desquamation.	Critic-Aid®, Pro-shield®, Sween®, Sween 24
	Barrier films: Use from first day of treatment until 2 weeks after treatment, or as long as skin intact.	Barrier film reduces friction and protects skin from water loss. Patients can shower. Film can remain in place for treatment.	Delays the onset of dermatitis, and minimizes moist desquamation	Cavilon™, Mepitel® film, Hydrofilm®
	Topical corticosteroids: Use daily from day 1 of treatment.	Steroids have a predominantly local anti-inflammatory effect to relieve itchy or burning feelings.	Reduces severity of dermatitis and pruritis and minimize discomfort	Hydrocortisone 1% cream or ointment, mometasone furoate 0.1%, betamethasone 0.1%
	Antimicrobial dressings: Use 24-7 from first day of treatment until 2 weeks post-treatment.	Dressings wick away excessive moisture and reduce friction, itchiness, and burning.	Delays the onset of dry or moist desquamation	InterDry® Ag
	InterDry Ag: Cover whole area and 2 cm beyond in each direction.	Use in areas with skin folds (e.g., inframammary, inguinal region).	Delays the onset of dry or moist desquamation	InterDry Ag
	Silver nylon dressing	Perineal area needs to remain moist.	Delays the onset of dry or moist desquamation	SilverClear®
Grade 1 • Follicular, faint to dull erythema/epilation and dry desquamation (dry, flaky, itchy skin) • Weeks 2–4 of treatment • Overwhelmed proliferating keratinocyte cells within basal layer, unable to sustain epidermal turnover • Impaired sweat and sebaceous glands	For follicular, faint, or dull erythema: Continue regular use of a hydrophilic and simple moisturizing lotions/creams, barrier creams/films, or antimicrobial dressing.	Interventions reduce friction, protect skin, and reduce excess moisture.	Skin remains intact; minimizes discomfort (same outcome for subsequent interventions)	Hydrocortisone cream 1% or ointment, mometasone furoate 0.1%, betamethasone 0.1% OR Critic-Aid, Pro-shield, Sween 24, Sween, OR Cavilon, Mepitel film, Hydrofilm
	For dry desquamation: If patient is symptomatic with pruritus or folliculitis, use topical corticosteroid (e.g., hydrocortisone 1% cream) 2–3 times/day. Use only on intact skin.	Steroids have a predominantly local anti-inflammatory effect to relieve itchy or burning feelings.		Hydrocortisone 1% cream
	Continue with barrier creams or films if using.	Barrier creams reduce friction, protects skin from water loss.		Cavilon, Mepitel film, Hydrofilm
	Saline soaks or sitz baths or Domeboro® soaks if perineum in treatment area	Soaks cool and soothe skin. Interventions do not replace washing.		Domeboro
	Silicone dressings	Dressings reduce friction and protect skin from water loss.		Mepilex® lite, Allevyn™, Biatain®

(Continued on next page)

Radiation Therapy Oncology Group Grade	Interventions or Self-Care Measures	Rationale	Expected Outcome	Product Examples
Grade 2 • Tender bright erythema, patchy moist desquamation, moderate edema • Moist, tender, red, weeping to crust forming exudate overlying exposed surface • Weeks 4–5 of treatment (peak 1–2 weeks post-treatment)	May need to use spray bottle or syringe to cleanse area. Continue with meticulous skin care: wash area, no rubbing.	Reduce friction and trauma.	Maintain skin cleanliness. Provide comfort and enhance moist wound healing environment; pain relief; sensitive skin is protected from clothing or where there is oozing/discharge (same outcome for subsequent interventions).	–
	Use room temperature or slightly warm normal saline soaks for 5–15 mins, 3–4 times daily. Leave to air dry 10–15 mins. Use sitz baths or Domeboro soaks to cleanse perianal areas. Stop using moisturizing creams in the open areas; apply only on intact skin.	Soaks cool and soothe skin; does not replace washing.		Domeboro
	Apply moisture-retentive protective barrier ointment after each saline soak. Avoid use close to the eyes.	Ointment provides moist wound-healing environment and barrier protection to prevent moisture loss. Ointment cools, soothes, and comforts. Soft silicones are chemically inert, provide a barrier, and prevent trauma to the skin/wound.		Silicone-based preparations, such as Proshield Plus Skin Protectant, StrataXrt, Sween 24, Critic-Aid
	Consider use of specialized ointments or low- and nonadherent dressings impregnated with dimethicone, secondary dressing, or light absorbency with Safetac®. Secondary dressings can be secured with stockinette or mesh. Monitor for signs of infection and consider the need to culture. Patients may require topical or systemic preparations in presence of infection. Use analgesics as required. Stress importance of nutrition.	Low- and nonadherent dressings can be removed easily and lessen risk of further damage to the tissues. Avoid tape to reduce irritation. Choice of dressing depends on exudate.		Adaptic™, Mepitel, Telfa™, Mepilex Lite, Mepilex Transfer, Mepilex Border, PolyMem®
Grade 3 • Confluent, moist desquamation • Risk of infection • Edema, bleeding, pain	Increase frequency of saline soaks. Monitor for signs of infection. Swab for culture and sensitivity as needed. Start or continue to apply specialized ointments and dressings.	Same as grade 2 rationale	–	–
	Consider use of other dressings, such as absorbent dressings and soft silicone dressings. Consider hydrocolloid dressings (post-treatment or during treatment based on individual situation).	Absorbent dressings are effective for drainage and do not stick to the wound. Hydrocolloid dressings promote autolytic cleansing of debris, may reduce healing time post-radiation, increase comfort reported by patients.	–	Safetac silicone foam dressings, impregnated dressings with analgesic, topical or systemic antimicrobial silver.
	Maintain moisture but prevent site from becoming too wet. Implement pain management measures: topical or systemic analgesics.		–	–

(Continued on next page)

Radiation Therapy Oncology Group Grade	Interventions or Self-Care Measures	Rationale	Expected Outcome	Product Examples
Grade 4 • Ulceration, hemorrhage, necrosis • Critical alert with patients	Wounds may be necrotic, bleeding, and/or infected during treatment; malignant wounds. Rule out infection. Wounds require individual assessment. Moist wound management may involve use of calcium alginates, absorbent dressings, silicone dressings, autolytic agents, and other specialized dressings depending on the goal of wound care (radiation skin reaction and/or malignant wounds). Topical or systemic antimicrobials can be administered. Team approach is required and may include physician, wound specialist, and plastics consult. Hyperbaric oxygen and surgical intervention with or without debridement may be implemented.	Determine goal of treatment (wound healing vs. prevention of complications, prevent infection, maintain hydration, ensure comfort).	–	–
Post-treatment skin care • 4–6-week resolution or progression to chronic wound	Avoid excessive sun exposure and trauma. Use of sunscreen and sun protection indefinitely in treated area; use SPF 30 or higher at all times.	Irradiated skin is more sensitive to sun exposure.	–	–
	Use of hydrophilic lotions, creams, or moisturizers.	Minimize dryness; rehydrate skin.		
	Monitor for late effects, telangiectasia, atrophy, vascular compromise, etc.	Community coordination may be required.		

Note. Based on information from Bauer et al., 2015; Baumann et al., 2018; Bensadoun et al., 2013; Bolderston et al., 2018; Bostock & Bryan, 2016; Bray et al., 2016; Brown & Pinnix, 2018; Fernández-Castro et al., 2017; Glover & Harmer, 2014; Haruna et al., 2017; Herst et al., 2014; Hindley et al., 2014; Kole et al., 2017; Laffin et al., 2015; Leventhal & Young, 2017; Lewis et al., 2014; Montpetit & Singh-Carlson, 2018; Morgan, 2014; Morley et al., 2014; Niazi et al., 2012; Schmeel et al., 2018; Shaw et al., 2015; Tse et al., 2016; Wong et al., 2013; Wooding, 2018; Yee et al., 2018.

From "Grading and Recommendations for Radiation Skin Reactions," by Ontario Radiation Therapy Skin Care Group, 2015. Copyright 2015 by Ontario Radiation Therapy Skin Care Group. Adapted with permission.

(c) Lanolin should be avoided in the treatment area, as it has the potential to cause irritation and allergic contact dermatitis. Products should be lanolin free (Bray et al., 2016).

(d) Products such as aloe vera, Biafine®, calendula, hyaluronic acid, sucralfate and its derivatives, and oral enzymes have insufficient evidence to recommend for use in reducing dermatitis (Chan et al., 2019; Fenton-Kerimian et al., 2015; Fisher et al., 2000; Gomes de Mensêses, Diniz dos Reis, Silva Guerra, De Luca Canto, & Barros Ferreira, 2018; Sharp et al., 2013; Wong et al., 2013; Yee et al., 2018).

(2) Topical steroids

(a) Prophylactic use of topical steroids, starting the first day of treatment, results in less dermatitis, and less moist desquamation.

(b) Several studies have been conducted in patients with breast cancer and head and neck cancer (Haruna et al., 2017; Hindley et al., 2014; Shaw et al., 2015; Wong et al., 2013; Yee et al., 2018; Zenda et al., 2018).

(c) Mometasone furoate (0.1%), betamethasone (0.1%), and hydrocortisone (1%) are topical steroids that have been studied, have similar results, and have been shown to significantly reduce pruritus (Ho et al., 2018).

(3) Semipermeable barriers and films

(a) Moisturizers are not needed when barriers or films are being used.

(b) Cavilon™ No Sting Barrier Film is an alcohol-free, nonsting, nonsticky film that can be applied by swab or spray (Herst, 2014; Kole, Kole, & Moran, 2017; Koukourakis, Kelekis, Kouvaris, Beli, & Kouloulias, 2010;

Micheli, Palese, Canzan, & Ambrosi, 2017; Shaw et al., 2015; Yee et al., 2018).

   i. This product reduces friction and protects skin from water loss.

   ii. It does not need to be washed off before RT.

   iii. Prophylactically, it can be applied daily for gynecologic cancers area and twice weekly for breast and head and neck cancers to reduce the severity of radiation dermatitis.

(c) Silicone dressings made with Safetac® technology, which is inert and adheres to dry skin and not the wound bed, are easy to remove without damaging the skin (Glover & Harmer, 2014).

(d) Prophylactic use of Mepitel® film dressing demonstrated reduced dermatitis in patients with breast and head and neck cancers. Patients can shower with the dressing applied, and the transparent film remains in place for the treatment (Fernández-Castro, Martín-Gil, Peña-García, López-Vallecillo, & García-Puig, 2017; Herst et al., 2014; Morgan, 2014; Narvaez et al., 2018; Wooding et al., 2018).

(e) Hydrofilm® used prophylactically from the beginning of RT reduced erythema, decreased the severity of radiation dermatitis, reduced sensation of itchiness and pain, and completely prevented moist desquamation in patients with breast cancer (Schmeel et al., 2018).

   i. The dressing can remain in place during RT because of minimal bolus effect.

   ii. Some patients may experience an allergic reaction to the dressing.

(f) Barrier creams (e.g., Critic-Aid®, Proshield®, Sween® 24 cream) reduce loss of moisture and form a barrier to reduce dermatitis when applied daily to treated areas (Kole et al., 2017; Laffin et al., 2015).

(g) Recent guidelines for recommendations of silicone-based film forming gel topical agents and semipermeable dressings are stated as weak or conditional with a low certainty of overall evidence because of concerns with risk of bias and imprecision (Gosselin et al., 2020; International Society of Nurses in Cancer Care, 2021; Wolf & Hong, 2019). Further research is recommended.

(4) Antimicrobial dressings

(a) InterDry® Ag is a textile dressing with an antimicrobial silver complex that wicks away excessive moisture and reduces friction, itchiness, and burning pain.

   i. It is intended for use in areas with skin folds (e.g., inframammary fold, axilla, inguinal region, pannus).

   ii. Patients who used this dressing did not require a prescription for the standard silver sulfadiazine cream (Montpetit & Singh-Carlson, 2018).

   iii. The dressing should be worn 24-7 from the start of RT, covering the affected area and 2 cm beyond. Patients should continue to wear it until two weeks after the end of treatment.

(b) Silver nylon dressings, which have antimicrobial properties, demonstrated a possible reduction of dermatitis when this dressing was worn prophylactically during RT affecting the perineum (Niazi et al., 2012).

d) Treatment of radiation-induced skin reactions (see Table 6)

(1) Treatment planning

(a) Infection should be ruled out in malignant, necrotic, or bleeding wounds.

(b) Providers should determine goals of treatment.

(c) Management requires a team approach including the radiation oncologist, nursing, wound specialists, and plastic surgery interventions. Dressings may include the use of calcium alginates, autolytic agents, silicone, or foam dressings depending on exudate and goals of care (Gove, Hampton, Smith, Hedger, & Topley, 2014).

(2) To cool and soothe skin irritation, saline compresses or soaks can be used three to four times a day. For the perineum, Domeboro® astringent soaks or sitz baths can be utilized (Leventhal & Young, 2017).

(3) Pruritus can be managed with moisturizing creams to hydrate and topical corticosteroids to decrease associated discomfort (Bauer, 2016; Haruna et al., 2017; Hindley et al., 2014; Leventhal & Young, 2017; Lucas et al., 2018; Morgan, 2014; Sio et al., 2016; Wong et al., 2013; Yee et al., 2018).

(4) For dry desquamation, applying a nonscented moisturizing cream or nonadherent silicone ointment or a foam dressing (e.g., Proshield, PolyMem®, Mepilex®) reduces friction (Bolderston et al., 2018; Cabrera & Karakashian 2018; Hegarty & Wong, 2014). Mepilex and Mepilex Lite thin foam dressings reduce friction to areas of dry dermatitis and reduce severity of dermatitis (Diggelmann et al., 2010; Kole et al., 2017; Zhong, Tang, Hu, & Feng, 2013).

(5) For moist desquamation, providers can promote healing and comfort by applying hydro-

philic creams or anti-inflammatory creams covered by a hydrogel or hydrocolloid dressing, or a silicone-based dressing (e.g., Mepilex Lite, Mepilex foam, PolyMem), depending on the amount of exudate (Bolderston et al., 2018; Gove et al., 2014; Kole et al., 2017; Leventhal & Young, 2017).

(6) If infection is present or suspected, an antimicrobial (e.g., silver sulfadiazine cream) may be added and covered by a nonadherent dressing.

    (a) A silicone-based dressing with silver may also be recommended.

    (b) If infection is suspected, the wound should be cultured. Topical or systemic antibiotics should be started based on results of culture (Bolderston et al., 2018; Glover, 2013; Gove et al., 2014; Hemati et al., 2012; Nherara, Trueman, Roberts, & Berg, 2017).

(7) All dressings should be nonadherent, and no adhesive tape products should be applied to the skin in the treated area.

e) RT techniques: Techniques such as IMRT, hypofractionated RT, accelerated partial breast irradiation, and prone positioning demonstrate decreased rates of dermatitis (Yee et al., 2018).

f) Long-term effects
  (1) Major late side effects
    (a) Telangiectasia, fibrosis, and necrosis can occur after receiving RT because of physiologic changes in the wound healing process.
    (b) The goal of treatment is to improve skin texture and elasticity.
  (2) Interventions and self-care after treatment
    (a) Skin can be kept moist and supple with moisturizing lotions.
    (b) Patients should protect their skin from ultraviolet A and ultraviolet B sunlight. Skin that has been exposed to prior radiation is more sensitive to the sun and has an increased risk of skin cancer (Bolderston et al., 2018).
    (c) Long-pulsed laser light therapy is used to treat telangiectasia (Yee et al., 2018).

5. Patient, caregiver, and family education
a) Studies support the use of multiple teaching strategies and tools to reinforce information on radiation-induced skin reactions and to empower patients in their self-care (Bauer, Laszewski, & Magnan, 2015; Bolderston et al., 2018; Cormier et al., 2016; Laszewski et al., 2016; Montpetit & Singh-Carlson, 2018).

b) Providers should teach patients, caregivers, and families care measures that can help minimize radiation-induced skin reactions (see Table 6).

c) Patients, caregivers, and families should be told what to expect related to radiation-induced skin reactions, including onset, how long reactions can last, and how to manage reactions depending on the severity of the reaction.

d) Providers should engage patients, caregivers, and families in the decision-making process, taking into consideration their comfort, the ease of application or use of the recommended products, and the cost associated with those products.

e) Providers must teach patients, caregivers, and families the signs and symptoms of infection to report to the treating RT team, as well as emphasize the importance of timely notification.

References

Archambeau, J.O., Pezner, R., & Wasserman, T. (1995). Pathophysiology of irradiated skin and breast. *International Journal of Radiation Oncology, Biology, Physics, 31,* 1171–1185. https://doi.org/10.1016/0360-3016(94)00423-I

Bauer, C. (2016). Understanding radiation dermatitis. *Wound Care Advisor, 5*(3), 21–24. https://woundcareadvisor.com/understanding-radiation-dermatitis

Bauer, C., Laszewski, P., & Magnan, M. (2015). Promoting adherence to skin care practices among patients receiving radiation therapy. *Clinical Journal of Oncology Nursing, 19,* 196–203. https://doi.org/10.1188/15.CJON.196-203

Baumann, B.C., Verginadis, I.I., Zeng, C., Bell, B., Koduri, S., Vachani, C., ... Mertz, J.M. (2018). Assessing the validity of clinician advice that patients avoid use of topical agents before daily radiotherapy treatments. *JAMA Oncology, 4,* 1742–1748. https://doi.org/10.1001/jamaoncol.2018.4292

Bensadoun, R.-J., Humbert, P., Krutman, J., Luger, T., Triller, R., Rougier, A., ... Dreno, B. (2013). Daily baseline skin care in the prevention, treatment, and supportive care of skin toxicity in oncology patients: Recommendations from a multinational expert panel. *Cancer Management and Research, 5,* 401–408. https://doi.org/10.2147/CMAR.S52256

Berthelet, E., Truong, P.T., Musso, K., Grant, V., Kwan, W., Moravan, V., ... Olivotto, I.A. (2004). Preliminary reliability and validity testing of a new skin toxicity assessment tool (STAT) in breast cancer patients undergoing radiotherapy. *American Journal of Clinical Oncology, 27,* 626–631. https://doi.org/10.1097/01.coc.0000138965.97476.0f

Bieck, T., & Phillips, S. (2010). Appraising the evidence for avoiding lotions or topical agents prior to radiation therapy. *Clinical Journal of Oncology Nursing, 14,* 103–105. https://doi.org/10.1188/10.CJON.103-105

Bolderston, A., Cashell, A., McQuestion, M., Cardoso, M., Summers, C., & Harris, R. (2018). A Canadian survey of the management of radiation-induced skin reactions. *Journal of Medical Imaging and Radiation Science, 49,* 164-172. https://doi.org/10.1016/j.jmir.2018.01.003

Bolderston, A., Lloyd, N.S., Wong, R.K.S., Holden, L., & Robb-Blenderman, L. (2006). The prevention and management of acute skin reactions related to radiation therapy: A systematic review and practice guideline. *Supportive Care in Cancer, 14,* 802–817. https://doi.org/10.1007/s00520-006-0063-4

Borrelli, M.R., Patel, R.A., Sokol, J., Nguyen, D., Momeni, A., Longaker, M.T., & Wan, D.C. (2019). Fat chance: The rejuvenation of irradiated skin. *Plastic and Reconstructive Surgery—Global Open, 7,* e2029. https://doi.org/10.1097/gox.0000000000002092

Bostock, S., & Bryan, J. (2016). Radiation-induced skin reactions: Assessment and management. *British Journal of Nursing, 25*(Suppl. 4), S18–S24. https://doi.org/10.12968/bjon.2016.25.4.S18

Bray, F.N., Simmons, B.J., Wolfson, A.H., & Nouri, N. (2016). Acute and chronic cutaneous reactions to ionizing radiation therapy. *Dermatology and Therapy, 6,* 185–206. https://doi.org/10.1007/s13555-016-0120-y

Broughton, G., II, Janis, J.E., & Attinger, C.E. (2006). The basic science of wound healing. *Plastic and Reconstructive Surgery, 117*(Suppl. 7), 12S–34S. https://doi.org/10.1097/01.prs.0000225430.42531.c2

Brown, S.A., & Pinnix, C.C. (2018). Avoiding topical agents before daily radiotherapy: Debunking dogma. *JAMA Oncology, 4,* 1748–1750. https://doi.org/10.1001/jamaoncol.2018.4291

Burris, H.A., III, & Hurtig, J. (2010). Radiation recall with anticancer agents. *Oncologist, 15,* 1227–1237. https://doi.org/10.1634/theoncologist.2009-0090

Cabrera, G., & Karakashian, A.L. (2018). Radiodermatitis. In D. Pravikoff (Ed.), *CINAHL nursing guide*. EBSCO Publishing.

Chan, R.J., Blades, R., Jones, L., Downer, T.-R., Peet, S.C., Button, E., ... Yates, P. (2019). A single-blind, randomized controlled trial of StrataXRT®—A silicone-based film-forming gel dressing for prophylaxis and management of radiation dermatitis in patients with head and neck cancer. *Radiotherapy and Oncology, 139*, 72–78. https://doi.org/10.1016/j.radonc.2019.07.014

Chao, K.S.C., Perez, C.A., & Wang, T.J.C. (Eds.). (2018). *Radiation oncology: Management decisions* (4th ed.). Wolters Kluwer.

Cohen, J.L., Jorizzo, J.L., & Kircik, L.H. (2007). Use of a topical emulsion for wound healing. *Journal of Supportive Oncology, 5*(10 Suppl. 5), 1–9.

Cormier, A.C., Drapek, L., Fahey, J., Rowen, B., Burns-Britton, B.A., Lavadinho-Lemos, M., & Hultman, T. (2016). When the patient seeks cure: Challenging chemotherapy and radiation side effects requiring creative solutions. *Clinical Journal of Oncology Nursing, 20*, 117–120. https://doi.org/10.1188/16.CJON.117-120

Cox, J.D., Stetz, J., & Pajak, T.F. (1995). Toxicity criteria of the Radiation Therapy Oncology Group (RTOG) and the European Organization for Research and Treatment of Cancer (EORTC). *International Journal of Radiation Oncology, Biology, Physics, 31*, 1341–1346. https://doi.org/10.1016/0360-3016(95)00060-c

Diggelmann, K.V., Zytkovicz, A.E., Tuaine, J.M., Bennett, N.C., Kelly, L.E., & Herst, P.M. (2010). Mepilex Lite dressings for the management of radiation-induced erythema: A systematic inpatient controlled clinical trial. *British Journal of Radiology, 83*, 971–978. https://doi.org/10.1259/bjr/62011713

Dormand, E.-L., Banwell, P.E., & Goodacre, T.E.E. (2005). Radiotherapy and wound healing. *International Wound Journal, 2*, 112–127. https://doi.org/10.1111/j.1742-4801.2005.00079.x

Evans, S.M., Schrlau, A.E., Chalian, A.A., Zhang, P., & Koch, C.J. (2006). Oxygen levels in normal and previously irradiated human skin as assessed by EF5 binding. *Journal of Investigative Dermatology, 126*, 2596–2606. https://doi.org/10.1038/sj.jid.5700451

Fackrell, D., Kirby, D., Sanghera, P., & Hartley, A. (2015). The effect of silver sulfadiazine and zinc oxide creams on dose distribution during radiotherapy. *Journal of Radiotherapy in Practice, 14*, 111–116. https://doi.org/10.1017/S1460396914000533

Feight, D., Baney, T., Bruce, S., & McQuestion, M. (2011). Putting Evidence Into Practice: Evidence-based interventions for radiation dermatitis. *Clinical Journal of Oncology Nursing, 15*, 481–492. https://doi.org/10.1188/11.CJON.481-492

Fenton-Kerimian, M., Cartwright, F., Peat, E., Florentino, R., Maisonet, O., Budin, W., ... Formenti, S. (2015). Optimal topical agent for radiation dermatitis during breast radiotherapy: A pilot study. *Clinical Journal of Oncology Nursing, 19*, 451–455. https://doi.org/10.1188/15.CJON.451-455

Fernández-Castro, M., Martín-Gil, B., Peña-García, I., López-Vallecillo, M., & García-Puig, M.E. (2017). Effectiveness of semi-permeable dressings to treat radiation-induced skin reactions. A systematic review. *European Journal of Cancer Care, 26*, e12685. https://doi.org/10.1111/ecc.12685

Fisher, J., Scott, C., Stevens, R., Marconi, B., Champion, L., Freedman, G.M., ... Wong, G. (2000). Randomized phase III study comparing best supportive care to biafine as a prophylactic agent for radiation-induced skin toxicity for women undergoing breast irradiation: Radiation therapy oncology group (RTOG) 97-13. *International Journal of Radiation Oncology, Biology, Physics, 48*, 1307–1310. https://doi.org/10.1016/S0360-3016(00)00782-3

Ghosh, G., Tallari, R., & Malviya, A. (2016). Toxicity profile of IMRT vs. 3D-CRT in head and neck cancer: A retrospective study. *Journal of Clinical and Diagnostic Research, 10*, XC01–XC03. https://doi.org/10.7860/jcdr/2016/21457.8583

Glover, D. (2013). The wound dressing maze: Selection made easy. *Dermatological Nursing, 12*(4), 29–34.

Glover, D., & Harmer, V. (2014). Radiotherapy-induced skin reactions: Assessment and management. *British Journal of Nursing, 23*(Suppl. 2), S28–S35. https://doi.org/10.12968/bjon.2014.23.Sup2.S28

Gomes de Mensêses, A., Diniz dos Reis, P.E., Silva Guerra, E.N., De Luca Canto, G., & Barros Ferreira, E. (2018). Use of trolamine to prevent and treat acute radiation dermatitis: A systematic review and meta-analysis. *Revista Latino-Americana de Enfermagem, 26*, e2929. https://doi.org/10.1590/1518-8345.2035.2929

Gosselin, T., Beamer, L., Ciccolini, K., Merritt, C., Omabegho, M., Shaffic, A., Skripnik, L. (2017). Symptom interventions: Radiodermatitis. https://www.ons.org/pep/radiodermatitis

Gosselin, T., Ginex, P.K., Backler, C., Bruce, S.D., Hutton, A., Marquez, C.M., ... Morgan, R.L. (2020). ONS Guidelines™ for cancer treatment–related radiodermatitis. *Oncology Nursing Forum, 47*(6), 654–670. https://doi.org/10.1188/20.ONF.654-670

Gove, J., Hampton, S., Smith, G., Hedger, C., & Topley, B. (2014). Using the exudate decision algorithm to evaluate wound dressings. *British Journal of Nursing, 23*(Suppl. 6), S24–S29. https://doi.org/10.12968/bjon.2014.23.Sup6.S24

Haruna, F., Lipsett, A., & Marignol, L. (2017). Topical management of acute radiation dermatitis in breast cancer patients: A systematic review and meta-analysis. *Anticancer Research, 37*, 5343–5353. https://doi.org/10.21873/anticanres.11960

Haubner, F., Ohmann, E., Pohl, F., Strutz, J., & Gassner, H.G. (2012). Wound healing after radiation therapy: Review of the literature. *Radiation Oncology, 7*, 162. https://doi.org/10.1186/1748-717x-7-162

Hegarty, F., & Wong, M. (2014). Polymeric membrane dressing for radiotherapy-induced skin reactions. *British Journal of Nursing, 23*(Suppl. 20), S38–S46. https://doi.org/10.12968/bjon.2014.23.Sup20.S38

Hemati, S., Asnaashari, O., Sarvizadeh, M., Motlagh, B.N., Akbari, M., Tajvidi, M., & Gookizadeh, A. (2012). Topical silver sulfadiazine for the prevention of acute dermatitis during irradiation for breast cancer. *Supportive Care in Cancer, 20*, 1613–1618. https://doi.org/10.1007/s00520-011-1250-5

Herst, P.M. (2014). Protecting the radiation-damaged skin from friction: A mini review. *Journal of Medical Radiation Sciences, 61*, 119–125. https://doi.org/10.1002/jmrs.46

Herst, P.M, Bennett, N.C., Sutherland, A.E., Peszynski, R.I., Paterson, D.B., & Jasperse, M.L. (2014). Prophylactic use of Mepitel Film prevents radiation-induced moist desquamation in an intra-patient randomised controlled clinical trial of 78 breast cancer patients. *Radiotherapy and Oncology, 110*, 137–143. https://doi.org/10.1016/j.radonc.2014.01.005

Hindley, A., Zain, Z., Wood, L., Whitehead, A., Sanneh, A., Barber, D., & Hornsby, R. (2014). Mometasone furoate cream reduces acute radiation dermatitis in patients receiving breast radiation therapy: Results of a randomized trial. *International Journal of Radiation Oncology, Biology, Physics, 90*, 748–755. https://doi.org/10.1016/j.ijrobp.2014.06.033

Ho, A.Y., Olm-Shipman, M., Zhang, Z., Siu, C.T., Wilgucki, M., Phung, A., ... Gelblum, D.Y. (2018). A randomized trial of mometasone furoate 0.1% to reduce high-grade acute radiation dermatitis in breast cancer patients receiving postmastectomy radiation. *International Journal of Radiation Oncology, Biology, Physics, 101*, 325–333. https://doi.org/10.1016/j.ijrobp.2018.02.006

International Society of Nurses in Cancer Care. (2021). *Evidence-based guidelines for the prevention of radiation dermatitis*. https://www.isncc.org/page/radiation-dermatitis

Iyama, A., Matsuyama, T., Matsumoto, E., Araki, T., Inokuchi, S., Yamashita, M., ... Oya, N. (2018). Effect of metal-containing topical agents on surface doses received during external irradiation. *Journal of Radiation Research, 59*, 794–799. https://doi.org/10.1093/jrr/rry078

Jo, I.Y., Kim, S.-W., & Son, S.H. (2017). Dosimetric evaluation of the skin-sparing effects of 3-dimensional conformal radiotherapy and intensity-modulated radiotherapy for left breast cancer. *Oncotarget, 8*, 3059–3063. https://doi.org/10.18632/oncotarget.13830

Kole, A.J., Kole, L., & Moran, M.S. (2017). Acute radiation dermatitis in breast cancer patients: Challenges and solutions. *Breast Cancer: Targets and Therapy, 9*, 313–323. https://doi.org/10.2147/BCTT.S109763

Koukourakis, G.V., Kelekis, N., Kouvaris, J., Beli, I.K., & Kouloulias, V.E. (2010). Therapeutics interventions with anti-inflammatory creams in post radiation acute skin reactions: A systematic review of most important clinical trials. *Recent Patents on Inflammation and Allergy Drug Discovery, 4*, 149–158. https://doi.org/10.2174/187221310791163099

Laffin, N., Smyth, W., Heyer, E., Fasugba, O., Abernethy, G., & Gardner, A. (2015). Effectiveness and acceptability of a moisturizing cream and a barrier cream during radiation therapy for breast cancer in the tropics: A randomized controlled trial. *Cancer Nursing, 38*, 205–214. https://doi.org/10.1097/NCC.0000000000000161

Laszewski, P., Zelko, R., Andriths, L., Vera Cruz, E., Bauer, C., & Magnan, M.A. (2016). Patient preference for instructional reinforcement regarding prevention of radiation dermatitis. *Clinical Journal of Oncology Nursing, 20*, 187–191. https://doi.org/10.1188/16.CJON.187-191

Leventhal, J., & Young, M.R. (2017). Radiation dermatitis: Recognition, prevention, and management. *Oncology, 31,* 885–899. https://www.cancernetwork.com/oncology-journal/radiation-dermatitis-recognition-prevention-and-management

Lewis, L., Carson, S., Bydder, S., Athifa, M., Williams, A.M., & Bremner, A. (2014). Evaluating the effects of aluminium-containing and non-aluminum containing deodorants on axillary skin toxicity during radiation therapy for breast cancer: A 3-armed randomized controlled trial. *International Journal of Radiation Oncology, Biology, Physics, 90,* 765–771. https://doi.org/10.1016/j.ijrobp.2014.06.054

Lucas, A.S., Lacouture, M.E., Thompson, J.A., & Schneider, S.M. (2018). Radiation dermatitis: A prevention protocol for patients with breast cancer. *Clinical Journal of Oncology Nursing, 22,* 429–437. https://doi.org/10.1188/18.CJON.429-437

McQuestion, M. (2006). Evidence-based skin care management in radiation therapy. *Seminars in Oncology Nursing, 22,* 163–173. https://doi.org/10.1016/j.soncn.2006.04.004

McQuestion, M. (2011). Evidence-based skin care management in radiation therapy: Clinical update. *Seminars in Oncology Nursing, 27,* e1–e17. https://doi.org/10.1016/j.soncn.2011.02.009

Micheli, C., Palese, A., Canzan, F., & Ambrosi, E. (2017). No Sting Barrier Film to protect skin in adult patients: Findings from a scoping review with implications for evidence-based practice. *Worldviews on Evidence-Based Nursing, 14,* 403–411. https://doi.org/10.1111/wvn.12232

Montpetit, C., & Singh-Carlson, S. (2018). Engaging patients with radiation related skin discomfort in self-care. *Canadian Oncology Nursing Journal, 28,* 191–211. https://doi.org/10.5737/23688076283191200

Morgan, K. (2014). Radiotherapy-induced skin reactions: Prevention and cure. *British Journal of Nursing, 23*(Suppl. 16), S24–S32. https://doi.org/10.12968/bjon.2014.23.Sup16.S24

Morley, L., Cashell, A., Sperduti, A., McQuestion, M., & Chow, J.C.L. (2014). Evaluating the relevance of dosimetric considerations to patient instructions regarding skin care during radiation therapy. *Journal of Radiotherapy in Practice, 13,* 294–301. https://doi.org/10.1017/S1460396913000241

Narvaez, C., Doemer, C., Idel, C., Setter, C., Olbrich, D., Ujmajuridze, Z., ... Rades, D. (2018). Radiotherapy related skin toxicity (RAREST_01): Mepitel® film versus standard care in patients with locally advanced head-and-neck cancer. *BMC Cancer, 18,* 197. https://doi.org/10.1186/s12885-018-4119-x

National Cancer Institute Cancer Therapy Evaluation Program. (2017). *Common terminology criteria for adverse events* [v.5.0]. https://ctep.cancer.gov/protocolDevelopment/electronic_applications/docs/CTCAE_v5_Quick_Reference_8.5x11.pdf

Nherara, L., Trueman, P., Roberts, C., & Berg, L. (2017). Silver delivery approaches in the management of partial thickness burns: A systematic review and indirect treatment comparison. *Wound Repair and Regeneration, 25,* 707–721. https://doi.org/10.1111/wrr.12559

Niazi, T.M., Vuong, T., Azoulay, L., Marijnen, C., Bujko, K., Nasr, E., ... Cummings, B. (2012). Silver clear nylon dressing is effective in preventing radiation-induced dermatitis in patients with lower gastrointestinal cancer: Results from a phase III study. *International Journal of Radiation Oncology, Biology, Physics, 84,* e305–e310. https://doi.org/10.1016/j.ijrobp.2012.03.062

Noble-Adams, R. (1999a). Radiation-induced skin reactions 2: Development of a measurement tool. *British Journal of Nursing, 8,* 1208–1211. https://doi.org/10.12968/bjon.1999.8.18.6490

Noble-Adams, R. (1999b). Radiation-induced skin reactions 3: Evaluating the RISRAS. *British Journal of Nursing, 8,* 1305–1312. https://doi.org/10.12968/bjon.1999.8.19.1305

Porock, D., Kristjanson, L., Nikoletti, S., Cameron, F., & Pedler, P. (1998). Predicting the severity of radiation skin reactions in women with breast cancer. *Oncology Nursing Forum, 25,* 1019–1029.

Ryan, J.L. (2012). Ionizing radiation: The good, the bad, and the ugly. *Journal of Investigative Dermatology, 132,* 985–993. https://doi.org/10.1038/jid.2011.411

Salvo, N., Barnes, E., van Draanen, J., Stacey, E., Mitera, G., Breen, D., ... De Angelis, C. (2010). Prophylaxis and management of acute radiation-induced skin reactions: A systematic review of the literature. *Current Oncology, 17,* 94–112. https://doi.org/10.3747/co.v17i4.493

Schmeel, L.C., Koch, D., Stumpf, S., Leitzen, C., Simon, B., Schüller, H., ... Wilhelm-Buchstab, T.M. (2018). Prophylactically applied Hydrofilm polyurethane film dressings reduce dermatitis in adjuvant radiation therapy of breast cancer patients. *Acta Oncologica, 57,* 908–915. https://doi.org/10.1080/0284186X.2018.1441542

Sekiguchi, K., Akahane, K., Ogita, M., Haga, C., Ito, R., Arai, S., ... Kawamori, J. (2018). Efficacy of heparinoid moisturizer as a prophylactic agent for radiation dermatitis following radiotherapy after breast-conserving surgery: A randomized controlled trial. *Japanese Journal of Clinical Oncology, 48,* 450–457. https://doi.org/10.1093/jjco/hyy045

Sharp, L., Finnilä, K., Johansson, H., Abrahamsson, M., Hatscheck, T., & Bergenmar, M. (2013). No differences between calendula cream and aqueous cream in the prevention of acute radiation skin reactions—Results from a randomized blinded trial. *European Journal of Oncology Nursing, 17,* 429–435. https://doi.org/10.1016/j.ejon.2012.11.003

Shaw, S.-Z., Nien, H.-H., Wu, C.-J., Lui, L.T., Su, J.-F., & Lang, C.-H. (2015). 3M Cavilon No-Sting Barrier Film or topical corticosteroid (mometasone furoate) for protection against radiation dermatitis: A clinical trial. *Journal of the Formosan Medical Association, 114,* 407–414. https://doi.org/10.1016/j.jfma.2013.04.003

Sievers, E.L., & Senter, P.D. (2013). Antibody-drug conjugates in cancer therapy. *Annual Review of Medicine, 64,* 15–29. https://doi.org/10.1146/annurev-med-050311-201823

Singh, M., Alavi, A., Wong, R., & Akita, S. (2016). Radiodermatitis: A review of our current understanding. *American Journal of Clinical Dermatology, 17,* 277–292. https://doi.org/10.1007/s40257-016-0186-4

Sio, T.T., Atherton, P.J., Birckhead, B.J., Schwartz, D.J., Sloan, J.A., Seisler, D.K., ... Miller, R.C. (2016). Repeated measures analyses of dermatitis symptom evolution in breast cancer patients receiving radiotherapy in a phase 3 randomized trial of mometasone furoate vs placebo (N06C4 [alliance]). *Supportive Care in Cancer, 24,* 3847–3855. https://doi.org/10.1007/s00520-016-3213-3

Straub, J.M., New, J., Hamilton, C.D., Lominska, C., Shnayder, Y., & Thomas, S.M. (2015). Radiation-induced fibrosis: Mechanisms and implications for therapy. *Journal of Cancer Research and Clinical Oncology, 141,* 1985–1994. https://doi.org/10.1007/s00432-015-1974-6

Tse, K., Morley, L., Cashell, A., Sperduti, A., McQuestion, M., & Chow, J.C.L. (2016). Dosimetric impacts on skin toxicity for patients using topical agents and dressings during radiation. *Journal of Radiotherapy in Practice, 15,* 314–321. https://doi.org/10.1017/S1460396916000285

Wolf, J.R., & Hong, A.M. (2019). Radiation dermatitis. In R. Corona (Ed.), *UpToDate.* Retrieved April 25, 2022, from https://www.uptodate.com/contents/radiation-dermatitis

Wong, R.K.S., Bensadoun, R.-J., Boers-Doets, C.B., Bryce, J., Chan, A., Epstein, J.B., ... Lacouture, M.E. (2013). Clinical practice guidelines for the prevention and treatment of acute and late radiation reactions from the MASCC Skin Toxicity Study Group. *Supportive Care in Cancer, 21,* 2933–2948. https://doi.org/10.1007/s00520-013-1896-2

Wooding, H., Yan, J., Yuan, L., Chyou, T.-Y., Gao, S., Ward, I., & Herst, P.M. (2018). The effect of Mepitel Film on acute radiation-induced skin reactions in head and neck cancer patients: A feasibility study. *British Journal of Radiology, 91,* 20170298. https://doi.org/10.1259/bjr.20170298

Yee, C., Wang, K., Asthana, R., Drost, L., Lam, H., Lee, J., ... Chow, E. (2018). Radiation-induced skin toxicity in breast cancer patients: A systematic review of randomized trials. *Clinical Breast Cancer, 18,* e825–e840. https://doi.org/10.1016/j.clbc.2018.06.015

Zenda, S., Yamaguchi, T., Yokota, T., Miyaji, T., Mashiko, T., Tanaka, M., ... Uchitomi, Y. (2018). Topical steroid versus placebo for the prevention of radiation dermatitis in head and neck cancer patients receiving chemoradiotherapy: The study protocol of J-SUPPORT 1602 (TOPICS study), a randomized double-blinded phase 3 trial. *BMC Cancer, 18,* 873. https://doi.org/10.1186/s12885-018-4763-1

Zhong, W.-H., Tang, Q.-F., Hu, L.-Y., & Feng, H.-X. (2013). Mepilex Lite dressing for managing acute radiation dermatitis in nasopharyngeal carcinoma patients: A systematic controlled clinical trial. *Medical Oncology, 30,* 761. https://doi.org/10.1007/s12032-013-0761-y

C. Pain
1. Pathophysiology
   a) For any patient, causes of pain may vary.
   b) The cancer itself may inflame or erode into bone, viscera, or nerves, causing pain (Bennett et al., 2019).
   c) RT may cause pain by damaging tissues or nerves.
   d) Nociceptive pain occurs as a result of tissue injury.
      (1) Causes of disease-related nociceptive pain include bone metastasis and obstruction of a hollow organ, such as with pancreatic cancer (Portenoy & Ahmed, 2018).
      (2) Causes of radiation-induced nociceptive pain include mucositis, skin reactions, enteritis, cystitis, proctitis, and chest wall pain (Chipko et al., 2019; Hauer-Jensen, Denham, & Andreyev, 2014; Portenoy & Ahmed, 2018; Radvansky, Pace, & Siddiqui, 2013; Serrano, Kalman, & Anscher, 2017; Sroussi et al., 2017). Pelvic RT increases the risk for insufficiency fractures, causing back and pelvis pain (Higham & Faithfull, 2015).
   e) Neuropathic pain results from nerve injury.
      (1) Causes of disease-related neuropathic pain include epidural spinal cord compression and tumor-induced plexopathies (Portenoy & Ahmed, 2018).
      (2) Causes of radiation-induced neuropathic pain include cervical, brachial, or lumbosacral plexopathies and polyneuropathies (Delanian, Lefaix, & Pradat, 2012; Portenoy & Ahmed, 2018).
   f) Procedure-related pain may occur in RT. Causes include frame placement for SRS, brachytherapy and fiducial placement for prostate cancer, and positioning during treatment exacerbating chronic pain (e.g., lumbar spine pain, shoulder pain).
   g) Patients with cancer may have comorbid conditions that cause pain, such as arthritis, diabetic neuropathy, or degenerative spine disease.
2. Incidence and prevalence
   a) In a recently updated systematic review and meta-analysis of literature published between September 2005 and January 2014, van den Beuken-van Everdingen, Hochstenbach, Joosten, Tjan-Heijnen and Janssen (2016) found that 55% of patients reported pain during anticancer therapy, 39% after curative treatment, and 66.4% in advanced, metastatic, or terminal disease.
   b) Moderate to severe pain (numerical rating scale score greater than 5) was reported by 38% of all patients (van den Beuken-van Everdingen, Hochstenbach, et al., 2016).
3. Assessment and screening
   a) Clinical guidelines recommend that clinicians should screen for pain at each encounter, using a quantitative or semiquantitative tool (NCCN, 2020; Paice et al., 2016).
   b) If new, worsening, or persistent pain is present, a comprehensive pain assessment and reassessment should be performed at regular intervals, individualized, and documented (Fink & Brant, 2018).
   c) Comprehensive pain assessment should include the following (Fink & Brant, 2018; Gallagher, Rogers, & Brant, 2017; Luckett et al., 2013; Paice et al., 2016).
      (1) In-depth interview exploring the multidimensional nature of pain
      (2) Pain descriptors (patient description of pain)
      (3) Intensity (pain intensity scale; verbal or nonverbal)
      (4) Location (one or multiple areas)
      (5) Onset and duration (persistent vs. breakthrough)
      (6) Aggravating and alleviating factors
      (7) Effect on function (ADLs, working)
      (8) Associated symptoms (e.g., loss of appetite, lack of sleep, depression)
      (9) Related social, psychosocial, psychiatric, and spiritual factors
      (10) Exploration of meaning of pain and its place in life (emotional, physical, and spiritual pain)
      (11) Current and past pain treatment therapies and outcomes
      (12) Past or current substance misuse or abuse (alcohol, illegal drugs, prescribed drugs)
      (13) Physical examination (general and focused based on assessment)
      (14) Appropriate diagnostic tests
      (15) Determination of pain as related to cancer, treatment, procedural, or exacerbation of chronic noncancer pain
      (16) Determination of pain type (Fink & Brant, 2018; Portenoy & Ahmet, 2018)
         (a) Acute: self-limiting, usually resolves in three months
         (b) Chronic: persistent, lasting longer than three months
         (c) Breakthrough: exacerbation of pain in presence of well-controlled background pain
   d) The following are potential barriers to pain assessment (Fink & Brant, 2018; Gallagher et al., 2017; Kwon, 2014; Luckett et al., 2013).
      (1) Communication (nonverbal patient or cognitive impairment)
      (2) Language (lack of common language to describe pain)
      (3) Cultural or age-related influences
      (4) Fear or misconceptions about addiction, tolerance, or disease progression
      (5) Fear of reporting pain (not wanting to bother staff, not wanting to delay treatment)

(6) Past or current substance misuse or abuse by patient or caregiver

4. Management

a) The goals of pain management are to enhance comfort, improve function, limit adverse effects, and ensure safety (Paice et al., 2016).

b) Pain management should involve an interprofessional team approach that clearly defines who is responsible for each aspect of care.

c) Providers must engage patients, families, and caregivers in all aspects of pain management.

d) Nonpharmacologic interventions can include the following.
   (1) Physical medicine and rehabilitation
   (2) Integrative therapies (e.g., massage, acupuncture, music) (Lu & Rosenthal, 2018)
   (3) Psychological approaches (e.g., cognitive behavioral therapy, distraction, mindfulness relaxation, guided imagery)

e) The following pharmacologic interventions may be used alone or in combination (Paice et al., 2016).
   (1) Nonopioid analgesics, such as acetaminophen, NSAIDs, and steroids
   (2) Adjuvant analgesics, such as antidepressants, and anticonvulsants (van den Beuken-van Everdingen, de Graeff, et al., 2016)
   (3) Topical therapies, such as NSAIDs and anesthetics
   (4) Opioids (short or long acting or combination) (Portenoy & Ahmed, 2014; Wickham, 2017; Wiffen, Wee, Derry, Bell, & Moore, 2017)
      (a) Depending on frequency of pain, schedule medications "around the clock" or as needed (e.g., prior to radiation treatment).
      (b) Combination with nonopioid medication and nonpharmacologic therapies
      (c) Risk assessment, mitigation, and management with opioid use (universal precautions) (Arthur & Hui, 2018; Choflet et al., 2016; Hande, 2017; NCCN, 2020; Paice, 2018)
         i. One in five patients with cancer may be at risk of opioid-use disorder (Carmichael, Morgan, & Del Fabbro, 2016). Silver et al. (2019) found that 50% of patients treated for oropharynx squamous cell cancer were chronic opioid users after treatment with RT.
         ii. Patients, family members, and caregivers may have a past or current substance abuse problem or addiction.
         iii. Initial assessment of risk factors for aberrant use of opioids should involve a detailed patient evaluation and screening tool, followed by

stratification into risk categories (low, moderate, or high) (Barclay, Owens, & Blackhall, 2014).
         iv. A patient–provider opioid agreement can be utilized.
         v. Urine drug tests can be used based on risk stratification.
         vi. Providers should check prescription drug monitoring programs prior to each new prescription.
         vii. Pill counts should be limited based on risk stratification.
         viii. Providers should use validated instruments to evaluate concurrent opioid misuse and abuse.
         ix. Providers should consider referral to substance abuse specialists to comanage pain in high-risk cases.
   (5) Medical cannabis depending on state regulations (Blake et al., 2017)

f) RT may be used to treat cancer-related pain, such as from bone metastases (Shiloh & Krishnan, 2018; van Dodewaard-de Jong et al., 2016; Zhang, Gilbo, Kohn, & Cox, 2018).

5. Documentation: Documentation of pain should include the following (Fink & Brant, 2018).

a) Results of pain screening from each visit

b) Findings from comprehensive pain assessment

c) Pain intensity rating from patient

d) Plan for pain management, including goals

e) Adherence to plan

f) Evaluation of plan effectiveness (outcomes)

g) Adverse effects

h) Education provided

6. Patient, caregiver, and family education

a) Lazarev et al. (2018) found the most common cause of premature discontinuation of curative radiation for head and neck cancer was "against medical advice," resulting in suboptimal survival. The authors emphasized the importance of patient and family education and optimization of symptom management.

b) Providers should discuss concerns about and differences in tolerance, physical dependence, and psychological addiction.

c) Providers should proactively manage potential side effects of the pain management plan, such as the following (Wickham, 2017).
   (1) Constipation
   (2) Sedation and drowsiness
   (3) Delirium
   (4) Nausea
   (5) Pruritus
   (6) Respiratory depression

d) Education includes information on the potential for misuse and abuse and responsible opioid use (de la Cruz et al., 2017; Hande, 2017; NCCN, 2020).

(1) Dangers of sharing medications with family or friends

(2) Proper storage (locked in a secure location)

(3) Dangers of combining with alcohol or illicit substances

(4) Importance of taking medication only as prescribed and contacting the provider if pain is not well managed

(5) Use of naloxone (if prescribed)

(6) Proper disposal of leftover medications

References

Arthur, J., & Hui, D. (2018). Safe opioid use: Management of opioid-related adverse effects and aberrant behaviors. *Hematology/Oncology Clinics of North America, 32,* 387–403. https://doi.org/10.1016/j.hoc.2018.01.003

Barclay, J.S., Owens, J.E., & Blackhall, L.J. (2014). Screening for substance abuse risk in cancer patients using the Opioid Risk Tool and urine drug screen. *Supportive Care in Cancer, 22,* 1883–1888. https://doi.org/10.1007/s00520-014-2167-6

Bennett, M.I., Kaasa, S., Barke, A., Korwisi, B., Rief, W., & Treede, R.-D. (2019). The IASP classification of chronic pain for *ICD-11*: Chronic cancer-related pain. *Pain, 160,* 38–44. https://doi.org/10.1097/j.pain.0000000000001363

Blake, A., Wan, B.A., Malek, L., DeAngelis, C., Diaz, P., Lao, N., ... O'Hearn, S. (2017). A selective review of medical cannabis in cancer pain management. *Annals of Palliative Medicine, 6*(Suppl. 2), S215–S222. https://doi.org/10.21037/apm.2017.08.05

Carmichael, A., Morgan, L., & Del Fabbro, E. (2016). Identifying and assessing the risk of opioid abuse in patients with cancer: An integrative review. *Substance Abuse and Rehabilitation, 7,* 71–79. https://doi.org/10.2147/SAR.S85409

Chipko, C., Ojwang, J., Gharai, L.R., Deng, X., Mukhopadhyay, N., & Weiss, E. (2019). Characterization of chest wall toxicity during long-term follow up after thoracic stereotactic body radiotherapy. *Practical Radiation Oncology, 9,* e338–e346. https://doi.org/10.1016/j.prro.2019.01.012

Choflet, A., Narang, A.K., Hoofring, L.H., Bonerigo, S., Mian, O.Y., Katulis, L., ... Appling, S. (2016). Prevalence of substance use in patients with cancer receiving radiation therapy. *Clinical Journal of Oncology Nursing, 20,* 397–402. https://doi.org/10.1188/16.cjon.397-402

de la Cruz, M., Reddy, A., Balankari, V., Epner, M., Frisbee-Hume, S., Wu, J., ... Bruera, E. (2017). The impact of an educational program on patient practices for safe use, storage, and disposal of opioids at a comprehensive cancer center. *Oncologist, 22,* 115–121. https://doi.org/10.1634/theoncologist.2016-0266

Delanian, S., Lefaix, J.-L., & Pradat, P.-F. (2012). Radiation-induced neuropathy in cancer survivors. *Radiotherapy and Oncology, 105,* 273–282. https://doi.org/10.1016/j.radonc.2012.10.012

Fink, R.M., & Brant, J.M. (2018). Complex pain assessment. *Hematology/Oncology Clinics of North America, 32,* 353–369. https://doi.org/10.1016/j.hoc.2018.01.001

Gallagher, E., Rogers, B.B., & Brant, J.M. (2017). Cancer-related pain assessment: Monitoring the effectiveness of interventions. *Clinical Journal of Oncology Nursing, 21*(Suppl. 3), 8–12. https://doi.org/10.1188/17.CJON.S3.8-12

Hande, K. (2017). Pain management: Strategies for screening and monitoring patients receiving chronic opioid therapy. *Clinical Journal of Oncology Nursing, 21,* 669–672. https://doi.org/10.1188/17.cjon.669-672

Hauer-Jensen, M., Denham, J.W., & Andreyev, H.J.N. (2014). Radiation enteropathy—Pathogenesis, treatment, and prevention. *Nature Reviews Gastroenterology and Hepatology, 11,* 470–479. https://doi.org/10.1038/nrgastro.2014.46

Higham, C., & Faithfull, S. (2015). Bone health and pelvic radiotherapy. *Clinical Oncology, 27,* 668–678. https://doi.org/10.1016/j.clon.2015.07.006

Kwon, J.H. (2014). Overcoming barriers in cancer pain management. *Journal of Clinical Oncology, 32,* 1727–1733. https://doi.org/10.1200/jco.2013.52.4827

Lazarev, S., Gupta, V., Ghiassi-Nejad, Z., Miles, B., Scarborough, B., Misiukiewicz, K.J., ... Bakst, R.L. (2018). Premature discontinuation of curative radiotherapy: Insights from head and neck irradiation. *Advances in Radiation Oncology, 3,* 62–69. https://doi.org/10.1016/j.adro.2017.10.006

Lu, W., & Rosenthal, D.S. (2018). Oncology acupuncture for chronic pain in cancer survivors: A reflection on the American Society of Clinical Oncology chronic pain guideline. *Hematology/Oncology Clinics of North America, 32,* 519–533. https://doi.org/10.1016/j.hoc.2018.01.009

Luckett, T., Davidson, P.M., Green, A., Boyle, F., Stubbs, J., & Lovell, M. (2013). Assessment and management of adult cancer pain: A systematic review and synthesis of recent qualitative studies aimed at developing insights for managing barriers and optimizing facilitators within a comprehensive framework of patient care. *Journal of Pain and Symptom Management, 46,* 229–253. https://doi.org/10.1016/j.jpainsymman.2012.07.021

National Comprehensive Cancer Network. (2020). *NCCN Clinical Practice Guidelines in Oncology (NCCN Guidelines®): Adult cancer pain* [v.1.2020]. https://www.nccn.org/professionals/physician_gls/pdf/pain.pdf

Paice, J. (2018). Navigating cancer pain management in the midst of the opioid epidemic. *Oncology, 32,* 386–390. https://www.cancernetwork.com/view/navigating-cancer-pain-management-midst-opioid-epidemic

Paice, J.A., Portenoy, R., Lacchetti, C., Campbell, T., Cheville, A., Citron, M., ... Bruera, E. (2016). Management of chronic pain in survivors of adult cancers: American Society of Clinical Oncology clinical practice guideline. *Journal of Clinical Oncology, 34,* 3325–3345. https://doi.org/10.1200/jco.2016.68.5206

Portenoy, R.K., & Ahmed, E. (2014). Principals of opioid use in cancer pain. *Journal of Clinical Oncology, 32,* 1662–1670. https://doi.org/10.1200/jco.2013.52.5188

Portenoy, R.K., & Ahmed, E. (2018). Cancer pain syndromes. *Hematology/Oncology Clinics of North America, 32,* 371–386. https://doi.org/10.1016/j.hoc.2018.01.002

Radvansky, L.J., Pace, M.B., & Siddiqui, A. (2013). Prevention and management of radiation-induced dermatitis, mucositis, and xerostomia. *American Journal Health-System Pharmacy, 70,* 1025–1032. https://doi.org/10.2146/ajhp120467

Serrano, N.A., Kalman, N.S., & Anscher, M.S. (2017). Reducing rectal injury in men receiving prostate cancer radiation therapy: Current perspectives. *Cancer Management and Research, 9,* 339–350. https://doi.org/10.2147/cmar.s118781

Shiloh, R., & Krishnan, M. (2018). Radiation for treatment of painful bone metastases. *Hematology/Oncology Clinics of North America, 32,* 459–468. https://doi.org/10.1016/j.hoc.2018.01.008

Silver, N., Dourado, J., Hitchcock, K., Fullerton, A., Fredenburg, K., Dziegielewski, P., ... Fillingim, R.B. (2019). Chronic opioid use in patients undergoing treatment for oropharyngeal cancer. *Laryngoscope, 129,* 2087–2093. https://doi.org/10.1002/lary.27791

Sroussi, H.Y., Epstein, J.B., Bensadoun, R.-J., Saunders, D.P., Lalla, R.V., Migliorati, C.A., ... Zumsteg, Z.S. (2017). Common oral complications of head and neck cancer radiation therapy: Mucositis, infections, saliva change, fibrosis, sensory dysfunctions, dental caries, periodontal disease, and osteoradionecrosis. *Cancer Medicine, 6,* 2918–2931. https://doi.org/10.1002/cam4.1221

van den Beuken-van Everdingen, M.H.J., de Graeff, A., Jongen, J.L.M., Dijkstra, D., Mostovaya, I., & Vissers, K. (2016). Pharmacological treatment of pain in cancer patients: The role of adjuvant analgesics, a systematic review. *Pain Practice, 17,* 409–419. https://doi.org/10.1111/papr.12459

van den Beuken-van Everdingen, M.H.J., Hochstenbach, L.M.J., Joosten, E.A.J., Tjan-Heijnen, V.C.G., & Janssen, D.J.A. (2016). Update on prevalence of pain in patients with cancer: Systematic review and meta-analysis. *Journal of Pain and Symptom Management, 51,* 1070–1090.e9. https://doi.org/10.1016/j.jpainsymman.2015.12.340

van Dodewaard-de Jong, J.M., Oprea-Lager, D.E., Hooft, L., de Klerk, J.M.H., Bloemendal, H., Verheul, H.M.W., ... van den Eertwegh, A. (2016). Radio-pharmaceuticals for palliation in bone pain in patients with castration-resistant prostate cancer metastatic to the bone. *European Urology, 70,* 416–426. https://doi.org/10.1016/j.eururo.2015.09.005

Wickham, R.J. (2017). Cancer pain management: Opioid analgesics, part 2. *Journal of the Advanced Practitioner in Oncology, 8,* 588–607. https://doi.org/10.6004/jadpro.2017.8.6.3

Wiffen, P.J., Wee, B., Derry, S., Bell, R.F., & Moore, R.A. (2017). Opioids for cancer pain—An overview of Cochrane reviews. *Cochrane Database of Systematic Reviews, 2017*(7). https://doi.org/10.1002/14651858.CD012592.pub2

Zhang, I., Gilbo, P., Kohn, N., & Cox, B. (2018). Clinical response to radium-223 dichloride in men with metastatic castrate-resistant prostate cancer. *Practical Radiation Oncology, 8,* 452–457. https://doi.org/10.1016/j.prro.2018.05.003

D. Distress and coping

1. Overview

   a) Distress ranges along a continuum that includes typical feelings of sadness, vulnerability, and fear to disabling depression and anxiety that can lead to social isolation and, for some, existential crisis. Distress is a natural part of dealing with a life-changing diagnosis; however, clinically significant levels of distress can have detrimental outcomes, making identification and management essential (NCCN, 2020).

   b) NCCN (2020) defines *distress* in the midst of cancer as "a multifactorial unpleasant experience of a psychological (i.e., cognitive, behavioral, emotional), social, spiritual, and/or physical nature that may interfere with one's ability to cope effectively with cancer, its physical symptoms, and its treatment" (p. DIS-2).

   c) Coping is internal and external attempts to manage stressful circumstances and the interpretation of what those circumstances mean to the individual (Maggi et al., 2019).

   d) Anxiety is an emotional and physiologic response to a stimulus that can range from normal stress to severe dysfunction. It is common among patients with cancer, and it can occur at any time during cancer care. Anxiety is usually highest shortly after diagnosis and decreases over time, but some continue to experience it after treatment completion (Cope et al., 2019).

2. Standards of care

   a) The American College of Surgeons Commission on Cancer (ACoS CoC, 2019) requires cancer programs to have a comprehensive screening program for psychosocial distress to receive accreditation. The requirement was implemented in 2015 as emerging research suggested that screening for and addressing distress can enhance quality of life and improve treatment outcomes.

   b) NCCN (2020) has published evidence-based standards of care for distress management, with guidance on interventions for mild distress and identifying patients that require referral to psychosocial resources.

   c) In a joint position statement on implementing screening for distress, the American Psychosocial Oncology Society, Association of Oncology Social Work, and ONS endorsed the Commission on Cancer standard on psychological distress screening, recognizing that it will help improve holistic cancer care through addressing unmet psychosocial needs (Pirl et al., 2014).

   d) Cancer advocacy organizations in Canada and the International Psycho-Oncology Society adopted the NCCN guidelines for distress management and named distress screening as the sixth vital sign among temperature, pulse, blood pressure, respiratory rate, and pain (Lazenby, 2014).

3. Risk factors

   a) Ethnicity

      (1) A large study of 4,664 distress screenings across 55 cancer treatment centers in the United States and Canada, including a significant proportion of ethnic minorities, found that average distress scores did not vary among ethnic groups overall (Carlson et al., 2019).

         (a) Results were surprising, considering prior studies have shown that patients with cancer of racial and ethnic minorities were more likely to report distress.

         (b) Factors to consider are access to health care, differences in educational needs, communication barriers, social support, health beliefs, and relationship with healthcare professionals.

         (c) Findings also suggested that the Distress Thermometer might be insufficient to detect differences in distress across racial and ethnic groups.

      (2) A study conducted at the Saskatchewan Cancer Agency in an RT department to determine if distress screening scores are associated with sex, age, treatment intent, or ethnicity, utilizing the Edmonton Symptom Assessment System (ESAS) combined with the Canadian Problem Checklist, found that Aboriginal or Métis participants reported higher scores for pain, depression, anxiety, and shortness of breath than non-Aboriginal or non-Métis participants (Bodnarchuk, Stavrou, & Gantefoer, 2014).

         (a) Aboriginal or Métis participants also reported more issues on the Canadian Problem Checklist, including finances, which may be the result of living in remote areas, causing concerns related to transportation, accommodation, and meals (Bodnarchuk et al., 2014).

(b) These results suggested that their region may benefit from a dedicated Native health service program or a Native health services patient navigator (Bodnarchuk et al., 2014).

b) Gender
   (1) Carlson et al. (2019) found that average distress was higher in women than in men, and women had more clinically significant distress.
      (a) Women with cancer were more likely to report depressive symptoms, but men were more likely to report somatic symptoms.
      (b) Men with prostate cancer were less distressed than men with other cancers.
      (c) Women with lung, head and neck, and pancreatic cancer were more likely to experience distress.
      (d) Women with gynecologic cancers were less likely to have distress than women with other cancers.
   (2) A study conducted to predict cues and symptoms of psychosocial distress revealed that distressed patients were younger, were female, and gave more verbal cues for distress (Sheldon, Blonquist, Hilaire, Hong, & Berry, 2015).
   (3) Bodnarchuk et al. (2014) found that women scored higher than men for distress factors such as pain, tiredness, and appetite on the ESAS.

c) Disease site and toxicities
   (1) Uncontrolled symptoms and severe comorbidities contribute to symptoms of distress in patients with cancer. Advances in treatment and early detection have increased survival rates, which is also associated with long-term physical and psychological side effects (NCCN, 2020).
   (2) Hess et al. (2015) found that distress was highest in patients with head and neck cancer, followed by lung cancer, genitourinary cancer, gastrointestinal cancers, palliative cases, and breast cancer.
   (3) Bodnarchuk et al. (2014) found that patients receiving palliative RT had higher scores for pain, tiredness, anxiety, drowsiness, appetite loss, and shortness of breath than patients treated with curative intent. The top reported issues relating to distress were tiredness, poor overall well-being, anxiety, and appetite.
   (4) Carlson et al. (2019) found that patients with lung cancer and pancreatic cancer were more likely to be distressed than those with other cancers. Severe physical symptoms, such as hemoptysis and shortness of breath, likely contribute to distress in patients with lung cancer. Patients with a history of smoking may feel guilt for their diagnosis, thus increasing distress.

d) Living situation
   (1) Hess et al. (2015) reported higher distress scores in patients living alone.
   (2) Social issues, such as family or caregiver conflicts, living alone, lack of social support, financial problems, younger age, history of trauma or abuse, or other stressors, can all contribute to distress (NCCN, 2020).

e) Health-related behaviors
   (1) Smoking is associated with high amounts of psychological distress (Choi, Chan, & Lehto, 2019).
   (2) Survivors with untreated distress are less compliant with surveillance screenings and are less likely to exercise and quit smoking (NCCN, 2020).

f) History of depression and anxiety (NCCN, 2020)
   (1) Depression is prevalent in patients with cancer and is associated with decreased cancer survival.
   (2) Patients with cancer and a history of psychiatric disorders, depression, a previous suicide attempt, and history of trauma or abuse have higher levels of distress.
   (3) Preexisting psychological or psychiatric conditions can influence the ability to cope with cancer.
   (4) Patients with depression have more issues with nonadherence to treatment than those with no history of depression.
   (5) The incidence of suicide among patients with cancer in the United States is twice that of the general population.
   (6) Pancreatic and head and neck cancers are associated with depression.

g) Socioeconomic status
   (1) The financial impact of cancer diagnosis can be an issue for many. Patients in treatment may experience loss of productivity and income because of limited ability to work. Survivors have been found to have more financial hardship when they are younger, are uninsured, and have a lower income (NCCN, 2020).
   (2) Habboush et al. (2017) found that out-of-pocket medical costs were the third most common cause of distress in patients undergoing RT, with finances as the sixth most common cause.

4. Incidence and prevalence: More than 40% of all patients with cancer will develop significant distress at some point during diagnosis, treatment, survivorship, progression of disease, palliative care, or end-of-life care (Cancer Care Ontario, 2018).

5. Assessment and screening
   a) National and international guidelines for distress screening
      (1) Screening for distress should be conducted a minimum of once or at pivotal medical visits.

Ideally, distress screenings should be administered at every medical visit, as well as, at minimum, during the initial visit, at appropriate intervals, and as clinically indicated with changes in disease status.

(2) Cancer programs should determine the mode of administration (NCCN, 2020).

　(a) Clinician-administered screening can be integrated into a review of systems to allow for immediate scoring and interpretation. Assessment of patient understanding of screening can take place immediately to clarify any confusion.

　(b) Patient-administered screening can be completed as paper or electronic questionnaires in the clinic waiting room.

　　i. Electronic administration of distress screening can provide immediate scoring and populate the health record in order to track patterns of distress over time.

　　ii. Some electronic health record systems can facilitate immediate triage, providing patients with referral information and education. This could automate referrals, thus streamlining processes for a busy setting.

　　iii. Completion of questionnaires remotely by mail or online can be used but requires processes to attend to responses quickly, especially if patients indicate they are in distress or in danger of self-harm.

(3) Facilities should use a standardized tool to screen for distress. Tools should identify the level and nature of distress (NCCN, 2020).

(4) Interprofessional committees should implement referral standards for distress management and follow clinical practice guidelines (NCCN, 2020).

　(a) Licensed mental health professionals and certified chaplains should be readily available or available by referral.

　(b) Caregivers should know that distress management is integral to total medical care and provided with information regarding psychosocial resources available within the treatment center and community.

b) Validated screening tools

(1) NCCN (2020) Distress Thermometer and Problem List measures distress similarly to pain on a 0–10 scale, with 0 being none and 10 being the worst.

　(a) The problem list enables patients to inform providers about specific concerns.

(b) Mild distress is indicated by a score of 0–3, and a score of 4 or greater indicates moderate to severe distress.

(2) The revised ESAS (ESAS-r) and Canadian Problem Checklist are tools designed to assist in the assessment of symptoms that are common in patients with cancer (Hui & Bruera, 2017).

　(a) Symptoms are rated on a 0–10 severity scale, with 0 being no symptoms and 10 being the worst possible.

　(b) A score of 0–3 indicates mild distress; 4–6 indicates moderate distress; and 7–10 indicates severe distress.

(3) CTCAE utilizes descriptive terminology for reporting adverse events with a grading scale for each event (NCI CTEP, 2017).

　(a) Grade 1 events are considered mild.

　(b) Grade 2 is moderate.

　(c) Grade 3 is severe or medically significant.

　(d) Grade 4 is life threatening.

　(e) Grade 5 indicates death related to the event.

(4) PRO-CTCAE is a measurement system of 78 symptomatic treatment toxicities, including anxiety, feeling discouraged, and sadness. Patients are asked to rate their symptoms over the past seven days as none, mild, moderate, severe, or very severe (NCI Division of Cancer Control and Population Sciences, 2020).

(5) The MD Anderson Symptom Inventory measures patient-reported outcomes, symptoms, and the degree to which they interfere with daily activities. A score of 0 means that symptoms did not interfere, and 10 indicates complete interference with daily activities (University of Texas MD Anderson Cancer Center, n.d.).

(6) Patient Health Questionnaire is a patient-reported diagnostic tool for mental health disorders for healthcare professionals (Holtzman, Pereira, & Yeung, 2018).

c) Patterns of distress

(1) Identifying patients at risk for distress can help nurses anticipate needs and utilize resources.

(2) Distress occurs at various times during cancer diagnosis and treatment, and it may be unrecognized if screening occurs only once (Pirl et al., 2014).

(3) It is imperative to respond to distress at the first opportunity because distress affects disease outcome and survival (Bodnarchuk et al., 2014).

(4) The following circumstances can increase vulnerability (NCCN, 2020).

　(a) Discovery and investigation of suspicious symptoms

(b) Diagnostic workups

(c) Diagnosis of cancer or diagnosis of advanced disease

(d) Genetic test results

(e) Awaiting treatment

(f) Increase in symptom burden

(g) Significant complications related to treatment

(h) Hospital admission and discharge

(i) Changes in treatment modality

(j) Treatment failure

(k) End of active treatment

(l) Medical follow-up and surveillance

(m) Transition to survivorship

(n) Recurrence and progression

(o) Transition to end-of-life care

(5) A pilot study examined the frequency of psychosocial distress screening in patients undergoing RT. Daily screenings were conducted utilizing the Distress Thermometer (Hess et al., 2015).

(a) Significant distress was reported at least once while receiving RT in 37% of patients (Hess et al., 2015).

(b) Weekly, every-other-week, monthly, and once at therapy onset screening models concluded that patients who were screened every other week identified nearly 90% of patients positively screened for distress by daily screening (Hess et al., 2015).

(c) Elevation of distress was noted near the fifth week of treatment, with lower levels of distress immediately after treatment onset.

(d) Data suggested that half of patients experiencing distress during treatment show improvement within six weeks of treatment completion (Hess et al., 2015).

(e) Screening at every-other-week intervals was determined to optimize efficiency and accuracy of screening efforts (Hess et al., 2015).

(6) A study conducted in a radiation oncology department at the Virginia Commonwealth University Health System assessed the association between distress scores and outcomes common in radiation oncology, such as admission during treatment, missed appointments, duration of time between consult and treatment, and weight loss during treatment (Anderson, Slade, McDonagh, Burton, & Fields, 2019).

(a) Individuals who reported severe distress scores (7–10) were more likely to miss appointments during their course of RT and were more likely to be admitted to the hospital, compared to patients with lower distress scores.

(b) Patients presenting with higher stages of disease were more likely to report higher distress scores.

(c) No correlation was found between patients with high distress scores and prolonged time between consult and treatment start or weight loss during treatment.

(7) A study to evaluate the association between patient-reported distress and survival found that higher distress before or during RT is associated with decreased survival. Findings showed that the top five causes of distress were how participants felt during treatment, fatigue, out-of-pocket expense, pain, and sleeping difficulties (Habboush et al., 2017).

(8) Fear of cancer recurrence or progression is a common type of distress in survivors. It is characterized by heightened health-related global anxiety, worries about risk of recurrence or progression, fear of a shortened life span, and symptom vigilance (Howell et al., 2015).

6. Management

a) Mild distress

(1) NCCN (2020) recommends that patients presenting with mild symptoms of distress or report a score less than 4 on a screening tool should be assessed for expected distress symptoms.

(a) Expected symptoms of distress include the following.

    i. Fear and worry about the future
    ii. Concerns about social role
    iii. Side effects of disease and treatment
    iv. Sadness about loss of health
    v. Anger
    vi. Loss of control
    vii. Poor sleep
    viii. Decreased appetite
    ix. Concentration problems
    x. Preoccupation with illness and death
    xi. Spiritual and existential concerns
    xii. Financial worries

(b) Clinicians should monitor, reevaluate, and offer continued support when distress is stable or decreased.

(c) If distress is persistent or increased, the guidelines for distress scores greater than 4 should be followed.

(2) The Canadian Association of Psychosocial Oncology has published algorithms for cancer-related distress, depression, and global anxiety. Mild distress is defined as a score less than 4 on the ESAS-r or Distress Thermometer, expected worries with effective coping skills, and symptoms that resolve gradually (Howell et al., 2015).

b) Moderate to severe distress
  (1) NCCN (2020) guidelines define moderate to severe distress as a score of 4 or more on a screening tool or clinical evidence of moderate to severe distress.
    (a) Clinicians should screen for family problems, practical problems, spiritual and religious concerns, physical problems, social issues, and emotional problems. High-risk patients with risk factors for distress should be assessed during periods of vulnerability.
    (b) Patients with unrelieved disease symptoms should be treated per disease-specific and supportive care guidelines. Referral for palliative care management should be considered.
    (c) Appropriate referrals should be made to social work, chaplaincy, and mental health professionals.
  (2) Canadian Association of Psychosocial Oncology guidelines define moderate distress and anxiety as a score of 4–6 on the ESAS-r or Distress Thermometer (Howell et al., 2015).
    (a) Clinicians should conduct a comprehensive assessment, focused on the most distressing symptoms, along with a focused assessment for depressive symptoms.
    (b) Clinicians can refer patients to psychosocial services as necessary. However, referral is required if any concerns about suicide or other risk factors are present.
  (3) Canadian Association of Psychosocial Oncology further defines severe distress and anxiety as a score of 7–9 on the ESAS-r or Distress Thermometer (Howell et al., 2015).
    (a) Clinicians must provide patients with a safe environment with one-on-one observation to reduce the risk of harm to self or others.
    (b) Urgent referrals to psychological services should be made for those that present with severe agitation, panic, delirium, or post-traumatic stress symptoms.
c) Interventions
  (1) Nurses routinely manage mild distress; however, measures can be taken for all patients, regardless of symptoms.
  (2) Grade 3 toxicities are associated with higher levels of distress, so interventions should address physical symptoms of disease and side effects of treatment (Hess et al., 2015).
    (a) ONS publishes resources for evidence-based interventions for physical symptoms, as well as anxiety (Cope et al., 2019).

  (b) The Pan-Canadian Oncology Symptom Triage and Remote Support team assembled clinical practice guidelines on appropriate practice for cancer-related symptoms, including anxiety and depression (Stacey et al., 2016).
(3) Nurses must acknowledge and validate a patient's distress (Smith, Loscalzo, Mayer, & Rosenstein, 2018).
  (a) Nurses can review distress scores with patients to ensure patient understanding of reporting and ensure scores are accurate.
  (b) Acknowledging and reviewing scores with patients lets them know that someone is paying attention and reinforces patient participation.
  (c) Assessing distress levels can help to normalize cancer distress screening and reduce stigma surrounding reporting adverse emotional reactions.
  (d) It is important for patients to be validated and know that distress is normal and expected.
(4) Effective communication is a method of support.
  (a) It is essential to clarify diagnosis, treatment options, and side effects; discuss advance care planning; and confirm patient understanding of disease and treatment options (NCCN, 2020).
  (b) Telephone contact with patients can be an effective tool to reduce anxiety.
  (c) In a study to assess the efficacy of telephone interventions by nurses to reduce anxiety scores of patients undergoing RT, anxiety was significantly reduced after telephone calls were conducted. Patients were asked about their feelings about treatment, provided with information on radiation, and given an opportunity to ask questions (Stamm, Girardon-Perlini, Pasqualoto, Beuter, & de Souza Magnago, 2018).
(5) Providing education can be a form of emotional support, as it can increase trust and communication, encourage hope, and provide patients with the control needed to deal with cancer and its treatment. Educating patients gives them the opportunity to make informed decisions.
  (a) RT can present many unknowns. Patients may fear that they will be radioactive or a danger to their loved ones. Education can lessen these fears and encourage trust (Fitch, 2018).
  (b) Nurses should review points of transition that may bring increased vulnerability to distress (NCCN, 2020).

(c) Nurses can provide information on signs and symptoms of worsening distress, as well as the need for additional support.

(d) Education should include nonpharmacologic strategies, such as exercise, mindfulness, and good nutrition. Clinicians can teach stress reduction strategies, such as relaxation and coping skills.

(e) Patients should be informed about support for issues such as transportation, medication assistance, and financial assistance.

(f) In a study of patients undergoing RT for prostate cancer, men who received nurse-led care reported fewer symptoms and felt satisfied and involved in their care (Long, 2017).

(g) Psychoeducational interventions conducted in group settings for patients and caregivers can provide information regarding treatments, symptoms, resources, and coping techniques. Booklets, videos, audio, computers, and interactive formats can be used (Cope et al., 2019).

(6) Cognitive and behavioral interventions can assist patients in identifying negative thoughts and beliefs that do not serve well-being and help them redirect energy in positive directions. Interactions that establish goals and develop coping skills increase the ability to solve problems and facilitate effective coping (Cope et al., 2019).

(a) Many patients will not want to see psychologists but will welcome psychosocial support from nurses. Nurses are perceived as approachable and trustworthy, giving them an opportunity to promote psychosocial care and interventions.

(b) Nurses should assess and strengthen coping strategies. Knowing and reinforcing helpful coping strategies can help patients deal with the distress that comes with diagnosis and treatment. Coping strategies can be especially useful in the event of disease progression or recurrence (Daem et al., 2019).

(c) Nurses should encourage activity as appropriate. Patients with cancer who have higher resilience are more physically active and have been shown to experience less psychosocial distress. Women with advanced breast cancer who were physically active for more than one hour a day at baseline had an increased likelihood of survival, compared to women who exercised less (Matzka et al., 2016; Palesh et al., 2018).

(d) Clinicians should offer support to patients who use tobacco. In a study aimed at examining differences in experience based on smoking status, current and former smokers had higher psychological distress (Choi et al., 2019).

i. Findings show a need for targeted interventions to reduce psychological distress and to promote adaptation in patients smoking at time of diagnosis.

ii. Nurses can provide support and resources, such as smoking cessation interventions, strategies to address nicotine cravings, emotion regulation, and adaptive coping skills.

iii. Assessing contributing factors for continued smoking can help to manage stress with a cancer diagnosis.

(7) Mindfulness-based stress reduction is a consciousness-based discipline based on Eastern philosophies. It focuses on being aware and present, as well as teaching the importance of feelings, thoughts, and sensations, to effectively deal with situations (Cope et al., 2019).

(8) Music therapy is the use of music to influence physiologic, psychological, and emotional functioning. It can increase relaxation. Music therapy has been shown to reduce anxiety during RT simulation and treatments (Cope et al., 2019; Hanedan Uslu, 2017; Rossetti et al., 2017).

(9) Art therapy has been shown to benefit patients receiving RT by reducing cancer-related anxiety and depression. Developmentally appropriate art activities can be of benefit to pediatric patients (Bultas, Saini, Marty, & Hendricks-Ferguson, 2017; Lee et al., 2017).

(10) Aromatherapy can promote emotional well-being, provide comfort, and alleviate certain physical symptoms (Allard & Katseres, 2018). In a study to assess the use of inhaled lavender in patients receiving RT, those using inhaled lavender showed a higher rate of improved distress scores than those who did not receive the intervention (Ohnikian, Dalcero, & Rutledge, 2016).

(11) Biofield therapy, such as healing touch and Reiki, are said to restore and balance energy field disturbances, encouraging the body's natural ability to heal.

(a) In a study to assess the use of healing touch and oncology massage on cancer pain, both modalities provided immediate pain relief (Gentile et al., 2018).

(b) A program evaluation on the use of Reiki for patients with cancer demonstrated a reduction of greater than 50% in symptoms of distress, anxiety, depression, pain, and fatigue in patients who received Reiki (Fleisher et al., 2014).

(12) Progressive muscle relaxation and guided imagery is the practice of alternately tensing and relaxing muscle groups in a sequence, often combined with guided imagery, using mental visualization and imagination relax (Cope et al., 2019).

(13) Spiritual interventions involve religious or existential aspects of care. Spiritual interventions have been shown to have effects on anxiety and depression. Nursing interventions that facilitate spiritual awareness and fulfill these needs can benefit spiritual and psychological outcomes (Oh & Kim, 2014).

(14) Clinicians should mobilize resources to ensure that social supports are in place for patients in need and follow up on the utilization and effectiveness of support. Support can include individual and caregiver support through internal and community resources, in-person and online support groups and conferences, internet resources, and help lines (NCCN, 2020).

(15) Support for professional development is important for nurses to feel confident in their abilities to help manage distress. Nurses should keep current and expand their competencies to address distress scores and provide evidence-based interventions (NCCN, 2020).

7. Documentation
   a) Screening data, referrals, provision of care, and follow-up should be documented in health records.
   b) Clinical outcomes measurement should include psychosocial assessment (NCCN, 2020).
   c) Data from screening programs can inform clinical care, patient education, program development, research, grant writing, and quality improvement (Smith et al., 2018).

8. Patient, caregiver, and family education: Numerous resources are available to help manage distress in patients with cancer. Clinicians should evaluate mobile applications and websites for accuracy and legitimacy prior to referring patients.
   a) NCCN guidelines
      (1) Clinicians: www.nccn.org/professionals/physician_gls/pdf/distress.pdf
      (2) Patients: www.nccn.org/patients/guidelines/distress/index.html
   b) American Cancer Society: www.cancer.org
   c) Alliance for Quality Psychosocial Care: www.wholecancerpatient.org; lists of psychosocial resources for patients, caregivers, and healthcare professionals in the United States, searchable by state
   d) Cancer Support Community
      (1) Cancer Support Helpline: 888-793-9355
      (2) Website: www.cancersupportcommunity.org
   e) Cancer*Care*: www.cancercare.org; online, telephone, and in-person support for patients
   f) ASCO Cancer.Net: www.cancer.net/coping-with-cancer
   g) Cancer Index : www.cancerindex.org/clinks5c.htm; information on resources available in Canada
   h) Twist Out Cancer: https://twistoutcancer.org
   i) ONS symptom interventions: www.ons.org/explore-resources?display=source&source=1506&ref=RO
   j) Pan-Canadian Oncology Symptom Triage and Remote Support clinical practice guidelines: https://ktcanada.ohri.ca/costars

References

Allard, M.E., & Katseres, J. (2018). Using essential oils to enhance nursing practice and for self-care. *Nurse Practitioner, 43*(5), 39–46. https://doi.org/10.1097/01.npr.0000531915.69268.8f

American College of Surgeons Commission on Cancer. (2019). *Optimal resources for cancer care: 2020 standards*. https://www.facs.org/quality-programs/cancer/coc/standards/2020

Anderson, J., Slade, A.N., McDonagh, P.R., Burton, W., & Fields, E.C. (2019). The long-lasting relationship of distress on radiation oncology-specific clinical outcomes. *Advances in Radiation Oncology, 4*, 354–361. https://doi.org/10.1016/j.adro.2018.11.001

Bodnarchuk, T., Stavrou, S., & Gantefoer, A. (2014). Screening for distress in the radiation therapy department: Distress incidence by sex, treatment intent, and ethnicity. *Journal of Medical Imaging and Radiation Sciences, 45*, 99–104. https://doi.org/10.1016/j.jmir.2014.02.001

Bultas, M.W., Saini, S.M., Marty, J., & Hendricks-Ferguson, V.L. (2017). Art making from the HEART: A pediatric case study about coping and distraction during oncology treatments. *Journal of Hospice and Palliative Nursing, 19*, 565–570. https://doi.org/10.1097/NJH.0000000000000389

Cancer Care Ontario. (2018). *Recommendations for the delivery of psychosocial oncology services in Ontario*. http://www.mhcwcancer.ca/Providers/whatsnew/Documents/CCO-PsychosocialOncologyReport.pdf

Carlson, L.E., Zelinski, E.L., Toivonen, K.I., Sundstrom, L., Jobin, C.T., Damaskos, P., & Zebrack, B. (2019). Prevalence of psychosocial distress in cancer patients across 55 North American cancer centers. *Journal of Psychosocial Oncology, 37*, 5–21. https://doi.org/10.1080/07347332.2018.1521490

Choi, S.H., Chan, R.R., & Lehto, R.H. (2019). Relationships between smoking status and psychological distress, optimism, and health environment perceptions at time of diagnosis of actual or suspected lung cancer. *Cancer Nursing, 42*, 156–163. https://doi.org/10.1097/ncc.0000000000000579

Cope, D.G., Coignet, H.C., Conley, S., Doherty, A., Drapek, L., Feldenzer, K., ... Walker, D.K. (2019, December 10). Symptom interventions: Anxiety. https://www.ons.org/pep/anxiety

Daem, M., Verbrugghe, M., Schrauwen, W., Leroux, S., Van Hecke, A., & Grypdonck, M. (2019). How interdisciplinary teamwork contributes to psychosocial cancer support. *Cancer Nursing, 42*, E11–E20. https://doi.org/10.1097/ncc.0000000000000588

Fitch, M.I. (2018). Programmatic approaches to psychosocial support. In N.J. Bush & L.M. Gorman (Eds.), *Psychosocial nursing care along the cancer continuum* (3rd ed., 509–530). Oncology Nursing Society.

Fleisher, K.A., Mackenzie, E.R., Frankel, E.S., Seluzicki, C., Casarett, D., & Mao, J.J. (2014). Integrative Reiki for cancer patients: A program evaluation. *Integrative Cancer Therapies, 13,* 62–67. https://doi.org/10.1177/1534735413503547

Gentile, D., Boselli, D., O'Neill, G., Yaguda, S., Bailey-Dorton, C., & Eaton, T.A. (2018). Cancer pain relief after healing touch and massage. *Journal of Alternative and Complementary Medicine, 24,* 968–973. https://doi.org/10.1089/acm.2018.0192

Habboush, Y., Shannon, R.P., Niazi, S.K., Hollant, L., Single, M., Gaines, K., ... Miller, R.C. (2017). Patient-reported distress and survival among patients receiving definitive radiation therapy. *Advances in Radiation Oncology, 2,* 211–219. https://doi.org/10.1016/j.adro.2017.03.004

Hanedan Uslu, G. (2017). Influence of music therapy on the state of anxiety during radiotherapy. *Turkish Journal of Oncology, 32,* 141–147. https://doi.org/10.5505/tjo.2017.1689

Hess, C.B., Singer, M., Khaku, A., Malinou, J., Juliano, J.J., Varlotto, J.M., ... Mackey, H.B. (2015). Optimal frequency of psychosocial distress screening in radiation oncology. *Journal of Oncology Practice, 11,* 298–302. https://doi.org/10.1200/jop.2014.003392

Holtzman, A.L., Pereira, D.B., & Yeung, A.R. (2018). Implementation of depression and anxiety screening in patients undergoing radiotherapy. *BMJ Open Quality, 7,* e000034. https://doi.org/10.1136/bmjoq-2017-000034

Howell, D., Keshavarz, H., Esplen, M.J., Hack, T., Hamel, M., Howes, J., ... Ali, M. (2015). *Pan-Canadian practice guideline: Screening, assessment and management of psychosocial distress, depression and anxiety in adults with cancer* (Version 2, 2015). Canadian Partnership Against Cancer. https://capo.ca/resources/Documents/Guidelines/3APAN-~1.PDF

Hui, D., & Bruera, E. (2017). The Edmonton Symptom Assessment System 25 years later: Past, present, and future developments. *Journal of Pain and Symptom Management, 53,* 630–643. https://doi.org/10.1016/j.jpainsymman.2016.10.370

Lazenby, M. (2014). The international endorsement of US distress screening and psychosocial guidelines in oncology: A model for dissemination. *Journal of the National Comprehensive Cancer Network, 12,* 221–227. https://doi.org/10.6004/jnccn.2014.0023

Lee, J., Choi, M.Y., Kim, Y.B., Sun, J., Park, E.J., Kim, J.H., ... Koom, W.S. (2017). Art therapy based on appreciation of famous paintings and its effect on distress among cancer patients. *Quality of Life Research, 26,* 707–715. https://doi.org/10.1007/s11136-016-1473-5

Long, K.-D.L. (2017). *Prostate cancer radiotherapy: Nursing interventions.* Joanna Briggs Institute Evidence-Based Practice Database.

Maggi, M., Gentilucci, A., Salciccia, S., Gatto, A., Gentile, V., Colarieti, A., ... Sciarra, A. (2019). Psychological impact of different primary treatments for prostate cancer: A critical analysis. *Andrologia, 51,* e13157. https://doi.org/10.1111/and.13157

Matzka, M., Mayer, H., Köck-Hódi, S., Moses-Passini, C., Dubey, C., Jahn, P., ... Eicher, M. (2016). Relationship between resilience, psychological distress and physical activity in cancer patients: A cross-sectional observation study. *PLOS ONE, 11,* e0154496. https://doi.org/10.1371/journal.pone.0154496

National Cancer Institute Cancer Therapy Evaluation Program. (2017). *Common terminology criteria for adverse events.* https://ctep.cancer.gov/protocolDevelopment/electronic_applications/docs/CTCAE_v5_Quick_Reference_8.5x11.pdf

National Cancer Institute Division of Cancer Control and Population Sciences. (2020). Patient Reported Outcomes Version of the Common Terminology for Adverse Events (PRO-CTCAE™). https://healthcaredelivery.cancer.gov/pro-ctcae

National Comprehensive Cancer Network. (2020). *NCCN Clinical Practice Guidelines in Oncology (NCCN Guidelines®): Distress management* [v.2.2020]. https://www.nccn.org/professionals/physician_gls/pdf/distress.pdf

Oh, P.-J., & Kim, S.H. (2014). The effects of spiritual interventions in patients with cancer: A meta-analysis. *Oncology Nursing Forum, 41,* E290–E301. https://doi.org/10.1188/14.ONF.E290-E301

Ohnikian, L., Dalcero, V., & Rutledge, J. (2016). The use of inhaled lavender for improving distress in radiation oncology patients. *International Journal of Radiation Oncology, 96*(Suppl. 2), E527–E528. https://doi.org/10.1016/j.ijrobp.2016.06.1950

Palesh, O., Kamen, C., Sharp, S., Golden, A., Neri, E., Spiegel, D., & Koopman, C. (2018). Physical activity and survival in women with advanced breast cancer. *Cancer Nursing, 41,* E31–E38. https://doi.org/10.1097/ncc.0000000000000525

Pirl, W.F., Fann, J.R., Greer, J.A., Braun, I., Deshields, T., Fulcher, C., ... Bardwell, W. (2014). Recommendations for the implementation of distress screening programs in cancer centers: Report from the American Psychosocial Oncology Society (APOS), Association of Oncology Social Work (AOSW), and Oncology Nursing Society (ONS) joint task force. *Cancer, 120,* 2946–2954. https://doi.org/10.1002/cncr.28750

Rossetti, A., Chadha, M., Torres, B.N., Lee, J.K., Hylton, D., Loewy, J.V., & Harrison, L.B. (2017). The impact of music therapy on anxiety in cancer patients undergoing simulation for radiation therapy. *International Journal of Radiation Oncology, Biology, Physics, 99,* 103–110. https://doi.org/10.1016/j.ijrobp.2017.05.003

Sheldon, L.K., Blonquist, T.M., Hilaire, D.M., Hong, F., & Berry, D.L. (2015). Patient cues and symptoms of psychosocial distress: What predicts assessment and treatment of distress by oncology clinicians? *Psycho-Oncology, 24,* 1020–1027. https://doi.org/10.1002/pon.3689

Smith, S.K., Loscalzo, M., Mayer, C., & Rosenstein, D.L. (2018). Best practices in oncology distress management: Beyond the screen. *American Society of Clinical Oncology Educational Book, 38,* 813–821. https://doi.org/10.1200/edbk_201307

Stacey, D., Ballantyne, B., Carley, M., Cummings, G., Green, E., Howell, D., ... Truant, T. (2016). *Remote symptom practice guides for adults on cancer treatments: Of the Pan-Canadian Oncology Symptom Triage and Remote Support (COSTaRS) team.* University of Ottawa School of Nursing, Ottawa Hospital Research Institute. https://ktcanada.ohri.ca/costars/Research/docs/COSTaRS_Pocket_Guide_March2016.pdf

Stamm, B., Girardon-Perlini, N.M.O., Pasqualoto, A.S., Beuter, M., & de Souza Magnago, T.S.B. (2018). Telephone intervention for anxiety management in oncology patients: A randomized clinical trial. *Acta Paulista de Enfermagem, 31,* 137–143. https://doi.org/10.1590/1982-0194201800021

University of Texas MD Anderson Cancer Center. (n.d.). The MD Anderson Symptom Inventory. https://www.mdanderson.org/research/departments-labs-institutes/departments-divisions/symptom-research/symptom-assessment-tools/md-anderson-symptom-inventory.html

E. Sexual function and dysfunction

1. Definition

   a) Depending on cause and condition, definitions of sexual dysfunction are broad.

   b) McCabe, Sharlip, Atalla, et al. (2016) wrote one of the most definitive compendia of definitions that serves as an important reference applicable to cancer.

   c) Definitions were based on *International Classification of Diseases* (10th edition) by the World Health Organization and *Diagnostic and Statistical Manual of Mental Disorders* (5th edition) by the American Psychiatric Association.

   d) Definitions are listed for the following gender-agnostic disorders and dysfunctions (McCabe, Sharlip, Atalla, et al., 2016).

   (1) Lack or loss of sexual desire

   (2) Sexual aversion

   (3) Lack of sexual enjoyment

   (4) Failure of sexual response

   (5) Orgasmic dysfunction

e) Definitions are listed for the following gender-specific dysfunctions (McCabe, Sharlip, Atalla, et al., 2016).
 (1) Female sexual interest/arousal disorder
 (2) Female orgasmic disorder
 (3) Genito-pelvic pain-penetration disorder
 (4) Male hypoactive sexual desire disorder
 (5) Erectile disorder
 (6) Premature (early) ejaculation
 (7) Delayed ejaculation
2. Pathophysiology
 a) General: Three phases of the sexual response cycle—desire, arousal, and orgasm—can be affected by cancer and cancer therapies (Krebs, 2014).
 (1) Sexual desire is an interest in sexual activity and is affected by factors such as anger, pain, body image, disease processes, and medications.
 (2) Sexual arousal is the perception of being "turned on" sexually. Subsequent to arousal, vasodilation and vasocongestion occur, leading to penile erection and vaginal lubrication. Impairment may result from surgery that cuts through the associated vessels or RT, which may cause sclerosis of vessels necessary for these functions.
 (3) Orgasm is the peak of sexual pleasure, usually characterized by strong feelings of pleasure and a series of involuntary contractions of the muscles of the genitals.
 (a) It is mediated by the sympathetic nervous system.
 (b) Therapies such as surgery, RT, and chemotherapy may have an adverse effect on the nerves involved in this portion of the sexual response cycle (Krebs, 2014).
 b) Acute effects on sexual function
 (1) Even with modern RT techniques, approximately 85% of all patients who receive RT will experience moderate to severe acute skin reactions within 90 days of treatment. Acute effects that interfere with sexual function include erythema, pain blistering, erosions, and, in some cases, ulceration (Bray, Simmons, Wolfson, & Nouri, 2016).
 (2) Cancer treatments may cause direct sexual organ toxicities or systemic toxicities, such as cognitive dysfunction, that may decrease libido and function. However, chemotherapy agents, particularly alkylating agents, and cancer-related pelvic surgeries, can cause high and permanent rates of gonadal damage (Torrealday, Kodaman, & Pal, 2017).
 (3) Even low doses of RT may be associated with premature ovarian insufficiency in premenopausal women or decreased testicular function in men.

 c) Late and long-term effects on sexual function
 (1) Late effects from cancer and cancer treatment may occur months or years after cancer treatment (NCI, n.d.).
 (2) Long-term effects are side effects that develop during treatment and do not resolve by treatment completion (i.e., are ongoing).
 (3) RT effects are progressive and may become symptomatic after a latent period, or a continuous progression may occur as acute edema, mucosal and submucosal inflammation, persistent ulceration, necrosis, and fibrosis (Jensen & Froeding, 2015).
 (4) Radiation-induced fibrosis of the skin and subcutaneous tissues may develop at any RT treatment site and may cause limited range of motion, contractures, and pain, all of which interfere with sexual function (Bray et al., 2016).
 (5) RT-related narrowing and obliteration of pelvic vasculature contributes to vaginal fibrosis and diminished lubrication.
 (6) Radiation-induced erectile dysfunction is multifactorial. Although literature is sparse in this topic, current mechanisms posited to result in radiation-induced erectile dysfunction in prostate cancer include damage to neuronal, vascular, and muscular processes that support male erection (Mahmood et al., 2016).
 (7) Men may experience dyspareunia immediately after ejaculation.
3. Incidence and prevalence
 a) Sociodemographic and cultural considerations
 (1) Sex
 (a) In general, studies of the U.S. population show that sexual dysfunction is more prevalent in women than men.
 (b) It is estimated that the rate of female sexual dysfunction in the general population is 40%–50%, with desire and arousal being the most commonly experienced types (McCabe, Sharlip, Lewis, et al., 2016).
 (c) Male sexual dysfunction tends to be a single type of dysfunction that worsens with age, with premature ejaculation (8%–30%, irrespective of age) and erectile dysfunction (20%–40% in men 60–69 years old) being the most common (McCabe, Sharlip, Lewis, et al., 2016).
 (2) Race and culture
 (a) Difference in sexual dysfunction by race and culture may exist, but data are sparse in cancer populations, especially related to RT.
 (b) General population studies suggest that, although African American women may

have lower quality of life after cancer therapies, they have higher sexual function (Addis et al., 2006; Hughes, Rostant, & Pelon, 2015). This is consistent with findings from pilot research studies examining women treated with pelvic RT for cervical and endometrial cancers (Bai et al., 2019).

    (c) Additional studies are needed to better understand the mechanism of these differences.

(3) Sexual and gender minority populations

    (a) A 2017 poll found that approximately 4.5% of U.S. adults identify as lesbian, gay, bisexual, transgender, queer, or questioning (LGBTQ). Individuals may identify as more than one of these distinctions (Newport, 2018).

    (b) Oncology specialists may be limited in their knowledge of LGBTQ health and cancer needs (Schabath et al., 2019).

    (c) Many members of the LGBTQ community have experienced unwelcoming healthcare experiences and may not present for routine cancer screening and medical care (Jabson & Kamen, 2016; Puechl, Russell, & Gray, 2019.)

    (d) When compared to their heterosexual counterparts, LGBTQ individuals have higher rates of health risk behaviors and are disproportionately affected by cancer, including anal, breast, cervical, colorectal, endometrial, lung, and prostate cancer diagnoses (Jackson, Agénor, Johnson, Austin, & Kawachi, 2016; Quinn et al., 2015).

    (e) Varying domains of sexual function and satisfaction have been shown to differ by sexual orientation in noncancer populations, highlighting the importance of culturally sensitive clinical assessment of sexual function that focuses on behaviors rather than labels (Flynn, Lin, & Weinfurt, 2017).

    (f) Limited research has examined the potential differences between sexual function based on sexual orientation and gender identity in cancer, particularly in studies focused on effects of RT.

b) General cancer considerations

(1) Sexual dysfunction does not occur in all patients with cancer (Hendren et al., 2005).

(2) Approximately 45% of patients treated for cancer experience altered sexual function that may decrease their quality of life and affect their significant other (Baker, Denniston, Smith, & West, 2005; Galbraith, Arechiga, Ramirez, & Pedro, 2005; Kadmon, Ganz, Rom, & Woloski-Wruble, 2008; Kendirci, Bejma, & Hellstrom, 2006).

(3) Women treated with pelvic irradiation for cancer, irrespective of modality, have a higher risk of sexual dysfunction when compared to healthy, age-matched controls and patients who receive surgery alone (Jensen & Froeding, 2015).

c) Breast cancer

(1) Most women with breast cancer treated with RT are also treated with other therapies, making it difficult to discern radiation-specific sexual side effects. However, women treated with RT for breast cancer have been found to have lower sexual well-being when compared to those without RT at three years after completion of therapy (Albornoz et al., 2014).

(2) Women treated with EBRT in combination with lumpectomy for breast cancer may experience disruption in sexual activity, most likely a result of effects of skin discomfort and fatigue (Krebs, 2014).

    (a) RT fibrosis most commonly occurs in patients with breast cancer treated in combination with surgery.

    (b) Side effects that influence sexual function include pain; skin retraction, induration, and color alterations; skin necrosis and ulcerations; restricted arm and neck movement; and lymphedema (Bray et al., 2016; Streicher & Simon, 2018).

(3) A literature review suggested that women with breast cancer who are treated with chemotherapy are at higher risk for sexual dysfunction than those who did not receive chemotherapy (Gilbert, Ussher, & Perz, 2010).

    (a) Chemotherapy is associated with dysfunctions related to arousal, lubrication, orgasm, and dyspareunia.

    (b) Radiation to the breast is associated with feeling medically "invaded" but is less likely to be associated with decreased sexual desire, as compared to chemotherapy.

(4) A systematic review identified that men with breast cancer often experience hot flashes and sexual dysfunction secondary to endocrine therapy. Researchers posited that these patients may have unique psychosocial responses to their diagnosis (Ruddy & Winer, 2013). However, little literature exists specific to experiences of men with breast cancer.

d) Human papillomavirus (HPV)-related head and neck cancer

(1) Between 1988 and 2004, HPV-negative, smoking-associated oropharyngeal cancer

declined by 50%, but HPV-positive cases, particularly in the oropharynx, have increased by 225% (NCI, 2020). This increase is largely thought to be attributable to sexual practice behavior changes that increase risk of HPV infection and HPV-related cancers (Rettig, Kiess, & Fakhry, 2015).

(2) A study that compared relationship outcomes between HPV-positive versus negative patients at diagnosis and at six-month follow-up found significant declines in the frequency of vaginal and oral sex in patients, regardless of HPV status. HPV-positive patients and their partners also reported guilt related to the cancer (Taberna et al., 2017).

(3) A small study of unmet needs in 44 partners of patients with head and neck cancer found that the highest unmet needs existed in the relationship domain, with 18.6% of partners indicating that they needed help addressing problems with their sex lives (Giuliani et al., 2017).

e) Vulvar cancer

(1) The rapid cell turnover of the vaginal and vulvar epithelium increases sensitivity to RT effects.

(2) Because vulvar cancers are relatively rare, few studies have been conducted on post-treatment sexual effects.

(3) One study reported that 50% of women with vulvar cancer had similar sexual function, as compared to pretreatment, and 42% had worse sexual function (Hazewinkel et al., 2012).

(4) Of note, treatment-related variables had limited influence on long-term sexual function, whereas a positive influence was found in those who had a partner, had good physical well-being, and were optimistic (Hazewinkel et al., 2012).

f) Cervical cancer

(1) Compared to surgery, RT generally has been associated with higher rates of sexual dysfunction in women treated for cervical carcinoma, but research has been sparse (Pieterse et al., 2013; Schover, Fife, & Gershenson, 1989).

(a) Vaginal stenosis has been reported in up to 88% of women treated with intracavitary RT for cervical cancer (Bruner et al., 1993; Mirabeau-Beale et al., 2015).

i. A wide range of incidence of vaginal stenosis has been reported, likely the result of a lack of a rigorous measurement system.

ii. Many studies use physician assessment of the vagina using the CTCAE grading system, with grade 1 defined as shortening or narrowing not interfering with function, grade 2 as interfering with function, and grade 3 as complete vaginal obliteration, not surgically correctable (NCI CTEP, 2017).

iii. This grading involves no objective measure nor patient-reported input on the interference with function.

iv. Physician inter-rater reliability of subjective items on the CTCAE have been documented as low, and physician report of assessments related to sexual function are well documented to differ substantially from patient self-report (Bruner, 2007; Damast et al., 2019).

(b) Further complicating clinical understanding of the true incidence and potential severity of vaginal stenosis is the inference that different RT doses and modalities have a differential effect on the vagina.

(c) Women with early-stage cervical cancer treated with RT plus surgery, versus surgery alone, experienced more sexual symptoms, particularly a higher prevalence of vaginal narrowing and shortening (35% vs. 13% at 12 months; 33% vs. 17% at 24 months) (Pieterse et al., 2013).

i. One early report indicated that surgery accounted for most of the risk of vaginal stenosis, as well as insufficient lubrication and reduced vaginal elasticity, when compared to RT (Bergmark, Åvall-Lundqvist, Dickman, Henningsohn, & Steineck, 1999).

ii. Another longitudinal study of women treated with RT found worse self-reported scores across domains of sexual functioning (sexual interest, satisfaction, lubrication, dyspareunia) compared to aged-matched controls (Jensen et al., 2003).

(d) Women aged 50 years and older may be at greater risk for vaginal stenosis (Brand, Bull, & Cakir, 2006).

(2) Surgical transposition of the ovaries has been attempted with varying degrees of success in protecting against premature ovarian insufficiency from pelvic irradiation in premenopausal women treated for cervical cancer.

(a) The ovaries (one or both) can be transposed outside the radiation field; however, success rates are higher in women younger than 35 years and are lower for women older than 35 years. In addition, rates of ovarian survival after transposition differ by therapy, including brachytherapy (63.6%–100%), EBRT (20%–100%), and concomitant chemoradiation (0%–69.2%) (Hoekman et al., 2019).

(b) Reasons for ovarian failure after transposition include scatter radiation and decreased blood flow to the ovaries due to bending of the vessels as a result of the transposition.

    i. At least one study recommended an optimal RT dose-volume limit of 7.5 Gy to less than 26% of the ovary to preserve ovarian function (Du & Qu, 2017).

    ii. Ovarian transposition is not without its own side effects and may include symptomatic ovarian cysts, reported in 0%–34% of women, and rare but possible ovarian metastases in transposed ovaries (Hoekman et al., 2018).

    iii. Whether transposing the ovaries prior to radiation is a safe and effective procedure remains an ongoing issue.

g) Endometrial cancer

(1) Limited research has been conducted to report the degree of sexual dysfunction after RT for endometrial cancer, and published research has consisted of small samples with mixed results.

(2) One study found that 81% of participants with early-stage endometrial cancer treated with adjuvant brachytherapy met criteria for sexual dysfunction (Damast et al., 2012).

(3) Another study reported that 68.6% of Chinese women with endometrial cancer experienced female sexual dysfunction, with older age and RT increasing odds of dysfunction (H. Gao, Xiao, Bai, & Zhang, 2017).

(4) A recent review of patient-reported outcomes among women with endometrial cancer found that sexual function outcomes varied by age and time since diagnosis. Additionally, physical activity was associated with improved sexual interest (Shisler et al., 2018).

(5) Another study of 395 Australian women with endometrial cancer found that surgery alone for endometrial cancer was associated with positive sexual well-being versus any adjuvant treatment, including RT (Rowlands, Lee, Beesley, & Webb, 2014).

(6) In a small study of Turkish women following endometrial cancer treatment, sexual enjoyment was poorer in women who had received EBRT versus those who had not (Karabuga et al., 2015).

(7) A small study found that the vaginal changes experienced by surgically treated women who had brachytherapy and were sexually active did not differ from the comparison group of women who did not receive brachytherapy (Quick, Seamon, Abdel-Rasoul, Salani, & Martin, 2012).

(8) According to one study, before RT, patients have demonstrated greater sexual dysfunction compared to healthy controls. By six months after RT, patients' sexual dysfunction was similar to controls (Bai et al., 2019).

h) Prostate cancer

(1) Reduced or absent semen production can occur with RT to the prostate.

(2) Although most studies have focused on erectile function, many other sexual side effects have been reported after RT for prostate cancer.

(3) In a systematic review, incidence of erectile dysfunction after RT for prostate cancer was 43%, compared to 86% after androgen deprivation therapy and 58% after radical prostatectomy (Wilt et al., 2008).

(4) One recent study of patient-reported sexual outcomes after RT demonstrated that 44% of men had decreased intensity of orgasms; 42% had penile length loss of more than 1 cm; 27% experienced decreased sensitivity in the penis; 15% experienced orgasm-related pain; 12% had curvature of the penis; 11% had anejaculation; and 4% reported anorgasmia (Frey et al., 2017).

i) Bladder cancer

(1) Very little research has been conducted on sexual dysfunction after treatment for bladder cancer.

(2) In a study of sexual function in men treated with RT for bladder cancer, 71% felt their sex life was worse after RT, and 56% were concerned about the deterioration (Little & Howard, 1998).

(3) A study of distressing symptoms after radical RT versus radical cystectomy for bladder cancer identified lower prevalence of sexual dysfunction in the patients treated with RT compared to the patients treated with radical cystectomy. However, of the 14 men treated with RT in this study, 36% were dissatisfied with their sex life, 75% had erectile dysfunction, and 43% lost ability to ejaculate. All of the 10 women treated with RT in this study had little to no sexual interest and were not sexually active during the study period (Henningsohn, Wijkström, Dickman, Bergmark, & Steineck, 2002).

(4) A recent systematic review of women who had received radical cystectomies for bladder cancer found inconsistent sexual function findings across a limited number of studies (Smith et al., 2017).

j) Testicular cancer

(1) A prospective Dutch study of short-term effects of orchiectomy and RT in 161 patients with testicular seminoma evaluated at pretreatment, three months, and six months found that 48% of men had fertility concerns. The study also found that 61% reported body changes after orchiectomy, which was associated with decreased sexual interest, pleasure, and erectile dysfunction. Additionally, although 91% of men remained sexually active, 45% reported that treatment had affected their sex lives in a negative way (Wortel, Alemayehu, & Incrocci, 2015).

(2) Another small study of men (mean age of 29 years) who presented with erectile dysfunction after treatment for testicular cancer found relatively normal erectile hemodynamics across cancer treatment types, indicating adrenaline-mediated dysfunction as the likely cause (Tal, Stember, Logmanieh, Narus, & Mulhall, 2014).

k) Anorectal cancer

(1) The ability to have an orgasm after multimodal therapy (preoperative RT followed by surgery) has been reported to be absent in 50% of both male and female patients. Orgasm may be absent in 45%–57% of patients after treatment for locally advanced primary or recurrent rectal cancer (Mannaerts et al., 2001).

(2) Prevalence rates for vaginal stenosis in women treated with intracavitary RT for anal canal cancer, across all grades of stenosis, have been reported as high as 87.6% (Mirabeau-Beale et al., 2015).

(3) In long-term follow-up, patients with anal carcinoma who were treated with RT were found to have acceptable overall quality-of-life scores but poor sexual function scores (Yerramilli et al., 2019).

(4) Preoperative RT and sphincter-preserving resection can lead to fecal urgency, which has been associated with lower sexual function (Ozgen et al., 2015).

(5) Men who have sex with men have an increased risk for anorectal cancer (Frisch, Smith, Grulich, & Johansen, 2003; Goldstone, Winkler, Ufford, Alt, & Palefsky, 2001).

l) Penile cancer

(1) The risk of male dyspareunia, or penile pain when having intercourse either vaginally or rectally, increases with treatments such as EBRT, which may cause thinning of penile skin, or laser treatment (Nishimoto & Mark, 2010; Windahl, Skeppner, Andersson, & Fugl-Meyer, 2004).

(2) For organ preservation, interstitial brachytherapy is preferred over partial penectomy in early-stage cases but may be associated with acute skin toxicity (Sharma et al., 2014).

m) Lung cancer

(1) Few studies have addressed sexuality as it relates to lung cancer.

(2) Patients with lung cancer may experience problems with sexual function throughout treatment, influenced by mood and social support, but limited findings to date do not support a difference between chemotherapy versus chemotherapy plus RT groups (Shell, Carolan, Zhang, & Meneses, 2008).

n) Hematologic malignancy

(1) TBI can induce gonadal dysfunction and tissue damage (e.g., sensitivity, scarring, atrophy).

(2) TBI has been negatively associated with sexual satisfaction and sexual function domains in men with hematologic malignancies receiving hematopoietic stem cell transplants and may lead to scarring in penile blood vessels (Wong et al., 2013; Yi & Syrjala, 2009).

4. Assessment

a) Baseline assessment

(1) Given the high prevalence of sexual dysfunction in the general population without a cancer diagnosis, it is imperative to obtain baseline assessments of sexual function prior to treatment to provide anticipatory guidance and to determine when to begin sexual rehabilitation in the treatment trajectory.

(2) Clinicians treating patients with pretreatment sexual dysfunction should begin discussions of the need for sexual counseling as soon as dysfunction is identified.

(3) Patients without preexisting dysfunction should be informed of the potential for treatment-related sexual dysfunction prior to beginning therapy and assured of management and referral strategies available as needed.

b) Risk factors: Pretreatment sexual activity, including presence of sexual dysfunction before diagnosis, may portend higher risks of post-treatment dysfunction.

c) Sexual history: For a comprehensive sexual history assessment tool, see Krebs (2014) and Lindau et al. (2016). Sexual history should include the following elements.

(1) Past medical history, including reproductive history, menopausal status for women, history of sexually transmitted infections, cancer, cancer treatments, and comorbidities

(2) Mental health status, including depression and anxiety and associated therapy or medical treatments

(3) Health behaviors, including use of alcohol, drug abuse, and sleep and exercise habits

(4) Cultural, racial, and ethnic background

    (a) Sexual values and norms vary widely among cultures, races, and ethnicities; however, well-designed studies on the topic are few (Meston & Ahrold, 2010).

    (b) Current literature suggests that Caucasian women with gynecologic cancer report more sexual dysfunction after cancer therapies when compared to African American women (Bai et al., 2019).

    (c) No difference in sexual functioning between African American, Caucasian, or Latino men was found in a large study of treatments of localized prostate cancer, as long as age and comorbidities were controlled (Tyson et al., 2017).

(5) History of sexual activity, including sexual orientation, age at first intercourse, number of partners, and problems with desire, arousal, or orgasm

(6) History of sexual abuse

    (a) An estimated 289,312 females and 46,121 males age 12 or older are forcibly raped or sexually assaulted in the United States each year (Morgan & Kena, 2018).

    (b) It has been estimated that 16% of women treated for gynecologic malignancies have been sexually abused (Bergmark et al., 1999).

    (c) Lifetime experience of sexual assault has also been associated with lower rates of cancer screening recommendations (Alcalá, Keim-Malpass, & Mitchell, 2018).

(7) Partner status, partner health, relationship quality, and sexual and intimacy issues: Couples who are mutually responsive, attend to each other's needs, and talk openly about their stress are more able to engage in effective sexual coping (Zunkel, 2002).

(8) Frequency of sexual activity over the past six months

(9) Satisfaction with sexual ability and frequency

(10) Medications that may interfere with sexual function (e.g., antihypertensives, antidepressants)

(11) Female issues

    (a) Dyspareunia

    (b) Vaginal dryness

    (c) Vaginal bleeding or spotting with and without intercourse

    (d) Vulvar or vaginal pain

(12) Male issues

    (a) Erectile ability

    (b) Retrograde ejaculation

    (c) Dyspareunia

    (d) Change in penile length or curvature

d) Physical examination

  (1) Female

    (a) Examination of skin over vulva and around anus for breakdown, lesions, fissures, or inflammation

    (b) Examination for scarring and vaginal stenosis

    (c) Examination for vaginal discharge or bleeding

  (2) Male

    (a) Examination of skin over the penis and scrotum for breakdown, lesions, or inflammation

    (b) Examination of anal area for breakdown, fissures, or lesions

5. Management of acute sexual affects

  a) Psychological

    (1) Prepare the patient and partner (as desired by patient) for possible treatment effects on sexual function. Culturally sensitive discussions should occur at the time of diagnosis and along the survivorship trajectory.

    (2) ASCO recommends offering psychosocial and psychosexual counseling to all patients with cancer. Dyad interventions may be especially efficacious for women with intimacy and body image concerns (Carter et al., 2018).

    (3) Sexual dysfunction may cause distress, which should be addressed in addition to the medical issues influencing dysfunction.

      (a) NCCN (2020) distress management guidelines recommend recognition, monitoring, documentation, and prompt treatment of distress as standard of care across the cancer trajectory and in all care settings.

      (b) Specific distress screening and treatment recommendations are available via the NCCN website (see Patient, caregiver, and family education).

  b) Behavioral

    (1) Clinicians should discuss safety and the importance of avoiding sex when patients' blood counts may put them at risk for infection and bleeding. They can encourage alternative forms of intimacy as the patient desires during these times (American Cancer Society, 2020).

    (2) Clinicians should encourage communication between patients and partners concerning fears about continued sexual function.

    (3) Clinicians should discuss the need for patients to preemptively manage symptoms (e.g., pain) before engaging in sexual activity.

c) Medical
(1) Identifying and treating any medical factors that may be influencing and contributing to sexual dysfunction is essential.
(2) Female-specific interventions
  (a) A review evaluating treatments for physical aspects of sexual dysfunction in women after pelvic RT found that topical estrogens and benzydamine have the strongest evidence of treatment benefit for acute radiation-induced vaginal changes (Denton & Maher, 2003).
  (b) Evidence also supports the use of vaginal dilators and intercourse to maintain vaginal patency (Denton & Maher, 2003).
  (c) The use of dilators should begin as soon as the patient can tolerate it to prevent adhesions (fibrous tissue) from forming.
    i. A patient can begin dilation during RT if it is tolerable.
    ii. A condom filled with cotton balls and tied at the bottom, used with ample lubricant, may make the experience more tolerable.
  (d) A systematic review found that flibanserin, a serotonin receptor agonist, has been demonstrated as safe and effective in trials used to treat hypoactive sexual disorder in women without cancer (Z. Gao, Yang, Yu, & Cui, 2015). ASCO lists this medication as an option for premenopausal women with cancer but notes that results have not yet been replicated in women with cancer or women on endocrine therapy (Carter et al., 2018).
  (e) Another systematic review that included any type of interventions for sexual dysfunction in women following cancer treatment yielded inconsistent findings and noted methodologic gaps preventing recommendations of particular interventions. The authors also highlighted a need for additional studies examining interventions in malignancies other than breast and gynecologic cancers (Candy, Jones, Vickerstaff, Tookman, & King, 2016).
(3) Male-specific interventions
  (a) Men may experience temporary pain with ejaculation, reduced semen, and irritated skin.
  (b) Penile implants, injectable medications, and vacuum devices introduced before or early after cancer treatment may benefit sexual response (i.e., erectile function) in some men. Vacuum devices used daily may prevent penile length loss (Carter et al., 2018).

  (c) Testosterone levels should be monitored and treated as indicated, even in men who do not have hormonally associated cancers.
6. Management of late and long-term sexual effects
a) Psychological
  (1) NCCN (2020) guidelines recommend recognition, monitoring, documentation, and prompt treatment of distress as standard of care across the cancer trajectory and in all care settings. Specific distress screening and treatment recommendations are available via the NCCN website (see Patient, caregiver, and family education).
  (2) Clinicians should support patients and their partners with concerns regarding sexual function.
  (3) Clinicians should refer patients with history of sexual abuse or marital problems to a social worker, family therapist, or sex counselor.
b) Behavioral
  (1) Clinicians should encourage communication between patients and partners concerning feelings regarding continued sexual function.
  (2) Clinicians can teach proper positioning for continued sexual activity to help prevent discomfort, depending on the therapy or problem (see Patient, caregiver, and family education).
  (3) Kegel exercises may decrease anxiety and discomfort and can lower urinary tract symptoms (Carter et al., 2018).
c) Medical
  (1) Female-specific interventions
    (a) Women need to continue to perform vaginal dilation with sexual intercourse, a vaginal dilator, or a vaginal vibrator at least three times per week for life to prevent vaginal shortening and narrowing.
    (b) Vaginal dryness can be addressed with water- and silicone-based lubricants for sexual activity and moisturizers for comfort (Huffman, Hartenbach, Carter, Rash, & Kushner, 2016).
    (c) Low-dose vaginal estrogen, lidocaine, dehydroepiandrosterone, and ospemifene may be appropriate in some cases for vaginal and vulvar atrophy symptoms (Carter et al., 2018). Risks and benefits of vaginal estrogen should be considered in women who have hormone-positive breast cancer.
      i. Limited data exists to support use of vaginal dehydroepiandrosterone in women with cancer or women on endocrine therapy.
      ii. Ospemifene is indicated for postmenopausal women without current

breast cancer or a history of breast cancer.

(d) For vasomotor symptoms, ASCO recommends hormone therapy as the most effective short-term intervention for vasomotor symptoms (e.g., hot flashes) (Carter et al., 2018).

i. Therapy should be evaluated at age 51 years and intermittently for indication of continued use.

ii. Systemic hormone therapy is contraindicated with hormone-sensitive breast cancer.

iii. Estrogen alone (oral, transdermal, or vaginal) is the preferred therapy for women after hysterectomy if not contraindicated.

iv. Alternative medical management options include paroxetine, venlafaxine, gabapentin, and clonidine. Paroxetine and fluoxetine are contraindicated in women with breast cancer taking tamoxifen. When discontinuing clonidine, the dose should be tapered to avoid hypertensive response.

v. Cognitive behavioral therapy and clinical hypnosis may reduce symptoms.

(e) For more complex issues, patients should be referred to appropriate providers, including the following.

i. Primary care

ii. Gynecology

iii. Urology (urinary incontinence)

iv. Colorectal surgery (fecal incontinence)

v. Psychology (individual and/or couples counseling)

vi. Sexual health specialist (e.g., pelvic floor physiotherapy)

(2) Male-specific interventions

(a) Approximately 40%–60% of men will experience erectile dysfunction after receiving radiation to the pelvic area, but impotence may develop over time (American Cancer Society, 2020).

(b) Phosphodiesterase type 5 (PDE5) inhibitors (e.g., sildenafil, tadalafil, vardenafil) should be first-line treatment for erectile dysfunction in men (Carter et al., 2018; Yafi, Sharlip, & Becher, 2018).

i. A systematic review found that PDE5 inhibitors are an effective treatment for erectile dysfunction following RT for prostate cancer (Miles et al., 2007).

ii. However, following treatment with concurrent androgen deprivation therapy and RT, less than 25% of men treated with sildenafil had improvement in erectile function (Bruner et al., 2011).

iii. Primary contraindications of PDE5 inhibitors include heart failure; uncontrolled hypertension; current use of nitrates (e.g., nitroglycerin); current use of cimetidine, ketoconazole, itraconazole, erythromycin, or ritonavir; moderate to severe renal insufficiency or end-stage renal disease; or severe hepatic impairment.

iv. The most common side effects are headache, flushing, dyspepsia, and nasal congestion. The risk of at least one side effect is approximately 30% for all PDE5 inhibitors. Most side effects are mild, and approximately 4% of men discontinue the drug because of adverse events (Tsertsvadze et al., 2009; Yafi et al., 2018).

v. PDE5 inhibitors improve genital vasocongestion but have shown little or no improvement in female self-report of sexual function; however, this has not been tested in women with sexual dysfunction related to cancer therapies (Chivers & Rosen, 2010).

(c) Vasomotor symptoms (e.g., hot flashes) may be medically managed with venlafaxine, medroxyprogesterone acetate, cyproterone acetate, and gabapentin. Cognitive behavioral and integrative therapies that have been shown to provide clinical benefit to women may also be offered to men (e.g., psychosocial counseling, acupuncture, slow breathing, hypnosis) (Carter et al., 2018).

(d) For more complex issues, clinicians should refer patients to appropriate providers, including the following.

i. Primary care

ii. Urology (urinary stress incontinence)

iii. Psychology (individual and/or couples counseling)

iv. Sexual health specialist

v. Physical therapy (exercises)

(e) For men who are not candidates for or who do not respond to PDE5 inhibitors, other potential treatments to improve erectile function include penile implants, injectable medications, or vacuum devices.

Positive patient-reported outcomes have been reported with some erectile aids (Dess et al., 2018).
  (3) Fertility issues after RT are beyond the scope of this section. See IV.F. Fertility for more detailed information.
7. Patient, caregiver, and family education
  a) Education should be tailored to address individuals' diagnoses and symptom experiences.
  b) Clinicians should counsel patients and partners on the potential impact of pelvic irradiation on sexual function, with the expected outcome being the ability of patients to verbalize an understanding of sexual dysfunction and discuss issues with their nurse or physician (Schover, 1999).
  c) Clinicians should teach patients and partners methods to minimize sexual discomfort or dysfunction.
    (1) The expected outcome is that patients and partners will comply with methods to minimize sexual dysfunction.
    (2) See Krebs (2014) for more in-depth instructions.
  d) Female patients should be taught to use a vaginal dilator to prevent vaginal stenosis after an intracavitary implant (Krebs, 2014).
    (1) Because maintaining vaginal health has been documented as a motivator for dilator adherence in women with endometrial cancer, patient education should include this emphasis (Hanlon et al., 2018).
    (2) The expected outcome of education is that the patient will maintain vaginal patency.
  e) Male patients should be taught to use erectile aids, with the expected outcome of patients maintaining erectile function.
  f) Discussion of when to resume intercourse and masturbation after therapy should occur with patients and partners. The expected outcome is that patients will not act too soon and risk incurring pain or performance anxiety, but also that they will not wait too long and build up a fear of returning to normal function.
  g) Clinicians should review patients' blood counts with them, teach them about cytopenias, and discuss safe ways to share intimacy with their partners during these times. The expected outcomes are that the patient will maintain safety while achieving desired intimacy.
  h) Patients and partners should be taught to report new or continued sexual dysfunction to a nurse or physician.
  i) Clinicians should assure patients that, if needed, they can be referred to specialists in sexual dysfunction, such as a urologist, psychologist, pelvic floor physical therapist, or sex therapist if physical, psychological, or relationship problems persist.

  j) Early web-based interventions for sexual dysfunction in patients with cancer are emerging.
    (1) A longitudinal, web-based intervention for sexual dysfunction in women with breast and gynecologic cancers and their partners showed positive results (Schover et al., 2013).
    (2) A psychoeducational, web-based clinical trial for sexual dysfunction in young patients with cancer is currently being tested (Lampic, Ljungman, Micaux Obol, Eriksson, & Wettergren, 2019).
8. Additional resources
  a) American Cancer Society
    (1) Fertility and sexual concerns: www.cancer.org/treatment/treatments-and-side-effects/physical-side-effects/fertility-and-sexual-side-effects.html
    (2) Managing female sexual problems related to cancer: www.cancer.org/treatment/treatments-and-side-effects/physical-side-effects/fertility-and-sexual-side-effects/sexuality-for-women-with-cancer/problems.html
    (3)
  b) LGBTQ health
    (1) Centers for Disease Control and Prevention (CDC): www.cdc.gov/lgbthealth/index.htm
    (2) National LGBT Cancer Network: https://cancer-network.org
    (3) National LGBTQIA+ Health Education Center: https://www.lgbthealtheducation.org
  c) NCCN guidelines and clinical resources, including sexual function, distress management, and sexual function during survivorship: https://www.nccn.org/professionals/physician_gls/default.aspx
  d) ASCO guidelines for sexual problems in people with cancer: https://www.asco.org/research-guidelines/quality-guidelines/guidelines/patient-and-survivor-care
  e) Alterowitz, R., & Alterowitz, B. (1999). *The Lovin' Ain't Over: The Couple's Guide to Better Sex After Prostate Disease*. Health Education Literary Publisher.
  f) Canadian Association of Nurses in Oncology. (2017). *Care for women after radiation to the pelvis.* https://cdn.ymaws.com/www.cano-acio.ca/resource/resmgr/Resources/Vaginal_Dilator_Booklet_LONG.pdf
  g) Katz, A. (2007). *Breaking the Silence on Cancer and Sexuality: A Handbook for Healthcare Providers.* Oncology Nursing Society.
  h) Katz, A. (2009). *Woman Cancer Sex.* Hygeia Media.
  i) Katz, A. (2010). *Man Cancer Sex.* Hygeia Media.
  j) Shaw, G.M. (2011). *Having Children After Cancer: How to Make Informed Choices Before and After Treatment and Build the Family of Your Dreams.* Celestial Arts.

References

Addis, I.B., Van Den Eeden, S.K., Wassel-Fyr, C.L., Vittinghoff, E., Brown, J.S., & Thom, D.H. (2006). Sexual activity and function in middle-aged and older women. *Obstetrics and Gynecology, 107,* 755–764. https://doi.org/10.1097/01.aog.0000202398.27428.e2

Albornoz, C.R., Matros, E., McCarthy, C.M., Klassen, A., Cano, S.J., Alderman, A.K., ... Pusic, A.L. (2014). Implant breast reconstruction and radiation: A multicenter analysis of long-term health-related quality of life and satisfaction. *Annals of Surgical Oncology, 21,* 2159–2164. https://doi.org/10.1245/s10434-014-3483-2

Alcalá, H.E., Keim-Malpass, J., & Mitchell, E.M. (2018). Sexual assault and cancer screening among men and women. *Journal of Interpersonal Violence.* Advance online publication. https://doi.org/10.1177/0886260518812797

American Cancer Society. (2020, February 1). How cancer and cancer treatment can affect sexuality. https://www.cancer.org/treatment/treatments-and-side-effects/physical-side-effects/fertility-and-sexual-side-effects/how-cancer-affects-sexuality.html

Bai, J., Belcher, S.M., Meador, R., Daniel, G., Shelton, J., Patel, P., ... Bruner, D.W. (2019). Comparisons of depression, sexual function, and quality of life between women with gynecological cancers and race-matched healthy controls. *Cancer Nursing, 44,* 116–124. https://doi.org/10.1097/NCC.0000000000000744

Baker, F., Denniston, M., Smith, T., & West, M.M. (2005). Adult cancer survivors: How are they faring? *Cancer, 104*(Suppl. 11), 2565–2576. https://doi.org/10.1002/cncr.21488

Bergmark, K., Åvall-Lundqvist, E., Dickman, P.W., Henningsohn, L., & Steineck, G. (1999). Vaginal changes and sexuality in women with a history of cervical cancer. *New England Journal of Medicine, 340,* 1383–1389. https://doi.org/10.1056/nejm199905063401802

Brand, A.H., Bull, C.A., & Cakir, B. (2006). Vaginal stenosis in patients treated with radiotherapy for carcinoma of the cervix. *International Journal of Gynecological Cancer, 16,* 288–293. https://doi.org/10.1111/j.1525-1438.2006.00348.x

Bray, F.N., Simmons, B.J., Wolfson, A.H., & Nouri, K. (2016). Acute and chronic cutaneous reactions to ionizing radiation therapy. *Dermatology and Therapy, 6,* 185–206. https://doi.org/10.1007/s13555-016-0120-y

Bruner, D.W. (2007). Should patient-reported outcomes be mandatory for toxicity reporting in cancer clinical trials? *Journal of Clinical Oncology, 25,* 5345–5347. https://doi.org/10.1200/jco.2007.13.3330

Bruner, D.W., James, J.L., Bryan, C.J., Pisansky, T.M., Rotman, M., Corbett, T., ... Berk, L. (2011). Randomized, double-blinded, placebo-controlled crossover trial of treating erectile dysfunction with sildenafil after radiotherapy and short-term androgen deprivation therapy: Results of RTOG 0215. *Journal of Sexual Medicine, 8,* 1228–1238. https://doi.org/10.1111/j.1743-6109.2010.02164.x

Bruner, D.W., Lanciano, R., Keegan, M., Corn, B., Martin, E., & Hanks, G. (1993). Vaginal stenosis and sexual function following intracavitary radiation for the treatment of cervical and endometrial carcinoma. *International Journal of Radiation Oncology, Biology, Physics, 27,* 825–830. https://doi.org/10.1016/0360-3016(93)90455-5

Candy, B., Jones, L., Vickerstaff, V., Tookman, A., & King, M. (2016). Interventions for sexual dysfunction following treatments for cancer in women. *Cochrane Database of Systematic Reviews, 2016*(2). https://doi.org/10.1002/14651858.cd005540.pub3

Carter, J., Lacchetti, C., Andersen, B.L., Barton, D.L., Bolte, S., Damast, S., ... Rowland, J.H. (2018). Interventions to address sexual problems in people with cancer: American Society of Clinical Oncology clinical practice guideline adaptation of Cancer Care Ontario Guideline. *Journal of Clinical Oncology, 36,* 492–511. https://doi.org/10.1200/jco.2017.75.8995

Chivers, M.L., & Rosen, R.C. (2010). Phosphodiesterase type 5 inhibitors and female sexual response: Faulty protocols or paradigms? *Journal of Sexual Medicine, 7,* 858–872. https://doi.org/10.1111/j.1743-6109.2009.01599.x

Damast, S., Alektiar, K.M., Goldfarb, S., Eaton, A., Patil, S., Mosenkis, J., ... Basch, E. (2012). Sexual functioning among endometrial cancer patients treated with adjuvant high-dose-rate intra-vaginal radiation therapy. *International Journal of Radiation Oncology, Biology, Physics, 84,* e187–e193. https://doi.org/10.1016/j.ijrobp.2012.03.030

Damast, S., Jeffery, D.D., Son, C.H., Hasan, Y., Carter, J., Lindau, S.T., & Jhingran, A. (2019). Literature review of vaginal stenosis and dilator use in radiation oncology. *Practical Radiation Oncology, 9,* 479–491. https://doi.org/10.1016/j.prro.2019.07.001

Denton, A.S., & Maher, J. (2003). Interventions for the physical aspects of sexual dysfunction in women following pelvic radiotherapy. *Cochrane Database of Systematic Reviews, 2003*(1). https://doi.org/10.1002/14651858.cd003750

Dess, R.T., Devasia, T.P., Aghdam, N., Jackson, W.C., Soni, P.D., Smith, C.P., ... Spratt, D.E. (2018). Patient-reported sexual aid utilization and efficacy after radiation therapy for localized prostate cancer. *International Journal of Radiation Oncology, Biology, Physics, 101,* 376–386. https://doi.org/10.1016/j.ijrobp.2018.01.055

Du, Z., & Qu, H. (2017). The relationship between ovarian function and ovarian limited dose in radiotherapy postoperation of ovarian transposition in young patients with cervical cancer. *Cancer Medicine, 6,* 508–515. https://doi.org/10.1002/cam4.924

Flynn, K.E., Lin, L., & Weinfurt, K.P. (2017). Sexual function and satisfaction among heterosexual and sexual minority U.S. adults: A cross-sectional survey. *PLOS ONE, 12,* e0174981. https://doi.org/10.1371/journal.pone.0174981

Frey, A., Pedersen, C., Lindberg, H., Bisbjerg, R., Sønksen, J., & Fode, M. (2017). Prevalence and predicting factors for commonly neglected sexual side effects to external-beam radiation therapy for prostate cancer. *Journal of Sexual Medicine, 14,* 558–565. https://doi.org/10.1016/j.jsxm.2017.01.015

Frisch, M., Smith, E., Grulich, A., & Johansen, C. (2003). Cancer in a population-based cohort of men and women in registered homosexual partnerships. *American Journal of Epidemiology, 157,* 966–972. https://doi.org/10.1093/aje/kwg067

Galbraith, M.E., Arechiga, A., Ramirez, J., & Pedro, L.W. (2005). Prostate cancer survivors' and partners' self-reports of health-related quality of life, treatment symptoms, and marital satisfaction 2.5–5.5 years after treatment. *Oncology Nursing Forum, 32,* E30–E41. https://doi.org/10.1188/05.ONF.E30-E41

Gao, H., Xiao, M., Bai, H., & Zhang, Z. (2017). Sexual function and quality of life among patients with endometrial cancer after surgery. *International Journal of Gynecological Cancer, 27,* 608–612. https://doi.org/10.1097/igc.0000000000000905

Gao, Z., Yang, D., Yu, L., & Cui, Y. (2015). Efficacy and safety of flibanserin in women with hypoactive sexual desire disorder: A systematic review and meta-analysis. *Journal of Sexual Medicine, 12,* 2095–2104. https://doi.org/10.1111/jsm.13037

Gilbert, E., Ussher, J.M., & Perz, J. (2010). Sexuality after breast cancer: A review. *Maturitas, 66,* 397–407. https://doi.org/10.1016/j.maturitas.2010.03.027

Giuliani, M., Milne, R., McQuestion, M., Sampson, L., Le, L.W., Jones, J., ... Ringash, J. (2017). Partner's survivorship care needs: An analysis in head and neck cancer patients. *Oral Oncology, 71,* 113–121. https://doi.org/10.1016/j.oraloncology.2017.06.011

Goldstone, S.E., Winkler, B., Ufford, L.J., Alt, E., & Palefsky, J.M. (2001). High prevalence of anal squamous intraepithelial lesions and squamous-cell carcinoma in men who have sex with men as seen in a surgical practice. *Diseases of the Colon and Rectum, 44,* 690–698. https://doi.org/10.1007/bf02234568

Hanlon, A., Small, W., Jr., Strauss, J., Lin, L.L., Hanisch, L., Huang, L., ... Bruner, D.W. (2018). Dilator use after vaginal brachytherapy for endometrial cancer: A randomized feasibility and adherence study. *Cancer Nursing, 41,* 200–209. https://doi.org/10.1097/ncc.0000000000000500

Hazewinkel, M.H., Laan, E.T.M., Sprangers, M.A.G., Fons, G., Burger, M.P.M., & Roovers, J.-P.W.R. (2012). Long-term sexual function in survivors of vulvar cancer: A cross-sectional study. *Gynecologic Oncology, 126,* 87–92. https://doi.org/10.1016/j.ygyno.2012.04.015

Hendren, S.K., O'Connor, B.I., Liu, M., Asano, T., Cohen, Z., Swallow, C.J., ... McLeod, R.S. (2005). Prevalence of male and female sexual dysfunction is high following surgery for rectal cancer. *Annals of Surgery, 242,* 212–223. https://doi.org/10.1097/01.sla.0000171299.43954.ce

Henningsohn, L., Wijkström, H., Dickman, P.W., Bergmark, K., & Steineck, G. (2002). Distressful symptoms after radical radiotherapy for urinary bladder cancer. *Radiotherapy and Oncology, 62,* 215–225. https://doi.org/10.1016/s0167-8140(01)00455-8

Hoekman, E.J., Broeders, E.A.B.J., Louwe, L.A., Nout, R.A., Jansen, F.W., & de Kroon, C.D. (2019). Ovarian function after ovarian transposition and additional pelvic radiotherapy: A systematic review. *European Journal of Surgical Oncology, 45,* 1328–1340. https://doi.org/10.1016/j.ejso.2019.02.017

Hoekman, E.J., Knoester, D., Peters, A.A.W., Jansen, F.W., de Kroon, C.D., & Hilders, C.G.J.M. (2018). Ovarian survival after pelvic radiation: Transposition until the age of 35 years. *Archives of Gynecology and Obstetrics, 298,* 1001–1007. https://doi.org/10.1007/s00404-018-4883-5

Huffman, L.B., Hartenbach, E.M., Carter, J., Rash, J.K., & Kushner, D.M. (2016). Maintaining sexual health throughout gynecologic cancer survivorship: A comprehensive review and clinical guide. *Gynecologic Oncology, 140,* 359–368. https://doi.org/10.1016/j.ygyno.2015.11.010

Hughes, A.K., Rostant, O.S., & Pelon, S. (2015). Sexual problems among older women by age and race. *Journal of Women's Health, 24,* 663–669. https://doi.org/10.1089/jwh.2014.5010

Jabson, J.M., & Kamen, C.S. (2016). Sexual minority cancer survivors' satisfaction with care. *Journal of Psychosocial Oncology, 34,* 28–38. https://doi.org/10.1080/07347332.2015.1118717

Jackson, C.L., Agénor, M., Johnson, D.A., Austin, S.B., & Kawachi, I. (2016). Sexual orientation identity disparities in health behaviors, outcomes, and services use among men and women in the United States: A cross-sectional study. *BMC Public Health, 16,* 807. https://doi.org/10.1186/s12889-016-3467-1

Jensen, P.T., & Froeding, L.P. (2015). Pelvic radiotherapy and sexual function in women. *Translational Andrology and Urology, 4,* 186–205. https://doi.org/10.3978/j.issn.2223-4683.2015.04.06

Jensen, P.T., Groenvold, M., Klee, M.C., Thranov, I., Petersen, M.A., & Machin, D. (2003). Longitudinal study of sexual function and vaginal changes after radiotherapy for cervical cancer. *International Journal of Radiation Oncology, Biology, Physics, 56,* 937–949. https://doi.org/10.1016/s0360-3016(03)00362-6

Kadmon, I., Ganz, F.D., Rom, M., & Woloski-Wruble, A.C. (2008). Social, marital, and sexual adjustment of Israeli men whose wives were diagnosed with breast cancer. *Oncology Nursing Forum, 35,* 131–135. https://doi.org/10.1188/08.ONF.131-135

Karabuga, H., Gultekin, M., Tulunay, G., Yuce, K., Ayhan, A., Yuce, D., & Yildiz, F. (2015). Assessing the quality of life in patients with endometrial cancer treated with adjuvant radiotherapy. *International Journal of Gynecological Cancer, 25,* 1526–1533. https://doi.org/10.1097/igc.0000000000000509

Kendirci, M., Bejma, J., & Hellstrom, W.J.G. (2006). Update on erectile dysfunction in prostate cancer patients. *Current Opinion in Urology, 16,* 186–195. https://doi.org/10.1097/01.mou.0000193407.05285.d8

Krebs, L.U. (2014). Altered body image and sexual health. In C.H. Yarbro, D. Wujcik, & B.H. Gobel (Eds.), *Cancer symptom management* (4th ed., pp. 507–540). Jones and Bartlett Learning.

Lampic, C., Ljungman, L., Micaux Obol, C., Eriksson, L.E., & Wettergren, L. (2019). A web-based psycho-educational intervention (Fex-Can) targeting sexual dysfunction and fertility-related distress in young adults with cancer: Study protocol of a randomized controlled trial. *BMC Cancer, 19,* 344. https://doi.org/10.1186/s12885-019-5518-3

Lindau, S.T., Abramsohn, E.M., Baron, S.R., Florendo, J., Haefner, H.K., Jhingran, A., ... Streicher, L. (2016). Physical examination of the female cancer patient with sexual concerns: What oncologists and patients should expect from consultation with a specialist. *CA: A Cancer Journal for Clinicians, 66,* 241–263. https://doi.org/10.3322/caac.21337

Little, F.A., & Howard, G.C.W. (1998). Sexual function following radical radiotherapy for bladder cancer. *Radiotherapy and Oncology, 49,* 157–161. https://doi.org/10.1016/s0167-8140(98)00109-1

Mahmood, J., Shamah, A.A., Creed, T.M., Pavlovic, R., Matsui, H., Kimura, M., ... Vujaskovic, Z. (2016). Radiation-induced erectile dysfunction: Recent advances and future directions. *Advances in Radiation Oncology, 1,* 161–169. https://doi.org/10.1016/j.adro.2016.05.003

Mannaerts, G.H.H., Schijven, M.P., Hendrikx, A., Martijn, H., Rutten, H.J.T., & Wiggers, T. (2001). Urologic and sexual morbidity following multimodality treatment for locally advanced primary and locally recurrent rectal cancer. *European Journal of Surgical Oncology, 27,* 265–272. https://doi.org/10.1053/ejso.2000.1099

McCabe, M.P., Sharlip, I.D., Atalla, E., Balon, R., Fisher, A.D., Laumann, E., ... Segraves, R.T. (2016). Definitions of sexual dysfunctions in women and men: A consensus statement from the Fourth International Consultation on Sexual Medicine 2015. *Journal of Sexual Medicine, 13,* 135–143. https://doi.org/10.1016/j.jsxm.2015.12.019

McCabe, M.P., Sharlip, I.D., Lewis, R., Atalla, E., Balon, R., Fisher, A.D., ... Segraves, R.T. (2016). Incidence and prevalence of sexual dysfunction in women and men: A consensus statement from the Fourth International Consultation on Sexual Medicine 2015. *Journal of Sexual Medicine, 13,* 144–152. https://doi.org/10.1016/j.jsxm.2015.12.034

Meston, C.M., & Ahrold, T. (2010). Ethnic, gender, and acculturation influences on sexual behaviors. *Archives of Sexual Behavior, 39,* 179–189. https://doi.org/10.1007/s10508-008-9415-0

Miles, C., Candy, B., Jones, L., Williams, R., Tookman, A., & King, M. (2007). Interventions for sexual dysfunction following treatments for cancer. *Cochrane Database of Systematic Reviews, 2007*(4). https://doi.org/10.1002/14651858.cd005540.pub2

Mirabeau-Beale, K., Hong, T.S., Niemierko, A., Ancukiewicz, M., Blaszkowsky, L.S., Crowley, E.M., ... Wo, J.Y. (2015). Clinical and treatment factors associated with vaginal stenosis after definitive chemoradiation for anal canal cancer. *Practical Radiation Oncology, 5*(3), e113–e118. https://doi.org/10.1016/j.prro.2014.09.003

Morgan, R.E., & Kena, G. (2018, October). Criminal victimization, 2016: Revised. https://www.bjs.gov/index.cfm?ty=pbdetail&iid=6427

National Cancer Institute. (n.d.). Late effect. In *NCI dictionary of cancer terms.* https://www.cancer.gov/publications/dictionaries/cancer-terms/def/late-effect

National Cancer Institute. (2020, January 27). Oropharyngeal cancer treatment (adult) (PDQ®) [Health professional version]. https://www.cancer.gov/types/head-and-neck/hp/adult/oropharyngeal-treatment-pdq#_397_toc

National Cancer Institute Cancer Therapy Evaluation Program. (2017). Common terminology criteria for adverse events [v.5.0]. https://ctep.cancer.gov/protocolDevelopment/electronic_applications/docs/CTCAE_v5_Quick_Reference_8.5x11.pdf

National Comprehensive Cancer Network. (2020). *NCCN Clinical Practice Guidelines in Oncology (NCCN Guidelines®): Distress management* [v.2.2020]. https://www.nccn.org/professionals/physician_gls/pdf/distress.pdf

Newport, F. (2018, May 22). *In U.S., estimate of LGBT population rises to 4.5%* [Press release]. https://news.gallup.com/poll/234863/estimate-lgbt-population-rises.aspx

Nishimoto, P.W., & Mark, D.D. (2010). Altered sexuality patterns. In C.G. Brown (Ed.), *A guide to oncology symptom management* (pp. 423–455). Oncology Nursing Society.

Ozgen, Z., Ozden, S., Atasoy, B.M., Ozyurt, H., Gencosmanoglu, R., & Imeryuz, N. (2015). Long-term effects of neoadjuvant chemoradiotherapy followed by sphincter-preserving resection on anal sphincter function in relation to quality of life among locally advanced rectal cancer patients: A cross-sectional analysis. *Radiation Oncology, 10,* 168. https://doi.org/10.1186/s13014-015-0479-4

Pieterse, Q.D., Kenter, G.G., Maas, C.P., de Kroon, C.D., Creutzberg, C.L., Trimbos, J.B.M.Z., & Ter Kuile, M.M. (2013). Self-reported sexual, bowel and bladder function in cervical cancer patients following different treatment modalities: Longitudinal prospective cohort study. *International Journal of Gynecological Cancer, 23,* 1717–1725. https://doi.org/10.1097/igc.0b013e3182a80a65

Puechl, A.M., Russell, K., & Gray, B.A. (2019). Care and cancer screening of the transgender population. *Journal of Women's Health, 28,* 761–768. https://doi.org/10.1089/jwh.2018.6945

Quick, A.M., Seamon, L.G., Abdel-Rasoul, M., Salani, R., & Martin, D. (2012). Sexual function after intracavitary vaginal brachytherapy for early-stage endometrial carcinoma. *International Journal of Gynecological Cancer, 22,* 703–708. https://doi.org/10.1097/igc.0b013e3182481611

Quinn, G.P., Sanchez, J.A., Sutton, S.K., Vadaparampil, S.T., Nguyen, G.T., Green, B.L., ... Schabath, M.B. (2015). Cancer and lesbian, gay, bisexual, transgender/transsexual, and queer/questioning (LGBTQ) populations. *CA: A Cancer Journal for Clinicians, 65,* 384–400. https://doi.org/10.3322/caac.21288

Rettig, E., Kiess, A.P., & Fakhry, C. (2015). The role of sexual behavior in head and neck cancer: Implications for prevention and therapy. *Expert Review of Anticancer Therapy, 15,* 35–49. https://doi.org/10.1586/14737140.2015.957189

Rowlands, I.J., Lee, C., Beesley, V.L., & Webb, P.M. (2014). Predictors of sexual well-being after endometrial cancer: Results of a national self-report survey. *Supportive Care in Cancer, 22,* 2715–2723. https://doi.org/10.1007/s00520-014-2263-7

Ruddy, K.J., & Winer, E.P. (2013). Male breast cancer: Risk factors, biology, diagnosis, treatment, and survivorship. *Annals of Oncology, 24,* 1434–1443. https://doi.org/10.1093/annonc/mdt025

Schabath, M.B., Blackburn, C.A., Sutter, M.E., Kanetsky, P.A., Vadaparampil, S.T., Simmons, V.N., ... Quinn, G.P. (2019). National survey of oncologists at National Cancer Institute-designated comprehensive cancer centers: Attitudes, knowledge, and practice behaviors about LGBTQ patients with cancer. *Journal of Clinical Oncology, 37,* 547–558. https://doi.org/10.1200/jco.18.00551

Schover, L.R. (1999). Counseling cancer patients about changes in sexual function. *Oncology, 13,* 1585–1591.

Schover, L.R., Fife, M., & Gershenson, D.M. (1989). Sexual dysfunction and treatment for early stage cervical cancer. *Cancer, 63,* 204–212. https://doi.org/10.1002/1097-0142(19890101)63:1<204::aid-cncr2820630133>3.0.co;2-u

Schover, L.R., Yuan, Y., Fellman, B.M., Odensky, E., Lewis, P.E., & Martinetti, P. (2013). Efficacy trial of an Internet-based intervention for cancer-related female sexual dysfunction. *Journal of the National Comprehensive Cancer Network, 11,* 1389–1397. https://doi.org/10.6004/jnccn.2013.0162

Sharma, D.N., Joshi, N.P., Gandhi, A.K., Haresh, K.P., Gupta, S., Julka, P.K., & Rath, G.K. (2014). High-dose-rate interstitial brachytherapy for T1–T2-stage penile carcinoma: Short-term results. *Brachytherapy, 13,* 481–487. https://doi.org/10.1016/j.brachy.2014.06.003

Shell, J.A., Carolan, M., Zhang, Y., & Meneses, K.D. (2008). The longitudinal effects of cancer treatment on sexuality in individuals with lung cancer. *Oncology Nursing Forum, 35,* 73–79. https://doi.org/10.1188/08.ONF.73-79

Shisler, R., Sinnott, J.A., Wang, V., Hebert, C., Salani, R., & Felix, A.S. (2018). Life after endometrial cancer: A systematic review of patient-reported outcomes. *Gynecologic Oncology, 148,* 403–413. https://doi.org/10.1016/j.ygyno.2017.11.007

Smith, A.B., Crowell, K., Woods, M.E., Wallen, E.M., Pruthi, R.S., Nielsen, M.E., & Lee, C.T. (2017). Functional outcomes following radical cystectomy in women with bladder cancer: A systematic review. *European Urology Focus, 3,* 136–143. https://doi.org/10.1016/j.euf.2016.05.005

Streicher, L., & Simon, J.A. (2018). Sexual function post-breast cancer. In W.J. Gradishar (Ed.), *Optimizing breast cancer management, volume 173* (pp. 167–189). https://doi.org/10.1007/978-3-319-70197-4_11

Taberna, M., Inglehart, R.C., Pickard, R.K.L., Fakhry, C., Agrawal, A., Katz, M.L., & Gillison, M.L. (2017). Significant changes in sexual behavior after a diagnosis of human papillomavirus-positive and human papillomavirus-negative oral cancer. *Cancer, 123,* 1156–1165. https://doi.org/10.1002/cncr.30564

Tal, R., Stember, D.S., Logmanieh, N., Narus, J., & Mulhall, J.P. (2014). Erectile dysfunction in men treated for testicular cancer. *BJU International, 113,* 907–910. https://doi.org/10.1111/bju.12331

Torrealday, S., Kodaman, P., & Pal, L. (2017). Premature ovarian insufficiency—An update on recent advances in understanding and management. *F1000Research, 6,* 2069. https://doi.org/10.12688/f1000research.11948.1

Tsertsvadze, A., Fink, H.A., Yazdi, F., MacDonald, R., Bella, A.J., Ansari, M.T., ... Wilt, T.J. (2009). Oral phosphodiesterase-5 inhibitors and hormonal treatments for erectile dysfunction: A systematic review and meta-analysis. *Annals of Internal Medicine, 151,* 650–661. https://doi.org/10.7326/0003-4819-151-9-200911030-00150

Tyson, M.D., Alvarez, J., Koyama, T., Hoffman, K.E., Resnick, M.J., Wu, X.-C., ... Barocas, D.A. (2017). Racial variation in patient-reported outcomes following treatment for localized prostate cancer: Results from the CEASAR Study. *European Urology, 72,* 307–314. https://doi.org/10.1016/j.eururo.2016.10.036

Wilt, T.J., MacDonald, R., Rutks, I., Shamliyan, T.A., Taylor, B.C., & Kane, R.L. (2008). Systematic review: Comparative effectiveness and harms of treatments for clinically localized prostate cancer. *Annals of Internal Medicine, 148,* 435–448. https://doi.org/10.7326/0003-4819-148-6-200803180-00209

Windahl, T., Skeppner, E., Andersson, S.-O., & Fugl-Meyer, K.S. (2004). Sexual function and satisfaction in men after laser treatment for penile carcinoma. *Journal of Urology, 172,* 648–651. https://doi.org/10.1097/01.ju.0000132891.68094.87

Wong, F.L., Francisco, L., Togawa, K., Kim, H., Bosworth, A., Atencio, L., ... Bhatia, S. (2013). Longitudinal trajectory of sexual functioning after hematopoietic cell transplantation: Impact of chronic graft-versus-host disease and total body irradiation. *Blood, 122,* 3973–3981. https://doi.org/10.1182/blood-2013-05-499806

Wortel, R.C., Alemayehu, W.G., & Incrocci, L. (2015). Orchiectomy and radiotherapy for stage I–II testicular seminoma: A prospective evaluation of short-term effects on body image and sexual function. *Journal of Sexual Medicine, 12,* 210–218. https://doi.org/10.1111/jsm.12739

Yafi, F.A., Sharlip, I.D., & Becher, E.F. (2018). Update on the safety of phosphodiesterase type 5 inhibitors for the treatment of erectile dysfunction. *Sexual Medicine Reviews, 6,* 242–252. https://doi.org/10.1016/j.sxmr.2017.08.001

Yerramilli, D., Drapek, L., Nipp, R.D., Horick, N., Moran, S.M.C., Noé, B., ... Wo, J. (2019). Sexual function, quality of life, and mood after radiation therapy in patients with anal cancer. *Journal of Gastrointestinal Cancer, 51,* 204–210. https://doi.org/10.1007/s12029-019-00233-w

Yi, J.C., & Syrjala, K.L. (2009). Sexuality after hematopoietic stem cell transplantation. *Cancer Journal, 15,* 57–64. https://doi.org/10.1097/ppo.0b013e318198c758

Zunkel, G. (2002). Relational coping processes: Couples' response to a diagnosis of early stage breast cancer. *Journal of Psychosocial Oncology, 20,* 39–55. https://doi.org/10.1300/J077v20n04_03

F. Fertility

1. Definition of oncofertility: Oncofertility is an interdisciplinary field to address the issue of gonadotoxicity (temporary or permanent damage to the ovaries or testes) associated with cancer therapies and to facilitate fertility preservation, if possible, prior to treatment exposure (Ronn & Holzer, 2013).
2. Clinical practice guidelines (Oktay et al., 2018)
   a) ASCO has published clinical practice guidelines to provide guidance on fertility preservation options for individuals with cancer.
   b) ASCO recommends that healthcare providers caring for adult and pediatric patients with cancer should address the possibility of infertility as early as possible prior to initiation of cancer treatment.
3. Risk of infertility
   a) Effect of RT on female fertility
      (1) RT is a common treatment proposed to adolescent and young adult (AYA) women (younger than 45 years old) in diseases such as, but not limited to, sarcomas, CNS tumors, gyneco-

logic cancers, lower gastrointestinal cancers, and hematologic malignancies (Marci et al., 2018).

    (a) Pelvic RT can be recommended in the case of cervical cancer, endometrial cancer, bladder cancer sarcomas, and lower gastrointestinal cancers (Marci et al., 2018).

    (b) Brachytherapy is often recommended in the case of cervical cancer (Biedka, Kuźba-Kryszak, Nowikiewicz, & Żyromska, 2016).

    (c) Craniospinal irradiation is used to treat CNS cancers (Marci et al., 2018).

    (d) TBI is often required before hematopoietic stem cell transplantation (HSCT) in hematologic malignancies (Marci et al., 2018).

(2) The effect of cancer treatment on female fertility is dependent on multiple factors, including tumor pathology, location, and presence or location of metastatic disease. Patient age and pretreatment ovarian function are also important factors (Hendershot et al., 2016; Marci et al., 2018; Rodriguez-Wallberg & Oktay, 2014).

    (a) Women have a nonrenewable pool of ovarian primordial follicles, the number of which declines through atresia and apoptosis over time. Approximately 1–2 million oocytes are present at birth, 30,000–50,000 at puberty, and 1,000 at 51 years (average age of menopause) (Marci et al., 2018; Wo & Viswanathan, 2009).

    (b) Genetics, lifestyle, and medical history (e.g., endometriosis, ovarian surgery, previous cancer diagnosis or treatment) can affect pretreatment ovarian function (Marci et al., 2018).

(3) Direct or indirect scatter radiation can affect reproductive organs. Damage to ovarian function can be progressive and irreversible, resulting in follicular atrophy and reduced ovarian reserve, early menopause, and infertility (Hendershot et al., 2016; Marci et al., 2018).

(4) Patients who require uterine irradiation may develop impaired uterine blood flow and damage to the endometrium, which can result in fibrosis, reduced uterine lining elasticity, and small uterine volumes, potentially leading to poor pregnancy outcomes (Hendershot et al., 2016).

(5) Craniospinal RT may also affect fertility as a result of its effect on the HPA axis, which is extremely vulnerable to radiation. Damage to the HPA axis can result in gonadotropin deficiency, which may lead to reduced pregnancies, amenorrhea (loss of menses), and infertility (Marci et al., 2018).

(6) It is common for patients to require multimodal treatments, which may have a synergistic effect on the disease, but also can further affect fertility (Loren et al., 2013).

(7) A female fertility risk chart and calculator are tools available through the Livestrong Foundation (n.d.-b) that can provide a general understanding of potential treatment risks but should not be used in place of a consultation with a healthcare professional.

b) Effect of RT on male fertility

(1) RT is a treatment option used for a number of cancers in male AYAs, including testicular tumors, hematologic malignancies, lower gastrointestinal cancers, bladder cancer, and soft tissue sarcomas (Hosni, Abd-Alkhalek, Foda, & Awad, 2016).

    (a) Direct RT to male reproductive organs is used in rare situations, such as with testicular tumors, testicular relapse of acute lymphoblastic leukemia, and testicular exposure in TBI in preparation for HSCT (Hosni et al., 2016).

    (b) Pelvic RT can be used in the treatment of lower gastrointestinal cancer, bladder cancer, pelvic lymph nodes (lymphoma and seminoma), adjacent soft tissue tumors (sarcoma of the thigh), and adjacent bony cancers (Hosni et al., 2016).

    (c) Cranial irradiation is used to treat pituitary tumors, CNS tumors, and head and neck cancer, as well as for prophylaxis of intracranial disease in patients with acute lymphoblastic leukemia (Hosni et al., 2016).

(2) Similar to female patients, the effect of cancer treatment on male fertility is dependent on tumor pathology and location, as well as presence or locations of metastases. However, in contrast to female patients, age is less significant in male patients, as regeneration of new spermatozoa is ongoing (Hendershot et al., 2016).

(3) Spermatogonia give rise to spermatocytes. Spermatogonia are very sensitive to radiation. As long as spermatogonia are not depleted and a population of germ cells remain, regeneration of spermatozoa can continue (Hosni et al., 2016; Rodriguez-Wallberg & Oktay, 2014).

(4) Recovery of spermatogenesis is dependent on the dose of RT. If damage or depletion of germinal stem cells occurs, this can result in

low sperm counts, abnormal sperm motility and morphology, decreased DNA integrity, or permanent azoospermia (absence of sperm) (Hosni et al., 2016; Wallace, Anderson, & Irvine, 2005).

(5) Leydig cells are located within the testis and produce testosterone. These cells are more resistant to RT; therefore, testosterone production can continue despite azoospermia (Rodriguez-Wallberg & Oktay, 2014).

(6) If the HPA axis falls within the radiation field, gonadotrophin deficiency can occur. Growth hormone is the most sensitive of the anterior pituitary hormones to RT, followed by gonadotropins (Hosni et al., 2016).

(7) A male fertility risk chart and calculator are tools available through the Livestrong Foundation (n.d.-a) that can provide a general understanding of potential treatment risks but should not be used in place of a consultation with a healthcare professional.

4. Fertility preservation and options

a) Fertility preservation options for female AYAs with cancer

(1) Oocyte cryopreservation (Oktay et al., 2018)

(a) Cryopreservation of oocytes (unfertilized eggs) is an option and may be especially appropriate for women who do not have a male partner or do not wish to use donor sperm.

(b) Oocyte cryopreservation requires a referral to a reproductive endocrinologist or fertility clinic.

(2) Embryo cryopreservation

(a) Embryo cryopreservation is an established fertility preservation method using in vitro fertilization to combine an oocyte and sperm in order to create an embryo prior to storage (Oktay et al., 2018).

(b) Embryo preservation requires a referral to a reproductive endocrinologist or fertility clinic.

(c) Procedures are often undertaken under light sedation through a transvaginal approach. Patients need to be medically fit to undergo the procedure (Srikanthan et al., 2018).

(d) Ovarian stimulation occurs with gonadotropins (hormones) prior to oocyte retrieval and requires daily subcutaneous injections for 9–13 days, as well as multiple transvaginal ultrasounds and blood tests. Random ovarian stimulation avoids women having to be at the beginning of their menstrual cycle in order to begin the fertility preservation process

(Hendershot et al., 2016; Srikanthan et al., 2018).

(e) Short-term exposure to high estrogen levels as a result of gonadotropins is an important safety concern for women with hormone sensitive disease (e.g., breast cancer). Alternative ovarian stimulation protocols involving tamoxifen or letrozole, which act as an antidote to the gonadotropins, should be used in this patient population (Lambertini et al., 2016).

(f) The cryopreservation process takes approximately two to three weeks and involves out-of-pocket costs for patients (Oktay et al., 2018).

(3) Ovarian transposition (oophoropexy)

(a) Ovarian transposition is the surgical relocation of ovaries to outside the radiation field.

(b) This procedure can reduce the risk of ovarian failure by approximately 50% (Lee et al., 2006).

(c) Radiation scatter and damage to the blood vessels supplying the ovaries can affect the success of this option, and patients should be counseled regarding this (Hendershot et al., 2016; Oktay et al., 2018; Srikanthan et al., 2018).

(4) Gonadotropin-releasing hormone (GnRH) agonists (Hendershot et al., 2016; Oktay et al., 2018; Srikanthan et al., 2018)

(a) Injectable GnRH agonists are prescribed to suppress and protect ovarian function in women receiving gonadotoxic chemotherapy.

(b) The literature remains mixed on the efficacy of GnRH agonists for fertility preservation.

(c) When proven fertility preservation methods such as oocyte, embryo, or ovarian tissue cryopreservation are not feasible, it is recommended that a GnRH agonist may be offered to patients in the hope of reducing the likelihood of chemotherapy-induced ovarian insufficiency.

(5) Ovarian tissue cryopreservation (Hendershot et al., 2016; Oktay et al., 2018; Srikanthan et al., 2018).

(a) Ovarian tissue cryopreservation is an experimental intervention that offers a fertility preservation option for prepubescent girls and for women who are unable to undergo oocyte or embryo cryopreservation.

(b) The ovarian cortical tissue is obtained through a laparoscopic surgical intervention under general anesthesia, and it is cryopreserved for future use.

(c) The tissue can be used in two ways.
  i. Tissue can be thawed and implanted at a later time to reinstate ovarian reserve.
  ii. Oocytes from the cortical strips can be harvested to use for in vitro fertilization.

b) Fertility preservation for male AYAs with cancer
  (1) Sperm cryopreservation (Hendershot et al., 2016; Oktay et al., 2018)
    (a) Cryopreservation of sperm is a proven and fairly inexpensive form of fertility preservation for postpubertal males receiving cancer treatment.
    (b) Individuals unable to produce a sperm sample through masturbation can be offered testicular sperm extraction or electroejaculation (stimulation of nerves resulting in ejaculation).
  (2) Testicular tissue cryopreservation (Hendershot et al., 2016; Oktay et al., 2018)
    (a) Cryopreservation of testicular tissue is an experimental intervention to preserve fertility in prepubescent boys that involves an open biopsy.
    (b) Research is being conducted to understand if the tissue can be used to do the following.
    (c) Testicular tissue can be implanted into the testicle with the goal of restoring spermatogenesis.
    (d) In vitro stimulation of the tissue into mature sperm can potentially be used for in vitro fertilization.

c) Fertility options following cancer treatment for female AYA survivors
  (1) Menstruation is not a reliable measure of fertility, and additional testing is necessary to assess female fertility status following cancer treatment (Barton et al., 2013).
  (2) The following measures can be used to assess fertility status (Hendershot et al., 2016).
    (a) Anti-Mullerian hormone
    (b) Antral follicle count
    (c) Routine hormones (luteinizing hormone, follicle-stimulating hormone, and estradiol)
  (3) A post-treatment ovarian function assessment provides the most accurate results approximately 12 months after the last administered dose of treatment or when it is thought the treatment is out of the individual's system (six months after therapy completion) (Lambertini et al., 2016).

    (a) For female patients at risk for premature ovarian failure, they may still have an opportunity to preserve oocytes or embryos following treatment (Hendershot et al., 2016).
    (b) It is critical that female patients are offered a referral to a reproductive endocrinologist following treatment.
  (4) When a woman is in premature ovarian failure, she can no longer conceive. However, pregnancy is possible for these patients if they have cryopreserved oocytes or embryos or have the financial resources to purchase donor oocytes (Hendershot et al., 2016).
  (5) Women with genetic mutations associated with their cancer diagnosis (e.g., *BRCA1*, *BRCA2*) have the option of sending their embryos for genetic testing prior to implantation at an additional cost.
  (6) Pregnancy after cancer should be considered safe, and it is generally not discouraged (Lambertini et al., 2016).
    (a) The proper timing of a pregnancy following cancer therapy remains unclear and should be individualized based on treatments received.
    (b) Two main issues should be considered (Lambertini et al., 2016).
      i. Risk of relapse
      ii. Cancer therapy leaving a patient's system

d) Fertility options following cancer treatment for male AYA survivors
  (1) Complete azoospermia is usually achieved approximately 18 weeks following RT or two months following gonadotoxic chemotherapy. Sperm production then ceases for the remainder of the treatment (Hendershot et al., 2016).
  (2) Following treatment, the highest chance for sperm recovery is within the first two years; however, it can take up to five years. Beyond five years, sperm recovery is less common (Hendershot et al., 2016).
  (3) Sperm recovery takes time and can be measured with a semen analysis on an annual basis to assess for sperm count, morphology, and motility recovery. Even if a semen analysis demonstrates a normal sperm sample, patients should not discard their frozen sperm until they are able to conceive naturally (Hendershot et al., 2016).
  (4) Patients who demonstrate prolonged azoospermia and have not banked sperm should be referred for a urology consultation, as these men may be candidates for microdissection tes-

ticular sperm extraction, which retrieves sperm produced in the testis that cannot travel to the ejaculate (Hendershot et al., 2016).

  (5) The safe time to conceive following treatment is still unclear; however, men should be advised to delay until cancer therapy has left their system (approximately six months after the final dose) (Lambertini et al., 2016).

5. Psychosocial considerations
  a) Approximately 40% of cancer survivors reported that they had no fertility counseling at the time of diagnosis. Fertility counseling is one of the most cited unmet needs among younger adult cancer survivors (Benedict, Shuk, & Ford, 2016; Marci et al., 2018).
  b) After treatment, AYA cancer survivors often have limited knowledge on their reproductive health, reporting false beliefs about their reproductive potential. Post-treatment infertility often comes as a surprise (Benedict et al., 2016).
  c) Cancer survivors are at increased risk for emotional distress, a reduced mental health state, and poor quality of life if they become infertile from their cancer treatment (Benedict et al., 2016; Hendershot et al., 2016).
  d) Fertility information and support for male and female patients across age groups should be offered across the cancer continuum, as this provides patients with the opportunity to express their concerns (Benedict et al., 2016).
  e) Counseling should include a balance between maintaining hope while fostering realistic expectations (Benedict et al., 2016).
6. Nursing implications (see Figure 13)
  a) Fertility counseling for patients at risk for infertility
    (1) According to NCCN guidelines for AYA patients, clinicians should discuss the risk of infertility due to cancer therapy with all patients at the time of diagnosis (Coccia et al., 2018).
    (2) This recommendation is supported by ASCO fertility guidelines, which further emphasize

that this discussion should take place as soon as possible prior to treatment initiation, and healthcare providers, including nurses, should be prepared to discuss infertility as a potential risk of therapy. A second fertility discussion should also take place following cancer therapy (Oktay et al., 2018).
    (3) Oncofertility counseling should be individualized, discussing the benefits of the proposed cancer treatment and the risk of infertility for each individual. Although treatment-related infertility can be difficult to estimate, factors to be considered include age, comorbidities, ovarian reserve in women, and sterilizing potential of the treatment (Lambertini et al., 2016).
    (4) Patients should be educated on established methods of fertility preservation (semen, oocyte, and embryo preservation) for postpubertal males and females. For prepubertal children, experimental options (if available) including ovarian and testicular tissue preservation, should be discussed (Oktay et al., 2018).
    (5) Discussion of associated costs is an important part of decision-making for patients regarding the feasibility of fertility preservation. Patients should be made aware of financial counseling services to support this component of decision-making (Oktay et al., 2018).
  b) Increasing patient access to a fertility clinic and psychosocial referral
    (1) Prior to treatment, fertility clinic referrals should be offered and initiated within 24 hours for all interested patients (Coccia et al., 2018).
    (2) Oncology teams should collaborate with local fertility clinics to establish fertility referral pathways in order to streamline the referral process for oncology teams and reduce patient wait times (Hendershot et al., 2016).
    (3) Patients and families should be referred to psychosocial services if they experience distress

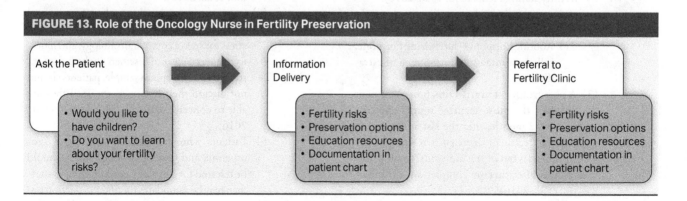

FIGURE 13. Role of the Oncology Nurse in Fertility Preservation

Ask the Patient
- Would you like to have children?
- Do you want to learn about your fertility risks?

Information Delivery
- Fertility risks
- Preservation options
- Education resources
- Documentation in patient chart

Referral to Fertility Clinic
- Fertility risks
- Preservation options
- Education resources
- Documentation in patient chart

related to potential infertility (Oktay et al., 2018).

7. Documentation: All fertility discussions held between oncology nurses and patients and families should be documented in the health record (Oktay et al., 2018).

8. Patient, caregiver, and family education: Patients prefer that information about fertility preservation is delivered to them by a healthcare professional and reinforced through written information, including a list of fertility clinics, resources to relieve financial burden, and statistics for patients to better understand the importance of fertility preservation (Tam et al., 2016).

9. Recommended resources
   a) Fertile Future: https://fertilefuture.ca
   b) Livestrong: www.livestrong.org/we-can-help/livestrong-fertility
   c) Oncofertility Consortium: http://oncofertility.northwestern.edu
   d) Oncofertility Referral Network (Canada): https://cancerkn.com/oncofertility-referral-network
   e) University Health Network Princess Margaret Cancer Centre AYA Oncology Program (Toronto, Ontario, Canada): www.uhn.ca/PrincessMargaret/Clinics/Adolescent_Young_Adult_Oncology

References

Barton, S.E., Najita, J.S., Ginsburg, E.S., Leisenring, W.M., Stovall, M., Weathers, R.E., ... Diller, L. (2013). Infertility, infertility treatment, and achievement of pregnancy in female survivors of childhood cancer: A report from the Childhood Cancer Survivor Study cohort. *Lancet Oncology, 14,* 873–881. https://doi.org/10.1016/S1470-2045(13)70251-1

Benedict, C., Shuk, E., & Ford, J.S. (2016). Fertility issues in adolescent and young adult cancer survivors. *Journal of Adolescent and Young Adult Oncology, 5,* 48–57. https://doi.org/10.1089/jayao.2015.0024

Biedka, M., Kuźba-Kryszak, T., Nowikiewicz, T., & Żyromska, A. (2016). Fertility impairment in radiotherapy. *Contemporary Oncology, 20,* 199–204. https://doi.org/10.5114/wo.2016.57814

Coccia, P.F., Pappo, A.S., Beaupin, L., Borges, V.F., Borinstein, S.C., Chugh, R., ... Matloub, Y. (2018). Adolescent and young adult oncology, version 2.2018. *Journal of the National Comprehensive Cancer Network, 16,* 66–97. https://doi.org/10.6004/jnccn.2018.0001

Hendershot, E., Maloney, A.-M., Fawcett, S., Sarvanantham, S., McMahon, E., Gupta, A., & Mitchell, L. (2016). Advanced practice nurses: Improving access to fertility preservation for oncology patients. *Canadian Oncology Nursing Journal, 26,* 40–45. https://doi.org/10.5737/236880762614045

Hosni, A., Abd-Alkhalek, S.E., Foda, M., & Awad, I. (2016). Potential risk of radiotherapy on fertility among male cancer survivors. *Cancer Therapy and Oncology International Journal, 1,* 555566. https://doi.org/10.19080/ctoij.2016.01.555566

Lambertini, M., Del Mastro, L., Pescio, M.C., Andersen, C.Y., Azim, H.A., Jr., Peccatori, F.A., ... Anserini, P. (2016). Cancer and fertility preservation: International recommendations from an expert meeting. *BMC Medicine, 14,* 1. https://doi.org/10.1186/s12916-015-0545-7

Lee, S.J., Schover, L.R., Partridge, A.H., Patrizio, P., Wallace, W.H., Hagerty, K., ... Oktay, K. (2006). American Society of Clinical Oncology recommendations on fertility preservation in cancer patients. *Journal of Clinical Oncology, 24,* 2917–2931. https://doi.org/10.1200/JCO.2006.06.5888

Livestrong Foundation. (n.d.-a). Fertility risks for men. https://prod-io.livestrong.org/sites/default/files/rs/images-email/pdfs/livestrong-fertility/LF_FertilityRiskCharts_Men.pdf

Livestrong Foundation. (n.d.-b). Fertility risks for women. https://prod-io.livestrong.org/sites/default/files/rs/images-email/pdfs/livestrong-fertility/LF_FertilityRiskCharts_Women.pdf

Loren, A.W., Mangu, P.B., Beck, L.N., Brennan, I., Magdalinski, A.J., Partridge, A.H., ... Oktay, K. (2013). Fertility preservation for patients with cancer: American Society of Clinical Oncology clinical practice guideline update. *Journal of Clinical Oncology, 31,* 2500–2510. https://doi.org/10.1200/JCO.2013.49.2678

Marci, R., Mallozzi, M., Di Benedetto, L., Schimberni, M., Mossa, S., Soave, I., ... Caserta, D. (2018). Radiations and female fertility. *Reproductive Biology and Endocrinology, 16,* 112. https://doi.org/10.1186/s12958-018-0432-0

Oktay, K., Harvey, B.E., Partridge, A.H., Quinn, G.P., Reinecke, J., Taylor, H.S., ... Loren, A.W. (2018). Fertility preservation in patients with cancer: ASCO clinical practice guideline update. *Journal of Clinical Oncology, 36,* 1994–2001. https://doi.org/10.1200/jco.2018.78.1914

Rodriguez-Wallberg, K.A., & Oktay, K. (2014). Fertility preservation during cancer treatment: Clinical guidelines. *Cancer Management and Research, 6,* 105–117. https://doi.org/10.2147/cmar.s32380

Ronn, R., & Holzer, H.E.G. (2013). Oncofertility in Canada: The impact of cancer on fertility. *Current Oncology, 20,* e338–e344. https://doi.org/10.3747/co.20.1358

Srikanthan, A., Amir, E., Bedard, P., Giuliani, M., Hodgson, D., Laframboise, S., ... Gupta, A. (2018). Fertility preservation in post-pubescent female cancer patients: A practical guideline for clinicians. *Molecular and Clinical Oncology, 8,* 153–158. https://doi.org/10.3892/mco.2017.1486

Tam, S., Puri, N., Stephens, D., Mitchell, L., Giuliani, M., Papadakos, J., & Gupta, A. (2016). Improving access to standardized fertility preservation information for older adolescents and young adults with cancer: Using a user-centered approach with young adult patients, survivors, and partners to refine fertility knowledge transfer. *Journal of Cancer Education, 33,* 528–535. https://doi.org/10.1007/s13187-016-1108-0

Wallace, W.H.B., Anderson, R.A., & Irvine, D.S. (2005). Fertility preservation for young patients with cancer: Who is at risk and what can be offered? *Lancet Oncology, 6,* 209–218. https://doi.org/10.1016/s1470-2045(05)70092-9

Wo, J.Y., & Viswanathan, A.N. (2009). The impact of radiotherapy on fertility, pregnancy, and neonatal outcomes of female cancer patients. *International Journal of Radiation Oncology, Biology, Physics, 73,* 1304–1312. https://doi.org/10.1016/j.ijrobp.2008.12.016

G. Treatment of patients who are pregnant
   1. Incidence
      a) Malignancy occurs in approximately 1 in 1,000 pregnancies (Stovall et al., 1995).
      b) The most common cancers that affect pregnant women are cancers of the breast, cervix, and uterus, as well as lymphomas and hematologic malignancies (Stovall et al., 1995; Vandenbroucke, Verheecke, Fumagalli, Lok, & Amant, 2017).
   2. General considerations
      a) It is generally advised that radiation should be avoided during pregnancy, but in some rare cases, RT is given during pregnancy.
      b) RT use in pregnancy poses special challenges because of the need to treat the mother but minimize dose and risk to both the mother and fetus. The risks to the fetus are dependent on gestational age.

c) Given the rarity of malignancy during pregnancy, research addressing RT during pregnancy is limited, and the existing literature is often case-based or summaries of what is available.

d) If at all possible, RT should be avoided during pregnancy, but if RT is deemed necessary, all measures should be taken to limit the fetal dose and limit side effects to the mother and fetus.

e) A woman may be exposed to radiation during pregnancy for several reasons (Williams & Fletcher, 2010).

   (1) Medical necessity

   (2) Unknown pregnancy at the time of diagnostic or therapeutic intervention

   (3) Workplace exposure

3. Fetal risk: Risks to a fetus are based on gestational age.

a) Organogenesis phase (weeks 2–7): Gross malformation and small head size, possibly with intellectual disabilities, can occur from radiation exposure. Extremely high doses of ionizing radiation will likely be deadly to an embryo (American College of Obstetricians and Gynecologists [ACOG], 2017; Mazzola et al., 2019; Nakagawa et al., 1997; Stovall et al., 1995).

b) First trimester (weeks 8–15): The brain is developing in the first trimester, and the resulting risks are small head size and intellectual disability. The risk of CNS effects is greatest during this time period (ACOG, 2017; Mazzola et al., 2019; Yonekura et al., 2014).

c) Second trimester (weeks 16–25): Second trimester risks are similar to those of the first trimester but also include cataracts, sterility, neurologic diseases, and development of secondary malignancies (Brent, 1983; Mazzola et al., 2019; Otake & Schull, 1984).

d) Third trimester (week 26 and beyond): The risks for intellectual disabilities and small head size may be minimal for exposures of less than 0.5 Gy (Miller & Mulvihill, 1976; Stovall et al., 1995).

4. Radiation protection: Fetal radiation exposure can be minimized with the following measures.

a) Use of lead shielding

b) Modification of RT techniques

   (1) Use of multileaf collimators (Luis, Christie, Kaminski, Kenny, & Peres, 2009; Stovall et al., 1995)

   (2) Reduction of field size (Luis et al., 2009; Stovall et al., 1995)

   (3) Modification of the beam energy (Luis et al., 2009; Stovall et al., 1995)

   (4) Proton beam therapy: Compared to conventional RT, proton beam therapy may be a safer option, as it is able to deliver the dose to a target area without theoretical harm to the fetus (Kalbasi et al., 2018).

c) Consultation with a dosimetry specialist for calculation of fetal radiation dose (Williams & Fletcher, 2010)

5. Safety counseling: Safety counseling should occur prior to starting any RT and should include anticipated fetal dosage and possible side effects (Williams & Fletcher, 2010).

6. Imaging studies

a) CT scans, nuclear studies, and x-rays in low doses performed during pregnancy have not been associated with fetal harm (ACOG, 2017).

b) Multiple x-rays rarely result in the same exposure as a high degree of ionizing radiation (ACOG, 2017).

c) MRI and ultrasound do not use ionizing radiation (Williams & Fletcher, 2010).

References

American College of Obstetricians and Gynecologists. (2017). Guidelines for diagnostic imaging during pregnancy and lactation. *Obstetrics and Gynecology, 130,* e210–e216. https://doi.org/10.1097/aog.0000000000002355

Brent, R.L. (1983). The effects of embryonic and fetal exposure to x-ray, microwaves, and ultrasound. *Clinical Obstetrics and Gynecology, 26,* 484–510. https://doi.org/10.1097/00003081-198306000-00030

Kalbasi, A., Kirk, M., Teo, B.-K.K., Diffenderfer, E., Ding, X., McDonough, J., ... Hill-Kayser, C. (2018). Proton craniospinal irradiation during the third trimester in pregnancy. *Practical Radiation Oncology, 8,* 213–216. https://doi.org/10.1016/j.prro.2017.09.005

Luis, S.A., Christie, D.R.H., Kaminski, A., Kenny, L., & Peres, M.H. (2009). Pregnancy and radiotherapy: Management options for minimizing risk, case series and comprehensive literature review. *Journal of Medical Imaging and Radiation Oncology, 53,* 559–568. https://doi.org/10.1111/j.1754-9485.2009.02124.x

Mazzola, R., Corradini, S., Eidemüeller, M., Figlia, V., Fiorention, A., Giaj-Levra, N., ... Alongi, F. (2019). Modern radiotherapy in cancer treatment during pregnancy. *Critical Reviews in Oncology/Hematology, 136,* 13–19. https://doi.org/10.1016/j.critrevonc.2019.02.002

Miller, R.W., & Mulvihill, J.J. (1976). Small head size after atomic irradiation. *Teratology, 14,* 355–358. https://doi.org/10.1002/tera.1420140311

Nakagawa, K., Aoki, Y., Kusama, T., Ban, N., Nakagawa, S., & Sasaki, Y. (1997). Radiotherapy during pregnancy: Effects on fetuses and neonates. *Clinical Therapeutics, 19,* 770–777. https://doi.org/10.1016/s0149-2918(97)80101-4

Otake, M., & Schull, W.J. (1984). *In utero* exposure to A-bomb radiation and mental retardation; A reassessment. *British Journal of Radiology, 57,* 409–414. https://doi.org/10.1259/0007-1285-57-677-409

Stovall, M., Blackwell, C.R., Cundiff, J., Novack, D.H., Palta, J.R., Wagner, L.K., ... Shalek, R.J. (1995). Fetal dose from radiotherapy with photon beams: Report of AAPM Radiation Therapy Committee Task Group No. 36. *Medical Physics, 22,* 63–82. https://doi.org/10.1118/1.597525

Vandenbroucke, T., Verheecke, M., Fumagalli, M., Lok, C., & Amant, F. (2017). Effects of cancer treatment during pregnancy on fetal and child development. *Lancet Child and Adolescent Health, 1,* 302–310. https://doi.org/10.1016/s2352-4642(17)30091-3

Williams, P.M., & Fletcher, S. (2010). Health effects of prenatal radiation exposure. *American Family Physician, 82,* 488–493. https://www.aafp.org/afp/2010/0901/p488.html

Yonekura, Y., Tsujii, H., Hopewell, J.W., Ortiz López, P.O., Cosset, J.-M., Paganetti, H., ... Nakamura, T. (2014). ICRP publication 127: Radiological protection in ion beam radiotherapy. *Annals of the ICRP, 43,* 5–113. https://doi.org/10.1177/0146645314559144

H. Nutritional issues

1. Overview

   a) Ensuring proper nutrition during cancer treatment is an important part of care. Malnutrition is common and can affect 20%–80% of patients diagnosed with cancer (Álvaro Sanz et al., 2019).

   b) The risk of malnutrition differs depending on tumor site, with highest risk in those with cancers of the head and neck, esophagus, stomach, colon, rectum, and pancreas (Virizuela et al., 2018).

   c) Malnutrition has been associated with reduced response to cancer treatment, increased treatment toxicity, delayed wound healing, and depression (Felder et al., 2015).

   d) It is the responsibility of all healthcare team members to ensure patients with cancer have their nutritional status monitored and evaluated.

      (1) Early nutrition intervention is essential.

      (2) Preventing weight loss can help to promote better tolerance to treatment and better quality of life (Escamilla & Jarrett, 2016; Lis, Gupta, Lammersfeld, Markman, & Vashi, 2012).

   e) When initiated early in treatment, nutrition interventions from a registered dietitian nutritionist (RDN) or registered dietitian (RD) can support weight maintenance and nutritional status maintenance, reduce malnutrition, shorten length of hospital stays and readmissions, improve patients' recovery, and reduce healthcare costs (Academy of Nutrition and Dietetics, n.d.-a; Dietitians of Canada, 2018).

   f) Cancer cachexia is a multifactorial syndrome marked by continual loss of skeletal muscle mass (with or without loss of adipose tissue), often seen in advanced stages of cancer. Unfortunately, cancer cachexia is not fully reversible by nutrition intervention via oral, enteral, or parenteral means (Fearon et al., 2011).

2. Malnutrition screening and assessment

   a) The Academy of Nutrition and Dietetics along with the American Society for Parenteral and Enteral Nutrition published a consensus statement in 2012 outlining six clinical characteristics to be assessed and used in documenting malnutrition and determining if malnutrition is severe or nonsevere. The organizations recommended considering the following six characteristics, along with clinical judgment, in determining if malnutrition is present (White, Guenter, Jensen, Malone, & Schofield, 2012).

      (1) Energy intake

      (2) Weight loss and its interpretation

      (3) Loss of subcutaneous fat

      (4) Loss of muscles mass

      (5) Fluid accumulation

      (6) Reduced hand grip strength

   b) The Global Leadership Initiative on Malnutrition convened in January 2016 with the purpose of developing a globally accepted malnutrition diagnostic criteria.

      (1) The organization is comprised of a core leadership committee with representatives from several of the global clinical nutrition societies: American Society of Parenteral and Enteral Nutrition; European Society for Clinical Nutrition and Metabolism; Latin American Federation of Nutritional Therapy, Clinical Nutrition and Metabolism; and Parenteral and Enteral Nutrition Society of Asia.

      (2) In 2018, the Global Leadership Initiative on Malnutrition published a consensus report, which outlined a two-step approach to diagnosing malnutrition (Cederholm et al., 2019).

         (a) Risk screening: Using a validated screening tool, clinicians should screen patients to identify those at risk.

         (b) Diagnostic assessment

            i. Phenotypic
               • Nonvolitional weight loss
               • Low body mass index
               • Reduced muscle mass
            ii. Etiologic
               • Reduced food intake or assimilation
               • Inflammation

      (3) For a diagnosis of malnutrition, at least one phenotypic criterion and one etiologic criterion must be present (Cederholm et al., 2019).

         (a) It was proposed by the authors that severity of malnutrition (moderate or severe) is determined based on phenotypic criteria, with specific ranges presented for percentage of weight loss, low body mass index, and reduced muscle mass.

         (b) The authors encourage further research to validate this approach.

   c) All patients with a newly diagnosed malignancy should be screened for risk of malnutrition (Academy of Nutrition and Dietetics, n.d.-b).

      (1) Any screening tool should be valid, reliable, and simple to administer.

      (2) Early screening identifies patients at malnutrition risk and can ensure a prompt referral to an RDN or RD.

      (3) Identification of malnourished patients or patients at risk of malnutrition using validated screening tools leads to early interventions and better outcomes for patients.

      (4) Rescreening should be conducted throughout treatment and should be completed at regular intervals for inpatients (Academy of Nutrition and Dietetics, n.d.-b).

      (5) Most screening tools suggest rescreening weekly to monitor for changes (Canadian Mal-

nutrition Task Force, 2014; Ferguson, Capra, Bauer, & Banks, 1999; Kondrup, Allison, Elia, Vellas, & Plauth, 2003).

(6) Completing malnutrition risk screening is a shared responsibility among all healthcare team members.

(7) Patients screened and determined to be at risk for malnutrition should be referred to an RDN or RD.

(8) Multiple valid and reliable screening tools are available for identifying malnutrition risk in adults with cancer in an outpatient setting (Academy of Nutrition and Dietetics, n.d.-b; Arribas et al., 2017; Cac-cialanza et al., 2016; Queensland Health, 2017).

　(a) Malnutrition Screening Tool (Ferguson et al., 1999)

　(b) Subjective Global Assessment Form (Canadian Malnutrition Task Force, 2017)

(9) Multiple valid and reliable screening tools are available for identifying malnutrition risk in adults with cancer in an inpatient setting (Academy of Nutrition and Dietetics, n.d.-b; Arribas et al., 2017; Caccialanza et al., 2016; Queensland Health, 2017).

　(a) Canadian Nutrition Screening Tool (Canadian Malnutrition Task Force, 2014)

　(b) Patient-Generated Subjective Global Assessment (Ottery, 2020)

　(c) Malnutrition Universal Screening Tool (British Association for Parenteral and Enteral Nutrition, 2018)

(10) Clinicians should consider a consult with an RDN or RD if patients have any of the criteria listed in Figure 14.

d) A nutrition assessment is the evaluation of all barriers to adequate nutrition and nutrition impact symptoms. Assessment also involves the creation of a plan to manage these barriers and improve or maintain nutritional status (Arends et al., 2017; Levin, 2013).

e) The Nutrition Care Process is a systematic approach for an RDN or RD to employ to ensure high quality nutrition care. It was created by the Academy of Nutrition and Dietetics (2017) and is recommended by the International Confederation of Dietetic Associations as a framework for dietetic practice. The Nutrition Care Process comprises four steps.

(1) Nutrition assessment: The following information is collected by an RDN or RD to determine a patient's overall nutritional status and needs (Academy of Nutrition and Dietetics, 2017).

　(a) Food and nutrition-related history (e.g., food and nutrient intake, medication, complementary and alternative medicine use)

　(b) Anthropometric measurements (e.g., height, weight, body mass index, weight history)

　(c) Biochemical data, medical tests, and procedures (e.g., resting metabolic rate, electrolytes, glucose)

　　i. Serum proteins (e.g., albumin, prealbumin, retinol-binding protein, transferrin, C-reactive protein) have been used historically to determine nutritional status (Bharadwaj et al., 2016).

FIGURE 14. When to Consult a Registered Dietitian

Nutrition Consult Criteria
- Weight loss
  - Greater than 5% in one month
  - Greater than 10% in six months
- BMI less than 19
- NPO for more than three days
- Pressure sores/decubitus ulcers/open wounds
- Nausea/vomiting for more than three days
- Chronic/severe constipation
- Chronic/severe diarrhea
- Cachexia
- Failure to thrive
- Severe food allergy/intolerance
- Small bowel obstruction/ileus
- Malabsorption/maldigestion
- Status post surgery to the head, face, or neck, including the oral cavity
- Status post gastrointestinal surgery (e.g., Whipple, gastrectomy, bowel resection, esophagectomy, ostomy)
- Decreased appetite/poor PO intake (more than three days) related to any of the following
  - Chemotherapy/radiation side effects
  - Dysphagia
  - Poor PO tolerance
  - Refusing PO
  - Mucositis/esophagitis
  - Dry mouth
  - Altered taste
  - Early satiety
  - Drug-nutrient interaction
  - Ascites/fluid overload/anasarca
  - Poor dentition/difficulty chewing
  - Anorexia
  - Head and neck surgery
  - Nausea/vomiting
- Patient is receiving or will receive chemotherapy and/or radiation therapy to the head, neck, face, abdomen, or pelvis.
- Patient has been diagnosed with cancer to any area of the gastrointestinal tract.
- Patient is currently receiving or would benefit from enteral nutrition support.
- Patient is currently receiving or would benefit from parenteral nutrition support.

BMI—body mass index; NPO—nothing by mouth; PO—oral

Note. Created by Maria C. Romano, MS, RD, CDN. From *Manual for Radiation Oncology Nursing Practice and Education* (4th ed., p. 87), by R.R. Iwamoto, M.L. Haas., T.K. Gosselin (Eds.), 2012, Oncology Nursing Society. Copyright 2012 by Oncology Nursing Society. Reprinted with permission.

ii. Albumin, an acute-phase visceral protein, can be altered during critical illness because of hydration status, disease state, and overall clinical condition (Marcason, 2017).

iii. Most studies show that using serum markers as determinants of protein-calorie malnutrition should not be considered, as these serum markers do not change when a change in nutritional intake occurs (Marcason, 2017).

iv. The major consensus in the literature is that laboratory markers are not reliable by themselves; therefore, they should only be used as a complement to findings from a thorough physical examination (Bharadwaj et al., 2016).

(d) Nutrition-focused physical findings (e.g., muscle and subcutaneous fat wasting, swallow function)

(e) Patient history (e.g., medical, health, family, social)

(2) Nutrition diagnosis

(a) An RDN or RD assesses the information collected in the nutrition assessment to create a statement that describes the nutrition problem.

(b) Statements are standardized to facilitate good communication and documentation of the nutrition care being provided.

(3) Nutrition intervention

(a) An RDN or RD develops a plan to address and improve the nutrition diagnosis or nutrition problem.

(b) Intervention may involve collaboration with the healthcare team.

(c) An RDN or RD provides a nutrition prescription, which is a calculation of a patient's estimated energy, protein, and fluid requirements using an appropriate predictive equation.

(d) Predictive equations consider a patient's age, weight, height, and fluid balance.

(4) Nutrition monitoring and evaluation

(a) An RDN or RD measures patient progress.

(b) Outcomes will be compared to goals and targets outlined during the nutrition intervention.

(c) New goals may be identified. An RDN or RD can provide encouragement and education on how to meet previously stated goals.

3. Nutrition-related effects of RT

a) Acute side effects

(1) Acute side effects of RT begin in approximately the second or third week of treatment. Symptoms peak approximately two-thirds of the way through treatment and may continue three to six weeks after treatment is completed (American Cancer Society, 2018; Canadian Cancer Society, 2018; see Table 7).

(2) Chronic radiation injury is also likely to adversely affect nutrition; however, chronic indications may not occur for months to years after treatment and can be irreversible (American Cancer Society, 2018; Canadian Cancer Society, 2018; Marian, Mattox, & Williams, 2017).

b) Late side effects: See Table 8.

4. Management of nutrition impact symptoms

a) Anorexia (Canadian Cancer Society, 2014; Cancer Care Ontario, 2012e; Marian et al., 2017)

(1) Definition: Anorexia is the loss of appetite or desire to eat.

(2) Potential secondary problems

(a) Weight loss

(b) Dehydration

(c) Electrolyte imbalances

(d) Malnutrition

(3) Nutrition interventions

(a) Eating small meals of high-calorie foods and fluids frequently throughout the day

(b) Eating in a pleasant atmosphere to avoid stress or feeling rushed at meals

(c) Eating at regular intervals, rather than waiting for appetite or hunger cues

TABLE 7. Possible Nutrition-Related Acute Side Effects of Radiation Therapy

Treatment Area	Acute Side Effects
Abdomen/pelvis: gastrointestinal system, reproductive organs, prostate, colon, rectum, testicles	Diarrhea, nausea and vomiting, anorexia
Central nervous system: brain, spinal cord, eye	Nausea and vomiting, anorexia, fatigue, elevated blood glucose from steroid medication
Head and neck: tongue, larynx, pharynx, oropharynx, nasopharynx, tonsils, salivary glands	Mouth changes (e.g., dysgeusia, oral mucositis, xerostomia, thick secretions), nausea and vomiting, throat changes (e.g., dysphagia, odynophagia, esophagitis), anorexia, fatigue
Thorax: esophagus, lung, possibly breasts if radiated field involves esophagus	Throat changes (e.g., dysphagia, odynophagia, esophagitis)

Note. Based on information from American Cancer Society, 2018; Canadian Cancer Society, 2018; Marian et al., 2017.

TABLE 8. Possible Nutrition-Related Late Side Effects of Radiation Therapy

Treatment Area	Late Side Effects
Central nervous system: brain, spinal cord, eye	Cognitive impairment and dementia leading to dysphagia
Esophagus	Esophageal stenosis, fibrosis, or necrosis
Gastrointestinal system	Diarrhea, malabsorption, chronic enteritis/colitis, intestinal changes (e.g., stricture, ulceration, obstruction, perforation, fistula)
Head and neck: tongue, larynx, pharynx, oropharynx, nasopharynx, tonsils, salivary glands	Trismus, permanent partial or complete xerostomia, permanent alterations in taste and smell, osteoradionecrosis of jaw

Note. Based on information from American Cancer Society, 2018; Canadian Cancer Society, 2018; Marian et al., 2017.

(d) Treating foods as medicine and as a part of treatment

(e) Drinking oral nutrition supplements (e.g., Ensure®, Boost®) when too tired to eat

(f) Engaging in light physical activity to stimulate appetite

(g) Considering foods that are easy to prepare and serve to save energy

(h) Eating more at times when feeling better

(4) Possible pharmacologic interventions

    (a) Corticosteroids (e.g., dexamethasone, prednisone)

    (b) Synthetic progestogens (e.g., medroxyprogesterone acetate, megestrol acetate)

    (c) Prokinetic agents (e.g., metoclopramide, domperidone)

    (d) Proton pump inhibitors (e.g., pantoprazole, rabeprazole)

b) Bloating, gas, and abdominal pain (Canadian Cancer Society, 2014; Peterson, Boers-Doets, Bensadoun, & Herrstedt, 2015)

(1) Causes: Bloating, gas, and abdominal pain may be the result of malabsorption caused by cancer treatment, medical conditions, or infections.

(2) Potential secondary problems

    (a) Cachexia

    (b) Steatorrhea

    (c) Weight loss

    (d) Dehydration

    (e) Fatigue

    (f) Malnutrition

    (g) Nutrient insufficiencies and deficiencies

(3) Nutrition interventions

    (a) Recording diet and symptom history to identify problem foods or eating habits

    (b) Eating small, frequent meals and snacks throughout the day

    (c) For bloating and gas, avoiding cruciferous vegetables, beans, and legumes

    (d) Limiting swallowed air by avoiding use of straws, carbonated beverages, and chewing gum, as well as eating slowly with mouth closed

    (e) For fatty, foul-smelling stools, avoiding high-fat foods

(4) Other possible interventions

    (a) Probiotics

    (b) Pancreatic enzymes

        i. Pancreatic enzymes may be required by patients with pancreatic cancer or bowel obstruction and those who have had pancreatic and gastric surgery (Berry, 2014).

        ii. Patients who have altered gastrointestinal function and require pancreatic enzymes should be referred to an RDN or RD for individualized counseling.

c) Constipation (American Cancer Society, 2018; Canadian Cancer Society, 2014; Cancer Care Ontario, 2012a; Larkin et al., 2018)

(1) Definition: Constipation is decreased frequency of bowel movements and difficulty in passing stools, which may be caused by dehydration, medications, or physiologic changes from cancer treatment.

(2) Potential secondary problems

    (a) Abdominal pain

    (b) Nausea

    (c) Vomiting

    (d) Early satiety

(3) Nutritional interventions

    (a) Educating patients on adequate hydration, fiber intake, and total food intake to help promote regular bowel movements

    (b) Eating at regular scheduled times throughout the day

    (c) Drinking 8 cups (2 L) of fluids every day and a slow increase of fiber to 25–35 g per day

    (d) Consuming hot beverages (e.g., hot prune juice), hot cereals, or high-fiber foods (e.g., bran, flaxseed, wheat germ) to create bulk and stimulate bowel movements

    (e) Including probiotics in food or supplements to help regulate bowel movements

    (f) Discussing how some medications can affect bowel function and using stool softeners and laxatives appropriately as needed

    (g) Establishing a schedule and adequate time for bowel movements

(4) Other possible interventions
   (a) First-line agents: oral colonic stimulant (e.g., senosides, bisacolyl) and oral colonic osmotic (e.g., lactulose, polyethylene glycol)
   (b) Second-line agents: suppositories (e.g., glycerin, bisacodyl) or enemas (e.g., phosphate enema)
   (c) Third-line agents: picosulfate sodium, magnesium oxide, and citric acid solution or methylnaltrexone (if patient is taking regular opioids)
   (d) Increasing physical activity as able can help relieve constipation.
(5) Other considerations
   (a) Patients should contact healthcare providers if they do not have bowel movement for two to three days.
   (b) Patients who have fluid restrictions or increased risk of bowel obstructions may need to be referred to an RDN or RD for individualized counseling.
   (c) Patients should speak to their oncologist prior to taking probiotics if they are receiving chemotherapy or immunotherapy or are participating in clinical trials.

d) Diarrhea (American Cancer Society, 2018; Bossi et al., 2018; Canadian Cancer Society, 2014; Cancer Care Ontario, 2012b)
(1) Definition: Diarrhea is an increase of three or more stools per day as compared to usual or an increase in liquidity of bowel movements. Diarrhea may be caused by diet, emotional stress, inflammation or irritation of the mucosa, certain medications and anticancer treatments (e.g., antibiotics), RT to the abdomen and pelvis, infections, and malabsorption syndrome from disease or antineoplastic treatment.
(2) Potential secondary problems
   (a) Dehydration
   (b) Electrolyte imbalances
   (c) Weight loss
   (d) Fatigue
   (e) Malnutrition
(3) Nutrition interventions
   (a) Recording diet and symptom history to identify problem foods or eating habits
   (b) Eating small, frequent meals throughout the day
   (c) Consuming a low-fat and bland diet by avoiding greasy, fried, spicy, or very rich foods while experiencing diarrhea
   (d) Consuming a low-insoluble-fiber diet (e.g., wheat bran, skins of fruit and vegetables, nuts and seeds, dark leafy greens, legumes)
   (e) Consuming a low-lactose diet if lactose intolerant
   (f) Avoiding caffeine and alcohol
   (g) Supplementing soluble fiber (e.g., applesauce, bananas, oatmeal, potatoes, rice) to diet at regular intervals throughout the day
   (h) Avoiding excessive amounts of sweetened beverages, such as fruit juice cocktails, fruit drinks, and soda, which can contribute to osmotic diarrhea
   (i) Avoiding sorbitol or other sugar alcohol–containing products (e.g., sugarless gum, candy)
   (j) Increasing fluid intake
   (k) Increasing consumption of high-potassium and high-sodium foods (e.g., potatoes, bananas, commercially prepared broths and soups) for severe diarrhea
(4) Possible pharmacologic and other interventions
   (a) First-line agent: loperamide
   (b) Second-line agents: diphenoxylate-atropine
   (c) Third-line agents: octreotide and opioids
   (d) Patients may need to be tested for *Clostridium difficile*. If positive, patients should be treated with metronidazole 500 mg orally three times daily for two weeks.

e) Dysgeusia (American Cancer Society, 2018; Canadian Cancer Society, 2014; Cancer Care Ontario, 2012c; Munankarmi, 2017)
(1) Definition: Dysgeusia is a change in sense of taste and may be caused by RT or chemotherapy.
   (a) Patients may experience little or no sense of taste and smell or heightened sense of metallic, bitter, salty, or sweet tastes.
   (b) It may take several months or up to a year after treatment for normal taste to return.
(2) Potential secondary problems
   (a) Decreased caloric intake
   (b) Nutrient insufficiencies and deficiencies
   (c) Weight loss
(3) Nutrition interventions
   (a) Maintaining good oral hygiene and rinsing mouth or brushing teeth before eating
   (b) Using fruit marinades, lemon, lime, herbs, spices, and pickles to season foods
   (c) Sucking on sugar-free lemon drops, gum, or mints to improve bad taste in mouth
   (d) Using bamboo or plastic utensils if food tastes metallic
   (e) Choosing alternative sources of protein (e.g., eggs, tofu, dairy, beans) if meats taste bitter or strange

(f) For bothersome odors, avoiding cooking areas during meal preparation, avoiding use of microwave ovens, using cup with a lid and straw to mask odors, and eating cold or raw foods (e.g., smoothies, crackers, cold sandwiches)

(4) Other possible interventions

(a) Rinsing with 1 teaspoon salt and 1 teaspoon baking soda in 1 L of water at least three to four times daily or more frequently if helpful

(b) Chewing xylitol gum or sucking on xylitol lozenges, up to 6 g per day

(c) Zinc gluconate and amifostine is not recommended for prevention of dysgeusia in patients with head and neck cancer.

f) Dysphagia (American Cancer Society, 2018; Canadian Cancer Society, 2014; De Felice et al., 2018)

(1) Definition: Dysphagia is difficulty swallowing due to extrinsic compression of the esophagus, mechanical obstruction, neurologic dysfunction, oral or esophageal candidiasis, severe mucositis, or esophagitis from chemotherapy or RT, resulting in decreased caloric intake.

(2) Potential secondary problems

(a) Dehydration
(b) Weight loss
(c) Nutrient insufficiencies
(d) Malnutrition

(3) Nutrition interventions for dysphagia

(a) Consulting with a speech-language pathologist

(b) Eating smaller, more frequent meals and snacks

(c) Consuming foods that have a uniform consistency

(d) Avoiding breads, cakes, cookies, and crackers or soaking them in milk, juice, gravy, or sauce before eating

(e) Avoiding distractions and limiting talking when eating

(4) Other possible interventions: using household or commercial thickeners (e.g., cornstarch, ThickenUp®, Thick & Easy®, Thick-It®) as instructed by a speech-language pathologist

g) Fatigue (American Cancer Society, 2018; Canadian Cancer Society, 2014; NCCN, 2020)

(1) Definition: *Fatigue* refers to lack of energy, tiredness, and mental fuzziness possibly caused by antineoplastic treatment, inadequate energy and protein intake, weight loss, pain, medications, dehydration, and sleep disturbances

(2) Potential secondary problems

(a) Poor oral intake
(b) Weight loss
(c) Depression

(3) Nutrition interventions

(a) Eating easy-to-prepare meals, snacks, prepared foods, and energy dense foods

(b) Keeping nonperishable snacks (e.g., trail mix) nearby

(c) Eating soft and easy-to-chew foods

(d) Eating small, frequent meals and snacks

(e) Eating well-balanced meals when feeling better

(f) Practicing energy saving (e.g., limiting errands or chores as much as possible)

(g) Taking a multivitamin or mineral supplement for anemia

(4) Other possible interventions

(a) Blood transfusion for anemia

(b) Light physical activity to help increase energy levels

h) Mucositis and esophagitis (American Cancer Society, 2018; Canadian Cancer Society, 2014; Cancer Care Ontario, 2012f; Peterson et al., 2015)

(1) Definition: Mucositis and esophagitis are inflammation of the mouth and esophagus, usually described as a painful, irritated throat, or the feeling of a lump in the throat. Accompanying symptoms can include indigestion, esophageal reflux, belching, feeling of fullness, and early satiety.

(2) Potential secondary problems

(a) Weight loss
(b) Nutrient insufficiencies and deficiencies
(c) Malnutrition

(3) Nutrition interventions

(a) Choosing foods lower in acidity; avoiding tomato products, citrus juices, and pickled foods

(b) Choosing less spicy foods; avoiding chili, chili powder, curry powder, cloves, black pepper, and hot sauces

(c) Choosing foods softer in texture (e.g., mashed potatoes, yogurt, egg, tofu); adding moisture (e.g., sauce, gravy)

(d) Serving foods cool or at room temperature

(e) Preparing smoothies with low-acid fruits (e.g., melons, bananas, peaches) and using yogurt, milk, or silken tofu for protein

(f) Avoiding alcohol and alcohol-containing mouthwashes

(g) Avoiding carbonated beverages

(4) Pharmacologic and other interventions

(a) Rinsing with 1 teaspoon salt and 1 teaspoon baking soda in 1L of water at least three to four times daily

(b) Applying topical anesthetics (e.g., viscous lidocaine, viscous xylocaine) before brushing teeth and before eating

(c) If topical anesthetics are not effective for pain relief, nonopioid or opioid analgesics may be required.

i) Nausea and vomiting (American Cancer Society, 2018; Canadian Cancer Society, 2014; Cancer Care Ontario, 2010; Hesketh et al., 2017; Roila et al., 2016)

(1) Causes: Nausea and vomiting may be caused by antineoplastic treatments, pain, dysgeusia, fatigue, thick oral secretions, constipation, psychological factors, and medication (e.g., antibiotics, narcotics).

(2) Potential secondary problems
   (a) Dehydration
   (b) Electrolyte imbalances
   (c) Weight loss
   (d) Nutrient insufficiencies and deficiencies

(3) Nutrition interventions
   (a) Eating small frequent meals, as hunger can make feelings of nausea stronger
   (b) Limiting exposure to food odors by avoiding food preparation areas
   (c) Eating cool, light foods with little odor
   (d) Avoiding greasy, high-fat foods
   (e) Consuming liquids between meals, rather than with meals, to maximize intake
   (f) Avoiding lying down for at least 30–60 minutes after eating
   (g) Eating dry, starchy, and salty foods (e.g., pretzels, saltines, potatoes, noodles, cooked cereals)
   (h) Eating hard candies (e.g., peppermints, lemon drops)

(4) Pharmacologic interventions
   (a) Metoclopramide or domperidone
   (b) Ondansetron
   (c) Lorazepam or oxazepam
   (d) Haloperidol
   (e) Dexamethasone

j) Oral candidiasis (American Cancer Society, 2018; Canadian Cancer Society, 2014; Cancer Care Ontario, 2012d; Peterson et al., 2015)

(1) Definition: Oral candidiasis may be an opportunistic infection seen as red or white patches in the mouth as a result of treatment or immunosuppression, causing taste changes, sore mouth, and coated tongue.

(2) Potential secondary problems
   (a) Sore mouth and throat
   (b) Decreased caloric intake
   (c) Weight loss
   (d) Malnutrition

(3) Nutrition interventions
   (a) Eating soft, moist foods with extra sauce, dressings, and gravies
   (b) Avoiding acidic and irritating ingredients (e.g., alcohol, caffeine, spicy foods, tomatoes, citrus, vinegar)
   (c) Consuming foods at room temperature or chilled
   (d) Using a straw to direct fluid away from painful parts of the mouth

(4) Pharmacologic and other interventions
   (a) Rinsing with 1 teaspoon salt and 1 teaspoon baking soda in 1 L of water at least three to four times daily
   (b) Chewing xylitol gum or sucking on xylitol lozenges, up to 6 g per day
   (c) Fluconazole
   (d) Applying topical anesthetics (e.g., viscous lidocaine, viscous xylocaine) before brushing and before eating
   (e) If topical anesthetics are not effective for pain relief, nonopioid or opioid analgesics may be required.

k) Xerostomia and thick saliva (American Cancer Society, 2018; Canadian Cancer Society, 2014; Cancer Care Ontario, 2012g; Peterson et al., 2015)

(1) Overview: Xerostomia is abnormal dryness of the mouth. Xerostomia and thick ropy saliva can cause difficulty eating and talking, as well as taste alterations.

(2) Potential secondary problems
   (a) Decreased oral intake
   (b) Nutrient insufficiencies and deficiencies
   (c) Weight loss

(3) Nutrition interventions
   (a) Eating frequent small meals
   (b) Adding broth, gravies, and sauces to meals and dunking dry foods in liquids
   (c) Sipping liquids or sucking on ice chips throughout the day
   (d) Sucking on sugarless hard candy, mints, and frozen grapes or melon balls
   (e) Avoiding caffeine, alcohol, and tobacco

(4) Pharmacologic and other interventions
   (a) Rinsing with 1 teaspoon salt and 1 teaspoon baking soda in 1 L of water at least three to four times daily
   (b) Using a cool mist humidifier at home to moisten air
   (c) Avoiding alcohol-containing mouth rinses
   (d) Artificial saliva products (e.g., Moi-Stir® spray, Biotene®) may be used for a brief course.
   (e) Acupuncture may stimulate gland secretion and alleviate xerostomia.

5. Nutrition support
   a) Oral intake issues
      (1) Side effects from RT, such as dysphagia, odynophagia, mucositis, anorexia, diarrhea, nau-

sea, and vomiting, can lead to inadequate oral intake (American Cancer Society, 2018; Marian et al., 2017).

(2) Oral intake should be encouraged and optimized with food and oral nutrition supplements as needed.

(3) If oral intake is not possible or suboptimal, nutrition support should be administered, with enteral nutrition being the preferred method (Doley & Phillips, 2017).

(a) Suboptimal oral intake can be defined as being unable to eat for more than one week or if overall intake is less than 60% of estimated energy requirements (Arends et al., 2017).

(b) Enteral nutrition bypasses the oral route and delivers nutrients into the digestive system.

(c) Enteral nutrition is preferred because it continues to use the gut, promoting more efficient metabolism and utilization of nutrients, maintaining gut integrity, and preventing translocation of bacteria (Doley & Phillips, 2017).

(d) Parenteral nutrition is the last resort to meet nutrition requirements, as there is limited evidence showing that it can improve treatment outcomes. It is significantly more costly than enteral nutrition; thus, the risks of providing parenteral nutrition support must be weighed against the benefits (Worthington et al., 2017).

b) Enteral nutrition

(1) Access

(a) Enteral access can be via nasogastric or nasoenteric tube or direct placement of a feeding tube into the stomach or jejunum.

(b) Short-term enteral nutrition (less than four weeks) can be administered via a nasally placed feeding tube (Boullata et al., 2017; Fang & Kinikini, 2017).

(c) For long-term enteral nutrition (longer than four to six weeks), a feeding tube should be inserted directly into the stomach or small bowel (Boullata et al., 2017; Fang & Kinikini, 2017).

(d) Determining feeding tube access depends on duration of use, gastric motility, risk of aspiration, altered digestive system anatomy, and any preexisting medical conditions (Fang & Kinikini, 2017).

(2) Delivery

(a) Enteral nutrition can be provided via continuous or bolus infusion or a combination of both methods.

(b) Along with patient input, an RDN or RD will determine the appropriate method of providing enteral nutrition and will take into consideration factors such as social history, feeding tube placement, and overall tolerance to enteral nutrition.

(3) Contraindications (Boullata et al., 2017; Doley & Phillips, 2017; Worthington et al., 2017)

(a) Nonoperative mechanical gastrointestinal obstruction

(b) Intractable vomiting or diarrhea refractory to medical management

(c) Severe short-bowel syndrome (less than 100 cm small bowel remaining)

(d) Paralytic ileus

(e) Distal high-output fistulas (too distal to bypass with feeding tube)

(f) Severe gastrointestinal bleed

(g) Severe gastrointestinal malabsorption (e.g., enteral nutrition failure as evidenced by progressive deterioration in nutritional status)

(h) Inaccessible gastrointestinal tract

(i) Need expected for less than five to seven days for malnourished adult patients or seven to nine days for adequately nourished adult patients

(j) Aggressive intervention not warranted or not desired

(4) Complications

(a) For common complications of enteral nutrition and suggested interventions, see Table 9 (Bischoff et al., 2020; Malone, Seres, & Lord, 2017).

(b) If complications cannot be resolved with suggestions, an RDN or RD should be consulted to assess changing formula type, rate, and method of delivery.

c) Parenteral nutrition

(1) Access (Ayers, Guenter, Holcombe, & Plogsted, 2014; Mirtallo, 2017)

(a) Parenteral nutrition is provided via peripheral IV infusion (i.e., peripheral parenteral nutrition) or through a central venous access device (i.e., central parenteral nutrition).

(b) Central parenteral nutrition is preferred for use in patients who will require support for longer than 7–14 days.

(c) Patients who require parenteral nutrition for at least five days but no more than two weeks and have good peripheral venous access can be considered for peripheral parenteral nutrition.

(d) An RDN or RD with an interprofessional team will determine the most appropriate route of infusion during the assessment.

TABLE 9. Common Complications of Enteral Nutrition and Suggested Interventions

Complication	Causes	Interventions
Aspiration, reflux	Flat head of bead resulting in incomplete closure of lower esophageal sphincter Large volume feeding boluses Delayed gastric motility	Elevate head of bed 30°–45°. Use small-bore feeding tube. Consider addition of prokinetic agents.
Clogged tube	Suboptimal flushing Improper medication administration	Change to liquid medications if possible. Flush with water between medications. Include use of a commercial declogging product if blockage cannot be cleared with water.
Constipation	Inadequate fluid intake Physical inactivity Medications Gastrointestinal obstruction, colonic dysmotility, ileus Inadequate or excessive fiber provision	Increase free water or fluid intake. Increase activity if possible. Minimize use of narcotics if possible. Recommend addition of laxatives. Evaluate and address underlying cause; enteral nutrition may need to be held.
Diarrhea	Medications Antibiotic-associated diarrhea Infectious etiology Bacterial contamination Malabsorption Steatorrhea Fiber-free formula or high-fiber formula	Rule out causes associated with medications or infections. Decrease feeding rate. Consider adding antidiarrheal agent.
Nausea, vomiting, abdominal distention, bloating	Large volume feeding boluses or rapid infusion of feedings Delayed gastric emptying	Consider addition of prokinetic agents. Consider change to postpyloric tube. Minimize use of narcotics if possible. Administer antiemetics.

(2) Considerations (Ayers et al., 2014; Mirtallo, 2017; Worthington et al., 2017)
  (a) Parenteral nutrition is more costly than enteral nutrition, so benefits should outweigh risks.
  (b) Parenteral nutrition should not be used solely based on medical diagnosis or disease state.
  (c) Use of parenteral nutrition should be carefully selected in palliative patients with an expected survival of two to three months and not be used to merely treat poor oral intake or cachexia associated with advanced malignancy.
  (d) Parenteral nutrition should be managed by the whole interprofessional team to ensure safety, reduce complications, and maximize cost effectiveness.
  (e) The interprofessional team should monitor and adjust the nutrition care plan as appropriate while patients are on parenteral nutrition to avoid or minimize complications.
(3) Indications (Ayers et al., 2014; Mirtallo, 2017; Worthington et al., 2017)
  (a) Nonfunctional or inaccessible gastrointestinal tract (e.g., bowel rest for ileus, bowel obstruction)
  (b) Severe nausea with vomiting (e.g., radiation enteritis, refractory short bowel syndrome)
  (c) Severe diarrhea or malabsorption
  (d) High-output gastrointestinal fistula (unless able to feed distal to fistula)
  (e) Severe acute necrotizing pancreatitis with inability to tolerate enteral nutrition
(4) Contraindications (Ayers et al., 2014; Mirtallo, 2017)
  (a) Functioning gastrointestinal tract
  (b) Well-nourished and inadequate enteral nutrition for less than seven days
  (c) Renal or hepatic compromise
  (d) Unstable hemodynamics
  (e) Aggressive intervention not warranted or desired
(5) Complications (Kumpf, 2017; Worthington et al., 2017)
  (a) Poor glycemic control
  (b) Essential fatty acid deficiency
  (c) Hypertriglyceridemia
  (d) Azotemia
  (e) Hepatobiliary complications (e.g., steatosis, cholestasis, gallbladder stasis)
  (f) Metabolic bone disease

6. Refeeding syndrome
   a) Refeeding syndrome is a potentially life-threatening complication that occurs when severely malnourished patients are rapidly initiated on nutrition support, usually enteral or parenteral nutrition (Friedli et al., 2018; McCray, 2016). Rapid delivery of nutrients can cause hypophosphatemia, hypokalemia, hypomagnesemia, and hyperglycemia, as well as metabolic shifts that can lead to respiratory, cardiac, and neurologic complications (Kaderbay et al., 2018).
   b) Patients are considered at risk for refeeding syndrome under the following circumstances (National Collaborating Centre for Acute Care, 2006).
      (1) Weight loss of 10% or more during the past six months
      (2) Physical signs of malnourishment (e.g., limited fat stores, muscle wasting)
      (3) Intake of 50% or less of usual diet for more than 7–10 days
      (4) Chronic alcohol use or abuse
   c) Enteral or parenteral nutrition should be started slowly and gradually advanced over the first week (Boland, Solanki, & O'Hanlon, 2013; National Collaborating Centre for Acute Care, 2006).
   d) Electrolytes (potassium, magnesium, phosphate) should be checked prior to feeding. During the first 7–10 days after initiation of feeding, electrolytes should be monitored and corrected until values are stable and normalized (Boland et al., 2013; National Collaborating Centre for Acute Care, 2006).
   e) Thiamine should be provided starting the day of enteral or parenteral initiation at a dose of 200–300 mg daily for 10 days (Boland et al., 2013; National Collaborating Centre for Acute Care, 2006).
   f) Weight should be monitored daily if fluid balance is a concern. Weight checks can occur weekly once fluid balance is stable (Boland et al., 2013; National Collaborating Centre for Acute Care, 2006).
7. Complementary and alternative medicine (CAM)
   a) CAM is used to describe therapies that are not part of standard cancer treatment (NCI, 2019).
      (1) Complimentary medicine is a treatment that is used in conjunction with standard treatments.
      (2) Alternative medicine is a treatment that is used in place of standard treatments.
      (3) Integrative medicine incorporates the use of standard treatments and CAM therapies.
   b) CAM includes products such as dietary supplements, herbal supplements, and vitamins (NCI, 2019).
      (1) Some CAM therapies have been shown to be effective and safe.
      (2) Not all CAM therapies are safe, and some may potentially be harmful. For example, taking megadoses of certain vitamins, minerals, and herbal supplements could interact with cancer treatments and medications.
   c) All patients considering CAM should be encouraged to speak to their healthcare team to ensure these therapies do not interact with cancer treatments and medications.
8. Special diets
   a) Many diets claim to improve patient outcomes.
      (1) Any diet that eliminates or restricts any of the macronutrients could lead to nutrient deficiencies in patients.
      (2) A healthy diet includes all types of foods and focuses on high intake of vegetables and fruits (U.S. Department of Health and Human Services & U.S. Department of Agriculture, 2015).
      (3) If patients are interested in a special diet, they should be referred to an RDN or RD, as some diets lack evidence of efficacy, may be overly restrictive, and eliminate key nutrients.
      (4) A referral to an RDN or RD can ensure patients get individualized diet education.
   b) At the beginning of treatment when patients are eating well without nutrition impact symptoms, they should be encouraged to follow a well-balanced diet without restrictions. For healthy eating guidelines, refer patients to one of the following resources for dietary guidance.
      (1) Canada's Food Guide: https://food-guide.canada.ca/en
      (2) Dietary Guidelines for Americans 2015–2020: https://health.gov/dietaryguidelines/2015/resources/2015-2020_Dietary_Guidelines.pdf
      (3) Managing Cancer Side Effects (Dana-Farber Cancer Institute): www.dana-farber.org/for-patients-and-families/care-and-treatment/support-services-and-amenities/nutrition-services/managing-cancer-side-effects
      (4) Planning Healthy Meals (Dana-Farber Cancer Institute): www.dana-farber.org/for-patients-and-families/care-and-treatment/support-services-and-amenities/nutrition-services/meal-planning
9. Survivorship
   a) The World Cancer Research Fund and American Institute for Cancer Research (2018) partnered with other organizations to evaluate the available evidence on cancer prevention to create a comprehensive report that includes diet recommendations for cancer prevention.
   b) The report recommended the following dietary measures for cancer prevention, which are applicable to cancer survivors (World Cancer Research Fund & American Institute for Cancer Research, 2018).
      (1) Healthy weight: Overweight and obesity are risk factors for different types of cancers, including but not limited to colorectal, breast, endometrial, and esophageal cancer.

(2) Regular physical activity: Including physical activity regularly can help ensure a healthy body weight.

(3) Diet rich in whole grains, vegetables, fruits, and beans: A diet rich in fruits, vegetables, beans, and whole grains may help maintain a healthy body weight and supplies vital nutrients.

(4) Limitation of consumption of fast-foods and other processed foods high in fat, starches, or sugars: Fast-food is a cause of overweight and obesity, and processed foods lack important nutrients.

(5) Limitation of consumption of red and processed meat: Intake of red meat and processed meat may increase risk of developing colorectal cancer.

(6) Limitation of consumption of sugar-sweetened drinks: Intake of sugar-sweetened drinks can cause weight gain, overweight, and obesity.

(7) Limitation of alcohol consumption: Alcohol increases the risk for many cancers, including but not limited to liver, colorectal, and mouth cancers.

(8) Avoidance of supplements for cancer prevention: Evidence is inconsistent regarding the use of high-dose supplements and reducing cancer risk. Most individuals can get all the nutrients they need from food.

(9) For mothers, breastfeeding if possible: Breastfeeding helps protect mothers against breast cancer, and breastfed babies have a lower risk of overweight and obesity.

(10) After a cancer diagnosis, adherence to American Institute for Cancer Research recommendations if possible: Following the cancer prevention recommendations may improve survival and reduce the risk of developing other health conditions or new primary cancers.

10. Patient, caregiver, and family education: Numerous resources are available to help patients with cancer achieve better nutrition and maintain a healthy diet.

a) Websites

(1) Academy of Nutrition and Dietetics: www.eatright.org; evidence-based nutrition recommendations, recipes, journal articles on nutrition-related studies, and a database of nutrition professionals for patient referral as needed

(2) American Cancer Society: www.cancer.org); tips for symptom management of nutrition-related problems

(3) American Institute for Cancer Research: www.aicr.org; recipes, information for cancer prevention and cancer survivors, serving size finder, and research updates

(4) ELLICSR: Health, Wellness, and Cancer Survivorship Centre: www.ellicsr.ca/en/clinics _programs/ellicsr_kitchen; recipes, information, and videos to support people touched by cancer

(5) National Center for Complementary and Integrative Health: http://nccam.nih.gov; evidence-based information about complementary and integrative health, including herbs and supplements

(6) NCI: www.cancer.gov; includes "Eating Hints: Before, During, and After Cancer Treatment," recipes and nutrition for patients with cancer (PDQ® documents with versions for patients and healthcare professionals), nutritional implications of cancer therapies, nutritional suggestions for symptom management, and a table on herbs and possible food–drug interactions

(7) Oncology Nutrition Dietetic Practice Group of the American Dietetic Association: www.oncologynutrition.org; evidence-based research information and nutrition tips

(8) Princess Margaret Cancer Foundation: https://thepmcf.ca/goesdowneasy/index.html; recipes and common challenges

(9) Support for People with Oral and Head and Neck Cancer: www.spohnc.org; patient-friendly website offering support to those with oral, head, or neck cancer. Patients are able to order educational materials free of charge and seek additional information about available clinical trials and current press releases related to their own cancer diagnosis.

b) Cookbooks

(1) Besser, J. (2016). *New Healthy Eating Cookbook: A Celebration of Food, Friends, and Healthy Living.* American Cancer Society.

(2) Bloch, A., Cassileth, B.R., Holmes, M.D., & Thomson, C.A. (Eds.). (2004). *Eating Well, Staying Well During and After Cancer.* American Cancer Society.

(3) Clegg, H., & Miletello, G. (2006). *Well Through Cancer: Easy Recipes and Recommendations During and After Treatment.* Favorite Recipes Press.

(4) Eldridge, B., & Hamilton, K. (2004). *Management of Nutrition Impact Symptoms in Cancer and Educational Handouts.* American Dietetic Association.

(5) Ghosh, K., Carson, L., & Cohen, E. (2011). *Betty Crocker Living With Cancer Cookbook.* John Wiley & Sons.

(6) Weihofen, D.L., Robbins, J., & Sullivan, P.A. (2002). *Easy-to-Swallow, Easy-to-Chew Cookbook: Over 150 Tasty and Nutritious Recipes for People Who Have Difficulty Swallowing.* John Wiley and Sons.

(7) Wilson, J.R. (2003). *I-Can't-Chew-Cookbook: Delicious Soft-Diet Recipes for People With Chewing, Swallowing, or Dry-Mouth Disorders.* Hunter House.

References

Academy of Nutrition and Dietetics. (n.d.-a). ONC: Nutrition status and outcomes in adult oncology patients (2013). https://www.andeal.org/topic.cfm?menu=5291&cat=4957

Academy of Nutrition and Dietetics. (n.d.-b). Recommendations summary: ONC: Oncology malnutrition screening tools for adult oncology patients 2013. https://www.andeal.org/template.cfm?template=guide_summary&key=4185

Academy of Nutrition and Dietetics. (2017). *Abridged nutrition care process terminology (NCPT) reference manual: Standardized terminology for the nutrition care process.* Author.

Álvaro Sanz, E., Garrido Siles, M., Rey Fernández, L., Villatoro Roldán, R., Rueda Domínguez, A., & Abilés, J. (2019). Nutritional risk and malnutrition rates at diagnosis of cancer in patients treated in outpatient settings: Early intervention protocol. *Nutrition, 57,* 148–153. https://doi.org/10.1016/j.nut.2018.05.021

American Cancer Society. (2018). *Nutrition for the person with cancer during treatment: A guide for patients and families.* https://www.cancer.org/content/dam/cancer-org/cancer-control/en/booklets-flyers/nutrition-for-the-patient-with-cancer-during-treatment.pdf

Arends, J., Bachmann, P., Baracos, V., Barthelemy, N., Bertz, H., Bozzetti, F., ... Preiser, J. (2017). ESPEN guidelines on nutrition in cancer patients. *Clinical Nutrition, 36,* 11–48. https://doi.org/10.1016/j.clnu.2016.07.015

Arribas, L., Hurtós, L., José Sendrós, M., Peiró, I., Salleras, N., Fort, E., & Sánchez-Migallón, J.M. (2017). NUTRISCORE: A new nutritional screening tool for oncological outpatients. *Nutrition, 33,* 297–303. https://doi.org/10.1016/j.nut.2016.07.015

Ayers, P., Guenter, P., Holcombe, B., & Plogsted, S. (Eds.). (2014). *A.S.P.E.N. parenteral nutrition handbook* (2nd ed.). American Society for Parenteral and Enteral Nutrition.

Berry, A.J. (2014). Pancreatic enzyme replacement therapy during pancreatic insufficiency. *Nutrition in Clinical Practice, 29,* 312–321. https://doi.org/10.1177/0884533614527773

Bharadwaj, S., Ginoya, S., Tandon, P., Gohel, T.D., Guirguis, J., Vallabh, H., ... Hanouneh, I. (2016). Malnutrition: Laboratory markers vs. nutritional assessment. *Gastroenterology Report, 4,* 272–280. https://doi.org/10.1093/gastro/gow013

Bischoff, S., Austin, P., Boeykens, K., Chourdakis, M., Cuerda, C., Jonkers-Schuitema, C., ... Pironi, L. (2020). ESPEN guideline on home enteral nutrition. *Clinical Nutrition, 39,* 5–22. https://doi.org/10.1016/j.clnu.2019.04.022

Boland, K., Solanki, D., & O'Hanlon, C. (2013, November). *IrSPEN Guideline document no. 1: Prevention and treatment of refeeding syndrome in the acute care setting.* https://www.irspen.ie/wp-content/uploads/2014/10/IrSPEN_Guideline_Document_No1.pdf

Bossi, P., Antonuzzo, A., Cherny, N.I., Rosengarten, O., Pernot, S., Trippa, F., ... Ripamonti, C.I. (2018). Diarrhoea in adult cancer patients: ESMO Clinical Practice Guidelines. *Annals of Oncology, 29*(Suppl. 4), iv126–iv142. https://doi.org/10.1093/annonc/mdy145

Boullata, J., Carrera, A.L., Harvey, L., Escuro, A.A., Hudson, L., Mays, A., ... Guenter, P. (2017). ASPEN safe practices for enteral nutrition therapy. *Journal of Parenteral and Enteral Nutrition, 41,* 15–103. https://doi.org/10.1177/0148607116673053

British Association for Parenteral and Enteral Nutrition. (2018). The 'MUST' toolkit. https://www.bapen.org.uk/screening-and-must/must/must-toolkit

Caccialanza, R., Pedrazzoli, P., Cereda, E., Gavazzi, C., Pinto, C., Paccagnella, A., ... Zagonel, V. (2016). Nutritional support in cancer patients: A position paper from the Italian Society of Medical Oncology (AIOM) and the Italian Society of Artificial Nutrition and Metabolism (SINPE). *Journal of Cancer, 7,* 131–135. https://doi.org/10.7150/jca.13818

Canadian Cancer Society. (2014). *Eating well when you have cancer.* http://www.procure.ca/wp-content/uploads/EN_Bien_manger_durant_un_cancer.pdf

Canadian Cancer Society. (2018). *Radiation therapy: A guide for people with cancer.* https://www.cancer.ca/~/media/cancer.ca/CW/publications/Radiation%20therapy/32056-1-NO.pdf

Canadian Malnutrition Task Force. (2014, March). *Canadian nutrition screening tool (CNST).* http://nutritioncareincanada.ca/sites/default/uploads/files/CNST.pdf

Canadian Malnutrition Task Force. (2017, April). Subjective global assessment form. http://nutritioncareincanada.ca/sites/default/uploads/files/SGA%20Tool%20EN%20colour_2017(1).pdf

Cancer Care Ontario. (2010, August). *Algorithm: Nausea and vomiting in adults with cancer: Screening and assessment.* https://www.cancercareontario.ca/system/files_force/symptoms/CCONauseaVomitAlgorithm.pdf

Cancer Care Ontario. (2012a). *Algorithm: Constipation symptoms in adults with cancer.* https://www.cancercareontario.ca/system/files_force/symptoms/CCOConstipationAlgorithm.pdf

Cancer Care Ontario. (2012b). *Algorithm: Diarrhea symptoms in adults with cancer.* https://www.cancercareontario.ca/system/files_force/symptoms/CCODiarrheaAlgorithm.pdf

Cancer Care Ontario. (2012c). *Algorithm: Dysgeusia in adults with cancer.* https://www.cancercareontario.ca/system/files_force/symptoms/CCOOralDysgeusiaAlgorithm.pdf

Cancer Care Ontario. (2012d). *Algorithm: Intra-oral infections in adults with cancer.* https://www.cancercareontario.ca/system/files_force/symptoms/CCOOralInfectionsAlgorithm.pdf

Cancer Care Ontario. (2012e). *Algorithm: Loss of appetite in adults with cancer: Screening and Assessment.* https://www.cancercareontario.ca/system/files_force/symptoms/CCOAppetiteAlgorithm.pdf

Cancer Care Ontario. (2012f). *Algorithm: Mucositis in adults with cancer: Screening and assessment.* https://www.cancercareontario.ca/system/files_force/symptoms/CCOOralMucositisAlgorithm.pdf

Cancer Care Ontario. (2012g). *Algorithm: Xerostomia in adults with cancer: Screening and assessment.* https://www.cancercareontario.ca/system/files_force/symptoms/CCOOralXerostomiaAlgorithm.pdf

Cederholm, T., Jensen, G.L., Correia, M.I.T.D., Gonzalez, M.C., Fukushima, R., Higashiguchi, T., ... Compher, C. (2019). GLIM criteria for the diagnosis of malnutrition—A consensus report from the global clinical nutrition community. *Clinical Nutrition, 38,* 1–9. https://doi.org/10.1016/j.clnu.2018.08.002

De Felice, F., de Vicentiis, M., Luzzi, V., Magliulo, G., Tombolini, M., Ruopolo, G., & Polimeni, A. (2018). Late radiation-associated dysphagia in head and neck cancer patients: Evidence, research and management. *Oral Oncology, 77,* 125–130. https://doi.org/10.1016/j.oraloncology.2017.12.021

Dietitians of Canada. (2018). *Dietitians in cancer care* [Brochure]. Author. https://www.dietitians.ca/DietitiansOfCanada/media/Documents/Resources/Dietitians-in-Cancer-Care-bilingual-handout.pdf

Doley, J., & Phillips, W. (2017). Overview of enteral nutrition. In C.M. Mueller, L.M. Lord, M. Marian, S.A. McClave, & S.J. Miller (Eds.), *The ASPEN adult nutrition support core curriculum* (3rd ed., pp. 213–225). American Society for Parenteral and Enteral Nutrition.

Escamilla, D.M., & Jarrett, P. (2016). The impact of weight loss on patients with cancer. *Nursing Times, 112,* 20–22.

Fang, J.C., & Kinikini, M. (2017). Enteral access devices. In C.M. Mueller, L.M. Lord, M. Marian, S.A. McClave, & S.J. Miller (Eds.), *The ASPEN adult nutrition support core curriculum* (3rd ed., pp. 251–264). American Society for Parenteral and Enteral Nutrition.

Fearon, K., Strasser, F., Anker, S.D., Bosaeus, I., Bruera, E., Fainsinger, R.L., ... Baracos, V.E. (2011). Definition and classification of cancer cachexia: An international consensus. *Lancet Oncology, 12,* 489–495. https://doi.org/10.1016/s1470-2045(10)70218-7

Felder, S., Lechtenboehmer, C., Bally, M., Fehr, R., Deiss, M., Faessler, L., ... Schuetz, P. (2015). Association of nutritional risk and adverse medical outcomes across different medical inpatient populations. *Nutrition, 31*, 1385–1393. https://doi.org/10.1016/j.nut.2015.06.007

Ferguson, M., Capra, S., Bauer, J., & Banks, M. (1999). Development of a valid and reliable malnutrition screening tool for adult acute hospital patients. *Nutrition, 15*, 458–464. https://doi.org/10.1016/s0899-9007(99)00084-2

Friedli, N., Stanga, Z., Culkin, A., Crook, M., Laviano, A., Sobotka, L., ... Schuetz, P. (2018). Management and prevention of refeeding syndrome in medical inpatients: An evidence-based and consensus-supported algorithm. *Nutrition, 47*, 13–20. https://doi.org/10.1016/j.nut.2017.09.007

Hesketh, P.J., Kris, M.G., Basch, E., Bholke, K., Barbour, S.Y., Clark-Snow, R.A., ... Lyman, G.H. (2017). Antiemetics: American Society of Clinical Oncology guidelines update. *Journal of Clinical Oncology, 35*, 3240–3261. https://doi.org/10.1200/jco.2017.74.4789

Kaderbay, A., Atallah, I., Fontaine, E., Chobert-Bakouline, M., Schmitt, S., Mitariu, P., & Righini, C.A. (2018). Malnutrition and refeeding syndrome prevention in head and neck cancer patients: From theory to clinical application. *European Archives of Oto-Rhino-Laryngology, 275*, 1049–1058. https://doi.org/10.1007/s00405-018-4935-2

Kondrup, J., Allison, S.P., Elia, M., Vellas, B., & Plauth, M. (2003). ESPEN guidelines for nutrition screening 2002. *Clinical Nutrition, 22*, 415–421. https://doi.org/10.1016/s0261-5614(03)00098-0

Kumpf, V. (2017). Complications of parenteral nutrition. In C.M Mueller, L.M. Lord, M. Marian, S.A. McClave, & S.J. Miller (Eds.), *The ASPEN adult nutrition support core curriculum* (3rd ed., pp. 345–360). American Society for Parenteral and Enteral Nutrition.

Larkin, P.J., Cherny, N.I., La Carpia, D., Guglielmo, M., Ostgathe, C., Scotté, F., & Ripamonti, C.I. (2018). Diagnosis, assessment and management of constipation in advanced cancer: ESMO clinical practice guidelines. *Annals of Oncology, 29*(Suppl. 4), iv111–iv125. https://doi.org/10.1093/annonc/mdy148

Levin, R. (2013). Nutrition risk screening and assessment of the oncology patient. In M. Lesser, N. Ledesma, S. Bergerson, & E. Trujillo (Eds.), In *Oncology nutrition for clinical practice* (pp. 25–32). Oncology Nutrition Dietetic Practice Group of the Academy of Nutrition and Dietetics.

Lis, C.G., Gupta, D., Lammersfeld, C.A., Markman, M., & Vashi, P.G. (2012). Role of nutritional status in predicting quality of life outcomes in cancer—A systematic review of the epidemiological literature. *Nutrition Journal, 11*, 27. https://doi.org/10.1186/1475-2891-11-27

Malone, A., Seres, D., & Lord, M.M. (2017). Complications of enteral nutrition. In C.M Mueller, L.M. Lord, M. Marian, S.A. McClave, & S.J. Miller (Eds.), *The ASPEN adult nutrition support core curriculum* (3rd ed., pp. 265–296). American Society for Parenteral and Enteral Nutrition.

Marcason, W. (2017). Should albumin and prealbumin be used as indicators for malnutrition? *Journal of the Academy of Nutrition and Dietetics, 117*, 1144. https://doi.org/10.1016/j.jand.2017.04.018

Marian, M., Mattox, M., & Williams, V. (2017). Cancer. In C.M. Mueller, L.M. Lord, M. Marian, S.A. McClave, & S.J. Miller (Eds.), *The ASPEN adult nutrition support core curriculum* (3rd ed., pp. 651–674). American Society for Parenteral and Enteral Nutrition.

McCray, S. (2016). Refeeding the malnourished patient: Lessons learned. *Practical Gastroenterology, 155*, 56–66. https://med.virginia.edu/ginutrition/wp-content/uploads/sites/199/2014/06/Parrish-September-16.pdf

Mirtallo, J.M. (2017). Overview of parenteral nutrition. In C.M Mueller, L.M Lord, M. Marian, S.A. McClave, & S.J. Miller (Eds.), *The ASPEN adult nutrition support core curriculum* (3rd ed., pp. 285–296). American Society for Parenteral and Enteral Nutrition.

Munankarmi, D. (2017). Management of dysgeusia related to cancer: A systematic review. *Journal of Lumbini Medical College, 5*, 3–12. https://doi.org/10.22502/jlmc.v5i1.110

National Cancer Institute. (2019). Complementary and alternative medicine. https://www.cancer.gov/about-cancer/treatment/cam

National Collaborating Centre for Acute Care. (2006). *Nutrition support for adults: Oral nutrition support, enteral tube feeding and parenteral nutri-*

tion. https://www.nice.org.uk/guidance/cg32/evidence/full-guideline-pdf-194889853

National Comprehensive Cancer Network. (2020). *NCCN Clinical Practice Guidelines in Oncology (NCCN Guidelines®): Cancer-related fatigue* [v.1.2020]. https://www.nccn.org/professionals/physician_gls/pdf/fatigue.pdf

Ottery, F.D. (2020). Scored patient-generated subjective global assessment (PG-SGA) [v4.3.2020]. http://pt-global.org/?page_id=6098

Peterson, D.E., Boers-Doets, C.B., Bensadoun, R.J., & Herrstedt, J. (2015). Management of oral and gastrointestinal mucosal injury: ESMO clinical practice guidelines for diagnosis, treatment, and follow-up. *Annals of Oncology, 26*(Suppl. 5), v139–v151. https://doi.org/10.1093/annonc/mdv202

Queensland Health. (2017, May). *Validated malnutrition screening and assessment tools: Comparison guide.* https://www.health.qld.gov.au/__data/assets/pdf_file/0021/152454/hphe_scrn_tools.pdf

Roila, F., Molassiotis, A., Herrstedt, J., Aapro, M., Gralla, R.J., Burera, E., ... van der Wetening, M. (2016). 2016 MASCC and ESMO guideline update for the prevention of chemotherapy- and radiotherapy-induced nausea and vomiting and of nausea and vomiting in advanced cancer patients. *Annals of Oncology, 27*(Suppl. 5), v119–v133. https://doi.org/10.1093/annonc/mdw270

U.S. Department of Health and Human Services & U.S. Department of Agriculture. (2015). *2015–2020 dietary guidelines for Americans* (8th ed.). https://health.gov/our-work/food-nutrition/2015-2020-dietary-guidelines/guidelines

Virizuela, J.A., Camblor-Álvarez, M., Luengo-Pérez, L.M., Grande, E., Álvarez-Hernández, J., Sendrós-Madrono, M.J., ... Ocón-Bretón, M.J. (2018). Nutritional support and parenteral nutrition in cancer patients: An expert consensus report. *Clinical and Translational Oncology, 20*, 619–629. https://doi.org/10.1007/s12094-017-1757-4

White, J.V., Guenter, P., Jensen, G., Malone, A., & Schofield, M. (2012). Consensus statement of the Academy of Nutrition and Dietetics/American Society for Parenteral and Enteral Nutrition: Characteristics recommended for the identification and documentation of adult malnutrition (undernutrition). *Journal of the Academy of Nutrition and Dietetics, 112*, 730–738. https://doi.org/10.1016/j.jand.2012.03.012

World Cancer Research Fund & American Institute for Cancer Research. (2018). *Diet, nutrition, physical activity and cancer: A global perspective: The third expert report.* https://www.wcrf.org/dietandcancer/resources-and-toolkit

Worthington, P., Balint, J., Bechtold, M., Bingham, A., Chan, L.-N., Durfee, S., ... Holcombe, B. (2017). When is parenteral nutrition appropriate? *Journal of Parenteral and Enteral Nutrition, 41*, 324–377. https://doi.org/10.1177/0148607117695251

I. Neutropenia

1. Overview
   a) Neutropenia is based on laboratory test results that indicate a decrease in the number of neutrophils in a blood specimen (NCI CTEP, 2017).
   b) Myelotoxicity, including neutropenia, is one of the most common treatment-related adverse events for patients receiving systemic antineoplastic therapy or RT to bone marrow–producing regions (Kurtin, 2012).
   c) Neutrophils comprise the proportion of white blood cells (WBCs) that are immature (banded neutrophils) and mature (segmented neutrophils) (O'Leary, 2015).
      (1) The absolute neutrophil count (ANC) represents the number of mature WBCs in circulation.

(2) ANC is calculated by multiplying the WBC count by the percentage of bands and segmented neutrophils and dividing by 100.

d) Neutropenia is generally defined as an ANC less than 1,500 cells/mm^3. Profound neutropenia (grade 4) usually is defined as an ANC less than 500 cells/mm^3, and this places the patient at great risk for infection (Aapro et al., 2011; NCI CTEP, 2017).

(1) Grade 1 neutropenia is defined as an ANC less than 8,000–1,500/mm^3.

(2) Grade 2 neutropenia is defined as an ANC less than 1,500–1,000/mm^3.

(3) Grade 3 neutropenia is defined as an ANC less than 1,000–500/mm^3.

(4) Grade 4 neutropenia is defined as an ANC less than 500/mm^3.

2. Pathophysiology

a) Neutrophils and monocytes stem from the colony-forming unit granulocyte-macrophage progenitor cell.

(1) The earliest identifiable cell of the neutrophil lineage is the myeloblast.

(2) Differentiation from a myeloblast to a segmented neutrophil takes 7–11 days. Healthy adult bone marrow produces approximately 100 billion neutrophils per kilogram each day (Roquiz, Al Diffalha, & Kini, 2016).

(3) A number of WBC subtypes are referred to as granulocytes, neutrophils being one. Neutrophils account for 60% of circulating WBCs and are the first responders to infection by bacteria, viruses, and other pathogens (O'Leary, 2015).

b) The bone marrow is the primary source for development of the components of blood (hematopoiesis). Hematopoiesis occurs primarily in the axial skeleton, with the majority of production taking place in the pelvis (70%–72%). Long bones such as the femurs, skull, sternum, ribs, and vertebral bodies also produce blood cells (Gatter & Brown, 2014).

c) Neutrophils divide rapidly and are susceptible to the cytotoxic effects of chemotherapy. Chemotherapy in combination with RT may also damage the bone marrow microenvironment, including the stroma and cytokine milieu (Carlesso & Cardoso, 2010).

(1) There are several potential mechanisms for RT effects on the bone marrow (Prabhu, Cassidy, & Landry, 2015).

(a) Direct damage to hematopoietic stem cells and reduction in their number and function

(b) Changes to the surrounding bone marrow stroma and microenvironment

(c) Injury to ancillary cell populations that serve to regulate the hematopoietic process

(2) Side effects and sequelae of RT are generally the result of the effect of radiation on healthy tissues. Early side effects are usually exhibited first by tissues with rapidly proliferating cells (e.g., gastrointestinal mucosa, bone marrow, skin). These tissues are considered acute-responding tissues (Ma, 2012).

d) Risk factors and impacting factors

(1) Patient related (Lyman et al., 2011; O'Leary, 2015)

(a) Advanced age

(b) Female sex

(c) Poor performance status

(d) Poor nutritional status

(e) Comorbid conditions

(f) Poor treatment health (previous neutropenia or decreased WBC count, hemoglobin, or serum albumin)

(2) Previous treatment: Factors associated with a high risk for chemotherapy-induced myelotoxicity include a previous history of radiation exposure (Kurtin, 2012).

(3) Concurrent treatment

(a) Any treatment regimen combining chemotherapy and RT must take into account the potential for increased dose-limiting marrow suppression (Mauch et al., 1995).

(b) With standard fields for pelvic irradiation, large areas of the bone marrow are exposed to radiation, causing a decrease in hematopoietic stem cells, which has the potential to cause increased toxicity, especially when given in conjunction with chemotherapy.

i. Some examples of concurrent chemotherapy drugs are the following. Concurrent cisplatin is indicated for cervical cancer and some high-risk endometrial cancer. 5-Fluorouracil and mitomycin are used for anal cancer. Capecitabine is used concurrently for rectal cancer.

ii. Extended-field radiation to treat para-aortic or common iliac nodes along with concurrent chemotherapy causes high rates of acute hematologic toxicity in patients with gynecologic cancers (Nicholas et al., 2017).

(4) Radiation field

(a) It has been recognized for decades that the radiation dose, site, and tissue volume all affect the acute response of bone marrow to therapy (Mauch et al., 1995).

i. When small radiation fields cover 10%–15% of the bone marrow, the unexposed bone marrow responds by increasing its population of progenitor cells to meet the demands for hematopoiesis.

ii. Treatment-limiting myelosuppression is rarely seen unless large areas containing a substantial portion of marrow are within the radiation fields. Approximately 40% of active bone marrow is in the pelvis.

(b) Radiation to bone marrow–producing regions (pelvis, ribs, sternum, skull, metaphyses of the long bones) may cause prolonged cytopenias (Metcalf, 2010).

(c) The effects on bone marrow are most likely to occur with large-volume irradiation of the pelvis or spine, as the primary site of functional bone marrow is the pelvis and vertebrae, which account for approximately 60% of total volume (Prabhu et al., 2015).

(d) Patients at the highest risk for developing cytopenias are those receiving concurrent chemoradiation, TBI, extended field (whole abdomen) radiation, and radiation to the spleen.
   i. Most radiation fields are designed to limit the amount of bone marrow exposed.
   ii. It may be necessary to reirradiate marrow-producing areas in high-risk patients, such as those who have been heavily pretreated (chemotherapy and/or RT) and those who have bony metastases that require RT for pain management (Dest, 2018).

(e) RT techniques for pelvic malignancy vary and include whole pelvis, low pelvis, organ-only, 3DCRT, IMRT, or brachytherapy. Hematologic toxicity may be associated with these types of therapies on the pelvis (Nicholas et al., 2017).

(f) Mell et al. (2017) reported a lower incidence of grade 3 or higher neutropenia in patients with cervical cancer treated with bone marrow–sparing IMRT.

(5) Radium-223

(a) Radium-223 dichloride is a bone-targeted, alpha-emitting radiopharmaceutical approved for the treatment of symptomatic bone metastases. When detected early in treatment, the impact of hematologic adverse effects can be minimized with appropriate precautions (Jacene, Gomella, Yu, & Rohren, 2018).

(b) For patients treated with radium-223 therapy, grade 3–4 neutropenia rates were not significantly different from placebo groups, but more neutropenia was observed with radiuim-223 compared to placebo for all grades. Grade 3 febrile neutropenia occurred in less than 1% of participants who received radium-223 (Vogelzang et al., 2017).

3. Incidence and prevalence

a) Myelosuppression occurs following RT when the treatment field involves marrow-producing tissue or with doses greater than 15 Gy. Even very low RT doses—as low as 0.3 Gy—can lead to measurable changes in peripheral blood counts owing to the exquisite radiosensitive nature of these cells (Prabhu et al., 2015).

b) Myelosuppression peaks in the third week of RT and often manifests as aplasia occurring simultaneously in all cell lines, rather than sequentially as seen with chemotherapy. The recovery period is less predictable because RT may be required for several additional weeks after the onset of marrow suppression (Kulkarni, Ghosh, Hauer-Jensen, & Kumar, 2010).

c) The incidence and severity of radiation-induced neutropenia is highly dependent on the volume of active bone marrow irradiated, dose received by that bone marrow, concurrent use of myelosuppressive chemotherapy, and other patient factors, such as age and comorbidities (Deek et al., 2016).

4. Assessment

a) A thorough patient history is important in assessing for the presence or risk of neutropenia (Braden, 2018).

b) Important diagnostic tools for assessing neutropenia include obtaining a complete blood count with differential and the respective ANC (O'Leary, 2015).

c) Physical examination of patients should focus on assessing for signs of infection.
   (1) In patients with decreased neutrophils, the number of mature neutrophils may not be sufficient to mount the response of usual signs of infection.
   (2) The usual objective signs of infection may be muted or absent because of the inhibition of phagocytic cells (Aapro et al., 2011).
      (a) In neutropenic patients, fever is the most common and, perhaps, the only response to infection (O'Leary, 2015).
      (b) Fever may be the only symptom of life-threatening infection.
      (c) Redness, purulence, and edema may be absent in febrile patients who are neutropenic (Adams, 2017).
   (3) The following are most common sites of infection in patients with neutropenia (Camp-Sorrell, 2018).
      (a) Respiratory tract
      (b) Gastrointestinal tract
      (c) Genitourinary tract, including the perineum and anus
      (d) Skin and mucous membranes
   (4) Febrile neutropenia is defined as a single temperature equivalent to 38.3°C (101°F) or

higher orally or 38°C (100.4°F) or higher orally over a one-hour period, along with neutropenia (ANC less than 500/mm³ or ANC less than 1,000/mm³ with a predicted decline to less than 500/mm³ during the next 48 hours) (NCCN, 2019).

    (a) Patients with febrile neutropenia generally present with fever and/or shaking chills.

        i. Low-risk patients may be asymptomatic and found to be neutropenic on routine laboratory evaluation.

        ii. Prompt implementation of institutional guidelines or standing orders for the management of neutropenic fevers, including antibiotic administration, is critical to prevent more serious complications (Kurtin, 2012).

    (b) Patients are at high risk for developing complications of febrile neutropenia related to any of the following factors (NCCN, 2019).

        i. Inpatient status when fever starts

        ii. Clinically unstable

        iii. Significant comorbidity

        iv. Allogeneic HSCT

        v. A prolonged and severe neutropenic episode (ANC less than 100/mm³ for seven days or more)

        vi. Hepatic insufficiency

        vii. Renal insufficiency

        viii. Uncontrolled or progressive cancer

        ix. Pneumonia or other complex infections at clinical presentation

        x. Grade 3–4 mucositis

  (5) When signs of infection are not recognized, patients are at risk for severe infection, which if left untreated, may lead to bacteremia, sepsis, end-organ damage, and death (O'Leary, 2015).

d) Providers should regularly assess for chemotherapy-related and RT-related side effects in the RT setting with patients receiving combined modality therapy. Complete blood cell counts should be evaluated throughout treatment (Gosselin, 2016; Russell, 2016).

5. Management

  a) Collaboration: Nurses collaborate with colleagues from other disciplines to ensure that all patient needs are met (Shaftic, 2017).

  b) Prevention of infection

    (1) Neutropenia predisposes patients to infection.

      (a) The severity and duration of neutropenia, together with host-related factors and secondary effects of the treatment regimen, contribute to the risk of more serious adverse events, including neutropenic fevers and bacteremia (Klastersky, Awada, Paesmans, & Aoun, 2011).

      (b) The risk of infection is associated with the degree and duration of neutropenia. More than 50% of patients with neutropenia can be expected to develop infection (Kyi, Hellmann, Wolchok, Chapman, & Postow, 2014).

      (c) Infections due to invasion and overgrowth of pathogenic microbes increase in frequency and severity as ANC decreases.

      (d) Because the major function of neutrophils is phagocytosis, neutropenia eliminates one of the body's prime defenses against bacterial infection.

    (2) Recommendations for practice include the following (Wilson et al., 2019).

      (a) Adherence to general infection control recommendations

      (b) Antibiotic and antifungal prophylaxis in at-risk patients

      (c) Antiviral prophylaxis in select at-risk patients

      (d) Catheter care bundle for prevention of central line–associated infection

      (e) Chlorhexidine skin prep

      (f) Colony-stimulating factors, including biosimilars, for at-risk patients

      (g) Contact precautions for resistant organisms; environmental interventions

      (h) Hand hygiene with alcohol sanitizer or soap and water

      (i) Influenza, pneumococcal, and meningococcal vaccination

    (3) Standard precautions represent the minimum infection prevention measures that apply to all patient care, regardless of suspected or confirmed infection status, in any healthcare setting. Standard precautions include the following (CDC, 2019a).

      (a) Hand hygiene

      (b) Use of personal protective equipment depending on anticipated exposure

      (c) Respiratory hygiene and cough etiquette

      (d) Safe injection practices

      (e) Safe handling of patient-contaminated equipment or surfaces in patient environment

  c) Monitoring of blood counts

    (1) The frequency of monitoring blood counts for patients at risk for neutropenia receiving RT varies by individual patient risk factors (Dest, 2018).

    (2) Patients undergoing pelvic irradiation with concurrent chemotherapy are monitored with weekly blood counts. For example, RT is held

when neutrophil counts decrease to 500/mm³ (Viswanathan et al., 2014).

(3) A hematologic evaluation should be performed before initiating radium-223 treatment. The required baseline parameters should include an ANC of 1,500/mm³ or more, platelet count of 100,000/mm³ or greater, and hemoglobin levels of 10 g/dl or greater (Dan et al., 2017).

(4) To monitor for possible myelosuppression during treatment, hematologic parameters (particularly hemoglobin, ANC, and platelet count) should be assessed before each intended cycle of radium-223. If ANC values diminish to less than 1,900/mm³ and do not recover within six to eight weeks despite supportive care, radium-223 should be discontinued (Dan et al., 2016).

d) Growth factors

(1) The prophylactic use of colony-stimulating factors can reduce the risk severity and duration of severe neutropenia and febrile neutropenia in adult and pediatric patients. Rather than stimulating the immune system to increase neutrophils, colony-stimulating factors accelerate the maturation of immature neutrophils that are already present (O'Leary, 2015).

(2) Types of colony-stimulating factors include the following (NCCN, 2019; Olsen, LeFebvre, & Brassil, 2019).

 (a) Granulocyte macrophage–colony-stimulating factor: sargramostim

 (b) Granulocyte–colony-stimulating factors
  i. Filgrastim
  ii. Pegfilgrastim

 (c) Biosimilars
  i. Tbo-filgrastim
  ii. Filgrastim-aafi
  iii. Filgrastim-sndz
  iv. Others as they become available

(3) Colony-stimulating factors can be used for the prevention of treatment-related febrile neutropenia. The choice of agent depends on convenience, cost, and the clinical situation (Smith et al., 2015).

(4) Colony-stimulating factors should be started more than 24 hours after chemotherapy and not within 24 hours before chemotherapy (NCCN, 2019).

(5) Use of colony-stimulating factors with RT should be considered carefully.

 (a) Colony-stimulating factors should be avoided in patients receiving concomitant chemotherapy and RT, particularly involving the mediastinum (Smith et al., 2015).

  i. Use of colony-stimulating factors has been associated with a higher incidence of thrombocytopenia and other complications when given with concurrent chemoradiation for head and neck or lung cancer.

  ii. In the absence of chemotherapy, therapeutic use of colony-stimulating factors may be considered in patients receiving RT alone if prolonged delays secondary to neutropenia are expected (Smith et al., 2015).

 (b) Growth factors supporting the development of all hematologic cell lines are seldom needed when RT is used as a single modality.

 (c) In combined modality therapy, growth factors are more commonly part of treatment regimens because of the increased risk of pancytopenia (Dest, 2018).

 (d) Use of hematopoietic growth factors has not been well defined for use in radiation-induced myelosuppression (Shelton, 2016).

 (e) No high-level evidence suggests that afebrile or asymptomatic neutropenia are contraindications for RT, but use of RT can preclude the ability to administer colony-stimulating factors, especially in the setting of mediastinal RT with concurrent chemotherapy (Prabhu et al., 2015).

e) Diet

(1) Current research suggests that dietary restrictions beyond customary food safety practices are unlikely to decrease the risk of infection. Safety practices include avoiding the following foods (U.S. Department of Agriculture & U.S. FDA, 2011).

 (a) Uncooked meats
 (b) Uncooked seafood
 (c) Uncooked eggs
 (d) Unwashed fruits and vegetables

(2) The American Cancer Society (2019) supports a change in practice focus that moves away from a traditional neutropenic diet to principles of safe food handling and patient education about food preparation and choices.

f) Hygiene

(1) One of the simplest and most effective interventions for reducing the risk of infection is hand hygiene (O'Leary, 2015).

(2) Oral care is an important aspect of caring for patients with neutropenia (Friefeld et al., 2011; Rogers, 2014).

(3) Hygiene should focus on preventing trauma to the skin and mucous membranes (Olsen et al., 2019).

g) Environment: Recommendations to prevent infection in the home for immunosuppressed patients and caregivers include the following (Thom, Kleinberg, & Roghmann, 2013).

   (1) Avoiding gardening or direct contact with soil or plants
   (2) Limiting contact with domestic pets and maintaining pet health
   (3) Avoiding contact with animal saliva, urine, and feces
   (4) Avoiding contact with exotic pets and wild animals

h) Vaccines

   (1) Clinicians should consider vaccination for influenza and pneumonia in patients with cancer (CDC, 2019b).
   (2) Patients with hematologic or solid tumor malignancies should receive an inactivated influenza vaccine annually. Pneumococcal vaccination is also recommended. All household members should be up to date with vaccines (NCCN, 2020).
   (3) Ideally, clinicians should administer vaccines to patients before initiation of cancer treatment (at least two weeks before cancer treatment), which includes chemotherapy, surgery, treatment with immunosuppressant drugs, RT, or splenectomy.

      (a) Inactivated or recombinant vaccines should be administered four weeks or more before cancer treatment and three months or more after chemotherapy. The inactivated influenza vaccine can be administered during cancer treatment.
      (b) Live viral vaccines can be administered four weeks or more before cancer treatment and three months or more after chemotherapy (NCCN, 2020).

   (4) Neutropenic patients should avoid contact with people who have been vaccinated with a live vaccine within the past 30 days (Olsen et al., 2019).

6. Patient, caregiver, and family education

   a) The best strategy for overall management of cancer- or treatment-induced neutropenia is prevention of infection.

      (1) Patients who are at risk for neutropenia or are predicted to develop it at any level are taught methods of preventing infection and how to recognize the early symptoms to ensure prompt, aggressive management of any infection that may occur.
      (2) Common infection prevention practices with a high level of scientific evidence include avoiding infection risks (e.g., avoiding exposures, good hygiene, food safety) and controlling environmental risks (e.g., hand hygiene, influenza vaccination) (Shelton, 2016).

   b) Food safety education for patients with weakened immune systems includes instruction on handling food safely, preventing cross-contamination when preparing food, and cooking foods to the proper temperature (American Cancer Society, 2019).

   c) Protective measures for neutropenic patients include the following (Olsen et al., 2019).

      (1) Reporting fever, chills, and other signs and symptoms of infection at onset
      (2) Maintaining personal hygiene
      (3) Washing hands frequently with soap and water or an antiseptic hand rub
      (4) Daily bathing
      (5) Avoiding activities that compromise skin integrity
      (6) Wearing gloves when working in the garden
      (7) Performing frequent oral assessment and care
      (8) Cleansing the perineal area from front to back after toileting
      (9) Avoiding exposure to people who are experiencing signs and symptoms of contagious conditions

References

Aapro, M.S., Bohlius, J., Cameron, D.A., Dal Lago, L., Donnelly, J.P., Kearney, N., ... Zielinski, C. (2011). 2010 update of EORTC guidelines for the use of granulocyte-colony stimulating factor to reduce the incidence of chemotherapy-induced febrile neutropenia in adults with lymphoproliferative disorders and solid tumours. *European Journal of Cancer, 47*, 8–22. https://doi.org/10.1016/j.ejca.2010.10.013

Adams, P.L. (2017). Hematologic issues. In J. Eggert (Ed.), *Cancer basics* (2nd ed., pp. 491–504). Oncology Nursing Society.

American Cancer Society. (2019). *Nutrition for the person with cancer during treatment: A guide for patients and families.* Author. https://www.cancer.org/content/dam/CRC/PDF/Public/6711.00.pdf

Braden, C.D. (2018, September 18). Neutropenia. Medscape. https://emedicine.medscape.com/article/204821-overview

Camp-Sorrell, D. (2018). Chemotherapy: Toxicities and management. In C.H. Yarbro, D. Wujcik, & B.H. Gobel (Eds.), *Cancer nursing: Principles and practice* (8th ed., pp. 497–554). Jones and Bartlett Learning.

Carlesso, N., & Cardoso, A.A. (2010). Stem cell regulatory niches and their role in normal and malignant hematopoiesis. *Clinical Opinions in Hematology, 17*, 281–286. https://doi.org/10.1097/moh.0b013e32833a25d8

Centers for Disease Control and Prevention. (2019a). Hand hygiene in healthcare settings. https://www.cdc.gov/handhygiene/index.html

Centers for Disease Control and Prevention. (2019b). Preventing infections in cancer patients. https://www.cdc.gov/cancer/preventinfections/index.htm

Dan, T.D., Doyle, L., Raval, A.J., Pridjlan, A., Gomella, L.G., & Den, R.B. (2016). Dosing, administration, and safety of radium-223: How I do it. *Canadian Journal of Urology International, 23*, 8301–8305. https://www.canjurol.com/abstract.php?ArticleID=&version=1.0&PMID=27347625

Dan, T.D., Eldredge-Hindy, H.B., Hoffman-Censits, J., Lin, J., Kelly, W.K., Gomella, L., ... Den, R.B. (2017). Hematologic toxicity of concurrent administration of radium-223 and next-generation antiandrogen therapies. *American Journal of Clinical Oncology, 40*, 342–347. https://doi.org/10.1097/coc.0000000000000181

Deek, M.P., Benenati, B., Kim, S., Chen, T., Ahmed, I., Zou, W., ... Jabbour, S.K. (2016). Thoracic vertebral body irradiation contributes to acute hematologic toxicity during chemoradiation therapy for non-small cell lung cancer. *International Journal of Radiation Oncology, Biology, Physics, 94,* 147–154. https://doi.org/10.1016/j.ijrobp.2015.09.022

Dest, V.M. (2018). Radiation therapy: Toxicities and management. In C.H. Yarbro, D. Wujcik, & B.H. Gobel (Eds.), *Cancer nursing: Principles and practice* (8th ed., pp. 333–374). Jones and Bartlett Learning.

Friefeld, A.G., Bow, E.J., Sepkowitz, K.A., Boeckh, M.J., Ito, J.I., Mullen, C.A., ... Wingard, J.R. (2011). Executive summary: Clinical practice guideline for the use of antimicrobial agents in neutropenic patients with cancer: 2010 update by the Infectious Diseases Society of America. *Clinical Infectious Diseases, 52,* 427–431. https://doi.org/10.1093/cid/ciq147

Gatter, K., & Brown, D. (2014). *Bone marrow diagnosis: An illustrated guide* (3rd ed.). Wiley-Blackwell.

Gosselin, T.K. (2016). Radiation therapy. In B.H. Gobel, S. Triest-Robertson, & W.H. Vogel (Eds.), *Advanced oncology nursing certification review and resource manual* (2nd ed., pp. 265–292). Oncology Nursing Society.

Jacene, H., Gomella, L., Yu, E.Y., & Rohren, E.M. (2018). Hematologic toxicity from radium-223 therapy for bone metastases in castration-resistant prostate cancer: Risk factors and practical considerations. *Clinical Genitourinary Cancer, 16,* E919–E925. https://doi.org/10.1016/j.clgc.2018.03.007

Klastersky, J., Awada, A., Paesmans, M., & Aoun, M. (2011). Febrile neutropenia: A critical review of the initial management. *Critical Reviews in Oncology/Hematology, 78,* 185–194. https://doi.org/10.1016/j.critrevonc.2010.03.008

Kulkarni, S., Ghosh, S.P., Hauer-Jensen, M., & Kumar, K.S. (2010). Hematological targets of radiation damage. *Current Drug Targets, 11,* 1375–1385. https://doi.org/10.2174/1389450111009011375

Kurtin, S. (2012). Myeloid toxicity of cancer treatment. *Journal of the Advanced Practitioner in Oncology, 3,* 209–223.

Kyi, C., Hellmann, M.D., Wolchok, J.D., Chapman, P.B., & Postow, M.A. (2014). Opportunistic infections in patients treated with immunotherapy for cancer. *Journal for Immunotherapy of Cancer, 2,* 19. https://doi.org/10.1186/2051-1426-2-19

Lyman, G.H., Kuderer, N.M., Crawford, J., Wolff, D.A., Culakova, E., Poniewerski, M.S., & Dale, D.C. (2011). Predicting individual risk of neutropenic complications in patients receiving cancer chemotherapy. *Cancer, 117,* 1917–1927. https://doi.org/10.1002/cncr.25691

Ma, C.-M.C. (2012). The practice of radiation oncology. In R.R. Iwamoto, M.L. Haas, & T.K. Gosselin (Eds.), *Manual for radiation oncology nursing practice and education* (4th ed., pp. 17–28). Oncology Nursing Society.

Mauch, P., Constine, L., Greenberger, J., Knospe, W., Sullivan, J., Liesveid, J., & Deeg, H.J. (1995). Hematopoietic stem cell compartment: Acute and late effects of radiation therapy and chemotherapy. *International Journal of Radiation Oncology, Biology, Physics, 31,* 1319–1339. https://doi.org/10.1016/0360-3016(94)00430-s

Mell, L.K., Sirák, I., Wei, L., Tarnawski, R., Mahantshetty, U., Yashar, C.M., ... Mundt, A.J. (2017). Bone marrow-sparing intensity modulated radiation therapy with concurrent cisplatin for stage IB-IVA cervical cancer: An international multicenter phase II clinical trial (INTERTECC-2). *International Journal of Radiation Oncology, Biology, Physics, 97,* 536–545. https://doi.org/10.1016/j.ijrobp.2016.11.027

Metcalf, D. (2010). The colony-stimulating factors and cancer. *Nature Reviews Cancer, 10,* 425–434. https://doi.org/10.1038/nrc2843

National Cancer Institute Cancer Therapy Evaluation Program. (2017). *Common terminology criteria for adverse events* [v. 5.0]. https://ctep.cancer.gov/protocolDevelopment/electronic_applications/docs/CTCAE_v5_Quick_Reference_5x7.pdf

National Comprehensive Cancer Network. (2019). *NCCN Clinical Practice Guidelines in Oncology (NCCN Guidelines®): Prevention and treatment of cancer-related infections* [v.1.2020]. https://www.nccn.org/professionals//physician_gls/PDF/infections.pdf

National Comprehensive Cancer Network. (2020). *NCCN Clinical Practice Guidelines in Oncology (NCCN Guidelines®): Survivorship* [v.1.2020]. https://www.nccn.org/professionals//physician_gls/PDF/survivorship.pdf

Nicholas, S., Chen, L., Choflet, A., Fader, A., Guss, Z., Hazell, S., ... Viswanathan, A.N. (2017). Pelvic radiation and normal tissue toxicity. *Seminars in Radiation Oncology, 27,* 358–369. https://doi.org/10.1016/j.semradonc.2017.04.010

O'Leary, C. (2015). Neutropenia and infection. In C.G. Brown (Ed.), *A guide to oncology symptom management* (pp. 483–504). Oncology Nursing Society.

Olsen, M.M., LeFebvre, K.B., & Brassil, K.J. (Eds.). (2019). *Chemotherapy and immunotherapy guidelines and recommendations for practice.* Oncology Nursing Society.

Prabhu, R.S., Cassidy, R.J., & Landry, J.C. (2015). Radiation therapy and neutropenia. *Current Problems in Cancer, 39,* 292–296. https://doi.org/10.1016/j.currproblcancer.2015.07.010

Rogers, B.B. (2014). Neutropenia. In D. Camp-Sorrell & R.A. Hawkins (Eds.), *Clinical manual for the oncology advanced practice nurse* (3rd ed., pp. 1027–1036). Oncology Nursing Society.

Roquiz, W., Al Diffalha, S., & Kini, A.R. (2016). Leukocyte development, kinetics, and function. In E.M. Keohane, J.L. Smith, & J.M. Walenga (Eds.), *Rodak's hematology: Clinical principles and applications* (5th ed., pp 149–166). Elsevier Saunders.

Russell, M.L. (2016). Nursing implications of radiation therapy. In J.K. Itano, J.M. Brant, F.A. Conde, & M.G. Saria (Eds.), *Core curriculum for oncology nursing* (5th ed., pp. 226–236). Elsevier.

Shaftic, A.M. (2017). Radiation therapy. In J. Eggert (Ed.), *Cancer basics* (2nd ed., pp. 173–195). Oncology Nursing Society.

Shelton, B.K. (2016). Myelosuppression and second malignancies. In B.H. Gobel, S. Triest-Robertson, & W.H. Vogel (Eds.), *Advanced oncology nursing certification review and resource manual* (2nd ed., pp. 451–490). Oncology Nursing Society.

Smith, T.J., Bohlke, K., Lyman, G.H., Carson, K.R., Crawford, J., Cross, S.J., ... Armitage, J.O. (2015). Recommendations for the use of WBC growth factors: American Society of Clinical Oncology clinical practice update. *Journal of Clinical Oncology, 33,* 3199–3212. https://doi.org/10.1200/jco.2015.62.3488

Thom, K.A., Kleinberg, M., & Roghmann, M.-C. (2013). Infection prevention in the cancer center. *Clinical Infectious Diseases, 57,* 579–585. https://doi.org/10.1093/cid/cit290

U.S. Department of Agriculture & U.S. Food and Drug Administration. (2011). *Food safety for people with cancer.* https://www.fda.gov/media/83710/download

Viswanathan, A.K., Lee, L.J., Eswara, J.R., Horowitz, N.S., Konstantinopoulos, P.A., Mirabeua-Beale, K.L., ... Wo, J.Y. (2014). Complications of pelvic radiation in patients treated for gynecologic malignancies. *Cancer, 24,* 3871–3883. https://doi.org/10.1002/cncr.28849

Vogelzang, N.J., Coleman, R.E., Michalski, J.M., Nilsson, S., O'Sullivan, J.M., Parker, C., ... Sartor, O. (2017). Hematologic safety of radium-223 dichloride: Baseline prognostic factors associated with myelosuppression in the ALSYMPCA trial. *Clinical Genitourinary Cancer, 15,* 42–52.e8. https://doi.org/10.1016/j.clgc.2016.07.027

Wilson, B.J., Ahmed, F., Crannell, C.E., Crego, W., Erb, C.H., Foster, J., ... Zitella, L. (2019, August 26). Symptom interventions: Prevention of infection: General. https://www.ons.org/pep/prevention-infection-general

J. Late effects of treatment

1. Overview
   a) Late effects can occur several months to years after treatment is completed, are usually permanent, and can worsen over time (Hall et al., 2016).
   b) The manifestation of long-term side effects differs depending on the site of treatment.
   c) See site-based sections for information on acute effects of treatment.
2. Brain and CNS

a) Radiation-induced cognitive decline: Radiation-induced cognitive decline has been difficult to study, as neurocognitive dysfunction is mainly seen in the hippocampus, affecting dependent functions of the brain, such as reduced learning and memory capacity, attention span, executive function, processing speed, and motor dexterity (Koontz, 2018; Pinkham, Sanghera, Wall, Dawson, & Whitfield, 2015; Saad & Wang, 2015).

(1) Pathophysiology

(a) Neurogenesis is the process of generating new brain cells.

  i. Neurogenesis occurs within specific regions of the brain or microenvironments, which includes the hippocampal dentate gyrus.

  ii. The hippocampus is the most active area of neurogenesis in humans and may be associated with new memory formation (Pinkham et al., 2015).

  iii. The hippocampus also coordinates learning, consolidation, and retrieval of information.

(b) Several theories may explain the causes of radiation-induced cognitive decline.

  i. Some data suggest that radiation injury in the hippocampus can cause impairment of functions, and it is theorized that as the underlying mechanisms become better understood, molecular targets and pathways can be altered to avoid radiation-induced toxicity (Pinkham et al., 2015; Saad & Wang, 2015).

  ii. Another theory suggests that cerebral white matter is sensitive to effects of RT, resulting in more demyelination and axonal damage in white matter when compared to gray matter.

  iii. Clinical evidence suggests that limited radiation-induced demyelination can cause neurocognitive impairments, including memory loss, decline in executive function, and decline in learning and attention span, with severe damage leading to dementia (Saad & Wang, 2015).

(c) Risk factors: Risk factors can be grouped into four categories: patient, treatment, tumor, and other.

  i. Patient factors that can influence neurocognitive function are age, gender, education, fatigue, depression, anxiety, and baseline cognitive function (Pinkham et al., 2015; Hansen & Roach, 2010).

  ii. Treatment factors include prior craniotomy or cranial radiation, chemotherapy or hormone therapy, and supportive therapies (e.g., opioids, antiepileptics, steroids).

  iii. Seizures, intracranial and extracranial disease burden, and paraneoplastic syndromes are tumor-related factors (Pinkham et al., 2015).

(2) Incidence

(a) The incidence of neurocognitive dysfunction is difficult to quantify because it may be related to disease progression or toxicity from treatment (Pinkham et al., 2015).

(b) Baseline neurocognitive assessment can detect up to 80% of neurocognitive deficits (Day et al., 2016).

(c) In patients receiving RT for brain tumors, more than 80% reported neurocognitive deficits, such as short-term memory loss and decreased mental acuity (Day et al., 2016).

(3) Assessment

(a) A comprehensive physical exam should include a detailed neurologic exam.

(b) Several validated neurocognitive function assessment tools can be used.

  i. The Hopkins Verbal Learning Test–Revised, Trail Making Test parts A and B, and Controlled Oral Word Association Test have been validated and used extensively with patients with brain metastasis (Pinkham et al., 2015).

  ii. The Mini-Mental State Examination, Montreal Cognitive Assessment, and Addenbrooke's Cognitive Examination are also commonly used.

  iii. These tools can be used to test speed and executive function, learning and memory, and verbal fluency (Day et al., 2016).

(c) Subjective assessment of patients is the most common assessment and provides information regarding everyday problems encountered by patients and caregivers.

  i. Day et al. (2016) recommended that the results of subjective measures should be taken with caution but noted the value to clinicians because patients with objective neurocognitive deficits and few subjective deficits may have poor insight into their condition and may not see the need to participate in rehabilitative services.

ii. The Cognitive Functioning Scale contains six items and has been used to measure the frequency of self-reported neurocognitive complaints in multiple studies (Day et al., 2016).

iii. Assessment of the patient may be affected by a multitude of factors, including patient willingness to participate in neurocognitive testing, fatigue, drowsiness, side effects of medications (e.g., steroids, antiepileptics, chemotherapy), or confounding patient conditions such as depression or anxiety (Day et al., 2016; Koontz, 2018).

(4) Documentation: Documentation should be according to facility requirements and standardized documentation sources, such as CTCAE.

(5) Collaborative management

(a) Interventions such as cognitive training can be used in various situations, including individual, in groups, or via computer.

(b) Cognitive training consists of a series or program of structured repeated activities administered on a regular basis.

(c) The goal of cognitive training is to improve, maintain, or restore mental function (Jansen et al., 2019).

(d) Memantine can be used daily during RT and continued for six months post treatment.

(e) Donepezil daily and the use of cognitive rehabilitation can preserve or improve patient's current cognition.

(f) Referral to a geriatrician and social work intervention may be appropriate (Koontz, 2018; Lynch, 2019; Pinkham et al., 2015; Saad & Wang, 2015).

(6) Patient, caregiver, and family education: Education should include the following.

(a) Side effects of therapy and possibility of cognitive decline

(b) Signs of worsening cognition

(c) Homecare services as needed

(d) Home safety measures

b) Radiation necrosis (cerebral)

(1) Pathophysiology

(a) Mechanisms

i. It is hypothesized that radiation necrosis is caused by vascular damage, which leads to an increase in vascular permeability, leading to vasogenic edema and ischemia, thus resulting in cell death.

ii. Immune-mediated mechanisms play a role in radiation necrosis by the pro-

duction of reactive oxygen species causing changes in cellular functions.

iii. These changes lead to the production of hypoxia-inducible factor (HIF-1α).

iv. HIF-1α upregulates the vascular endothelial growth factor (VEGF), which is secreted by astrocytes and endothelial cells (Loganadane et al., 2018).

v. The presence of VEGF exacerbates edema, vascular permeability, microbleeding, and local hypoxia (X. Jiang et al., 2014; Koontz, 2018; Yoritsune et al., 2014).

(b) Risk factors

i. High total dose or high dose per fraction increases risk for radiation necrosis.

ii. Radiation necrosis is usually not seen in standard fractionated whole-brain irradiation.

iii. For patients treated with partial brain irradiation, a direct dose–toxicity relationship exists. RT with higher total dose or dose per fraction increases the likelihood of radiation necrosis (Koontz, 2018).

(2) Incidence

(a) Radiation necrosis is a dose-limiting toxicity of RT to the brain.

(b) Incidence of radiation necrosis for patients receiving hypofractionated RT for brain metastases is estimated to be 10%–15% (Masucci, 2018).

(c) Incidence can be as high as 25%–30% for asymptomatic radiation necrosis found on imaging scan (Loganadane et al., 2018).

(3) Assessment

(a) Radiation necrosis is difficult to diagnose and can be mistaken for tumor progression (Koontz, 2018).

(b) Serial imaging using MRI and magnetic resonance perfusion is recommended and should be evaluated by neuroradiologists.

(c) In rare cases, biopsy may be needed to differentiate between tumor progression or necrosis from RT.

(d) Monitoring for new or worsening symptoms or neurologic deficits is essential.

(4) Documentation: Documentation should adhere to facility requirements and standardized documentation sources, such as CTCAE.

(5) Collaborative management

(a) Radiation necrosis may be managed conservatively with observation if the patient is asymptomatic.

(b) Initial treatment for symptomatic patients includes systemic therapies, such as corticosteroids to reduce cerebral edema for symptom management. Steroids can be tapered as symptoms improve (Loganadane et al., 2018).

(c) The next line of treatment includes systemic treatment with bevacizumab or local interventions, including minimally invasive laser interstitial thermal ablation or surgical resection (Koontz, 2018; Loganadane et al., 2018).

(6) Patient, caregiver, and family education: Education should involve information on side effects of therapy and instruction to contact the healthcare provider for new or worsening neurologic symptoms.

c) Radiation myelopathy of cranial nerves
(1) Pathophysiology
(a) Koontz (2018) noted radiation myelopathy is rare and defined it as, "symptomatic peripheral sensory or motor deficits caused by radiation treatment that results in pain, paresthesia, sensory deficits, paralysis, Brown-Sequard syndrome and bowel/bladder incontinence" (p. 13).

(b) Radiation to the spine causes disruption of the blood–spinal cord barrier as a result of the destruction of vascular endothelial cells, resulting in demyelination and tissue necrosis (C.S. Wong, Fehlings, & Sahgal, 2015).

(c) Risk factors for radiation myelopathy include fractionation size, technique (e.g., SBRT, conventional fractionation with 3DCRT, IMRT), total dose, comorbidities, prior radiation to the spinal cord, and concomitant chemotherapy (Koontz, 2018; C.S. Wong et al., 2015).

(2) Incidence
(a) Radiation myelopathy usually occurs between six months and three years after RT.

(b) Kirkpatrick, van der Kogel, and Schultheiss (2010) analyzed dose–volume data on radiation-induced myelopathy in humans and found that when using conventional fractionation of 1.8–2 Gy per fraction to the full-thickness cord, the estimated risk of myelopathy is less than 1% at 54 Gy and less than 10% at 61 Gy, with a calculated strong dependence on dose per fraction (a/b = 0.87 Gy.)

(c) Reirradiation data suggest partial repair of RT-induced subclinical damage becoming

evident approximately six months after RT and increasing over the next two years.

(d) Reports of myelopathy from SRS to spinal lesions appear rare (less than 1%) when the maximum spinal cord dose is limited to the equivalent of 13 Gy in a single fraction or 20 Gy in three fractions.

(3) Assessment
(a) Radiation myelopathy is a diagnosis of exclusion and is based on clinical and radiographic findings.

(b) Physical examination should include a comprehensive neurologic examination.

(c) Notation should be made for the appearance of signs and symptoms of sensory or motor deficits, loss of function, or pain (Kirkpatrick et al., 2010).

(d) Diagnosis can be confirmed by MRI of the spinal cord, which typically demonstrates areas of low signals on T1-weighted images, high signals on T2, and focal enhancement.

(e) Quantitative MRI techniques, such as apparent diffusion coefficients, magnetization transfer, and diffusion tensor imaging, may provide useful longitudinal, structural, and functional information in the assessment of spinal cord injury after radiation.

(f) PET scans obtained with contrast (fluorodeoxyglucose) show increased activity and uptake in the area of the irradiated spinal cord that is understood to be damaged by irradiation (C.S. Wong et al., 2015).

(4) Collaborative management
(a) There is no effective treatment that can reverse radiation-induced myelopathy.

(b) Medical management includes steroids, pentoxifylline, and hyperbaric oxygen (Koontz, 2018; C.S. Wong et al., 2015).

(c) Patients may require evaluation by urology and pain management.

(d) A bowel management program and referral for home care may be necessary.

(5) Patient, caregiver, and family education
(a) Education includes information on new or worsening neurologic symptoms and pain.

(b) Bowel management regimen should be reviewed.

(c) Clinicians should provide specialized instructions as needed for management of pain and bowel or bladder incontinence (e.g., urinary catheterization, bowel regimen, epidural catheter for pain control).

d) Cranial nerve neuropathies (predominantly visual and auditory)

  (1) Pathophysiology

    (a) Radiation-induced optic neuropathy (RION) can result in permanent partial or complete visual field loss.

      i. RION usually presents with subacute, painless, progressive, and profound vision loss months to years after RT.

      ii. RION may be caused by radiation-induced microangiopathy associated with endothelial cell loss, leading to demyelination in the anterior visual pathway (Doroslovački et al., 2018; W. Wang et al., 2016).

    (b) Radiation-induced sensorineural hearing loss (SNHL) is described as an extensive degeneration of outer hair cells in the organ of Corti and atrophy or damage of the audiovestibular nerve (cranial nerve VIII) (Dinh et al., 2015; Koontz, 2018).

      i. Cochlear fibrosis caused by radiation can also cause progressive of hearing loss several years after treatment (Lambert, Gunn, & Gidley, 2016).

      ii. SNHL is permanent and progressive over time.

      iii. Patients can also experience cataracts and brain stem injury (Zheng et al., 2015).

  (2) Incidence

    (a) RION is rare.

      i. Data obtained from mostly Asian populations showed that risk factors include comorbidities (diabetes mellitus), total radiation dose, female sex, tumor compression on the optic nerve, and chemotherapy.

      ii. The maximum dose point is 54–55 Gy using 1.8–2 Gy fractions, with doses greater than 60 Gy increasing the risk of RION.

      iii. Most cases are diagnosed at approximately two years after treatment (Brecht et al., 2019; Doroslovački et al., 2018).

    (b) SNHL occurs in 27%–95% of patients treated for cancers of the head and neck (Dinh et al., 2015).

      i. A mean dose of 45 Gy to the cochlea is associated with a 30% rate of hearing loss.

      ii. In single fraction radiosurgery, doses less than 4 Gy are associated with lower rates of hearing loss (25% or less) (Koontz, 2018).

      iii. Risk factors include higher dose to the cochlea, chemotherapy (especially concurrent platinum-based regimens), older age, post-irradiation otitis media with effusion, and baseline hearing loss (de Oliveira et al., 2017; Theunissen et al., 2015).

  (3) Assessment

    (a) RION is usually diagnosed based on physical examination to include visual field and visual acuity. Diagnosis also involves gadolinium-enhanced MRI, which shows contrast enhancement of the affected optic nerve on T1-weighted images in the absence of recurrent tumor or other lesions (Brecht et al., 2019).

    (b) SNHL is assessed using pure tone audiometry and speech discrimination.

  (4) Documentation: Documentation should adhere to facility requirements and standardized documentation sources, such as CTCAE.

  (5) Collaborative management

    (a) There is no known effective treatment for RION; however, the use of hyperbaric oxygen, pentoxifylline, steroids, and bevacizumab has been reported in the literature as showing minimal improvement of vision in patients (Doroslovački et al., 2018).

    (b) Because of the loss of high-frequency hearing, SNHL is managed with the placement of cochlear implants, if the damage to cranial nerve VIII is minimal, or an auditory brain stem implant, which bypasses the cochlea and cranial nerve VIII (Koontz, 2018).

  (6) Patient, caregiver, and family education

    (a) Clinicians should provide information regarding support services, including long-term disability and home care.

    (b) Instruction should include components of home safety (e.g., furniture and rug placement, use of assistive devices).

e) Radiation vasculopathy

  (1) Definition

    (a) Radiation vasculopathy is a term used to describe a heterogeneous and poorly defined complex of radiation-induced vessel injury or abnormalities, including carotid stenosis, intracranial stenosis, and vascular anomalies (e.g., cavernous malformations, aneurysms) (Twitchell, Karsy, Guan, Couldwell, & Taussky, 2019).

    (b) Patterns of radiation-induced vascular change are atypical and are dissimilar to vascular changes found with standard ath-

erosclerosis (N.M. Rao, Vitners, & Saver, 2017).

(2) Pathophysiology

    (a) Radiation vasculopathy is characterized by connective tissue proliferation, medial thinning, adventitial fibrosis, and dense hyalinization of the vessel wall.

    (b) The damage to the endothelial cells leads to progressive cellular dysfunction and lack of blood supply, resulting in diminished arterial wall circulation and stenosis.

    (c) The lack of blood supply to the irradiated vessels is associated with extensive collateral vasculature, which is a unique property of irradiated vessels (N.M. Rao et al., 2017).

    (d) Vasculopathy may lead to the development of cavernomas, hemorrhagic and ischemic cerebrovascular accidents, arteriovenous malformation (AVM), hemorrhages, and moyamoya syndrome.

(3) Incidence

    (a) The exact incidence of radiation vasculopathy is unknown.

    (b) The incidence of carotid stenosis within the radiation field is 20%–50% and is dependent on the type of RT technique, age at onset, comorbid atherosclerotic risk factors, and time from RT to evaluation (N.M. Rao et al., 2017).

    (c) Development of modern RT techniques has led to improvement in survival, but an increased incidence of occlusive vasculopathies is now being seen years after initial RT (E.S. Murphy et al., 2015; N.M. Rao et al., 2017).

(4) Assessment

    (a) A physical examination should include a thorough neurologic examination.

    (b) Examination should assess for new onset or worsening of neurologic symptoms, such as headaches, syncope, nausea, numbness, weakness, confusion, dizziness, vomiting, or seizures.

    (c) Radiologic evaluation of vessels with an ultrasound, MRI, or magnetic resonance angiography may reveal greater vessel wall thickness and extensive collateralization of adjacent vessels (N.M. Rao et al., 2017).

    (d) Patients treated for radiation vasculopathy likely have hypercoagulability because of their underlying cancer history.

    (e) Clinicians should obtain coagulation profiles, blood chemistries, liver function tests, and complete blood counts as needed.

(5) Documentation: Documentation should adhere to facility requirements and standardized documentation sources, such as CTCAE.

(6) Collaborative management

    (a) Treatment is aimed at correcting the underlying cause and correction of coagulopathies.

    (b) The treatment guidelines for cerebrovascular accident in patients with radiation vasculopathy have been extrapolated from the management of cerebrovascular accident, which includes tissue plasminogen activator, aspirin, heparin, low-molecular-weight heparin, surgery, embolization, angioplasty, and stenting (E.S. Murphy et al., 2015).

    (c) Associated symptoms, such as cerebral edema, can be managed with steroids.

(7) Patient, caregiver, and family education: Education should include information on the signs of thrombosis and cerebrovascular accident (shortness of breath, swelling of the extremities or neck, headaches, facial asymmetry, and change in mental status).

f) Second primary tumors

(1) Radiation to the brain rarely causes the formation of a second primary tumor; however, the most common are meningiomas and gliomas (Yamanaka, Hayano, & Kanayama, 2017).

(2) Koontz (2018) reported the incidence 25 years after therapy as 25%.

(3) Yamanaka et al. (2017) reported the latency period between treatment and the development of a meningioma was 22.9 ± 11.4 years when they conducted a systematic review of radiation-induced meningiomas.

(4) Risk factors for radiation-induced meningioma are increased total dose, younger age at time of treatment, and large volume of the brain treated. Stereotactic RT and proton therapy seem to be less associated, but the incidence may increase as long-term follow-up accumulates (C.S. Chung et al., 2013).

(5) Assessment and management include routine imaging and physical examination, including a comprehensive neurologic examination.

(6) Patient, caregiver, and family education should involve reviewing the side effects of therapy, including the possibility of second primary tumor formation, as well as stressing the importance of routine, lifelong follow-up.

g) Endocrine disorders

(1) Pathophysiology

    (a) Irradiation of the HPA can cause direct damage to the cells and affect the hypo-

thalamus, thyroid, pineal gland, pituitary gland, and adrenal glands.
- (b) The hypothalamus is more sensitive to the effects of radiation when compared to the pituitary (Koontz, 2018).
- (2) Incidence
  - (a) Endocrine disorders can occur in patients who receive radiation to the base of the skull or nasopharynx, as well as TBI (Koontz, 2018).
  - (b) Irradiation of the neck can result in 20%–50% incidence of post-treatment hypothyroidism (VanKoevering et al., 2020).
  - (c) Hypopituitarism secondary to RT is associated with a 55% increase in mortality, particularly in patients who do not receive replacement therapy (VanKoevering et al., 2020).
  - (d) Lamba et al. (2019) reviewed the data from 74 patients with meningioma who received sellar or perisellar region irradiation and reported the median time to develop adrenal insufficiency was 32 months.
  - (e) The risk of hypothyroidism after RT appears to be dose dependent and can occur many years after therapy (Lamba et al., 2019).
- (3) Assessment
  - (a) A physical examination should include a comprehensive neurologic examination.
  - (b) Neuroradiologic imaging can be used to rule out hemorrhage, tumor progression, or cerebral edema.
- (4) Documentation: Documentation should adhere to facility requirements and standardized documentation sources, such as CTCAE.
- (5) Collaborative management
  - (a) Hormone replacement therapies can be prescribed.
  - (b) Reproductive assessment should be performed for patients of childbearing years.
  - (c) Patients should receive an early referral to endocrinology for monitoring and adjustment of hormone replacement therapy.
- (6) Patient, caregiver, and family education: Education should provide information regarding support for acute and long-term effects of therapy, reproductive abilities, and sexual dysfunction.
- 3. Head and neck
  - a) Dysphagia
    - (1) Pathophysiology
      - (a) *Dysphagia* is defined as difficulty swallowing. It can cause a sensation of choking or a globus sensation (i.e., feeling a lump in the throat without pain) (Koontz, 2018).
      - (b) Irradiation leads to the production of reactive oxygen and nitrogen species, causing oxidative damage and genetic changes. This results in the accelerated fibroblast production and increased collagen content ending in fibrosis and atrophy.
      - (c) *Radiation-induced dysphagia* is an umbrella term for a group of mechanical, structural, and neurologic deficits.
      - (d) Dysphagia involves the combination of reduced retraction of base of the tongue, poor epiglottic retroflexion, reduced laryngeal elevation, delay in pharyngeal transit, and poor coordination of swallowing muscles (King, Dunlap, Tennant, & Pitts, 2016).
      - (e) The dose of radiation to the pharyngeal constrictor muscles, glottis, and supraglottic larynx is directly related to the development of severe late dysphagia (Deschuymer et al., 2018).
      - (f) Dysphagia is associated with aspiration pneumonia and gastrointestinal tube placement, which can occur more than five years after treatment (Koontz, 2018; Siddiqui & Movsas, 2017).
    - (2) Incidence
      - (a) Dysphagia can begin during treatment and persist 6–12 months after treatment or more than two years after treatment without early symptoms.
      - (b) It has been estimated that 46%–63% of head and neck cancer survivors demonstrate some degree of late dysphagia (N. Jiang, Zhang, Li, Zhao, & Eisele, 2016).
      - (c) L. Jiang et al. (2018) conducted a study of 134 patients diagnosed with nasopharyngeal cancer, and 53% reported mild to moderate late dysphagia.
      - (d) There is a significant portion of patients with head and neck cancers who present with dysphagia due to tumor involvement. This should not be considered radiation-induced dysphagia (Siddiqui & Movsas, 2017).
      - (e) Increased dysphagia has been associated with cancer of the hypopharynx (N. Jiang et al., 2016).
    - (3) Assessment
      - (a) Clinicians should perform baseline and ongoing oral examination, including evaluation of range of motion of lips, tongue, and jaw.
      - (b) Clinicians should perform a baseline speech and swallowing evaluation prior to treatment and evaluation at regular inter-

vals after treatment (Koontz, 2018; Siddiqui & Movsas, 2017).

    (c) Patients should be monitored for signs of aspiration and assessed for risks of aspiration (Rodriguez & Foxhall, 2019).

    (d) Nutritional assessment should be performed, and patients should be referred to an RDN or RD as needed.

    (e) Painful swallowing (odynophagia) may be a sign of infection or tumor recurrence in the setting of late-term follow-up.

(4) Documentation

    (a) Documentation should adhere to facility requirements and standardized documentation sources, such as CTCAE and RTOG/EORTC scoring systems, which are scored by the provider.

    (b) Other patient-reported assessment scales can be used for documentation (Deschuymer et al., 2018; L. Jiang et al., 2018).

      i. EORTC Quality of Life questionnaire

      ii. MD Anderson dysphagia intervention scoring (global, emotional, functional, and physical subscales)

(5) Collaborative management

    (a) Dysphagia can be evaluated with fiberoptic endoscopy and videofluoroscopy studies.

    (b) Patients can be referred to a speech and swallowing pathologist for clinical swallowing evaluation, as well as physical and occupational therapy (Balusik, 2014).

    (c) If stricture formation causes dysphagia, dilatation as needed may be appropriate (Siddiqui & Movsas, 2017).

    (d) If possible, pretreatment promotion of swallowing exercises, Mendelsohn maneuvers, Shaker exercises, tongue hold, tongue resistance, and Falsetto phonation can decrease post-treatment swallowing difficulty.

    (e) Individualized rehabilitation plans can improve functionality, health outcomes, and quality of life (Greco et al., 2018; Sobecki-Ryniak & Krouse, 2013).

(6) Patient, caregiver, and family education (Sobecki-Ryniak & Krouse, 2013)

    (a) Instruction includes the importance of maintaining nutritional status and performing swallowing exercises daily.

    (b) Patients, caregivers, and family should know when to contact a healthcare provider, in the event of worsening dysphagia, throat or neck pain, or inability to maintain nutritional intake.

    (c) Clinicians should educate on the importance of good oral hygiene.

    (d) Education should include the importance of routine follow-up with members of the healthcare team (e.g., speech pathologist, medical and radiation oncologist, surgeon, dietitian).

    (e) Clinicians should provide reassurance and education on self-care practices, in addition to helping patients adjust to reentering social circles of family and community.

b) Xerostomia

(1) Pathophysiology

    (a) Xerostomia is the sensation of having a dry mouth, characterized by a marked decrease in the production of and change in the composition of saliva (Buglione et al., 2016).

    (b) Many factors influence xerostomia.

      i. Irradiation of the salivary glands results in lower pH of saliva, causing the saliva to become thick with decreased buffering capacity. This decreased buffering inhibits the ability to prevent plaque and accelerates demineralization, resulting in prolonged low pH and dental caries through the promotion of cariogenic oral flora (Buglione et al., 2016).

      ii. Other factors are gender, age, smoking, use of alcohol-containing mouthwash, concurrent platinum-containing chemotherapy, and medications.

      iii. The effects are proportional to radiation dose (Koontz, 2018; Strojan et al., 2017).

    (c) Patients complain of thick ropy saliva that is difficult to expectorate, which can cause a choking sensation.

    (d) Patients also experience dysgeusia or taste changes, halitosis, difficulty speaking, oral or salivary retrograde infection, difficulty eating and swallowing, pain, polydipsia, and dental caries (Buglione et al., 2016; Koontz, 2018; Siddiqui & Movsas, 2017).

    (e) Xerostomia is a subjective complaint but can significantly impact quality of life. It can begin as an acute toxicity and progress to subacute and continue to be a late toxicity (Siddiqui & Movsas, 2017).

(2) Incidence

    (a) The rate and severity of xerostomia has declined with the advent of modern RT techniques, such as IMRT, which can reduce the dose to the contralateral parotid and submandibular glands.

(b) The incidence decreased from 60%–70% with two-dimensional RT to approximately 40% with IMRT (Siddiqui & Movsas, 2017; Strojan et al., 2017).

(c) The severity decreases gradually over time and can stabilize within four years. In some cases, xerostomia scores can worsen five or more years after radiation (Strojan et al., 2017; Zheng et al., 2015).

(3) Assessment

(a) Clinicians should examine the oral cavity and neck routinely, as well as monitor weight and nutritional status.

(b) Assessment should use validated provider scoring tools (e.g., CTCAE, RTOG, Late Effects of Normal Tissue–Somatic, Objective, Management, Analytic [LENT-SOMA] scale) and patient-reported scales (e.g., EORTC scoring) at baseline and to track changes in severity.

(4) Documentation

(a) Documentation should adhere to facility requirements and standardized documentation sources, such as CTCAE and RTOG/EORTC scoring systems, which are scored by the provider.

(b) Patient-reported assessment scales can be used for documentation (Deschuymer et al., 2018; L. Jiang et al., 2018).

  i. EORTC Quality of Life questionnaire

  ii. MD Anderson dysphagia intervention scoring (global, emotional, functional, and physical subscales)

(5) Collaborative management

(a) The use of IMRT can reduce the severity of xerostomia. A mean dose less than 26 Gy to the parotid gland and mean dose less than 35 Gy to the submandibular gland may reduce the severity of xerostomia (Jensen, 2016).

(b) Amifostine is a thiol metabolite that scavenges reactive oxygen species generated by ionizing radiation. It is an IV medication administered daily prior to therapy and has been shown to reduce the rate of acute and late xerostomia in patients treated with RT alone. However, amifostine has not shown benefit for patients treated with concurrent chemotherapy and RT (Siddiqui & Movsas, 2017).

(c) Cholinergic stimulants act on the postganglionic cells that innervate smooth muscles and exocrine glands, such as salivary and sweat glands (Buglione et al., 2016).

  i. Studies comparing cholinergic stimulants to placebo have shown improvement in global xerostomia in 53.5% of patients treated with pilocarpine and 47.4% of those treated with cevimeline (Strojan et al., 2017).

  ii. Side effects of this class of drug include bronchospasm, bradycardia, vasodilation, sweating, urinary symptoms, flu-like syndrome, and diarrhea (Strojan et al., 2017).

(d) Salivary stimulation

  i. Other forms of salivary stimulation, such as chewing gum and sucking hard candy (acidic or bitter flavors) that contains xylitol to prevent tooth decay, may increase saliva production. If the salivary gland stimulation is ineffective, saliva substitutes or oral lubricants in the form of sprays, gels, and mouthwashes can be used.

  ii. Acupuncture and acupuncture-like transcutaneous electrical nerve stimulation (ALTENS) have been evaluated in five randomized clinical trials and have shown an increase in whole saliva secretion and improvement in subjective relief of symptoms with a low toxicity profile (Strojan et al., 2017; Trinh, Graham, Irnich, Cameron, & Forget, 2016). Systematic reviews of acupuncture have not identified sufficient evidence of efficacy, but a randomized prospective trial found that ALTENS was as effective as pilocarpine and had fewer side effects (Koontz, 2018).

  iii. Hyperbaric oxygen therapy has been studied in radiation-induced xerostomia. A systematic review by Fox et al. (2015) reported that hyperbaric oxygen therapy is useful in the treatment of radiation-induced xerostomia, and patients reported long-term improvement on subjective assessments.

(e) Patients should regularly see a dentist for routine follow-up.

(f) Patients can be referred to an RDN or RD to discuss food choices to maintain weight and oral health.

(6) Patient, caregiver, and family education

(a) Education should include the importance of good daily oral care, including brushing and flossing before and after each meal and at bedtime.

(b) Patients should increase intake of water or sugar-free, low-acid fluids to promote hydration.

(c) Education should include the importance of maintaining nutritional status.

(d) Patients should avoid alcohol intake and alcohol-containing mouthwashes.

(e) Frequent rinsing with baking soda, salt, and water solution may relieve symptoms of xerostomia (Siddiqui & Movsas, 2017).

(f) Use of room humidification, especially while sleeping, can be helpful (Buglione et al., 2016).

c) Compromised dental integrity

(1) Pathophysiology

(a) Ionizing radiation to the oral cavity damages cancer cells directly and through the production of free radicals.

(b) Salivary gland dysfunction leads to reduced production and consistency (xerostomia) of saliva, which leads to bacteria remaining in the mouth.

(c) Acidic saliva can cause demineralization of the teeth, resulting in dental caries (Dawes et al., 2015).

(d) Radiation-induced caries are highly destructive and progressive, beginning in the cervical and incisal edges and quickly progressing to involve the pulp, causing a weakening of dentin and enamel, as well as shear fracturing of the teeth (Gupta et al., 2015; Velo et al., 2018).

(2) Incidence

(a) Location of the tumor and RT technique used affect the incidence of compromised dental integrity.

(b) Dental caries can appear as soon as three months after treatment (Gupta et al., 2015).

(c) More than 50% of patients treated with RT for head and neck cancer experience dental decay.

(d) A higher incidence of subsequent dental caries has been noted with parotid gland RT doses exceeding 26 Gy and a maximum dose of 70 Gy. A mean dose of 40 Gy to the mandible was predictive of post-RT dental extractions (Kufta, Forman, Swisher-McClure, Sollecito, & Panchal, 2018).

(3) Assessment

(a) Assessment involves a complete dental examination, including clinical examination and radiographs.

(b) Tooth viability should be assessed prior to treatment.

(c) Caries should be treated, and teeth in poor condition should be removed.

(4) Documentation: Documentation should adhere to facility requirements and standardized documentation sources, such as CTCAE.

(5) Collaborative management

(a) Patients should be referred to a dentist who specializes in the management of oral care of patients after irradiation to the head and neck. If a specialist is not available, a community dentist should be educated on the management of oral disease after RT.

(b) Prevention of dental caries and the preservation of teeth can safeguard dignity and increase quality of life (Frydrych, Slack-Smith, & Parsons, 2017; Jensen, 2016).

(c) Patients are required to use daily fluoride trays for the rest of their lives.

(d) Patients can be referred to an RDN or RD to discuss dietary modifications to reduce or eliminate sugary, carbonated, and other acidic foods or drinks.

(6) Patient, caregiver, and family education

(a) Clinicians should encourage daily flossing and brushing (morning, night, and after eating).

(b) Education should include information on comprehensive daily oral hygiene, including daily use of pH neutral fluoride gels in trays, fluoride toothpaste, flossing, remineralization mouth rinses, and artificial saliva preparations.

(c) Clinicians should discuss the importance of following dentist instructions, including the use of fluoride trays.

(d) Major dental work, including extractions, should be avoided immediately after head and neck radiation because of the risks associated with delayed healing and osteoradionecrosis.

d) Dysgeusia

(1) Pathophysiology

(a) Dysgeusia is one of a combination of taste disorders. It is defined as an alteration in taste: ageusia is a loss of taste, and hypergeusia is heightened taste sensitivity. It may present as a variety of complaints, including metallic, bitter, sour, salty, or more rarely, sweet taste, that may be triggered, reduced, or not affected by eating and can lead to decreased nutritional intake and weight loss (Epstein & Barasch, 2010).

(b) The mechanisms by which information is passed between the different cells within the taste bud itself remain obscure. Nonetheless, it is understood that, within the taste bud, signals are passed between the type I, II, and III cells and one of three cranial nerves (facial, glossopharyngeal, and vagus), which serve to conduct afferent signals to the CNS.

(c) The effects of RT can ultimately lead to taste receptor damage, synaptic uncoupling, and other neurologic damage (Irune, Dwivedi, Nutting, & Harrington, 2014).

(d) The facial nerve (cranial nerve VII) participates in gustatory function; the glossopharyngeal nerve (cranial nerve IX) supplies the posterior one-third of the tongue; and the vagus nerve (cranial nerve X) innervates the taste fields within the epithelia of the pharynx and larynx (via the superior laryngeal nerve).

   i. Damage to any of these nerves can result in loss of function of the taste receptor tissue it innervates.

   ii. This loss may be mitigated by the compensatory action of the other functioning nerves, as they intensify their taste responses.

(e) All four basic taste sensations (sweet, bitter, salty, and sour) and umami (savory) are affected during RT to the oral cavity. The sweet sensation is typically lost first, resulting in reports of increased bitter and salty tastes. Subsequently, patients will experience general abnormal taste and reduction in taste acuity (Epstein & Barasch, 2010).

(f) RT is thought to cause a loss of taste buds through a direct cytotoxic and antiproliferative effect on tissues within the irradiated volume (Irune et al., 2014).

(g) According to Irune et al. (2014), "some researchers suggest that xerostomia, as a consequence of [RT], may also contribute to taste receptor dysfunction as a direct effect of hyposalivation and failure of taste stimuli to dissolve in thickened saliva and to be adequately transported to receptor cells" (p. 1107).

(2) Incidence

(a) Taste complaints have been reported in up to 75% of patients irradiated for head and neck cancer (Koontz, 2018).

   i. Taste complaints are often present prior to treatment as a consequence of the malignancy.

   ii. A review noted that up to 89% of patients have taste disturbance prior to RT (Epstein & Barasch, 2010).

   iii. Before RT, subjective assessment has reported changes in bitter (35%), salty (18%), and sweet (6%) sensations (Epstein & Barasch, 2010).

(b) RT to the head and neck commonly affects saliva production and taste receptor function, typically after 10–14 days of treatment, consistent with the taste receptor turnover (Epstein & Barasch, 2010).

   i. After RT, taste sensation may improve over several months as mucosal damage heals.

   ii. Taste change may persist as a result of hyposalivation and receptor damage. Changes can last one to two years before a patient has reached maximal recovery and sensation of moisture in the mouth.

(c) Patients often experience radiation-induced xerostomia, dysphagia, and dysgeusia together, which is a major cause of the malnutrition (Irune et al., 2014).

(3) Assessment

(a) Severity of dysgeusia should be assessed using a validated patient-reported outcome tool, such as the EORTC Quality of Life Questionnaire or the University of Washington questionnaire.

(b) Physical examination should include an extensive oral exam.

(c) Weight should be monitored.

(4) Documentation: Documentation should adhere to facility requirements and standardized documentation sources, such as CTCAE.

(5) Collaborative management

(a) Dietary management should involve working with patients, caregivers, and families to determine patient preferences.

(b) Attempts to decrease xerostomia may lessen the severity of taste alterations.

(c) Evidence surrounding the use of zinc supplementation is inconclusive (Koontz, 2018).

(d) Patients can be referred to an RDN or RD as needed.

(6) Patient, caregiver, and family education

(a) Clinicians can encourage frequent oral hygiene, including the use of baking soda, salt, and water rinses, as well as mouthwashes, to promote oral hydration.

(b) Patients can use hard sugar-free candy or gum.

e) Changes in voice quality

(1) Pathophysiology

(a) Irradiation of the head and neck, specifically the larynx, causes the acute changes of mucosal edema, necrosis, and sloughing of tissue, which contribute to acute dysfunction (Johns et al., 2012).

    i. As acute inflammation resolves, collagen deposition occurs and progresses to tissue fibrosis in the vocal folds.

    ii. Fibrosis causes a loss of vocal fold flexibility.

    iii. Patients with radiation-induced fibrosis experience hoarseness, inability to be heard over noise, and vocal strain with speaking.

(b) The extent of vocal cord damage is correlated to the RT dose to the larynx.

    i. The combination of chemotherapy and RT magnifies these negative effects on patients' speech, ADLs, and quality of life.

    ii. Voice problems years after RT, with or without chemotherapy, may be attributed to impaired vocal fold vibration with incomplete closure as a result of dryness of the laryngeal mucosa, muscle atrophy, fibrosis, hyperemia, and erythema (Kraaijenga et al., 2015).

    iii. Damage to cranial nerves X and XII can lead to speech difficulties and can appear several years after RT (Koontz, 2018).

(2) Incidence: Adequately controlled and randomized data on voice outcomes are scarce, and the available studies often utilized different diagnostic tests to assess voice quality (Kraaijenga et al., 2015; Naunheim et al., 2019).

(3) Assessment

(a) Physical examination includes direct and indirect laryngoscopy to evaluate vocal cord edema, movement, or erythema.

(b) Assessment should note voice quality and level of hoarseness.

(c) Clinicians should inquire about a patient's ability to communicate in person and the effect of voice quality on work, socializing, or telephone use.

(d) Patient-reported scoring tools, such as the Voice Handicap Index and the Voice-Related Quality of Life survey, can also be used (J.I. Chang, Bevans, & Schwartz, 2012).

(4) Documentation

(a) Hoarseness and aphonia can be documented using CTCAE with the following grades (NCI CTEP, 2017).

    i. Grade 1 hoarseness: mild or intermittent voice change; fully understandable; self-resolves

    ii. Grade 2 hoarseness: moderate or persistent voice changes; may require occasional repetition but understandable on telephone; medical evaluation indicated

    iii. Grade 3 hoarseness: severe voice changes, including predominantly whispered speech

    iv. Grade 3 aphonia: voicelessness; inability to speak

(b) Documentation should include resolution, improvement, or worsened symptoms of dysphonia, as well as change in quality of life, in patients with dysphonia after treatment or observation (Stachler et al., 2018).

(5) Collaborative management: Treatment can include the following.

(a) Injection laryngoplasty: vocal fold medicalization procedure that can improve speech quality in patients with unilateral vocal cord paralysis

(b) Referral to speech pathologist for evaluation and voice rehabilitation services

(c) Avoidance of straining voice to decrease vocal cord irritation

(d) Avoidance of alcohol, tobacco, and spicy and acidic foods, which may contribute to gastric reflux disease and affect voice quality

(e) Maintenance of oral hygiene and gargling with warm salt water

(f) Humidifier use at home, especially while sleeping

(6) Patient, caregiver, and family education

(a) Instruction includes measures to maintain or improve voice quality.

(b) Instruction includes information on symptoms of cancer recurrence or infection.

f) Hearing changes: See previous information on cranial nerve neuropathies.

g) Osteoradionecrosis

(1) Pathophysiology

(a) Osteoradionecrosis is defined as an area of exposed necrotic bone in a previously irradiated area that does not heal over a period of three to six months and is characterized by radiation-induced activation and dysregulation of fibroblastic activity that causes inflammation, vascular fibrosis, and thrombosis (Nadella, Kodali, Guttikonda, & Jonnalagadda, 2015; Owosho et al., 2017).

(b) Blood flow to the mandible is supplied by the inferior alveolar artery, which when damaged by radiation, causes ischemic

necrosis in the atrophic tissue because of poor vascularization due to occlusion of capillaries by small thrombi that obliterate the vascular lumen.

(c) The absence of collateral blood supply leads to symptomatic necrosis, especially in the premolar, molar, and retromolar regions (De Felice, Musio, & Tombolini, 2016; Nadella et al., 2015).

(d) Severely damaged capillary beds and arterioles impair the blood supply to the irradiated bone, resulting in hypoxia and ischemic necrosis of the bone (Siddiqui & Movsas, 2017).

(e) Osteoradionecrosis is characterized by exposed bone in the area that does not heal spontaneously, persists for several months, and slowly worsens in the absence of primary tumor, recurrence, or metastasis (Siddiqui & Movsas, 2017).

(f) Osteoradionecrosis can lead to infection and pathologic fracture.

(2) Incidence

(a) The incidence of osteoradionecrosis has been decreasing over the past 20 years because of the use of IMRT rather than conventional RT techniques, as well as understanding of the importance of dental health (Brennan, Bradley, & Brands, 2017).

(b) Studies have placed the incidence at 2%–22% (Strojan et al., 2017).

(c) The incidence has been reduced to 0%–6% with the use of IMRT and delineation of the mandible in treatment planning. In one study, incidence of osteoradionecrosis was 96% when the dose to the mandible was greater than 60 Gy (Brennan et al., 2017; Siddiqui & Movsas, 2017).

(d) An emphasis on dental health prior to the initiation of therapy is a factor related to lower incidence (Brennan et al., 2017).

(e) The following risk factors are associated with the development of osteoradionecrosis (De Felice et al., 2016; Nadella et al., 2015).

   i. Tumor location
   ii. Radiation dose greater than 60 Gy
   iii. Brachytherapy
   iv. Dental extractions after RT
   v. Poor dental hygiene
   vi. Poor dentition
   vii. Mandibular injury
   viii. Infection
   ix. Malnutrition or poor nutrition
   x. Concurrent chemotherapy and RT
   xi. Long history of alcohol and tobacco use

(3) Assessment: Assessment should include a detailed oral examination.

(4) Documentation: Documentation should adhere to facility requirements and standardized documentation sources, such as CTCAE.

(5) Collaborative management

(a) Wounds can be irrigated with saline solution or chlorohexidine (0.2%).

(b) Systemic antibiotics should be administered as needed for infection.

(c) Patients with early and limited osteoradionecrosis can be referred to surgery for debridement.

(d) Resection may be needed for pathological fracture.

(e) Patients can receive hyperbaric oxygen therapy.

(f) Oral medications, including pentoxifylline 400 mg twice a day with tocopherol (vitamin E) 1,000 IU daily, with or without clodronate, can be prescribed (Koontz, 2018).

(g) Patients should follow up with a dentist every three to six months.

(h) Patients should avoid tooth extractions for two years after RT.

(6) Patient, caregiver, and family education

(a) Education should consist of information about the risk factors and signs and symptoms of osteoradionecrosis.

(b) Patients should avoid irritants, such as tobacco, alcohol, or dentures.

(c) Instruction should include information on comprehensive oral hygiene at least twice daily with gentle brushing and flossing.

h) Trismus

(1) Pathophysiology

(a) Trismus is defined as restricted mouth opening or jaw movement due to the disorder of temporomandibular joint (TMJ). It is most likely caused by the proliferation of fibroblasts and infiltrating inflammatory cells, resulting in radiation fibrosis.

(b) Radiation damage to the mandible and TMJ and denervation atrophy of the joint muscles result in contractures in masticatory muscles and decreased degree of movement of the TMJ (Wu & Lam, 2016).

(c) Measurement of the maximal interincisal distance, which is the distance from the edge of the maxillary incisor and the mandibular incisors, determines degree of trismus.

i. For edentulous patients, measure the distance between the maxillary and mandibular alveolar ridges.

ii. Dijkstra trismus criterion of a maximal interincisal distance less than 35 mm is commonly used (Astradsson et al., 2018).

(2) Incidence

(a) Trismus can impair ability to chew, swallow, and speak. It can be detrimental to oral health, dental integrity, and overall quality of life (Heijnen et al., 2016; Lee et al., 2018; Rapidis et al., 2015).

(b) Psychological difficulties can include low self-esteem, depression, and suicidal tendencies (Lee et al., 2018; Rapidis et al., 2015).

(c) Mouth opening after RT decreases on average by 18%–32% compared to mouth opening prior to RT. In the first year after RT, Rapidis et al. (2015) reported that mouth opening on average decreases 2.4% per month, and by the second year, the rate decreases to 0.2% per month, then down to 0.1% per month in the third and fourth year.

i. A higher radiation dose to the relevant tissues correlates to greater the decrease in mouth opening.

ii. Functional impairment can be caused by doses as low as 15 Gy (Rapidis et al., 2015).

(d) A recent study suggested that the incidence of trismus was not influenced by different RT regimens when curative dose to the areas of the masticatory muscles and ligaments of the TMJ are used (Rapidis et al., 2015).

(3) Assessment

(a) Trismus can also be a sign of recurrent disease, so assessment and quick determination as post-treatment changes or recurrent disease may affect patient survival and treatment outcomes.

(b) Clinical examination should monitor TMJ range of motion and pain on movement.

(c) Clinicians should perform a physical examination of the oral cavity and range of motion of the TMJ.

(d) Using the LENT-SOMA score (normal mouth opening greater than 30 mm), the measurement should be taken twice. The greater value should be documented (Rapidis et al., 2015).

(e) CT or MRI can also be utilized.

(4) Documentation

(a) Documentation should adhere to facility requirements and standardized documentation sources, such as CTCAE and RTOG/EORTC.

(b) LENT-SOMA can be used promote standardized documentation of trismus. Grades 3 and 4 are considered severe.

i. Grade 1: maximum interincisal distance 20–30 mm

ii. Grade 2: maximum interincisal distance 10–20 mm

iii. Grade 3: maximum interincisal distance 5–10 mm

iv. Grade 4: maximum interincisal distance less than 5 mm

(5) Collaborative management

(a) The prevention of trismus is most important because it is irreversible and can be progressive.

(b) If possible, IMRT should be used to reduce the dose to critical structures and muscles.

(c) Pain control with NSAIDs can be prescribed as needed.

(d) Injections of voltage-dependent sodium channel blockers (e.g., oxcarbazepine, lamotrigine) at trigeminal or other nerves and pterygoid muscles, as well as botulinum toxin into the TMJ region, can be administered. These treatments do not improve trismus but are used for pain control.

(e) Physiotherapy and microcurrent therapy have also been used.

(f) Hyperbaric oxygen and pentoxifylline are not effective treatments (Rapidis et al., 2015).

(g) Patients should be referred to rehabilitation services, including Speech Language Pathology, for mouth opening and jaw movement exercises and mechanical devices such as Therabite® or conventional tools (e.g., stacked tongue depressor) to help stretch the jaw and increase maximum interincisal distance.

(h) If possible, patients should begin exercises during RT and continue after treatment.

(i) Surgical intervention, such as coronoidectomy and forced mouth opening under general anesthesia, are used if other treatments are unsuccessful (Wu & Lam, 2016). If fibrosis occurs in the other masticatory muscles and other subcutaneous tissues, the coronoidectomy will not be effective.

(j) Patients should be referred to an RDN or RD, as needed, if they are unable to maintain nutritional status.

(6) Patient, caregiver, and family education
- (a) Patients, caregivers, and families should understand the importance of exercises. Adherence is essential to prevent worsening of trismus.
- (b) Instruction of exercises should include return demonstration by the patient.

i) Shoulder mobility impairment
- (1) Pathophysiology
  - (a) Shoulder mobility impairment is usually caused by damage to the spinal accessory nerve, which innervates the trapezius and sternocleidomastoid muscles.
  - (b) Radiation-induced nerve damage is not clearly understood but is thought to begin with endothelial cell dysfunction and vascular dysfunction that result in microvascular necrosis and local ischemia, leading to fibroblast activation and damage to the connective tissue cells. These changes over time, coupled with demyelination and poorly vascularized tissue, lead to fibrosis (Stubblefield, 2017).
  - (c) Secondary effects of musculoskeletal impairment include adhesive capsulitis and myofascial pain in the upper trapezius, levator scapulae, and rhomboid muscles.
  - (d) Although less frequent, shoulder morbidity may also develop as a result of RT (B.A. Murphy & Deng, 2015).
  - (e) Nerve injury can result in pain, sensory dysfunction, and weakness and interfere with ADLs (Stubblefield, 2017).
- (2) Incidence
  - (a) The incidence of radiation-induced accessory nerve neuropathy is approximately 12% (Stubblefield, 2017).
  - (b) As it relates to musculoskeletal effects, Ghiam et al. (2017) stated, "Prominent late toxicities include functional deficiencies related to speech, swallowing, general functional impairment due to weakness and deconditioning, and musculoskeletal impairment" (p. 2085).
  - (c) Head and neck cancer survivors commonly encounter musculoskeletal impairment of the neck and shoulder, causing limitations in the neck.
  - (d) Data indicate that neck dissection or RT may result in chronic shoulder dysfunction in a significant portion of head and neck survivors (Ghiam et al., 2017).
- (3) Assessment
  - (a) Physical examination should assess shoulder function for strength, range of motion, symmetry, and signs of impingement.
  - (b) Assessment should also include imaging, laboratory evaluation, and electrodiagnostic testing.
  - (c) Patients should be referred to rehabilitation services for pain, disability, and range-of-motion issues.
- (4) Documentation: Documentation should adhere to facility requirements and standardized documentation sources, such as the following.
  - (a) Shoulder Pain and Disability Index (13-item questionnaire that assesses shoulder pain and shoulder disability on a numerical scale)
  - (b) Vanderbilt Head and Neck Symptom Survey
  - (c) General Symptom Survey (61-item instrument that measures acute and late symptoms of head and neck cancer)
- (5) Collaborative management
  - (a) Neuropathic agents are commonly prescribed to manage musculoskeletal impairment–associated pain. Antispasmodics and botulinum toxin are used to ameliorate muscle spasms.
  - (b) Clinical experience and small nonrandomized or randomized trials indicate that interventions such as Pilates and yoga may enhance functional outcomes in the short term.
  - (c) Physical therapy using traditional techniques, such as stretching, strengthening exercises, resistance training, and myofascial release, are recommended to minimize functional loss due to neck and shoulder fibrosis.
  - (d) Physical therapy and therapeutic exercise after surgical intervention and chemoradiation have been reported to improve quality of life, alleviate upper extremity pain, enhance upper extremity strength, improve shoulder abduction, augment fitness, and enhance functional capacity (Su et al., 2017).
- (6) Patient, caregiver, and family education: Clinicians should educate patients, caregivers, and families on the importance of consistency in performing exercises because retention of optimal musculoskeletal function requires lifelong maintenance therapy (Su et al., 2017).

j) Hypothyroidism
- (1) Pathophysiology
  - (a) Fujiwara et al. (2015) indicated that "the mechanisms underlying the development of thyroid disorders after [RT] are thought to include vascular damage, capsular fibro-

sis, iodine insufficiency due to an inadequate diet, and direct parenchymal damage, but the details remain unclear" (p. 579).

    (b) Radiation-induced thyroiditis is considered as the primary damage to the thyroid gland when the follicular epithelial cells and blood vessels are damaged, leading to hypothyroidism as a late effect.

    (c) The actual mechanism of radiation-induced thyroid damage is still unclear, and other causes, including autoimmune reactions and parenchymal cell damages, have been reported (Z. Lin et al., 2018).

    (d) Damage to the HPA axis may result in hypothyroidism, with overt symptoms of weight gain, dry skin, hair loss, cold intolerance, general weakness, muscle cramps, depression, irritability, and memory loss.

    (e) Hypothyroidism can also lead to coagulopathy, diastolic hypertension, dyslipidemia, and atherosclerosis, which, in turn, increase the risk of cardiovascular events and mortality (Fan et al., 2017; B.A. Murphy & Deng, 2015).

(2) Incidence

    (a) The incidence of radiation-induced hypothyroidism in head and neck cancers ranges from 17%–53% in some studies (Fujiwara et al., 2015; Harris et al., 2016).

        i. Hypothyroidism after RT develops at a median interval of 1.4–1.8 years (range 0.3–7.2 years) (Boomsma, Bijl, & Langendijk, 2011).

        ii. Risk factors for the development of hypothyroidism include the type of RT technique. IMRT without thyroid dose constraints can result in increased thyroid damage.

        iii. When using IMRT, it is important to use thyroid dose constraints, which result in a lower median thyroid dose (Rønjom et al., 2013).

    (b) The majority of radiation-induced hypothyroidism cases are subclinical, which are asymptomatic and can only be detected by thyroid hormone study showing elevated thyroid-stimulating hormone level (Z. Lin et al., 2018).

(3) Assessment (Boomsma et al., 2011)

    (a) Hypothyroidism can be easily diagnosed by laboratory tests, including serum thyrotropin-releasing hormone, thyroid-stimulating hormone, triiodothyronine, and free thyroxin.

    (b) Clinical hypothyroidism is generally defined as a high serum thyroid stimulating hormone concentration with serum thyroxin beyond normal limits and presence of clinical symptoms, such as fatigue, weakness, cold intolerance, weight gain, cognitive dysfunction, constipation, dry skin, hoarseness, edema, decreased hearing, myalgia and paresthesia, depression, menorrhagia, and arthralgia.

    (c) Subclinical hypothyroidism is generally defined as increased thyroid-stimulating hormone without symptoms; serum thyroxin concentration could be low or within normal limits.

(4) Documentation: Documentation should adhere to facility requirements and standardized documentation sources, such as CTCAE and RTOG/EORTC scoring systems.

(5) Collaborative management

    (a) Thyroid-stimulating hormone level should be checked prior to starting RT, routinely at six months after treatment, then every 6–12 months (NCCN, 2020a).

    (b) Treatment with levothyroxine is recommended, and the dose should be adjusted according to thyroid function test and patient symptoms (Rønjom et al., 2013)

(6) Patient, caregiver, and family education (Z. Lin et al., 2018)

    (a) Education should include information on the late effects of radiation to the head and neck.

    (b) Education should include information on the signs and symptoms of hypothyroidism, such as weakness, fatigue, weight gain, cold intolerance, hair changes, poor wound healing, depression, dry skin, and constipation.

k) Increased risk of cerebrovascular accident (stroke)

(1) Pathophysiology

    (a) It is hypothesized that the arterial injury caused by RT accelerates atherosclerosis, through which radiation-induced damage of the cerebrovascular and carotid artery disease can develop (Arthurs, Hanna, Zaza, Peng, & Hall, 2016; Plummer, Henderson, O'Sullivan, & Read, 2011).

    (b) Risk factors for cerebrovascular accident as it relates to RT include concomitant chemotherapy, hypertension, hypercholesterolemia, diabetes, smoking, younger age at the time of head and neck irradiation, and history of cerebrovascular accident or transient ischemic attack.

(c) RT may accelerate atherosclerotic changes in the vasculature, leading to large vessel stenosis or occlusion (Demeestere & Thijs, 2016).

(2) Incidence

(a) Patients with head and neck squamous cell carcinoma treated with RT have an increased risk of carotid stenosis, transient ischemic attack, and general carotid injury (Arthurs et al., 2016; Plummer et al., 2011).

(b) Arthurs et al. (2016) conducted a retrospective population-based cohort study of 14,069 patients and found that treatment with RT was associated with a 46% higher hazard of cerebrovascular accident. With RT as the sole treatment modality, there was 70% increased risk of stroke compared to surgery alone.

(3) Assessment

(a) Physical examination includes routine comprehensive neurologic evaluation.

(b) Patients should be monitored for changes in neurologic function.

(c) Clinicians should obtain medical history and monitor patients with risk factors.

(d) Clinicians should assess for new or worsening of neurologic symptoms, such as headaches, syncope, nausea and vomiting, numbness, weakness, confusion, dizziness, or seizures.

(e) Radiologic evaluation of vessels with an ultrasound, MRI, or magnetic resonance angiography may reveal greater vessel wall thickness and extensive collateralization of adjacent vessels (N.M. Rao et al., 2017).

(f) Patients treated for radiation vasculopathy likely have hypercoagulability due to their underlying cancer history. Coagulation profiles, blood chemistries, liver function tests, and complete blood counts should be obtained as needed.

(4) Documentation: Documentation should adhere to facility requirements and standardized documentation sources, such as CTCAE.

(5) Collaborative management

(a) Clinicians should employ carotid artery screening and preventive strategies.

(b) Carpenter et al. (2018) recommended that patients with head and neck cancer be screened for asymptomatic carotid artery stenosis two to five years after RT completion.

(c) The treatment guidelines for cerebrovascular accident in these patients have been extrapolated from standard management, which includes tissue plasminogen activator, aspirin, heparin, low-molecular-weight heparin, surgery, embolization, angioplasty, and stenting (E.S. Murphy et al., 2015).

(6) Patient, caregiver, and family education (Carpenter et al., 2018)

(a) Patients, caregivers, and families should know the signs and symptoms of cerebrovascular accident and when to contact a healthcare provider.

(b) Patients should understand the importance of managing comorbidities that may increase risk of transient ischemic attack and cerebrovascular accident, such as hypertension, diabetes, and hypercholesterolemia.

l) External lymphedema and fibrosis

(1) Pathophysiology

(a) Radiation to the head and neck can result in inflammation and eventual fibrosis of vasculature in the subcutaneous and deep tissues of the face, neck, and shoulders. This leads to decreased drainage and overload of the lymphatic system in the head and neck region. The result is swelling, tightness, decreased range of motion, and discomfort (Koontz, 2018).

(b) Although the etiology of head and neck lymphedema varies, common causes include surgery that removes lymph nodes or impairment of lymphatic vessel contractility (lymphangiomotoricity) associated with RT or surgery. Additionally, the tumor itself may cause vessel obstruction (Koontz, 2018; Smith et al., 2015).

(c) If left untreated, chronic edema coupled with permanent fibrosis may result in significant long-term cosmetic, functional, and psychosocial consequences that are often irreversible, including discomfort and problems associated with speech, respiration, voice, and swallowing (Smith et al., 2015).

(2) Incidence

(a) External lymphedema and fibrosis can occur at three months or years after treatment, and up to 50% of patients can experience some degree of external lymphedema (Koontz, 2018; Smith et al., 2015).

(b) Severity increases over time. External lymphedema and fibrosis may not be preventable in many patients, as combination of bilateral neck dissection and RT significantly increases the probability of this toxicity (Koontz, 2018).

(3) Assessment
  (a) Clinicians should monitor for patient reports of neck pain, stiffness, or decreased range of motion.
  (b) Physical examination should note changes in head and neck area. Measurement of this area may not be useful because of fluctuation of fluid and lack of reproducible landmarks.
(4) Documentation: Documentation should adhere to facility requirements and standardized documentation sources, such as CTCAE.
(5) Collaborative management: When possible, patients should be referred to a certified lymphedema specialist or lymphedema rehabilitation program for complete decongestive therapy (CDT), including manual lymph drainage.
  (a) CDT has been shown to decrease lymphedema in 60% of patients and remains the gold standard for treatment (Smith et al., 2015).
  (b) The contraindications to CDT include hyperthyroidism, more than 50% internal carotid artery blockage, upper quadrant deep-vein thrombosis, acute radiation dermatitis, acute renal failure, or a history of multiple cerebrovascular accidents or transient ischemic attacks (Smith et al., 2015).
  (c) CDT is a two-phased, six-component treatment regimen. The first phase aims to reduce the size of the affected area and emphasizes proper skin care. Once maximum fluid volume reduction has been reached, the second phase (maintenance) begins and requires lifelong self-maintenance.
  (d) Although there is no cure for lymphedema, it can be successfully managed with CDT (C.J. Chang & Cormier, 2013).
  (e) Pentoxifylline 800 mg daily and vitamin E 1,000 mg daily should be prescribed for at least six months (Koontz, 2018).
(6) Patient, caregiver, and family education
  (a) Education includes the importance of exercises and massage therapy performed at home, as prescribed by the therapist.
  (b) Clinicians should instruct on the use of compression garments or pads.
4. Lymphedema (primary and secondary)
  a) Pathophysiology
    (1) Lymphedema is an accumulation of lymph fluid in the interstitial tissue that causes swelling of a limb or other areas, such as the neck, trunk, or genitals.
    (2) It can occur as a toxicity of treatment, appearing on the same side of the body as the cancer treatment.

(3) Lymphedema is caused by obstruction or disruption of the lymphatic circulation, which leads to the accumulation of protein-rich fluid in the interstitial tissues, thus leading to edema, which can lead to impaired function of the affected limb or area, pain, discomfort, loss of sensation, chronic infections, and decreased quality of life.
(4) Lymphedema is classified as primary or secondary.
  (a) Primary lymphedema is caused by a congenital dysfunction or abnormality of the lymphatic system.
  (b) Secondary lymphedema results from obstruction or disruption of the normal lymph flow because of tumors or damage to lymphatic channels.
  (c) In the United States, treatment for breast cancer is the leading cause of secondary lymphedema (C.J. Chang & Cormier, 2013).
b) Incidence: The incidence for patients treated with axillary RT is 31%–65% and 29%–65% for RT to the chest wall and regional lymph nodes after mastectomy and irradiation of the axilla (Kenyon, Mayer, & Owens, 2014).
c) Assessment
  (1) A comprehensive physical examination should focus on areas of edema, such as the neck and extremities.
  (2) The affected areas should be measured to monitor for changes in circumference.
  (3) Examination should assess perfusion in the affected limb, including warmth, color, and pitting or nonpitting edema.
  (4) Assess for signs of recurrences such as adenopathy.
  (5) Prompt detection of lymphedema is important because treatment is most effective during stages 0 and 1, which are reversible, and therapy results in fewer complications (C.J. Chang & Cormier, 2013).
d) Documentation: Documentation should adhere to facility requirements and standardized documentation sources, such as CTCAE.
e) Collaborative management
  (1) Patients can experience psychological distress as a result of lymphedema; therefore, emotional support and referral for counseling when appropriate should be provided (NCI, 2019).
  (2) Gradient pressure garments and CDT can be prescribed.
  (3) Axillary reverse mapping, exercise, weight management, and prevention and early intervention protocols are likely to be effective (Armer et al., 2017).

(4) Low-level laser therapy may be useful for pain and edema (Smoot, Chiavola-Larson, Lee, Manibusan, & Allen, 2015).

(5) Refer to V.B. Head and neck cancer for additional information.

f) Patient, caregiver, and family education

(1) Patients, caregivers, and families should be instructed to inform a provider if they notice swelling, tightness, heaviness, numbness, or pain in the limb on the affected side.

(2) NCI recommends that patients take the following measures to manage lymphedema (Asdourian et al., 2016; NCI, 2019).

(a) Continuing a moderate exercise program

(b) Maintaining nail and skin hygiene to avoid infection, which can lead to cellulitis

(c) Routinely visiting a podiatrist to prevent ingrown toenails and infections

(d) Using moisturizers and antibiotic ointments on small breaks in the skin

(e) Using the unaffected limb to test temperatures (e.g., bath water, cooking)

(f) Avoiding pooling of blood in the involved limb

i. NCI does not recommend blood draws in the affected arm.

ii. Studies have shown that special precautions, such as avoiding venipuncture, blood pressure measurement, and air travel, are not supported by high-level evidence (Asdourian et al., 2016).

5. Radiation-induced second primary malignancy

a) Definition: Radiation-induced second primary malignancy (second malignancy) is defined as a malignancy that "falls within the primary or secondary radiation beam, has a different histology than the primary cancer, has a latency period of several years, not present at the time of initial diagnosis and the patient is not part of a cancer-prone syndrome" (Koontz, 2018, p. 277). Ionizing radiation is a potential carcinogen and the development of secondary cancers related to irradiation is rare.

b) Incidence

(1) The risk of developing a second malignancy is multifactorial and directly related to the RT technique, mean dose to the site, field site and size, patient age, and combination with chemotherapy. Malignancy can manifest more than 10 years after irradiation (Bazire, De Rycke, Asselain, Fourquet, & Kirova, 2017; Braunstein & Cahlon, 2018; Hoekstra et al., 2018; Koontz, 2018).

(2) A retrospective single institution study of 17,745 women treated with adjuvant RT with or without chemotherapy (81.8%) compared to those who did not receive RT with or without chemotherapy (18.2%) found the frequency of second malignancy for women treated with RT alone was significantly greater at 14%, compared to those who did not receive adjuvant RT at 11% (Bazire et al., 2017).

(3) Other researchers have found a much lower rate reported as 0.2% at 10 years or slightly higher rates of lung cancer for smokers (Kenyon et al., 2014).

(4) The most common second malignancies were lung cancer, esophageal cancer, contralateral breast cancer, and sarcomas (Bazire et al., 2017; Koontz, 2018).

(5) C.S. Chung et al. (2013) reported there was not a significant difference in the incidence of second malignancies between patients treated with proton therapy when compared to photon therapy at one-year post-therapy.

c) Collaborative management

(1) Clinicians should follow NCCN and American Cancer Society guidelines for survivorship.

(2) Patients should be referred for smoking cessation.

(3) Clinicians should encourage routine follow-up with a primary care provider (PCP).

(4) Clinicians should provide psychological support and refer for psychosocial evaluation as needed.

(5) RT technique should be used to reduce the dose to the internal mammary and supraclavicular lymph nodes if not contraindicated.

d) Patient, caregiver, and family education

(1) Education includes the importance of smoking cessation.

(2) Patients should understand signs and symptoms of new cancer or recurrence, including skin changes, pain, unintentional weight loss, dysphagia, recurrent dyspepsia, masses or lumps, chest pain, arm swelling, arm or shoulder pain, shortness of breath, wheezing, hoarseness, fatigue, loss of appetite, recurrent lung infections (e.g., bronchitis, pneumonia).

(3) Education includes the importance of maintaining a healthy diet and weight.

(4) Patients, caregivers, and families should understand the importance of decreasing psychological distress and promotion of well-being.

6. Thorax

a) Radiation fibrosis: See previous information on external lymphedema and fibrosis.

b) Radiation myelopathy: See previous information on radiation myelopathy.

c) Radiation pneumonitis

(1) Pathophysiology

(a) Irradiation of tumors in the thorax initiates a chain of events beginning with the release of damage-associated molecular patterns (DAMPs), cytokines (TNF-α, interleukin-6, interleukin-1α), and chemokines, leading to an immune response with increased capillary permeability and leukocytic infiltration in the surrounding healthy tissue.

(b) An increase in proinflammatory immune cells resulting in pneumonitis occurs in healthy tissue (Simone, 2017; Wirsdörfer, de Leve, & Jendrossek, 2019).

(c) Pneumonitis can begin to develop at one month to one year after irradiation and is characterized by severe or worsening dyspnea, nonproductive cough, low-grade fevers, pleuritic chest pain, weight loss, fatigue, and malaise (Koontz, 2018; Simone, 2017).

(d) The symptoms can be severe and result in acute respiratory distress syndrome, a life-threatening condition. Symptoms must be differentiated from other diagnoses, such as tumor progression, pneumonia, or chronic obstructive pulmonary disease exacerbation (Simone, 2017).

(e) Pneumonitis causes inflammation, which can result in permanent lung damage or radiation fibrosis over time (X. Lin & Corcoran, 2019).

(f) Risk factors include median dose to the lung of 60 Gy, daily fraction size of greater than 2 Gy, poor pulmonary function, tumor size and location (lower lobe lung tumors), advanced age, concurrent chemotherapy combination of carboplatin and paclitaxel, history of smoking, gender, and radiation dose to the heart (Simone, 2017).

(g) It is unclear if treatment with concurrent RT and immune checkpoint inhibitors causes an increased incidence of pneumonitis, but radiation recall pneumonitis has been reported in patients receiving immune checkpoint inhibitors previously treated with thoracic RT (Schoenfeld et al., 2019; C.R. Sears et al., 2019).

(h) Shimokawaji et al. (2020) performed a retrospective study of 669 patients with non-small cell lung cancer (NSCLC) treated with nivolumab and found previous thoracic RT was not a significant risk factor for radiation recall pneumonitis (Shimokawaji et al., 2020).

(2) Incidence: The incidence of pneumonitis in patients with lung or breast cancer is 13%–36% (Wirsdörfer et al., 2019).

(3) Assessment: Assessment involves physical examination, comprehensive respiratory evaluation, and thoracic imaging (chest x-ray or chest CT).

(4) Documentation: Documentation should adhere to facility requirements and utilize standardized tools, such as CTCAE.

(5) Collaborative management

(a) Treatment can include prednisone 60 mg daily for two weeks with taper by 10 mg every one to two weeks, oxygen therapy, and supportive medications (antitussives) (Koontz, 2018; Simone, 2017).

(b) Treatment with antioxidants, amifostine, and pentoxifylline is being studied (Simone, 2017).

(c) Patients should be referred to a pulmonologist.

(6) Patient, caregiver, and family education

(a) Clinicians should educate patients, caregivers, and families on signs and symptoms of pneumonitis.

(b) Clinicians should educate patients, caregivers, and families on the importance of taking medications as prescribed to aid in management of cough and shortness of breath. Patients should contact healthcare providers if they experience new or worsening pulmonary symptoms.

(c) Education should include information on management of activities to prevent fatigue.

(d) Clinicians should provide and review written instructions on how to taper steroids.

d) Cardiac injury: Refer to IV.K. Cardiac toxicity and cardiac implantable electronic devices for information on radiation-related cardiotoxicities.

(1) Pathophysiology

(a) Irradiation of heart muscle results in damage to the endothelial cells that cause ischemia, inflammation causing microvascular and macrovascular damage to the myocytes, and myocardial cell death, which over time results in fibrosis and accelerated atherosclerosis (Koontz, 2018; Nitsche, Pahl, Huber, Eilf, & Dunst, 2015).

(b) Radiation-induced cardiac injury can lead to disease, such as congestive heart failure, constrictive pericarditis, pericardial effusion, valvular disease, and coronary artery disease. These typically occur at least 10 years after irradiation (Jain, Russell, Schwartz, Panjrath, & Aronow, 2017).

(2) Incidence

(a) Studies published before 2000 showed an increased risk in cardiovascular mortality after RT for breast cancer on the left side. For example, the Early Breast Cancer Trialists' Collaborative Group reported a 30% increase in death due to cardiac disease in women treated with RT for breast cancer (Leung, Chan, & Muo, 2016; Taylor & Kirby, 2015).

   (b) Leung et al. (2016) studied women with early breast cancer and compared those who received adjuvant RT to no RT and did not find a significant difference (p = 0.13) in overall cardiac morbidity and mortality between the groups.

   (c) Risk factors for cardiac toxicity are volume of heart irradiated, history of ischemic heart disease, diabetes, hypertension, smoking, hyperlipidemia, and myocardial infarction. Treatment with anthracyclines and anti-HER2 antibodies and older age are also risk factors (Cao, Zhu, Wagar, & Meng, 2017; Jain et al., 2017; Koontz, 2018; Taylor & Kirby, 2015).

(3) Collaborative management

   (a) Patients should be referred to a cardiologist for evaluation.

   (b) Clinicians should perform routine echocardiograms to evaluate left ventricular function and myocardial perfusion imaging (Jain et al., 2017).

   (c) Clinicians should perform routine imaging, including cardiac MRI and equilibrium radionuclide angiocardiography (multigated acquisition), in patients who are treated with chemotherapy and RT (Cao et al., 2017).

   (d) If possible, clinicians should use treatment techniques such as breath holding, prone breast, or IMRT to decrease the dose to the heart (Russell et al., 2016).

(4) Patient, caregiver, and family education: Patients, caregivers, and families should understand signs and symptoms of radiation-induced cardiotoxicity, such as chest pain, fatigue, shortness of breath, or difficulty lying flat.

e) Radiation-induced esophageal stricture

(1) Pathophysiology

   (a) Radiation-induced esophageal stricture is caused by fibrosis of the esophagus. The esophagus is sensitive to the damage caused by RT, as it has a high turnover of cells (Agarwalla, Small, Mendelson, Scott, & Kochman, 2015).

   (b) Irradiation causes an immune response within the tissue leading to inflammation and vasculature changes, such as obliterative endarteritis and ischemia of the esophageal wall. This results in irrevers-

ible tissue changes with the formation of collagen within the tissue matrix, as well as fibrosis, leading to stricture or stenosis of the esophagus with accompanying decreased or dysfunctional esophageal motility (Agarwalla et al., 2015; Francis et al., 2014; Park et al., 2018).

   (c) The median time to occurrence of radiation-induced esophageal stricture is six months (range 3–8 months) after RT, but it can also occur several years after treatment (Agarwalla et al., 2015; Park et al., 2018).

   (d) Risk factors for stricture include the following (Francis et al., 2014).

      i. Radiation dose to the esophagus, larynx, or constrictor muscles

      ii. Radiation fractionation and technique

      iii. Multimodal therapy with chemotherapy, specifically taxanes, and RT

      iv. Female sex

      v. Severe mucositis (head and neck cancer)

      vi. Gastrotomy or nasogastric tube placement prior to initiation of therapy

(2) Incidence

   (a) Radiation-induced esophageal stricture is a common occurrence for patients who receive radiation to the chest for cancers of the breast, esophagus, head and neck, or lung (Agarwalla et al., 2015).

   (b) Park et al. (2018) reported the estimated risk increases as the dose to chest increases.

      i. For example, the risk is less than 2% if a patient receives less than 50 Gy to the chest, and risk increases to 15% if the dose is 60 Gy or more (Park et al., 2018).

      ii. Other studies have reported an overall incidence rate of 3.3%–23% (Francis et al., 2014; J.J. Wang, Goldsmith, Holman, Cianchetti, & Chan, 2012).

   (c) Agarwalla et al. (2015) reported a recurrence rate of 33% for patients who were treated with esophageal dilation, and one-third of patients will have recurrent dysphagia within the first year after dilation (Agarwalla et al., 2015; van Boeckel & Siersema, 2015).

(3) Assessment

   (a) Assessment should check for clinical changes, such as weight loss, chest pain, dysphagia, or hemoptysis.

   (b) Patients should be referred for upper endoscopy.

(4) Documentation: Documentation should adhere to facility requirements and standardized documentation sources, such as CTCAE and RTOG/EORTC scoring systems.

(5) Collaborative management

    (a) Patients can be referred for possible fluoroscopic or endoscopic balloon dilation.

        i. This method is preferred because it is less invasive than surgical intervention.

        ii. Although dilation is safe and effective, serious complications, such as esophageal rupture, vocal cord palsy, and fistulas between the esophagus and trachea, can arise (Agarwalla et al., 2015; Park et al., 2018).

    (b) Strictures can recur and may require multiple dilations (Agarwalla et al., 2015).

    (c) Clinicians should evaluate patients for surgical intervention (esophageal resection) or esophageal dilation (Park et al., 2018).

    (d) Patients should be referred to an RDN or RD.

    (e) Patients should be referred for speech and swallowing evaluation.

    (f) Clinicians should monitor for aspiration and pneumonia.

(6) Patient, caregiver, and family education

    (a) Patients, caregivers, and families should understand the importance of maintaining nutritional status. Patients should report new or worsening dysphagia.

    (b) Clinicians should review speech and swallowing exercises with patients. Patients, caregivers, and families should understand the importance of performing exercise daily to maintain or improve swallowing function.

f) Brachial plexopathy (breast cancer)

(1) Pathophysiology

    (a) Brachial plexopathy is a disorder characterized by regional paresthesia of the brachial plexus, marked discomfort and muscle weakness, and limited movement in the arm or hand. It is also characterized by paresthesias in the hand and arm, shoulder and upper arm pain and atrophy, and loss of deep tendon reflexes on the affected side (Koontz, 2018; NCI CTEP, 2017).

    (b) The brachial plexus is a collection of nerves that innervates the arm and involves the spinal roots formed at the anterior rami of the four most inferior cervical roots (C5, C6, C7, and C8) and the most superior thoracic nerve root (T1) (Stone & DeAngelis, 2016).

    (c) Irradiation of the brachial plexus causes tissue damage, inflammation, and microvasculature injury resulting in fibrosis (C.Y. Wong et al., 2017).

(2) Incidence

    (a) Brachial plexopathy is not a common toxicity of breast irradiation but can have a significant effect on quality of life. It usually occurs 8–12 months after treatment (Koontz, 2018).

    (b) Stubblefield (2017) stated that standard protocol for RT to the breast and chest wall is 50 Gy administered as 25 fractions of 2 Gy.

        i. With this dose and fractionation, the reported risk of brachial plexus injury is less than 1%.

        ii. The dose per fraction can safely be increased to 2.2–2.5 Gy if the total dose is reduced to 34–40 Gy.

        iii. If the dose per fraction is increased to 2.2–4.58 Gy and the total dose is increased to 43.5–60 Gy, then the risk of brachial plexopathy rises sharply to 1.7%–73%.

(3) Assessment

    (a) Upon physical examination, brachial plexopathy may present with the following symptoms (Baima, Silver, & Most, 2018; Chia & Master, 2018; Warade, Jha, Pattankar, & Desai, 2019).

        i. Numbness

        ii. Pain

        iii. Sensory loss

        iv. Weakness

        v. Paresthesias

        vi. Dysesthesia

        vii. Depressed or absent reflexes

        viii. Swelling of the upper extremity

        ix. Weakness in hand, wrist, or arm

        x. Muscle atrophy

        xi. Decreased motor strength

    (b) Providers should obtain PET or MRI of the brachial plexus (prior to treatment if possible) to distinguish between cancer recurrence and radiation-induced plexopathy.

        i. On MRI, neoplastic changes will be characterized by a mass, and radiation-induced plexopathy is characterized by T2 hyperintensity of the affected nerve.

        ii. Fibrosis due to radiation is isointense to hypointense relative to muscle on T2-weighted images.

        iii. In contrast, tumor infiltration of the brachial plexus appears as a mass lesion that is hyperintense on T2-weighted sequences; however, the vascularized fibrous scar tissues appear hyperintense on T2-weighted images, thereby making diagnosis extremely difficult (Warade et al., 2019).

(c) The role of electromyography in diagnosis is not clear. Stubblefield (2017) stated that electromyography is useful in identifying peripheral nerve disorders resulting from radiation, but Koontz (2018) stated electromyography may reveal fasciculations more pronounced than clinical symptoms and is of little diagnostic benefit.

(d) Myokymia (localized quivering muscle) is present in 60% of radiation-induced plexopathy cases and less often in cancer-induced plexopathy (Koontz, 2018).

(4) Documentation: Documentation should adhere to facility requirements and standardized documentation sources, such as CTCAE for brachial plexopathy grading (NCI CTEP, 2017, p. 98).

(a) Grade 1: asymptomatic; clinical or diagnostic observations only; intervention not indicated

(b) Grade 2: moderate symptoms; limiting instrumental ADLs

(c) Grade 3: severe symptoms; limiting self-care ADLs

(5) Collaborative management: Treatment is supportive and aimed at alleviating symptoms.

(a) Gabapentin 300–1,200 mg three times daily or pregabalin 75–150 mg twice daily for neuropathic pain

(b) Benzodiazepines (e.g., diazepam 2–10 mg three to four times daily) for paresthesias (Koontz, 2018)

(c) Referral for physical therapy

(d) Referral for transcutaneous electrical nerve stimulation to treat neuropathic pain

(e) Psychological counseling related to the chronicity of pain (Warade et al., 2019)

(6) Patient, caregiver, and family education

(a) Education includes signs of worsening nerve damage and when to contact a provider.

(b) Education includes possible accommodations for neurologic weakness needed in the home to perform ADLs and employment duties.

(c) Patients, caregivers, and families should understand the importance of early and continuing occupational therapy to maintain functional status.

7. Gastrointestinal tract and abdomen
   a) Chronic gastritis and enteritis
      (1) Pathophysiology
         (a) Irradiation of tumors in the gastrointestinal tract initiate a cascade of events beginning with the release of damage-associated molecular patterns, cytokines (TNF-α, interleukin-6, interleukin-1α), and chemokines. This leads to an immune response with increased capillary permeability and leukocytic infiltration in the surrounding healthy tissue.

         (b) The consequence in normal tissue is an increase in proinflammatory immune cells resulting in gastritis. This leads to chronic inflammation of the stomach, intestines, and bladder, with telangiectasia and bleeding (Najafi et al., 2018; Simone, 2017; Wirsdörfer et al., 2019).

         (c) Chronic enteritis can result in ulceration, hemorrhage, intestinal stenosis, intestinal fistula, and perforation (Shen, Liu, & Zhu, 2018).

      (2) Incidence
         (a) Kalaiselvan et al. (2014) reported an incidence rate of 20%.

         (b) Radiation-induced gastritis can occur at doses higher than 50 Gy (Yahyapour et al., 2018).

      (3) Assessment
         (a) Physical examination involves medical history and symptoms, including abdominal or acute epigastric pain alone or associated with nausea, vomiting, anorexia, dyspepsia, or anemia (Sangro et al., 2017).

         (b) Patients can be referred for upper and lower endoscopy.

      (4) Documentation: Documentation should adhere to facility requirements and standardized documentation sources, such as CTCAE.

      (5) Collaborative management
         (a) Medical management includes steroids, pentoxifylline, metronidazole, and antidiarrheals (Koontz, 2018; Nicholas et al., 2017; Shen et al., 2018; C.S. Wong et al., 2015).

         (b) Hyperbaric oxygen is used to treat chronic gastrointestinal radiation-induced toxicities, but the data from randomized controlled trials are conflicting (Nicholas et al., 2017).

         (c) Antioxidant therapy with vitamins A, E, and C can be effective in alleviating diarrhea, urgency, and hemorrhage for patients with proctitis (Najafi et al., 2018).

(d) Patients can be referred for argon plasma coagulation (Yun, Kim, Kim, & Lim, 2015).

(e) The use of radiofrequency ablation, which uses a thermal effect to coagulate and necrose affected tissue, is becoming more common (Shen et al., 2018).

(f) Patients may require evaluation by gastroenterology, nutrition, and pain management. Clinicians should monitor for malabsorption and dehydration.

(6) Patient, caregiver, and family education

   (a) Clinicians should initiate a bowel management program.

   (b) Clinicians should review dietary changes, including fiber intake and probiotics. Patients can be referred for home care as needed.

   (c) Patient, caregivers, and families should know when to contact the provider for new or worsening symptoms, such as abdominal pain and bloating, rectal bleeding and pain, diarrhea, and fever.

b) Radiation-induced proctitis

(1) Pathophysiology

   (a) Radiation-induced proctitis (chronic radiation proctopathy or pelvic radiation disease) can occur after treatment of pelvic cancers such as anus, rectum, bladder, prostate, gynecologic organs (uterus, ovaries, cervix, and vagina), and small bowel (van de Wetering et al., 2016).

   (b) The process of proctitis begins with acute inflammation, edema, and endothelial injury, followed by loss of the epithelial lining, leading to the deposition of extracellular matrix, and can end with normal cellular repair of some tissue and fibrosis, ulceration, arteriolar endarteritis, vascular sclerosis, strictures, rectal bleeding, tenesmus (cramping rectal pain), diarrhea, and ischemia in other tissues (Alashkham, Paterson, Rauchhaus, & Nabi, 2016; Bansal, Soni, Kaur, Chauhan, & Kaushal, 2016; Mintet et al., 2015).

   (c) Patients with chronic proctitis can present with persistent rectal bleeding, diarrhea, rectal fistulas, incontinence, excessive flatulence, and intestinal strictures. In rare cases, cancerous changes can occur (Bansal et al., 2016; Koontz, 2018).

(2) Incidence

   (a) The reported incidence of radiation proctitis in patients irradiated to the pelvic organs is between 5% and 65% (Bansal et al., 2016; van de Wetering et al., 2016; Weiner et al., 2016).

   (b) Risk factors include the following (Bansal et al., 2016; Koontz, 2018; Nicholas et al., 2017; van de Wetering et al., 2016; Vanneste et al., 2015; Weiner et al., 2016).

     i. Diabetes mellitus

     ii. Colitis

     iii. Inflammatory bowel disease

     iv. Hypertension

     v. Peripheral vascular disease

     vi. Collagen vascular disease (systemic lupus erythematosus, scleroderma)

     vii. Prior abdominal surgery

     viii. Concurrent chemotherapy

   (c) The severity and incidence of proctitis is correlated to the volume of rectum receiving more than 70 Gy. A larger volume of rectum treated with RT leads to increased proctitis.

   (d) The use of IGRT, IMRT, or rectum spacers and balloons can reduce the dose to the rectum and affect the severity of radiation-induced proctitis (Vanneste et al., 2015).

(3) Assessment

   (a) Assessment involves comprehensive physical examination and medical history, including surgeries (e.g., bowel surgeries), history of colitis or pelvic inflammatory disease, cardiovascular disease, smoking, collagen vascular disease (e.g., systemic lupus erythematosus, scleroderma), diabetes mellitus, changes in bowel habits, and weight loss.

   (b) Laboratory testing includes blood chemistry and hemoglobin.

   (c) Endoscopy should be used to determine extent of chronic proctitis. Degrees of severity are as follows (Vanneste et al., 2015).

     i. Inflammation-predominant form (edema, mucosal pallor, and ulcer)

     ii. Bleeding-predominant form (friability, spontaneous hemorrhage, and telangiectasia)

     iii. Mixed form (features of bleeding and inflammation forms)

(4) Documentation: Documentation should adhere to facility requirements and standardized documentation sources, such as CTCAE (NCI CTEP, 2017, p. 35).

   (a) Grade 1: rectal discomfort, intervention not indicated

   (b) Grade 2: symptomatic (e.g., rectal discomfort, passing blood or mucus), medical intervention indicated; limiting instrumental ADLs

   (c) Grade 3: severe symptoms; fecal urgency or stool incontinence; limiting self-care ADLs *(d)* Grade 4: life-threatening consequences; urgent intervention indicated

(5) Collaborative management

(a) Treatment has not been standardized. Medical treatments include antidiarrheals, pentoxifylline, vitamin A, hydrocortisone suppositories, anti-inflammatories (sulfasalazine, mesalamine), metronidazole added to an anti-inflammatory regimen, short-chain fatty acid enema, corticosteroid enema, and sucralfate enema.

(b) For more severe proctitis, patients may undergo endoscopy, argon plasma coagulation, and hyperbaric oxygen therapy. Surgical intervention is used to repair fistulas (Bansal et al., 2016; Koontz, 2018; van de Wetering et al., 2016).

(c) Clinicians should avoid rectal biopsies, unless carcinoma is suspected, as rectal biopsy or treatment with formalin coagulation can result in fistula formation (Koontz, 2018).

(d) Monitor for signs of dehydration and malnutrition.

(e) Formalin therapy had been used in the past but is now associated with increased incidence of fistula formation and worsening fecal incontinence (Koontz, 2018).

(f) Patients should be referred to an RDN or RD.

(g) Acupuncture has been shown to be effective for pain from radiation-induced proctitis for patients treated for cervical and endometrial cancer (Lu & Rosenthal, 2018).

(6) Patient, caregiver, and family education

(a) Education includes information on side effects of therapy.

(b) Patients should monitor diet modifications, such as maintaining a low-residue diet, avoiding fatty foods and lactose products, and reducing fiber and spicy foods, as instructed by an RDN or RD.

(c) Patients should maintain adequate hydration and monitor weight.

(d) Clinicians should educate patients, caregivers, and families on signs of infection (e.g., fever, chills, pain) and when to contact a healthcare provider, such as with change in stools, hematochezia, abdominal cramping and pain, and worsening or new diarrhea.

(e) Clinicians should provide instruction on skin care, including cleansing the perineum with warm water and mild soap, using sitz baths, and using moisture barrier ointments or creams.

8. Bladder

a) Overview

(1) The severity of toxicities for bladder and pelvic irradiation can be affected negatively by treatment modality, dose, and treatment field size.

(2) Men with prostate cancer who received brachytherapy experienced worse lower urinary tract symptoms, such as urinary irritation and obstructive symptoms, when compared to those treated with EBRT (Nicholas et al., 2017).

(3) Obesity and smoking in patients with cervical cancer can worsen bladder toxicities. Hematuria is increased with the use of anticoagulants (Nicholas et al., 2017).

(4) According to Raup et al. (2016), RT may lead to widespread tissue damage, which puts patients at higher risk for spontaneous development of fistulae as a result of devascularization and necrosis. Pelvic irradiation increases the risk of bladder outlet dysfunction (bladder neck contracture or stress urinary incontinence), which adds to the morbidity of fistulae.

b) Bladder dysfunction: lower urinary tract symptoms (urinary frequency, urgency, hematuria, and incontinence)

(1) Pathophysiology

(a) Lower urinary tract symptoms and overactive bladder syndrome both consist of urgency with or without urinary incontinence, hesitancy, weakened urinary stream, frequency, and nocturia (Miyake et al., 2015; Thiruchelvam et al., 2015).

(b) These symptoms can be caused by bladder inflammation due to RT, resulting in decreased functional bladder capacity (Leddy, 2018; Miyake et al., 2015).

(c) Lower urinary tract symptoms can be categorized as storage symptoms, such as frequency, urgency, and nocturia, or symptoms associated with bladder irritation, such as difficulty emptying, weak stream, hesitancy, and intermittency (Onishi et al., 2019).

(2) Incidence

(a) Higher rates of urinary obstruction and urgency can occur in men receiving RT for prostate cancer and men receiving doses greater than 70 Gy to the bladder (Thor et al., 2016).

(b) The incidence of lower urinary tract symptoms in women treated for pelvic cancer can range from 26% to greater than 60% at 5–11 years after RT (Leddy, 2018; Nicholas et al., 2017).

(c) The exact incidence of lower urinary tract symptoms after RT to the pelvis in men and women is unknown (Lobo et al., 2018).

(3) Assessment
    (a) Assessment includes physical examination of pelvis and detailed history: onset, severity, and duration of symptoms (e.g., urinary retention, frequency, urgency, hesitancy, nocturia, stranguria, incontinence, pelvic pain) (Leddy, 2018).
    (b) The severity of lower urinary tract symptoms and overactive bladder syndrome should be assessed using validated standardized surveys.
        i. Overactive Bladder Symptom Score or Overactive Bladder Questionnaire for general symptoms
        ii. Specific forms, such as International Prostate Symptom Score
    (c) Evaluation may include more invasive procedures including urodynamic studies and cystoscopy (Leddy, 2018).

(4) Documentation: Documentation should adhere to facility requirements and standardized documentation sources, such as CTCAE, Overactive Bladder Symptom Score, Overactive Bladder Questionnaire, and International Prostate Symptom Score.

(5) Collaborative management
    (a) Initial management can include behavioral modifications, such as decreased intake of urinary irritants (caffeine), elimination of fluid intake prior to sleep, pelvic floor exercises (e.g., Kegel exercises), and use of a 72-hour voiding journal (Leddy, 2018).
    (b) Medical management is the first line of treatment for lower urinary tract symptoms.
        i. Alpha-blockers, such as naftopidil, tamsulosin, or silodosin, and anticholinergics, such as trospium chloride, have been shown to improve urinary symptoms.
        ii. Other antimuscarinics (urinary antispasmodics), such as oxybutynin, and beta 3 adrenergic receptor agonists, such as mirabegron) are also effective (Thiruchelvam et al., 2015; Yan et al., 2017).
        iii. These medications can be used as monotherapy, and some may be used in combination.
    (c) The second or third line of therapy is more invasive and may include botulinum toxin A, percutaneous tibial nerve stimulation,

sacral nerve stimulation, or sacral neuromodulation (Leddy, 2018; Thiruchelvam et al., 2015).
    (d) Surgical interventions, such as urethroplasty, can also improve stress incontinence when the urethra is reconstructed and an artificial urinary sphincter is placed (P.H. Chung, Esposito, Wessells, & Voelzke, 2018).

c) Fistula formation
(1) Pathophysiology
    (a) Fistula formation can occur when any of the organs of the pelvis, vagina, prostate, pelvic bone, bladder, and lower intestinal tract are irradiated.
    (b) Fistulae may result from radiation, but in many instances, subsequent manipulation of irradiated tissue may result in fistula formation.
    (c) Bugeja, Ivaz, Frost, Andrich, and Mundy (2016) noted that fistula formation may result from dilation, incision, or resection of a previously irradiated area.

(2) Incidence
    (a) The incidence of fistulae can vary according to the area irradiated.
    (b) In prostate cancer RT, the incidence has increased to 52.6%, up from 3.8% in 1977. Ureterovaginal and vesicovaginal fistulas caused by focal high-dose RT to the pelvis are rare (Bugeja et al., 2016).
    (c) Factors such as increased depth of tumor invasion of genitourinary structures are more likely to result in fistulae (Nicholas et al., 2017).

(3) Assessment
    (a) Assessment includes physical examination, urine culture and analysis, and urine cytology.
    (b) Cystoscopy can be performed.

(4) Documentation: Documentation should adhere to facility requirements and standardized documentation sources, such as CTCAE.

(5) Collaborative management
    (a) Conservative measures include management of symptoms, pain, and leakage of urine (Bugeja et al., 2016).
    (b) Surgical repair of the fistula is not recommended because of poor vasculature and wound healing caused by irradiation, low rates of success, and patients having persistent urinary dysfunction despite surgical intervention.
        i. Surgery may be an option in tertiary settings with experienced surgeons, as corrective surgery is complex with

a higher likelihood of sepsis (Bugeja et al., 2016).

  ii. In one study, 42.5% of patients ultimately required a urinary diversion after pelvic irradiation (Nicholas et al., 2017; Raup et al., 2016).

  iii. Surgical interventions include fistula tract excision and repair of small fistulas or temporary or permanent urinary diversion.

  iv. The need for permanent urinary or bowel diversion has been reported as high as 100% if surgical intervention is needed (Bugeja et al., 2016).

  v. Surgical intervention should involve the members of the interprofessional team, including social workers, physical therapists, and psychiatrists.

  d) Hemorrhagic cystitis

    (1) Pathology

      (a) Hemorrhagic cystitis refers to a combination of symptoms that includes hematuria, lower urinary tract symptoms, and urothelial damage caused by damage to the epithelium of the bladder (Farrington & Murphy, 2019; Goucher, Saad, Lukka, & Kapoor, 2019).

      (b) See previous information on chronic gastritis and enteritis.

    (2) Incidence

      (a) Hemorrhagic cystitis can occur months to years after RT.

      (b) The incidence for patients treated with 3DCRT to the pelvic area was approximately 5% (Nicholas et al., 2017).

      (c) Older studies by Levenback, Eifel, Burke, Morris, and Gershenson (1994) of patients with cervical cancer treated with combination intracavitary RT and EBRT reported an incidence of 6.5%.

      (d) Hemorrhagic cystitis can occur in up to 9% of patients treated with pelvic irradiation (Leddy, 2018).

    (3) Assessment

      (a) Laboratory assessment includes urine analysis, cytology, and culture, as well as complete blood counts.

      (b) Cystoscopy can be performed.

      (c) Clinicians should monitor for possible bladder neoplasm.

    (4) Documentation: Documentation should adhere to facility requirements and standardized documentation sources, such as CTCAE.

    (5) Collaborative management

      (a) Conservative measures, such as the administration of analgesics, bladder irrigation, hydration, antibiotics for infection, and blood transfusions, are used.

      (b) Other treatments include hyperbaric oxygen therapy, installation of intravesical agents, or systemic agents.

      (c) Transarterial embolization may be used in refractory cases (Goucher et al., 2019; Nicholas et al., 2017).

      (d) Severe refractory cystitis may require urinary diversion using percutaneous nephrostomy tubes or cystectomy (Leddy, 2018).

    (6) Patient, caregiver, and family education

      (a) Clinicians should educate patients on signs and symptoms of hematuria and anemia.

      (b) Education should include information on medications that may increase bleeding. Patients may require skin care management (Farrington & Murphy, 2019).

  e) Urethral stricture or fibrosis (radiation-induced urethral stricture)

    (1) Pathophysiology

      (a) Treatment is challenging because of the effects of irradiation: decreased vascularization resulting in poor wound healing (P.H. Chung et al., 2018).

      (b) Refer to previous information on radiation-induced esophageal stricture.

    (2) Incidence

      (a) RTOG studies have reported that, in patients with prostate cancer and grade 3 genitourinary toxicity, the incidence of urethral stricture is 50% (Nicholas et al., 2017).

      (b) The rate of stricture is related to therapy used.

        i. Patients treated with radical prostatectomy had a 8.4% incidence, and patients treated with brachytherapy and EBRT had a 5.2% incidence (P.H. Chung et al., 2018).

        ii. The incidence can increase with combination therapy of brachytherapy and EBRT (5.2%), compared to brachytherapy alone (1.8%) or EBRT alone (1.7%) for men with prostate cancer (P.H. Chung et al.,2018).

      (c) Urethra stricture is most common in men undergoing HDR brachytherapy, with an incidence of 31.6%, compared to 3% of patients with gynecologic cancers who are treated with brachytherapy (P.H. Chung et al., 2018; Nicholas al., 2017).

    (3) Assessment: Assessment includes physical examination and cystoscopy.

(4) Documentation: Documentation should adhere to facility requirements and standardized documentation sources, such as CTCAE.
(5) Collaborative management
   (a) The most common treatment is urethral dilation.
   (b) Surgical interventions include posterior excision and primary anastomotic urethroplasty, which is the more common procedure, and urethral substitution with grafts and flaps, which is used less frequently (P.H. Chung et al., 2018).

9. Male pelvic region and prostate
   a) Proctitis: See previous information on radiation-induced proctitis.
   b) Sexual dysfunction: See IV.E. Sexual function and dysfunction.
   c) Erectile dysfunction: See IV.E. Sexual function and dysfunction.
   d) Infertility
      (1) Pathophysiology
         (a) The testes are sensitive to the effects of irradiation, and effects are dose dependent.
         (b) Low doses of radiation result in testicular failure.
            i. N. Rao, Shridhar, and Hoffe (2014) stated that fractions of 2 Gy can cause permanent sterility, and fractions of less than 1 Gy are low enough for complete recovery of spermatogenesis.
            ii. Alterations in the hypothalamic–pituitary–gonadal axis can be an indirect cause of impaired spermatogenesis (Halpern, Hill, & Brannigan, 2020).
      (2) Assessment
         (a) Clinicians should initiate discussion with patient and partner regarding plans for reproduction.
         (b) Patients should be referred to a fertility specialist or reproductive urologist (Halpern et al., 2020).
      (3) Collaborative management
         (a) The Ethics Committee of the American Society for Reproductive Medicine (2018) stated that the only approved options for cryopreservation of spermatozoa are by ejaculation or surgical sperm retrieval.
         (b) Testicular tissue cryopreservation and testicular tissue reimplantation or grafting should be offered to a patient only as part of a clinical trial (Oktay et al., 2018).
         (c) Patients should be referred to a psychologist and reproductive specialist.
         (d) Treatment planning optimizes testicular shielding.
         (e) If sperm quality is inadequate, then reproduction techniques such as intracytoplasmic sperm injection can be used to enhance sperm production and quality (Ethics Committee of the American Society for Reproductive Medicine, 2018).
      (4) Patient, caregiver, and family education
         (a) Patients and partners should understand the effect of RT on fertility and options for sperm preservation and banking.
         (b) The optimal time to begin fertility preservation counseling is prior to cancer therapy (N. Rao et al., 2014).

10. Female pelvic region
    a) Vaginal stenosis, including fibrosis and dryness
       (1) Pathophysiology
          (a) Radiation-induced vaginal stenosis can result from vaginal transformation, which is caused by fibrosis, decreased elasticity, decreased vaginal lubrication, decreased genital sensation, and increased friability.
          (b) These changes lead to vaginal narrowing, which affects sexual function and speculum insertion during gynecologic examination (Pessi et al., 2016).
          (c) In the longer term, vaginal wall thinning, adhesions, atrophy, and fibrosis may occur and are often followed by decreased vaginal elasticity, narrowing, shortening, and, ultimately, total vaginal stenosis (Incrocci & Jensen, 2013).
          (d) Vaginal dryness is a late-term toxicity of pelvic region irradiation (Nicholas et al., 2017).
          (e) Irradiation of the pelvic region in women can result in inflammation, as well as desquamation of the vaginal walls leading to thinning of the vaginal walls and increased friability, resulting in decreased vaginal lubrication and atrophy (Incrocci & Jensen, 2013).
       (2) Incidence
          (a) Vaginal stenosis is a common late complication in women treated definitively with chemoradiation to the pelvic region.
          (b) Younger age, higher tumor radiation dose, and earlier year of treatment were associated with increased degree of vaginal stenosis (Mirabeau-Beale et al., 2015).
          (c) In a study of 233 women treated with pelvic irradiation, women reported vaginal stenosis was a significant post-treatment toxicity that represented with a cluster of symptoms, including dyspareunia, vagi-

nal pain, dryness, and bleeding (Kachnic, Bruner, Qureshi, & Russo, 2017).

    (d) One study of 252 women treated with pelvic irradiation, EBRT, or brachytherapy reported significant sexual dysfunction (57%), vaginal adhesions (53%), telangiectasia (60%), and vaginal stenosis (54.7%) (Incrocci & Jensen, 2013; Nunns, Williamson, Swaney, & Davy, 2000).

(3) Assessment: Assessment includes physical examination of the external genitalia and vagina to assess for lubrication, vaginal perineal lesions, erythema, or discharge.

(4) Documentation: Documentation should adhere to facility requirements and standardized documentation sources, such as CTCAE and LENT-SOMA.

(5) Collaborative management

    (a) Vaginal dilators can be prescribed.

    (b) Nonhormonal vaginal lubricants should be recommended. Over-the-counter products, such as water-based lubricants (e.g., K-Y® jelly), hyaluronic acid–based vaginal gel (e.g., Hyalofemme®), and polycarbophil-based vaginal moisturizers (e.g., Replens®), have been shown to improve vaginal dryness and decrease irritation and dyspareunia when used consistently.

    (c) Nonhormonal moisturizers may not be effective for severe chronic vaginal dryness or stenosis (C.S. Sears, Robinson, & Walker, 2018).

    (d) Estrogen-based creams may be effective to treat vaginal dryness and may improve vaginal stenosis. The use of estrogen-based treatments is not recommended for patients with hormone-dependent gynecologic cancers; therefore, the use of these medications in this population remains controversial (C.S. Sears et al., 2018).

    (e) Intravaginal administration of dehydroepiandrosterone has been shown in a randomized controlled trial to improve vaginal dryness, lubrication, and sexual desire (C.S. Sears et al., 2018). NCCN (2020b) recommends that survivors of estrogen-dependent cancers use dehydroepiandrosterone with caution. The safety of vaginal estrogen and vaginal testosterone in this patient population has not been established.

    (f) Patients can be referred for pelvic floor physiotherapy.

    (g) Preliminary results from several studies have shown that treatment with microab-lative fractional carbon dioxide lasers may improve vaginal atrophy. Patients tolerated the treatment well, and additional studies with long-term follow-up are needed (C.S. Sears et al., 2018).

(6) Patient, caregiver, and family education

    (a) Clinicians should inform patients on the options for vaginal dilation (vaginal dilator, prosthetic silicone rubber penis, or sexual intercourse).

    (b) Clinicians can provide directions on use and maintenance of a vaginal dilator and using a lubricant. Clinicians can recommend that the dilator be warmed in water prior to use and that using dilator should be done in a calm, relaxed environment.

    (c) A partner may facilitate the use of a vaginal dilator.

    (d) Clinicians should educate patients on the use of vaginal lubricants and moisturizers.

    (e) Clinicians should educate patients on the difference between hormonal and nonhormonal moisturizers and lubricants.

b) Bladder irritation, ulceration, fistula formation, and stricture: See previous information on bladder effects.

c) Sexual dysfunction: See IV.E. Sexual function and dysfunction.

d) Radiation-induced proctitis: See previous information on radiation-induced proctitis.

e) Infertility and menopause: See IV.F. Fertility.

11. Skin

    a) Alopecia

        (1) Pathophysiology

            (a) Radiation-induced alopecia is clinically apparent decreased hair density in the radiation field and is considered permanent if it persists more than six months after RT.

            (b) Alopecia can occur in any hair-bearing area that undergoes irradiation, such as the face, neck, or extremities (Bresters et al., 2017; Freites-Martinez et al., 2019).

            (c) Irradiation will also inhibit the proliferation of matrix cells in the base of a growing hair. This may be transient, leading to hair thinning, or this can produce alopecia or epilation, with the eventual regrowth of hair (Martin, Vulin, & Hendry, 2016).

            (d) Permanent alopecia is thought to be caused by destruction of hair follicle stem cells (Bresters et al., 2017).

               i. Irradiation of the skin causes severe damage to the skin, resulting in loss of hair follicles and sebaceous glands resulting in alopecia (Bray, Simmons, Wolfson, & Nouri, 2016).

ii. It is hypothesized that irradiation of the hair follicles causes damage to the highly mitotic cells, but the molecular mechanism of the damage remains unclear (Yue & Xu, 2017).

iii. Severity and permanence are related to the dose of radiation and use of scalp-sparing RT techniques (Barisano et al., 2018).

iv. Permanent alopecia can occur at dose greater than 7 Gy (Koontz, 2018).

(2) Incidence

(a) Alopecia is also a common outcome for children and adults who receive cranial RT for primary or metastatic cancer of the brain and meninges (Ahmad, Sardana, Chufal, & Bhatt, 2018).

(b) Hair loss is one of the most stressful side effects for patients undergoing oncologic treatment with either chemotherapy or cranial irradiation (Lawenda et al., 2004).

(c) An analysis of radiation dose–response relationship reported that a dose of 36 Gy (2 Gy per fraction, five days per week) was reported to cause permanent alopecia in 0%–80% of patients (median risk 5%) and that a dose of 45 Gy resulted in a risk of 5%–100% (median risk 15%) of permanent alopecia (Lawenda et al., 2004).

(3) Assessment: Assessment involves physical examination of involved areas for edema, erythema, intact skin, and signs of infection.

(4) Documentation: Documentation should adhere to facility requirements and standardized documentation sources, such as CTCAE and the Severity of Alopecia Tool with a scale of 0 (no hair loss) to 100 (complete alopecia).

(5) Collaborative management

(a) Existing clinical strategies to manage alopecia have been largely ineffective (Soref & Fahl, 2015).

(b) RT techniques to decrease dose to the scalp should be used.

(c) For mild alopecia, topical minoxidil foam (5%) twice daily can be prescribed.

(d) Botulinum toxin A can be prescribed at 5 units per 0.1 ml every three months for 12 months for grade 2 alopecia.

(e) Scalp reconstruction, including excision or tissue expansion, can be performed.

(f) Patients can be referred for hair transplantation (Freites-Martinez et al., 2019).

(g) Clinicians can suggest cosmetic options, including powders, scalp micropigmentation or tattoo, and hairstyle changes.

(6) Patient, caregiver, and family education

(a) Clinicians should educate patients, caregivers, and families on the psychological changes that can occur due to alopecia. Patients should be made aware of counseling services.

(b) Patients with treatment-induced alopecia report poorer quality of life, lower self-esteem, and heightened self-consciousness (Ahmad et al., 2018).

(c) Patients should avoid exposing scalp to the sun.

(d) Clinicians should educate patients on hair care techniques, such as gentle brushing, washing, and styling.

i. Patients should avoid bleaching, coloring, blow dryers, hot rollers, and curling and straightening irons.

ii. Clinicians should provide information on organizations that provide hats or wigs.

b) Radiation-induced fibrosis: See also IV.B. Skin reactions, and Williams et al. (2017).

(1) Pathophysiology

(a) Chronic cutaneous reactions result in radiation-induced fibrosis.

(b) In healthy cells, transforming growth factor-beta regulates cellular proliferation and differentiation, wound healing, activation of fibroblasts, and extracellular matrix protein synthesis (Bray et al., 2016; Straub et al., 2015).

(c) Fibroblasts play a crucial role in wound healing by deposing and remodeling collagen fibers, and in the irradiated tissue, the structure of these fibers becomes disorganized, possibly the result of dysregulation of matrix metalloproteases (Agishev et al., 2018).

(d) Irradiation of the skin leads to collateral obliteration of microvasculature and hypoxia, resulting in dermal and subcutaneous fibrosis, especially in the capillary endothelium (Luan et al., 2016).

(e) At first, radiation-induced fibrosis manifests as functional pathology of microcirculation and hypoxia in the irradiated tissue. Subsequently, it leads to morphologic changes in cells and formation of late manifestations in the form of fibrosis and sclerosis, which directly cause increasing hypoxia in the damaged area creating a positive feedback loop (Agishev et al., 2018).

i. The skin can become dry, scaly, and hyperkeratotic. These changes can progress to persistent dyspigmentation, atrophy, telangiectasia, ulceration, and necrosis.

    ii. Alopecia due to loss of hair follicles and sebaceous glands can also occur (Kawashima et al., 2016).

    iii. Telangiectasia is the dilation of small vessels under the skin or mucosal surface, commonly referred as "spider veins" (Soriano, Calpena, Souto, & Clares, 2019).

    iv. Chronic radiation dermatitis can be permanent and progressive and can develop years after treatment is completed.

    v. Risk factors are related to total dose, technique, and patient characteristics (Bray et al., 2016).

  (f) Radiation-induced fibrosis may manifest as skin induration and thickening, muscle shortening and atrophy, limited joint mobility, lymphedema, mucosal fibrosis, ulceration, fistula, hollow organ stenosis, and pain (Straub et al., 2015).

(2) Incidence

  (a) Radiation-induced fibrosis is prevalent and has a significant impact on quality of life in patients who receive RT.

  (b) Fibrosis usually occurs 4–12 months after RT, progresses over several years, and affects almost every part of the body that is exposed to radiation (Straub et al., 2015).

  (c) Risk factors for fibrosis are radiation dose and volume of tissue irradiated, but radiation-induced fibrosis is not associated with and is not preceded by acute radiation dermatitis (Soriano et al., 2019).

(3) Assessment

  (a) Assessment includes checking for atrophy, fibrosis, changes in pigmentation, and telangiectasias.

  (b) Assessment also includes checking for nonhealing wounds, ulcerations, and evidence of local cancer recurrence.

(4) Documentation: Documentation should adhere to facility requirements and standardized documentation sources. The RTOG/EORTC scale addresses grading for acute and late skin toxicities.

(5) Collaborative management

  (a) IMRT is the recommended treatment technique if possible.

  (b) Routine skin hygiene to the radiation portal, which is the use of mild soaps, moistur-

izers, and deodorant, may be used (Gosselin et al., 2017).

  (c) In a breast cancer setting, treatment with pentoxifylline and vitamin E has been shown to improve tissue compliance in patients with radiation-induced fibrosis (Jacobson et al., 2013).

  (d) Chronic cutaneous reactions, such as telangiectasias, can be treated with laser therapy.

  (e) Treatment of chronic ulcerations and wounds can involve silver-based and tetrachlorodecaoxide dressings, laser therapy (pulsed-dye laser), and growth factors (e.g., platelet-derived growth factors, fibroblast growth factors).

  (f) Skin fibrosis can be treated with the following interventions (Soriano et al., 2019).

    i. Physical therapy (deep massage and exercise of the limb or area)

    ii. Laser therapy alone or in combination with epidermal grafting

    iii. Systemic therapies (pentoxifylline in combination with vitamin E)

    iv. Antioxidant superoxide dismutase in systemic or topical form

  (g) The benefits of hyperbaric oxygen therapy and cytokines (interferon gamma) for skin fibrosis have not been proven (Soriano et al., 2019).

(6) Patient, caregiver, and family education

  (a) Patients should use protective measures, such as avoiding sun exposure and tanning booths and beds, as well as using sunscreen of SPF 30 or greater.

  (b) Patients should use moisturizing lotions and creams daily and avoid products that dry the skin, such as perfumes, harsh chemicals, and alcohol-containing products.

12. Bone

  a) Fractures

    (1) Pathophysiology

      (a) Irradiation of the bone leads to radiation-induced osteopenia due to the loss of functional osteoblasts in the radiation field.

      (b) Radiation inhibits cell cycle progression of osteoclasts, thus changing their ability to differentiate and sensitizing them to apoptosis signals (Chandra et al., 2015).

      (c) Late effects can range from mild osteopenia to osteoradionecrosis.

    (2) Incidence

      (a) Fracture developments are dose dependent (Jawad et al., 2016).

(b) Vertebral compression fractures can occur after stereotactic RT to the spine, but the contributing factors are not completely understood (Boyce-Fappiano et al., 2017).

(c) Rich et al. (2018) completed a systematic review of palliative RT for bone metastasis, reporting that the rate of pathologic fracture was 4% with single fraction and 3% with multiple fractions.

(d) Fractures can result in impaired mobility, pain, and detrimental effects on quality of life, especially for older adult patients with pelvis fractures (Chandra et al., 2015).

(e) Ramlov et al. (2017) assessed 101 women with locally advanced cervical cancer treated with definitive chemotherapy, IMRT, and brachytherapy and reported that 20% of the patients were diagnosed with pelvic insufficiency fractures on MRI, and approximately half were asymptomatic.

(3) Assessment

(a) Comprehensive examination includes the musculoskeletal and neurologic systems.

(b) Examination includes assessment for pain on palpation, difficulty weight bearing, or decreased range of motion due to pain, edema, or weakness.

(c) Imaging assessment can include x-ray, CT, MRI, or PET.

(d) Evaluation should involve an interprofessional team (radiation oncology, medical oncology, orthopedics, neurosurgery, pain management, and rehabilitation) (Sharif & Qadeer, 2016).

(4) Documentation: Documentation should adhere to facility requirements and standardized documentation sources such as CTCAE, including pain scores.

(5) Collaborative management

(a) Pain management can include analgesics and dexamethasone as needed.

(b) Treatment planning should include members of the interprofessional team. Treatment may involve multiple modalities with surgery.

(c) Patients should be evaluated for tumor progression.

(d) Clinicians should monitor for psychosocial distress and refer patients for counseling.

(e) Clinicians should consult with rehabilitative services.

(6) Patient, caregiver, and family education

(a) Instruction includes information on management of pain.

(b) Clinicians should explain signs and symptoms of progressive disease, such as weakness or worsening pain.

(c) Clinicians should provide psychosocial support.

(d) Clinicians should provide information on community support services.

(e) Clinicians should discuss physical changes in the household that may be required to promote patient safety (e.g., removal of rugs, installation of assistive devices).

b) Radiation-induced rib fracture

(1) Pathophysiology: See previous information on fractures.

(2) Incidence

(a) Rib fractures and chest wall pain have been reported after conventional RT. Patients present with chest wall pain or may be asymptomatic (Okoukoni et al., 2017).

(b) Nicholls, Gorayski, and Harvey (2015) reported that the incidence of radiation-induced rib fracture in patients with breast cancer treated with RT is 0.1%–5%.

(c) Other researchers estimate the incidence at 1%–19% (Chandra, Park, & Pignolo, 2019).

(d) Risk factors for radiation-induced rib fracture in breast cancer are radiation dose, fractionation and field size, preexisting osteoporosis, and postmenopausal status (Harris et al., 2016; Nicholls et al., 2015).

(3) Collaborative management

(a) Chest x-ray and rib series, as well as additional imaging, should be used to exclude recurrence or a second primary cancer.

(b) Physical examination of the chest should check for tenderness or pain on palpation of ribs, spine, or sternum.

(c) Assessment should check for changes in respiratory status.

(d) Pain should be managed with analgesics.

(4) Patient, caregiver, and family education: Clinicians should educate patients, caregivers, and families on signs of worsening toxicity, including chest or chest wall pain, difficulty or painful breathing, pain with cough, pain with movement, new or worsening rib pain, rib swelling, or change in the shape of the chest or thorax.

References

Agarwalla, A., Small, A.J., Mendelson, A.H., Scott, F.I., & Kochman, M.L. (2015). Risk of recurrent or refractory strictures and outcome of endoscopic dilation for radiation-induced esophageal strictures. *Surgical Endoscopy, 29,* 1903–1912. https://doi.org/10.1007/s00464-014-3883-1

Agishev, T.T., Topuzov, E.E., Krasnozhon, D.A., Petrachkov, A.O., Pavlov, R.V., & Doniyarov, S.H. (2018). Determination of oxygen perfusion in the area of radiation-induced fibrosis of the skin in patients with breast cancer and its role in pathogenesis of late radiation injury. *Experimental Oncology, 40,* 235–238. http://exp-oncology.com.ua/article/11591

Ahmad, I., Sardana, K., Chufal, K.S., & Bhatt, C.P. (2018). Radiation induced alopecia: An under-appreciated side effect of whole brain radiotherapy and strategies to ameliorate it. *Journal of Nuclear Medicine and Radiation Therapy, 9,* 002. https://doi.org/10.4172/2155-9619.S9-002

Alashkham, A., Paterson, C., Rauchhaus, P., & Nabi, G. (2016). Can angiotensin-converting enzyme inhibitors reduce the incidence, severity, and duration of radiation proctitis? *International Journal of Radiation Oncology, Biology, Physics, 94,* 93–101. https://doi.org/10.1016/j.ijrobp.2015.09.013

Armer, J.M., Beck, M., Burns, B.R., Deng, J., Fu, M.R., Lockwood, S., ... Poage, E.G. (2017). Symptom interventions: Lymphedema. https://www.ons.org/pep/lymphedema

Arthurs, E., Hanna, T.P., Zaza, K., Peng, Y., & Hall, S.F. (2016). Stroke after radiation therapy for head and neck cancer: What is the risk? *International Journal of Radiation Oncology, Biology, Physics, 96,* 589–596. https://doi.org/10.1016/j.ijrobp.2016.07.007

Asdourian, M.S., Skolny, M.N., Brunelle, C., Seward, C.E., Salama, L., & Taghian, A.G. (2016). Precautions for breast cancer-related lymphoedema: Risk from air travel, ipsilateral arm blood pressure measurements, skin puncture, extreme temperatures, and cellulitis. *Lancet Oncology, 17,* e392–e405. https://doi.org/10.1016/S1470-2045(16)30204-2

Astradsson, T., Laurell, G., Ahlberg, A., Nikolaidis, P., Johansson, H., & Ehrsson, Y.T. (2018). Trismus in patients with head and neck cancer and 5-year overall survival. *Acta Oto-Laryngologica, 138,* 1123–1127. https://doi.org/10.1080/00016489.2018.1511059

Baima, J.A., Silver, J.K., & Most, M. (2018). Neuromuscular dysfunction in the cancer patient: Evaluation and treatment. *Muscle and Nerve, 58,* 335–343. https://doi.org/10.1002/mus.26103

Balusik, B. (2014). Management of dysphagia in patients with head and neck cancer. *Clinical Journal of Oncology Nursing, 18,* 149–150. https://doi.org/10.1188/14.CJON.149-150

Bansal, N., Soni, A., Kaur, P., Chauhan, A.K., & Kaushal, V. (2016). Exploring the management of radiation proctitis in current clinical practice. *Journal of Clinical and Diagnostic Research, 10*(6), XE01–XE06. https://doi.org/10.7860/JCDR/2016/17524.7906

Barisano, G., Bergamaschi, S., Acharya, J., Rajamohan, A., Gibbs, W., Kim, P., ... Law, M. (2018). Complications of radiotherapy and radiosurgery in the brain and spine. *Neurographics, 8,* 167–187. https://doi.org/10.3174/ng.1700066

Bazire, L., De Rycke, Y., Asselain, B., Fourquet, A., & Kirova, Y.M. (2017). Risks of second malignancies after breast cancer treatment: Long-term results. *Cancer/Radiothérapie, 21,* 10–15. https://doi.org/10.1016/j.canrad.2016.07.101

Boomsma, M.J., Bijl, H.P., & Langendijk, J.A. (2011). Radiation-induced hypothyroidism in head and neck cancer patients: A systematic review. *Radiotherapy and Oncology, 99,* 1–5. https://doi.org/10.1016/j.radonc.2011.03.002

Boyce-Fappiano, D., Elibe, E., Schultz, L., Ryu, S., Siddiqui, M.S., Chetty, I., ... Siddiqui, F. (2017). Analysis of the factors contributing to vertebral compression fractures after spine stereotactic radiosurgery. *International Journal of Radiation Oncology, Biology, Physics, 97,* 236–245. https://doi.org/10.1016/j.ijrobp.2016.09.007

Braunstein, L.Z., & Cahlon, O. (2018). Potential morbidity reduction with proton radiation therapy for breast cancer. *Seminars in Radiation Oncology, 28,* 138–149. https://doi.org/10.1016/j.semradonc.2017.11.009

Bray, F.N., Simmons, B.J., Wolfson, A.H., & Nouri, K. (2016). Acute and chronic cutaneous reactions to ionizing radiation therapy. *Dermatology and Therapy, 6,* 185–206. https://doi.org/10.1007/s13555-016-0120-y

Brecht, S., Boda-Heggemann, J., Budjan, J., Siebenlist, K., Stieler, F., Steil, V., ... Buergy, D. (2019). Radiation-induced optic neuropathy after stereotactic and image guided intensity-modulated radiation therapy (IMRT). *Radiotherapy and Oncology, 134,* 166–177. https://doi.org/10.1016/j.radonc.2019.02.003

Brennan, P.A., Bradley, K.L., & Brands, M. (2017). Intensity-modulated radiotherapy in head and neck cancer—An update for oral and maxillofacial surgeons. *British Journal of Oral and Maxillofacial Surgery, 55,* 770–774. https://doi.org/10.1016/j.bjoms.2017.07.019

Bresters, D., Wanders, D.C.M., Louwerens, M., Ball, L.M., Fiocco, M., & Van Doorn, R. (2017). Permanent diffuse alopecia after haematopoietic stem cell transplantation in childhood. *Bone Marrow Transplantation, 52,* 984–988. https://doi.org/10.1038/bmt.2017.15

Bugeja, S., Ivaz, S., Frost, A., Andrich, D.E., & Mundy, A.R. (2016). Complex fistula disease in the pelvic malignancy cancer survivor who has been treated with radiation. *Current Bladder Dysfunction Reports, 11,* 113–119. https://doi.org/10.1007/s11884-016-0358-3

Buglione, M., Cavagnini, R., Di Rosario, F., Maddalo, M., Vassalli, L., Grisanti, S., ... Magrini, S.M. (2016). Oral toxicity management in head and neck cancer patients treated with chemotherapy and radiation: Xerostomia and trismus (part 2). Literature review and consensus statement. *Critical Reviews in Oncology/Hematology, 102,* 47–54. https://doi.org/10.1016/j.critrevonc.2016.03.012

Cao, L., Zhu, W., Wagar, E.A., & Meng, Q.H. (2017). Biomarkers for monitoring chemotherapy-induced cardiotoxicity. *Critical Reviews in Clinical Laboratory Sciences, 54,* 87–101. https://doi.org/10.1080/10408363.2016.1261270

Carpenter, D.J., Mowery, Y.M., Broadwater, G., Rodrigues, A., Wisdom, A.J., Dorth, J.A., ... Brizel, D.M. (2018). The risk of carotid stenosis in head and neck cancer patients after radiation therapy. *Oral Oncology, 80,* 9–15. https://doi.org/10.1016/j.oraloncology.2018.02.021

Chandra, A., Lin, T., Zhu, J., Tong, W., Huo, Y., Jia, H., ... Qin, L. (2015). PTH1–34 blocks radiation-induced osteoblast apoptosis by enhancing DNA repair through canonical Wnt pathway. *Journal of Biological Chemistry, 290,* 157–167. https://doi.org/10.1074/jbc.M114.608158

Chandra, A., Park, S.S., & Pignolo, R.J. (2019). Potential role of senescence in radiation-induced damage of the aged skeleton. *Bone, 120,* 423–431. https://doi.org/10.1016/j.bone.2018.12.006

Chang, C.J., & Cormier, J.N. (2013). Lymphedema interventions: Exercise, surgery, and compression devices. *Seminars in Oncology Nursing, 29,* 28–40. https://doi.org/10.1016/j.soncn.2012.11.005

Chang, J.I., Bevans, S.E., & Schwartz, S.R. (2012). Otolaryngology clinic of North America: Evidence-based practice: Management of hoarseness/dysphonia. *Otolaryngologic Clinics of North America, 45,* 1109–1126. https://doi.org/10.1016/j.otc.2012.06.012

Chia, B.S.H., & Master, Z. (2018). Pitfalls in lung stereotactic body radiotherapy—A review of organ toxicities and dose constraints. *Journal of Xiangya Medicine, 3,* 36. https://doi.org/10.21037/jxym.2018.09.04

Chung, C.S., Yock, T.I., Nelson, K., Xu, Y., Keating, N.L., & Tarbell, N.J. (2013). Incidence of second malignancies among patients treated with proton versus photon radiation. *International Journal of Radiation Oncology, Biology, Physics, 87,* 46–52. https://doi.org/10.1016/j.ijrobp.2013.04.030

Chung, P.H., Esposito, P., Wessells, H., & Voelzke, B.B. (2018). Incidence of stress urinary incontinence after posterior urethroplasty for radiation-induced urethral strictures. *Urology, 114,* 188–192. https://doi.org/10.1016/j.urology.2017.11.024

Dawes, C., Pedersen, A.M.L., Villa, A., Ekström, J., Proctor, G.B., Vissink, A., ... Wolff, A. (2015). The functions of human saliva: A review sponsored by the World Workshop on Oral Medicine VI. *Archives of Oral Biology, 60,* 863–874. https://doi.org/10.1016/j.archoralbio.2015.03.004

Day, J., Gillespie, D.C., Rooney, A.G., Bulbeck, H.J., Zienius, K., Boele, F., & Grant, R. (2016). Neurocognitive deficits and neurocognitive rehabilitation in adult brain tumors. *Current Treatment Options in Neurology, 18,* 22. https://doi.org/10.1007/s11940-016-0406-5

De Felice, F., Musio, D., & Tombolini, V. (2016). Osteoradionecrosis and intensity modulated radiation therapy: An overview. *Critical Reviews in Oncology/Hematology, 107,* 39–43. https://doi.org/10.1016/j.critrevonc.2016.08.017

de Oliveira, P.F., Santos, R.G.S., Carneiro, T.C., Taguchi, C.K., Rocha, G.R., Silva, P.P., ... De Moraes Baldrighi, E.Z. (2017). Effects in hearing thresholds in subjects receiving radiotherapy as treatment for head and neck cancer. *Otolaryngology, 7,* 299. https://doi.org/10.4172/2161-119X.1000299

Demeestere, J., & Thijs, V. (2016). Radiation therapy and stroke. In A. Tsiskaridze, A. Lindgren, & A. Qureshi (Eds.), *Treatment-related stroke: Including iatrogenic and in-hospital strokes* (pp. 113–122). Cambridge University Press.

Deschuymer, S., Nevens, D., Duprez, F., Laenen, A., Dejaeger, E., De Neve, W., ... Nuyts, S. (2018). Clinical factors impacting on late dysphagia following radiotherapy in patients with head and neck cancer. *British Journal of Radiology, 91,* 1088. https://doi.org/10.1259/bjr.20180155

Dinh, C., Chen, S., Padgett, K., Dinh, J., Telischi, F., Elsayyad, N., ... Van De Water, T. (2015). Dexamethasone protects against radiation-induced loss of auditory hair cells in vitro. *Otology and Neurotology, 36,* 1741–1747. https://doi.org/10.1097/MAO.0000000000000850

Doroslovački, P., Tamhankar, M.A., Liu, G.T., Shindler, K.S., Ying, G.-S., & Alonso-Basanta, M. (2018). Factors associated with occurrence of radiation-induced optic neuropathy at "safe" radiation dosage. *Seminars in Ophthalmology, 33,* 581–588. https://doi.org/10.1080/08820538.2017.1346133

Epstein, J.B., & Barasch, A. (2010). Taste disorders in cancer patients: Pathogenesis, and approach to assessment and management. *Oral Oncology, 46,* 77–81. https://doi.org/10.1016/j.oraloncology.2009.11.008

Ethics Committee of the American Society for Reproductive Medicine. (2018). Fertility preservation and reproduction in patients facing gonadotoxic therapies: An ethics committee opinion. *Fertility and Sterility, 110,* 380–386. https://doi.org/10.1016/j.fertnstert.2018.05.034

Fan, C.-Y., Lin, C.-S., Chao, H.-L., Huang, W.-Y., Su, Y.-F., Lin, K.-T., ... Kao, C.-H. (2017). Risk of hypothyroidism among patients with nasopharyngeal carcinoma treated with radiation therapy: A population-based cohort study. *Radiotherapy and Oncology, 123,* 394–400. https://doi.org/10.1016/j.radonc.2017.04.025

Farrington, N., & Murphy, C. (2019). Bladder management in palliative care. In B.R. Ferrell & J.A. Paice (Eds.), *Oxford textbook of palliative nursing* (5th ed., pp. 230–237). Oxford University Press.

Fox, N.F., Xiao, C., Sood, A.J., Lovelace, T.L., Nguyen, S.A., Sharma, A., & Day, T.A. (2015). Hyperbaric oxygen therapy for the treatment of radiation-induced xerostomia: A systematic review. *Oral Surgery, Oral Medicine, Oral Pathology and Oral Radiology, 120,* 22–28. https://doi.org/10.1016/j.oooo.2015.03.007

Francis, D.O., Hall, E., Dang, J.H., Vlacich, G.R., Netterville, J.L., & Vaezi, M.F. (2015). Outcomes of serial dilation for high-grade radiation-related esophageal strictures in head and neck cancer patients. *The Laryngoscope, 125,* 856–862. https://doi.org/10.1002/lary.24987

Freites-Martinez, A., Shapiro, J., van den Hurk, C., Goldfarb, S., Jimenez, J.J., Rossi, A.M., ... Lacouture, M.E. (2019). Hair disorders in cancer survivors. *Journal of the American Academy of Dermatology, 8,* 1179–1196. https://doi.org/10.1016/j.jaad.2018.03.056

Frydrych, A.M., Slack-Smith, L.M., & Parsons, R. (2017). Compliance of post-radiation therapy head and neck cancer patients with caries preventive protocols. *Australian Dental Journal, 62,* 192–199. https://doi.org/10.1111/adj.12491

Fujiwara, M., Kamikonya, N., Odawara, S., Suzuki, H., Niwa, Y., Takada, Y., ... Hirota, S. (2015). The threshold of hypothyroidism after radiation therapy for head and neck cancer: A retrospective analysis of 116 cases. *Journal of Radiation Research, 56,* 577–582. https://doi.org/10.1093/jrr/rrv006

Ghiam, M.K., Mannion, K., Dietrich, M.S., Stevens, K.L., Gilbert, J., & Murphy, B.A. (2017). Assessment of musculoskeletal impairment in head and neck cancer patients. *Supportive Care in Cancer, 25,* 2085–2092. https://doi.org/10.1007/s00520-017-3603-1

Gosselin, T., Beamer, L., Ciccolini, K., Merritt, C., Omabegho, M., Shaftic, A., & Lucas, A.S. (2017). Symptom interventions: Radiodermatitis. https://www.ons.org/pep/radiodermatitis

Goucher, G., Saad, F., Lukka, H., & Kapoor, A. (2019). Canadian Urological Association best practice report: Diagnosis and management of radiation-induced hemorrhagic cystitis. *Canadian Urological Association Journal, 13*(2), 15–23. https://doi.org/10.5489/cuaj.5788

Greco, E., Simic, T., Ringash, J., Tomlinson, G., Inamoto, Y., & Martino, R. (2018). Dysphagia treatment for patients with head and neck cancer undergoing radiation therapy: A meta-analysis review. *International Journal of Radiation Oncology, Biology, Physics, 101,* 421–444. https://doi.org/10.1016/j.ijrobp.2018.01.097

Gupta, N., Pal, M., Rawat, S., Grewal, M.S., Garg, H., Chauhan, D., ... Devnani, B. (2015). Radiation-induced dental caries, prevention and treatment—A systematic review. *National Journal of Maxillofacial Surgery, 6,* 160–166. https://doi.org/10.4103/0975-5950.183870

Hall, S., Rudrawar, S., Zunk, M., Bernaitis, N., Arora, D., McDermott, C., & Anoopkumar-Dukie, S. (2016). Protection against radiotherapy-induced toxicity. *Antioxidants, 5,* 22. https://doi.org/10.3390/antiox5030022

Halpern, J.A., Hill, R., & Brannigan, R.E. (2020). Guideline based approach to male fertility preservation. *Urologic Oncology: Seminars and Original Investigations, 38,* 31–35. https://doi.org/10.1016/j.urolonc.2019.02.009

Hansen, E.K., & Roach, M., III. (Eds.). (2018). *Handbook of evidence-based radiation oncology* (3rd ed.). Springer. https://doi.org/10.1007/978-3-319-62642-0

Harris, J., Almarzouki, H., Barber, B., Scrimger, R., Romney, J., O'Connell, D., ... Seikaly, H. (2016). Free thyroid transfer: A novel procedure to prevent radiation-induced hypothyroidism. *International Journal of Radiation Oncology, Biology, Physics, 96,* 42–45. https://doi.org/10.1016/j.ijrobp.2016.04.004

Heijnen, B.J., Speyer, R., Kertscher, B., Cordier, R., Koetsenruijter, K.W.J., Swan, K., & Bogaardt, H. (2016). Dysphagia, speech, voice, and trismus following radiotherapy and/or chemotherapy in patients with head and neck carcinoma: Review of the literature. *BioMed Research International, 2016,* 6086894. https://doi.org/10.1155/2016/6086894

Hoekstra, N., Fleury, E., Lara, T.R.M., van der Baan, P., Bahnerth, A., Struik, G., ... Pignol, J.-P. (2018). Long-term risks of secondary cancer for various whole and partial breast irradiation techniques. *Radiotherapy and Oncology, 128,* 428–433. https://doi.org/10.1016/j.radonc.2018.05.032

Incrocci, L., & Jensen, P.T. (2013). Pelvic radiotherapy and sexual function in men and women. *Journal of Sexual Medicine, 10*(Suppl. 1), 53–64. https://doi.org/10.1111/jsm.12010

Irune, E., Dwivedi, R.C., Nutting, C.M., & Harrington, K.J. (2014). Treatment-related dysgeusia in head and neck cancer patients. *Cancer Treatment Reviews, 40,* 1106–1117. https://doi.org/10.1016/j.ctrv.2014.06.011

Jacobson, G., Bhatia, S., Smith, B.J., Button, A.M., Bodeker, K., & Buatti, J. (2013). Randomized trial of pentoxifylline and vitamin E vs standard follow-up after breast irradiation to prevent breast fibrosis, evaluated by tissue compliance meter. *International Journal of Radiation Oncology, Biology, Physics, 85,* 604–608. https://doi.org/10.1016/j.ijrobp.2012.06.042

Jain, D., Russell, R.R., Schwartz, R.G., Panjrath, G.S., & Aronow, W. (2017). Cardiac complications of cancer therapy: Pathophysiology, identification, prevention, treatment, and future directions. *Current Cardiology Reports, 19,* 36. https://doi.org/10.1007/s11886-017-0846-x

Jansen, C.E., Von Ah, D., Allen, D.H., Mayo, S., Merriman, J.D., & Myers, J.S. (2019). Symptom interventions: Cognitive impairment. https://www.ons.org/pep/cognitive-impairment

Jawad, M.S., Fahim, D.K., Gersztenkorn, P.C., Flickinger, J.C., Sahgal, A., Grills, I.S., ... Guckenberger, M. (2016). Vertebral compression fractures after stereotactic body radiation therapy: A large, multi-institutional, multinational evaluation. *Journal of Neurosurgery: Spine, 24,* 928–936. https://doi.org/10.3171/2015.10.SPINE141261

Jensen, S.B. (2016). AAOM clinical practice statement: Subject: Clinical management of cancer therapy-induced salivary gland hypofunction and xerostomia. *Oral Surgery, Oral Medicine, Oral Pathology, and Oral Radiology, 122,* 310–312. https://doi.org/10.1016/j.oooo.2016.04.015

Jiang, L., Huang, C., Gan, Y., Wu, T., Tang, X., Wang, Y., ... Zhang, Y. (2018). Radiation-induced late dysphagia after intensity-modulated radiotherapy in nasopharyngeal carcinoma patients: A dose–volume effect analysis. *Scientific Reports, 8,* 16396. https://doi.org/10.1038/s41598-018-34803-y

Jiang, N., Zhang, L.-J., Li, L.-Y., Zhao, Y., & Eisele, D.W. (2016). Risk factors for late dysphagia after (chemo)radiotherapy for head and neck cancer: A systematic methodological review. *Head and Neck, 38,* 792–800. https://doi.org/10.1002/hed.23963

Jiang, X., Engelbach, J.A., Yuan, L., Cates, J., Gao, F., Drzymala, R.E., ... Garbow, J.R. (2014). Anti-VEGF antibodies mitigate the development of radiation necrosis in mouse brain. *Clinical Cancer Research, 20,* 2695–2702. https://doi.org/10.1158/1078-0432.CCR-13-1941

Johns, M.M., Kolachala, V., Berg, E., Muller, S., Creighton, F.X., & Branski, R.C. (2012). Radiation fibrosis of the vocal fold: From man to mouse. *Laryngoscope, 122*(Suppl. 5), SS107–SS125. https://doi.org/10.1002/lary.23735

Kachnic, L.A., Bruner, D.W., Qureshi, M.M., & Russo, G.A. (2017). Perceptions and practices regarding women's vaginal health following radiation therapy: A survey of radiation oncologists practicing in the United States. *Practical Radiation Oncology, 7*, 356–363. https://doi.org/10.1016/j.prro.2017.02.003

Kalaiselvan, R., Theis, V.S., Dibb, M., Teubner, A., Anderson, I.D., Shaffer, J.L., ... Lal, S. (2014). Radiation enteritis leading to intestinal failure: 1994 patient-years of experience in a national referral centre. *European Journal of Clinical Nutrition, 68*, 166–170. https://doi.org/10.1038/ejcn.2013.251

Kawashima, M., Nozaki, M., Komazaki, K., Yamamuro, R., Ishizuna, K., & Kojima, M. (2016). Quantitative assessment of chronic skin reactions including erythema and pigmentation after breast conserving therapy. *Advances in Breast Cancer Research, 5*, 121–128. https://doi.org/10.4236/abcr.2016.53014

Kenyon, M., Mayer, D.K., & Owens, A.K. (2014). Late and long-term effects of breast cancer treatment and surveillance management for the general practitioner. *Journal of Obstetric, Gynecologic and Neonatal Nursing, 43*, 382–398. https://doi.org/10.1111/1552-6909.12300

King, S.N., Dunlap, N.E., Tennant, P.A., & Pitts, T. (2016). Pathophysiology of radiation-induced dysphagia in head and neck cancer. *Dysphagia, 31*, 339–351. https://doi.org/10.1007/s00455-016-9710-1

Kirkpatrick, J.P., van der Kogel, A.J., & Schultheiss, T.E. (2010). Radiation dose–volume effects in the spinal cord. *International Journal of Radiation Oncology, Biology, Physics, 76*(Suppl. 3), S42–S49. https://doi.org/10.1016/j.ijrobp.2009.04.095

Koontz, B.F. (Ed.). (2018). *Radiation therapy treatment effects: An evidence-based guide to managing toxicity.* Springer.

Kraaijenga, S.A.C., van der Molen, L., Jacobi, I., Hamming-Vrieze, O., Hilgers, F.J.M., & van den Brekel, M.W.M. (2015). Prospective clinical study on long-term swallowing function and voice quality in advanced head and neck cancer patients treated with concurrent chemoradiotherapy and preventive swallowing exercises. *European Archives of Oto-Rhino-Laryngology, 272*, 3521–3531. https://doi.org/10.1007/s00405-014-3379-6

Kufta, K., Forman, M., Swisher-McClure, S., Sollecito, T.P., & Panchal, N. (2018). Pre-radiation dental considerations and management for head and neck cancer patients. *Oral Oncology, 76*, 42–51. https://doi.org/10.1016/j.oraloncology.2017.11.023

Lamba, N., Bussiere, M.R., Niemierko, A., Abedi, P., Fullerton, B.C., Loeffler, J.S., ... Shih, H.A. (2019). Hypopituitarism following cranial irradiation for meningiomas: A single-institution experience. *Practical Radiation Oncology, 9*, e266–e273. https://doi.org/10.1016/j.prro.2019.01.009

Lambert, E.M., Gunn, G.B., & Gidley, P.W. (2016). Effects of radiation on the temporal bone in patients with head and neck cancer. *Head and Neck, 38*, 1428–1435. https://doi.org/10.1002/hed.24267

Lawenda, B.D., Gagne, H.M., Gierga, D.P., Niemierko, A., Wong, W.M., Tarbell, N.J., ... Loeffler, J.S. (2004). Permanent alopecia after cranial irradiation: Dose–response relationship. *International Journal of Radiation Oncology, Biology, Physics, 60*, 879–887. https://doi.org/10.1016/j.ijrobp.2004.04.031

Leddy, L.S. (2018). Management of lower urinary tract symptoms after pelvic radiation in females. *Current Urology Reports, 19*, 106. https://doi.org/10.1007/s11934-018-0848-2

Lee, R., Yeo, S.T., Rogers, S.N., Caress, A.L., Molassiotis, A., Ryder, D., ... Slevin, N. (2018). Randomized feasibility study to compare the use of Therabite® with wooden spatulas to relieve and prevent trismus in patients with cancer of the head and neck. *British Journal of Oral and Maxillofacial Surgery, 56*, 283–291. https://doi.org/10.1016/j.bjoms.2018.02.012

Leung, H.W.C., Chan, A.L.F., & Muo, C.-H. (2016). Late cardiac morbidity of adjuvant radiotherapy for early breast cancer—A population-based study. *Journal of Cardiology, 67*, 567–571. http://dx.doi.org/10.1016/j.jjcc.2015.07.009

Levenback, C., Eifel, P.J., Burke, T.W., Morris, M., & Gershenson, D.M. (1994). Hemorrhagic cystitis following radiotherapy for stage Ib cancer of the cervix. *Gynecologic Oncology, 55*, 206–210. https://doi.org/10.1006/gyno.1994.1278

Lin, X., & Corcoran, S. (2019). CE: Caring for survivors of Hodgkin lymphoma. *American Journal of Nursing, 119*, 32–41. https://doi.org/10.1097/01.NAJ.0000553181.82330.d4

Lin, Z., Yang, Z., He, B., Wang, D., Gao, X., Tam, S.-Y., & Wu, V.W.C. (2018). Pattern of radiation-induced thyroid gland changes in nasopharyngeal carcinoma patients in 48 months after radiotherapy. *PLOS ONE, 13*, e0200310. https://doi.org/10.1371/journal.pone.0200310

Lobo, N., Kulkarni, M., Hughes, S., Nair, R., Khan, M.S., & Thurairaja, R. (2018). Urologic complications following pelvic radiotherapy. *Urology, 122*, 1–9. https://doi.org/10.1016/j.urology.2018.07.017

Loganadane, G., Dhermain, F., Louvel, G., Kauv, P., Deutsch, E., Le Péchoux, C., & Levy, A. (2018). Brain radiation necrosis: Current management with a focus on non-small cell lung cancer patients. *Frontiers in Oncology, 8*, 336. https://doi.org/10.3389/fonc.2018.00336

Lu, W., & Rosenthal, D.S. (2018). Oncology acupuncture for chronic pain in cancer survivors: A reflection on the American Society of Clinical Oncology chronic pain guideline. *Hematology/Oncology Clinics of North America, 32*, 519–533. https://doi.org/10.1016/j.hoc.2018.01.009

Luan, A., Duscher, D., Whittam, A.J., Paik, K.J., Zielins, E.R., Brett, E.A., ... Wan, D.C. (2016). Cell-assisted lipotransfer improves volume retention in irradiated recipient sites and rescues radiation-induced skin changes. *Stem Cells, 34*, 668–673. https://doi.org/10.1002/stem.2256

Lynch, M. (2019). Preservation of cognitive function following whole brain radiotherapy in patients with brain metastases: Complications, treatments, and the emerging role of memantine. *Journal of Oncology Pharmacy Practice, 25*, 657–662. https://doi.org/10.1177/1078155218798176

Martin, M.T., Vulin, A., & Hendry, J.H. (2016). Human epidermal stem cells: Role in adverse skin reactions and carcinogenesis from radiation. *Mutation Research/Reviews in Mutation Research, 770*, 349–368. https://doi.org/10.1016/j.mrrev.2016.08.004

Masucci, G.L. (2018). Hypofractionated radiation therapy for large brain metastases. *Frontiers in Oncology, 8*, 379. https://doi.org/10.3389/fonc.2018.00379

Mintet, E., Rannou, E., Buard, V., West, G., Guipaud, O., Tarlet, G., ... François, A. (2015). Identification of endothelial-to-mesenchymal transition as a potential participant in radiation proctitis. *American Journal of Pathology, 185*, 2550–2562. https://doi.org/10.1016/j.ajpath.2015.04.028

Mirabeau-Beale, K., Hong, T.S., Niemierko, A., Ancukiewicz, M., Blaszkowsky, L.S., Crowley, E.M., ... Wo, J.Y. (2015). Clinical and treatment factors associated with vaginal stenosis after definitive chemoradiation for anal canal cancer. *Practical Radiation Oncology, 5*, e113–e118 https://doi.org/10.1016/j.prro.2014.09.003

Miyake, M., Tanaka, N., Asakawa, I., Tatsumi, Y., Nakai, Y., Anai, S., ... Konishi, N. (2015). Changes in lower urinary tract symptoms and quality of life after salvage radiotherapy for biochemical recurrence of prostate cancer. *Radiotherapy and Oncology, 115*, 321–326. https://doi.org/10.1016/j.radonc.2015.04.026

Murphy, B.A., & Deng, J. (2015). Advances in supportive care for late effects of head and neck cancer. *Journal of Clinical Oncology, 33*, 3314–3321. https://doi.org/10.1200/JCO.2015.61.3836

Murphy, E.S., Xie, H., Merchant, T.E., Yu, J.S., Chao, S.T., & Suh, J.H. (2015). Review of cranial radiotherapy-induced vasculopathy. *Journal of Neuro-Oncology, 122*, 421–429. https://doi.org/10.1007/s11060-015-1732-2

Nadella, K.R., Kodali, R.M., Guttikonda, L.K., & Jonnalagadda, A. (2015). Osteoradionecrosis of the jaws: Clinico-therapeutic management: A literature review and update. *Journal of Maxillofacial and Oral Surgery, 14*, 891–901. https://doi.org/10.1007/s12663-015-0762-9

Najafi, M., Motevaseli, E., Shirazi, A., Geraily, G., Rezaeyan, A., Norouzi, F., ... Abdollahi, H. (2018). Mechanisms of inflammatory responses to radiation and normal tissues toxicity: Clinical implications. *International Journal of Radiation Biology, 94*, 335–356. https://doi.org/10.1080/09553002.2018.1440092

National Cancer Institute. (2019). Lymphedema (PDQ®) [Health professional version]. https://www.cancer.gov/about-cancer/treatment/side-effects/lymphedema/lymphedema-hp-pdq

National Cancer Institute Cancer Therapy Evaluation Program. (2017). *Common toxicity criteria for adverse events* [v.5.0.]. https://ctep.cancer.gov/protocolDevelopment/electronic_applications/docs/CTCAE_v5_Quick_Reference_8.5x11.pdf

National Comprehensive Cancer Network. (2020a). *NCCN Clinical Practice Guidelines in Oncology (NCCN Guidelines*): Head and neck cancers* [v.1.2020]. https://www.nccn.org/professionals/physician_gls/pdf/head-and-neck.pdf

National Comprehensive Cancer Network. (2020b). *NCCN Clinical Practice Guidelines in Oncology (NCCN Guidelines*): Survivorship* [v.1.2020]. https://www.nccn.org/professionals/physician_gls/pdf/survivorship.pdf

Naunheim, M.R., Garneau, J., Park, C., Carroll, L., Goldberg, L., & Woo, P. (2019). Voice outcomes after radiation for early-stage laryngeal cancer. *Journal of Voice*. Advance online publication. https://doi.org/10.1016/j.jvoice.2018.11.007

Nicholas, S., Chen, L., Choflet, A., Fader, A., Guss, Z., Hazell, S., ... Viswanathan, A.N. (2017). Pelvic radiation and normal tissue toxicity. *Seminars in Radiation Oncology, 27*, 358–369. https://doi.org/10.1016/j.semradonc.2017.04.010

Nicholls, L., Gorayski, P., & Harvey, J. (2015). Osteoradionecrosis of the ribs following breast radiotherapy. *Case Reports in Oncology, 8*, 332–338. https://doi.org/10.1159/000438786

Nitsche, M., Pahl, R., Huber, K., Eilf, K., & Dunst, J. (2015). Cardiac toxicity after radiotherapy for breast cancer: Myths and facts. *Breast care, 10*, 131–135. https://doi.org/10.1159/000376560

Nunns, D., Williamson, K., Swaney, L., & Davy, M. (2000). The morbidity of surgery and adjuvant radiotherapy in the management of endometrial carcinoma. *International Journal of Gynecological Cancer, 10*, 233–238. https://doi.org/10.1046/j.1525-1438.2000.010003233.x

Okoukoni, C., Farris, M., Hughes, R.T., McTyre, E.R., Helis, C.A., Munley, M.T., & Willey, J.S. (2017). Radiation-induced bone toxicity. *Current Stem Cell Reports, 3*, 333–341. https://doi.org/10.1007/s40778-017-0099-z

Oktay, K., Harvey, B.E., Partridge, A.H., Quinn, G.P., Reinecke, J., Taylor, H.S., ... Loren, A.W. (2018). Fertility preservation in patients with cancer: ASCO clinical practice guideline update. *Journal of Clinical Oncology, 36*, 1994–2001. https://doi.org/10.1200/JCO.2018.78.1914

Onishi, K., Tanaka, N., Miyake, M., Nakai, Y., Anai, S., Torimoto, K., ... Fujimoto, K. (2019). Changes in lower urinary tract symptoms after iodine-125 brachytherapy for prostate cancer. *Clinical and Translational Radiation Oncology, 14*, 51–58. https://doi.org/10.1016/j.ctro.2018.11.001

Owosho, A.A., Tsai, C.J., Lee, R.S., Freymiller, H., Kadempour, A., Varthis, S., ... Estilo, C.L. (2017). The prevalence and risk factors associated with osteoradionecrosis of the jaw in oral and oropharyngeal cancer patients treated with intensity-modulated radiation therapy (IMRT): The Memorial Sloan Kettering Cancer Center experience. *Oral Oncology, 64*, 44–51. https://doi.org/10.1016/j.oraloncology.2016.11.015

Park, J.-H., Kim, K.Y., Song, H.-Y., Cho, Y.C., Kim, P.H., Tsauo, J., ... Kim, J.H. (2018). Radiation-induced esophageal strictures treated with fluoroscopic balloon dilation: Clinical outcomes and factors influencing recurrence in 62 patients. *Acta Radiologica, 59*, 313–321. https://doi.org/10.1177/0284185117713351

Pessi, M.R., Kassulke Feuerchutte, K., Martins da Rosa, L., de Almeida Hammerschmidt, K.S., Radünz, V., & Alvarez, A.M. (2016). Prevention of vaginal stenosis after brachytherapy: Nursing intervention. *Journal of Nursing UFPE On Line, 10*, 3495–3502. https://periodicos.ufpe.br/revistas/revistaenfermagem/article/view/11433

Pinkham, M.B., Sanghera, P., Wall, G.K., Dawson, B.D., & Whitfield, G.A. (2015). Neurocognitive effects following cranial irradiation for brain metastases. *Clinical Oncology, 27*, 630–639. https://doi.org/10.1016/j.clon.2015.06.005

Plummer, C., Henderson, R.D., O'Sullivan, J.D., & Read, S.J. (2011). Ischemic stroke and transient ischemic attack after head and neck radiotherapy. *Stroke, 42*, 2410–2418. https://doi.org/10.1161/STROKEAHA.111.615203

Ramlov, A., Pedersen, E.M., Røhl, L., Worm, E., Fokdal, L., Lindegaard, J.C., & Tanderup, K. (2017). Risk factors for pelvic insufficiency fractures in locally advanced cervical cancer following intensity modulated radiation therapy.

International Journal of Radiation Oncology, Biology, Physics, 97, 1032–1039. https://doi.org/10.1016/j.ijrobp.2017.01.026

Rao, N., Shridhar, R., & Hoffe, S.E. (2014). Late effects of pelvic radiation for rectal cancer and implications for survivorship. *Seminars in Colon and Rectal Surgery, 25*, 38–43. https://doi.org/10.1053/j.scrs.2013.09.008

Rao, N.M., Vinters, H.V., & Saver, J.L. (2017). Radiation vasculopathy. In L.R. Caplan, J. Biller, M.C. Leary, E.H. Lo, A.J. Thomas, M. Yenari, & J.H. Zhang (Eds.), *Primer on cerebrovascular diseases* (2nd ed., pp. 579–583). Elsevier Academic Press.

Rapidis, A.D., Dijkstra, P.U., Roodenburg, J.L.N., Rodrigo, J.P., Rinaldo, A., Strojan, P., ... Ferlito, A. (2015). Trismus in patients with head and neck cancer: Etiopathogenesis, diagnosis and management. *Clinical Otolaryngology, 40*, 516–526. https://doi.org/10.1111/coa.12488

Raup, V.T., Eswara, J.R., Geminiani, J., Madison, K., Heningburg, A.M., & Brandes, S.B. (2016). Gracilis muscle interposition flap repair of urinary fistulae: Pelvic radiation is associated with persistent urinary incontinence and decreased quality of life. *World Journal of Urology, 34*, 131–136. https://doi.org/10.1007/s00345-015-1597-1

Rich, S.E., Chow, R., Raman, S., Zeng, K.L., Lutz, S., Lam, H., ... Chow, E. (2018). Update of the systematic review of palliative radiation therapy fractionation for bone metastases. *Radiotherapy and Oncology, 126*, 547–557. https://doi.org/10.1016/j.radonc.2018.01.003

Rodriguez, M.A., & Foxhall, L.E. (Eds.). (2019). *Handbook of cancer survivorship care.* Demos Medical.

Rønjom, M.F., Brink, C., Bentzen, S.M., Hegedüs, L., Overgaard, J., & Johansen, J. (2013). Hypothyroidism after primary radiotherapy for head and neck squamous cell carcinoma: Normal tissue complication probability modeling with latent time correction. *Radiotherapy and Oncology, 109*, 317–322. https://doi.org/10.1016/j.radonc.2013.06.029

Russell, R.R., Alexander, J., Jain, D., Poornima, I.G., Srivastava, A.V., Storozynsky, E., & Schwartz, R.G. (2016). The role and clinical effectiveness of multimodality imaging in the management of cardiac complications of cancer and cancer therapy. *Journal of Nuclear Cardiology, 23*, 856–884. https://doi.org/10.1007/s12350-016-0538-8

Saad, S., & Wang, T.J.C. (2015). Neurocognitive deficits after radiation therapy for brain malignancies. *American Journal of Clinical Oncology, 38*, 634–640. https://doi.org/10.1097/COC.0000000000000158

Sangro, B., Martínez-Urbistondo, D., Bester, L., Bilbao, J.I., Coldwell, D.M., Flamen, P., ... Sharma, R.A. (2017). Prevention and treatment of complications of selective internal radiation therapy: Expert guidance and systematic review. *Hepatology, 66*, 969–982. https://doi.org/10.1002/hep.29207

Schoenfeld, J.D., Nishino, M., Severgnini, M., Manos, M., Mak, R.H., & Hodi, F.S. (2019). Pneumonitis resulting from radiation and immune checkpoint blockade illustrates characteristic clinical, radiologic and circulating biomarker features. *Journal for Immunotherapy of Cancer, 7*, 112. https://doi.org/10.1186/s40425-019-0583-3

Sears, C.R., Peikert, T., Possick, J.D., Naidoo, J., Nishino, M., Patel, S.P., ... Rivera, M.P. (2019). Knowledge gaps and research priorities in immune checkpoint inhibitor–related pneumonitis. An official American Thoracic Society research statement. *American Journal of Respiratory and Critical Care Medicine, 200*, e31–e43. https://doi.org/10.1164/rccm.201906-1202ST

Sears, C.S., Robinson, J.W., & Walker, L.M. (2018). A comprehensive review of sexual health concerns after cancer treatment and the biopsychosocial treatment options available to female patients. *European Journal of Cancer Care, 27*, e12738. https://doi.org/10.1111/ecc.12738

Sharif, S., & Qadeer, M. (2016). Metastatic spine—A review. *World Spinal Column Journal, 7*, 58–63.

Shen, X.-J., Liu, L., & Zhu, J.-Y. (2018). Radiofrequency ablation in a patient with radiation enteritis: A case report. *Medicine, 97*, e13328. https://doi.org/10.1097/MD.0000000000013328

Shimokawaji, T., Narita, S., Naito, T., Udagawa, H., Goto, K., Miyawaki, T., ... Horinouchi, H. (2020). Clinical characteristics of nivolumab-induced radiation recall pneumonitis in patients with non-small cell lung cancer: A multicenter real-world analysis of 669 patients [Abstract]. *Journal of Clinical Oncology, 38*(Suppl. 5), 88. https://doi.org/10.1200/JCO.2020.38.5_suppl.88

Siddiqui, F., & Movsas, B. (2017). Management of radiation toxicity in head and neck cancers. *Seminars in Radiation Oncology, 27,* 340–349. https://doi.org/10.1016/j.semradonc.2017.04.008

Simone, C.B., II. (2017). Thoracic radiation normal tissue injury. *Seminars in Radiation Oncology, 27,* 370–377. http://dx.doi.org/10.1016/j.semradonc.2017.04.009

Smith, B.G., Hutcheson, K.A., Little, L.G., Skoracki, R.J., Rosenthal, D.I., Lai, S.Y., & Lewin, J.S. (2015). Lymphedema outcomes in patients with head and neck cancer. *Otolaryngology—Head and Neck Surgery, 152,* 284–291. https://doi.org/10.1177/0194599814558402

Smoot, B., Chiavola-Larson, L., Lee, J., Manibusan, H., & Allen, D.D. (2015). Effect of low-level laser therapy on pain and swelling in women with breast cancer-related lymphedema: A systematic review and meta-analysis. *Journal of Cancer Survivorship, 9,* 287–304. https://doi.org/10.1007/s11764-014-0411-1

Sobecki-Ryniak, D., & Krouse, H.J. (2013). Head and neck cancer: Historical evolution of treatment and patient self-care requirements. *Clinical Journal of Oncology Nursing, 17,* 659–663. https://doi.org/10.1188/13.CJON.659-663

Soref, C.M., & Fahl, W.E. (2015). A new strategy to prevent chemotherapy and radiotherapy-induced alopecia using topically applied vasoconstrictor. *International Journal of Cancer, 136,* 195–203. https://doi.org/10.1002/ijc.28961

Soriano, J.L., Calpena, A.C., Souto, E.B., & Clares, B. (2019). Therapy for prevention and treatment of skin ionizing radiation damage: A review. *International Journal of Radiation Biology, 95,* 537–553. https://doi.org/10.1080/09553002.2019.1562254

Stachler, R.J., Francis, D.O., Schwartz, S.R., Damask, C.C., Digoy, G.P., Krouse, H.J., ... Nnacheta, L.C. (2018). Clinical practice guideline: Hoarseness (dysphonia)(update) executive summary. *Otolaryngology—Head and Neck Surgery, 158,* 409–426. https://doi.org/10.1177/0194599817751031

Stone, J.B., & DeAngelis, L.M. (2016). Cancer-treatment-induced neurotoxicity—Focus on newer treatments. *Nature Reviews Clinical Oncology, 13,* 92–105. https://doi.org/10.1038/nrclinonc.2015.152

Straub, J.M., New, J., Hamilton, C.D., Lominska, C., Shnayder, Y., & Thomas, S.M. (2015). Radiation-induced fibrosis: Mechanisms and implications for therapy. *Journal of Cancer Research and Clinical Oncology, 141,* 1985–1994. https://doi.org/10.1007/s00432-015-1974-6

Strojan, P., Hutcheson, K.A., Eisbruch, A., Beitler, J.J., Langendijk, J.A., Lee, A.W.M., ... Ferlito, A. (2017). Treatment of late sequelae after radiotherapy for head and neck cancer. *Cancer Treatment Reviews, 59,* 79–92. https://doi.org/10.1016/j.ctrv.2017.07.003

Stubblefield, M.D. (2017). Neuromuscular complications of radiation therapy. *Muscle and Nerve, 56,* 1031–1040. https://onlinelibrary.wiley.com/doi/10.1002/mus.25778

Su, T.-L., Chen, A.-N., Leong, C.-P., Huang, Y.-C., Chiang, C.-W., Chen, I.-H., & Lee, Y.-Y. (2017). The effect of home-based program and outpatient physical therapy in patients with head and neck cancer: A randomized, controlled trial. *Oral Oncology, 74,* 130–134. https://doi.org/10.1016/j.oraloncology.2017.10.002

Taylor, C.W., & Kirby, A.M. (2015). Cardiac side-effects from breast cancer radiotherapy. *Clinical Oncology, 27,* 621–629. https://doi.org/10.1016/j.clon.2015.06.007

Theunissen, E.A.R., Bosma, S.C.J., Zuur, C.L., Spijker, R., van der Baan, S., Dreschler, W.A., ... Rasch, C.R.N. (2015). Sensorineural hearing loss in patients with head and neck cancer after chemoradiotherapy and radiotherapy: A systematic review of the literature. *Head and Neck, 37,* 281–292. https://doi.org/10.1002/hed.23551

Thiruchelvam, N., Cruz, F., Kirby, M., Tubaro, A., Chapple, C.R., & Sievert, K.-D. (2015). A review of detrusor overactivity and the overactive bladder after radical prostate cancer treatment. *BJU International, 116,* 853–861. https://doi.org/10.1111/bju.13078

Thor, M., Olsson, C., Oh, J.H., Petersen, S.E., Alsadius, D., Bentzen, L., ... Deasy, J.O. (2016). Urinary bladder dose–response relationships for patient-reported genitourinary morbidity domains following prostate cancer radiotherapy. *Radiotherapy and Oncology, 119,* 117–122. https://doi.org/10.1016/j.radonc.2016.01.013

Trinh, K., Graham, N., Irnich, D., Cameron, I.D., & Forget, M. (2016). Acupuncture for neck disorders. *Cochrane Database of Systematic Reviews, 2016*(5). https://doi.org/10.1002/14651858.CD004870.pub4

Twitchell, S., Karsy, M., Guan, J., Couldwell, W.T., & Taussky, P. (2019). Sequelae and management of radiation vasculopathy in neurosurgical patients. *Journal of Neurosurgery, 130,* 1889–1897. https://doi.org/10.3171/2017.12.JNS172635

van Boeckel, P.G.A., & Siersema, P.D. (2015). Refractory esophageal strictures: What to do when dilation fails. *Current Treatment Options in Gastroenterology, 13,* 47–58. https://doi.org/10.1007/s11938-014-0043-6

van de Wetering, F.T., Verleye, L., Andreyev, H.J.N., Maher, J., Vlayen, J., Pieters, B.R., ... Scholten, R.J.P.M. (2016). Non-surgical interventions for late rectal problems (proctopathy) of radiotherapy in people who have received radiotherapy to the pelvis. *Cochrane Database of Systematic Reviews, 2016*(4). https://doi.org/10.1002/14651858.CD003455.pub2

VanKoevering, K.K., Sabetsarvestani, K., Sullivan, S.E., Barkan, A., Mierzwa, M., & McKean, E.L. (2020). Pituitary dysfunction after radiation for anterior skull base malignancies: Incidence and screening. *Journal of Neurological Surgery Part B: Skull Base, 8,* 75–81. https://doi.org/10.1055/s-0039-1679893

Vanneste, B.G.L., Van De Voorde, L., de Ridder, R.J., Van Limbergen, E.J., Lambin, P., & van Lin, E.N. (2015). Chronic radiation proctitis: Tricks to prevent and treat. *International Journal of Colorectal Disease, 30,* 1293–1303. https://doi.org/10.1007/s00384-015-2289-4

Velo, M.M.D.A.C., Farha, A.L.H., da Silva Santos, P.S., Shiota, A., Sansavino, S.Z., Souza, A.T., ... Wang, L. (2018). Radiotherapy alters the composition, structural and mechanical properties of root dentin in vitro. *Clinical Oral Investigations, 22,* 2871–2878. https://doi.org/10.1007/s00784-018-2373-6

Wang, J.J., Goldsmith, T.A., Holman, A.S., Cianchetti, M., & Chan, A.W. (2012). Pharyngoesophageal stricture after treatment for head and neck cancer. *Head and Neck, 34,* 967–973. https://doi.org/10.1002/hed.21842

Wang, W., Yang, H., Guo, L., Su, H., Wei, S., & Zhang, X. (2016). Radiation-induced optic neuropathy following external beam radiation therapy for nasopharyngeal carcinoma: A retrospective case-control study. *Molecular and Clinical Oncology, 4,* 868–872. https://doi.org/10.3892/mco.2016.787

Warade, A.C., Jha, A.K., Pattankar, S., & Desai, K. (2019). Radiation-induced brachial plexus neuropathy: A review. *Neurology India, 67,* 47. https://doi.org/10.4103/0028-3886.250704

Weiner, J.P., Wong, A.T., Schwartz, D., Martinez, M., Aytaman, A., & Schreiber, D. (2016). Endoscopic and non-endoscopic approaches for the management of radiation-induced rectal bleeding. *World Journal of Gastroenterology, 22,* 6972. https://doi.org/10.3748/wjg.v22.i31.6972

Williams, L., Ciccolini, K., Johnson, L.A., Robison, J., Shelton, G., & Lucas, A.S. (2017). Symptom interventions: Skin reactions. https://www.ons.org/pep/skin-reactions

Wirsdörfer, F., de Leve, S., & Jendrossek, V. (2019). Combining radiotherapy and immunotherapy in lung cancer: Can we expect limitations due to altered normal tissue toxicity? *International Journal of Molecular Sciences, 20,* 24. https://doi.org/10.3390/ijms20010024

Wong, C.S., Fehlings, M.G., & Sahgal, A. (2015). Pathobiology of radiation myelopathy and strategies to mitigate injury. *Spinal Cord, 53,* 574–580. https://doi.org/10.1038/sc.2015.43

Wong, C.Y., Wong, S.C., Lee, Y.P.E., Sze, C.K., Ngai, W.T., & Yeung, M.W. (2017). Brachial plexus metastasis masquerading as radiation-induced brachial plexopathy. *Hong Kong Journal of Radiology, 20,* e7–e11. https://doi.org/10.12809/hkjr1716806

Wu, V.W.C., & Lam, Y.-N. (2016). Radiation-induced temporo-mandibular joint disorder in post-radiotherapy nasopharyngeal carcinoma patients: Assessment and treatment. *Journal of Medical Radiation Sciences, 63,* 124–132. https://doi.org/10.1002/jmrs.145

Yahyapour, R., Amini, P., Rezapour, S., Cheki, M., Rezaeyan, A., Farhood, B., ... Najafi, M. (2018). Radiation-induced inflammation and autoimmune diseases. *Military Medical Research, 5,* 9. https://doi.org/10.1186/s40779-018-0156-7

Yamanaka, R., Hayano, A., & Kanayama, T. (2017). Radiation-induced meningiomas: An exhaustive review of the literature. *World Neurosurgery, 97,* 635–644.e8. https://doi.org/10.1016/j.wneu.2016.09.094

Yan, M., Xue, P., Wang, K., Gao, G., Zhang, W., & Sun, F. (2017). Does combination therapy with tamsulosin and trospium chloride improve lower urinary tract symptoms after SEEDS brachytherapy for prostate cancer compared with tamsulosin alone? *Strahlentherapie und Onkologie, 193,* 714–721. https://doi.org/10.1007/s00066-017-1162-5

Yoritsune, E., Furuse, M., Kuwabara, H., Miyata, T., Nonoguchi, N., Kawabata, S., ... Miyatake, S.-I. (2014). Inflammation as well as angiogenesis may participate in the pathophysiology of brain radiation necrosis. *Journal of Radiation Research, 55,* 803–811. https://doi.org/10.1093/jrr/rru017

Yue, Z., & Xu, B. (2017). The feather model for chemo- and radiation therapy-induced tissue damage. In G. Sheng (Ed.), *Methods in molecular biology: Vol. 1650. Avian and reptilian developmental biology: Methods and protocols.* Humana Press. https://doi.org/10.1007/978-1-4939-7216-6_20

Yun, H.G., Kim, H.Y., Kim, D.Y., & Lim, Y.J. (2015). Successful treatment of intractable bleeding caused by radiation-induced hemorrhagic gastritis using oral prednisolone: A case report. *Cancer Research and Treatment, 47,* 334–338. https://doi.org/10.4143/crt.2013.114

Zheng, Y., Han, F., Xiao, W., Xiang, Y., Lu, L., Deng, X., ... Zhao, C. (2015). Analysis of late toxicity in nasopharyngeal carcinoma patients treated with intensity modulated radiation therapy. *Radiation Oncology, 10,* 17. https://doi.org/10.1186/s13014-014-0326-z

K. Cardiac toxicity and cardiac implantable electronic devices

1. Overview
   a) As a result of advances in early detection and treatment in a growing and aging population, the number of cancer survivors in the United States continues to increase (Miller et al., 2019).
      (1) As of January 2019, more than 16.9 million cancer survivors were living in the United States, and this number is projected to rise to 22.1 million by 2030 (Miller et al., 2019).
      (2) More than 60% of cancer survivors are alive at 5 years and more than 40% are alive at 10 years or longer after the end of treatment.
      (3) This growing population includes aging survivors living with risks for long-term treatment-related toxicities and other medical issues (de Moor et al., 2013).
      (4) Aging cancer survivors are more likely to have multiple comorbidities and poorer physical functioning than younger cancer survivors (Avis & Deimling, 2008; Bellizzi, Mustian, Palesh, & Diefenbach, 2008).
   b) Cancer is the second leading cause of death in the United States, with cardiovascular disease as the greatest cause of mortality in the United States and around the world (Benjamin et al., 2019; Miller et al., 2019).
      (1) The risk for cardiovascular disease in some cancer survivors, particularly those with a history of breast cancer, lung cancer, lymphoma, multiple myeloma, or childhood malignancy, may be greater than that of the general population as a result of cancer treatment (Aleman et al., 2014; Armenian et al., 2016; Findlay, Gill, Plummer, DeSantis, & Plummer, 2019; Lipshultz, Cochran, Franco, & Miller, 2013; Strongman et al., 2019).
      (2) For postmenopausal breast cancer survivors, mortality related to cardiovascular disease exceeds the likelihood of mortality related to cancer recurrence. This risk is most notable at seven years after breast cancer diagnosis (Bradshaw et al., 2016).
      (3) Improving cardiovascular disease risk factors, screening, and early intervention is critical to minimizing the risk of advanced heart disease.
      (4) High cardiovascular disease risk in people with cancer is multifactorial and may be attributed to overlapping baseline risk factors for both conditions, including obesity, smoking, and longer survival, as well as the effect of cancer treatment modalities with potential for cardiovascular toxicity, such as chemotherapy, molecular targeted therapies, and RT (Mehta et al., 2018).
      (5) Advancing atherosclerosis, hypertension, left ventricular dysfunction, and, ultimately, heart failure are potential cardiovascular toxicities of common oncologic therapies (Bloom et al., 2016).
      (6) Newer targeted therapies, such as tyrosine kinase inhibitors, VEGF signaling inhibitors, immune checkpoint inhibitors, and trastuzumab (humanized monoclonal antibody targeting HER2) may impart risks such as arrhythmia and vascular or metabolic disruptions (Moslehi, 2016).
      (7) Cardiac considerations in cancer treatment should begin prior to the time of treatment and should remain a consideration for all healthcare team members involved in the care of a patient throughout survivorship (Hamo & Bloom, 2017).
   c) For radiation oncology team members, cardiac considerations should include an assessment of the cardiac risk factors that may be associated with the planned radiation course, baseline cardiovascular risk factors of a patient, and cardiac risks associated with other cancer treatment modalities previously used and planned for use to treat a patient.
      (1) Interprofessional coordination through cardio-oncology is often highly valuable for patients with oncologic cardiotoxicity risks and high baseline cardiac risk factors (Hayek et al., 2019).
      (2) Following clinical consideration of these elements, discussion and shared decision-making between the radiation oncologist, the patient, caregivers, and other specialists should occur.
2. Pathophysiology
   a) Mechanism
      (1) Mechanisms of radiation-induced heart disease have been studied for many years.

(2) Radiation-induced heart disease results from long-term changes related to the affect of ionizing radiation and resulting endothelial damage, microvascular damage, and a proinflammatory state (Hendry et al., 2008).

(3) Radiation-induced cardiac changes are a result of downstream changes related to fibrosis, including myocyte ischemia and injury, inflammation, oxidative stress, and microvascular dysfunction (Mehta et al., 2018).

    (a) The initial insult occurs as radiation causes cell injury, damage to the endothelium, activation of the acute inflammatory response, and recruitment of profibrotic inflammatory cytokines to the site of irradiation.

    (b) As a result of this damage and inflammation, microvascular and macrovascular changes occur, leading to pericardial changes, myocardial fibrosis, or coronary artery disease. Valvular disease may occur but is least likely (Darby et al., 2010).

b) Historical perspectives on radiation exposure

   (1) Atomic bombs

    (a) Some of the earliest literature on radiation exposure extends from cohort studies such as the Life Span Study and the subsequent Adult Health Study involving the survivors of the Hiroshima and Nagasaki atomic bombings who experienced total body radiation exposure (Shimizu et al., 2010; Shimizu, Pierce, Preston, & Mabuchi, 1999).

    (b) This population was found to have excess relative risk of 14% (6%–23%, p < 0.001) higher than the background rate (no radiation exposure) for all heart disease (Shimizu et al., 1999).

    (c) This analysis was essentially unchanged (0.1%) by accounting for potential confounding factors with independent associations for heart disease, including smoking, alcohol intake, education, type of occupation, obesity (body mass index), and diabetes (Shimizu et al., 2010).

    (d) Studies in this cohort have also identified a persistent increased inflammatory state. Survivors were found to have high circulating levels of interleukin-6, C-reactive protein, and TNF-α more than 60 years beyond exposure, indicating that radiation exposure and natural aging enhance the persistent inflammatory state over time (Hayashi et al., 2012).

    (e) When considering the cardiovascular disease burden in this cohort, it is important to note that these data relate to TBI; therefore, this cohort also has an increased risk of cancer and other causes of morbidity and mortality.

   (2) Hodgkin lymphoma

    (a) Another group who historically received large fields of radiation exposure in the area of the heart were those with Hodgkin lymphoma who were treated with mantle field radiation or larger nodal irradiation to regions such as the mediastinum and left chest.

    (b) This treatment approach yielded higher cure rates; however, patients were found to have significantly increased incidence of cardiac toxicity following treatment, in addition to pulmonary disease and second malignancies, including breast and thyroid cancer.

    (c) The heart dose for these patients often exceeded 30 Gy (Boivin, Hutchison, Lubin, & Mauch, 1992; R.T. Hoppe, 1997; Swerdlow et al., 2007).

   (3) Breast cancer

    (a) The understanding of radiation-related heart changes has also significantly grown from the large body of literature reporting outcomes for breast cancer survivors who received RT as a component of their treatment.

    (b) Early reports, including a review by Cuzick et al. (1988), concluded that breast cancer survivors who received RT had an increased excess risk of noncancer–related mortality after 10 years.

      i. Women who received left-sided postmastectomy RT were two to three times more likely to develop cardiovascular disease. This risk was increased in patients who received radiation to the internal mammary nodes. Paszat et al. (1998) provided the first quantitatively convincing evidence of an increased rate of myocardial infarction after breast cancer RT.

      ii. Reanalysis five years later confirmed that the risk of death from heart disease was 44% higher in women with left-sided compared with right-sided breast cancer. Risk of death from recurrent breast cancer was the same regardless of the side treated (Darby, McGale, Taylor, & Peto, 2005).

    (c) A landmark population-based case-control study including patients who completed RT for breast cancer between 1958 and

2001 in Sweden and Denmark concluded the following (Darby et al., 2013).

   i. The rate of major coronary events increased by 7.4% per 1 Gy in the mean radiation dose delivered to the heart (95% CI, 2.9–14.5; p < 0.001).

   ii. This risk was similar for women with and without a cardiac risk factor at the time of diagnosis. However, for women with baseline cardiac risks, the absolute risks were greater. Notably, for mean heart doses less than 2 Gy, no significantly increased event rates were seen.

   iii. Mean heart dose for modern RT plans is now aimed to be 2 Gy or less (Darby et al., 2013).

c) Types of radiation-induced heart disease

  (1) Acute pericardial disease

    (a) Acute pericarditis occurs most commonly in patients receiving mediastinal radiation for thoracic or esophageal tumors.

    (b) Patients present with chest pain and can have increased acute phase reactants on laboratory values, including neutrophil count, C-reactive protein, and erythrocyte sedimentation rate (Darby et al., 2010).

    (c) The mainstay of treatment for this condition is anti-inflammatory therapy, which may include NSAIDs, such as ibuprofen, aspirin, or indomethacin, with gastrointestinal protection (proton pump inhibitor), in combination with colchicine.

      i. NSAID treatment should continue until resolution of symptoms or normalization of C-reactive protein, followed by tapering over a few weeks (approximately two to four weeks).

      ii. The duration of colchicine treatment should be three months (Adler et al., 2015).

  (2) Chronic pericarditis

    (a) Chronic pericarditis can occur within 10 years or more following RT and may present as a pericardial effusion, potentially progressing to overt cardiac tamponade. This is often associated with other radiation-induced cardiac lesions (Groarke et al., 2014).

    (b) Cardiac echocardiogram is essential for diagnosis. Chronic pericarditis only occurs in patients who have received large doses of radiation to the heart (Groarke et al., 2014). A small number of patients may progress to constrictive pericarditis requir-

ing resection of the parietal pericardium for treatment (Darby et al., 2010).

  (3) Coronary artery disease

    (a) Coronary artery disease related to RT is the result of injury to the intima of the coronary arteries. This injury promotes activation of the inflammatory process that results in atherosclerosis.

    (b) RT may accelerate the pathway of age-related atherosclerosis, leading to clinical coronary artery disease at a younger age. Additionally, microvascular damage from radiation to the myocardium may reduce cardiac tolerance for infarction, thereby increasing the lethality of ischemic events (Darby et al., 2010).

    (c) RT regimens mainly affect the left anterior descending artery for patients with breast cancer and the right coronary artery and basal structures for patients with mediastinal tumors (Groarke et al., 2014; Lind et al., 2003).

      i. Radiation-related atherosclerosis and resultant coronary artery disease is the most common cause of radiation-related cardiac death.

      ii. The ischemic events may be accompanied by classic angina symptoms or sudden cardiac death, or they may be "silent." Silent or asymptomatic myocardial ischemia is more likely for patients who have received radiation to the mediastinum and have the potential for resultant nerve damage locally (Donnellan et al., 2016).

  (4) Valvular disease

    (a) Valvular disease can result from radiation, but the incidence is low: 0.5%–4% of patients who receive RT with exposure to the heart (Donnellan et al., 2016).

    (b) The leaflets of the valves may undergo fibrosis and calcification.

    (c) Valvular disease has a longer latent period of approximately 10–20 years and is more common in valves on the left side of the heart, mainly the aortic valve (Darby et al., 2010; Donnellan et al., 2016).

  (5) Myocardial disease

    (a) Myocardial disease occurs as a result of microvascular injury and resulting in chronic ischemia and fibrosis.

    (b) This is seen more often in patients receiving high doses of radiation (mediastinal doses of 30 Gy or higher) and in patients who are receiving cardiotoxic systemic

agents such as anthracyclines (Donnellan et al., 2016; Mehta et al., 2018).

(6) Arrhythmias

    (a) Conduction abnormalities are the least common radiation-related heart changes.

    (b) Arrhythmias result following fibrosis in the cells of the myocardium associated with the heart rhythm conduction pathways.

    (c) Incidences of radiation-related conduction abnormalities are most often seen in patients who have received RT to the mediastinum.

    (d) The resulting rhythm changes seen most commonly include infranodal and right bundle branch block (Donnellan et al., 2016; Yusuf, Venkatesulu, Mahadevan, & Krishnan, 2017).

d) Proton beam therapy

(1) Proton beam therapy has the potential to reduce the dose to the heart, as this modality may decrease radiation dose to healthy tissue.

(2) A recent comparative analysis of proton beam therapy for mediastinal Hodgkin lymphoma demonstrated dosimetric benefits to the heart, lungs, and breast using involved-node proton beam therapy versus photon treatment with 3DCRT and IMRT (B.S. Hoppe et al., 2012).

(3) In a review of studies published on proton therapy for breast cancer, authors presented information from 13 studies that showed reduced heart dose with proton therapy versus 3DCRT and IMRT (Kammerer et al., 2018). However, more long-term data are necessary to understand the cardioprotective ability of this therapy.

e) Cardiac risks with systemic therapy

(1) Half of patients with cancer will receive RT for curative or symptomatic treatment (Baskar, Lee, Yeo, & Yeoh, 2012). RT is often given in combination with other treatment modalities, including many neoadjuvant or adjuvant systemic agents that also increase or potentiate risk for cardiotoxicity.

(2) Radiation oncology team members should consider exposure to all cardiotoxic modalities for their patients as multiple oncology cardiotoxicity risk factors may warrant consideration with treatment planning, as well as screening and surveillance for cardiotoxicity during and after treatment.

(3) Cardiac dysfunction following cancer treatment regimens, including anthracycline therapy (e.g., doxorubicin, epirubicin, daunorubicin) is well documented (Curigliano et al., 2012; Volkova & Russell, 2011).

    (a) Anthracycline therapy is frequently used in pediatric chemotherapy regimens and in breast cancer treatment regimens.

    (b) Risk of cardiotoxicity increases with dose of anthracyclines and concomitant treatment with other chemotherapy agents, and it is worsened by baseline cardiovascular risk factors (Bloom et al., 2016).

(4) Alkylating agents, such as cyclophosphamide, can also be cardiotoxic; however, toxicity occurs at higher doses than those used for most regimens, including those for breast cancer.

(5) Taxanes can have cardiotoxic effects, but the greater concern with these agents is related to their ability to potentiate the risk of cardiotoxicity of other agents, such as anthracyclines.

(6) Trastuzumab, a HER2-targeted therapy (often administered for HER2-positive breast cancer) carries a risk for left ventricular dysfunction (14%) and heart failure (4%). This risk is increased with concomitant or prior use of anthracyclines, which are part of breast cancer chemotherapy regimens. Patients on trastuzumab receive cardiac screening prior to, during, and following completion of this treatment with noninvasive imaging (echocardiogram preferred) (Bloom et al., 2016; Volkova & Russell, 2011).

(7) 5-Fluorouracil is an antimetabolite commonly used in the treatment of gastrointestinal tumors.

    (a) 5-Fluorouracil is often used in combination with RT, as it possesses radiation sensitization properties.

    (b) Cardiotoxicity is a known adverse effect of 5-fluorouracil, and incidence rates range 1%–18% (Van Cutsem, Hoff, Blum, Abt, & Osterwalder, 2002).

    (c) Cardiotoxicity associated with 5-fluorouracil includes acute onset of symptoms (within two to five days of therapy initiation), angina being most commonly reported.

    (d) Other toxicity findings reported include cardiac arrhythmias, congestive heart failure, myocardial infarction, dilatative cardiomyopathy, cardiogenic shock, cardiac arrest, or sudden death syndrome. Coronary artery thrombosis, arteritis, and vasospasm are proposed as the most likely underlying mechanisms of this acute toxicity (Curigliano et al., 2012; Van Cutsem et al., 2002).

(8) Androgen deprivation therapy is used to decrease testosterone in the treatment of prostate cancer. These medications are recommended as adjuvant therapy, alongside RT, for definitive treatment of higher risk disease, and they are also used to treat metastatic prostate cancer.

(a) Although the exact mechanism of the effect on the cardiovascular system has not been determined definitively, studies have shown an increase in cardiac events including myocardial infarction, nonfatal cardiovascular disease, and stroke, as well as an increased risk of cardiovascular mortality in patients with prior heart disease.

(b) After completion of therapy, changes in patients' metabolic states can occur, including hyperinsulinemia and hypercholesterolemia. Changes in body composition, which may lead to cardiovascular disease, can also occur.

(c) The American Cancer Society, American Urological Association, and American Heart Association recommend caution for patients with preexisting heart disease and risk factor modification and management for patients receiving this androgen deprivation therapy. This was also endorsed by ASTRO (Levine et al., 2010).

(d) Bhatia et al. (2016) proposed the ABCDE approach to reduce cardiovascular disease in this population. It can be deployed in the radiation oncology clinic setting. The acronym stands for the following.

  i. Awareness and aspirin
  ii. Blood pressure
  iii. Cholesterol and cigarettes (smoking cessation)
  iv. Diet and diabetes (monitoring blood glucose)
  v. Exercise

(9) The use of immune checkpoint inhibitors as first-line or adjuvant therapy is becoming more common in treatment of melanoma, lung cancer, renal cell carcinoma, and urothelial cancer.

(a) Immune checkpoint inhibitors are associated with significant immune-related adverse events, including cardiovascular events (e.g., myocarditis) (Moslehi, 2016).

(b) In a recent analysis by investigators of the World Health Organization pharmacovigilance database, investigators identified 122 patients with immune checkpoint inhibitor–associated myocarditis, resulting in death for 50% of cases (Salem et al., 2018).

(c) Further research is needed to characterize incidence of immune-related cardiovascular adverse events for patients receiving immunotherapy with other potentially cardiotoxic treatment modalities, including RT.

3. Cardiac implantable electronic device (CIED) concerns
  a) Overview

(1) Any implanted device within the planned RT field is considered and accounted for in treatment planning.

(2) Very serious consideration and concern is necessary when RT is discussed for patients with CIEDs, which include permanent pacemakers, implantable cardioverter defibrillators, or cardiac resynchronization therapy pacemakers or defibrillators.

b) Modes of CIED failure

(1) Electromagnetic interference may affect device sensing, switches, triggering, function, and reprogramming. Electromagnetic interference has been difficult to isolate from other causes. It is of lower concern because the reported malfunctions have been minimal and transient in nature, occurring only when the interference is present (Beinart & Nazarian, 2013).

(2) Magnetic fields may cause current induction, heating, movement, parameter reset, unpredictable pacing (e.g., inhibition of pacing, asynchronous pacing), and battery depletion.

  (a) Many CIEDs are considered contraindications to MRI (Beinart & Nazarian, 2013; Indik et al., 2017).

  (b) Though modern devices are now MRI-conditional, every CIED should be reviewed by a safety protocol with the department of radiation safety prior to consideration of magnetic field exposure.

(3) Dose-rate effects occur when high-frequency (Gy/minute) x-rays cause interference or "noise" that confuses the CIED, resulting in transient interference during irradiation.

  (a) The majority of these effects have been found to be mild; however, serious consequences may include changes to the electrical signal, such as signal amplitude and transient and permanent silencing, which may be lethal in patients who are pacing dependent (Hudson, Coulshed, D'Souza, & Baker, 2010).

    i. In a report by Grant et al. (2015), three signal interference noise events occurred in the 249 courses of RT—a 1.2% risk per course. These did not result in a clinical effect.

    ii. The theoretical risk of signal interference in an implantable cardioverter defibrillator is high, given that accidental discharge during RT would be severe.

  (b) Pacemakers are also subject to failures resulting from a dose-rate effect.

    i. Mouton, Haug, Bridier, Dodinot, and Eschwege (2002) tested 97 pacemakers at varying dose-rates and total doses and found the threshold for no dose rate effect to be 0.2 Gy/minute.

    ii. The assessment of risk for dose-rate effects is not well understood for contemporary devices based on different treatment regimens, but it is thought to increase with increased dose-rate (Mouton et al., 2002).

(4) High LET interference from neutrons has been shown to cause single-event upsets in CIEDs for proton and high-energy (greater than 10 MV) photon therapy.

    (a) Interference clinically manifests as changes in the processor circuity, resulting in memory loss or resets that do not cause physical damage. The single-event upsets may also lead to loss of device functionality (Miften et al., 2019).

    (b) In a single institution retrospective analysis, 42 patients with CIEDs received treatment with proton beam therapy for thoracic, prostate, liver, or base of skull tumors, from March 2009 through July 2012 (Gomez et al., 2013).

        i. Five patients had a single incidence of a device reset (two pacemakers and three defibrillators), a total reset rate of 0.36% over the 1,352 total fractions or 12% per course.

        ii. Resets were more common in those with thoracic tumors and those who received a high estimated neutron dose to the device.

    (c) Grant et al. (2015) conducted a similar review of patients with CIEDs receiving photon RT to the abdomen, brain, chest, head and neck, and pelvis, as well as TBI, from August 2005 through January 2014.

        i. This series included 247 patients and recorded 15 single-event upsets in neutron-producing RT (15 MV or 18 MV photon beams).

        ii. This was reported as a 21% incidence of device reset per course or 1.2% incidence per neutron-producing fraction.

        iii. The results indicated a risk of 34% for implantable cardioverter defibrillators, 10% for permanent pacemakers, and 7% overall incidence among all courses (Grant et al., 2015).

    (d) As a result of the potential for significant effects of CIEDs, reports and guidelines advise avoidance of energy greater than 10

MV for patients with CIEDs (Gelblum & Amols, 2009; Grant et al., 2015).

(5) Cumulative dose is the most serious of the five failure modes.

    (a) Early evidence confirmed external beam ionizing radiation to be destructive to CIED electrical components when the device is within the path of the beam. Devices were found to be potentially altered at cumulative doses as low as 2 Gy with potential for failure occurring at 10 Gy or more (Marbach, Sontag, Van Dyk, & Wolbarst, 1994; Viganego, Singh, & Fradley, 2016).

    (b) Cumulative dose includes direct and peripheral dose for the CIED. Sources of peripheral dose include leakage; scatter from collimators, wedges, and beam modifiers; within-patient scatter; and neutron production.

    (c) The contribution of nonpatient scatter is highest when the CIED is within 10 cm of the field edge.

    (d) Alternatively, leakage makes up a larger majority of the peripheral dose when the device is 20 cm or more from the field edge. Leakage can be reduced with shielding.

    (e) The effect of peripheral dose increases with treatment field size and is more pronounced near the beam edge because of scatter within the patient from the beam.

    (f) Neutron contribution to the peripheral dose increases with increasing distance from the beam and with increasing energy up to 20 MV. Radiation insult occurs to the device as radiation-produced thermal neutrons scatter throughout the vault, encounter the circuitry of the CIED, and disrupt the electrical charge. This can cause damage to the random-access memory of the device and ultimately lead to data and memory errors or device reset.

c) Guidelines and clinical practice recommendations

(1) Viganego et al. (2016) published a review of CIED effects from RT and included a summary of the evidence and considerations and recommendations that are CIED specific.

    (a) Defibrillators have been found to be more sensitive to radiation damage than pacemakers because of device design, and for these devices, the result can be prolonged charge times, delays in implantable cardioverter defibrillator shock delivery, and inappropriate detection of events.

(b) For patients who are pacemaker dependent, risk is also present. Any risk for damage in pacemaker-dependent patients is of grave concern, as the consequence of malfunction would be fatal.

(c) It is critically important to verify a patient's pacemaker dependence prior to treatment planning with medical record confirmation or electrophysiology consultation.

(2) The Heart Rhythm Society published an expert consensus statement on treatment of patients with CIEDs (Indik et al., 2017).

(a) The statement recommended avoiding neutron-producing beams (e.g., photon energy greater than 10 MV, protons) and considered a 5 Gy dose threshold. Indik et al. (2017) were ultimately unable to make a recommendation concerning cumulative dose risks.

(b) During discussions of all alternatives for prevention of damage to a CIED that is within the planned treatment field, moving the device may be a consideration. However, this is a very high-risk procedure for the patient and may increase mortality risk significantly.

(c) Depending on individual patient risk factors, device pocket reentry procedures introduce significant risk for infection, and a CIED infection is associated with a staggeringly high 20% increased risk of mortality.

(d) Removal and redirecting the associated leads also present multiple challenges.

(e) Device removal and manipulation should be avoided at all costs, and considerations for minimizing risk to CIEDs with careful radiation planning is preferred (Tarakji, Ellis, Defaye, & Kennergren, 2016).

(3) Guidelines from the American Association of Physicists in Medicine Task Group 34 for managing patients with pacemakers were published in 1994 (Marbach et al., 1994). These recommendations have been variably utilized and do not cover defibrillators, newer device technology, and novel RT delivery methods (Lenarczyk et al., 2017; Miften et al., 2019; Solan, Solan, Bednarz, & Goodkin, 2004).

(4) Evidence-based consensus guidelines by the Dutch Society of Radiotherapy and Oncology proposed risk-based management for RT patients with CIEDs (Hurkmans et al., 2012).

(5) American Association of Physicists in Medicine Task Group 203 published recommendations for treatment planning to reduce device and patient risk. Recommendations include the following (Miften et al., 2019).

(a) Avoiding prolonged (more than three seconds) irradiation of the device

(b) Utilizing lower dose rates

(c) Keeping treatment and imaging field edge to more than 5 cm from generator and maximizing this distance through beam angle selection

(d) Utilizing in vivo dosimetry for the first treatment fraction for devices within 10 cm of field edge

(e) Estimating cumulative dose based on distance from the field edge

(f) Keeping the cumulative dose less than 5 Gy or manufacturer's recommended limit

(g) Implementing and closely following a risk-based monitoring plan for patients (see Figure 15)

(h) Avoiding external lead shielding of CIEDs during RT

(i) Confirming MRI device compatibility if magnetic resonance simulation is considered

(6) Other recommendations

(a) For medium- and high-risk patients, available support should include audiovisual monitoring, pulse oximetry, electrocardiogram monitoring, cardiac resuscitation cart, and temporary transcutaneous pacing with staff trained in its use.

(b) For patients with implantable cardioverter defibrillators, clinicians should consult with an electrophysiologist to determine if antitachyarrythmia therapy should be deactivated during RT sessions through programming or magnet use.

(c) For all patients with CIEDs, device interrogations should occur prior to and at the completion of RT, with mid-course checks recommended for medium-risk patients and weekly checks when dose exceeds 5 Gy for high-risk patients (Miften et al., 2019).

(d) All radiation oncology team members should be aware of the hazards that exist for patients undergoing RT with CIEDs in place. Most critically, coordination between medical physicists, cardiac specialists, and radiation oncologists is recommended during treatment planning, with attention to the most recent available literature and guideline updates.

(e) Individual devices have specifications regarding RT.

   i. Given the variability among specifications for devices, no safe thresh-

FIGURE 15. Radiation Therapy Patient Management Checklist

Patient Information _____

Date: _____

1. Initial Consultation

    a. CIED alert added to patient's chart _____

    b. Copy of CIED card made and filed in patient's chart _____

    c. Appointment with Cardiac Electrophysiology (EP) scheduled if needed_____

    d. Determine from cardiologist whether magnet is required _____

2. Simulation stage

    a. Patient was evaluated to verify dependence on device _____

    b. Verify CIED alert added to patient's chart _____

    c. Verify treatment planning directive completed by physician_____

    d. Note added to planning directive to only use photons ≤10 MV and avoid physical wedges where possible_____

    e. Contact vendor for dose threshold recommendations _____

3. Planning stage

    a. Verify only ≤10 MV photons used for treatment _____

    b. Estimate dose/fraction and cumulative dose_____

    c. Verify proximity of treatment fields to device

        i. If edge of field > 10 cm, then no further action necessary.

        ii. If edge of field <10 cm, then continue with checklist. _____

    d. If necessary, add note to patient's chart to place in vivo dosimeter on fraction #1

    e. Verify/adjust imaging fields do not irradiate device.

        i. If device is in imaging field, use kV imaging where possible.

        ii. If fields adjusted, add note in chart to indicate appropriate field size for imaging.

4. First day of treatment delivery

    a. Place in vivo dosimeter on CIED at closest approach to treatment field area _____

    b. Verify imaging field does not irradiate CIED_____

    c. Read dosimeter and generate summary of reading for physician _____

5. Dose to CIED

< 2 Gy (Low-Risk)	2–5 Gy (Medium-Risk)	> 5 Gy or neutrons (High-Risk)
• Resuscitation protocol. • Pacemaker magnet, pulse oximetry, and AED available at treatment unit. • Close monitoring of the CIED patient with an audio-visual system during treatment. • Communication with cardiology/electrophysiology. • ICD patients: consult with cardiology/electrophysiology on setting program tachycardia OFF or the use of magnet. • CIED interrogation before 1st fraction and after last fraction.	*Low-Risk requirements* *AND* • Formal consultation with cardiology/electrophysiology. • Pacing-dependent: consult with • cardiology/electrophysiology on the use of magnet and pulse oximetry. • Appropriate cardiac support available to manage complications from potential CIED malfunctions. • CIED technologist to interrogate the device at midtreatment.	*Medium-Risk requirements* *AND* • ECG weekly monitoring. • Trained staff examines ECG. • Cardiologist/pacemaker technologist should be available, if needed. • CIED technologist to interrogate the device weekly once the device receives > 5 Gy.

Note. From "Management of Radiotherapy Patients With Implanted Cardiac Pacemakers and Defibrillators: A Report of the AAPM TG-203," by M. Miften, D. Mihailidis, S.F. Kry, C. Reft, C. Esquivel, J. Farr, … J. Wilkinson, 2019, *Medical Physics, 46,* p. e779 (https://doi.org/10.1002/mp.13838). Copyright 2019 by American Association of Physicists in Medicine. Reprinted with permission.

old or modality can be recommended for RT for any patient with a CIED.

ii. Radiation oncology care teams should screen all patients at consultation for CIEDs in patient history, and each department should have a management policy in place for risk-based management for patients with CIEDs.

iii. This policy should be developed by an interprofessional team, including radiation oncologists, medical physicists, dosimetrists, radiation oncology therapists, radiation oncology nurses, electrophysiology physicians, and cardio-oncology physician experts.

4. Prevention, screening, and surveillance
   a) Prevention
      (1) Prevention is accomplished through radiation planning and treatment delivery, as well as working with patients to minimize their baseline cardiac risk factors.
      (2) Baseline cardiovascular risks that should be considered include hypertension, diabetes, tobacco use, underlying left ventricular dysfunction or heart failure, coronary artery disease, older age, female sex, postmenopausal status, and genetic polymorphisms.
      (3) The risk for radiation-induced heart disease is highest when the treatment field is within proximity to the heart.
      (4) Treatment planning for thoracic disease types, including lung, esophageal, and breast cancer, as well as Hodgkin lymphoma, considers minimizing heart dose.
      (5) Modern RT techniques are incorporated into treatment planning to minimize risk for cardiac effects from treatment (Groarke et al., 2014; Piroth et al., 2019).
         (a) Shielding techniques
         (b) Limiting the mean heart dose to 2 Gy when possible
         (c) Limiting the dose per fraction to approximately 2 Gy per day with fractionation regimens whenever possible
      (6) For patients with breast cancer, multiple techniques may spare the heart.
         (a) For patients with tumors in the left upper outer quadrant, radiation oncologists may utilize a heart block with three-dimensional treatment planning to spare the heart and lower inner quadrant breast tissue. Studies have not shown an increased risk of in-breast recurrence with this technique (Yue et al., 2014).
         (b) Prone breast treatment may be appropriate and may decrease the dose of radiation to the heart. This technique is limited to patients based on body habitus and tumor location, as studies have shown benefits of reducing heart dose and decreasing coverage of axillary fields in women with larger breasts (Beck et al., 2014).
         (c) Novel treatment delivery techniques, including deep inspiratory breath hold, for patients receiving treatment to the left chest will decrease the mean heart dose further. Limited to patients who can physically tolerate holding their breath for at least 20 seconds, deep inspiratory breath hold moves the heart into a more medial position (Aznar et al., 2015).
      (7) IMRT allows the radiation oncologist to create the desired dose variation inside the radiation field. This is utilized with IGRT, including regular image checks during treatment to more closely approximate the radiation dose to the tumor and the allowable margin.
      (8) SBRT is used to deliver a high dose of radiation to a small area of tissue with minimal margin, utilizing advanced imaging to ensure that the disease target is within field while sparing the healthy tissue.
      (9) Mean heart dose and coronary artery dose volume information can be analyzed through treatment planning systems during RT planning (Garibaldi et al., 2017).
      (10) Partial-breast RT techniques utilize brachytherapy with shielding to deliver radiation through a source directly into the cavity (Coles et al., 2017).
         (a) This technique limits exposure of radiation to breast tissue, eliminating dose to the heart or lungs.
         (b) It is an attractive option because it eliminates the burden of an extended course of RT following surgery, as it is performed at the time of breast conservation surgery.
         (c) This course is associated with overall lower toxicity to the skin and healthy tissue.
         (d) Though trials have proven noninferiority in outcomes compared to whole-breast irradiation, this option is only available to patients with lower-risk tumors with appropriate margins at the time of lumpectomy.
   b) Surveillance
      (1) Surveillance for cardiotoxicity following RT facilitates earlier diagnosis of radiation-related cardiac injury, thus reducing morbidity and mortality related to heart failure (Groarke et al., 2014).

(2) Providers should emphasize a complete cardiac review of systems and physical exam and have a low threshold for use of noninvasive imaging for detection of cardiac dysfunction.

(3) Noninvasive cardiac screening may include echocardiogram (preferred), cardiac perfusion imaging, stress testing, and coronary calcium score by CT if the coronary arteries received 35 Gy or higher during the treatment course.

(4) Screening generally is most appropriate beginning five years after radiation exposure.

(5) As valvular heart disease presents later than coronary artery disease, repeat screening 10 years after exposure is appropriate, depending on treatment location and dose.

(6) Screening threshold should be lowered in patients with baseline cardiac risk factors, including tobacco use, hyperlipidemia, hypertension, and diabetes, as well as exposure to adjuvant systemic treatments associated with cardiotoxicity, such as anthracyclines (Darby et al., 2010; Darby et al., 2013).

c) Guidelines for prevention, screening, and surveillance

(1) The short- and long-term risk for cardiac dysfunction in survivors of childhood cancers treated with anthracycline or RT to the chest is well addressed in medical literature (Lipshultz et al., 2013; Oeffinger et al., 2006). Correspondingly, guidelines for surveillance and prevention of cardiomyopathy in this population have been established (Armenian et al., 2015).

(2) Until recently, comparable consensus screening and prevention guidelines for survivors of adult-onset cancers were not in place. However, as a result of the growing body of literature on this topic and the critical need for guidance on the prevention of heart failure in cancer survivors, ASCO convened an expert panel to conduct a systematic evidence review of available literature and developed clinical practice guideline recommendations for key areas of cardiac consideration in oncology clinical practice (Armenian et al., 2017).

(a) The guidelines addressed questions related to the following (Armenian et al., 2017).

i. Which patients are most at risk for developing cardiace dysfunction based on baseline risk factors and treatment modalities

ii. Preventive strategies to minimize risk prior to and during administration of potentially cardiotoxic therapies

iii. Preference for surveillance and monitoring during and after treatment in patients at risk for cardiac dysfunction

(b) At-risk patients were identified as those who received the following treatments (Armenian et al., 2017).

i. High radiation dose (greater than 30 Gy) with the heart in the treatment field

ii. Low radiation dose (less than 30 Gy) with the heart in the treatment field, in combination with lower-dose anthracycline treatment (e.g., doxorubicin less than 250 mg/m², epirubicin less than 600 mg/m²).

(c) Risk reduction recommendations for patients receiving mediastinal or breast radiation included deep-inspiratory breath holding and IMRT (Armenian et al., 2017).

(d) Screening and surveillance recommendations were included for all patients and those at an increased risk for cardiac dysfunction. Recommendations include but are not limited to the following (Armenian et al., 2017).

i. Thorough cardiac history and physical examination before, during, and following treatment

ii. Cardiac risk factor modification before, during, and following treatment

iii. Echocardiography 6–12 months after treatment for those at increased risk

iv. Referral to a cardio-oncology expert for patients with asymptomatic cardiac dysfunction during or following treatment

5. Collaboration with cardio-oncology

a) Cardio-oncology has emerged as a new specialty field and refers to an approach involving cardiologists, oncologists, and hematologists collaborating on prevention, early detection, and management of cardiovascular disease in patients with cancer throughout all stages of cancer therapy and survivorship (Hayek et al., 2019).

b) Interprofessional collaboration with these specialists will be invaluable as cancer therapies, such as multimodal treatment and immune checkpoint inhibitors, impose greater risk for cardiotoxicity.

c) Collaboration with cardio-oncology specialists and electrophysiologists is also of high value when a patient presents with a CIED near the planned area for treatment, when a patient is pacing dependent, or when high-energy beams (greater than 10 MV) are preferred for a patient with a CIED.

d) Given their understanding of the electrophysiology concerns for a patient and the specific utility of a CIED, as well as the unique pathophysiology of cardiac diseases in the setting of malignancy and any cardiac risks associated with other oncologic treatment modalities planned, cardio-oncologists can partner with other healthcare providers to develop strategies for appropriately preventing and managing CIED complications (Hayek et al., 2019; Indik et al., 2017; Miften et al., 2019).

6. Survivorship concerns

a) For patients who receive RT, radiation-related cardiotoxicity and radiation-induced heart disease are most commonly late effects of treatment.

(1) This circumstance will be increasingly relevant for the aging population of survivors alive today.

(2) Long-term follow-up care in the oncology setting should consider the cardiac implications of all cancer treatment modalities in light of a patient's baseline cardiac risks.

(3) Cardiac health should be emphasized in survivorship care.

(4) Specialty oncology-embedded survivorship programs emphasize education around cardiac risks in addition to assessment for cardiac risks and appropriate surveillance.

b) All healthcare team members should be aware of the heart risks associated with RT and the important considerations during and following care for patients with CIEDs in place.

c) Although younger age at the time of RT increases a patient's overall lifetime risk for experiencing radiation-induced heart disease, with advances in treatment and longer survival for aging patients with cancer, cardiotoxicity should be a consideration for all patients in the radiation oncology setting if they receive treatment to the left chest or mediastinal area.

d) With new RT modalities, including SBRT for early-stage NSCLC, research is needed to understand the influence of these treatment modalities on acute and late cardiac risks.

References

Adler, Y., Charron, P., Imazio, M., Badano, L., Barón-Esquivias, G., Bogaert, J., ... Tomkowski, W. (2015). 2015 ESC guidelines for the diagnosis and management of pericardial diseases: The Task Force for the Diagnosis and Management of Pericardial Diseases of the European Society of Cardiology (ESC); Endorsed by: The European Association for Cardio-Thoracic Surgery (EACTS). *European Heart Journal, 36,* 2921–2964. https://doi.org/10.1093/eurheartj/ehv318

Aleman, B.M.P., Moser, E.C., Nuver, J., Suter, T.M., Maraldo, M.V., Specht, L., ... Darby, S.C. (2014). Cardiovascular disease after cancer therapy. *European Journal of Cancer Supplements, 12,* 18–28. https://doi.org/10.1016/j.ejcsup.2014.03.002

Armenian, S.H., Hudson, M.M., Mulder, R.L., Chen, M.H., Constine, L.S., Dwyer, M., ... Kremer, L.C.M. (2015). Recommendations for cardiomyopathy surveillance for survivors of childhood cancer: A report from the International Late Effects of Childhood Cancer Guideline Harmonization Group. *Lancet Oncology, 16,* E123–E136. https://doi.org/10.1016/s1470-2045(14)70409-7

Armenian, S.H., Lacchetti, C., Barac, A., Carver, J., Constine, L.S., Denduluri, N., ... Lenihan, D. (2017). Prevention and monitoring of cardiac dysfunction in survivors of adult cancers: American Society of Clinical Oncology clinical practice guideline. *Journal of Clinical Oncology, 35,* 893–911. https://doi.org/10.1200/jco.2016.70.5400

Avis, N.E., & Deimling, G.T. (2008). Cancer survivorship and aging. *Cancer, 113*(Suppl. 12), 3519–3529. https://doi.org/10.1002/cncr.23941

Aznar, M.C., Maraldo, M.V., Schut, D.A., Lundemann, M., Brodin, N.P., Vogelius, I.R., ... Petersen, P.M. (2015). Minimizing late effects for patients with mediastinal Hodgkin lymphoma: Deep inspiration breath-hold, IMRT, or both? *International Journal of Radiation Oncology, Biology, Physics, 92,* 169–174. https://doi.org/10.1016/j.ijrobp.2015.01.013

Baskar, R., Lee, K.A., Yeo, R., & Yeoh, K.-W. (2012). Cancer and radiation therapy: Current advances and future directions. *International Journal of Medical Sciences, 9,* 193–199. https://doi.org/10.7150/ijms.3635

Beck, R.E., Kim, L., Yue, N.J., Haffty, B.G., Khan, A.J., & Goyal, S. (2014). Treatment techniques to reduce cardiac irradiation for breast cancer patients treated with breast-conserving surgery and radiation therapy: A review. *Frontiers in Oncology, 4,* 327. https://doi.org/10.3389/fonc.2014.00327

Beinart, R., & Nazarian, S. (2013). Effects of external electrical and magnetic fields on pacemakers and defibrillators: From engineering principles to clinical practice. *Circulation, 128,* 2799–2809. https://doi.org/10.1161/circulationaha.113.005697

Bellizzi, K.M., Mustian, K.M., Palesh, O.G., & Diefenbach, M. (2008). Cancer survivorship and aging: Moving the science forward. *Cancer, 113*(Suppl. 12), 3530–3539. https://doi.org/10.1002/cncr.23942

Benjamin, E.J., Muntner, P., Alonso, A., Bittencourt, M.S., Callaway, C.W., Carson, A.P., ... Virani, S.S. (2019). Heart disease and stroke statistics—2019 update: A report from the American Heart Association. *Circulation, 139,* e56–e528. https://doi.org/10.1161/CIR.0000000000000659

Bhatia, N., Santos, M., Jones, L.W., Beckman, J.A., Penson, D.F., Morgans, A.K., & Moslehi, J. (2016). Cardiovascular effects of androgen deprivation therapy for the treatment of prostate cancer: ABCDE steps to reduce cardiovascular disease in patients with prostate cancer. *Circulation, 133,* 537–541. https://doi.org/10.1161/CIRCULATIONAHA.115.012519

Bloom, M.W., Hamo, C.E., Cardinale, D., Ky, B., Nohria, A., Baer, L., ... Butler, J. (2016). Cancer therapy–related cardiac dysfunction and heart failure: Part 1: Definitions, pathophysiology, risk factors, and imaging. *Circulation: Heart Failure, 9,* e002661. https://doi.org/10.1161/circheartfailure.115.002661

Boivin, J.-F., Hutchison, G.B., Lubin, J.H., & Mauch, P. (1992). Coronary artery disease mortality in patients treated for Hodgkin's disease. *Cancer, 69,* 1241–1247. https://doi.org/10.1002/cncr.2820690528

Bradshaw, P.T., Stevens, J., Khankari, N., Teitelbaum, S.L., Neugut, A.I., & Gammon, M.D. (2016). Cardiovascular disease mortality among breast cancer survivors. *Epidemiology, 27,* 6–13. https://doi.org/10.1097/ede.0000000000000394

Coles, C.E., Griffin, C.L., Kirby, A.M., Titley, J., Agrawal, R.K., Alhasso, A., ... Bliss, J.M. (2017). Partial-breast radiotherapy after breast conservation surgery for patients with early breast cancer (UK IMPORT LOW trial): 5-year results from a multicentre, randomised, controlled, phase 3, non-inferiority trial. *Lancet, 390,* 1048–1060. https://doi.org/10.1016/S0140-6736(17)31145-5

Curigliano, G., Cardinale, D., Suter, T., Platanitotis, G., de Azambuja, E., Sandri, M.T., ... Roila, F. (2012). Cardiovascular toxicity induced by chemotherapy, targeted agents and radiotherapy: ESMO clinical practice guidelines. *Annals of Oncology, 23*(Suppl. 7), vii155–vii166. https://doi.org/10.1093/annonc/mds293

Cuzick, J., Stewart, H.J., Peto, R., Baum, M., Fisher, B., Host, H., ... Wallgren, A. (1988). Overview of randomized trials of postoperative adjuvant radiotherapy in breast cancer. In H. Scheurlen, R. Kay, & M. Baum (Eds.), *Recent results in cancer research: Vol. 111. Cancer clinical trials: A critical appraisal* (pp. 108–129). Springer. https://doi.org/10.1007/978-3-642-83419-6_15

Darby, S.C., Cutter, D.J., Boerma, M., Constine, L.S., Fajardo, L.F., Kodama, K., ... Shore, R.E. (2010). Radiation-related heart disease: Current knowledge and future prospects. *International Journal of Radiation Oncology, Biology, Physics, 76*, 656–665. https://doi.org/10.1016/j.ijrobp.2009.09.064

Darby, S.C., Ewertz, M., McGale, P., Bennet, A.M., Blom-Goldman, U., Brønnum, D., ... Hall, P. (2013). Risk of ischemic heart disease in women after radiotherapy for breast cancer. *New England Journal of Medicine, 368*, 987–998. https://doi.org/10.1056/nejmoa1209825

Darby, S.C., McGale, P., Taylor, C.W., & Peto, R. (2005). Long-term mortality from heart disease and lung cancer after radiotherapy for early breast cancer: Prospective cohort study of about 300,000 women in US SEER cancer registries. *Lancet Oncology, 6*, 557–565. https://doi.org/10.1016/s1470-2045(05)70251-5

de Moor, J.S., Mariotto, A.B., Parry, C., Alfano, C.M., Padgett, L., Kent, E.E., ... Rowland, J.H. (2013). Cancer survivors in the United States: Prevalence across the survivorship trajectory and implications for care. *Cancer Epidemiology, Biomarkers and Prevention, 22*, 561–570. https://doi.org/10.1158/1055-9965.epi-12-1356

Donnellan, E., Phelan, D., McCarthy, C.P., Collier, P., Desai, M., & Griffin, B. (2016). Radiation-induced heart disease: A practical guide to diagnosis and management. *Cleveland Clinic Journal of Medicine, 83*, 914–922. https://doi.org/10.3949/ccjm.83a.15104

Findlay, S.G., Gill, J.H., Plummer, R., DeSantis, C., & Plummer, C. (2019). Chronic cardiovascular toxicity in the older oncology patient population. *Journal of Geriatric Oncology, 10*, 685–689. https://doi.org/10.1016/j.jgo.2019.01.018

Garibaldi, C., Jereczek-Fossa, B.A., Marvaso, G., Dicuonzo, S., Rojas, D.P., Cattani, F., ... Ricotti, R. (2017). Recent advances in radiation oncology. *Ecancermedicalscience, 11*, 785. https://doi.org/10.3332/ecancer.2017.785

Gelblum, D.Y., & Amols, H. (2009). Implanted cardiac defibrillator care in radiation oncology patient population. *International Journal of Radiation Oncology, Biology, Physics, 73*, 1525–1531. https://doi.org/10.1016/j.ijrobp.2008.06.1903

Gomez, D.R., Poenisch, F., Pinnix, C.C., Sheu, T., Chang, J.Y., Memon, N., ... Dougherty, A.H. (2013). Malfunctions of implantable cardiac devices in patients receiving proton beam therapy: Incidence and predictors. *International Journal of Radiation Oncology, Biology, Physics, 87*, 570–575. https://doi.org/10.1016/j.ijrobp.2013.07.010

Grant, J.D., Jensen, G.L., Tang, C., Pollard, J.M., Kry, S.F., Krishnan, S., ... Rozner, M.A. (2015). Radiotherapy-induced malfunction in contemporary cardiovascular implantable electronic devices: Clinical incidence and predictors. *JAMA Oncology, 1*, 624–632. https://doi.org/10.1001/jamaoncol.2015.1787

Groarke, J.D., Nguyen, P.L., Nohria, A., Ferrari, R., Cheng, S., & Moslehi, J. (2014). Cardiovascular complications of radiation therapy for thoracic malignancies: The role for non-invasive imaging for detection of cardiovascular disease. *European Heart Journal, 35*, 612–623. https://doi.org/10.1093/eurheartj/eht114

Hamo, C.E., & Bloom, M.W. (2017). Cancer and heart failure: Understanding the intersection. *Cardiac Failure Review, 3*, 66–70. https://doi.org/10.15420/cfr.2016:24:2

Hayashi, T., Morishita, Y., Khattree, R., Misumi, M., Sasaki, K., Hayashi, I., ... Nakachi, K. (2012). Evaluation of systemic markers of inflammation in atomic-bomb survivors with special reference to radiation and age effects. *FASEB Journal, 26*, 4765–4773. https://doi.org/10.1096/fj.12-215228

Hayek, S.S., Ganatra, S., Lenneman, C., Scherrer-Crosbie, M., Leja, M., Lenihan, D.J., ... Ky, B. (2019). Preparing the cardiovascular workforce to care for oncology patients: JACC review topic of the week. *Journal of the American College of Cardiology, 73*, 2226–2235. https://doi.org/10.1016/j.jacc.2019.02.041

Hendry, J.H., Akahoshi, M., Wang, L.S., Lipshultz, S.E., Stewart, F.A., & Trott, K.R. (2008). Radiation-induced cardiovascular injury. *Radiation and Environmental Biophysics, 47*, 189–193. https://doi.org/10.1007/s00411-007-0155-7

Hoppe, B.S., Flampouri, S., Su, Z., Morris, C.G., Latif, N., Dang, N.H., ... Mendenhall, N.P. (2012). Consolidative involved-node proton therapy for stage IA–IIIB mediastinal Hodgkin lymphoma: Preliminary dosimetric outcomes from a phase II study. *International Journal of Radiation Oncology, Biology, Physics, 83*, 260–267. https://doi.org/10.1016/j.ijrobp.2011.06.1959

Hoppe, R.T. (1997). Hodgkin's disease: Complications of therapy and excess mortality. *Annals of Oncology, 8*(Suppl. 1), S115–S118. https://doi.org/10.1093/annonc/8.suppl_1.s115

Hudson, F., Coulshed, D., D'Souza, E., & Baker, C. (2010). Effect of radiation therapy on the latest generation of pacemakers and implantable cardioverter defibrillators: A systematic review. *Journal of Medical Imaging and Radiation Oncology, 54*, 53–61. https://doi.org/10.1111/j.1754-9485.2010.02138.x

Hurkmans, C.W., Knegjens, J.L., Oei, B.S., Maas, A.J.J., Uiterwaal, G.J., van der Borden, A.J., ... van Erven, L. (2012). Management of radiation oncology patients with a pacemaker or ICD: A new comprehensive practical guideline in the Netherlands. *Radiation Oncology, 7*, 198. https://doi.org/10.1186/1748-717x-7-198

Indik, J.H., Gimbel, J.R., Abe, H., Alkmim-Teixeira, R., Birgersdotter-Green, U., Clarke, G.D., ... Woodard, P.K. (2017). 2017 HRS expert consensus statement on magnetic resonance imaging and radiation exposure in patients with cardiovascular implantable electronic devices. *Heart Rhythm, 14*, e97–e153. https://doi.org/10.1016/j.hrthm.2017.04.025

Kammerer, E., Le Guevelou, J., Chaikh, A., Danhier, S., Geffrelot, J., Levy, C., ... Thariat, J. (2018). Proton therapy for locally advanced breast cancer: A systematic review of the literature. *Cancer Treatment Reviews, 63*, 19–27. https://doi.org/10.1016/j.ctrv.2017.11.006

Lenarczyk, R., Potpara, T.S., Haugaa, K.H., Deharo, J.-C., Hernandez-Madrid, A., del Carmen Exposito Pineda, M., ... Dagres, N. (2017). Approach to cardio-oncologic patients with special focus on patients with cardiac implantable electronic devices planned for radiotherapy: Results of the European Heart Rhythm Association survey. *EP Europace, 19*, 1579–1584. https://doi.org/10.1093/europace/eux195

Levine, G.N., D'Amico, A.V., Berger, P., Clark, P.E., Eckel, R.H., Keating, N.L., ... Zakai, N. (2010). Androgen-deprivation therapy in prostate cancer and cardiovascular risk: A science advisory from the American Heart Association, American Cancer Society, and American Urological Association: Endorsed by the American Society for Radiation Oncology. *Circulation, 121*, 833–840. https://doi.org/10.1161/CIRCULATIONAHA.109.192695

Lind, P.A., Pagnanelli, R., Marks, L.B., Borges-Neto, S., Hu, C., Zhou, S.-M., ... Hardenbergh, P.H. (2003). Myocardial perfusion changes in patients irradiated for left-sided breast cancer and correlation with coronary artery distribution. *International Journal of Radiation Oncology, Biology, Physics, 55*, 914–920. https://doi.org/10.1016/s0360-3016(02)04156-1

Lipshultz, S.E., Cochran, T.R., Franco, V.I., & Miller, T.L. (2013). Treatment-related cardiotoxicity in survivors of childhood cancer. *Nature Reviews Clinical Oncology, 10*, 697–710. https://doi.org/10.1038/nrclinonc.2013.195

Marbach, J.R., Sontag, M.R., Van Dyk, J., & Wolbarst, A.B. (1994). Management of radiation oncology patients with implanted cardiac pacemakers: Report of AAPM Task Group No. 34. *Medical Physics, 21*, 85–90. https://doi.org/10.1118/1.597259

Mehta, L.S., Watson, K.E., Barac, A., Beckie, T.M., Bittner, V., Cruz-Flores, S., ... Volgman, A.S. (2018). Cardiovascular disease and breast cancer: Where these entities intersect: A scientific statement from the American Heart Association. *Circulation, 137*, e30–e66. https://doi.org/10.1161/cir.0000000000000556

Miften, M., Mihailidis, D., Kry, S.F., Reft, C., Esquivel, C., Farr, J., ... Wilkinson, J. (2019). Management of radiotherapy patients with implanted cardiac pacemakers and defibrillators: A report of the AAPM TG-203. *Medical Physics, 46*, e757–e788. https://doi.org/10.1002/mp.13838

Miller, K.D., Nogueira, L., Mariotto, A.B., Rowland, J.H., Yabroff, K.R., Alfano, C.M., ... Siegel, R.L. (2019). Cancer treatment and survivorship statistics, 2019. *CA: A Cancer Journal for Clinicians, 69*, 363–385. https://doi.org/10.3322/caac.21565

Moslehi, J.J. (2016). Cardiovascular toxic effects of targeted cancer therapies. *New England Journal of Medicine, 375,* 1457–1467. https://doi.org/10.1056/NEJMra1100265

Mouton, J., Haug, R., Bridier, A., Dodinot, B., & Eschwege, F. (2002). Influence of high-energy photon beam irradiation on pacemaker operation. *Physics in Medicine and Biology, 47,* 2879–2893. https://doi.org/10.1088/0031-9155/47/16/304

Oeffinger, K.C., Mertens, A.C., Sklar, C.A., Kawashima, T., Hudson, M.M., Meadows, A.T., ... Robison, L.L. (2006). Chronic health conditions in adult survivors of childhood cancer. *New England Journal of Medicine, 355,* 1572–1582. https://doi.org/10.1056/NEJMsa060185

Paszat, L.F., Mackillop, W.J., Groome, P.A., Boyd, C., Schulze, K., & Holowaty, E. (1998). Mortality from myocardial infarction after adjuvant radiotherapy for breast cancer in the Surveillance, Epidemiology, and End-Results cancer registries. *Journal of Clinical Oncology, 16,* 2625–2631. https://doi.org/10.1200/jco.1998.16.8.2625

Piroth, M.D., Baumann, R., Budach, W., Dunst, J., Feyer, P., Fietkau, R., ... Sauer, R. (2019). Heart toxicity from breast cancer radiotherapy: Current findings, assessment, and prevention. *Strahlentherapie und Onkologie, 195,* 1–12. https://doi.org/10.1007/s00066-018-1378-z

Salem, J.-E., Manouchehri, A., Moey, M., Lebrun-Vignes, B., Bastarache, L., Pariente, A., ... Moslehi, J.J. (2018). Cardiovascular toxicities associated with immune checkpoint inhibitors: An observational, retrospective, pharmacovigilance study. *Lancet Oncology, 19,* 1579–1589. https://doi.org/10.1016/s1470-2045(18)30608-9

Shimizu, Y., Kodama, K., Nishi, N., Kasagi, F., Suyama, A., Soda, M., ... Shore, R.E. (2010). Radiation exposure and circulatory disease risk: Hiroshima and Nagasaki atomic bomb survivor data, 1950–2003. *BMJ, 340,* b5349. https://doi.org/10.1136/bmj.b5349

Shimizu, Y., Pierce, D.A., Preston, D.L., & Mabuchi, K. (1999). Studies of the mortality of atomic bomb survivors. Report 12, Part II. Noncancer mortality: 1950–1990. *Radiation Research, 152,* 374–389. https://doi.org/10.2307/3580222

Solan, A.N., Solan, M.J., Bednarz, G., & Goodkin, M.B. (2004). Treatment of patients with cardiac pacemakers and implantable cardioverter-defibrillators during radiotherapy. *International Journal of Radiation Oncology, Biology, Physics, 59,* 897–904. https://doi.org/10.1016/j.ijrobp.2004.02.038

Strongman, H., Gadd, S., Matthews, A., Mansfield, K.E., Stanway, S., Lyon, A.R., ... Bhaskaran, K. (2019). Medium and long-term risks of specific cardiovascular diseases in survivors of 20 adult cancers: A population-based cohort study using multiple linked UK electronic health records databases. *Lancet, 394,* 1041–1054. https://doi.org/10.1016/S0140-6736(19)31674-5

Swerdlow, A.J., Higgins, C.D., Smith, P., Cunningham, D., Hancock, B.W., Horwich, A., ... Linch, D.C. (2007). Myocardial infarction mortality risk after treatment for Hodgkin disease: A collaborative British cohort study. *Journal of the National Cancer Institute, 99,* 206–214. https://doi.org/10.1093/jnci/djk029

Tarakji, K.G., Ellis, C.R., Defaye, P., & Kennergren, C. (2016). Cardiac implantable electronic device infection in patients at risk. *Arrhythmia and Electrophysiology Review, 5,* 65–71. https://doi.org/10.15420/aer.2015.27.2

Van Cutsem, E., Hoff, P.M., Blum, J.L., Abt, M., & Osterwalder, B. (2002). Incidence of cardiotoxicity with the oral fluoropyrimidine capecitabine is typical of that reported with 5-fluorouracil. *Annals of Oncology, 13,* 484–485. https://doi.org/10.1093/annonc/mdf108

Viganego, F., Singh, R., & Fradley, M.G. (2016). Arrhythmias and other electrophysiology issues in cancer patients receiving chemotherapy or radiation. *Current Cardiology Reports, 18,* 52. https://doi.org/10.1007/s11886-016-0730-0

Volkova, M., & Russell, R. (2011). Anthracycline cardiotoxicity: Prevalence, pathogenesis and treatment. *Current Cardiology Reviews, 7,* 214–220. https://doi.org/10.2174/157340311799960645

Yue, N.J., Goyal, S., Park, J.H., Jones, S., Xu, X., Khan, A., ... Chen, T. (2014). Optimization of heart block in the left-sided whole breast radiation treatments. *Frontiers in Oncology, 4,* 342. https://doi.org/10.3389/fonc.2014.00342

Yusuf, S.W., Venkatesulu, B.P., Mahadevan, L.S., & Krishnan, S. (2017). Radiation-induced cardiovascular disease: A clinical perspective. *Frontiers in Cardiovascular Medicine, 4,* 66. https://doi.org/10.3389/fcvm.2017.00066

L. Bone metastases

1. Pathophysiology

   a) The majority of bone metastases are hematogenous and spread by arterial or venous routes. The axial skeleton is seeded more than the appendicular skeleton because of persistence of red bone marrow (Macedo et al., 2017).

   (1) Bone metastases are thought to be caused by overstimulation of osteoclasts or osteoblasts, causing a lytic or blastic lesion.

   (2) Either lesion can cause bone pain, but lytic lesions are associated with a higher rate of pathologic fracture.

   b) The appearance of bone metastases on imaging depends on primary tumor histology (von Moos, Costa, Ripamonti, Niepel, & Santini, 2017).

   (1) Prostate cancer produces blastic metastases.

   (2) Lung and breast cancers are predominantly lytic but can be mixed or blastic.

   (3) Renal cancer produces lytic metastases.

   c) Cancer-related bone pain has several possible mechanisms (Mantyh, 2014).

   (1) Alteration of equilibrium between osteoblasts and osteoclasts can result in structural degradation of the bone.

   (2) Direct invasion of tumor cells into nerve route and release of chemical mediators can stimulate nerve fibers.

   (3) Muscles can spasm in an attempt to maintain skeletal stability.

2. Incidence

   a) Depending on primary tumor site, the incidence of bone metastases varies extensively with patients with breast, prostate, or lung cancer, accounting for over 85% of patients with metastatic disease (De Felice, Piccioli, Musio, & Tombolini, 2017).

   b) Although they are usually found after treatment for primary disease, in 20% of patients bone metastases are the presenting symptom at time of diagnosis (De Felice et al., 2017).

3. Prognosis (De Felice et al., 2017)

   a) Bone metastases are usually associated with a poor prognosis, with life expectancy limited to several months.

   b) However, significant progress in systemic and supportive therapies have increased life expectancy. As a result, more patients are living longer with bone metastases, and survival rates are variable.

   c) Local control of bone metastases is important to improve pain and quality of life for those living with metastatic bone disease.

d) Skeletal metastases most commonly occur in the bones of the axial skeleton (thoracic and lumbar spine, pelvis, ribs, and long bones in upper and lower extremities).

4. Assessment: CT, MRI, and bone scans can be used to detect and assess bone metastases.

    a) CT scan is an excellent modality for detailed imaging.

    b) MRI can be used for soft tissue resolution.

    c) Bone scan is the method of choice for detecting osseous metastasis during initial staging. It is more sensitive than specific for detection of bone metastasis.

5. Management

    a) Interprofessional and holistic approach to care

    (1) Holistic assessment of patients within an interprofessional team is crucial in order to provide the best approach to pain control in patients with symptomatic bone metastases.

    (a) Taking time to listen to patients' concerns and understanding their goals will allow the team to tailor therapy after considering the risks and benefits associated with the proposed treatment.

    (b) Assessment of the social, emotional, and functional aspects of patients is considered, and nurses play a vital role in this realm (von Moos et al., 2017).

    (2) The ESAS is a tool for screening multiple symptoms such as pain, fatigue, and anxiety and is used initially at consultation and following any intervention (Bruera, Kuehn, Miller, Selmser, & Macmillan, 1991).

    b) RT

    (1) In the setting of metastatic cancer to the bone, RT is a major element of symptom management. RT provides successful palliation of painful bone metastases, as it is time efficient and associated with few side effects (Lutz, Jones, & Chow, 2014).

    (2) The beneficial effects of RT on bone pain are mainly related to its ability to produce ossification.

    (a) Radiation diminishes osteoclast activation and kills tumor cells, resulting in the reduction in tumor volume and discomfort in adjacent nerves (Goblirsch, Zwolak, & Clohisy, 2006).

    (b) RT can be used to relieve pain, prevent impending pathologic fracture, and promote healing of pathologic fracture. RT can be successful in improving pain in 60%–70% of patients with bone metastases, but it may take up to a month to see full effect (Lutz et al., 2017).

    (3) Fractionation schedules

    (a) Literature has shown that a single fraction of RT has the same response rate as multiple fractions in the management of bone metastases. However, the rate of retreatment required after single fraction is higher, and this retreatment may occur any time after one month following initial treatment (Lutz et al., 2017).

    (b) A single fraction of radiation (8 Gy) provides noninferior pain relief when compared to a more prolonged RT course in painful spinal sites and is convenient and reasonable for patients with limited life expectancy (Lutz et al., 2017).

    (c) Although the efficacy of multifractionated RT is well-documented, the literature continues to suggest that single-fraction RT should be widely adopted for painful uncomplicated bone metastases because it is cost efficient, reduces burden for patients, and is equally effective (R. Chow et al., 2017).

    (d) A multifractionated RT strategy should be used for pain relief in complicated bone metastases, such as with pathologic fracture or spinal cord compression, in patients with reasonable performance status and life expectancy (R. Chow et al., 2017).

    (e) The 2014 ASTRO Choosing Wisely guidelines recommended 10 or fewer fractions of RT or a single fraction for patients with poor prognosis (Wallace et al., 2018).

    i. Wallace et al. (2018) disclosed that uptake of this recommendation is variable across the world despite strong evidence.

    ii. The highest uptake of single-fraction RT is found in Australia (75%) and Canada (65%), and the lowest is in the United States (less than 20%). This may be related to the method of remuneration for radiation oncologists (Wallace et al., 2018).

    (f) Despite publication of clinical practice guidelines, single-fraction RT is internationally underutilized (McDonald, Chow, Lam, Rowbottom, & Soliman, 2014).

    c) Bone-targeted agents

    (1) Bone-targeted agents are recommended for all patients with metastatic bone disease because these medications may delay not only the onset of skeletal-related events but also the onset of bone pain. In metastatic cancer, the efficacy of bisphosphonates for reducing pain has been well demonstrated, and they may delay

time to pain progression and to regular use of analgesics (Coleman, Body, Aapro, Hadji, & Herrstedt, 2014).

(2) Although RT is the treatment of choice for localized bone pain, many patients have widespread pain that is difficult to localize. Bisphosphonates provide an additional treatment approach for the relief of bone pain that can be useful across a range of primary tumor types (Coleman et al., 2014).

(3) Osteonecrosis of the jaw is more common with IV bisphosphonates, which are administered monthly.

 (a) Osteonecrosis of the jaw is less commonly seen with a less intensive administration frequency.

 (b) Treatment is mainly conservative, with one-third of patients having complete healing.

 (c) Risk factors include history of tooth extraction, poor oral hygiene, and use of dental appliances (Macedo et al., 2017).

d) Surgery

 (1) Surgery may be appropriate in selected cases involving spinal cord compression or bone stabilization.

 (2) Mirels' classification is an objective scoring system for predicting fracture risk in the setting of metastatic disease to bone (Jawad & Scully, 2010).

 (a) This system is based on four criteria: site of lesion, nature of lesion, size of lesion, and pain. Each is weighted with 1–3 points, with the total score linked to fracture risk and recommendations for prophylactic surgical treatment.

 (b) A score of 9 or greater predicts an impending pathologic fracture for which prophylactic stabilization is recommended (Jawad & Scully, 2010).

 (3) Spinal Instability Neoplastic Score (SINS) is used to facilitate the diagnosis of spinal instability based on a combination of radiographic criteria and pain characteristics.

 (a) According to the SINS classification, patients with a score of 7 or more are considered to be at risk for spinal instability and warrant surgical consultation.

 (b) SINS measures the following factors (Fisher et al., 2010).

 i. Global spine location of tumor
 ii. Pain
 iii. Bone lesion quality
 iv. Spinal alignment
 v. Vertebral body collapse
 vi. Posterior involvement

 (c) SINS is a reliable and valuable tool to judge spinal instability and to assist oncologists regarding the timing of referral to spinal surgery for further evaluation and management of spinal metastases (Fox, Spiess, Hnenny, & Fourney, 2017).

 (4) When vertebral compression fracture causes pain, percutaneous vertebral augmentation—vertebroplasty (kyphoplasty) with or without polymethyl methacrylate—should be considered (Laredo, Chiras, Kemel, Taihi, & Hamze, 2018).

 (a) This interventional technique may be used to improve the mechanical stability of the vertebra, as well as improve pain from compression fracture.

 (b) Vertebral augmentation has been shown to improve pain and quality of life alone or in conjunction with RT.

 (c) Vertebral augmentation is generally reserved for patients without epidural disease or retropulsion of bone fragments into the spinal canal.

e) Radiopharmaceuticals

 (1) According to Cancer Care Ontario (2015) guidelines, radiopharmaceuticals (strontium-89 and samarium-153) may be used as an option for the palliation of multiple sites of bone pain from metastatic prostate cancer. These patients represented 80% of those who benefited in clinical trials in which histology was specified.

 (2) Strontium-89 and samarium-153 may also be used in the setting of lung and breast cancers.

 (3) Use of radiopharmaceutical therapy should consider the following patient factors.

 (a) Bone marrow function
 (b) Performance status
 (c) Recent use of other bone marrow suppression agents (chemotherapy or RT)
 (d) Appropriateness of alternative palliative interventions (e.g., wide-field or local-field RT, hormone therapy, chemotherapy, bisphosphonates)
 (e) Anticipated life expectancy

 (4) The decision to administer radiopharmaceutical therapy should be based on an interprofessional assessment involving radiation oncology, nuclear medicine, medical oncology, and palliative care.

6. Side effects of RT for bone metastases

 a) Pain flare

 (1) Pain flare is a transient increase in the severity of pain typically occurring 24–48 hours after RT. It is a common event, occurring in nearly 40% of patients who receive palliative RT for symp-

tomatic bone metastases (Gomez-Iturriaga et al., 2015).

(2) The pathophysiology of pain flare is largely unknown. It has been suggested that it occurs through edema of the periosteum of the irradiated bone, resulting in nerve compression or a release of inflammatory cytokines.

(3) Dexamethasone may prevent or reduce the occurrence of pain flare through anti-inflammatory actions (Gomez-Iturriaga et al., 2015).

(4) A randomized, double-blind, placebo-controlled trial in patients treated in Canadian cancer centers examined the efficacy of dexamethasone on pain flare (E. Chow et al., 2015).

(a) Patients received a single-fraction 8 Gy dose to bone metastases and 8 mg dexamethasone on the day of treatment and for four subsequent days.

(b) Dexamethasone improved quality of life by reducing nausea and increasing functional activity and appetite, without serious adverse effects.

(c) Results confirmed that a low-dose steroid is efficacious in prophylaxis of radiation-induced pain flare (E. Chow et al., 2015).

(5) Niglas et al. (2017) maintained that the decision to use dexamethasone for prophylaxis of radiation-induced pain flare should be individualized and should consider the risk of pain flare (e.g., higher risk with spine RT) and patient comorbidities, such as medical contraindications to steroids (e.g., uncontrolled diabetes, uncontrolled hypertension, active peptic ulcer).

b) Fatigue

(1) Although fatigue is a common symptom for many patients with advanced cancer, RT for bone metastases can contribute to overall increase in fatigue during treatment and often for weeks afterward.

(2) As fatigue is often correlated with depression and reduced quality of life, it is important to prepare patients for this potential side effect.

(3) Baseline performance status should be determined prior to treatment, as it may affect treatment decisions and feasibility of RT (Cheon et al., 2015).

c) Hypercalcemia (Goldner, 2016; Mallik, Mallik, Macabulos, & Dorigo, 2016)

(1) Hypercalcemia is a potential oncologic emergency that may occur in up to 30% of all patients at some point in the disease course, but it is most commonly seen during advanced stages (Goldner, 2016).

(2) Life expectancy of patients with hypercalcemia is weeks to months, as it is considered a poor prognostic sign.

(3) Hypercalcemia is a result of abnormalities in the bone formation and degradation cycle.

(a) Bone mineralization is a well-balanced cycle of bone formation stimulated by osteoblasts and bone resorption.

(b) Osteolysis from invasion of stroma by skeletal metastases causes activation of the receptor activator of nuclear factor-kappa B pathway, thus stimulating bone resorption while inhibiting calciuria in the kidneys.

(4) Signs and symptoms include dehydration from diabetes insipidus (polyuria, polydipsia, constipation), abdominal pain, nausea, and cognitive changes (e.g., reduced level of consciousness, electrocardiogram abnormalities).

(5) Treatment is based on etiology and includes increasing calciuresis via IV fluids; reducing bone resorption via IV bisphosphonates, subcutaneous calcitonin, and denosumab; reducing intestinal absorption of calcium via glucocorticoids; and reducing parathyroid hormone via calcitonin.

7. Patient, caregiver, and family education: Coleman et al. (2014) highlighted lifestyle modification strategies for prevention of bone loss in patients at risk of pathologic fractures.

a) Increased weight-bearing exercises

b) Smoking cessation

c) Reduction of alcoholic beverage consumption

d) Adequate calcium intake

e) Supplementary vitamin D

References

Bruera, E., Kuehn, N., Miller, M.J., Selmser, P., & Macmillan, K. (1991). The Edmonton Symptom Assessment System (ESAS): A simple method for the assessment of palliative care patients. *Journal of Palliative Care, 7,* 6–9. https://doi.org/10.1177/082585979100700202

Cancer Care Ontario. (2015). *Radiopharmaceuticals for the palliation of painful bone metastases: Practice guideline report 14-1.* https://www.cancercareontario.ca/en/guidelines-advice/types-of-cancer/2251

Cheon, P.M., Pulenzas, N., Zhang, L., Mauti, E., Wong, E., Thavarajah, N., ... Chow, E. (2015). Fatigue scores in patients receiving palliative radiotherapy for painful bone metastases. *Supportive Care in Cancer, 23,* 2097–2103. https://doi.org/10.1007/s00520-014-2561-0

Chow, E., Meyer, R.M., Ding, K., Nabid, A., Chabot, P., Wong, P., ... Wong, R. (2015). Dexamethasone in the prophylaxis of radiation-induced pain flare after palliative radiotherapy for bone metastases: A double blind, randomised placebo-controlled, phase 3 trial. *Lancet Oncology, 16,* 1463–1472. https://doi.org/10.1016/s1470-2045(15)00199-0

Chow, R., Hoskin, P., Chan, S., Mesci, A., Hollenberg, D., Lam, H., ... Chow, E. (2017). Efficacy of multiple fraction conventional radiation therapy for painful uncomplicated bone metastases: A systematic review. *Radiotherapy and Oncology, 122,* 323–331. https://doi.org/10.1016/j.radonc.2016.12.031

Coleman, R., Body, J.J., Aapro, M., Hadji, P., & Herrstedt, J. (2014). Bone health in cancer patients: ESMO clinical practice guidelines. *Annals of Oncology, 25*(Suppl. 3), iii24–iii37. https://doi.org/10.1093/annonc/mdu103

De Felice, F., Piccioli, A., Musio, D., & Tombolini, V. (2017). The role of radiation therapy in bone metastases management. *Oncotarget, 8,* 25691–25699. https://doi.org/10.18632/oncotarget.14823

Fisher, C.G., DiPaola, C.P., Ryken, T.C., Bilsky, M.H., Shaffrey, C.I., Berven, S.H., ... Fourney, D.R. (2010). A novel classification system for spinal instability in neoplastic disease: An evidence-based approach and expert consensus from the Spine Oncology Study Group. *Spine, 35,* E1221–E1229. https://doi.org/10.1097/BRS.0b013e3181e16ae2

Fox, S., Spiess, M., Hnenny, L., & Fourney, D.R. (2017). Spinal instability neoplastic score (SINS): Reliability among spine fellows and resident physicians in orthopedic surgery and neurosurgery. *Global Spine Journal, 7,* 744–748. https://doi.org/10.1177/2192568217697691

Goblirsch, M.J., Zwolak, P.P., & Clohisy, D.R. (2006). Biology of bone cancer pain. *Clinical Cancer Research, 12*(Suppl. 20), 6231s–6235s. https://doi.org/10.1158/1078-0432.ccr-06-0682

Goldner, W. (2016). Cancer-related hypercalcemia. *Journal of Oncology Practice, 12,* 426–431. https://doi.org/10.1200/JOP.2016.011155

Gomez-Iturriaga, A., Cacicedo, J., Navarro, A., Morillo, V., Willisch, P., Carvajal, C., ... Bilbao, P. (2015). Incidence of pain flare following radiotherapy for painful bone metastases: Multicentre prospective observational study. *BMC Palliative Care, 14,* 48. https://doi.org/10.1186/s12904-015-0045-8

Jawad, M.U., & Scully, S.P. (2010). Mirels' classification: Metastatic disease in long bones and impending pathologic fracture. *Clinical Orthopaedics and Related Research, 468,* 2825–2827. https://doi.org/10.1007/s11999-010-1326-4

Laredo, J.-D., Chiras, J., Kemel, S., Taihi, L., & Hamze, B. (2018). Vertebroplasty and interventional radiology procedures for bone metastases. *Joint Bone Spine, 85,* 191–199. https://doi.org/10.1016/j.jbspin.2017.05.005

Lutz, S., Balboni, T., Jones, J., Lo, S., Petit, J., Rich, S., ... Hahn, C. (2017). Palliative radiation therapy for bone metastases: Update of an ASTRO evidence-based guideline. *Practical Radiation Oncology, 7,* 4–12. https://doi.org/10.1016/j.prro.2016.08.001

Lutz, S.T., Jones, J., & Chow, E. (2014). Role of radiation therapy in palliative care of the patient with cancer. *Journal of Clinical Oncology, 32,* 2913–2919. https://doi.org/10.1200/jco.2014.55.1143

Macedo, F., Ladeira, K., Pinho, F., Saraiva, N., Bonito, N., Pinto, L., & Gonçalves, F. (2017). Bone metastases: An overview. *Oncology Reviews, 11,* 43–49. https://doi.org/10.4081/oncol.2017.321

Mallik, S., Mallik, G., Macabulos, S.T., & Dorigo, A. (2016). Malignancy associated hypercalcaemia-responsiveness to IV bisphosphonates and prognosis in a palliative population. *Supportive Care in Cancer, 24,* 1771–1777. https://doi.org/10.1007/s00520-015-2962-8

Mantyh, P.W. (2014). Bone cancer pain: From mechanism to therapy. *Current Opinion in Supportive Palliative Care, 8,* 83–90. https://doi.org/10.1097/spc.0000000000000048

McDonald, R., Chow, E., Lam, H., Rowbottom, L., & Soliman, H. (2014). International patterns of practice in radiotherapy for bone metastases: A review of the literature. *Journal of Bone Oncology, 3,* 96–102. https://doi.org/10.1016/j.jbo.2014.10.003

Niglas, M., Raman, S., Rodin, D., Detsky, J., DeAngelis, C., Soliman, H., ... Tsao, M. (2017). Should dexamethasone be standard in the prophylaxis of pain flare after palliative radiotherapy for bone metastases?—A debate. *Annals of Palliative Medicine, 7,* 279–283. https://doi.org/10.21037/apm.2017.04.08

von Moos, R., Costa, L., Ripamonti, C.I., Niepel, D., & Santini, D. (2017). Improving quality of life in patients with advanced cancer: Targeting metastatic bone pain. *European Journal of Cancer, 71,* 80–94. https://doi.org/10.1016/j.ejca.2016.10.021

Wallace, A.S., Fiveash, J.B., Williams, C.P., Kvale, E., Pisu, M., Jackson, B.E., & Rocque, G.B. (2018). Choosing wisely at end of life: Use of shorter courses of palliative radiation therapy for bone metastasis. *International Journal of Radiation Oncology, Biology, Physics, 102,* 320–324. https://doi.org/10.1016/j.ijrobp.2018.05.061

V. Site-Specific Management

A. Brain and central nervous system
1. Tumor categories (Louis et al., 2016)
   a) The 2016 World Health Organization categories for CNS tumors are based on molecular parameters (genetic alteration) along with histology (morphologic and immunohistochemical) (Huse & Holland, 2010; Louis et al., 2016).
   b) Grading criteria include cellular atypia, mitotic activity, vascular proliferation, and necrosis.
   c) The added specificity to tumor classifications is expected to provide greater diagnostic, prognostic, and treatment-response accuracy and ultimately improve patient management.
   d) The following CNS tumor types are commonly treated with varying modes of RT. Refer to Louis et al. (2016) for further description of World Health Organization CNS tumor categories.
      (1) Astrocytic tumors (Newton & Shroff, 2018; Splittgerber, 2019)
         (a) Malignant cells derive from astrocytes that undergo abnormal growth and cellular transformation.
         (b) Astrocytes provide physical and biochemical support, insulation of the receptive surface of neurons, and interactions with capillary endothelial cells in the establishment and maintenance of the blood–brain barrier.
         (c) Glioblastoma multiforme tumors derive from astrocytes.
         (d) Common astrocytoma distinctions are associated with isocitrate dehydrogenase and *TP53* mutations, as well as *ATRX* loss.
         (e) Common glioblastoma multiforme mutations are *TERT* promoter, *TP53*, *ATRX*, *PTEN*, and *EGFR* amplification.
      (2) Oligodendroglial tumors (Newton & Shroff, 2018; Simonetti, Gaviani, Botturi, Innocenti, & Silvani, 2015; Splittgerber, 2019)
         (a) Oligodendroglial tumors derive from oligodendrocytes, whose principal function is the production and maintenance of the CNS myelin.
         (b) Common mutations include isocitrate dehydrogenase and 1p/19q codeletions.
      (3) Ependymomas (Newton & Shroff, 2018)
         (a) Ependymomas are abnormal growths of ependymal cells that line the ventricular walls and spinal cord.
         (b) Ependymomas commonly present with hydrocephalus secondary to obstruction of the fourth ventricle.
         (c) Depending on location, ependymomas are difficult to completely excise.
      (4) Choroid plexus tumors (Newton & Shroff, 2018; Splittgerber, 2019)
         (a) Choroid plexus tumors are composed of cuboid epithelial cells, which provide a continuous layer with ependymal cells, which produce cerebrospinal fluid (CSF).
         (b) The cuboid epithelial lining acts as a brain–CSF barrier, preventing toxic substances from entering the ventricular system.
      (5) Embryonal tumors (Newton & Shroff, 2018)
         (a) Embryonal tumors are rapidly growing masses from embryonic or fetal cells.
         (b) Medulloblastoma, CNS primitive neuroectodermal tumors, and atypical teratoid rhabdoid tumors are types of embryonal tumors.
         (c) Common mutations include *WNT*, *SHH*, and *TP53*.
      (6) Tumors of the cranial and paraspinal nerves (Montano et al., 2016)
         (a) Cranial and paraspinal nerve tumors derive from cellular and extracellular support structures to cranial or spinal nerves.
         (b) These tumors are usually slow growing and benign, but a small subset is malignant.
      (7) Meningioma: A meningioma is a tumor arising from the meninges (lining of the brain), usually the arachnoid mater (Brastianos et al., 2019; Newton & Shroff, 2018).
      (8) Metastatic tumors (Nayak, Lee, & Wen, 2012; Newton & Shroff, 2018).
         (a) Histology of the primary cancer is the most important risk factor for the development of metastases.
         (b) Brain metastasis most commonly arises from lung, breast, melanoma, colorectal, and renal cell carcinomas and accounts for 67%–80% of all metastatic lesions.
         (c) Intramedullary spinal metastasis most commonly arises from breast, lung, and prostate cancers and lymphomas.
      (9) Leptomeningeal metastasis: Leptomeningeal metastasis is most commonly associated with leukemia and lymphoma, but it may also occur with breast and gastrointestinal carcinomas.
2. Incidence and epidemiology (Ostrom et al., 2018; Siegel, Miller, & Jemal, 2018)
   a) For 2019, malignant and nonmalignant brain and CNS tumors were estimated at 86,970 new cases (Ostrom et al., 2018).
      (1) Malignant diagnoses account for 26,170 cases (30.9%), with glioblastoma multiforme accounting for 47.7% of malignant CNS tumors. Malignant CNS tumors are more common in men, at 55.4% of diagnoses.

(2) Nonmalignant diagnoses account for 60,800 cases (67.2%), with meningioma accounting for 53.1% of nonmalignant CNS tumors.

b) Incidence of brain tumors increases with age.

c) From 2008 to 2011, malignant CNS tumors accounted for 77,375 deaths and represented an average mortality rate of 4.37 cases per 100,000 (Ostrom et al., 2018).

d) Five-year survival rate for malignant CNS tumors is 35% and decreases with age (Ostrom et al., 2018).

    (1) Survival for ages 0–19 years is 74.1%.

    (2) Survival for ages 75 years and older is 6.1%.

e) Several risk factors are associated with an increased risk of developing CNS tumors (Chang, Mehta, Vogelbaum, Taylor, & Ahluwalia, 2018; Dorsey et al., 2020).

    (1) The only environmental factor unequivocally associated with the increased risk of developing primary CNS tumors is prior exposure to ionizing radiation.

    (2) Cell phone use has not been associated with glioma development, but electromagnetic fields from power lines are being studied for long-term effects on health and cancer risk.

    (3) Several genetic disorders may increase risk for developing CNS tumors (Schoemaker et al., 2010).

        (a) Neurofibromatosis type 1, caused by changes to the *NF1* gene, can lead to the development of neurofibromas, schwannomas, meningiomas, and gliomas.

        (b) Neurofibromatosis type 2, caused by changes to the *NF2* gene, can lead to development of vestibular schwannomas, meningiomas, and spinal cord ependymomas.

        (c) Tuberous sclerosis, caused by changes to *TSC1* or *TSC2* genes, can lead to development of subependymal giant cell astrocytomas.

        (d) Von Hippel-Lindau disease, caused by changes in the *VHL* gene, can lead to the development of hemangioblastomas in the brain and spine.

        (e) Li-Fraumeni syndrome, caused by changes in the *TP53* gene, can lead to the development of gliomas.

3. RT standard of care

a) The standard of RT administration falls into two categories: combined modality and single modality.

b) Radiation-specific treatments are dependent on tumor pathology, molecular profile, histology, and radiosensitivity (see Table 10).

c) Typically, higher-grade CNS tumors require combined-modality therapy involving optimal surgical resection, followed by fractionated conformal partial brain RT and concurrent or adjuvant chemotherapy (NCCN, 2020).

    (1) In a study of patients with glioblastoma, daily administration of temozolomide during RT was found to be superior for survival compared to RT alone (Stupp et al., 2009).

        (a) At two years, combined-modality therapy had a survival rate of 27.2%, versus 10.9% with RT as a single modality.

        (b) At three years, combined-modality therapy had a survival rate of 16%, versus 4.4% for RT as a single modality.

        (c) At four years, combined-modality therapy had a survival rate of 12.1%, versus 3% for RT as a single modality.

        (d) At five years, combined-modality therapy had a survival rate of 9.8%, versus 1.9% for RT as a single modality.

    (2) Tumor-treating fields involve the use of alternating electric fields, which have antimitotic activity, delivered through transducers applied to the scalp. In a study of patients who previously received standard chemoradiation for glioblastoma, patients treated with tumor-treating fields and temozolomide had a median overall survival of 20 months, compared to 16 months in patients who received temozolomide alone (Stupp et al., 2015).

d) Treatment for benign CNS tumors (World Health Organization grade I–II) generally includes optimal surgical resection as indicated, followed by fractionated conformal partial brain RT as a single modality (NCCN, 2020).

4. Side effects

a) Assessment

    (1) Neurologic symptoms and deficits are based on the region of affected CNS.

    (2) Clinicians should perform a thorough neurologic and physical examination. See Table 11 for the parameters of a normal neurologic examination.

    (3) See Table 12 for localized symptoms according to brain structure involvement.

b) Documentation: Documentation should adhere to facility requirements. See Figure 16 for standard documentation sources.

c) Acute side effects: Acute side effects are toxicities that occur during treatment and manifest four to six weeks after treatment (Alentorn, Hoang-Xuan, & Mikkelsen, 2016; Kotecha, Gondi, Ahulwalia, Brastianos, & Mehta, 2018; Lovely et al., 2013; Schiff et al., 2015).

    (1) Focal symptoms

        (a) Pathophysiology: Focal symptoms involve transient worsening of pretreatment deficits localized to tumor location within the brain parenchyma or spine. The cause of focal symptoms is a multifactorial process

Tumor Type and WHO Grade	General RT Recommendations	Modifications to Treatment	Histology-Specific Modifications to Treatment
Malignant glioma, WHO grade III	Treat with 60 Gy in 2 Gy fractions or 59.4 Gy in 1.8 Gy fractions. Lower doses can be applied when tumor volumes are large or when brain stem or spinal cord are involved.	For KPS < 60, hypofractionated accelerated course can be considered to complete treatment in 3–4 weeks (e.g., 34 Gy in 10 fractions, 40.5 Gy in 15 fractions, 50 Gy in 20 fractions). For age > 70 years, shorter fractionated course may be considered (e.g., 25 Gy in 5 fractions).	For anaplastic astrocytoma, anaplastic oligodendroglioma, or mixed anaplastic oligoastrocytoma, specific histological features of 1p/19q are considered. For mixed histology and no molecular data or disease containing both oligoastrocytoma and astrocytoma regions with 1p/19q codeletion, options include the following. • Fractionated brain RT followed by adjuvant temozolomide • Fractionated brain RT with concurrent and adjuvant temozolomide • Fractionated brain RT and neoadjuvant or adjuvant PCV For anaplastic oligodendroglioma with 1p/19q codeletion, options include the following. • Fractionated brain RT followed by adjuvant temozolomide • Fractionated brain RT with concurrent and adjuvant temozolomide • Fractionated brain RT and neoadjuvant or adjuvant PCV
Recurrent local resectable anaplastic glioma, WHO grade III	Consider reirradiation (SRS or fractionated), particularly if a long interval has passed since prior RT and/or a patient had a good response to prior RT.	–	–
Malignant glioma, WHO grade IV	Treat with 60 Gy in 2 Gy fractions or 59.4 Gy in 1.8 Gy fractions. Lower doses can be applied when tumor volumes are large or when brain stem or spinal cord are involved.	For KPS < 60, hypofractionated accelerated course can be considered to complete treatment in 3–4 weeks (e.g., 34 Gy in 10 fractions, 40.5 Gy in 15 fractions, 50 Gy in 20 fractions). For age > 70 years, shorter fractionated course may be considered (e.g., 25 Gy in 5 fractions).	For GBM, RT recommendations depend on age, KPS, and MGMT promoter methylation status. For age ≤ 70 years, KPS ≥ 60, and methylated MGMT, options include the following. • Standard brain RT with concurrent temozolomide, followed by adjuvant temozolomide and alternating electric field therapy • Standard brain RT with concurrent temozolomide, followed by adjuvant temozolomide For age < 70 years, KPS > 60, and unmethylated or indeterminate MGMT, options include the following. • Standard brain RT with concurrent temozolomide, followed by adjuvant temozolomide and alternating electric field therapy • Standard brain RT with concurrent temozolomide, followed by adjuvant temozolomide • Standard brain RT For age < 70 years and KPS < 60, provide hypofractionated brain RT with or without concurrent or adjuvant temozolomide. For age > 70 years, KPS > 60, and methylated MGMT, options include the following. • Hypofractionated brain RT with concurrent and adjuvant temozolomide

(Continued on next page)

Tumor Type and WHO Grade	General RT Recommendations	Modifications to Treatment	Histology-Specific Modifications to Treatment
Malignant glioma, WHO grade IV *(cont.)*			• Standard brain RT with concurrent temozolomide, followed by adjuvant temozolomide and alternating electric field therapy • Standard brain RT with concurrent temozolomide, followed by adjuvant temozolomide • Hypofractionated brain RT only For age > 70 years, KPS > 60, and unmethylated or indeterminate MGMT, options include the following. • Hypofractionated brain RT with concurrent and adjuvant temozolomide • Standard brain RT with concurrent temozolomide, followed by adjuvant temozolomide and alternating electric field therapy • Standard brain RT with concurrent temozolomide, followed by adjuvant temozolomide • Hypofractionated brain RT only For age > 70 years and KPS < 60, provide hypofractionated brain RT only.
Recurrent GBM, WHO grade IV	Consider reirradiation (SRS or fractionated), particularly if a long interval has passed since prior RT and/or a patient had a good response to prior RT.	For diffuse or multiple lesions, consider alternating electric field therapy.	–
Low-grade glioma, WHO grade I or II	Treat with 45–54 Gy in 1.8–2 Gy fractions or 59.4 Gy in 1.8 Gy fractions. RT dose can be increased to 59.4–60 Gy for wild-type IDH low-grade gliomas.	For new diagnosis, options include the following. • RT with adjuvant PCV • RT with adjuvant temozolomide • RT with concurrent and adjuvant temozolomide For recurrent or progressive disease and previous RT, consider reirradiation with conformal RT with or without chemotherapy if progression-free survival is > 2 years after RT, a new lesion is outside target of prior RT, and recurrence is small and geometrically favorable. For recurrent or progressive disease and no prior RT, options include the following. • RT with adjuvant PCV • RT with adjuvant temozolomide • RT with concurrent and adjuvant temozolomide • Fractionated RT	–

(Continued on next page)

Tumor Type and WHO Grade	General RT Recommendations	Modifications to Treatment	Histology-Specific Modifications to Treatment
Ependymoma, WHO grades I–III	Treatment is based on tumor location. Cranial RT dosing is 54–59.5 Gy in 1.8–2 Gy fractions. Spinal RT dosing is 45–54 Gy in 1.8 Gy fractions. Craniospinal dosing is 36 Gy in 1.8 Gy fractions, followed by limited field to spine lesions to 45 Gy. Tumors below the conus medullaris may require higher doses of 54–60 Gy. Consider using IMRT or proton therapy to reduce toxicity.	For new diagnosis or recurrence of intracranial or spinal ependymoma with no evidence of metastasis in the spine or CSF, consider limited-field fractionated RT. For new diagnosis or recurrence of intracranial or spinal ependymoma with evidence of metastasis in the spine or CSF, consider craniospinal RT	–
Medulloblastoma, WHO grade IV	Craniospinal RT dosing recommendations are 30–36 Gy with boost to primary brain site to 54–55.8 Gy, with or without chemotherapy.	If treating with adjuvant chemotherapy, reduce craniospinal RT dose to 23.4 Gy. Treat those with high risk for recurrence with increased craniospinal RT dose, up to 36 Gy. Treat localized recurrence with additional RT, such as SRS.	–
Primary CNS lymphoma	Low-dose whole-brain RT based on response to chemotherapy For complete response, limit whole-brain RT to 23.4 Gy in 1.8 Gy fractions. For partial or incomplete response, provide whole-brain RT 30–36 Gy followed by a limited field to the gross disease site to 45 Gy or focal RT to residual disease.	If no chemotherapy is administered, provide 24–36 Gy followed by a boost to area of gross disease to a total of 45 Gy. For relapse or recurrence, options include the following. • Focal RT if prior whole-brain RT was performed • Whole-brain RT or involved-field RT for those unresponsive to high-dose methotrexate and no prior RT • Whole-brain RT or involved-field RT for those unresponsive to high-dose chemotherapy with stem cell rescue	–
Meningioma, WHO grades I–III	SRS or fractionated SRS is preferred. Highly conformal fractionated RT is recommended to spare brain tissues and structures. Doses are based on patient status, tumor status and treatability, and potential for neurologic deficits.	For recurrence, provide RT if not previously performed or consider reirradiation.	–
Meningioma, WHO grade I	Treatment options include the following. • Fractionated brain RT at 45–54 Gy • SRS dose of 12–16 Gy as a single fraction • Hypofractionated SRT at 25 Gy in 5 fractions	–	–

(Continued on next page)

Tumor Type and WHO Grade	General RT Recommendations	Modifications to Treatment	Histology-Specific Modifications to Treatment
Meningioma, WHO grade II	Treat with brain RT at 54–60 Gy in 1.8–2 Gy fractions and limit margin expansion (1–2 cm) into brain parenchyma if there is no evidence of disease extension.	–	–
Meningioma, WHO grade III	Treat with brain RT 59.4–60 GY in 1.8–2 Gy fractions with 2–3 cm margins.	–	–
Vestibular schwannoma (acoustic neuroma), WHO grade I–II	Small lesions may be treated with SRS (12 Gy in 1 fraction), which has less morbidity than surgery, including preservation of facial function and hearing.	For larger lesions or adjacent to brain stem, consider SRT to 54 Gy in 1.8 Gy fractions.	–
Primary spinal cord tumors, including spinal meningioma, neurofibroma, schwannoma, ependymoma, astrocytoma	RT recommendations are based on tumor location and intramedullary or extramedullary involvement. Symptomatic patients should undergo RT. Recurrence of disease requires reirradiation (likely SBRT). Treat with spinal RT to 45–54 Gy in 1.8 Gy fractions.	Tumors below the conus medullaris may require higher doses to 60 Gy.	–
Brain metastases	Recommendations for whole-brain RT and SRS are based on histology, number, size, and location of metastases. Treat with whole-brain RT at 20–40 Gy in 5–20 fractions and consider hippocampal-sparing whole-brain RT or SRS at 15–24 Gy based on tumor volume. For solitary lesion or dominant and symptomatic lesion, consider surgical resection if possible, followed by SRS to cavity for decreased acute side effects and effect on cognitive function as compared to whole-brain RT.	For 1–3 brain lesions, options include the following. • SRS preferred • Whole-brain RT at 30–45 Gy in 1.8–2 fractions • Whole-brain RT with or without SRS For > 3 brain lesions, treat with SRS or whole-brain RT. Those with KPS < 60 and noncandidates for SRS, it is recommended to provide whole-brain RT at 20 Gy in 5 fractions. For larger volume lesions, consider fractionated SRS at 27 Gy in 3 fractions or 30 Gy in 5 fractions.	–
Metastatic spinal cord tumors	Dose depends on KPS, spinal stability, presence of epidural disease, intent of treatment, and tumor histology regarding degree of radioresistance. RT is performed after spinal stabilization. Common doses are 8 Gy in 1 fraction, 20 Gy in 5 fractions, or 30 Gy in 10 fractions.	Consider SBRT at 15–24 Gy in 1 fraction, 24 Gy in 2 fractions, 24–27 Gy in 3 fractions, or standard RT 30–35 Gy in 5 fractions.	–

(Continued on next page)

TABLE 10. Radiation Therapy Recommendations for Central Nervous System Tumors *(Continued)*

Tumor Type and WHO Grade	General RT Recommendations	Modifications to Treatment	Histology-Specific Modifications to Treatment
Leptomeningeal metastasis	Dose depends on volume and extent of disease, KPS, and primary disease.	For KPS ≥ 60, treat with whole-brain RT with the option to add involved-field RT to control for bulky disease and reduce symptoms (pain, neurologic compromise, and neuropathies). For KPS < 60, treat with involved-field RT to control for bulky disease and reduce symptoms (pain, neurologic compromise, and neuropathies).	–

CNS—central nervous system; CSF—cerebrospinal fluid; GBM—glioblastoma multiforme; IDH—isocitrate dehydrogenase; IMRT—intensity-modulated radiation therapy; KPS—Karnofsky Performance Status; MGMT—O^6-methylguanine-DNA-methyltransferase; PCV—procarbazine, lomustine, and vincristine; RT—radiation therapy; SBRT—stereotactic body radiation therapy; SRS—stereotactic radiosurgery; SRT—stereotactic radiation therapy; WHO—World Health Organization

Note. Based on information from Bovi, 2018; Brastianos et al., 2019; Brown et al., 2017; Brown et al., 2016; Chang et al., 2018; Forst et al., 2014; Grommes et al., 2018; Hamel-Perreault et al., 2010; Mariş, Nica et al., 2014; National Comprehensive Cancer Network, 2020; Nead & Swisher-McClure, 2019; Tsao et al., 2012; van Linge et al., 2018; Zarnett et al., 2014.

TABLE 11. Components of Neurologic Assessment

Component	Assessment
Balance	Romberg (standing with eyes closed)
Coordination	Point-to-point (finger to nose, heel to shin) Rapid alternating movements (hand or feet tapping)
Cranial nerves	Olfactory (I): smell Optic (II): central and peripheral vision Oculomotor (III): pupil constriction and eye movement Trochlear (IV): medial eye movement Trigeminal (V): sensory function of face, jaw clenching Abducens (VI): lateral eye movement Facial (VII): motor function of face, taste anterior two-thirds of tongue Acoustic (VIII): hearing, balance Glossopharyngeal (IX): gag, taste posterior one-third of tongue Vagus (X): swallow, palate elevation Spinal accessory (XI): neck and shoulder movement Hypoglossal (XII): tongue movement
Gait	Normal walking Tandem gait
Mental status	Level of consciousness, orientation, affect
Motor function	Hand grips, dorsiflexion and plantar flexion, individual muscular movements Pronator drift Deep tendon reflexes
Sensory function	Light touch, temperature discrimination, proprioception Vibratory sensation
Speech	Expressive (fluency) Receptive (follows commands)

Note. Based on information from Catsman-Berrevoets & Patay, 2018; Splittgerber, 2019; Wilson-Pauwels et al., 2010.

TABLE 12. Localized Symptoms Based on Primary and Metastatic Tumor Location

Structure	Symptom
Brain Stem and Spine	
Medulla oblongata	Increased intracranial pressure (headache, stiff neck, vital function failure, and paralysis of cranial nerves IX–XII)
	Herniation (resulting from significant increased intracranial pressure displacing the medulla and cerebellar tonsils downward through foramen magnum)
Midbrain	Ipsilateral cranial nerve II–III deficit (dilated nonreactive pupil; upward, downward, and inward gaze paralysis)
	Contralateral cranial nerve IV paralysis of superior oblique muscle; hydrocephalus (blocked cerebral aqueduct)
Pons	Ipsilateral cranial nerve V–VIII paralysis
	Contralateral hemiparesis
Spinal cord	Ipsilateral dysfunction in motor or sensory areas (dermatome charts useful)
	Radiation-induced Lhermitte syndrome (rare)
Cerebral Cortex	
Frontal	Difficulty performing skilled movements
	Paralysis of contralateral body parts
	Seizures
	Muscle spasm
	Abnormal eye movements or deviation
	Altered smell
	Expressive or global aphasia (Broca's area)
	Loss of initiative
	Poor judgment
	Emotional changes
	Loss of inhibition
Occipital	Visual field deficits
	Contralateral inability to recognize objects
Parietal	Contralateral sensory disturbance
	Contralateral astereognosis
Temporal	Bilateral hearing loss
	Acoustic verbal agnosia
	Receptive or global aphasia (Wernicke's area)
Limbic System and Central Brain	
Basal ganglia	Severe motor or sensory symptoms
Cerebellum	Altered gait (wide-based, stiff-legged), ipsilateral dysdiadochokinesia (difficulty with rapid alternating movements), dysarthria (altered articulation), prolonged deep tendon reflexes, nystagmus, and hypotonia
	Tremor with fine motor movements and vermis syndrome (head and trunk muscle incoordination, fall forward or backward)
Corpus callosum	Altered memory and contralateral sensory discrimination
Hippocampal formation	Inability to form memory
	Amnesia
Hypothalamus	Genital hypoplasia
	Diabetes insipidus
	Obesity
	Sleep disturbances
	Irregular pyrexia
	Emaciation
Internal capsule	Widespread effects on contralateral body

(Continued on next page)

TABLE 12. Localized Symptoms Based on Primary and Metastatic Tumor Location *(Continued)*

Structure	Symptom
Lateral and third ventricle	Hydrocephalus
Optic chiasm	Bilateral blindness
Pineal gland	Severe alteration of reproductive function
Thalamus	Contralateral impairment of light touch, tactile localization, and discrimination Loss of appreciation of joint movements

Note. Based on information from Catsman-Berrevoets & Patay, 2018; Splittgerber, 2019; Wilson-Pauwels et al., 2010.

related to tumor and therapy effects, which results in localized peritumoral edema from vasogenic and cytotoxic edema.

  i. Vasogenic edema is the result of tumor effects from gliomas or brain metastases, resulting in the disruption of the blood–brain barrier, allowing passage of fluid into the extracellular space of the brain parenchyma. Production of angiogenic factors, such as VEGF, promotes tumor angiogenesis of permeable vessels that increases the surrounding edema. RT causes further injury to vascular endothelial structures, increasing leakiness and edema, hypoxia, and reactive gliosis.

  ii. Cytotoxic edema results from cytotoxic effects of RT, thus causing cellular swelling, which increases intracellular compartments and leads to cellular death.

  iii. Localized peritumoral edema from radiation-induced injury is dependent on multiple factors, including total dose, doses per fraction, treatment volume, and specific target cell population.

  iv. Edema is more prevalent with partial brain RT than whole-brain RT because of the higher dose provided in partial brain irradiation.

  v. Disruption of the blood–brain barrier and edema often present as early T2 signal abnormality on MRI.

(b) Collaborative management (Lovely et al., 2013; Ryken et al., 2010)

  i. Steroid therapy is given in the management of focal symptoms caused by localized peritumoral edema. Steroids reduce capillary permeability as soon as one hour after a single dose.

  ii. Dexamethasone or methylprednisolone therapy may be initiated or increased to alleviate focal symptoms. Dexamethasone often is used because it has relatively little mineralocorticoid activity. Dexamethasone is a strong inducer of the cytochrome P450 (CYP) 3A4 pathway; thus, drug interactions require monitoring for dose adjustment. Hepatic microsomal enzyme inducers can increase the metabolism of glucocorticoids, requiring dose adjustments.

  iii. Symptoms not fully alleviated by steroid therapy may require additional management. Pain medications or antiepileptic medications may be used in management of headaches, restless legs, muscular spasms, sleep disorders, and mood disorders.

  iv. Patients should be monitored when receiving new medications for tolerance and side effects.

  v. Nonpharmacologic interventions, such as relaxation techniques, can be considered as appropriately indicated.

FIGURE 16. Standardized Documentation Sources

- Common Terminology Criteria for Adverse Events for treatment-related side effects
- Graded Prognostic Assessment for brain metastasis (Sperduto et al., 2012)
- *Oncology Nursing: Scope and Standards of Practice* (Lubejko & Wilson, 2019)
- Performance status
  - Eastern Cooperative Oncology Group Scale: 0 (perfect health[a]) to 5 (death)
  - Karnofsky Performance Scale: 0 (death) to 100 (perfect health[a])

[a] Perfect health is defined as the ability to perform full activities of daily living with no restrictions on activities.

(c) Patient, caregiver, and family education

    i. Education should include information on the many side effects of corticosteroid therapy (Lovely et al., 2013; Schiff et al., 2015).

- Dermatologic: acne, impaired wound healing, hirsutism, thin and fragile skin, atrophy, petechiae, and bruising
- Endocrine: increased blood sugar (requires close monitoring of diabetic patients), cushingoid state, growth retardation, menstrual irregularities, and decreased carbohydrate tolerance
- Fluid and electrolyte disturbances: sodium retention, potassium loss, hypertension, and moon face
- Gastrointestinal: stomach irritation and abdominal distension; patient instruction on the use of medications as prescribed, which may include proton pump inhibitors, H_2 receptor antagonists, or antacids to prevent peptic ulcers (Narum, Westergren, & Klemp, 2014)
- Infection: increased susceptibility, especially to *Candida* and *Pneumocystis*; may mask signs of infection, such as fever
- Musculoskeletal: proximal steroid myopathy (especially in thigh muscles, then upper arms) and osteoporosis
- Nervous system: mood swings, restlessness, insomnia, vertigo, psychoses, headaches, euphoria, intracerebral hemorrhage, cataracts, and increased intraocular pressure

    ii. Written and verbal instructions should elucidate the signs and symptoms of peritumoral edema.

    iii. Written and verbal instructions should include the use of steroid and antiepileptic medication with particular emphasis on the importance of maintaining the medication schedule and risks involved in abrupt, unsupervised cessation of either drug, which could result in withdrawal side effects. Both medications require supervised tapering according to individual symptom responses to achieve desired outcomes (Krumholz et al., 2015).

    iv. Long-term steroid use affects a patient's quality of life and self-image as a result of fluid retention, weight gain, leg weakness, insomnia, diabetes, and delayed wound healing.

    v. Clinicians can provide literature regarding support programs; see Figure 17 for more information.

(2) Headache

    (a) Pathophysiology: Headache results from increases in edema caused by blood–brain barrier disruption, capillary permeability, and increased intracranial pressure from primary tumor, metastatic growth, or treatment-related effects that distort nerve endings in the pain-sensitive dura (Armstrong et al., 2016; Lovely et al., 2013; Schiff et al., 2015).

    (b) Risk factors and incidence

        i. Incidence increases with higher RT doses per fraction. Prevalence is higher with whole-brain RT than in partial brain RT because of the greater volume treated (Kepka et al., 2018; Krayenbuehl, Di Martino, Guckenberger, & Andratschke, 2017).

        ii. Steroid prophylaxis may reduce occurrence.

        iii. Edema may occur if steroids are tapered quickly.

        iv. Headaches may develop as a presenting symptom or during the course of the disease, particularly in the early morning. Headaches may recur more commonly in patients for whom headache was a presenting symptom; therefore, these patients should be evaluated for disease progression (Lovely et al., 2013).

    (c) Focal assessment

        i. Assessment should include headache history.

- Current cancer treatment plan and history
- History of presenting symptoms, including precipitating factors, headache frequency, duration, intensity, location, time of day, initial presentation, and changes in symptoms over time

---

FIGURE 17. Resources for People With Central Nervous System Cancers

- American Brain Tumor Association: www.abta.org
- American Cancer Society: www.cancer.org
- National Brain Tumor Society: www.braintumor.org
- National Cancer Institute: www.cancer.gov

- Associated symptoms, including nausea, vomiting, syncope, visual changes, and fatigue
- Prodromal signs, including feeling tired, clumsy, or thirsty, and light or sound sensitivity
- Pharmacologic and nonpharmacologic interventions that have been tried and the results
- Any recent changes in medications, specifically steroid therapy

ii. Sudden severe headache may indicate late signs of increased intracranial pressure and may be associated with a widening pulse pressure, bradycardia, and severe hypertension (Catsman-Berrevoets & Patay, 2018).

(d) Collaborative management (Catsman-Berrevoets & Patay, 2018)

i. Steroid therapy of dexamethasone or methylprednisolone can be initiated or increased. See information on focal symptoms.

ii. Pain medications, such as nonsteroidal medications, may provide symptomatic relief.

iii. Nonpharmacologic interventions, such as relaxation techniques, may be useful.

(e) Patient, caregiver, and family education

i. Development of new or worsening headaches, including precipitating and alleviating factors, frequency, duration, intensity, location, and associated symptoms, needs to be reported to the healthcare team.

ii. Written and verbal instructions should be provided for the use of steroid therapy and any additional pharmacologic agents, such as nonsteroidal medications. Refer to previous section on steroid management of focal symptoms.

iii. Literature regarding support programs should be provided; see Figure 17 for more information.

(3) Seizures

(a) Pathophysiology: A seizure is a sudden excessive abnormal electrical stimulation in the brain that alters neurologic function, including motor, sensory, and autonomic visceral function, as well as mental status. It may constitute the presenting symptom for diagnosis or disease progression and recurrence in 30%–90% of patients (Englot, Change, & Vecht, 2016;

J.W. Lee et al., 2010; Schiff et al., 2015; Yan et al., 2016).

i. The mechanism of how brain tumors cause seizures is not well understood but may be related to focal irritation.

ii. Tumor locations more frequently associated with seizures include temporal lobes, frontal lobes and their motor cortices, and parietal lobes and their sensory cortices.

iii. Low-grade primary brain tumors presenting with seizures usually are larger than those presenting with other symptoms, whereas high-grade primary tumors presenting with seizures are likely to be smaller than those presenting with other symptoms (Kahlenberg et al., 2012).

(b) Risk factors and incidence

i. Seizures occur more often in patients with primary tumors than metastases. Seizures are more likely to occur in those with low-grade primary brain tumors than those with high-grade tumors.

ii. Seizures are a presenting symptom in 30%–50% of patients with primary brain tumors (J.W. Lee et al., 2010) and 15%–20% of patients with brain metastases (Maschio et al., 2010). In both groups, a similar proportion of patients will eventually develop seizures after diagnosis.

(c) Focal assessment (Catsman-Berrevoets & Patay, 2018; Krumholz et al., 2015)

i. Assessment includes seizure history.
- Current cancer treatment plan and history
- History of presenting symptoms, including precipitating factors, frequency, duration, intensity, location, time of day, initial presentation, and changes in symptoms over time
- Precipitating signs or aura, including sensing unusual odor, tastes, or sounds, visual disturbances, or feelings of flushing
- Associated symptoms, including nausea, headache, or weakness
- Pharmacologic and nonpharmacologic interventions that have been tried and the results
- Any recent changes in medications, specifically steroid therapy

ii. Laboratory profiles, such as blood chemistries, liver function tests, complete blood counts, and appropriate drug levels if on antiepileptic drugs, should be obtained.

iii. Neuroradiologic tests to rule out hemorrhage, tumor progression or new lesion, and increased cerebral edema, should be obtained.

iv. CSF can be collected to rule out infection. Lumbar puncture should only be performed if absence of increased intracranial pressure is confirmed. Clinicians should assess craniotomy site for potential source of infection if applicable.

v. Clinicians should obtain an electroencephalogram within 24 hours of an event or if altered mental status persists.

(d) Collaborative management

i. Multiple studies have demonstrated that prophylactic antiepileptics are not effective in preventing seizures in those newly diagnosed with brain tumors, but those with a first seizure are at 50% risk of having a second seizure. Definitive recommendations for initiating prophylaxis have not been established (Krumholz et al., 2015).

ii. Antiepileptics are appropriate in patients who have experienced a seizure.

iii. Multiple older antiepileptics (phenytoin, carbamazepine, oxcarbazepine, phenobarbital, primidone) are CYP450 enzyme inducers; thus, drugs such as corticosteroids and chemotherapy agents require monitoring interactions (Catsman-Berrevoets & Patay, 2018).

iv. Multiple newer antiepileptics, such as levetiracetam, gabapentin, pregabalin, and lamotrigine, are not CYP450 enzyme inducers.

v. Patients with primary brain tumors or brain metastases treated with antiepileptic therapy have the same overall survival; however, better overall survival was observed when administering carbamazepine (p = 0.02), lamotrigine (p = 0.015), levetiracetam (p = 0.03), and valproic acid (p = 0.009) (Cacho-Diaz, San-Juan, Salmeron, Boyzo, & Lorenzana-Mendoza, 2018).

vi. Antiepileptic therapy should be monitored with serum drug levels for agents with narrow pharmacologic therapeutic index. Blood chemistries, liver function, and complete blood counts should be monitored.

vii. Clinicians should refer to a neurologist for refractory seizure management.

(e) Patient, caregiver, and family education (Krumholz et al., 2015)

i. Patients with primary brain tumors are at increased risk for developing dermatologic reactions to antiepileptics (greater than 20%). This includes development of Stevens-Johnson syndrome.

ii. All reactions need to be reported to the healthcare team, as 20% of patients with primary brain tumors on antiepileptic therapy have reported severe reactions warranting discontinuation.

iii. If a patient is on a CYP450-inducing antiepileptic, clinicians should alert the patient, caregiver, and family to potential drug interactions and monitoring parameters.

iv. Clinicians should provide information regarding the importance for drug adherence, as antiepileptics should not be stopped abruptly.

v. Clinicians should advise patients regarding state-mandated driving regulations and restrictions for patients who have had any seizure activity within the past six months. Some states have mandatory healthcare reporting.

vi. Literature regarding support programs should be provided; see Figure 17 for more information.

(4) Nausea and vomiting (J. Lee et al., 2018; Lovely et al., 2013)

(a) Pathophysiology: The mechanism of nausea and vomiting is a multifactorial process involving neural structures and neurotransmitters, which can be affected by tumor location and treatment.

i. The vomiting center lies within the lateral reticular formation of the medulla, near the floor of the fourth ventricle, and is activated by several mechanisms: cerebral cortex, vestibular apparatus, chemoreceptor trigger zone, and visceral and vagal afferent pathways of the gastrointestinal tract. Tumor location, an increase in intracranial pressure or cerebral edema, and disruption of these structures can activate the complex processes involved in nausea and vomiting.

ii. Neurotransmitters are sensitive to many chemical toxins within the blood and CNS: dopamine, serotonin, neurokinin-1, muscarinic, substance P, and histamine. Disruption of the blood–brain barrier and the normal receptor-transmitter actions will cause nausea and vomiting.

iii. Although several cancer therapies for patients with brain tumors may not be considered highly emetogenic, persistent nausea or nausea with emesis may exist, requiring additional support. Anticipatory nausea may ensue as a result of the overwhelming persistence of previous uncontrolled nausea.

(b) Risk factors and incidence

i. Tumor location near or adjacent to the vomiting center, fourth ventricle, or medulla, as well as known increased cerebral edema affecting those locations, can lead to nausea and vomiting.

ii. RT targeted to the neural structures of the vomiting center can cause nausea and vomiting.

(c) Focal assessment

i. Assessment includes detailed history (J. Lee et al., 2018).

- Current cancer treatment plan and history
- History of presenting symptoms, including precipitating factors, onset and duration, descriptors of the vomitus, prior experiences with nausea and vomiting, smell or odor sensitivities, and interference with daily life
- Associated symptoms, including increased salivation, diaphoresis, retching, dysphagia, thirst, tachycardia, diarrhea, loss of appetite, and anxiety
- Assessment for other symptoms, including cachexia, anemia, endocrine dysfunction, pain, fluid and electrolyte disturbances, seizures, and infection
- Pharmacologic and nonpharmacologic interventions that have been tried and the results

- Any recent changes in medications, including steroid therapy and antiepileptics

ii. Laboratory profiles, such as blood chemistries, liver function tests, complete blood counts, and appropriate drug levels if on antiepileptics, should be obtained.

(d) Collaborative management (J. Lee et al., 2018)

i. A serotonin receptor (5-HT$_3$) antagonist can be administered. Dose can be maximized, as necessary.

ii. Steroid therapy can be initiated or adjusted dosage.

iii. Use of a neurokinin-1 receptor antagonist may be beneficial for concurrent chemotherapy administration.

iv. Benzodiazepines may be useful for those with anticipatory nausea; however, the sedative side effect can alter mental status.

v. Additional pharmacologic agents include phenothiazines and anticholinergics, but sedative side effects require monitoring in this patient population.

vi. Adding cannabinoids or synthetic cannabinoids to daily regimen can be considered. These agents are safe with a low toxicity profile in patients with primary brain tumors (D.H. Allen, 2019).

vii. Nonpharmacologic interventions, such as relaxation therapy, diversion or attention distraction, hypnosis, and imagery, may be beneficial.

(e) Patient, caregiver, and family education

i. Patients should record episodes of nausea and vomiting to assess for precipitating factors and adjust interventions as necessary.

ii. Clinicians should provide information regarding side effects of pharmacologic agents and drug interactions.

iii. Clinicians should provide literature regarding support programs; see Figure 17 for more information.

(5) Acute alopecia and scalp dermatitis (Bray, Simmons, Wolfson, & Nouri, 2016)

(a) Pathophysiology: Hair follicles and glands are more susceptible to radiation damage because of the relatively rapid growth and proliferation.

i. Radiation causes premature conversion of hair follicle cells from the anagen (active) phase to the telogen (resting) phase, which results in new hairs being shed at an increased rate.

    ii. The scalp is sensitive to dose-dependent radiation damage ranging from mild to severe (Bray et al., 2016); see IV.B. Skin reactions.

(b) Risk factors and incidence (Bray et al., 2016)

    i. Temporary alopecia occurs with doses as low as 5 Gy; temporary dermatitis occurs with doses as low as 2 Gy.

    ii. Whole-brain RT of 30 Gy (300 cGy per fraction) can result in permanent vertex alopecia caused by dose accumulation.

    iii. After partial brain RT, patchy alopecia occurs in scalp areas receiving approximately 45 Gy (180–200 cGy per fraction).

    iv. Higher doses (45 Gy or greater) may produce permanent alopecia or delayed regrowth for more than a year; scalp desquamation or ulceration can last for weeks.

(c) Focal assessment: Scalp evaluation includes examination for complications of acute side effects of brain irradiation.

    i. Dry scalp

    ii. Radiation dermatitis

    iii. Hyperpigmentation

    iv. Alopecia

    v. Delayed wound healing (e.g., craniotomy or burr hole sites)

(d) Collaborative management

    i. Patients should gently wash hair with mild shampoo one to two times a week and use a water-soluble lubricant on scalp.

    ii. Patients should use a soft-bristle brush on hair to diminish follicular injury.

    iii. Patients should avoid sun exposure to the scalp by wearing a hat or covering. They may apply a sunscreen with SPF 30 or greater.

    iv. The area behind auricles should be checked for moist desquamation, as radiation dose may concentrate in skin folds.

    v. Patients should avoid hair dyes and permanent hair treatments.

    vi. Surgical reconstruction can be considered for appropriate cases.

(e) Patient, caregiver, and family education

    i. Clinicians should inform patients about the areas in which radiation alopecia is expected to occur related to the calculated scalp dose.

    ii. Alopecia is expected to begin two to three weeks after initiation of treatment; regrowth takes three to six months after completion of treatment.

    iii. Hair regrowth may be of a different color or consistency.

    iv. Some hair loss may be permanent, depending on RT dose (e.g., whole-brain RT of 30 Gy, partial brain RT of 45 Gy).

    v. Clinicians should provide literature regarding wigs (types, where to purchase, insurance reimbursement, wig alternatives) and reconstructive interventions if appropriate (see Figure 17).

(6) Fatigue: See IV.A. Fatigue.

d) Subacute side effects: Subacute side effects are toxicities that develop from four weeks to six months following RT (Day et al., 2016; Loughan, Allen, Baumstarck, et al., 2018).

  (1) Persistent fatigue: See IV.A. Fatigue.

  (2) Cranial neuropathies (predominantly visual and auditory)

(a) Pathophysiology (Delanian, Lefaix, & Pradat, 2012; Rong, Tang, Chen, Lu, & Peng, 2012)

    i. Focal irritation to ocular apparatus or cochlea causes temporary visual (changes in acuity) or auditory (ringing) disturbances.

    ii. Inflammation to the external ear canal causes increased cerumen production, resulting in difficulties hearing.

(b) Risk factors and incidence (Delanian et al., 2012; Rong et al., 2012)

    i. RT field proximity to the optic chiasm, optic nerves, optic globes, acoustic nerve, and cochlear areas increases risk.

    ii. Damage to the lacrimal gland can lead to dry eye and corneal injury.

    iii. Cataract formation may occur with doses exceeding 35 Gy.

    iv. Risk of damage to the optic chiasm and nerves is dose dependent, at 0.3% for dose fractions below 2 Gy versus 4% for dose fractions at 2 Gy or greater.

    v. For single-fraction SRS, injury to optic apparatus causing optic neuropathy is dose dependent. Incidence is 78% for doses greater than 14 Gy, 27% for doses of 10–15 Gy, and minimal incidence with doses less than 10 Gy.

vi. Most cranial neuropathies are temporary and reported at 13% incidence, with only 8% being permanent, for doses up to 40 Gy.

(c) Focal assessment

i. Assessment should check for visual acuity disturbances (Mayo et al., 2010).
- Current cancer treatment plan and history
- History of presenting symptoms, including precipitating factors, time of day that disturbance is worse or better, interference with daily life, and light sensitivity
- Assessment for scleral and conjunctival irritation
- Consideration of infectious processes
- Consideration of neuroradiographic evaluations to rule out hemorrhage, tumor progression or new lesion, and increasing cerebral edema
- Pharmacologic and nonpharmacologic interventions that have been tried and the results
- Any recent changes in medications, specifically steroid therapy

ii. Assessment should check for auditory disturbances (Bhandare et al., 2010).
- Current cancer treatment plan and history
- History of presenting symptoms, including precipitating factors, time of day that disturbance is worse or better, interference with daily life, and sound sensitivity
- Assessment of ear canal for infection, desquamation, and cerumen impaction
- Weber and Rinne tests for conductive hearing loss and SNHL
- Consideration of infectious processes
- Pharmacologic and nonpharmacologic interventions that have been tried and the results
- Any recent changes in medications, specifically steroid therapy

iii. Laboratory profiles, such as blood chemistries, liver function tests, com-

plete blood counts, and appropriate drug levels if on antiepileptics, should be obtained.

(d) Collaborative management

i. Management of visual acuity disturbances includes the following.
- Referral to have corrective lenses adjusted to promote safety with gait, driving, and performing other ADLs
- Adjustment of medications, particularly steroid therapy, as appropriate
- Consideration of neuro-ophthalmology referral if disturbance persists

ii. Management of auditory disturbances includes the following.
- Removal of cerumen blockage if appropriate; routine management of cerumen
- Treatment of infection if underlying cause
- Consideration of formal auditory testing and evaluation if disturbance persists; recommendations for surgical options or hearing aids

(e) Patient, caregiver, and family education

i. Clinicians should inform patients that these disturbances are usually short in duration.

ii. Patient should inform providers if symptoms persist or worsen over time.

(3) Somnolence syndrome (Harjani, Gururajachar, & Krishnaswamy, 2016)

(a) Pathophysiology: Somnolence syndrome is a radiation-induced brain injury characterized by somnolence ranging from mild drowsiness to overwhelming exhaustion, low-grade fever, nausea, vomiting, and headache. Symptoms typically occur one to four months after completion of RT.

(b) Risk factors and incidence: This syndrome is typically encountered after whole-brain RT in children. Although occurrence is rare, it also is reported in adults.

(c) Focal assessment

i. Clinicians should consider neuroradiographic evaluations to rule out hemorrhage, tumor progression or new lesion, and increased cerebral edema.

ii. Laboratory profiles, such as blood chemistries, liver function tests, complete blood counts, and appropriate drug levels if on antiepileptics, should be obtained.

(d) Collaborative management: Symptoms are transient and resolve within several weeks. Corticosteroid therapy may be useful.

(e) Patient, caregiver, and family education
   i. Clinicians should inform patients and caregivers that these disturbances are usually short in duration.
   ii. Patients and caregivers should inform providers if symptoms persist or worsen over time.

e) Late effects
   (1) Overview (Boele et al., 2015)
      (a) Late effects are usually irreversible and progressive sequelae to RT occurring from six months to years after treatment.
      (b) Possible etiology is white matter damage from vascular injury, demyelination, and necrosis. Vascular injury involves damage to the endothelium, leading to platelet aggregation and thrombus formation, followed by endothelial proliferation and intraluminal collagen formation.
      (c) Late effects often have significant impacts in health-related quality of life.
   (2) Radiation necrosis (Chung, Bryant, & Brown, 2018)
      (a) Pathophysiology: Radiation necrosis is a severe brain injury to white matter resulting in perivascular necrosis, and mimics recurrent tumor on MRI and CT, with the shared characteristics of location close to original tumor site, contrast enhancement, edema, growth over time, and exertion of mass effect.
      (b) Risk factors and incidence: Extensive review of the literature has recently been undertaken to determine dose-volume predictors of developing radiation necrosis (Lawrence et al., 2010).
         i. For partial brain RT, a dose-response relationship exists. At 2 Gy per fraction, incidence of necrosis is 5% at average 72 Gy (range 60–84 Gy) and 10% at average 90 Gy (range 84–102 Gy).
         ii. For twice-daily fractionation, a steep increase in toxicity occurs with dose greater than 62.5 Gy.
         iii. For large fraction size (greater than 2.5 Gy), the incidence and severity of toxicity are unpredictable.
         iv. Factors affecting the risk of developing radiation necrosis include total dose, dose per fraction, and volume of brain treated.
         v. Suggested risk factors for radiation necrosis include chemotherapy, dose variance within the volume treated, shorter overall treatment time, older age, and diabetes mellitus.
         vi. Median appearance is one to two years following therapy.
      (c) Focal assessment: Signs of radiation necrosis can be clinically observed as reappearance or worsening of initial symptoms and neurologic deficits.
      (d) Collaborative management
         i. Initial treatment is corticosteroid therapy
         ii. Surgical excision of mass lesions or drainage of cystic lesions can significantly improve neurologic symptoms if conservative management fails (Chung et al., 2018).
      (e) Patient, caregiver, and family education
         i. Neurologic symptoms or changes need to be reported immediately to the healthcare team.
         ii. Instruction includes management of side effects and risks of corticosteroid therapy.
         iii. Clinicians should explore support services needed for worsening functional deficits (e.g., speech, physical or occupational therapy) and provide literature regarding support programs (see Figure 17).
   (3) Radiation myelopathy (Kirkpatrick, van der Kogel, & Schultheiss, 2010)
      (a) Pathophysiology: Radiation myelopathy is a rare radiation-induced severe spinal cord injury that may result in pain, paresthesias, paralysis, sensory deficits, Brown-Séquard syndrome, and bowel and bladder incontinence. Most cases occur within three years after RT but rarely before six months after treatment.
      (b) Risk factors and incidence: Extensive review of the literature was undertaken to determine dose-volume predictors of developing radiation-related sequelae (Kirkpatrick et al., 2010).
         i. With conventional fractionation of 1.8–2 Gy to full-thickness spinal cord, the estimated risk of myelopathy (defined as CTCAE grade 2 or higher) is less than 1% at 54 Gy and less than 10% at 61 Gy.
         ii. Reirradiation data suggest partial repair of radiation-induced subclinical damage at approximately six

months after treatment and increasing over two years.

    iii. Risk effect with concurrent chemotherapy is unknown.

(c) Neuroimaging diagnostics: MRI shows hypointensity on T1-weighted images, hyperintensity on T2-weighted images, and hyperintensity on T1 gadolinium diethylenetriamine penta-acetic acid–contrasted images (Kirkpatrick et al., 2010).

(d) Collaborative management

    i. Patients may require specialized pain management.

    ii. Urology evaluation should be included for management of bladder incontinence.

    iii. A bowel management program should be initiated.

(e) Patient, caregiver, and family education

    i. Patients and caregivers should be educated regarding neurologic symptoms, including back or extremity pain, weakness, numbness or tingling, and bowel or bladder incontinence, which need to be reported immediately to the healthcare team, as these could be symptoms of spinal cord compression requiring emergent intervention.

    ii. The home environment should be assessed for safety issues if a patient has altered extremity strength or sensation.

    iii. Specialized instruction is needed for management of pain and bowel or bladder incontinence (e.g., urinary catheterization, bowel regimen, epidural catheter for pain control).

    iv. Clinicians should explore support services needed for worsening functional deficits and provide literature regarding support programs (see Figure 17).

(4) Cranial neuropathies (RION and SNHL)

(a) Pathophysiology

    i. RION usually presents as painless visual loss, with vasculature injury thought to be the most significant contributing cause. Field of vision loss depends on location of injury. Visual symptoms generally develop within three years of RT (Mayo et al., 2010).

    ii. SNHL is caused by damage to the cochlea or acoustic nerve, producing a clinically significant increase in bone conduction threshold at the key human speech frequencies (0.5–4 kHz). After fractionated RT, this

rarely occurs as early as three months, with a median latency of 1.5–2 years (Bhandare et al., 2010).

(b) Risk factors and incidence

    i. Mayo et al. (2010) determined dose-volume predictors of developing RION. Total dose and fraction size are the most important treatment-related risk factors. Age older than 70 years is a patient-related risk factor (Mayo et al., 2010).

    ii. Incidence of RION for conventionally fractionated RT is near zero with doses up to 50 Gy, unusual for doses less than 55 Gy, 3%–7% with doses of 55–60 Gy, and 7%–20% for doses greater than 60 Gy (Mayo et al., 2010).

    iii. The mean dose to the cochlea should be limited to 45 Gy or less for conventionally fractionated RT to minimize risk of developing radiation-induced SNHL after treatment of head and neck cancer and vestibular schwannoma (Bhandare et al., 2010).

(c) Focal assessment

    i. For RION, visual acuity and visual fields are assessed.

    ii. For SNHL, pure-tone audiometry and speech discrimination are assessed.

(d) Collaborative management

    i. For RION, patients are referred to a neuro-ophthalmologist or low-vision ophthalmologist.

    ii. For SNHL, patients are referred to otolaryngology or auditory specialists.

    iii. Patients should be referred to disability specialists for special needs regarding low vision, blindness, or deafness.

(e) Patient, caregiver, and family education

    i. Clinicians should provide information regarding support for patients and families, as these effects are long-term disabilities and special accommodations may be required (see Figure 17).

    ii. Patients should consider home safety evaluation for visual and auditory assistive devices.

    iii. An occupational therapy driving evaluation for visual losses may be needed to assess for safety.

(5) Neuroendocrinopathies (Gan et al., 2015)

(a) Pathophysiology: HPA axis damage and organ dysfunction may induce neuroendo-

crinopathies, such as panhypopituitarism, hypothyroidism, adrenal insufficiency, and sex hormone dysfunction.

(b) Incidence and risk factors

i. Involvement of pituitary gland within RT field increases long-term risk of diabetes insipidus.

ii. Pediatric patients are susceptible to long-term neuroendocrine deficiencies. In 166 children followed 30 years after RT for optic gliomas, the following neuroendocrine deficiencies were observed.

- Growth hormone deficiency (40.3%)
- Central precocious puberty (26%)
- Gonadotropin deficiency (20.4%)
- Thyroid-stimulating hormone deficiency (13.3%)
- Adrenocorticotropic hormone deficiency (13.3%)

(c) Focal assessment

i. Neuroradiographic evaluations can rule out hemorrhage, tumor progression or new lesion, and increased cerebral edema.

ii. Laboratory profiles, such as endocrine function tests, blood chemistries, liver function tests, complete blood counts, and appropriate drug levels if on antiepileptics, should be obtained.

(d) Collaborative management

i. Replacement therapies for endocrine disorders should be monitored for effects. Referral to a neuroendocrinologist may be necessary.

ii. Clinicians should perform a reproductive assessment and planning for patients of childbearing years.

iii. Patients should be referred to a neuroendocrinologist for long-term follow-up.

(e) Patient and family education

i. Clinicians should provide information regarding support for the patients and families, as this is a long-term disability and special accommodations may be required.

ii. Clinicians should provide information regarding potential effects on reproductive abilities and sexual functioning.

(6) Neurocognitive impairment: Cognitive function is the result of healthy brain performance and entails several cognitive domains that relay information for optimal performance through subcortical pathways. These domains include attention, executive function, information processing speed, visuospatial skill, motor function, language, and memory. Neurocognitive impairment, frequently referred to as *cognitive impairment* or *cognitive dysfunction*, is defined as a decline in function in one or more cognitive domains (B.D. Allen et al., 2018; D.H. Allen & Loughan, 2018).

(a) Pathophysiology: Precise mechanisms of neurocognitive impairments observed beyond tumor location are not fully understood but are most likely multifactorial. Some of these factors may include the following (D.H. Allen & Loughan, 2018; Loughan, Allen, Von Ah, & Braun, 2018):

i. Cellular DNA damage from RT to the cerebral cortex and subcortical pathways used in cognitive function

ii. Structural damage to axons and myelin in the cerebral white matter from RT

iii. Cytokine release in response to prolonged inflammation of the HPA axis

(b) Risk factors (D.H. Allen & Loughan, 2018; Loughan, Allen, Von Ah, & Braun, 2018; Raghubar et al., 2018)

i. Whole-brain RT has been associated with increased risk.

ii. Total dose of partial brain RT and field location have been associated with cognitive decline.

iii. Doses as low as 18 Gy have resulted in neurocognitive deficits in pediatric patients.

iv. Hippocampal stem cells promoting neurogenesis for memory function may be sensitive to a dose as low as 5 Gy.

v. Specific areas of cognitive impairments from RT may include slowed information processing speed, alterations in executive function, impaired memory, impaired sustained attention, and dysfunction of motor coordination.

vi. Cognitive decline occurs with aging.

vii. Cortical synaptic plasticity has been associated with radiation-related, age-dependent changes in cognitive function (Zhang et al., 2018).

viii. Presence of apolipoprotein E epsilon 4 allele has been associated with cognitive decline in long-term cancer survivors; areas of specific decline pertained to visual memory and visuospatial skills.

 ix. Premorbid intelligence and educational attainment may offer a protective component in the development of cognitive impairment.

 x. Individuals undergoing concurrent RT and high-dose chemotherapy may be at higher risk for developing cognitive impairment (Habets et al., 2014).

 xi. If whole-brain RT is utilized, clinicians may consider hippocampal sparing techniques to reduce long-term sequalae (Kepka et al., 2018; Krayenbuehl et al., 2017).

(c) Focal assessment

 i. Global neurocognitive assessment can be performed for trending change over time with instruments such as the Mini-Mental State Examination. However, global cognitive assessments are limited in discerning mild cognitive impairments (Von Ah, Jansen, & Allen, 2014).

 ii. Neuropsychological measurement batteries have established age-based and education-based norms for healthy populations.

 iii. Subjective cognitive instruments assess a patient's perspective of cognitive function, such as the following (Von Ah et al., 2014).
- Attentional Function Index
- Cognitive Failures Questionnaire
- Functional Assessment of Cancer Therapy–Cognitive
- Patient's Assessment of Own Functioning Inventory
- Perception of Cognition Questionnaire

 iv. Neuroradiographic evaluations can rule out vascular-related dementia.

 v. Laboratory profiles, such as blood chemistries, liver function tests, and complete blood counts, should be obtained.

(d) Collaborative management (D.H. Allen & Loughan, 2018; Andrade, 2016; Von Ah et al., 2014)

 i. Monitoring for changes in subjective and global cognitive function measures is useful over time.

 ii. Referral to a neuropsychologist for a complete neuropsychological evaluation should be considered if changes are observed.

 iii. A baseline evaluation of cognitive function early in the diagnosis is helpful in order to objectively monitor for changes over time.

 iv. Patients should be monitored for effects of stimulants, and doses should be adjusted as needed.

 v. Pharmacologic and nonpharmacologic interventions should be considered.

 vi. Methylphenidate and dexmethylphenidate, modafinil and armodafinil, memantine, and donepezil have been suggested as being useful in improving cognitive impairment. Study limitations warrant further research.

 vii. Cognitive training programs also have demonstrated some benefit in improving cognitive function yet need further research.

 viii. Use of erythropoietin-stimulating agents is not recommended because of FDA warnings.

(e) Patient, caregiver, and family education

 i. Caregivers should monitor for signs of cognitive change over time. The healthcare team should be contacted if changes are observed.

 ii. Clinicians should provide information on available cognitive training programs.

 iii. Clinicians should provide information regarding support for patients and families, as this is a long-term disability and special accommodations may be required (see Figure 17).

(7) Post-RT vasculopathy

(a) Pathophysiology: Inflammation of intracranial and extracranial vessels creates vascular irregularities (Mamlouk, Handwerker, Ospina, & Hasso, 2013; Neu et al., 2018).

(b) Incidence: Adult survivors of primary brain tumors treated with standard RT have incurred hemorrhagic foci, large confluent areas of white matter change, and lacunar white matter lesions. Increasing age influences lesion severity.

(c) Focal assessment

 i. Assessment includes onset of symptoms, such as headache, syncope, and other stroke-like symptoms.

 ii. Neuroradiographic evaluations can determine the type of vascular impairment and associated cerebral edema.

 iii. Laboratory profiles, such as coagulation profiles, blood chemistries, liver function tests, and complete blood counts, should be obtained.

(d) Collaborative management
  i. Treatment is aimed at correction of the underlying cause and correction of coagulopathies.
  ii. Management of associated symptoms includes steroid therapy for cerebral edema.

(e) Patient, caregiver, and family education
  i. Clinicians should provide information regarding support for patients and families for long-term disability and special accommodations that may be required (see Figure 17).
  ii. Clinicians should provide information regarding persistent risk for recurrent vascular events and monitoring for recurrent events or stroke symptoms.

(8) RT-induced leukoencephalopathy
  (a) Pathophysiology: A distinct pathogenesis is unknown but may be related to oligodendroglial demyelination, gliosis, coagulation necrosis, small vessel disease or vascular injury, and edema (Bompaire et al., 2018; Mamlouk et al., 2013).
  (b) Risk factors and incidence
    i. Leukoencephalopathy is associated with severe cognitive dysfunction negatively affecting quality of life.
    ii. MRI demonstrates diffuse supratentorial white matter abnormalities with fluid-attenuated inversion recovery (FLAIR) white matter hyperintensities. No differentiation was found between whole-brain and focal RT for 40 patients demonstrating extensive FLAIR abnormalities (68%), brain atrophy (87%), and intraparenchymal cysts (21%). All 40 patients presented with severe cognitive dysfunction, 68% had gait difficulties, and 38% had urinary incontinence (Bompaire et al., 2018).
    iii. Severe cases may involve necrotizing leukoencephalopathy. Patients experience a shorter latency period with increased vascular injury leading to disseminated coagulation necrosis (Mamlouk et al., 2013)
  (c) Focal assessment
    i. Neuroradiographic evaluations can rule out hemorrhage, tumor progression or new lesion, and increased cerebral edema.
    ii. Neuropsychological assessment is performed to determine cognitive function.

(d) Collaborative management
  i. Treatment is aimed at correction of the underlying cause and correction of coagulopathies.
  ii. Management of associated symptoms includes steroid therapy for cerebral edema.

(e) Patient, caregiver, and family education
  i. Clinicians should provide information regarding support for patients and families for long-term disability and special accommodations that may be required (see Figure 17).
  ii. Clinicians should provide information regarding persistent risk for recurrent vascular events and monitoring for recurrent events or stroke symptoms.

References

Alentorn, A., Hoang-Xuan, K., & Mikkelsen, T. (2016). Presenting signs and symptoms in brain tumors. In M.S. Berger & M. Weller (Eds.), *Handbook of Clinical Neurology: Vol. 134. Gliomas* (pp. 19–26). Elsevier. https://doi.org/10.1016/B978-0-12-802997-8.00002-5

Allen, B.D., Acharya, M.M., Lu, C., Giedzinski, E., Chmielewski, N.N., Quach, D., ... Limoli, C.L. (2018). Remediation of radiation-induced cognitive dysfunction through oral administration of the neuroprotective compound NSI-189. *Radiation Research, 189,* 345–353. https://doi.org/10.1667/RR14879.1

Allen, D.H. (2019). Dronabinol therapy: Central nervous system adverse events in adults with primary brain tumors. *Clinical Journal of Oncology Nursing, 23,* 23–26. https://doi.org/10.1188/19.CJON.23-26

Allen, D.H., & Loughan, A.R. (2018). Impact of cognitive impairment in patients with gliomas. *Seminars in Oncology Nursing, 34,* 528–546. https://doi.org/10.1016/j.soncn.2018.10.010

Andrade, C. (2016). A method for deciding about the possible safety of modafinil and armodafinil in patients with seizure disorder. *Journal of Clinical Psychiatry, 77,* e25–e28. https://doi.org/10.4088/JCP.15f10580

Armstrong, T.S., Vera-Bolanos, E., Acquaye, A.A., Gilbert, M.R., Ladha, H., & Mendoza, T. (2016). The symptom burden of primary brain tumors: Evidence for a core set of tumor- and treatment-related symptoms. *Neuro-Oncology, 18,* 252–260. https://doi.org/10.1093/neuonc/nov166

Bhandare, N., Jackson, A., Eisbruch, A., Pan, C.C., Flickinger, J.C., Antonelli, P., & Mendenhall, W. (2010). Radiation therapy and hearing loss. *International Journal of Radiation Oncology, Biology, Physics, 76*(Suppl. 3), S50–S57. https://doi.org/10.1016/j.ijrobp.2009.04.096

Boele, F.W., Douw, L., Reijneveld, J.C., Robben, R., Taphoorn, M.J.B., Aaronson, N.K., ... Klein, M. (2015). Health-related quality of life in stable, long-term survivors of low-grade glioma. *Journal of Clinical Oncology, 33,* 1023–1029. https://doi.org/10.1200/JCO.2014.56.9079

Bompaire, F., Lahutte, M., Buffat, S., Soussain, C., Ardisson, A.E., Terziev, R., ... Ricard, D. (2018). New insights in radiation-induced leukoencephalopathy: A prospective cross-sectional study. *Supportive Care in Cancer, 26,* 4217–4226. https://doi.org/10.1007/s00520-018-4296-9

Bovi, J.A. (2018). Prevention of brain metastases. *Frontiers in Neurology, 9,* 758. https://doi.org/10.3389/fneur.2018.00758

Brastianos, P.K., Galanis, E., Butowski, N., Chan, J.W., Dunn, I.F., Goldbrunner, R., ... Raleigh, D.R. (2019). Advances in multidisciplinary therapy for meningiomas. *Neuro-Oncology, 21*(Suppl. 1), i18–i31. https://doi.org/10.1093/neuonc/noy136

Bray, F.N., Simmons, B.J., Wolfson, A.H., & Nouri, K. (2016). Acute and chronic reactions to ionizing radiation therapy. *Dermatology and Therapy, 6,* 185–206. https://doi.org/10.1007/s13555-016-0120-y

Brown, P.D., Ballman, K.V., Cerhan, J.H., Anderson, S.K., Carrero, X.W., Whitton, A.C., ... Roberge, D. (2017). Postoperative stereotactic radiosurgery compared with whole brain radiotherapy for resected metastatic brain disease (NCCTG N107C/CEC-3): A multicentre, randomised, controlled, phase 3 trial. *Lancet Oncology, 18,* 1049–1060. https://doi.org/10.1016/S1470-2045(17)30441-2

Brown, P.D., Jaeckle, K., Ballman, K.V., Farace, E., Cerhan, J.H., Anderson, S.K., ... Asher, A.L. (2016). Effect of radiosurgery alone vs radiosurgery with whole brain radiation therapy on cognitive function in patients with 1 to 3 brain metastases: A randomized clinical trial. *JAMA, 316,* 401–409. https://doi.org/10.1001/jama.2016.9839

Cacho-Diaz, B., San-Juan, D., Salmeron, K., Boyzo, C., & Lorenzana-Mendoza, N. (2018). Choice of antiepileptic drugs affects the outcome in cancer patients with seizures. *Clinical and Translational Oncology, 20,* 1571–1576. https://doi.org/10.1007/s12094-018-1892-6

Catsman-Berrevoets, C., & Patay, Z. (2018). Cerebellar mutism syndrome. In M. Manto & T.A.G.M. Huisman (Eds.), *Handbook of clinical neurology: Vol. 155. The cerebellum: Disorders and treatment* (pp. 273–288). Elsevier. https://doi.org/10.1016/B978-0-444-64189-2.00018-4

Chang, S.M., Mehta, M.P., Vogelbaum, M.A., Taylor, M.D., & Ahluwalia, M.S. (2018). Neoplasms of the central nervous system. In V.T. DeVita, Jr., T.S. Lawrence, & S.A. Rosenberg (Eds.), *DeVita, Hellman, and Rosenberg's cancer: Principles and practice of oncology* (11th ed.). Wolters Kluwer.

Chung, C., Bryant, A., & Brown, P.D. (2018). Interventions for the treatment of brain radionecrosis after radiotherapy or radiosurgery. *Cochrane Database of Systematic Reviews, 2018*(7). https://doi.org/10.1002/14651858.CD011492.pub2

Day, J., Yust-Katz, S., Cachia, D., Wefel, J., Katz, L.H., Tremont, I.W., ... Rooney, A.G. (2016). Interventions for the management of fatigue in adults with a primary brain tumour. *Cochrane Database of Systematic Reviews, 2016*(4). https://doi.org/10.1002/14651858.CD011376.pub2

Delanian, S., Lefaix, J.-L., & Pradat, P.-F. (2012). Radiation-induced neuropathy in cancer survivors. *Radiotherapy and Oncology, 105,* 273–282. https://doi.org/10.1016/j.radonc.2012.10.012

Dorsey, J.F., Salinas, R.D., Dang, M., Alonso-Basanta, M., Judy, K.D., Maity, A., ... Pruitt, A.A. (2020). Cancer of the central nervous system. In J.E. Niederhuber, J.O. Armitage, J.H. Doroshow, M.B. Kastan, & J.E. Tepper (Eds.), *Abeloff's clinical oncology* (6th ed., pp. 906–967). Elsevier.

Englot, D.J., Change, E.F., & Vecht, C.J. (2016). Epilepsy and brain tumors. In M.S. Berger & M. Weller (Eds.), *Handbook of Clinical Neurology: Vol. 134. Gliomas* (pp. 267–285). Elsevier. https://doi.org/10.1016/B978-0-12-802997-8.00016-5

Forst, D.A., Nahed, B.V., Loeffler, J.S., & Batchelor, T.T. (2014). Low-grade gliomas. *Oncologist, 19,* 403–413. https://doi.org/10.1634/theoncologist.2013-0345

Gan, H.-W., Phipps, K., Aquilina, K., Gaze, M.N., Hayward, R., & Spoudeas, H.A. (2015). Neuroendocrine morbidity after pediatric optic gliomas: A longitudinal analysis of 166 children over 30 years. *Journal of Clinical Endocrinology and Metabolism, 100,* 3787–3799. https://doi.org/10.1210/jc.2015-2028

Grommes, C., Rubenstein, J.L., DeAngelis, L.M., Ferreri, A.J.M., & Batchelor, T.T. (2018). Comprehensive approach to diagnosis and treatment of newly diagnosed primary CNS lymphoma. *Neuro-Oncology, 21,* 296–305. https://doi.org/10.1093/neuonc/noy192

Habets, E.J.J., Taphoorn, M.J.B., Nederend, S., Klein, M., Delgadillo, D., Hoang-Xuan, K., ... Reijneveld, J.C. (2014). Health-related quality of life and cognitive functioning in long-term anaplastic oligodendroglioma and oligoastrocytoma survivors. *Journal of Neuro-Oncology, 116,* 161–168. https://doi.org/10.1007/s11060-013-1278-0

Hamel-Perreault, E., Mathieu, D., & Masson-Cote, L. (2019). Factors influencing the outcome of stereotactic radiosurgery in patients with five or more brain metastases. *Current Oncology, 26,* e64–e69.

Harjani, R.R., Gururajachar, J.M., & Krishnaswamy, U. (2016). Comprehensive assessment of somnolence syndrome in patients undergoing radiation to the brain. *Reports of Practical Oncology and Radiotherapy, 21,* 560–566. https://doi.org/10.1016/j.rpor.2016.08.003

Huse, J.T., & Holland, E.C. (2010). Targeting brain cancer: Advances in the molecular pathology of malignant glioma and medulloblastoma. *Nature Reviews Cancer, 10,* 319–331. https://doi.org/10.1038/nrc2818

Kahlenberg, C.A., Fadul, C.E., Roberts, D.W., Thadani, V.M., Bujarski, K.A., Scott, R.C., & Jobst, B.C. (2012). Seizure prognosis of patients with low-grade tumors. *Seizure, 21,* 540–545. https://doi.org/10.1016/j.seizure.2012.05.014

Kepka, L., Tyc-Szczepaniak, D., Osowiecka, K., Sprawka, A., Trąbska-Kluch, B. & Czeremszynska, B. (2018). Quality of life after whole brain radiotherapy compared with radiosurgery of the tumor bed: Results from a randomized trial. *Clinical and Translational Oncology, 20,* 150–159. https://doi.org/10.1007/s12094-017-1703-5

Kirkpatrick, J.P., van der Kogel, A.J., & Schultheiss, T.E. (2010). Radiation dose–volume effects in the spinal cord. *International Journal of Radiation Oncology, Biology, Physics, 76*(Suppl. 3), S42–S49. https://doi.org/10.1016/j.ijrobp.2009.04.095

Kotecha, R., Gondi, V., Ahluwalia, M.S., Brastianos, P.K., & Mehta, M.P. (2018). Recent advances in managing brain metastasis. *F1000Research, 7,* 1772. https://doi.org/10.12688/f1000research.15903.1

Krayenbuehl, J., Di Martino, M., Guckenberger, M., & Andratschke, N. (2017). Improved plan quality with automated radiotherapy planning for whole brain with hippocampus sparing: A comparison to the RTOG 0933 trial. *Radiation Oncology, 12,* 161. https://doi.org/10.1186/s13014-017-0896-7

Krumholz, A., Wiebe, S., Gronseth, G.S., Gloss, D.S., Sanchez, A.M., Kabir, A.A., ... French, J.A. (2015). Evidence-based guideline: Management of an unprovoked first seizure in adults: Report of the Guideline Development Subcommittee of the American Academy of Neurology and the American Epilepsy Society. *Neurology, 84,* 1705–1713. https://doi.org/10.1212/WNL.0000000000001487

Lawrence, Y.R., Li, X.A., el Naqa, I., Hahn, C.A., Marks, L.B., Merchant, T.E., & Dicker, A. (2010). Radiation dose–volume effects in the brain. *International Journal of Radiation Oncology, Biology, Physics, 76*(Suppl. 3), S20–S27. https://doi.org/10.1016/j.ijrobp.2009.02.091

Lee, J., Cherwin, C., Czaplewski, L.M., Dabbour, R., Lewis, C., Selm-Orr, D.L., ... Whiteside, S. (2018). Symptom interventions: Chemotherapy-induced nausea and vomiting—Adult. https://www.ons.org/pep/chemotherapy-induced-nausea-and-vomiting-adult

Lee, J.W., Wen, P.Y., Hurwitz, S., Black, P., Kesari, S., Drappatz, J., ... Broomfield, E.B. (2010). Morphological characteristics of brain tumors causing seizures. *Archives of Neurology, 67,* 336–342. https://doi.org/10.1001/archneurol.2010.2

Loughan, A.R., Allen, D.H., Baumstarck, K., Boyer, L., Auquier, P., Lanoye, A., & Braun, S. (2018). Quality of life in neuro-oncology. In H.B. Newton (Ed.), *Handbook of brain tumor chemotherapy, molecular therapeutics, and immunotherapy* (2nd ed., pp. 767–781). Elsevier. https://doi.org/10.1016/B978-0-12-812100-9.00061-9

Loughan, A.R., Allen, D.H., Von Ah, D., Braun, S. (2018). Neuropsychology of chemotherapy in brain tumor patients. In H.B. Newton (Ed.), *Handbook of brain tumor chemotherapy, molecular therapeutics, and immunotherapy* (2nd ed., pp. 783–809). Elsevier. https://doi.org/10.1016/B978-0-12-812100-9.00062-0

Louis, D.N., Perry, A., Reifenberger, G., von Deimling, A., Figarella-Branger, D., Cavenee, W.K., ... Ellison, D.W. (2016). The 2016 World Health Organization classification of tumors of the central nervous system: A summary. *Acta Neuropathologica, 131,* 803–820. https://doi.org/10.1007/s00401-016-1545-1

Lovely, M.P., Stewart-Amidei, C., Page, M., Mogensen, K., Arzbaecher, J., Lupica, K., & Maher, M.E. (2013). A new reality: Long-term survivorship with a malignant brain tumor. *Oncology Nursing Forum, 40,* 267–274. https://doi.org/10.1188/13.ONF.267-274

Lubejko, B., & Wilson, B. (2019). *Oncology nursing: Scope and standards of practice.* Oncology Nursing Society.

Mamlouk, M.D., Handwerker, J., Ospina, J., & Hasso, A.N. (2013). Neuroimaging findings of the post-treatment effects of radiation and chemotherapy of primary glial neoplasms. *Neuroradiology Journal, 26,* 396–412. https://doi.org/10.1177/197140091302600405

Mariş, D., Nica, D., Mohan, D., Moisa, H., & Ciurea, A.V. (2014). Multidisciplinary management of adult low grade gliomas. *Chirurgia, 109,* 590–599. http://revistachirurgia.ro/pdfs/2014-5-590.pdf

Maschio, M., Dinapoli, L., Gomellini, S., Ferraresi, V., Sperati, F., Vidiri, A., ... Jandolo, B. (2010). Antiepileptics in brain metastases: Safety, efficacy and impact on life expectancy. *Journal of Neuro-Oncology, 98,* 109–116. https://doi.org/10.1007/s11060-009-0069-0

Mayo, C., Martel, M.K., Marks, L.B., Flickinger, J., Nam, J., & Kirkpatrick, J. (2010). Radiation dose–volume effects of optic nerves and chiasm. *International Journal of Radiation Oncology, Biology, Physics, 76*(Suppl. 3), S28–S35. https://doi.org/10.1016/j.ijrobp.2009.07.1753

Montano, N., D'Alessandris, Q.G., D'Ercole, M., Lauretti, L., Pallini, R., Di Bonadventura, R., ... Fernandez, E. (2016). Tumors of the peripheral nervous system: Analysis of prognostic factors in a series with long-term follow-up and review of the literature. *Journal of Neurosurgery, 125,* 363–371. https://doi.org/10.3171/2015.6.JNS15596

Narum, S., Westergren, T., & Klemp, M. (2014). Corticosteroids and risk of gastrointestinal bleeding: A systematic review and meta-analysis. *BMJ Open, 4,* e004587. https://doi.org/10.1136/bmjopen-2013-004587

National Comprehensive Cancer Network. (2020). *NCCN Clinical Practice Guidelines in Oncology (NCCN Guidelines®): Central nervous system cancers* [v.2.2020]. http://www.nccn.org/professionals/physician_gls/PDF/cns.pdf

Nayak, L., Lee, E.Q., & Wen, P.Y. (2012). Epidemiology of brain metastases. *Current Oncology Reports, 14,* 48–54. https://doi.org/10.1007/s11912-011-0203-y

Nead, K.T., & Swisher-McClure, S. (2019). Utilization of hypofractionated radiation therapy in older glioblastoma patients. *Journal of Geriatric Oncology, 10,* 155–158. https://doi.org/10.1016/j.jgo.2018.06.006

Neu, M.A., Tanyildizi, Y., Wingerter, A., Henninger, N., El Malki, K., Alt, F., ... Faber, J. (2018). Susceptibility-weighted magnetic resonance imaging of cerebrovascular sequelae after radiotherapy for pediatric brain tumors. *Radiotherapy and Oncology, 127,* 280–286. https://doi.org/10.1016/j.radonc.2018/03/010

Newton, H.B., & Shroff, S. (2018). Overview of brain tumor epidemiology and histopathology. In H.B. Newton (Ed.), *Handbook of brain tumor chemotherapy, molecular therapeutics, and immunotherapy* (2nd ed., pp. 3–20). Elsevier. https://doi.org/10.1016/B978-0-12-812100-9.00001-2

Ostrom, Q.T., Gittleman, H., Truitt, G., Boscia, A., Kruchko, C., & Barnholtz-Sloan, J.S. (2018). CBTRUS statistical report: Primary brain and other central nervous system tumors diagnosed in the United States in 2011–2015. *Neuro-Oncology, 20*(Suppl. 4), iv1–iv86. https://doi.org/10.1093/neuonc/noy131

Raghubar, K.P., Lamba, M., Cecil, K.M., Yeates, K.O., Mahone, E.M., Limke, D., ... Ris, M.D. (2018). Dose–volume metrics and their relation to memory performance in pediatric brain tumor patients: A preliminary study. *Pediatric Blood and Cancer, 65,* e27245. https://doi.org/10.1002/pbc.27245

Rong, X., Tang, Y., Chen, M., Lu, K., & Peng, Y. (2012). Radiation-induced cranial neuropathy in patients with nasopharyngeal carcinoma: A follow-up study. *Strahlentherapie und Onkologie, 188,* 282–286. https://doi.org/10.1007/s00066-011-0047-2

Ryken, T.C., McDermott, M., Robinson, P.D., Ammirati, M., Andrews, D.W., Asher, A.L., ... Kalkanis, S.N. (2010). The role of steroids in the management of brain metastases: A systematic review and evidence-based clinical practice guideline. *Journal of Neuro-Oncology, 96,* 103–114. https://doi.org/10.1007/s11060-009-0057-4

Schiff, D., Lee, E.Q., Nayak, L., Norden, A.D., Reardon, D.A., & Wen, P.Y. (2015). Medical management of brain tumors and the sequelae of treatment. *Neuro-Oncology, 17,* 488–504. https://doi.org/10.1093/neuonc/nou304

Schoemaker, M.J., Robertson, L., Wigertz, A., Jones, M.E., Hosking, F.J., Feychting, M., ... Swerdlow, A. (2010). Interaction between 5 genetic variants and allergy in glioma risk. *American Journal of Epidemiology, 171,* 1165–1173. https://doi.org/10.1093/aje/kwq075

Siegel, R.L., Miller, K.D., & Jemal, A. (2018). Cancer statistics, 2018. *CA: A Cancer Journal for Clinicians, 68,* 7–30. https://doi.org/10.3322/caac.21442

Simonetti, G., Gaviani, P., Botturi, A., Innocenti, A., & Silvani, A. (2015). Clinical management of grade III oligodendroglioma. *Cancer Management and Research, 7,* 213–223. https://doi.org/10.2147/CMAR.S56975

Sperduto, P.W., Kased, N., Roberge, D., Xu, Z., Shanley, R., Luo, X., ... Mehta, M. (2012). Summary report on the graded prognostic assessment: An accurate and facile diagnosis-specific tool to estimate survival for patients with brain metastases. *Journal of Clinical Oncology, 30,* 419–425. https://doi.org/10.1200/JCO.2011.38.0527

Splittgerber, R. (2019). *Snell's clinical neuroanatomy* (8th ed.). Wolters Kluwer.

Stupp, R., Hegi, M.E., Mason, W.P., van den Bent, M.J., Taphoorn, M.J.B., Janzer, R.C., ... Mirimanoff, R.-O. (2009). Effects of radiotherapy with concomitant and adjuvant temozolomide versus radiotherapy alone on survival in glioblastoma in a randomised phase III study: 5-year analysis of the EORTC-NCIC trial. *Lancet Oncology, 10,* 459–466. https://doi.org/10.1016/S1470-2045(09)70025-7

Stupp, R., Taillibert, S., Kanner, A.A., Kesari, S., Steinberg, D.M., Toms, S.A., ... Ram, Z. (2015). Maintenance therapy with tumor-treating fields plus temozolomide vs. temozolomide alone for glioblastoma: A randomized clinical trial. *JAMA, 314,* 2535–2543. https://doi.org/10.1001/jama.2015.16669

Tsao, M.N., Rades, D., Wirth, A., Lo, S.S., Danielson, B.L., Gaspar, L.E., ... Chang, E.L. (2012). Radiotherapeutic and surgical management for newly diagnosed brain metastasis(es): An American Society for Radiation Oncology evidence-based guideline. *Practical Radiation Oncology, 2,* 210–225. https://doi.org/10.1016/j.prro.2011.12.004

van Linge, A., van Os, R., Hoeskstra, N., Heijmen, B., Stienstra, L., Dallenga, A., ... Mendez Romero, A. (2018). Progression of hearing loss after LINAC-based stereotactic radiotherapy for vestibular schwannoma is associated with cochlear dose, not with pre-treatment hearing level. *Radiation Oncology, 13,* 253. https://doi.org/10.1186/s13014-018-1202-z

Von Ah, D., Jansen, C.E., & Allen, D.H. (2014). Evidence-based interventions for cancer- and treatment-related cognitive impairment. *Clinical Journal of Oncology Nursing, 18,* 17–25. https://doi.org/10.1188/14.CJON.S3.17-25

Wilson-Pauwels, L., Stewart, P.A., Akesson, E.J., & Spacey, S.D. (2010). *Cranial nerves: Function and dysfunction* (3rd ed.). People's Medical Publishing House.

Yan, P., Liang, T., Zhang, C., Cai, J., Zhang, W., Chen, B., ... Jiang, T. (2016). Clinicopathological factors predictive of postoperative seizures in patients with gliomas. *Seizure, 35,* 93–99. https://doi.org/10.1016/j.seizure.2015.12.013

Zarnett, O.J., Sahgal, A., Gosio, J., Perry, J., Berger, M.S., Chang, S., & Das, MS. (2014). Treatment of elderly patients with glioblastoma: A systematic evidence-based analysis. *JAMA Neurology, 72,* 589–596. https://doi.org/10.1001/jamaneurol.2014.3739

Zhang, D., Zhou, W., Lam, T.T., Weng, C., Bronk, L., Ma, D., ... Grosshans, D.R. (2018). Radiation induces age-dependent deficits in cortical synaptic plasticity. *Neuro-Oncology, 20,* 1207–1214. https://doi.org/10.1093/neuonc/noy052

B. Head and neck

1. Incidence
   a) Historically, head and neck cancer has been linked with excessive alcohol and tobacco use.
      (1) Over the past few decades, however, epidemiologic studies have also linked oncogenic viruses, such as HPV and Epstein-Barr virus, and industrial toxins to head and neck cancer.
      (2) According to CDC (2019), in the United States in 2016, the latest year for which incidence data are available, 45,543 new cases of

cancer of the oral cavity and pharynx were reported, and 10,170 people died from cancer of the oral cavity and pharynx cancer.

(3) For every 100,000 people, 12 new cases of and 3 deaths from cancer of the oral cavity and pharynx were reported (CDC, 2019).

b) Studies of incidence by site have shown an increase in the incidence of oropharynx and salivary gland cancers and a decrease in hypopharynx and larynx cancers (Mifsud et al., 2017).

(1) The oropharynx is now the most common site for head and neck cancer and is most common in developed countries, such as Australia, Canada, Japan, Norway, and the United States.

(2) More than 60% of oropharynx cancers are related to HPV.

(3) The oropharynx consists of the tonsillar pillars, base of tongue, pharyngeal tonsils, glossotonsillar sulcus, anterior soft palate, and uvula.

c) Except for salivary gland cancers, the incidence of head and neck cancers is higher in men than in women (Mifsud et al., 2017).

2. HPV association

a) As of 2015, HPV-associated oropharynx cancer was the most common HPV–associated cancer in the United States (Mulcahy, 2018).

b) Given the favorable prognosis of HPV-related cancers, when compared to non-HPV–related counterparts, the American Joint Committee on Cancer (AJCC) modified the staging system of head and neck cancers to reflect this component as a prognostic indicator (Lydiatt et al., 2017).

(1) Prevention

(a) Routine vaccination series (HPV 9-valent vaccine) is recommended to start in children 9–12 years old for prevention of cervical, vulvar, vaginal, and anal cancers caused by HPV (U.S. FDA, 2020).

(b) Additionally, in 2018, FDA approved vaccination in adults up to age 45 if previously unvaccinated.

(c) HPV vaccination may help to prevent other HPV-related cancers, such as oropharyngeal cancers; however, studies are needed to further refine guidelines as applicable to head and neck cancers (U.S. FDA, 2018).

(2) Outcomes

(a) HPV-related head and neck cancer is associated with better sensitivity to chemoradiation and improved progression-free and overall survival.

(b) More than 90% of HPV-related cancers of the oropharynx are associated with HPV-16 (Candotto et al., 2018).

(c) AJCC recently updated the staging of head and neck cancers to reflect high

incidence of HPV-related cancer. Staging now includes a separate algorithm for HPV-related cancers (Lydiatt et al., 2017).

3. Histopathology

a) Squamous cell carcinoma remains the predominant histopathology of head and neck cancers.

b) The most common sites of head and neck cancer are oropharynx, oral cavity, nasopharynx, hypopharynx, larynx, paranasal sinuses, salivary gland, and thyroid gland (Amin et al., 2018).

4. Treatment options

a) Treatment varies and depends on tumor location, pathologic features, and staging.

(1) Most patients require an interprofessional approach with individualized single or multimodal treatment consisting of RT, chemotherapy, and surgery.

(2) The use of higher radiation doses, sophisticated techniques, and radiosensitizing chemotherapy have improved survival and local control.

b) Immunotherapy

(1) Immunotherapy also has a role in head and neck cancer treatment, with agents such as nivolumab and pembrolizumab used for management of recurrence or metastasis.

(2) Future studies seek to determine whether immunotherapy agents have a role in treatment modality prior to primary treatment failure (NCI, 2019).

5. Side effects of head and neck RT

a) Mucositis

(1) Pathophysiology

(a) Mucositis is damage to the mucosa of the alimentary tract, occurring as a result of chemotherapy and RT.

(b) Mucositis is commonly referred to as *stomatitis*, *esophagitis*, and *pharyngitis*.

(c) Pathogenesis is composed of four phases (Maria, Eliopoulos, & Muanza, 2017).

i. In the initial inflammatory phase, the radiation-injured tissues release cytokines (interleukin-1β, prostaglandins, and TNF-α), which increase inflammation.

ii. Within a week, the epithelial phase is initiated by the cytotoxic and apoptotic effects of radiation on proliferating basal cells. Epithelial turnover is the determent of the recovery period.

iii. The painful ulcerative and bacteriologic phase begins with epithelial breakdown exposing nerve endings at the lamina propria. Neutropenia and secondary infection with Gram-negative bacteria, yeast, and bacterial exotoxins aggravate the inflammatory reaction by causing tissues to release nitric oxide, interleukin-1β, and TNF-α.

    iv. The healing phase is composed of matrix signaling to basal epithelial cells, which migrate, proliferate, and differentiate throughout the healing process (see Figure 18).

(2) Risk factors and incidence

    (a) Patients with radiation-induced oral mucositis can experience several side effects and sequelae, including oral pain (69%); dysphagia (56%); opioid use (53%); weight loss of 3–7 kg, feeding tube insertion, and hospital or intensive care unit admission (15%); and treatment modification or interruption (11%–16%) (Maria et al., 2017).

    (b) Although the anatomic distribution of mucositis is predominantly related to the radiation dose distribution, nonkeratinized oral tissues (buccal mucosa, lateral tongue, soft palate, floor of mouth) are more susceptible to mucositis than keratinized oral tissues.

    (c) For patients with head and neck cancer receiving concurrent chemotherapy and RT, oral mucositis may be more severe, appear earlier in the treatment course, and last longer (Sroussi et al., 2017).

    (d) Patient risk factors include the following; however, because of limited studies and controversial results, there is still no clear consensus on the evaluation of risk for RT-induced oral mucosal reactions in patients with head and neck cancer (Tao et al., 2017).

       i. Poor oral hygiene and periodontal disease, chronic alcohol consumption, cigarette smoking, hyposalivation, low body mass index (less than 18.5), and comorbidities (e.g., diabetes mellitus)

       ii. Age, sex, and therapeutic regimen (suggested)

       iii. High cytokine levels, decreased renal function, and previous cancer treatment (e.g., RT, chemotherapy, HSCT)

(3) Assessment (Sroussi et al., 2017)

    (a) The overall goal of assessment is to identify and track patient changes to personalize interventions.

    (b) Although many tools are available for assessment, for consistency, the same tool should be used throughout the course of treatment. The most commonly used grading tools are as follows.

       i. World Health Organization

       ii. RTOG

       iii. Western Consortium for Cancer Nursing Research

       iv. CTCAE

    (c) Prior to beginning treatment, patients should have a baseline oral assessment and a dental evaluation. Findings of inadequate oral hygiene should be addressed and improved prior to treatment.

    (d) Throughout treatment, weekly oral assessments should be performed. Increased frequency of assessing the oral cavity should occur if the patient is experiencing oral lesions, dysphagia, weight loss, pain, diffi-

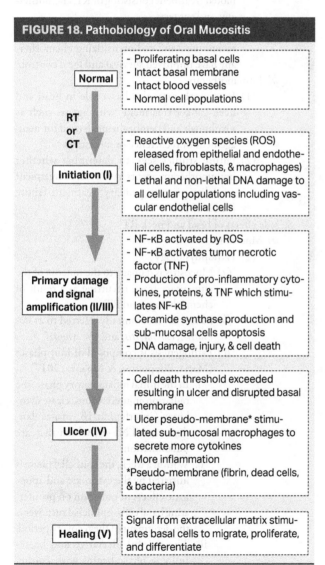

FIGURE 18. Pathobiology of Oral Mucositis

Normal
- Proliferating basal cells
- Intact basal membrane
- Intact blood vessels
- Normal cell populations

RT or CT

Initiation (I)
- Reactive oxygen species (ROS) released from epithelial and endothelial cells, fibroblasts, & macrophages)
- Lethal and non-lethal DNA damage to all cellular populations including vascular endothelial cells

Primary damage and signal amplification (II/III)
- NF-κB activated by ROS
- NF-κB activates tumor necrotic factor (TNF)
- Production of pro-inflammatory cytokines, proteins, & TNF which stimulates NF-κB
- Ceramide synthase production and sub-mucosal cells apoptosis
- DNA damage, injury, & cell death

Ulcer (IV)
- Cell death threshold exceeded resulting in ulcer and disrupted basal membrane
- Ulcer pseudo-membrane* stimulated sub-mucosal macrophages to secrete more cytokines
- More inflammation
*Pseudo-membrane (fibrin, dead cells, & bacteria)

Healing (V)
- Signal from extracellular matrix stimulates basal cells to migrate, proliferate, and differentiate

CT—chemotherapy; NF-κB—nuclear factor-kappa B; RT—radiation therapy

Note. From "Radiation-Induced Oral Mucositis," by O.M. Maria, N. Eliopoulos, and T. Muanza, 2017, *Frontiers in Oncology, 7,* 89, p. 2 (https://doi.org/10.3389/fonc.2017.00089). Copyright 2017 by O.M. Maria, N. Eliopoulos, and T. Muanza. Licensed under Creative Commons Attribution 4.0 International (CC BY 4.0; https://creativecommons.org/licenses/by/4.0).

culty eating, changes in speech, taste, xerostomia, increased secretions, fever, or halitosis.

  (e) Physical examination should assess the entire oral cavity (lips, tongue, mucosa, and gingiva) for moisture, ulcers or lesions, color, signs of infection, and integrity.

  (f) Functional examination should assess mouth opening, range of tongue mobility, and patient report of difficulty with speech, swallowing, or eating.

(4) Documentation

  (a) Use of a standardized oral mucositis grading system is advantageous to consistency of assessment.

  (b) Documentation should include the oral mucositis grading scores, as well as a comprehensive pain assessment; degree of xerostomia, dysphagia, and secretions; and presence or absence of infection.

    i. Pain at rest (not talking, eating, or swallowing) and pain with talking, eating, or swallowing on a standard 0–10 pain scale

    ii. Assessment of the type of analgesia used and its effectiveness

    iii. Degree of xerostomia and type and amount of secretions

    iv. Signs and symptoms of infection (redness, ulcers, lesions, bleeding, and thrush)

(5) Collaborative management

  (a) Prevention

    i. No FDA-approved intervention exists for prevention of radiation-induced mucositis.

    ii. Early identification of patients at increased risk and provision of needed interventions to decrease their overall risk is of high importance.

  (b) Interventions (Maria et al., 2017)

    i. Dental evaluation and all dental interventions should be completed prior to RT.

    ii. Collaboration with radiation oncologists and radiation therapists is necessary to address the possible need for dental guards to increase spacing from the buccal mucosa to lessen radiation scatter.

    iii. Collaboration with medical oncologists is necessary to discuss choice of chemotherapy sensitizer agent for patients at high risk for mucositis.

    iv. Early inclusion of a nutritionist and speech and swallowing therapist on a patient's treatment team can address potential needs.

    v. Clinicians should assess a patient's coping ability and involve psychosocial team members into the treatment team to assist with coping skills and suggest coping strategies.

(6) Patient, caregiver, and family education

  (a) Education should stress the importance of twice-daily dental care and improved oral hygiene, such as the following measures (Maria et al., 2017).

    i. Meticulous brushing and flossing at least twice daily with a soft toothbrush; no flossing while platelet count is less than $50,000/mm^3$ or ANC less than $1,000/mm^3$

    ii. Salt and soda rinses four to six times daily and especially after eating

    iii. Use of fluoride trays (if dentist prescribed) and use of fluoride toothpaste

    iv. Decreased use of dentures and ill-fitting dentures

    v. Continued increased oral hygiene and ongoing dental care during and after treatment

  (b) Patients, caregivers, and families should understand nutrition and diet changes that may decrease irritation of mucositis. An RDN or RD can provide guidance, resources, and support (Maria et al., 2017).

    i. Avoidance of spicy, high-acid foods

    ii. Avoidance of alcohol, smoking, and mouth rinses with alcohol

    iii. Avoidance of crunchy or sharp foods that increase abrasion to the oral mucosa

    iv. Adequate hydration

  (c) Patients should understand that increased oral cavity moisture will decrease discomfort from mucositis. See item c) Xerostomia for further information.

  (d) Education includes the importance of topical and systemic pain management.

    i. Topical numbing agents are frequently used for temporary relief of mucositis pain to aide in eating. Although still widely used, they are no longer recommended for practice by ONS (Eilers et al., 2019).

    ii. Systemic pain management is an integral part of care. Education topics include the following.

      • Initial topical numbing agents and systemic pain management as mucositis increases

- Pain management for maintaining adequate hydration and nutrition to prevent complications and hospitalization
- Name, dose, frequency, and route of the medication
- Side effects, side effects management, potential interactions, and safety precautions
- Dose escalations, as needed, to maintain proper pain levels for continued nutrition and hydration
- Safe storage and disposal of medications
- Working with speech and swallowing therapist and compliance with exercises

b) Dysphagia
  (1) Pathophysiology
    (a) Dysphagia is any difficulty with swallowing.
    (b) Dysphagia has many causes; therefore, it may be experienced prior to treatment, during treatment, or after treatment.
    (c) For patients with head and neck cancer, the oropharyngeal phase of swallowing is most affected.
    (d) The oropharyngeal phase of swallowing consists of three main parts: oral preparatory, oral, and pharyngeal phases.
      i. During the oral preparatory phase, saliva and mastication are used to break down the food into a soft bolus. For adequate bolus formation, the tongue must seal across the hard palate and lateral alveolus.
      ii. The oral phase lasts only 1–1.5 seconds and begins when the food bolus moves posteriorly from the oral cavity into the pharynx with the squeeze from the tongue.
      iii. The pharyngeal phase includes muscular movements that propel the food into the esophagus: closure of velopharynx, stabilization of the hyoid with the suprahyoid and infrahyoid muscles, tilt of epiglottis, and closure of vocal folds, as well as pharyngeal wall contraction and movement of the base of tongue, ending with the upper esophageal sphincter opening for food to pass through.
    (e) Understanding the anatomic and physiologic mechanism for normal swallowing aids in understanding the dysphagia that

many patients with head and neck cancer may experience (Logemann & Larsen, 2012).
  (2) Risk factors and incidence
    (a) Overall incidence is difficult to categorize because of the variability in presentation and models for screening. A range of 6%–94% of patients with head and neck cancer develop dysphagia at some point during their disease course (Moayer & Sinha, 2013).
    (b) Dysphagia may present prior to treatment.
      i. Tumor burden itself can cause dysphagia.
      ii. Size and location of the tumor, as it affects any of the physiologic functions related to swallowing, will cause some degree of dysphagia.
      iii. Dysphagia may result in coughing or choking while eating, nasal speech or regurgitation, residual food in the oral cavity or pharynx, and change in dietary habit (Reddy & Priyadharshini, 2017).
      iv. Trismus, or reduced opening of the jaw, is often found in patients with head and neck cancer with invasion into muscles of mastication and similarly affects the oral preparatory phase of normal swallow function (Rapidis et al., 2015).
      v. Surgical resection may disrupt normal tissue, nerves, cartilage, and musculature prior to RT, thus leading to dysphagia (Denaro, Merlano, & Russi, 2013).
    (c) Dysphagia can present during treatment.
      i. RT to the head and neck may cause acute toxicities, such as mucositis and related pain, as well as xerostomia, sialorrhea, and ropey secretions that disrupt normal swallow function (de Souza Tolentino et al., 2011).
      ii. Chemotherapy, high-dose RT, and lack of participation in swallowing exercises throughout treatment contribute to dysphagia during treatment (Denaro et al., 2013).
    (d) Dysphagia may appear after treatment (Denaro et al., 2013).
      i. Late effects, such as fibrosis, lymphedema, nerve injury, xerostomia, tooth decay, muscle atrophy, and trismus (as a result of fibrosis rather than tumor burden), can continue to cause dysphagia.

    ii. Dysphagia as a late effect can not only hinder quality of life but can lead to increased risk for morbidity and mortality, such as with aspiration pneumonia.

(e) Other risk factors include the following (Denaro et al., 2013).

    i. Intensification of treatment with chemotherapy

    ii. Increased age, female sex, decreased performance status, and baseline swallowing function

    iii. Dysphagia at baseline presentation

    iv. Increased tumor and node stage

    v. Increased volume of tissue treated

    vi. Involvement of the hypopharynx

    vii. Bilateral neck irradiation

(3) Assessment

(a) Factors that affect dysphagia should be assessed at baseline, throughout treatment, and in the post-treatment setting.

(b) Instrumental assessment should include video-fluoroscopic modified barium swallow and fiber-optic endoscopic evaluation with a speech and language pathologist. These assessments aid in understanding and identifying structural and functional abnormalities in swallowing and allow for compensatory and dietary recommendations (Denaro et al., 2013).

(c) Vital signs, laboratory values, and frequent weight checks are useful for evaluating nutritional status and acute changes that may occur with worsening dysphagia.

(4) Documentation: Documentation should adhere to standardized sources.

(a) CTCAE (NCI CTEP, 2017, p. 27)

    i. Grade 1: symptomatic, able to eat regular diet

    ii. Grade 2: symptomatic and altered eating/swallowing

    iii. Grade 3: severely altered eating and swallowing; tube feeding, [total parental nutrition], or hospitalization indicated

    iv. Grade 4: life-threatening consequences; urgent intervention indicated

(b) High-quality patient-reported outcome tools for measuring oropharyngeal dysphagia include the Sydney Swallow Questionnaire and Swallowing Quality of Life questionnaire (Patel et al., 2017).

(5) Collaborative management

(a) Symptoms should be managed by the clinical team to prevent worsening dysphagia. Possible symptoms include but are not limited to the following.

    i. Odynophagia

    ii. Mucositis

    iii. Lymphedema

    iv. Fibrosis

    v. Trismus

    vi. Xerostomia

(b) Patients should also see an RDN or RD before treatment, as needed throughout treatment, and in the post-treatment setting.

(c) Acute side effects

    i. Enteral support either with nasogastric tube or gastrostomy tube may be needed because of acute dysphagia causing malnutrition and dehydration throughout treatment. Lower body mass index, male sex, pretreatment swallowing difficulties, nodal disease, and bilateral neck irradiation are associated with increased need for enteral support (van der Linden et al., 2016).

    ii. Gastrostomy tube placement remains controversial, as does timing for placement within treatment (prophylactic vs. reactive).

    iii. When a gastronomy tube is used prophylactically, quality of life tends to be greater at six months after treatment, but this is associated with long-term tube dependence.

    iv. With enteral support, nutritional status, as measured by body weight throughout treatment, also remains more stable, but average weight loss parallels those patients with reactive tube placement after treatment (McLelland, Andrews, Chaudry, Teckie, & Goenka, 2018).

    v. Gastrostomy tube placement is associated with greater risk of esophageal toxicity than nasogastric tube placement and is also associated with higher costs and without noted improvement in survival. There are no guidelines for the type or timing of enteral support; therefore, it should be individualized with a careful evaluation of risks and benefits for each patient (Nugent, Parker, & McIntyre, 2010).

(d) Long-term effects (De Felice et al., 2018)

    i. Late dysphagia appears as three marked signs: enteral support (either via nasogastric or gastrostomy tube), aspiration or stricture noted on videofluoroscopy, or aspiration pneumonia that occurs two months after treatment.

    ii. Choking, coughing, anxiety, and discomfort while swallowing in the post-treatment time frame are also signs of late dysphagia.

    iii. Late dysphagia is best managed through an interprofessional team approach, including surgery, speech-language pathology, radiation oncology, medical oncology, radiology, and maxillofacial prosthodontics.

    iv. Patients should be seen by a speech-language pathologist before and after for evaluation and management of dysphagia on a routine basis, as rehabilitation is vital for adjustment and improvement of treatment-related anatomical and physiologic changes. Adjustments include postural changes, and modification of initiation of food speed and bolus volume and consistency.

    v. Prosthetics may be of use in patients with cancer of the oral cavity.

    vi. In the future, the use of proton therapy may demonstrate reduction in radiation dose to critical organ structures that otherwise aid in maintaining normal swallow function. There is currently no literature that analyzes this as a functional outcome at this time.

(6) Patient, caregiver, and family education (De Felice et al., 2018)

    (a) Swallowing and range-of-motion exercises should be completed at a minimum of 10 times daily.

    (b) Patients, caregivers, and families should be educated on the signs and symptoms of worsening dysphagia. Education should also include the importance of managing acute and late toxicities to aid in avoiding worsening of dysphagia.

c) Xerostomia

(1) Pathophysiology (Pinna, Campus, Cumbo, Mura, & Milia, 2015)

    (a) Xerostomia is defined as perceived dry mouth due to hyposalivation and alteration in salivary composition.

    (b) Healthy people may produce up to 1,500 ml of saliva per day, whereas those with history of head and neck RT with severe xerostomia may produce less than 500 ml of saliva per day.

    (c) The submandibular gland and the parotid gland contribute to 90% of salivary flow, whereas other minor salivary glands present in the oral cavity and pharynx contribute the other 10%.

    (d) The parotid gland, however, is more radiosensitive than the submandibular gland.

    (e) Radiation causes dysfunction of salivary secretion in two ways: damaging secretory cells or damaging membrane components critical to intracellular signaling.

    (f) Early changes at the tissue level include interstitial fibrosis, progressive loss of the fine vasculature, and vacuolization of serous acinar cells.

    (g) Serous acinar cells seem to be more readily affected by radiation, compared to the mucous cells, presumably because of the relatively rapid turnover rate and profuse vasculatures of serous cells. As such, saliva is more acidic and viscous with less buffering capacity.

    (h) During the late stages of RT, glands become progressively fibrotic, leading to almost complete loss of acinar elements and the striated duct system. Ultimately, no saliva may be present.

(2) Incidence and risk factors

    (a) Even small doses of radiation can lead to decreased salivary function. Patients who receive 20–40 Gy may have undetectable salivary function, and it is estimated that 1 Gy of radiation to a salivary gland is responsible for up to 5% reduction in functional output.

    (b) The following factors increase risk (da Silva, Kupek, & Peres, 2017).

      i. Patients with chronic diseases (e.g., Sjögren syndrome, diabetes) and medication usage (including chemotherapy) are at an increased risk for developing xerostomia.

      ii. Age is also thought to be a contributing factor but has not been studied extensively enough to draw definitive conclusions.

      iii. Larger treatment volumes that include the submandibular and parotid gland and bilateral treatment of these glands increase risk.

    (c) The following factors may reduce incidence (Tariq, Jamshaid, & Majeed, 2015).

      i. Prevention of xerostomia, if possible, is key.

ii. The salivary glands, especially the parotid, should be spared by the radiation oncologist whenever possible.

iii. If the mean radiation dose is less than 20 Gy to one or both glands, severe xerostomia may be avoided.

iv. IMRT and proton therapy are two commonly used RT techniques that allow for partial volume radiation to the major salivary glands and may preserve salivary flow.

(3) Assessment

   (a) Xerostomia may cause sore throat and dysphagia that may subsequently lead to dietary changes, weight loss, and malnutrition.

   (b) Other complications of xerostomia include halitosis, plaque accumulation, mucosal injury, nocturnal oral discomfort, enamel erosion and dental caries, periodontal disease, and dysgeusia (Tariq et al., 2015).

   (c) Physical examination should include the following (Pinna et al., 2015).

      i. Constitutional: monitoring for weight loss, dietary changes, and dysphagia

      ii. Oral cavity: monitoring for dry or cracked mucous membranes and lips, ulceration, signs of mucosal trauma, tenderness, or signs of infection

(4) Documentation: Clinician and patient-reported outcome tools are available to document xerostomia.

   (a) The University of Michigan Xerostomia Questionnaire is a validated patient-report outcome tool.

   (b) CTCAE and RTOG scales are common clinician tools (Kamal et al., 2018; NCI CTEP, 2017).

   (c) When measuring salivary flow, patient reported-outcome tools are more accurate than clinician tools for capturing degree of xerostomia in patients with head and neck cancer (Memtsa et al., 2017).

(5) Collaborative management (Tariq et al., 2015)

   (a) When xerostomia develops, management is mainly focused on symptom control and reducing related complications.

   (b) Excellent oral care and dental follow-up before and after RT is imperative for reducing the incidence of gingivitis, dental plaques, and caries.

   (c) Sialagogues (salivary stimulants) can be used for comfort.

      i. Nonpharmacologic agents: gums, sprays, or oils

      ii. Pharmacologic agents: pilocarpine and cevimeline.

   (d) Acupuncture may be used to stimulate saliva function as well.

   (e) Unfortunately, clinical practice varies from country to country, and thus clinician to clinician, rendering treatment effect variable.

   (f) Collaborating with an RDN or RD for individualized recommendations is useful when patients are struggling to maintain their weight.

(6) Patient, caregiver, and family education: Patients should be educated on the importance of practicing good oral hygiene, following up with a specialized dentist regularly, and knowing signs and symptoms of oral cavity infection and when to see a specialist.

d) Compromised dental integrity

(1) Pathophysiology

   (a) RT to the head and neck has an increased effect for the risk of decreased quality in a patient's overall dentition, with the side effects of dental caries, periodontitis, xerostomia, trismus, increased risk of oral infection, and osteoradionecrosis (Kim, Yang, & Sung, 2016).

   (b) Patients are at increased risk of dental caries following RT primarily because of hyposalivation (Sroussi et al., 2017).

      i. Saliva has essential functions in maintaining tooth structure by control of pH, remineralization, and antimicrobial and tooth-cleansing effects.

      ii. Dental caries results from a loss of equilibrium in tooth demineralization and remineralization, culminating in mineral loss. This leads to damage of the organic phase of tooth structures, resulting in cavitation.

      iii. Demineralization first appears as increased white lesions involving gumline regions and cusp tips of the teeth.

      iv. Untreated caries can progress rapidly and require more extensive treatment, making prevention and early detection of mineral loss essential.

      v. Sequelae include pain, infection of the jawbone, and potentially the need for tooth extraction. In patients who have high-dose RT to the region, risk of osteoradionecrosis is present.

   (c) Periodontitis is a highly prevalent and chronic microbial and inflammatory disease characterized by the loss of tooth-supporting tissue inclusive of the alveolar bone (Sroussi et al., 2017).

    i. Periodontitis may culminate in pain, infection of the jawbone around dental roots, and tooth loss.

    ii. The effects of xerostomia, changes in the oral microflora, mucositis, and history of periodontitis put patients with head and neck cancer at higher risk.

(d) Xerostomia contributes to compromised dental integrity. See previous information on xerostomia.

(e) Trismus is a well-known complication defined as an inability to open the mouth or difficulty with mouth opening secondary to spasm of the muscles of mastication (Bensadoun et al., 2010; Melchers et al., 2009). See subsequent information on trismus.

(f) Damage to the lining of the mouth and weakened immune system allow for infections to occur. A systemic review indicated that the weighted mean prevalence of clinical oral candidiasis during head and neck RT is 37.4%. Factors promoting clinical fungal infection in this population include the following (Devi & Singh, 2014).

    i. Hyposalivation caused by radiation damage to the salivary gland

    ii. Tissue damage from radiation-induced oral mucositis

    iii. Dietary deficiency

    iv. Inability to maintain oral hygiene

(g) Osteoradionecrosis compromises dental integrity. See subsequent information on osteoradionecrosis.

(2) Incidence and risk factors

(a) Treatment-related risks

    i. Radiation-induced hyposalivation makes enamel surface more susceptible to demineralization and multiple dental caries (Walker, Wichman, Cheng, Coster, & Williams, 2011).

    ii. Smooth surface enamel in the cervical region of teeth that is usually less susceptible to caries becomes discolored and friable. Compromise to the integrity of the tooth structure is progressive.

    iii. Advanced radiation-induced dental caries may lead to tooth fracture, dental abscess, tooth loss, and osteoradionecrosis (Turner, Mupparapu, & Akintoye, 2013).

    iv. Radiation dose of 30–60 Gy puts patients at greater risk for tooth damage, which is likely related to salivary gland effects (Walker et al., 2011).

    v. Chemotherapy causes neutropenia, neutrophil dysfunction, and impaired inflammatory response, which further delay tissue healing and consequent loss of more periodontal tissues (Turner et al., 2013).

(b) Oral cavity risks: Oral cavity risks include poor dental hygiene, need for extractions, or significant dental work (e.g., root canals, deep dental caries, broken or fractured teeth, significant gum disease with exposed dental roots).

(c) Patient risk factors: Age, general oral hygiene, use of fluoride and pretreatment dental care, smoking, and good overall nutrition are all factors that affect a patient's risk for compromised dentition after head and neck RT (Maria et al., 2017).

(3) Assessment (Sroussi et al., 2017)

(a) A dentist should perform an oral cavity assessment prior to treatment and every three months for early detection of oral disease.

(b) Dental hygiene instruction should be a part of patient assessment.

(4) Collaborative management (Sroussi et al., 2017)

(a) Dental work should be completed prior to treatment, as healing after treatment may be slowed with a higher risk of possible complications.

(b) The treating dentist should be provided with a letter template stating the items to be assessed prior to the start of therapy.

(c) Fluoride trays and oral gel should be prescribed.

(d) A fluoride toothpaste should be prescribed. Patients should use it twice daily for their lifetime.

(e) In case of fungal infection, topical antifungal agents (e.g., nystatin rinse or pastilles, clotrimazole troches) can be effective. Patients should avoid eating, drinking, and rinsing for at least 30 minutes after use. For persistent lesions, systemic agents (e.g., fluconazole) can be prescribed.

(f) Bacterial infection can be treated by maintenance of oral hygiene, oral antibiotics or systemic antibiotic, and maintenance of nutritional status.

(g) Oral hygiene and dental care instruction are part of patient education at the end of

RT. Clinicians can assist with obtaining a dental provider if needed.

(5) Patient, caregiver, and family education

    (a) Patients should understand the need for a dental assessment prior to beginning RT.

    (b) Clinicians should inform patients that if any significant dental work or extractions are recommended, it should take place at least two weeks prior to the start of RT to allow for healing.

    (c) If patients are in financial need or do not have dental coverage, clinicians should provide resources for reduced-cost or free dental care.

e) Taste changes

(1) Pathophysiology

    (a) The sense of taste is mediated by taste buds in the oral cavity. Taste buds are multicellular receptor organs containing 60–100 cells, which are continually renewed by progenitor cells located at the basement membrane and along the lateral margins of buds (Nguyen, Reyland, & Barlow, 2012).

    (b) There are three types of taste cells.

      i. Type I for salt taste transportation

      ii. Type II for sweet, bitter, and salt tastes

      iii. Type III for sour tastes and umami (savory tastes)

    (c) Three models have been proposed to explain irradiation-triggered taste dysfunction (Nguyen et al., 2012).

      i. Neurites that innervate sensory organs are radiosensitive, thus, disruption of the contact between taste cells and nerves leads to taste cell death.

      ii. Irradiation directly damages differentiated taste cells.

      iii. Irradiation targets proliferating progenitors, interrupting production of new taste cells.

    (d) Taste sensation has three main functions: pleasure, defense, and sustenance.

    (e) Taste is regulated by the brain stem, mainly through cranial nerves VII (facial nerve) and IX (glossopharyngeal). The taste receptor cells on the taste buds contain nerve endings of cranial nerve VII or IX that detect chemical stimuli and transmit it to the brain stem, which then interprets it (Deshpande et al., 2018).

(2) Incidence and risk factors

    (a) It was found that the majority of patients (70%–100%) experienced partial or total taste loss during RT. Impairment was observed in all five tastes (Deshpande et al., 2018).

      i. Irrespective of RT to the tip of the tongue, bitter and salty tastes were found to be most severely affected, and sweet taste was least affected.

      ii. All tastes declined in the fourth to fifth week after the start of RT and improved in the 11th week.

      iii. Regardless of the taste quality, maximum impairment in taste was seen in patients during the fourth to sixth week.

    (b) Risk factors for taste disorder range from complete loss (ageusia) to a range of loss (hypogeusia).

      i. Many patients with head and neck cancer also have comorbidities that add additional risk factors to their taste disorders.

- Age
- Diabetes
- Hypothyroidism
- Obesity
- Hypertension
- Smoking
- Poor oral health and dentition
- Respiratory infections
- Medications

      ii. Patients with head and neck cancer are at increased risk of chemosensory dysfunction related to RT alone or chemoradiation treatment. Chemosensory dysfunction is frequently associated with anticancer therapies.

      iii. RT reduces the number of taste buds, and tongue exposure is related to taste impairment.

      iv. Chemotherapy commonly causes changes in sensory function, with 56%–76% of patients reporting dysgeusia or taste alterations in some form (Kershaw & Mattes, 2018).

(3) Assessment

    (a) Assessment of clinical manifestations should involve the following.

      i. Patient report of experiencing changes in taste

      ii. Assessment of the specific type of taste change experience (sweet, bitter, salt, sour, and umami tastes)

      iii. Assessment of foods and nutrient types a patient is avoiding

    (b) Physical examination should involve the following (Deshpande et al., 2018).

i. Weekly weight monitoring

ii. Examination of oral cavity

iii. Blood laboratory values

(4) Documentation: Documentation of taste changes should include the following (Deshpande et al., 2018).

(a) Altered degree of overall taste and specific type (sweet, bitter, salt, sour, and umami tastes)

(b) Presence of unpleasant taste (e.g., metallic taste)

(c) Change in dietary intake

(d) Assessment for depression and food aversion

(5) Collaborative management

(a) Self-care dietary strategies by patients to minimize alterations in taste include the following (Einarsson, Laurell, & Ehrsson, 2019).

i. Changing food habits by adding new recipes

ii. Increasing food palatability by adding artificial flavors

iii. Adding more fats and sauces

iv. Eating smaller and more frequent meals

v. Using more condiments

vi. Eating blander foods

vii. Adding sweetness to meats

viii. Sucking on hard candy

ix. Eating more boiled foods

x. Avoiding beef

(b) Additional strategies include the following (Kershaw & Mattes, 2018).

i. Eating room temperature food or precooked foods

ii. Using plastic utensils to minimize metallic tastes

iii. Chewing mint gum and using hard candy and lemon-flavored candy to mask tastes

iv. Collaborating with psychology professionals for symptoms of depression or food aversion

(6) Patient, caregiver, and family education (Einarsson et al., 2019)

(a) Clinicians should inform patients, caregivers, and family of taste changes prior to beginning treatment to assist with mental readiness. They should understand when to expect changes to occur and how long changes will last.

(b) Patients, caregivers, and family should be taught self-care strategies as mentioned previously.

(c) Clinicians should emphasize good oral hygiene during and after RT.

(d) Clinicians should discuss patients' most effective coping mechanism for taste changes.

(e) Rinsing with baking soda (1 teaspoon) and salt (1 teaspoon) in 500 ml of water before and after each meal may help with taste changes and improve oral health.

(f) Patients should understand alternative sources of protein to ensure adequate nutrition. Suggestions may include yogurt, eggs, peanut butter, fish, beans, hummus, and protein shakes.

f) Change in voice quality

(1) Pathophysiology

(a) An individual's voice is a unique sound signature used as a primary means to communicate thoughts, needs, and wants.

(b) The human vocal system comprises the lungs and the lower airway, which supply air pressure; the vocal folds, which vibrate to modulate the airflow and produce voice source; and the vocal tract, which modifies the voice source, thus creating specific output sounds (Zhang, 2016).

i. The vocal folds are located in the larynx and form a constriction to the airway.

ii. Each vocal fold is approximately 11–15 mm long in adult women and 17–21 mm in men. Folds stretch across the larynx along the anterior–posterior direction, attaching anteriorly to the thyroid cartilage and posteriorly to the anterolateral surface of the arytenoid cartilages.

(2) Incidence and risk factors

(a) Voice disorders negatively impact quality of life, job performance, and job attendance, costing the United States approximately $2.67 billion in lost wages, physicians' visits, and treatment expenses (Craig et al., 2015).

(b) Dysphonia is frequently noted in patients with head and neck cancer (Rinkel et al., 2016).

i. The tumor site, treatment type (amount of radiation and chemotherapy), and presence of lymphedema or inflammation are significant factors in changes to a patient's voice.

ii. Age, alcohol use, gastroesophageal reflux disease, smoking, xerostomia, and fibrosis are also factors.

(3) Assessment

(a) Recognition of the importance of patient-reported outcome measures in voice disorders has sparked rapid growth in their number and construct diversity (e.g., quality of life, coping) since the first patient-reported outcome measure was introduced in 1984 (Linear Analog Scale of Assessment–Voice Quality) (Francis et al., 2017).

(b) Swallowing and speech problems were significantly related to each other, indicating that many patients who experience swallowing problems also experience speech problems (Francis et al., 2017).

(c) Clinicians should assess a patient's baseline voice quality (pitch, hoarseness, and projection) prior to treatment. Clinicians should monitor for changes with ongoing assessments throughout treatment. Assessment of voice quality changes is part of ongoing aftercare.

(d) In a physical examination, vocal folds can be assessed with direct flexible laryngoscopy for movement, edema, and inflammation.

(e) In psychosocial assessment, clinicians should determine how a patient's voice quality has affected daily life.

    i. Ability and increased effort to communicate with others in public or loud situations

    ii. Ability to be heard over the phone

    iii. Effects on job performance

    iv. Ability to participate in conversation or to socialize

(4) Documentation: The degree of voice change can be described in the following ways (Villari & Courey, 2015).

(a) Mild: Voice changes in pitch or projection are minimal and resolve after completion of treatment. Changes do not affect ability to communicate.

(b) Moderate: Persistent voice changes require the patient to repeat or write to be understood. The patient cannot communicate via telephone and depends on written text to be understood.

(c) Dysphonia: The patient has severe voice changes and must use written text to communicate. The patient uses significant effort to produce a whispered voice.

(d) Aphonia: The patient is unable to speak.

(5) Collaborative management (Craig et al., 2015)

(a) A speech and swallowing therapist should be consulted before, during, and after treatment to provide ongoing assessment and management.

(b) A lymphedema therapist can assist with management.

(c) An RDN or RD can assess nutrition needs and educate on foods to avoid (e.g., spicy, acidic).

(d) Patients should be monitored for pain management needs.

(6) Patient, caregiver, and family education (Reiter, Hoffman, Pickhard, & Brosch, 2015)

(a) Patients should understand the importance of adherence to speech and swallowing exercises.

(b) Patients should cease using alcohol and tobacco products.

(c) Patients should understand the importance of compliance with and ongoing management of lymphedema.

(d) Clinicians should provide resources for impaired speech communication (see www.nidcd.nih.gov/health/assistive-devices-people-hearing-voice-speech-or-language-disorders).

(e) Nurses should encourage rest of vocal folds, use of a humidifier, and use of saline gargles.

g) Hearing changes

(1) Pathophysiology

(a) Ototoxicity may occur as a result of RT, and damage to the cochlea directly from radiation is the main cause of hearing loss in this population.

(b) A correlation exists between radiation dose to the cochlea and hearing loss, with greatest negative effect noted on high-frequency hearing (Hajisafari et al., 2018).

(c) Radiation effects to surrounding structures may cause Eustachian tube dysfunction and recurrent otitis media, possibly leading to hearing loss (Schmitt & Page, 2017).

(2) Incidence and risk factors

(a) Radiation dose greater than 40 Gy increases the risk of SNHL, with approximately one-third of patients who receive 60 Gy to the cochlea developing permanent SNHL (Havle, Ahmed, Vihapure, Khairmode, & Tripti, 2019).

(b) Highest risk for hearing loss is in patients with a primary tumor in the nasopharynx, skull base, or paranasal sinuses.

(c) Concurrent treatment with cisplatin or carboplatin increases risk of ototoxicity (Schmitt & Page, 2017).

(d) Additional risks for hearing loss include the following (Lee et al., 2015; U.S. Preventive Services Task Force, 2013).

i. Cardiovascular factors (smoking, history of cardiovascular disease, diabetes)
ii. Male sex
iii. History of noise exposure
iv. Previous recurrent inner ear infections
v. Advanced age
vi. Lower socioeconomic status

(3) Assessment
  (a) Review of systems
    i. Clinicians should ask patients, caregivers, and family members if they have noticed decreased hearing in one or both ears.
    ii. A single-item screening question such as "Do you have difficulty or change in hearing?" is an acceptable screening method (Oosterloo et al., 2020).
  (b) Physical examination
    i. The whisper test, finger rub, Weber test, and Rinne test are useful for evaluating hearing loss and determining if hearing loss is unilateral or bilateral. Rinne test may be used to assess air and bone conduction, and it can discern if the hearing loss is conductive or sensorineural in nature (Selby, 2011).
    ii. The ear should be inspected both externally and with an otoscope for signs of debris, cerumen impaction, discharge, foreign bodies, erythema, swelling, or middle ear effusions ("Head, eyes, and ears," 2014).

(4) Documentation: CTCAE outlines descriptions of hearing loss for patients not enrolled in a monitoring program (NCI CTEP, 2017, p. 12).
  (a) Grade 1: subjective change in hearing in the absence of documented hearing loss
  (b) Grade 2: hearing loss with hearing aid or intervention not indicated; limiting instrumental ADLs
  (c) Grade 3: hearing loss with hearing aid or intervention indicated; limiting self-care ADLs

(5) Collaborative management (Oosterloo et al., 2020)
  (a) Clinicians should counsel patients on the usefulness of audiograms.
  (b) Referral for a hearing aid may be warranted.
  (c) Referral to otolaryngologist may be warranted for chronic middle ear effusions, cerumen impaction, or sudden acute hearing loss.

(6) Patient, caregiver, and family education
  (a) Clinicians should educate patients about the risk for hearing loss as a treatment-related effect.
  (b) Patients, caregivers, and family should monitor for signs of hearing loss.
  (c) Clinicians should advise patients to report any changes in hearing at routine follow-up if subtle and immediately if acute.

h) Osteoradionecrosis
  (1) Pathophysiology (Sroussi et al., 2017)
    (a) Osteoradionecrosis is the result of ischemic necrosis of the bones associated with soft tissue necrosis without the presence of tumor.
    (b) Histopathologic changes occur in three phases.
      i. Prefibrotic phase with increased endothelial cell activity and inflammation
      ii. Subsequent phase characterized by abnormal fibroblastic activity
      iii. Final phase with characteristic fibro-atrophic remodeling and loss of osteocytes in bone
    (c) Other histopathologic findings include initial hyperemia, endarteritis, and thrombosis, followed by cell loss, hypovascularity, increase in bone marrow fat, and fibrosis.
    (d) The histomorphometric analysis was statistically significant for hypocellularity, hypovascularity, and fibrosis.
  (2) Incidence and risk factors
    (a) Osteoradionecrosis, by most reports, has been substantively reduced in the modern RT era by use of IMRT for mandibular dose reduction and careful dental management. There is a suggestion that osteoradionecrosis may represent a "historical" toxicity (De Felice, Musio, & Tombolini, 2015).
    (b) Treatment-related risk factors include the total radiation dose, fraction, and volume. Surgical intervention and chemotherapy are also factors.
    (c) Patients with HPV-related oropharyngeal carcinoma are comparatively more curable and may have decades of risk for post-RT sequelae, such as osteoradionecrosis, to develop (MD Anderson Head and Neck Cancer Symptom Working Group, 2017).
    (d) A 2018 study of the risk factors showed that patients with oropharyngeal cancer developed osteoradionecrosis earlier compared to those with oral cavity cancer (Chronopoulos, Zarra, Ehrenfeld, & Otto, 2018).

i. Osteoradionecrosis can occur spontaneously without any precipitating dentoalveolar trauma.

ii. Radiation dose to the jaw greater than 60 Gy, poor periodontal status, and alcohol use after RT are significantly related to the risk of developing osteoradionecrosis.

(3) Assessment: Assessment should include the following (Sroussi et al., 2017).

   (a) Comprehensive patient history to evaluate risk factors

   (b) Ongoing clinical assessment for pain (mandibular, face, or mouth)

   (c) Physical examination to assess teeth and gums for chronic wounds and repeat infections

(4) Documentation: Staging systems for osteoradionecrosis have been developed by Schwartz and Kagan (2002) and Notani et al. (2003).

   (a) The system developed by Schwartz and Kagan (2002) is based on clinical and radiologic findings.

   (b) Notani et al. (2003) divided the cases into three grades based on the extent of the osteoradionecrosis lesion (Chronopoulos et al., 2018).

      i. Grade I osteoradionecrosis is limited to alveolar bone.

      ii. Grade II osteoradionecrosis is limited to the alveolar bone and/or the mandible above the level of the mandibular alveolar canal.

      iii. Grade III osteoradionecrosis extends to the mandible under the level of the mandibular alveolar canal, and a skin fistula and/or a pathologic fracture is present.

(5) Collaborative management (acute and long term)

   (a) Prevention

      i. Despite efforts to reduce risk of oral complications, no standard of care exists for preventive dental care before RT in patients with head and neck cancer (Schuurhuis et al., 2015).

      ii. An ongoing multicenter, prospective cohort study found that the majority of participants in this head and neck cancer cohort presented with some level of dental disease at the start of RT, which may increase the risk of poor outcomes (Brennan et al., 2017).

      iii. Given the current findings of a high rate of carious teeth (37%) and peri-odontal disease (47%), a pre-RT dental assessment is needed to address active dental disease prior to the start of RT (Schuurhuis et al., 2015).

      iv. Patients should be referred to their dentist prior to RT for an overall assessment of the oral health and possible need for significant dental work or extractions.

      v. If dental extractions or significant dental work are needed, hyperbaric oxygen therapy can be used to decrease the risk of osteoradionecrosis.

      vi. Clinicians should ensure good oral care and prescribe fluoride toothpaste for prevention of caries.

      vii. Patients should maintain a well-balanced diet with good nutritional status (Nadella, Kodali, Guttikonda, & Jonnalagadda, 2015).

   (b) Medical intervention

      i. Pentoxifylline increases erythrocyte flexibility to optimize the microcirculatory flow and is tolerated clinically up to 60 weeks. It also has anti–TNF-α effects, causes vasodilation, inhibits human dermal fibroblast proliferation and extracellular matrix production, and increases collagenase activity.

      ii. Tocopherol is a fat-soluble antioxidant with vitamin E activity that protects cell membranes from lipid peroxidation and can inhibit transforming growth factor-β1 and procollagen gene expression (Fan et al., 2014).

      iii. Clodronate is a newer-generation, non-nitrogenous bisphosphonate that reduces osteoclast numbers and activity to minimize bone resorption, increases bone formation, and reduces the fibroblast proliferation (McCaul, 2014).

      iv. Glicksman, Khalili, Fung, Parnes, and Agrawal (2015) observed a clinical benefit after administering a combination of pentoxifylline, tocopherol, and clodronate therapy for osteoradionecrosis of the temporal bone.

      v. The addition of a bisphosphonate to a pentoxifylline and tocopherol regimen may provide an increased efficacy (Ceponis, Keilman, Guerry, & Freiberger, 2016; McLeod, Pratt, Mellor, & Brennan, 2012).

(c) Medical and surgical intervention

 i. Previous studies evaluated ultrasound to revascularize areas of osteoradionecrosis (Nadella et al., 2015).

 ii. The patients were treated with ultrasound (3 MHz, pulsed 1:4, 1 W/cm) for 40 sessions of 15 minutes per day (Nadella et al., 2015).

 iii. One study reported that 10 of 21 (48%) cases showed healing when treated with debridement and ultrasound alone; 11 cases remained unhealed after ultrasound therapy and after debridement were covered with a local flap; and only one case needed mandibular resection and reconstruction (Nadella et al., 2015).

 iv. The goal of hyperbaric oxygen in radiation tissue damage is to revascularize irradiated tissues and to improve the fibroblastic cellular density, thus limiting the amount of nonviable tissue to be surgically removed. This enhances wound healing and prepares the tissues for reconstruction when indicated.

 v. Marx and Ames first outlined a standard approach to the treatment of established osteonecrosis of the jaw with adjunctive hyperbaric oxygen therapy. They proposed an approach known as the Wilfred-Hall protocol, which consists of three stages (Kaur, Hay, Macdonald, & Rich, 2009).

  • Stage I: Therapy starts with 30 consecutive treatments. If the wound shows no definitive clinical improvement, a further 10 exposures are given (40 exposures). For failure to heal after three months, the patient is advanced to stage II.

  • Stage II: The exposed bone is removed by alveolar sequestrectomy, and 20 further treatments are given (60 exposures). If wound dehiscence or failure to heal occurs, the patient is advanced to stage III.

  • Stage III: The criteria for this category are failure of stage II, pathologic fracture, orocutaneous fistula, or radiographic evidence of resorption to the inferior border of the mandible.

 vi. Recommended management commences with the 30-exposure protocol, along with surgical resection to bleeding bone and bony reconstruction, followed by soft tissue coverage. An additional 10 treatments are recommended. If healing fails, additional surgery is performed and 10 further exposures to hyperbaric oxygen are given at that time (Strojan et al., 2017).

(d) Surgical intervention

 i. In advanced or refractory cases of osteoradionecrosis (pathologic fracture, orocutaneous fistula), surgical treatment, at present, remains the only treatment option available (Rice, Polyzois, Ekanayake, Omer, & Stassen, 2015).

 ii. Major advances in the surgical management of osteoradionecrosis are related to reconstructive surgery.

 iii. The use of myocutaneous flaps and microvascular free bone flaps have allowed for substantial modifications in the decision-making process of the extent of the surgical ablation of extensive osteoradionecrosis.

 iv. The replacement of the dead bone with a vascularized bone-containing flap will not only allow for restoration of the mandibular continuity but also bring nonirradiated soft tissue coverage with intact blood supply.

 v. Commonly used flaps are the fibular flap, ileac crest flap, and scapular-parascapular flaps (Nadella et al., 2015).

(6) Patient, caregiver, and family education

(a) Clinicians should stress the importance of ongoing meticulous oral hygiene and regular dental visits.

(b) Clinicians should inform patients of signs and symptoms to report (e.g., pain, swelling, repeat oral infections).

(c) Patients should have an oral surgeon or dentist contact the radiation oncologist prior to any significant dental work or extraction to obtain the radiation dose and recommendations.

i) Trismus

(1) Pathophysiology

(a) Trismus is a well-known complication defined as an inability to open the mouth or difficulty with mouth opening secondary to spasm of the muscles of mastication (Bensadoun et al., 2010).

(b) Maximal interincisal opening is the maximal distance between the edges of the

upper and lower incisors. In the general population, it is 40–60 mm. Measurements of 35 mm or less are considered to be trismus (Dijkstra, Huisman, & Roodenburg, 2006; Owosho et al., 2016).

(c) Significant trismus affects a patient's daily life functions, posing difficulty with eating, daily dental care, professional dental care, speech, pain, and overall general discomfort.

(d) Trismus affects the foods patients are able to eat as a result of decreased mouth opening and chewing abilities.

(e) Many are discouraged to eat socially because of the increased length of time needed to finish a meal.

(f) Patients are less compliant with dental care due to the pain and difficulty involved.

(2) Incidence and risk factors

(a) Reported incidences of trismus in patients with oral and oropharyngeal cancer treated with IMRT can be 4%–77.3% (Chao et al., 2004; Gomez et al., 2009; Hsieh et al., 2014; Ingle et al., 2010; Rao et al., 2015).

(b) The risk of developing trismus can be attributed to a multitude of factors—namely age and gender of the patient, tumor location, pre-RT maximal interincisal opening measurements, radiation dose to the primary tumor, and radiation doses to the muscles of mastication (Kamstra, Dijkstra, van Leeuwen, Roodenburg, & Langendijk, 2015; Lindblom et al., 2014; Rao et al., 2015; Teguh et al., 2008; van der Molen et al., 2013).

(c) Surgical intervention contributes to the risk of developing trismus.

(d) Post-treatment trismus is unpredictable in frequency and severity. It usually develops three to six months after RT and often becomes a lifelong problem.

(3) Assessment

(a) Clinical manifestations of trismus can include the following (Johnson et al., 2012; Owosho et al., 2016).

  i. Patients report experiencing stiffness and difficulty when opening the mouth wide.

  ii. Patients report difficulty and discomfort with chewing.

  iii. Patients change their diet or food choices to soft and liquid foods because of difficulty chewing.

  iv. Using the Gothenburg trismus questionnaire, five of eight patients with trismus reported significant changes in their quality of life. Patients with significant changes in their quality of life all reported moderate to very severe difficulty with feeding and jaw opening (Johnson et al., 2012).

(b) Physical examination in cases of trismus should take the following into account (Loh, Mcleod, & Elhassen, 2017).

  i. Normal mouth opening varies between individuals, within a range of 40–60 mm.

  ii. Men generally display greater mouth opening than women.

  iii. Maximal interincisal opening is widely used to objectively measure trismus.

  iv. For edentulous patients, the distance from one alveolar ridge to the opposing side vertically can be used instead.

(4) Documentation

(a) The severity of trismus can be classified into three grades measured by the maximal interincisal opening in adults (Wu & Lam, 2016).

  i. Grade 1: 40–25 mm

  ii. Grade 2: 25–10 mm

  iii. Grade 3: less than 10 mm

(b) Dijkstra et al. (2006) defined 35 mm as the functional cutoff point for trismus in patients with head and neck cancer, on the basis of significant mandibular function impairment and perceived restriction in mouth opening.

(c) A later study conducted by Scott, Butterworth, Lowe, and Rogers (2008) also supported this cutoff level (Wu & Lam, 2016).

(5) Collaborative prevention and management

(a) Prevention (Loh et al., 2017)

  i. Prevention of trismus is preferable to treating it.

  ii. As soon as they start RT, patients at risk of trismus should be given home exercises to maintain maximum mouth opening and jaw mobility.

(b) Physical therapy and exercise (Loh et al., 2017)

  i. Patients who develop trismus require an intensive exercise program, and if necessary, combined with physiotherapy to improve mouth opening.

  ii. Clinicians should collaborate with a physical therapist specializing in speech and swallowing before RT begins, throughout treatment, and after completion to provide continued assessment and specific exercises to the patient.

iii. Many products are available to treat trismus. Stacked tongue depressors can be used to encourage gradual opening without overstressing the fibrotic tissue.

(c) Medication

i. Medications, such as superoxide dismutase and pentoxifylline, mainly slow the progression of trismus or allow regression by reducing free radicals and improving vasculature in soft tissues, hence promoting the repair processes in injured tissues.

ii. Superoxide dismutase catalyzes free radicals, converting them to less active species to slow the radiation-induced damage in healthy tissues.

iii. Pentoxifylline has immunomodulatory properties that delay the progression of trismus by downregulating the production of cytokines, which account for the pathogenesis of radiation-induced fibrosis. Pentoxifylline can increase erythrocyte deformability for decreasing blood viscosity and increasing oxygen release from erythrocytes, hence improving microcirculation and tissue oxygenation, favoring the repair processes. A mean increase of at least 4 mm in maximal interincisal opening and symptomatic relief after RT in patients experiencing severe trismus have been reported (Wu & Lam, 2016).

(d) Clinicians should consult with an RDN or RD to evaluate overall diet and nutritional needs.

(6) Patient, caregiver, and family education (Wu & Lam, 2016)

(a) A physical therapist should teach and reinforce exercises prior to starting treatment.

(b) Clinicians should emphasize that prevention of trismus is the best course of management.

(c) Clinicians should instruct patients on the benefits and importance of compliance with exercises throughout treatment and afterward.

j) Shoulder mobility

(1) Pathophysiology (Eickmeyer et al., 2014)

(a) Shoulder dysfunction is common after neck dissection in head and neck cancer survivors and, as survival times increase, may contribute to significant morbidity in this population.

(b) Neck surgery can damage the spinal accessory nerve (cranial nerve XI) and denervate the trapezius and sternocleidomastoid muscles.

(c) Loss of muscle function can compromise shoulder movement and lead to secondary sequelae, such as adhesive capsulitis, rotator cuff impingement, and myofascial pain.

(d) Damage to the cervical plexus can cause neuropathic pain in the neck region, typically involving the C2–C4 dermatomes.

(e) All of these impairments may contribute to reduced range of motion, particularly abduction and flexion; lead to decreased performance of ADLs; and contribute to chronic pain.

(f) Subjective complaints of shoulder dysfunction and pain have a major effect on quality of life.

(2) Incidence and risk factors

(a) Up to 80% of patients with head and neck cancer treated with neck lymph node dissection experienced shoulder pain that led to impaired shoulder function. It is most profound in the patients that have been surgically treated with a radical neck or modified neck dissection (Wang et al., 2013).

(b) Shoulder range of motion and quality-of-life measures demonstrate the best function in patients not treated with surgery, intermediate function in those treated with nerve-sparing surgery, and the worst function in those treated with nerve-sacrificing surgery (Eickmeyer et al., 2014).

(c) Shoulder range of motion did not correlate with the presence or absence of RT (Eickmeyer et al., 2014).

(d) Age, previous injuries, presence of arthritis, and overall general health are also considerations.

(3) Assessment: Pretreatment assessment, along with shoulder range-of-motion measurements during and after treatment, should be performed by a physical therapist.

(4) Documentation (Wang et al., 2013)

(a) The full degree of motion should be documented: active and passive flexion, extension, abduction, adduction, and internal and external rotation.

(b) It has been noted that decreased shoulder mobility affects a patient's overall quality of life; therefore, documentation using a standardized quality-of-life assessment tool is recommended.

(5) Collaborative management (Wang et al., 2013)
 (a) Assessment by a physical therapist prior to treatment is essential. Treatment of shoulder mobility problems extends through cancer therapy and aftercare to survivorship.
 (b) Clinicians should identify barriers to adherence to exercises (e.g., lack of motivation, time constraints, emotional issue affecting ability to focus or remember, overall decreased physical condition) and assist patients to make necessary adjustments to overcome barriers.
(6) Patient, caregiver, and family education
 (a) Clinicians should provide resources for patients to locate and obtain the needed physical therapy.
 (b) Clinicians should stress the importance of adherence to ongoing physical therapy.
k) Hypothyroidism
 (1) Pathophysiology (Ling et al., 2016)
  (a) Treatment for head and neck cancers often includes radiation to the thyroid gland.
  (b) The absolute mechanism of thyroid dysfunction after RT in head and neck cancer is not fully understood, but possible causes include fibrosis of thyroid glandular cells, abnormal vascular proliferation, and autoimmune dysfunction of the thyroid gland.
 (2) Incidence and risk factors
  (a) Though hypothyroidism affects 5%–10% of the general population, those who have received head and neck RT are at an increased risk (Sandoni, Rodolico, Pappalardo, Portaro, & Benvenga, 2016).
  (b) Risk factors for hypothyroidism include use of chemotherapy and female sex. Increased age is an independent risk factor (Ling et al., 2016).
  (c) Although a radiation dose of 30 Gy to the thyroid is generally accepted as a risk factor for developing hypothyroidism, controversial study results have not clarified what dose is directly associated with increased incidence (Laway et al., 2012).
  (d) A transient change in thyroid function may occur and resolve within the first three months, thus not representing an accurate permanent abnormality (Laway et al., 2012).
  (e) Although hypothyroidism is the most commonly seen thyroid dysfunction after treatment, clinicians should be aware that hyperthyroidism has also developed (Ling et al., 2016).

(3) Assessment
 (a) Thyroid-stimulating hormone levels are used to diagnose primary hypothyroidism.
 (b) Patients who received RT to the thyroid gland should have their thyroid-stimulating hormone levels checked every 6–12 months after treatment (Haddad & Limaye, 2019).
 (c) Signs and symptoms of hypothyroid may include, but are not limited to, fatigue, weight gain, cold intolerance, dry skin, constipation, or myalgias (Gaitonde, Rowley, & Sweeney, 2012).
(4) Documentation: CTCAE can be used as a standardized documentation source (NCI CTEP, 2017, p. 15).
 (a) Grade 1: asymptomatic; clinical or diagnostic observations only; intervention not indicated
 (b) Grade 2: symptomatic; thyroid replacement indicated; limiting instrumental ADL
 (c) Grade 3: severe symptoms; limiting self-care ADL; hospitalization indicated
 (d) Grade 4: life-threatening consequences; urgent intervention indicated
 (e) Grade 5: death
(5) Collaborative management: Pharmacologic thyroid hormone replacement therapy, thyroxine, is usually needed for life. Nurses should know the signs and symptoms of hypothyroidism and assess for and document medication adherence at follow-up visits (Gaitonde et al., 2012).
(6) Patient, caregiver, and family education: Patients should be educated to take the medication on an empty stomach (Gaitonde et al., 2012).
l) Vascular changes
 (1) Pathophysiology
  (a) There is evidence to support that head and neck RT is a risk factor for developing carotid artery disease that may result in carotid injury, stenosis, and transient ischemic attacks.
  (b) This increased risk may result from stenosis of the artery, damage to the intima–media layer (thus accelerating atherosclerosis), or damage to the adventitia layer (causing change in normal blood supply) (Plummer, Henderson, O'Sullivan, & Read, 2011).
  (c) With these changes comes an increased risk for ischemic stroke, which occurs when thrombus restricts blood flow and oxygen to the brain.

(d) Occlusion results in irreversible cell death within the brain (Galloway & Lakin, 2017).

(2) Incidence and risk factors

   (a) The extent to which ischemic stroke may affect this population is largely unknown, likely because variations in study design, but estimates suggest risk of 1%–10%. Other large studies found that 12%–19% of patients are at increased risk, and still others suggest up to 50% of patients are at increased risk (Arthurs, Hanna, Zaza, Peng, & Hall, 2016; Smith et al., 2008).

   (b) Patients treated with RT alone had a 70% higher risk of ischemic stroke, compared to surgery alone (Arthurs et al., 2016).

   (c) A large study of 6,862 patients with head and neck cancer found the 10-year incidence of cardiovascular-related events to be 34% in those treated with definitive RT and 25% in those treated with surgery and RT (Smith et al., 2008).

   (d) HPV status may be an independent risk factor for development of ischemic stroke or a transient ischemic attack after treatment. With the prevalence of HPV-related head and neck cancers on the rise, further investigation of HPV-status as it relates to risk for stroke is needed (Addison et al., 2017).

   (e) Risk for ischemic stroke is highest in those with risk factors, such as smoking, alcohol use, diabetes, atrial fibrillation, dyslipidemia, sedentary lifestyle, poor diet, hypertension, and obesity. Nonmodifiable risk factors include advanced age, male sex, lower socioeconomic status, and Afro-Caribbean and Asian ethnicity (Galloway & Lakin, 2017).

(3) Assessment (Galloway & Lakin, 2017; Smith et al., 2008)

   (a) Studies have suggested screening for asymptomatic carotid stenosis is cost-effective.

   (b) Means for surveillance include routine carotid bruit assessment and imaging (CT angiography, MRI, or ultrasound) in the years following treatment.

   (c) Patients should be assessed for hypertension, diabetes, dyslipidemia, atrial fibrillation, smoking, alcohol use, sedentary lifestyle, poor diet, hypertension, obesity, and adherence to medications during routine office visits.

(4) Documentation: A medication compliance assessment, thorough history, and neurologic assessment should be documented.

(5) Collaborative management and education

   (a) Prevention of vascular issues through education and healthy lifestyle is key.

   (b) Patients, caregivers, and family should be educated on modifiable risk factors and lifestyle recommendations (Galloway & Lakin, 2017).

     i. Reducing saturated fat

     ii. Limiting alcohol, processed foods, and sugary drinks

     iii. Consuming less than 6 g salt per day

     iv. Exercising at least 150 minutes per week

     v. Consuming five portions of fruits and vegetables per day

     vi. Smoking cessation

   (c) Patients, caregivers, and family should be educated on the signs of an ischemic stroke (Internet Stroke Center, 2019).

     i. Weakness on one side of the body

     ii. Sudden numbness on one side of the body

     iii. Sudden confusion or trouble speaking

     iv. Sudden dizziness and loss of coordination

     v. Sudden severe headache

     vi. Sudden trouble seeing

m) Lhermitte sign and transient radiation myelopathy

(1) Pathophysiology

   (a) Lhermitte sign is a transient, often painful sensory phenomenon that is described as an electric shock traveling down the back and into the arms and legs when flexing the neck.

   (b) Although the underlying pathophysiology is not well understood, it is thought to occur because of demyelination of the cervical nerves in those who have been treated with head and neck RT (Teoli, Cabrero, & Ghassemzadeh, 2019).

   (c) The demyelinated axons are sensitive to irritation from neck flexion, causing ascending sensory shock sensation (Pak, Vineberg, Feng, Ten Haken, & Eisbruch, 2012).

(2) Risk factors and incidence

   (a) Incidence ranges 3.6%–21% in patients with head and neck cancer treated with RT (Pak et al., 2012).

   (b) Risk factors may include unilateral neck irradiation and radiation dose greater than 30 Gy to the spinal cord. History of diabetes did not appear to be a risk factor, but evidence is variable between studies (Laidley et al., 2018).

(3) Assessment
  (a) Although Lhermitte sign is referred to as a "sign," it is a symptom that a patient may report.
  (b) The best assessment is to inquire if a patient feels a shock-like sensation when flexing the neck (Teoli et al., 2019).
(4) Collaborative management
  (a) Specifically within the post-RT head and neck cancer population, there is no known cure.
  (b) Gabapentin or carbamazepine may decrease the severity of symptoms (Teoli et al., 2019).
  (c) A neck brace or collar can be used to reduce exacerbation of symptoms because Lhermitte sign is worsened with neck movement.
  (d) Deep breathing, muscle relaxation, and active and passive stretching may offer some relief.
(5) Patient, caregiver, and family education: Patients who develop Lhermitte sign should be educated that, in many cases, the symptoms are self-limiting and resolve within 12 months (Khare & Seth, 2015).

References

Addison, D., Seidelmann, S.B., Janjua, S.A., Emami, H., Staziaki, P.V., Hallett, T.R., ... Neilan, T.G. (2017). Human papillomavirus status and the risk of cerebrovascular events following radiation therapy for head and neck cancer. *Journal of the American Heart Association, 6,* e006453. https://doi.org/10.1161/JAHA.117.006453

Amin, M.B., Edge, S., Greene, F., Byrd, D.R., Brookland, R.K., Washington, M.K., ... Gershenwald, J.E. (Eds.). (2018). *AJCC cancer staging manual* (8th ed.). Springer.

Arthurs, E., Hanna, T.P., Zaza, K., Peng, Y., & Hall, S.F. (2016). Stroke after radiation therapy for head and neck cancer: What is the risk? *International Journal of Radiation Oncology, Biology, Physics, 96,* 589–596. https://doi.org/10.1016/j.ijrobp.2016.07.007

Bensadoun, R.-J., Risenbeck, D., Lockhart, P.B., Elting, R.S., Spijkervert, F.K.L., & Brennen, M.T. (2010). A systematic view of trismus induced by cancer therapies in head and neck cancer patients. *Supportive Care in Cancer, 18,* 133–138. https://doi.org/10.1007/s00520-010-0847-4

Brennan, M.T., Treister, N.S., Sollecito, T.P., Schmidt, B.L., Patton, L.L., Mohammadi, K., ... Lalla, R.V. (2017). Dental disease before radiotherapy in patients with head and neck cancer: Clinical registry of dental outcomes in head and neck cancer patients. *Journal of the American Dental Association, 148,* 868–877. https://doi.org/10.1016/j.adaj.2017.09.011

Candotto, V., Gargari, M., Gaudio, R.M., Cura, F., Baggi, L., Arcuri, C., ... Carinci, F. (2018). HPV related head and neck carcinoma: A short literature review on treatments. *ORAL and Implantology, 11,* 72–76. https://www.oimplantology.org/index.php?PAGE=articolo_dett&ID_ISSUE=1008&id_article=8603

Centers for Disease Control and Prevention. (2019). United States cancer statistics: Data visualizations. http://www.cdc.gov/cancer/dataviz

Ceponis, P., Keilman, C., Guerry, C., & Freiberger, J.J. (2016). Hyperbaric oxygen therapy and osteonecrosis. *Oral Diseases, 23,* 141–151. https://doi.org/10.1111/odi.12489

Chao, K.S.C., Ozyigit, G., Blanco, A.I., Thorstad, W.L., Deasy, J.O., Haughey, B.H., ... Sessions, D., (2004). Intensity-modulated radiation therapy for oropharyngeal carcinoma: Impact of tumor volume. *International Journal of Radiation Oncology, Biology, Physics, 59,* 43–50. https://doi.org/10.1016/j.ijrobp.2003.08.004

Chronopoulos, A., Zarra, T., Ehrenfeld, M., & Otto, S. (2018). Osteoradionecrosis of the jaws: Definition, epidemiology, staging and clinical and radiological findings. A concise review. *International Dental Journal, 68,* 22–30. https://doi.org/10.1111/idj.12318

Craig, J., Tomlinson, C., Stevens, K., Kotagal, K., Fornadley, J., Jacobson, B., ... Francis, D.O. (2015). Combining voice therapy and physical therapy: A novel approach to treating muscle tension dysphonia. *Journal of Communication Disorders, 58,* 169–178. https://doi.org/10.1016/j.jcomdis.2015.05.001

da Silva, L., Kupek, E., & Peres, K.G. (2017). General health influences episodes of xerostomia: A prospective population-based study. *Community Dentistry and Oral Epidemiology, 45,* 153–159. https://doi.org/10.1111/cdoe.12271

De Felice, F., de Vincentiis, M., Luzzi, V., Magliulo, G., Tombolini, M., Ruoppolo, G., & Polimeni, A. (2018). Late radiation-associated dysphagia in head and neck cancer patients: Evidence, research and management. *Oral Oncology, 77,* 125–130. https://doi.org/10.1016/j.oraloncology.2017.12.021

De Felice, F., Musio, D., & Tombolini, V. (2015). Osteoradionecrosis: An old toxicity in the EMRT era? *Oral Oncology, 51,* e60–e61. https://doi.org/10.1016/j.oraloncology.2015.03.002

Denaro, N., Merlano, M.C., & Russi, E.G. (2013). Dysphagia in head and neck cancer patients: Pretreatment evaluation, predictive factors, and assessment during radio-chemotherapy, recommendations. *Clinical and Experimental Otorhinolaryngology, 6,* 117–126. https://doi.org/10.3342/ceo.2013.6.3.117

Deshpande, T.S., Blanchard, P., Wang, L., Foote, R.L., Zhang, X., & Frank, S.J. (2018). Radiation-related alterations of taste function in patients with head and neck cancer: A systematic review. *Current Treatment Options in Oncology, 19,* 72. https://doi.org/10.1007/s11864-018-0580-7

de Souza Tolentino, E., Stuchi Centurion, B., Caetano Ferreira, L.H., Pereira de Souza, A., Damante, J.H., & Rubira-Bullen, I.R.F. (2011). Oral adverse effects of head and neck radiotherapy: Literature review and suggestion of a clinical oral care guideline for irradiated patients. *Journal of Applied Oral Science, 19,* 448–454. https://doi.org/10.1590/s1678-77572011000500003

Devi, S., & Singh, N. (2014). Dental care during and after radiotherapy in head and neck cancer. *National Journal of Maxillofacial Surgery, 5,* 117–125. https://doi.org/10.4103/0975-5950.154812

Dijkstra, P.U., Huisman, P.M., & Roodenburg, J.L.N. (2006). Criteria for trismus in head and neck oncology. *International Journal of Oral and Maxillofacial Surgery, 35,* 337–342. https://doi.org/10.1016/j.ijom.2005.08.001

Eickmeyer, S.M., Walczak, C.K., Myers, K.B., Lindstrom, D.R., Layde, P., & Campbell, B.H. (2014). Quality of life, shoulder range of motion, and spinal accessory nerve status in 5-year survivors of head and neck cancer. *PM&R, 6,* 1073–1080. https://doi.org/10.1016/j.pmrj.2014.05.015

Eilers, J.G., Asakura, Y., Blecher, C.S., Burgoon, D., Chiffelle, R., Ciccolini, K., ... Valinski, S. (2019). Symptom interventions: Mucositis. https://www.ons.org/pep/mucositis

Einarsson, S., Laurell, G., & Ehrsson, Y.T. (2019). Experiences and coping strategies related to food and eating up to two years after the termination of treatment in patients with head and neck cancer. *European Journal of Cancer Care, 28,* e12964. https://doi.org/10.1111/ecc.12964

Fan, H., Kim, S.M., Cho, Y.J., Eo, M.Y., Lee, S.K., & Woo, K.M. (2014). New approach for the treatment of osteoradionecrosis with pentoxifylline and tocopherol. *Biomaterials Research, 18,* 13. https://doi.org/10.1186/2055-7124-18-13

Francis, D.O., Daniero, J.J., Hovis, K.L., Sathe, N., Jacobson, B., Penson, D.F., ... McPheeters, M.L. (2017). Voice-related patient-reported outcome measures: A systematic review of instrument development and validation. *Journal of Speech, Language, and Hearing Research, 60,* 62–88. https://doi.org/10.1044/2016_jslhr-s-16-0022

Gaitonde, D.Y., Rowley, K.D., & Sweeney, L.B. (2012). Hypothyroidism: An update. *American Family Physician, 86,* 244–251. https://www.aafp.org/afp/2012/0801/p244.html

Galloway, T., & Lakin, A. (2017). Assessing and tackling risk factors for stroke. *Practice Nurse, 47*(6), 32–37.

Glicksman, J.T., Khalili, S., Fung, K., Parnes, L.S., & Agrawal, S.K. (2015). Pentoxifylline-tocopherol-clodronate combination: A novel treatment for osteoradionecrosis of the temporal bone. *Head and Neck, 37,* E191–E193. https://doi.org/10.1002/hed.24057

Gomez, D.R., Zhung, J.E., Gomez, J., Chan, K., Wu, A.J., Wolden, S.L., ... Lee, N.Y. (2009). Intensity-modulated radiotherapy in postoperative treatment of oral cavity cancers. *International Journal of Radiation Oncology, Biology, Physics, 73,* 1096–1103. https://doi.org/10.1016/j.ijrobp.2008.05.024

Haddad, R., & Limaye, S. (2019). Overview of approach to long-term survivors of head and neck cancer. In S. Shaw (Ed.), *UpToDate.* Retrieved March 23, 2020, from https://www.uptodate.com/contents/overview-of-approach-to-long-term-survivors-of-head-and-neck-cancer

Hajisafari, A., Bakhshandeh, M., Aghamiri, S.M.R., Houshyari, M., Rakhsha, A., Bolokat, E.R., & Rezazadeh, A. (2018). Prospective evaluation of the early effects of radiation on the auditory system frequencies of patients with head and neck cancers and brain tumors after radiotherapy. *Ear, Nose and Throat Journal, 97*(3), E10–E17.

Havle, A.D., Ahmed, M.D.F., Vihapure, G.M., Khairmode, G.S., & Tripti. (2019). Evaluation of sensorineural hearing loss as a consequence of conventional radiotherapy in head and neck cancer. *Journal of Clinical and Diagnostic Research, 13,* MC01–MC04. https://www.jcdr.net/article_abstract.asp?issn=0973-709x&year=2019&volume=13&issue=2&page=MC01&issn=0973-709x&id=12632

Head, eyes, and ears. (2014). In *Bates' visual guide to physical examination.* Wolters Kluwer. https://batesvisualguide.com/multimedia.aspx?categoryId=21787#21774

Hsieh, L.-C., Chen, J.W., Wang, L.-Y., Tsang, Y.-M., Shueng, P.-W., Liao, L.-J., ... Hsieh, C.-H. (2014). Predicting the severity and prognosis of trismus after intensity-modulated radiation therapy for oral cancer patients by magnetic resonance imaging. *PLOS ONE, 9,* e92561. https://doi.org/10.1371/journal.pone.0092561

Ingle, C.J., Yip, K., Caskie, V., Dyson, C., Ford, A., & Scrase, C.D. (2010). Intensity modulated radiotherapy (IMRT) in the management of locally advanced oropharyngeal squamous cell carcinomata (SCC): Disease control and functional outcome using the therapy outcome measure (TOM) score—Report from a single U.K. institution. *Head and Neck Oncology, 28.* https://doi.org/10.1186/1758-3284-2-28

Internet Stroke Center. (2019). Warning signs. http://www.strokecenter.org/patients/about-stroke/warning-signs-of-stroke

Johnson, J., Carlsson, S., Johansson, M., Pauli, N., Rydén, A., Fagerberg-Mohlin, B., & Finizia, C. (2012). Development and validation of the Gothenburg trismus questionnaire (GTQ). *Oral Oncology, 8,* 730–736. https://doi.org/10.1016/j.oraloncology.2012.02.013

Kamal, M., Rosenthal, D.I., Volpe, S., Goepfert, R.P., Garden, A.S., Hutcheson, K.A., ... Gunn, G.B. (2018). Patient reported dry mouth: Instrument comparison and model performance for correlation with quality of life in head and neck cancer survivors. *Radiotherapy and Oncology, 126,* 75–80. https://doi.org/10.1016/j.radonc.2017.10.037

Kamstra, J.I., Dijkstra, P.U., van Leeuwen, M., Roodenburg, J.L.N., & Langendijk, J.A. (2015). Mouth opening in patients irradiated for head and neck cancer: A prospective repeated measures study. *Oral Oncology, 5,* 548–555. https://doi.org/10.1016/j.oraloncology.2015.01.016

Kaur, J., Hay, K.D., Macdonald, H., & Rich, A.M. (2009). Retrospective audit of the use of the Marx protocol for prophylactic hyperbaric oxygen therapy in managing patients requiring dental extractions following radiotherapy to the head and neck. *New Zealand Dental Journal, 105*(2), 47–50.

Kershaw, J.C., & Mattes, R.D. (2018). Nutrition and taste and smell dysfunction. *World Journal of Otorhinolaryngology—Head and Neck Surgery, 4,* 3–10. https://doi.org/10.1016/j.wjorl.2018.02.006

Khare, A., & Seth, D. (2015). Lhermitte's sign: The current status. *Annals of Indian Academy of Neurology, 18,* 154–156. https://doi.org/10.4103/0972-2327.150622

Kim, R.H.-K., Yang, P., & Sung, E.C. (2016). Managing intraoral lesions in oral cancer patients in a general dental practice: An overview. *Journal of the California Dental Association, 44*(2), 85–92.

Laidley, H.M., Noble, D.J., Barnett, G.C., Forman, J.R., Bates, A.M., Benson, R.J., ... Burnet, N.G. (2018). Identifying risk factors for L'hermitte's sign after IMRT for head and neck cancer. *Radiation Oncology, 13,* 84. https://doi.org/10.1186/s13014-018-1015-0

Laway, B.A., Shai, K.M., Majid, S., Lone, M.M., Afroz, F., Khan, S., & Roohi, R. (2012). Incidence of primary hypothyroidism in patients exposed to therapeutic external beam radiation, where radiation portals include a part or whole of the thyroid gland. *Indian Journal of Endocrinology and Metabolism, 16*(Suppl. 2), S329–S331.

Lee, J.S., Choi, H.G., Jang, J.H., Sim, S., Hong, S.K., Lee, H.-J., ... Kim, H.-J. (2015). Analysis of predisposing factors for hearing loss in adults. *Journal of Korean Medical Science, 30,* 1175–1182. https://doi.org/10.3346/jkms.2015.30.8.1175

Lindblom, U., Gärskog, O., Kjellén, E., Laurell, G., Jaghagen, E.L., Wahlberg, P., ... Nilsson, P. (2014). Radiation-induced trismus in the ARTSCAN head and neck trial. *Acta Oncologica, 5,* 620–627. https://doi.org/10.3109/0284186x.2014.892209

Ling, S., Bhatt, A.D., Brown, N.V., Nguyen, P., Sipos, J.A., Chakravarti, A., & Rong, Y. (2016). Correlative study of dose to thyroid and incidence of subsequent dysfunction after head and neck radiation. *Head and Neck, 39,* 538. https://doi.org/10.1002/hed.24643

Logemann, J.A., & Larsen, K. (2012). Oropharyngeal dysphagia: Pathophysiology and diagnosis for the anniversary issue of *Diseases of the Esophagus. Diseases of the Esophagus, 25,* 299–304. https://doi.org/10.1111/j.1442-2050.2011.01210.x

Loh, S.Y., Mcleod, R.W.J., & Elhassan, H.A. (2017). Trismus following different treatment modalities for head and neck cancer: A systematic review of subjective measures. *European Archives of Oto-Rhino-Laryngology, 274,* 2695–2707. https://doi.org/10.1007/s00405-017-4519-6

Lydiatt, W.M., Patel, S.G., O'Sullivan, B., Brandwein, M.S., Ridge, J.A., Migliacci, J.C., ... Shah, J. (2017). Head and neck cancers—Major changes in American Joint Committee on Cancer eighth edition Cancer Staging Manual. *CA: A Cancer Journal for Clinicians, 67,* 122–137. https://doi.org/10.3322/caac.21389

Maria, O.M., Eliopoulos, N., & Muanza, T. (2017). Radiation-induced oral mucositis. *Frontiers in Oncology, 7,* 89. https://doi.org/10.3389/fonc.2017.00089

McCaul, J.A. (2014). Pharmacologic modalities in the treatment of osteoradionecrosis of the jaw. *Oral and Maxillofacial Surgery Clinics of North America, 26,* 247–252. https://doi.org/10.1016/j.coms.2014.02.002

McLelland, S., III, Andrews, J.Z., Chaudry, H., Teckie, S., & Goenka, A. (2018). Prophylactic versus reactive gastrostomy tube placement in advanced head and neck cancer treatment with definitive chemoradiotherapy: A systematic review. *Oral Oncology, 87,* 77–81. https://doi.org/10.1016/j.oraloncology.2018.10.028

McLeod, N.M., Pratt, C.A., Mellor, T.K., & Brennan, P.A. (2012). Pentoxifylline and tocopherol in the management of patients with osteoradionecrosis, the Portsmouth experience. *British Journal of Oral Maxillofacial Surgery, 50,* 41–44. https://doi.org/10.1016/j.bjoms.2010.11.017

MD Anderson Head and Neck Cancer Symptom Working Group. (2017). Dose-volume correlates of mandibular osteoradionecrosis in oropharynx cancer patients receiving intensity-modulated radiotherapy: Results from a case-matched comparison. *Radiotherapy and Oncology, 124,* 232–239. https://doi.org/10.1016/j.radonc.2017.06.026

Melchers, L.J., Van Weert, E., Beurskens, C.H.G., Reintsema, H., Slagter, A.P., Roodenburg, J.L., & Dijkstra, P.U. (2009). Exercise adherence in patients with trismus due to head and neck oncology: A qualitative study into the use of the Therabite®. *International Journal of Oral Maxillofacial Surgery, 3,* 947–954. https://doi.org/10.1016/j.ijom.2009.04.003

Memtsa, P.-T., Tolia, M., Tzitzikas, I., Bizakis, J., Pitevou-Gombaki, K., Charalambidou, M., ... Kyrgias, G. (2017). Assessment of xerostomia and its impact on quality of life in head and neck cancer patients undergoing radiation therapy. *Molecular and Clinical Oncology, 6,* 789–793. https://doi.org/10.3892/mco.2017.1200

Mifsud, M., Eskander, A., Irish, J., Gullane, P., Gilbert, R., Brown, D., ... Goldstein, D. (2017). Evolving trends in head and neck cancer epidemiology:

Ontario, Canada 1993–2010. *Head and Neck, 39.* https://doi.org/10.1002/hed.24829

Moayer, R., & Sinha, U. (2013). Dysphagia in head and neck cancer: A review. *Open Journal of Stomatology, 3,* 486–491. https://doi.org/10.4236/ojst.2013.39079

Mulcahy, N. (2018, August 23). CDC: Top HPV-associated cancer is now oropharyngeal. https://www.medscape.com/viewarticle/901122

Nadella, K.R., Kodali, R.M., Guttikonda, L.K., & Jonnalagadda, A. (2015). Osteoradionecrosis of the jaws: Clinico-therapeutic management: A literature review and update. *Journal of Maxillofacial and Oral Surgery, 14,* 891–901. https://doi.org/10.1007/s12663-015-0762-9

National Cancer Institute. (2019, May 16). Drugs approved for head and neck cancer. https://www.cancer.gov/about-cancer/treatment/drugs/head-neck

National Cancer Institute Cancer Therapy Evaluation Program. (2017). *Common terminology criteria for adverse events* [v.5.0]. https://ctep.cancer.gov/protocoldevelopment/electronic_applications/docs/CTCAE_v5_Quick_Reference_8.5x11.pdf

Nguyen, H.M., Reyland, M.E., & Barlow, L.A. (2012). Mechanisms of taste bud cell loss after head and neck irradiation. *Journal of Neuroscience, 32,* 3474–3484. https://doi.org/10.1523/jneurosci.4167-11.2012

Notani, K.-I., Yamazaki, Y., Kitada, H., Sakakibara, N., Fukuda, H., Omori, K., & Nakamura, M. (2003). Management of mandibular osteoradionecrosis corresponding to the severity of osteoradionecrosis and the method of radiotherapy. *Head and Neck, 25,* 181–186. https://doi.org/10.1002/hed.10171

Nugent, B., Parker, M.J., & McIntyre, I.A. (2010). Nasogastric tube feeding and percutaneous endoscopic tube feeding in patients with head and neck cancer. *Journal of Human Nutrition and Dietetics, 23,* 277–284. https://doi.org/10.1111/j.1365-277X.2010.01047.x

Oosterloo, B.C., Homans, N.C., de Jong, R.J.B., Ikram, M.A., Nagtegaal, A.P., & Goedegebure, A. (2020). Assessing hearing loss in older adults with a single question and person characteristics: Comparison with pure tone audiometry in the Rotterdam Study. *PLOS ONE, 15,* e0228349. https://doi.org/10.1371/journal.pone.0228349

Owosho, A.A., Pedreira Ramalho, L.M., Rosenberg, H.I., Yom, S.K., Drill, E., Riedel, E., ... Estilo, C.L. (2016). Objective assessment of trismus in oral and oropharyngeal cancer patients treated with intensity-modulated radiation therapy (IMRT). *Journal of Cranio-Maxillofacial Surgery, 44,* 1408–1413. https://doi.org/10.1016/j.jcms.2016.06.008

Pak, D., Vineberg, K., Feng, F., Ten Haken, R.K., & Eisbruch, A. (2012). Lhermitte sign after chemo-IMRT of head-and-neck cancer: Incidence, doses, and potential mechanisms. *International Journal of Radiation Oncology, Biology, Physics, 83,* 1528–1533. https://doi.org/10.1016/j.ijrobp.2011.10.052

Patel, D.A., Sharda, R., Hovis, K.L., Nichols, E.E., Sathe, N., Penson, D.F., ... Francis, D.O. (2017). Patient-reported outcome measures in dysphagia: A systematic review of instrument development and validation. *Diseases of the Esophagus, 30*(5), 1–23. https://doi.org/10.1093/dote/dow028

Pinna, R., Campus, G., Cumbo, E., Mura, I., & Milia, E. (2015). Xerostomia induced by radiotherapy: An overview of the physiopathology, clinical evidence, and management of the oral damage. *Therapeutics and Clinical Risk Management, 11,* 171–188. https://doi.org/10.2147/tcrm.s70652

Plummer, C., Henderson, R., O'Sullivan, J.D., & Read, S.J. (2011). Ischemic stroke and transient ischemic attack after head and neck radiotherapy: A review. *Stroke, 42,* 2410–2418. https://doi.org/10.1161/STROKEAHA.111.615203

Rao, S.D., Saleh, Z.H., Setton, J., Tam, M., McBride, S.M., Riaz, N., ... Lee, N.Y. (2015). Dose-volume factors correlating with trismus following chemoradiation for head and neck cancer. *Acta Oncologica, 55,* 99–104. https://doi.org/10.3109/0284186x.2015.1037864

Rapidis, A.D., Dijkstra, P.U., Roodenburg, J.L.N., Rodrigo, J.P., Rinaldo, A., Strojan, P., ... Ferlito, A. (2015). Trismus in patients with head and neck cancer: Etiopathogenesis, diagnosis and management. *Clinical Otolaryngology, 40,* 516–526. https://doi.org/10.1111/coa.12488

Reddy, S.S., & Priyadharshini, R. (2017). Oropharyngeal dysphagia: Understanding the etiology. *Journal of Otolaryngology Research, 1*(1), 115. https://www.scientificliterature.org/otolaryngology-volume1issue1.html

Reiter, R., Hoffman, T., Pickhard, A., & Brosch, S. (2015). Hoarseness—Causes and treatments. *Deutsches Ärzteblatt International, 112,* 329–337. https://doi.org/10.3238/arztebl.2015.0329

Rice, N., Polyzois, I., Ekanayake, K., Omer, O., & Stassen, L.F.A. (2015). The management of osteoradionecrosis of the jaws—A review. *Surgeon, 13,* 101–109. https://doi.org/10.1016/j.surge.2014.07.003

Rinkel, R.N., Verdonck-de Leeuw, I.M., Doornaert, P., Buter, J., de Bree, R., Langendijk, J.A., ... Leemans, C.R. (2016). Prevalence of swallowing and speech problems in daily life after chemoradiation for head and neck cancer based on cut-off scores of the patient-reported outcome measures SWAL-QOL and SHI. *European Archives of Oto-Rhino-Laryngology, 273,* 1849–1855. https://doi.org/10.1007/s00405-015-3680-z

Sandoni, A., Rodolico, C., Pappalardo, M.A., Portaro, S., & Benvenga, S. (2016). Hypothyroid myopathy: A peculiar clinical presentation of thyroid failure. Review of the literature. *Reviews in Endocrine and Metabolic Disorders, 17,* 499–519. https://doi.org/10.1007/s11154-016-9357-0

Schmitt, N.C., & Page, B.R. (2017). Chemoradiation-induced hearing loss remains a major concern for head and neck cancer patients. *International Journal of Audiology, 57*(Suppl. 4), S48–S53. https://doi.org/10.1080/14992027.2017.1353710

Schuurhuis, J.M., Stokman, M.A., Witjes, M.J.H., Dijkstra, P.U., Vissink, A., & Spijkervet, F.K.L. (2015). Evidence supporting pre-radiation elimination of oral foci of infection in head and neck cancer patients to prevent oral sequelae. A systematic review. *Oral Oncology, 51,* 212–220. https://doi.org/10.1016/j.oraloncology.2014.11.017

Schwartz, H.C., & Kagan, A.R. (2002). Osteoradionecrosis of the mandible: Scientific basis for clinical staging. *American Journal of Clinical Oncology, 25,* 68–171. https://doi.org/10.1097/00000421-200204000-00013

Scott, B., Butterworth, C., Lowe, D., & Rogers, S.N. (2008). Factors associated with restricted mouth opening and its relationship to health-related quality of life in patients attending a maxillofacial oncology clinic. *Oral Oncology, 44,* 430–438. https://doi.org/10.1016/j.oraloncology.2007.06.015

Selby, M. (2011). Assessing the ear. *Practice Nurse, 41*(14), 40–45.

Smith, G.L., Smith, B.D., Buchholz, T.A., Giordano, S.H., Garden, A.S., Woodward, W.A., ... Rosenthal, D.I. (2008). Cerebrovascular disease risk in older head and neck cancer patients after radiotherapy. *Journal of Clinical Oncology, 26,* 5119–5125. https://doi.org/10.1200/jco.2008.16.6546

Sroussi, H.Y., Epstein, J.B., Bensadoun, R.-J., Saunders, D.P., Lalla, R.V., Migliorati, C.A., ... Zumsteg, Z.S. (2017). Common oral complications of head and neck cancer radiation therapy: Mucositis, infections, saliva change, fibrosis, sensory dysfunctions, dental caries, periodontal disease, and osteoradionecrosis. *Cancer Medicine, 6,* 2918–2931. https://doi.org/10.1002/cam4.1221

Strojan, P., Hutcheson, K.A., Eisbruch, A., Beitler, J.J., Langendijk, J.A., Lee, A.W.M., ... Ferlito, A. (2017). Treatment of late sequelae after radiotherapy for head and neck cancer. *Cancer Treatment Reviews, 59,* 79–92. https://doi.org/10.1016/j.ctrv.2017.07.003

Tao, Z., Gao, J., Qian, L., Huang, Y., Zhou, Y., Yang, L., ... Zhang, Y. (2017). Factors associated with acute oral mucosal reaction induced by radiotherapy in head and neck squamous cell carcinoma: A retrospective single-center experience. *Medicine, 96,* e8446. https://doi.org/10.1097/md.0000000000008446

Tariq, A., Jamshaid, M., & Majeed, I. (2015). Xerostomia: Post radiation management strategies. *International Journal of Pharmaceutical Research and Allied Sciences, 4*(3), 35–47. https://ijpras.com/en/article/xerostomia-post-radiation-management-strategies

Teguh, D.N., Levendag, P.C., Voet, P., van der Est, H., Noever, I., de Kruijf, W., ... Heijman, B. (2008). Trismus in patients with oropharyngeal cancer: Relationship with dose in structures of mastication apparatus. *Head and Neck, 30,* 622–630. https://doi.org/10.1002/hed.20760

Teoli, D., Cabrero, F.R., & Ghassemzadeh, S. (2019). Lhermitte sign. *StatPearls.* https://www.ncbi.nlm.nih.gov/books/NBK493237

Turner, L., Mupparapu, M., & Akintoye, S.O. (2013). Review of the complications associated with treatment of oropharyngeal cancer: A guide for the dental practitioner. *Quintessence International, 44,* 267–279. https://doi.org/10.3290/j.qi.a29050

U.S. Food and Drug Administration. (2018, October 5). FDA approves expanded use of Gardasil 9 to include individuals 27 through 45 years old [Press release]. https://www.fda.gov/newsevents/newsroom/pressannouncements/ucm622715.htm

U.S. Food and Drug Administration. (2020, February 21). Gardasil. https://www.fda.gov/vaccines-blood-biologics/vaccines/gardasil-9

U.S. Preventive Services Task Force. (2013). Screening for hearing loss in older adults: Recommendation statement from USPSTF. (2013). *American Family Physician, 87*(2). https://www.aafp.org/afp/2013/0115/od1.html

van der Linden, N.C., Kok, A., Leermakers-Vermeer, M.J., de Roos, N.M., de Bree, R., van Cruijsen, H., & Terhaard, C.H.J. (2016). Indicators for enteral nutrition use and prophylactic percutaneous endoscopic gastrostomy placement in patients with head and neck cancer undergoing chemoradiotherapy. *Nutrition in Clinical Practice, 32,* 225–232. https://doi.org/10.1177/0884533616682684

van der Molen, L., Heemsbergen, W.D., de Jong, R., van Rossum, M.A., Smeele, L.E., Rasch, C.R.N., & Hilgers, F.J.M. (2013). Dysphagia and trismus after concomitant chemo-intensity-modulated radiation therapy (chemo-IMRT) in advanced head and neck cancer: Dose–effect relationships for swallowing and mastication structures. *Radiotherapy and Oncology, 106,* 364–369. https://doi.org/10.1016/j.radonc.2013.03.005

Villari, C.R., & Courey, M.S. (2015). Management of dysphonia after radiation therapy. *Otolaryngologic Clinics of North America, 48,* 601–609. https://doi.org/10.1016/j.otc.2015.04.006

Walker, M.P., Wichman, B., Cheng, A.-L., Coster, J., & Williams, K.B. (2011). Impact of radiotherapy dose on dentition breakdown in head and neck cancer patients. *Practical Radiation Oncology, 1,* 142–148. https://doi.org/10.1016/j.prro.2011.03.003

Wang, H.-L., Keck, J.F., Weaver, M.T., Mikesky, A., Bunnell, K., Buelow, J.M., & Rawl, S.M. (2013). Shoulder pain, functional status, and health-related quality of life after head and neck cancer surgery. *Rehabilitation Research and Practice, 2013,* 601768. https://doi.org/10.1155/2013/601768

Wu, V.W.C., & Lam, Y.-N. (2016). Radiation-induced temporo-mandibular joint disorder in post-radiotherapy nasopharyngeal carcinoma patients: Assessment and treatment. *Journal of Medical Radiation Sciences, 63,* 124–132. https://doi.org/10.1002/jmrs.145

Zhang, Z. (2016). Mechanics of human voice production and control. *Journal of the Acoustical Society of America, 140,* 2614–2635. https://doi.org/10.1121/1.4964509

C. Breast

1. Incidence

   a) Breast cancer is one of the most common cancers, as the Surveillance, Epidemiology, and End Results (SEER) cancer registry estimated 276,480 new cases of female breast cancer with 42,170 deaths in 2020 (NCI, 2020).

   b) Female breast cancer accounted for 15.3% of all new cancer cases in 2018 (NCI, 2020).

   c) Breast cancer in men occurs at a much lower incidence. The American Cancer Society (2020) estimated the incidence of male breast cancer to be 2,620 new cases and 520 deaths in 2020.

   d) It was estimated that more than 3.5 million women were living with breast cancer in 2017. Some patients with breast cancer may shift treatment goals from curative to living with a chronic disease or to palliative care during their lifetime while living with this disease (NCI, 2020).

   e) Radiation oncology nurses can play a vital role in caring for this group of patients as they navigate the trajectory of their cancer.

2. Staging

   a) Staging is conducted using the AJCC system, which accounts for tumor size, nodal involvement, and the presence of metastasis—noted as tumor-node-metastasis (TNM).

      (1) The most recent version of this system incorporates clinical prognostic factors into the staging for each newly diagnosed patient with breast cancer.

      (2) Recent changes include the addition of prognostic information in staging—the clinical prognostic stage, which accounts for the biology of the tumor.

      (3) The clinical prognostic staging can cause classical staging to be upgraded or downgraded based on grade of tumor, estrogen, and progesterone and HER2 status of the tumor (Shao et al., 2019).

      (4) Initial staging assignments stay with the patient even if the disease progresses to metastatic.

      (5) The challenge in radiation oncology is that the evidence used to make treatment recommendations are largely based on the historical anatomic stage, but many aspects of care are changing to make decisions based on type of surgery, chemotherapy sequencing, and the need and type of radiation.

   b) Treatment decisions are based on the stage of disease. Staging takes place two ways: clinical and pathologic.

      (1) Clinical staging occurs prior to any definitive surgery and is frequently used for patients receiving neoadjuvant therapy or for those with metastatic or inoperable tumors. Clinical staging is denoted with c before TNM.

      (2) Pathologic staging is used after definitive surgery to the breast. Pathologic staging is denoted with p before the TNM.

3. Treatment goals

   a) Overview

      (1) The goal of RT may be defined as adjuvant, curative, or palliative, as well as for the purposes of stimulating the immune system with a combination of drugs.

      (2) It is essential for nurses to understand the intention of treatment to properly educate patients about goals, outcomes, and potential side effects and to address psychosocial needs. This is the first step to providing a comprehensive care plan.

   b) Adjuvant RT

      (1) NCI (n.d.) defines adjuvant therapy as additional cancer treatment given after the primary treatment to lower the risk that the cancer will recur.

      (2) Adjuvant RT for breast cancer is most commonly given as part of breast-conserving surgery.

(3) The goal of adjuvant RT is to prevent recurrence of breast cancer by destroying any cancer cells left behind within the breast, the chest wall, and the nodes draining into the lymphatics after surgery, in order to reduce the chance of local recurrence and improve overall survival (Taghian, 2020).

(4) After breast-conserving surgery, RT to the conserved breast decreases the rate at which the disease recurs by one-half and reduces the breast cancer death rate by approximately one-sixth (Darby et al., 2011).

(5) The combined modality of surgical removal and adjuvant RT offers the best curative cancer rates.

c) Curative RT

(1) Adjuvant RT can also be targeted to the breast and lymph nodes with a curative intent when it is suspected that the tumor has been left in place after surgery, such as with locally advanced breast cancer or inflammatory breast cancer.

(2) Curative RT may be used if a patient is unable to undergo surgery to the breast because of the size of the tumor or adherence of the tumor to the skin or vessels nearby (Tryfonidis, Senkus, Cardoso, & Cardoso, 2015).

(3) This type of radiation may be applied to operative tumors that are node negative but with high-risk features such as the following (Taghian, 2020).

   (a) T3, T4, as well as T2 with limited axillary dissection (less than 10 nodes)

   (b) High-grade histology

   (c) Estrogen receptor negative

   (d) Lymphovascular invasion

d) Palliative RT

(1) Palliative RT may be used to halt bleeding or shrink a large vascular tumor with the goals of improving quality of life, halting chronic or acute bleeding, and shrinking a tumor so that a less morbid surgery may be attempted after partial regression or shrinkage.

(2) Patients with breast cancer may also undergo palliative RT when they have metastasis or local recurrence.

   (a) This may occur more than once over a patient's lifetime.

   (b) It is important to keep a careful accounting of each course of RT, even if it occurred at another facility.

   (c) Overlap of previous radiation fields needs to be carefully considered for risks and benefits.

   (d) Regarding reirradiation near the original site of prior breast RT, Grann and Haffty (2019) noted that although previous RT increases the risk of toxicities (e.g., rib fractures, chest wall fibrosis, reconstruction complications), the risk is acceptable.

   (e) On reirradiation after initial treatment, Nieder, Langendijk, Guckenberger, and Grosu (2018) wrote, "If the interval to the next [RT] course was relatively short, i.e., 6–12 months, only 25% more was allowed, and no increase was permitted with intervals shorter than six months. The safety of this policy is difficult to judge from the available evidence. However, it might be a starting point from which more, ideally prospectively documented data can be derived. Even in the setting of first reirradiation, dose constraints are only beginning to emerge" (p. 309).

   (f) RT can be used to relieve symptoms of painful, bleeding, or obstructive sites of metastatic disease in bones, lungs, brain, skin, and lymph nodes (Grewal, Freedman, Jones, & Taunk, 2019).

e) Immunotherapy

(1) At the time of this publication, many trials are underway to explore radiation's ability to be an immune stimulatory tool for patients with breast cancer and other cancers, when used in combination with various checkpoint inhibitors or costimulatory drugs.

(2) Historically, radiation was thought to be immunosuppressive; however, new data have shown that RT using different radiation doses can help to stimulate the immune system to eliminate cancer (Ye & Formenti, 2018). See X.C. Immunotherapy for more information.

4. Targeted tissue and radiation field

a) RT can target a portion of the breast, the whole breast or chest wall, and surrounding regional lymph nodes. However, organs surrounding these intended targets may receive radiation doses.

b) Knowledge of dose distribution at the initiation of treatment is essential to developing an appropriate care plan and to educate a patient of the expected side-effects. See discussion of side effects, acute and late toxicities.

(1) Whole-breast RT will target the entire breast and may include a higher dose additionally targeted at the tumor bed (boost) after surgical removal (Deseyne et al., 2017).

   (a) This is the most common type of breast RT for early-stage disease.

   (b) Methods on how to spare healthy tissue will be discussed later in this section.

   (c) Common side effects are skin reactions, cosmetic changes to the breast, and fatigue.

(d) A targeted boost may also be used where margins are close or where residual tumor persists.

(2) Partial breast RT will only treat the surgically resected cavity in appropriately selected early-stage cases, with a margin of healthy tissue. Side effects are the same as whole-breast RT but can be minimized with a smaller treatment volume (Formenti et al., 2012).

(3) Comprehensive breast RT will include the whole breast or mastectomy chest wall and may include a tumor bed boost or scar boost (Deseyne et al., 2017).

    (a) Targeted nodal RT will treat all or some of the at-risk lymph nodes. These will include the level 1, 2, and 3 lymph nodes, as well as supraclavicular nodes.

    (b) The side effect profile is similar to whole-breast RT but also includes greater cardiac risk, pneumonitis, esophagitis, lymphedema, brachial plexopathy, and a small relative risk of second malignancies in the future.

    (c) The inclusion of the internal mammary nodes may be considered in advanced cases or when these lymph nodes are detected to be involved at baseline imaging.

    (d) Treating the internal mammary nodes will place the heart and lungs into the field of treatment, thus carrying more risk to these structures.

5. Radiation dosages and fractionation

    a) Hypofractionated whole-breast irradiation

      (1) Hypofractionation is the technique of using larger doses (higher Gy) of radiation given across fewer daily treatments (fractions).

      (2) Accelerated hypofractionated whole-breast RT includes a dose fractionation scheme of administering 40–42.5 Gy with or without a boost (Taghian, 2020).

      (3) The initial whole-breast hypofractionation trials excluded patients with node-positive breast cancer, tumors larger than 5 cm, breast width of 25 cm or more at the posterior border of the medial and lateral tangential beams, high-grade tumors, and ductal carcinoma in situ (DCIS) (Hopwood et al., 2010; Lymberis et al., 2012; Whelan et al., 2010).

      (4) All of these prior exclusions to hypofractionated RT for breast cancer have since or are being further studied with promising results in support of wider use of a whole-breast hypofractionated irradiation approach (Lymberis et al., 2012; Osa et al., 2014; Shin et al., 2016).

      (5) Use of hypofractionated RT resulted in lower acute skin toxicity rates compared with conventional fractionated RT. Breast volume greater than 1,000 cm³ was associated with lower acute grade 2 toxicity with the use of hypofractionated RT despite achieving similar dosimetry to conventional fractionated RT (Butler-Xu, Marietta, Zahra, TenNapel, & Mitchell, 2018).

    b) Boost

      (1) Traditionally, for invasive cancers, a boost (extra dose) is delivered sequentially after whole-breast RT to the tumor bed, with a daily dose of 2 Gy or 2.5 Gy for five to seven days (Taghian, 2020).

        (a) Other studies of large groups of women receiving 40.5 Gy to the whole breast with a *concurrent* tumor bed boost (0.5 Gy daily for 15 days) *concurrent* with whole-breast RT have shown excellent control rates (Osa et al., 2014).

        (b) Strong evidence has shown the benefit of both sequential and concurrent boosts with hypofractionated whole-breast RT (Taghian, 2020).

      (2) In a trial of more than 1,300 women, treatment with hypofractionated RT for three weeks with a concurrent boost has proven to be safe and effective at a median follow-up of five years (Shaikh et al., 2018).

        (a) Cosmetic outcome was rated as good to excellent, as assessed by clinicians and patients.

        (b) The local recurrence-free survival rate was 97.7%.

        (c) Included in this cohort were 348 women younger than 50 years old, with equivalent results (Shaikh et al., 2018).

      (3) Smaller studies have proven the feasibility and safety of giving nodal RT and chest wall RT in a hypofractionated schedule for three weeks to patients who underwent mastectomy.

        (a) The study by Shin et al. (2016) used a smaller sample size and had a shorter median follow-up time to measure disease-free survival.

        (b) Hypofractionated RT seems to be equally efficacious and no more toxic when compared with conventional RT in carcinoma of the breast, even in the previously unselected subgroup of patients who were previously excluded from the original three-week hypofractionated trial (Mishra, Khurana, Mishra, & Hadi, 2016).

        (c) Other smaller series have also demonstrated the safety of hypofractionated RT in patients who underwent mastectomy and patients with higher stages of disease requiring nodal irradiation.

(d) Shin et al. (2016) concluded that prone hypofractionated breast, chest wall, and nodal RT are safe and well tolerated.

(e) Although the initial pattern of local and regional control is encouraging, longer follow-up is warranted for efficacy and late toxicity assessment, particularly of the brachial plexus.

c) Conventional and historical dosage and fractions

(1) Traditionally, patients diagnosed with DCIS and early-stage invasive cancer received 2 Gy per fraction in 25 fractions for a total dose of 50 Gy.

(2) An additional 10 Gy in five fractions is delivered to the volume of breast surrounding the excision site (tumor bed boost), but different fractionation schedules may be prescribed.

(3) For patients with close surgical margins, the operative bed may receive a boost of up to 14 Gy in seven fractions.

(4) Others have used 46 Gy in 23 fractions to the whole breast with 14 Gy boost in seven fractions (Raza et al., 2012).

d) Safely omitting RT in some patients

(1) Some older patients diagnosed with DCIS may wish to forgo RT with accepting a higher risk of recurrence.

(2) Some studies have shown that the risk of DCIS recurrence decreases with advanced age, supporting the argument that older women (75 years and older) may choose observation after lumpectomy (Cronin, Olese, Patil, Morrow, & Van Zee, 2016).

(3) These data for risk of local recurrence and mortality risk have been reported from two pivotal studies (Wapnir et al., 2011).

(a) National Surgical Adjuvant Breast and Bowel Project B17 and B24 trials demonstrated that after 15 years, the rate of breast tumor recurrence was 19.4% for patients with DCIS treated with only lumpectomy and 8.5% for patients treated with lumpectomy, RT, and tamoxifen.

(b) These pivotal studies demonstrated that the risk of recurrence of DCIS decreases with age. This effect is particularly strong at the extremes of age and is independent of other clinical pathologic factors.

(c) In these studies, the oldest women had low risk of recurrence, and the youngest women had a higher overall risk. The youngest women were at higher risk for invasive recurrence, but mortality remained low.

(d) If the recurrence was invasive, it was associated with increased mortality, but that increase was not observed for patients with

DCIS, allowing for the option of omitting RT in patients older than 75 years.

(4) Although patients with DCIS may have a lower risk of mortality when forgoing RT, clinicians should discuss that RT can prevent recurrences with patients.

(a) A study of 3,762 women who had breast-conserving surgery for DCIS with or without RT demonstrated a 10-year recurrence rate of 20% in participants who did not receive RT and 12.7% in participants who received RT (Ratovich et al., 2013).

(b) The same study showed that the rate of invasive recurrence was 10% in the non-RT group versus 7% in the RT group, and the rate of recurrence of DCIS was 10% in the non-RT group versus 6.1% in the RT group (Ratovich et al., 2013).

6. RT techniques

a) EBRT

(1) EBRT is a local therapy in which high doses of radiation are administered over a period of time from a linear accelerator delivering radiation through medial and lateral tangential beams.

(2) EBRT can be directed to the whole breast, only a portion of the breast (partial breast irradiation), to the mastectomy reconstruction or chest wall, and the regional lymph nodes.

(3) Multiple adjacent treatment fields must be carefully matched to avoid geographic overdosage (hot spots) or geographic underdosage (cold spots) (McBride, Withers, & Schaue, 2019).

(a) Geographic overdosage can result in decreased range of motion, fibrosis, telangiectasia, and necrosis of the treated tissue.

(b) Geographic underdosage can result in locoregional recurrence following RT when an area of tissue harboring residual disease receives a subtherapeutic dose of radiation.

b) Partial breast EBRT

(1) Partial breast EBRT will include treatment to the lumpectomy cavity and a margin around the lumpectomy cavity (1–5 cm).

(2) Many single-institution studies have tested partial breast RT for efficacy and safety, with mild fluctuations in dosage and method.

(3) One of the most accepted methods is external beam partial breast RT. Treatment can be given in 30 Gy over five fractions for appropriate patients (Formenti et al., 2012).

(4) Excluding a portion of the breast tissue may not be appropriate for all cases of early-stage breast cancer.

(5) Studies on partial breast EBRT have led ASTRO to issue a consensus statement regard-

ing which patients are appropriate candidates for partial breast RT.

    (a) The suitable category would include women aged 50 years and older, stage T1, or DCIS (screen-detected, low to intermediate nuclear grade, size less than 2.5 cm, margins negative to at least 3 mm) (Correa et al., 2017).

    (b) The advantages of this method of partial breast RT are superb imaging, decreased time of treatment delivery, decreased dose to healthy organs, and minimal side effects.

c) Nodal irradiation

  (1) The regional lymph nodes are at risk in patients diagnosed with locally advanced breast carcinoma.

    (a) For patients who have undergone breast-conserving surgery, the RT fields should be modified to include these node-bearing regions in addition to the glandular breast.

    (b) Traditionally, RT would be added to the regional lymph nodes if more than three axillary lymph nodes were involved at the time of sentinel lymph node dissection and axillary lymph node dissection.

  (2) A 10-year follow-up of the ACoS Oncology Group Z0011 study has upheld that despite the potential for residual axillary disease after sentinel node dissection, sentinel node dissection without axillary node dissection offers excellent regional control for selected patients with early lymph node metastasis in breast cancer treated with breast-conserving therapy and adjuvant systemic therapy (Giuliano et al., 2016).

  (3) The Z0011 study has led to a change in the surgical practice of not completing an axillary dissection when the sentinel nodes are positive (Giuliano et al., 2016).

    (a) This practice leaves radiation oncologists with incomplete information to guide treatment field selection; it would be unknown if more than three lymph nodes are involved.

    (b) Many radiation oncologists would choose to cover the lymph nodes because most women in the Z00111 study received RT.

  (4) The effect of off-protocol nodal irradiation on rates of regional control cannot be determined (Giuliano et al., 2016).

    (a) Based on the subset of 335 patients for whom detailed RT information was available, 51% of the patients in this study received high tangents with treatment to within 2 cm of the humeral head, which may merely reflect a radiation oncologist's preference.

    (b) However, 15% of the patients were treated with a prohibited third field, and only 11% of the patients received no radiation at all.

    (c) No difference was seen in patient characteristics or outcomes among those who received nodal irradiation and those who did not, and no difference in locoregional recurrence was seen by applying a prohibited third field.

    (d) The high tangents included definitively level 1 and level 2 axillary nodes. The third field would cover even more lymph nodes.

    (e) Although there was no difference between sentinel node biopsy-positive without additional axillary node dissection and sentinel node biopsy-positive with node dissection, it should be noted that the majority of patients received RT within both groups through the reported third field.

d) Neoadjuvant treatment (chemotherapy, antihormonal, or targeted biologics)

  (1) Neoadjuvant chemotherapy is defined as chemotherapy that is administered before breast cancer surgery.

    (a) Neoadjuvant therapy may also now include the addition of targeted therapies, such as anti-HER2 therapies (e.g., trastuzumab, pertuzumab) and endocrine therapies (e.g., tamoxifen, anastrozole).

    (b) Patients have a preoperative c-TNM staging performed.

    (c) Once the treatment with chemotherapy or targeted agents has been given, definitive breast surgery is usually performed to fully assess the remaining cancer that persisted in the breast and regional lymph nodes.

    (d) Patients then undergo p-TNM staging.

  (2) Neoadjuvant chemotherapy for breast cancer is increasingly being used in women with operable breast cancer in addition to its established role for inoperable, locally advanced, or inflammatory breast cancer.

  (3) Achieving a pathologic complete response, defined as eradication of all invasive disease in the breast and lymph nodes, is predictive of improved survival.

  (4) The magnitude of the benefit of pathologic complete response is strongest in women with triple-negative breast cancer and women with HER2-positive and estrogen/progesterone hormone receptor–negative breast cancers (Cortazar et al., 2014).

    (a) Traditionally, for patients who received neoadjuvant chemotherapy and subsequent surgery for locally advanced breast cancer, the standard radiation fields should encompass the original extent of disease.

(b) In 2019, ongoing clinical trials are questioning whether this should be the current standard for RT after neoadjuvant chemotherapy and neoadjuvant targeted therapies, especially when complete responses are achieved (Arnaout et al., 2018).

(c) After completing the neoadjuvant drug therapy and surgery, the staging is denoted as *yp-TNM* to denote that full surgical staging has occurred after neoadjuvant therapy.

(d) At the time of this publication, clinical questions still exist regarding whether to treat all initial sites of disease with RT in patients treated with neoadjuvant therapies who achieve pathologic complete response.

e) Postmastectomy RT

(1) Postmastectomy RT may be indicated based on tumor size of greater than 5 cm, involvement of more than three lymph nodes, or close or positive margins.

(2) As previously discussed, based on study Z0011, patients with fewer than three positive lymph nodes at sentinel biopsy may be considered for postmastectomy RT.

(3) The radiation field would include the axilla if an axillary node dissection was not completed to verify that fewer than three lymph nodes are involved.

(4) Women with early-stage breast cancer who had a mastectomy in the adjuvant setting, with no lymph node involvement and clean surgical margins, are not offered RT.

(5) A recent meta-analysis of more than 5,000 women compared breast conservation to mastectomy in terms of overall survival (Onitilo, Engel, Stankowski, & Doi, 2015).

(a) When breast-conserving surgery plus RT was compared to mastectomy alone, overall survival was 96.5% versus 93.4% at 3 years, 92.9% versus 88.3% at 5 years, and 80.9% versus 67.2% at 10 years.

(b) These analyses suggest that survival benefit is not related only to the surgery itself but that the prognostic advantage of breast-conserving surgery plus RT over mastectomy may also be related to the addition of adjuvant RT.

(c) This conclusion requires prospective confirmation in randomized trials.

(6) Postmastectomy RT has an important role in reducing the risk of recurrence in patients diagnosed with locally advanced breast cancer (McBride et al., 2019).

(a) The entire volume of the mastectomy flaps must be included in the treatment field. This comprises the entire length of the mastectomy scar, any clips, and drain sites.

(b) Traditionally, the dose has been 50 Gy in 25 fractions. An additional boost can be considered for the scar or any region with positive margins.

(c) As previously discussed, studies are exploring hypofractionation in a three-week period in this population.

(d) The side effect profile is the same as whole-breast RT.

i. The lungs and heart may have more exposures in postmastectomy RT.

ii. The side effects of nodal irradiation may also occur at a higher rate (e.g., lymphedema if the lymph nodes are included).

f) Brachytherapy

(1) Brachytherapy was one of the first types of delivery methods to attempt partial breast irradiation.

(a) Patient inconvenience, risk for infection, and local pain are difficult to justify when partial breast EBRT methods are now readily available.

(b) It should be noted that many European health agencies still advocate for this method of partial breast RT.

(2) Recommendations issued by ASTRO for the use of intraoperative RT for breast cancer include counseling patients regarding the higher risk of ipsilateral breast tumor recurrence with intraoperative RT compared with whole-breast RT; the need for prospective monitoring of long-term local control and toxicity with low-energy radiograph intraoperative RT given limited follow-up; and restriction of intraoperative RT to women with invasive cancer considered suitable (Correa et al., 2017).

(3) The American Brachytherapy Society has issued a consensus statement on accelerated partial breast irradiation (Shah et al., 2018).

(a) Regarding RT techniques, the strongest evidence supports the use of interstitial brachytherapy and IMRT accelerated partial breast irradiation.

(b) Moderate evidence supports use of applicator brachytherapy or 3DCRT accelerated partial breast irradiation.

(c) Intraoperative RT and electronic brachytherapy should not be offered regardless of technique outside of clinical trial.

g) Techniques for treatment optimization and immobilization

  (1) RT techniques

    (a) IMRT

    (b) IGRT

    (c) Cone beam CT scan

    (d) SBRT

  (2) Deep inspiration breath hold

    (a) Deep inspiration breath hold is a technique that takes advantage of a more favorable position of the heart during inspiration to minimize heart dose over a course of RT.

    (b) Respiratory motion is monitored during deep inspiration breath hold, and patients are instructed to hold their breath at certain points in the breathing cycle.

    (c) The Varian real-time position management system can be used with this technique (Bergom, Currey, Desai, Tai, & Strauss, 2018).

      i. A device is placed on the patient's chest, and vertical displacement throughout the respiratory cycle provides data to track the patient's breathing.

      ii. In this method, clinicians coach the patient, and the patient must voluntarily learn to hold breathing in cycles.

      iii. The treatment beam is gated to stop treatment if the breathing signal is outside a preset threshold.

      iv. This type of gating in deep inspiration breath hold should be differentiated from standard respiratory gating, in which the patient is breathing freely, and the beam is repeatedly turned off during a predetermined portion of the respiratory cycle.

      v. Unlike deep inspiration breath hold, respiratory gating with free breathing is not usually an effective method for cardiac sparing because the heart does not move away drastically from the chest wall or breast during the standard respiratory cycle.

  (3) Proton beam therapy (National Association for Proton Therapy, 2019)

    (a) The major advantage of proton therapy treatment over standard RT is that protons slowly deposit their energy as they travel toward the cancerous tumor.

    (b) Because of a unique physical characteristic known as the Bragg Peak, protons deposit the majority of the radiation dose directly in the tumor and travel no further through the body.

    (c) The characteristics of proton beam therapy result in fewer healthy tissues and organs receiving unnecessary radiation, thereby reducing unwanted complications and side effects.

    (d) To date, most studies have shown that the benefit of proton beam therapy in breast cancer is primarily seen in patients receiving internal mammary node irradiation.

    (e) When patients receive whole-breast or chest wall RT alone or in conjunction with the supraclavicular nodes but not the internal mammary nodes, there is only a limited benefit to proton beam therapy (Braunstein & Cahlon, 2018).

    (f) As more centers begin to offer proton therapy, clinicians can expect to see more clinical trials testing its utility in breast cancer.

    (g) See the National Association for Proton Therapy website (www.proton-therapy.org) for more information.

  (4) Immobilization and positioning (Fenton-Kerimian, Maisonet, & Formenti, 2013; Osa et al., 2014)

    (a) RT for breast cancer has traditionally been administered with patients in the supine position with immobilization of the arms in a wing board and the torso in a vacuum-formed cushion (Vac-Lok™).

    (b) When patients have more skin folds, more radiation will be deposited in the skin and a bolus effect can occur, leading to more skin reactions.

    (c) With patients in the supine position, tangential beams may deposit more radiation into the lungs and heart.

    (d) Many centers prefer to treat the breast, especially pendulous breasts, in the prone position. Gravity allows the breast to hang and move away from the heart and lungs.

7. Risk factors during RT

  a) A patient's medical comorbidities and environmental exposures need to be taken into consideration at the initiation of RT. Nurses should remain vigilant for potentially heightened side effects in patients with comorbidities, which may affect their risk during RT.

  b) Patients with autoimmune diseases may be more sensitive to the damaging effects of radiation.

    (1) A 16-year study demonstrated that autoimmune disease was a potential predictor of infection incidence in post-treatment patients with breast cancer after adjusting for clinical confounding factors (Chen, Ho, Chen, Hsu, & Chen, 2019).

    (2) This should be reflected in the care plan with more frequent follow-up after treatment.

(3) Some examples of autoimmune diseases to monitor for are Sjögren syndrome, rheumatoid arthritis, and systemic lupus erythematosus. There are many other more obscure autoimmune diseases, and radiation oncology nurses should be aware of this prior to treatment.

c) Several patient-related risk factors are associated with higher grades of radiation dermatitis (McQuestion, 2011).

(1) Chronic sun exposure
(2) Comorbidities that affect wound healing (e.g., diabetes, renal failure)
(3) Collagen vascular disease
(4) Seroma drainage prior to or during RT
(5) Dehiscence or infection of surgical wound
(6) Older age
(7) Breast size
(8) Smoking
(9) Poor nutrition

d) Treatment-related factors, such as the following, also affect outcomes and side effects (McQuestion, 2011).

(1) Cumulative dose delivered
(2) Location of treatment field
(3) Fraction size and schedule
(4) Techniques employed
(5) Larger treatment field
(6) Duration of treatment
(7) Use of bolus material

8. Genetics

a) Tumor genetics

(1) A 2015 meta-analysis summarized the number of articles published about the various genetic tests for further prognostic predictions based on the genetics of breast tumors (Rouzier et al., 2013).

(2) In addition to looking for microassays to predict outcomes of chemotherapy treatment, some companies seek to validate assays for other clinical decisions.

(3) Specifically, Oncotype DX® Breast DCIS Score has been developed to identify patients with DCIS who may have a lower risk of recurrence.

(a) The final 12-gene panel includes seven cancer-related and five reference genes.

(b) The score is scaled numerically 0–100 and classified into three risk categories: low risk (less than 39), intermediate risk (39–54), and high risk (55 and greater).

(c) The Oncotype DX Breast DCIS Score was designed to quantify the 10-year risk of any ipsilateral breast event (local or invasive recurrence) after breast-conserving surgery for pure DCIS without RT (Nofech-Mozes, Hanna, & Rakovitch, 2019).

(d) Long-term follow-up is needed before sufficient evidence can extrapolate whether low-risk patients could forgo RT without increasing long-term risk of recurrence (Nofech-Mozes et al., 2019).

(e) The one large validation study still found a 10-year risk of local recurrence in the breast of 9.7%, even for women with a low recurrence score, clear margins, and non-multifocal DCIS (Ratovich et al., 2015).

b) Patient genetics

(1) The genetic information on actionable mutations is expanding very quickly.

(2) The *BRCA1* and *BRCA2* gene mutations are known to pose an increased risk of breast cancer and other cancers. *BRCA1* and *BRCA2* test results may direct patient decisions on the aggressiveness of cancer treatment.

(3) Unlike the microassays that may test the tumor's genetics, genetic testing examines genetic variants and mutations that may alert patients or their relatives to a higher risk of developing certain cancers.

(4) This testing is performed with a blood or saliva sample and should involve visiting with a genetic counselor to address recommendations for cancer surveillance and appropriate family screening.

(5) Clinicians should recommend patients with breast cancer for genetic testing and counseling for any of the following reasons.

(a) History of breast cancer at age younger than 50 years
(b) History of ovarian cancer
(c) Relatives with breast, ovarian, pancreatic, or prostate cancer
(d) Any male family members with breast cancer
(e) Ashkenazi Jewish ancestry
(f) Any family members with *BRCA1* or *BRCA2* mutation

(6) Increased toxicity to RT has been reported in patients with ataxia-telangiectasia syndrome and heterozygous carriers of *ATM* mutations, most likely because of defective DNA repair and genomic instability in healthy tissues. However, heterozygous germ-line mutations apparently do not contribute to second primary cancers following RT (Choi, Kipps, & Razelle, 2016).

9. Side effects

a) Acute side effects

(1) Acute side effects of radiation are those side effects that typically occur during the first one to three months after the start of RT.

(2) Acute side effects from RT for breast cancer include breast edema, pain, tenderness, infection, and fatigue. A small transient decrease in

blood counts can occur, especially if larger fields that include significant bone marrow are used or if patients have been heavily pretreated with chemotherapy.

(3) The most prevalent and expected acute side effect of breast irradiation is radiation dermatitis.
  (a) It can present as erythema and progress to skin desquamation.
  (b) Breast cancer can recur in the skin of the breast and is included in the target; therefore, some level of skin changes can be expected.
  (c) Skin side effects are usually not severe but cause much discomfort for patients.
  (d) Education should include informing patients that a skin reaction will occur to help them cope with the visible changes that will emerge during treatment.
  (e) Refer to IV.B. Skin reactions for more information.

b) Late side effects
  (1) Overview
    (a) Late side effects of breast RT are those that occur three months and up to several years after treatment. These side effects are expected depending on field size.
    (b) Late side effects are rarer than acute side effects.
  (2) Lymphedema
    (a) Lymphatic disruption
      i. Lymphatic disruption can result from surgical removal of lymph nodes or other cancer treatments (e.g., RT) that inhibit the normal function of lymph nodes.
      ii. The disruption can cause a backup of lymphatic fluid in the interstitial spaces between cells, which then causes visible swelling.
      iii. If the undamaged portion of the lymphatic system is unable to remove fluid from that portion of the body, the protein-rich fluids continue to build up, resulting in lymphedema.
    (b) Incidence (McDuff et al., 2019)
      i. The timing of lymphedema is important for screening and care plan development.
      ii. A study of more than 2,000 women at risk for lymphedema found that women receiving axillary node dissection and regional nodal irradiation had the highest five-year incidence of lymphedema (31.2%).
      iii. Women who underwent axillary node dissection without regional node irradiation had a 24.6% chance of developing lymphedema. Women who underwent sentinel node biopsy with regional node irradiation had a 12.2% risk.
      iv. Because of the high risk of lymphedema, surgeons often support avoiding axillary node dissection in women. This reflects the results of the Z0011 study, which advocates against axillary node dissection after positive sentinel node biopsy.
      v. Although lymphedema can occur at any time during the cancer care trajectory, certain time points predict when the risk may be the highest. Risk peaked at 12–30 months postoperatively. Earliest onset was associated with axillary node dissection. For those treated with regional nodal irradiation, risk peaked at 18–24 months with axillary node dissection and at 36–48 months with sentinel node biopsy (McDuff et al., 2019).
      vi. The predictive information gleaned from this study is important for monitoring patients in these time frames for lymphedema, reinforcement of prevention education, and referral to appropriate therapies.
    (c) Risk factors: Factors affecting lymphedema risk include the following (McDuff et al., 2019).
      i. Higher preoperative body mass index
      ii. Axillary lymph node dissection
      iii. Regional lymph node irradiation
    (d) Interventions
      i. Patients should be taught how to prevent lymphedema.
      ii. Baseline measurements of the arm should be taken for comparison to postsurgery arm circumference.
      iii. At the first occurrence of lymphedema, detailed measurements should be taken (with a tape measure) of the affected limb at consistent points for reproducibility.
      iv. With the first occurrence, it is necessary to rule out other possible causes, such as axillary recurrence of cancer or cellulitis.
      v. Patients should be referred to a certified lymphedema therapist for combination therapy or CDT, which includes manual lymphatic drainage, compression, exercise,

and skin care (Johns Hopkins Medicine, n.d.).

    vi. For sudden onset of chills and fever; patients should be prescribed antibiotics (e.g., penicillin, amoxicillin, cefazolin). For patients with a penicillin allergy, cephalosporin can be prescribed (Auwaerter, 2019).

    vii. Patients can use compression garments, pumps, and bandaging to reduce swelling and help stagnant fluid in the arm to move into functioning lymphatic passageways. Pressure on the outside of the arm decreases internal pressure in the lymphatic system and maximizes the effects of the muscles pumping lymph throughout the body.

    viii. Exercise should include flexing and curling of the hand and arm; stretching to maintain or restore range of motion, increase flexibility, improve lymphatic flow, and reduce fibrosis; aerobic activity to encourage lymphatic flow through muscular contraction; and strength training to protect muscles from fatigue, which will stimulate lymphatic fluid production.

    ix. Newer surgical techniques have emerged to help overcome lymphedema and its complications. The two most common surgical interventions are vascularized lymph node transfer and lymphovenous anastomosis, both of which can effectively treat primary lymphedema (Cheng, Loh, & Lin, 2018).

    x. The reduction of above-knee circumference, body weight, and episodes of cellulitis was significantly greater in vascularized lymph node transfer, compared to lymphovenous anastomosis (Cheng et al., 2018).

    xi. See the National Lymphedema Network website (https://lymphnet.org) for a directory of lymphedema therapists.

(3) Second primary malignancy

    (a) Second primary malignancies (second malignancies) are cancers caused by treatment with RT or chemotherapy. These cancers are usually of a different type from the original diagnosis and should not be confused with recurrence, metastasis, or new primaries of different types of breast cancer.

    (b) Patients who received chemotherapy will have a higher risk of second malignancy when treated with RT, depending on which drugs were received (Smith, 2003).

      i. Patients treated with doxorubicin and cyclophosphamide with intensified doses of cyclophosphamide requiring granulocyte–colony-stimulating factor support had increased rates of treatment-related acute myeloid leukemia and myelodysplastic syndrome, even though the incidence was slight relative to breast cancer relapse.

      ii. In-breast RT appeared to be associated with an increased risk of acute myeloid leukemia and myelodysplastic syndrome.

    (c) Information about second malignancies is often reflective of older treatment methods.

      i. Follow-up for second malignancies is often a challenge, largely because of the need to follow patients for 10–20 years.

      ii. It is difficult to estimate the relative risk of second malignancy in current patients.

    (d) A large meta-analysis of 762,468 patients attempted to identify the risk of second malignancy after breast cancer RT (all types) (Grantzau & Overgaard, 2015).

      i. More than five years after therapy, the relative risk of a second nonbreast cancer was measured at 1.12.

      ii. The following types of cancers were associated with previous breast RT.
  - Lung (relative risk 1.39)
  - Esophagus (relative risk 1.53)
  - Sarcoma (relative risk 2.53)

      iii. RT for breast cancer is associated with an increased risk of second nonbreast cancers, overall and in organs adjacent to previous treatment fields.

    (e) A study of 755 women with DCIS or stage I–II breast cancer who underwent breast-conserving surgery followed by whole-breast RT found the 15-year age-adjusted probability of developing any second malignancy to be 12%, which was close to the SEER rate of 12.1% for a nonbreast malignancy incidence in the general population (Kushner, Hwang, Wang, Solin, & Vapiwala, 2018).

      i. The second malignancy was likely unrelated to treatment, and the risk of cancer was similar to control groups.

    ii. This information can be used when teaching patients about the risk for second malignancy. Patients with early-stage breast cancer undergoing breast-conserving treatment are at similar risk for malignancy as the general population.

  (f) Patient education should include information on surveillance and prevention.

    i. Patients should be educated to report symptoms such as cough, unexplained weight loss, difficulty eating, and difficulty completing ADLs.

    ii. Clinicians should encourage patients to have regular survivorship follow-up care.

    iii. A meta-analysis of modern radiation literature (2010–2015) estimated the risk of lung cancer with modern RT techniques to be 4% for long-term continuing smokers and 0.3% for nonsmokers and former smokers (Taylor et al., 2017).

    iv. The carcinogenic effects of cigarette smoke can be synergized by RT and increase risk of lung cancer. Smoking cessation should be strongly encouraged (Iyer & Jhingran, 2006).

(4) Radiation pneumonitis

  (a) Radiation pneumonitis can occur as a direct result of radiation fields used to treat the chest affecting a portion of the lung. It presents as inflammation of the lung without an infectious etiology.

  (b) Radiation pneumonitis can occur between six weeks and six months after completion of RT and tends to be related to the volume of lung included in the radiation treatment field, the cumulative dose, and treatment technique.

  (c) Risk of pneumonitis is greater in patients treated with comprehensive chest wall RT than those who received whole-breast RT.

  (d) The initial hallmark signs of radiation pneumonitis are dry cough, shortness of breast, low-grade fever, pain, malaise, and chest tightness. Patients should be taught to report these symptoms.

  (e) Chest x-ray or CT is used to confirm diagnosis of radiation pneumonitis and rule out other causes. Scans show patchy consolidation within the area of the high-dose radiation field, and lung tissue does not con-

form to normal lobar anatomy (Bledsoe, Nath, & Decker, 2017).

  (f) High-dose steroids, such as prednisone, are the backbone of treatment to reduce inflammation and symptoms. Radiation pneumonitis can lead to bacterial infection, which is treated with antibiotics. Oxygen therapy may be indicated for chronic radiation pneumonitis (Bledsoe et al., 2017).

  (g) With better imaging, incidence has been declining; however, some newer immunotherapies can increase the risk of pneumonitis for patients who also receive RT. Previous exposure to certain agents, such as the following, prior to RT may increase the likelihood of lung injury (Huang, Fan, Li, & Du, 2019; Jain & Berman, 2018; Palma et al., 2013).

    i. Cyclophosphamide

    ii. Taxanes

    iii. Methotrexate

    iv. Therapies targeting mechanistic target of rapamycin (mTOR), cytotoxic T-lymphocyte antigen 4 (CTLA-4), programmed cell death protein 1 (PD-1), or programmed cell death-ligand 1 (PD-L1)

(5) Brachial plexopathy

  (a) Brachial plexopathy is a rare late complication of RT characterized by severe neurologic pain with worsening sensory motor deficits in the arm on the treated side of the body (Warade, Jha, Pattanker, & Desai, 2019).

  (b) Nurses should assess for pain and numbness, especially in the fourth and fifth digits of the treated side; paresthesia; dysesthesia; swelling of the upper arm, hand, or wrist; arm weakness; inability to extend and lift the wrist; and possible muscle atrophy (Kamenova et al., 2009).

  (c) Total radiation dose, fractionation dose, treatment technique, overlapping treatment fields, increased dose to the axilla and supraclavicular lymph nodes, concurrent chemotherapy, and the premorbid state of the irradiated nerves can contribute to the development of brachial plexopathy (Gosk, Rutowski, Reichert, & Rabczyński, 2007; Kamenova et al., 2009).

  (d) Clinicians should obtain CT or MRI of the brachial plexus to diagnose brachial plexopathy. A diffuse, ill-defined loss of tissue plane is consistent with

radiation-induced injury to the brachial plexus.

(e) The use of tricyclic antidepressants, SNRIs, calcium channel alpha-2-delta ligands, topical lidocaine, opioid analgesics, and tramadol may be useful in the treatment of neuropathic pain (Gosk et al., 2007; Dworkin et al., 2010).

(f) For intractable pain, clinicians should refer patients for consideration of a transcutaneous electrical nerve stimulation unit or dorsal column stimulator.

(g) Patients should be referred to physical therapy to prevent deconditioning.

(h) Delayed damage to these plexuses may be slowly progressive over many years. This is thought to be related to damage of the Schwann cells. Unfortunately, late injury is usually permanent and disabling (Stone & DeAngelis, 2016).

(6) Bone toxicity and rib fracture

(a) RT doses do not typically result in profound acute injury to bony structures (Hoebers, Ferguson, & O'Sullivan, 2011).

(b) Late effects of RT include damage to osteoblasts, decreased matrix formation, and osteopenia within the previous treatment field. These can be seen on radiograph one year following the completion of treatment (Hoebers et al., 2011; Iyer & Jhingran, 2006).

(c) Rib fracture increases in incidence with a higher total radiation dose, hypofractionation, low machine energy, and larger volume of rib or chest wall included in the RT fields (Hoebers et al., 2011).

(d) Many patients with breast cancer are on aromatase inhibitors (e.g., anastrozole, letrozole), which have an additive risk of osteopenia and osteoporosis that may predispose women to a higher risk of rib fracture.

(e) If rib fracture is suspected, a rib x-ray should be obtained to confirm and rule out metastasis.

(7) Cardiac and vascular toxicity

(a) As cancer survivors live longer, radiation-induced heart disease has become more understood.

(b) Radiation-induced heart disease can affect the pericardial sac, coronary arteries, myocardium, and heart valves (Filopei & Frishman, 2012).

(c) Estimated absolute risks of cardiac mortality from modern RT were approximately 1% for smokers and 0.3% for non-

smokers and former smokers (Taylor et al., 2017).

(d) A meta-analysis studying mean heart dose during 2003–2013 found that the mean heart dose was 4.2 Gy and varied with target tissue. When internal mammary nodes were treated, the mean heart dose was 8 Gy (Taylor et al., 2015).

(e) Refer to IV.K. Cardiac toxicity and cardiac implantable electronic devices for more information.

(8) Radiation recall

(a) Radiation recall reaction is an erythematous, scaly, tender, or painless localized rash confined to a previous radiation field, presenting months to years after radiation. It usually results from exposure to chemotherapy or other agents (Bourgeois, Grisoli, Soine, & Rosen, 2017).

(b) The rash has an appearance similar to severe sunburn.

(c) It is a rare late effect and must be distinguished from other differential diagnoses, including infection or cancer recurrence.

(d) A punch biopsy of the skin and a careful drug exposure history will help to make the diagnosis.

(e) Treatment generally consists of corticosteroids to reduce inflammation and, rarely, delay of chemotherapy until the skin heals (Burris & Hurtig, 2010).

(9) Effects on lactation

(a) The inability to lactate from the treated breast is common after breast irradiation.

(b) The treated breast may produce no or limited milk; however, the contralateral breast should increase production if a patient becomes pregnant years after treatment.

(c) Patients should be counseled that the unaffected breast may become engorged with milk, and the treated breast will appear smaller until breastfeeding is completed.

(d) Breastfeeding after breast cancer local therapy (surgery and RT) can be challenging but should not be discouraged (De Simone & Pagani, 2017).

(10) Pregnancy after breast cancer (De Simone & Pagnani, 2017)

(a) De Simone and Pagani (2017) wrote that all the available retrospective data confirm that pregnancy after breast cancer is safe for the mother and offspring, as well as women with hormone receptor–positive disease.

(b) Timing of conception after the cancer is still a matter of debate, especially in women receiving adjuvant endocrine therapy.

(c) A worldwide perspective trial is currently assessing safety of interrupting endocrine treatment to allow conception.

(11) Cosmetic changes

(a) Radiation fibrosis and shrinkage of the treated breast can occur as a late effect after RT (Kaidar-Person, Marks, & Jones, 2018).

   i. The fibrous tissue in the breast can thicken, leading to changes such as retraction and asymmetry. This is usually painless.

   ii. Radiation fibrosis can occur in 13% of women receiving breast RT.

   iii. This cosmetic asymmetry can be improved with the use of pentoxifylline and vitamin E.

(b) Capsular contracture is a tightening of the tissue around a breast implant.

   i. Capsular contracture can cause shrinking and tightening of the mass of scar tissue around a breast implant because the immune system reacts to the foreign body.

   ii. Capsular contracture is usually associated with pain or poor cosmetic symmetry and occurs even without RT in some reconstructed breasts.

   iii. Capsular contracture occurs more frequently when immediate breast reconstruction is associated with postmastectomy RT.

   iv. A meta-analysis demonstrated that regardless of timing, postmastectomy RT applied to implant-based breast reconstruction was associated with high risk of reconstructive failure and capsular contracture (Ricci et al., 2017).

   v. The combination of pentoxifylline and vitamin E can prevent severe contracture and implant losses, allowing for immediate reconstruction with implant or tissue expansion, even if post-mastectomy RT is planned (Cooke et al., 2016).

References

American Cancer Society. (2020). Key statistics for breast cancer in men. https://www.cancer.org/cancer/breast-cancer-in-men/about/key-statistics.html

Arnaout, A., Lee, J., Gelmon, K., Poirier, B., Lu, F.I., Akra, M., ... Grenier, D. (2018). Neoadjuvant therapy for breast cancer: Updates and proceedings from the seventh annual meeting of the Canadian Consortium for Locally Advanced Breast Cancer. *Current Oncology, 25,* e490–e498. https://doi.org/10.3747/co.25.4153

Auwaerter, P. (2019). Lymphangitis. In J.G. Bartlett, P.G. Auwaerter, & P. Pham (Eds.), *Johns Hopkins ABX guide.* Unbound Medicine. http://www.hopkinsguides.com/hopkins/ub

Bergom, C., Currey, A., Desai, N., Tai, A., & Strauss, J.B. (2018). Deep inspiration breath hold: Techniques and advantages for cardiac sparing during breast cancer irradiation. *Frontiers in Oncology, 8,* 87. https://doi.org/10.3389/fonc.2018.00087

Bledsoe, T.J., Nath, S.K., & Decker, R.H. (2017). Radiation pneumonitis. *Clinics in Chest Medicine, 38,* 201–208. https://doi.org/10.1016/j.ccm.2016.12.004

Bourgeois, A., Grisoli, S.B., Soine, E.J., & Rosen, L.B. (2017). Tamoxifen-induced radiation recall dermatitis. *Dermatology Online Journal, 23,* 4. https://escholarship.org/uc/item/1d38c9c7

Braunstein, L.Z., & Cahlon, O. (2018). Potential morbidity reduction with proton radiation therapy in breast cancer. *Seminars in Radiation Oncology, 28,* 138–149. https://doi.org/10.1016/j.semradonc.2017.11.009

Burris, H.A., III, & Hurtig, J. (2010). Radiation recall with anticancer agents. *The Oncologist, 15,* 1227–1237. https://doi.org/10.1634/theoncologist.2009-0090

Butler-Xu, Y.S., Marietta, M., Zahra, A., TenNapel, M., & Mitchell, M. (2018). The effect of breast volume on toxicity using hypofractionated regimens for early stage breast cancer for patients. *Advances in Radiation Oncology, 4,* 261–267. https://doi.org/10.1016/j.adro.2018.10.005

Chen, C.C., Ho, W.L., Chen, H.H., Hsu, C.Y., & Chen, J.P. (2019). The association between infection incidence and autoimmune diseases in breast cancer patients after anti-cancer treatment. *Journal of Cancer, 10,* 829–835. https://doi.org/10.7150/jca.27970

Cheng, M., Loh, C., & Lin, C. (2018). Outcomes of vascularized lymph node transfer and lymphovenous anastomosis for treatment of primary lymphedema. *Plastic and Reconstructive Surgery–Global Open, 6,* e2056. https://doi.org/10.1097/gox.0000000000002056

Choi, M., Kipps, T., & Razelle, K. (2016). ATM mutations in cancer: Therapeutic implications. *Molecular Cancer Therapeutics, 15,* 1781–1791. https://doi.org/10.1158/1535-7163.mct-15-0945

Cooke, M., Johnson, N., Zegzula, H.D., Schray, M., Glissmeyer, M., & Sorenson, L. (2016). Prophylactic use of pentoxifylline (Trental) and vitamin E to prevent capsular contracture after implant reconstruction in patients requiring adjuvant radiation. *American Journal of Surgery, 211,* 854–859. https://doi.org/10.1016/j.amjsurg.2016.01.006

Correa, C., Harris, E.E., Leonardi, M.C., Smith, B.D, Taghian, A.G., Thompson, A.M., ... Harris, J.R. (2017). Accelerated partial breast irradiation: Executive summary for the update of an ASTRO evidence-based consensus statement. *Practical Radiation Oncology, 7,* 73–79. https://doi.org/10.1016/j.prro.2016.09.007

Cortazar, P., Zhang, L., Untch, M., Mehta, K., Costantino, J.P., Wolmark, N., ... von Minckwitz, G. (2014). Pathological complete response and long-term clinical benefit in breast cancer: The CTNeoBC pooled analysis. *Lancet, 384,* 164–172. https://doi.org/10.1016/s0140-6736(13)62422-8

Cronin, P.A., Olese, C., Patil, S., Morrow, M., & Van Zee, K.J. (2016). Impact of age on risk of recurrence of ductal carcinoma in situ: Outcomes of 2996 women treated with breast-conserving surgery over 30 years. *Annals of Surgical Oncology, 23,* 2816–2824. https://doi.org/10.1245/s10434-016-5249-5

Darby, S., McGale, P., Correa, C., Taylor, C., Arriagada, R., Clarke, M., ... Peto, R. (2011). Effect of radiotherapy after breast-conserving surgery on 10-year recurrence and 15-year breast-cancer death: Meta-analysis of individual patient data for 10,801 women in 17 randomised trials. *Lancet, 378,* 1707–1716. https://doi.org/10.1016/s0140-6736(11)61629-2

Deseyne, P., Speleers, B., De Neve, W., Boute, B., Paelinck, L., Van Hoof, T., ... Veldeman, L. (2017). Whole breast and regional nodal irradiation in prone versus supine position in left sided breast cancer. *Radiation Oncology, 12,* 89. https://doi.org/10.1186/s13014-017-0828-6

De Simone, V., & Pagani, O. (2017). Pregnancy after breast cancer: Hope after the storm. *Minerva Ginecologica, 69,* 597–607. https://doi.org/10.23736/S0026-4784.17.04113-2

Dworkin, R.H., O'Connor, A.B., Audette, J., Baron, R., Gourlay, G.K., Haanpää, M.L., ... Wells, C.D. (2010). Recommendations for the pharmacological management of neuropathic pain: An overview and literature update. *Mayo Clinic Proceedings, 85*(Suppl. 3), S3–S14. https://doi.org/10.4065/mcp.2009.0649

Fenton-Kerimian, M., Maisonet, O., & Formenti, S.C. (2013). Changes in breast radiotherapy: Prone positioning and hypofractionation. *Clinical Journal of Oncology Nursing, 17,* 550–553. https://doi.org/10.1188/13.cjon.550-553

Filopei, J., & Frishman, W. (2012). Radiation-induced heart disease. *Cardiology in Review, 20,* 184–188. https://doi.org/10.1097/crd.0b013e3182431c23

Formenti, S.C., Hsu, H., Fenton-Kerimian, M., Roses, D., Guth, A., Jozsef, G., ... Dewyngaert, J.K. (2012). Prone accelerated partial breast irradiation after breast-conserving surgery: Five-year results of 100 patients. *International Journal of Radiation Oncology, Biology, Physics, 84,* 606–611. https://doi.org/10.1016/j.ijrobp.2012.01.039

Giuliano, A.E., Ballman, K., McCall, L., Beitsch, P., Whitworth, P.W., Blumencranz, P., ... Hunt, K.K. (2016). Locoregional recurrence after sentinel lymph node dissection with or without axillary dissection in patients with sentinel lymph node metastases: Long-term follow-up from the American College of Surgeons Oncology Group (Alliance) ACOSOG Z0011 randomized trial. *Annals of Surgery, 264,* 413–420. https://doi.org/10.1097/sla.0000000000001863

Gosk, J., Rutowski, R., Reichert, P., & Rabczyński, J. (2007). Radiation-induced brachial plexus neuropathy—Aetiopathogenesis, risk factors, differential diagnostics, symptoms and treatment. *Folia Neuropathologica, 45,* 26–30. https://www.termedia.pl/Review-article-Radiation-induced-brachial-plexus-neuropathy-8211-aetiopathogenesis-risk-factors-differential-diagnostics-symptoms-and-treatment,20,7662,1,1.html

Grann, A., & Haffty, B.G. (2019). Excision and reirradiation for local recurrence in previously treated patient. *International Journal of Radiation Oncology, Biology, Physics, 105,* 473. https://doi.org/10.1016/j.ijrobp.2019.08.043

Grantzau, T., & Overgaard, J. (2015). Risk of second non-breast cancer after radiotherapy for breast cancer: A systematic review and meta-analysis of 762,468 patients. *Radiotherapy and Oncology, 114,* 56–65. https://doi.org/10.1016/j.radonc.2014.10.004

Grewal, A.S., Freedman, G.M., Jones, J.A., & Taunk, N.K. (2019). Hypofractionated radiation therapy for durable palliative treatment of bleeding, fungating breast cancers. *Practical Radiation Oncology, 9,* 73–76. https://doi.org/10.1016/j.prro.2018.11.003

Hoebers, F.J.P., Ferguson, P.C., & O'Sullivan, B. (2011). Bone. In D.C. Shrieve & J.S. Loeffler (Eds.), *Human radiation injury* (pp. 481–498). Lippincott Williams and Wilkins.

Hopwood, P., Haviland, J.S., Sumo, G., Mills, J., Bliss, J.M., & Yarnold, J.R. (2010). Comparison of patient-reported breast, arm, and shoulder symptoms and body image after radiotherapy for early breast cancer: 5-year follow-up in the randomized standardization of breast radiotherapy (START) trials. *Lancet Oncology, 11,* 231–240. https://doi.org/10.1016/s1470-2045(09)70382-1

Huang, Y., Fan, H., Li, N., & Du, J. (2019). Risk of immune-related pneumonitis for PD1/PD-L1 inhibitors: Systematic review and network meta-analysis. *Cancer Medicine, 8,* 2664–2674. https://doi.org/10.1002/cam4.2104

Iyer, R., & Jhingran, A. (2006). Radiation injury: Imaging findings in the chest, abdomen and pelvis after therapeutic radiation. *Cancer Imaging, 6,* S131–S139. https://doi.org/10.1102/1470-7330.2006.9095

Jain, V., & Berman, A.T. (2018). Radiation pneumonitis: Old problem, new tricks. *Cancers, 10,* 222. https://doi.org/10.3390/cancers10070222

Johns Hopkins Medicine. (n.d.). Treating lymphedema. https://www.hopkinsmedicine.org/health/treatment-tests-and-therapies/treating-lymphedema

Kaidar-Person, O., Marks, L.B., & Jones, E.L. (2018). Pentoxifylline and vitamin E for treatment or prevention of radiation-induced fibrosis in patients with breast cancer. *Breast Journal, 24,* 816–819. https://doi.org/10.1111/tbj.13044

Kamenova, B., Braverman, A.A., Schwartz, M., Sohn, C., Lange, C., Efiom-Ekaha, D., ... Yoon, H. (2009). Effective treatment of the brachial plexus syndrome in breast cancer patients by early detection and control of locoregional metastases with radiation or systemic therapy. *International Journal of Clinical Oncology, 14,* 219–224. https://doi.org/10.1007/s10147-008-0838-3

Kushner, C.J., Hwang, W.-T., Wang, S., Solin, L.J., & Vapiwala, N. (2018). Long-term risk of second malignancies in women after breast conservation therapy for ductal carcinoma in situ or early-stage breast cancer. *Breast Cancer Research and Treatment, 170,* 45–53. https://doi.org/10.1007/s10549-018-4729-7

Lymberis, S., DeWyngaert, J.K., Parhar, P., Chhabra, A., Fenton-Kerimian, M., Chang, J., ... Formenti, S.C. (2012). Prospective assessment of optimal individual position (prone versus supine) for breast radiotherapy: Volumetric and dosimetric correlations in 100 patients. *International Journal of Radiation Oncology, Biology, Physics, 84,* 902–909. https://doi.org/10.1016/j.ijrobp.2012.01.040

McBride, W.H., Withers, H.R., & Schaue, D. (2019). Biologic basis of radiation therapy. In E.C. Halperin, D.E. Wazer, C.A. Perez, & L.W. Brady (Eds.), *Perez and Brady's principles and practice of radiation oncology* (7th ed., pp. 87–111). Wolters Kluwer.

McDuff, S.G.R., Mina, A.I., Brunelle, C.L., Salama, L., Warren, L.E.G., Abouegylah, M., ... Taghian, A.G. (2019). The timing of lymphedema after treatment for breast cancer: When are patients most at risk? *International Journal of Radiation, Biology, Physics, 103,* 62–70. https://doi.org/10.1016/j.ijrobp.2018.08.036

McQuestion, M. (2011). Evidence-based skin care management in radiation therapy: Clinical update. *Seminars in Oncology Nursing, 27,* e1–e17. https://doi.org/10.1016/j.soncn.2011.02.009

Mishra, R., Khurana, R., Mishra, H., & Hadi, R. (2016). Retrospective analysis of efficacy and toxicity of hypo-fractionated radiotherapy in breast carcinoma. *Journal of Clinical and Diagnostic Research, 10,* XC01–XC03. https://doi.org/10.7860/jcdr/2016/20769.8350

National Association for Proton Therapy. (2019). How does proton therapy work? https://www.proton-therapy.org/science

National Cancer Institute. (n.d.). Adjuvant therapy. In *NCI dictionary of cancer terms.* https://www.cancer.gov/publications/dictionaries/cancer-terms/def/adjuvant-therapy

National Cancer Institute. (2020). Cancer stat facts: Female breast cancer. https://seer.cancer.gov/statfacts/html/breast.html

Nieder, C., Langendijk, J.A., Guckenberger, M., & Grosu, A.L. (2018). Second re-irradiation: A narrative review of the available clinical data. *Acta Oncologica, 57,* 305–310. https://doi.org/10.1080/0284186x.2017.1409433

Nofech-Mozes, S., Hanna, W., & Rakovitch, E. (2019). Molecular evaluation of breast carcinoma *in situ* with oncotype DX DCIS. *American Journal of Pathology, 31,* 975–980. https://doi.org/10.1016/j.ajpath.2018.12.003

Onitilo, A.A., Engel, J.M., Stankowski, R.V., & Doi, S.A.R. (2015). Survival comparisons for breast conserving surgery and mastectomy revisited: Community experience and the role of radiation therapy. *Clinical Medicine and Research, 13,* 65–73. https://doi.org/10.3121/cmr.2014.1245

Osa, E.-O.O., DeWyngaert, K., Roses, D., Speyer, J., Guth, A., Axelrod, D., ... Formenti, S.C. (2014). Prone breast intensity modulated radiation therapy: 5-year results. *International Journal of Radiation Oncology, Biology, Physics, 89,* 899–906. https://doi.org/10.1016/j.ijrobp.2014.03.036

Palma, D.A., Senan, S., Tsujino, K., Barriger, R.B., Rengan, R., Moreno, M., ... Rodrigues, G. (2013). Predicting radiation pneumonitis after chemoradiation therapy for lung cancer: An international individual patient data meta-analysis. *International Journal of Radiation Oncology Biology and Physics, 85,* 444–450. https://doi.org/10.1016/j.ijrobp.2012.04.043

Ratovich, E., Nofech-Mozes, S., Hanna, W., Baehner, F.L., Saskin, R., Butler, S.M., ... Paszat, L. (2015). A population-based validation study of the DCIS score predicting recurrence risk in individuals treated by breast-conserving surgery alone. *Breast Cancer Research and Treatment, 152,* 389–398. https://doi.org/10.1007/s10549-015-3464-6

Ratovich, E., Nofech-Mozes, S., Narod, S.A., Hanna, W., Thiruchelvam, D., Saskin, R., ... Paszat, L. (2013). Can we select individuals with low risk ductal carcinoma in situ (DCIS)? A population-based outcome analysis. *Breast Cancer Research and Treatment, 138,* 581–590. https://doi.org/10.1007/s10549-013-2455-8

Raza, S., Lymberis, S.C., Ciervide, R., Axelrod, D., Fenton-Kerimian, M., Magnolfi, C., ... Formenti, S.C. (2012). Comparison of acute and late toxicity of two regimens of 3- and 5-week concomitant boost prone IMRT to standard 6-week breast radiotherapy. *Frontiers in Oncology, 2,* 44. https://doi.org/10.3389/fonc.2012.00044

Ricci, J.A., Epstein, S., Momoh, A.O., Lin, S.J., Singhal, D., & Lee, B.T. (2017). A meta-analysis of implant-based breast reconstruction and timing of adjuvant radiation therapy. *Journal of Surgical Research, 218,* 108–116. https://doi.org/10.1016/j.jss.2017.05.072

Rouzier, R., Pronzato, P., Chéreau, E., Carlson, J., Hunt, B., & Valentine, W.J. (2013). Multigene assays and molecular markers in breast cancer: A systematic review of health economic analyses. *Breast Cancer Research and Treatment, 139,* 621–637. https://doi.org/10.1007/s10549-013-2559-1

Shah, C., Vicini, F., Shaitelman, S.F., Hepel, J., Keisch, M., Arthur, D., ... Wazer, D.E. (2018). The American Brachytherapy Society consensus statement for accelerated partial-breast irradiation. *Brachytherapy, 17,* 154–170. https://doi.org/10.1016/j.brachy.2017.09.004

Shaikh, F., Chew, J., Hochman, T., Purswani, J., Maisonet, O., Peat, E., ... Gerber, N.K. (2018). Hypofractionated whole-breast irradiation in women less than 50 years old treated on 4 prospective protocols. *International Journal of Radiation Oncology, Biology, Physics, 101,* 1159–1167. https://doi.org/10.1016/j.ijrobp.2018.04.034

Shao, N., Xie, C., Shi, Y., Ye, R., Long, J., Shi, H., ... Lin, Y. (2019). Comparison of the 7th and 8th edition of American Joint Committee on Cancer (AJCC) staging systems for breast cancer patients: A Surveillance, Epidemiology and End Results (SEER) analysis. *Cancer Management and Research, 11,* 1433–1442. https://doi.org/10.2147/cmar.s185212

Shin, S.M., No, H.S., Vega, R.M., Fenton-Kerimian, M., Maisonet, O., Hitchen, C., ... Formenti, S.C. (2016). Breast, chest wall, and nodal irradiation with prone set-up: Results of a hypofractionated trial with a median follow-up of 35 months. *Practical Radiation Oncology, 6,* e81–e88. https://doi.org/10.1016/j.prro.2015.10.022

Smith, R.E. (2003). Risk for the development of treatment-related acute myelocytic leukemia and myelodysplastic syndrome among patients with breast cancer: Review of the literature and the National Surgical Adjuvant Breast and Bowel Project experience. *Clinical Breast Cancer, 4,* 273–279. https://doi.org/10.3816/cbc.2003.n.032

Stone, J.B., & DeAngelis, L.M. (2016). Cancer-treatment–induced neurotoxicity—Focus on newer treatments. *Nature Reviews Clinical Oncology, 13,* 92–105. https://doi.org/10.1038/nrclinonc.2015.152

Taghian, A. (2020, May 7). Adjuvant radiation therapy for women with newly diagnosed, non-metastatic breast cancer. In S.R. Vora (Ed.), *UpToDate.* Retrieved May 19, 2020, from https://www.uptodate.com/contents/adjuvant-radiation-therapy-for-women-with-newly-diagnosed-non-metastatic-breast-cancer

Taylor, C., Correa, C., Duane, F.K., Aznar, M.C., Anderson, S.J., Bergh, J., ... McGale, P. (2017). Estimating the risks of breast cancer radiotherapy: Evidence from modern radiation doses to the lungs and heart and from previous randomized trials. *Journal of Clinical Oncology, 35,* 1641–1649. https://doi.org/10.1200/jco.2016.72.0722

Taylor, C.W., Wang, Z., Macaulay, E., Jagsi, R., Duane, F., & Darby, S.C. (2015). Exposure of the heart in breast cancer radiation therapy: A systemic review of heart doses published during 2003 to 2013. *International Journal of Radiation Oncology, Biology, Physics, 93,* 845–853. https://doi.org/10.1016/j.ijrobp.2015.07.2292

Tryfonidis, K., Senkus, E., Cardoso, M.J., & Cardoso, F. (2015). Management of locally advanced breast cancer—Perspectives and future directions. *Nature Reviews Clinical Oncology, 12,* 147–162. https://doi.org/10.1038/nrclinonc.2015.13

Wapnir, I.L., Dignam, J.J., Fisher, B., Mamounas, E., Anderson, S.J., Julian, T.B., ... Wolmark, N. (2011). Long-term outcomes of invasive ipsilateral breast tumor recurrences after lumpectomy in NSABP B-17 and B-24 randomized clinical trials for DCIS. *Journal of the National Cancer Institute, 103,* 478–488. https://doi.org/10.1093/jnci/djr027

Warade, A.C., Jha, A.K., Pattanker, S., & Desai, K. (2019). Radiation-induced brachial plexus neuropathy: A review. *Neurology India, 67*(Suppl. 1), 47–52. https://doi.org/10.4103/0028-3886.250704

Whelan, T.J., Pignol, J.-P., Levine, M.N., Julian, J.A., MacKenzie, R., Parpia, S., ... Freeman, C. (2010). Long-term results of hypofractionated radiation therapy for breast cancer. *New England Journal of Medicine, 362,* 513–520. https://doi.org/10.1056/nejmoa0906260

Ye, J.C., & Formenti, S.C. (2018). Integration of radiation and immunotherapy in breast cancer—Treatment implications. *Breast, 38,* 66–74. https://doi.org/10.1016/j.breast.2017.12.005

D. Thorax

1. Indications

   a) NSCLC

      (1) NSCLC accounts for 84% of all lung cancer cases. There are three major subtypes of NSCLC (American Cancer Society, 2020).

         (a) Adenocarcinoma (approximately 40%), which forms in the cells that line the alveoli

         (b) Squamous cell (epidermoid; 25%–30%), which originates from the cells lining the airways

         (c) Undifferentiated large cell (10%–15%), which has an unknown origin cell

      (2) The TNM staging system provides common language to describe the extent of disease and define prognosis. The most recent revision of the system (8th edition), published by AJCC and the Union for International Cancer Control, became the worldwide standard as of January 1, 2018 (Detterbeck, Boffa, Kim, & Tanoue, 2017).

      (3) Surgery remains the standard of care for medically operable stage I–II NSCLC. ASTRO guidelines on SBRT for early-stage NSCLC note that technological developments have provided support for the use of SBRT in challenging clinical situations; however, randomized controlled trials are needed for stronger recommendations to be made (Videtic et al., 2017).

      (4) In 1998, a Medical Research Council (United Kingdom) meta-analysis noted that overall survival decreased with postoperative RT (or PORT) in patients with NSCLC. In 2005 and 2010, the PORT Meta-Analysist Trialists Group added new clinical data without significant change to the conclusions, except to note a 24% decrease in local recurrence in stage III (N2) NSCLC treated with postoperative RT (Burdett et al., 2016).

      (5) Patients with medically inoperable early-stage NSCLC can be treated with definitive RT.

         (a) Medically inoperable patients include those with poor respiratory status, as evidenced by pulmonary function testing; severe pulmonary hypertension; end organ disease; severe cerebral, cardiac,

or peripheral vascular disease; or severe chronic cardiac disease (Timmerman et al., 2018).

(b) Conventional RT can be delivered in 2 Gy fractions (60–70 Gy total), or SBRT can be delivered in 1–10 fractions (25–70 Gy total).

(6) Patients with locally advanced unresectable NSCLC may receive chemoradiation, or if they are unable to tolerate chemotherapy, then receive RT alone, with a minimum dose of 60 Gy in 2 Gy fractions as the standard of care for conventional radiation (Rodrigues et al., 2015b).

(7) Concomitant chemoradiation shows improved patient survival, local control, and disease response rate over sequential chemoradiation (Rodrigues et al., 2015a).

(8) The effectiveness of adjuvant and neoadjuvant RT and chemoradiation remain an area of ongoing interest to researchers because of advances in surgical techniques and RT delivery (Rodrigues et al., 2015a).

(9) Palliative concurrent treatment, moderately hypofractionated RT, and chemoradiation are indicated for incurable stage III NSCLC (Moeller et al., 2018).

(10) For stage IV disease, RT is effective for palliation of symptoms including pain, airway obstruction, hemoptysis, and SVCS.

(a) Patients with stage IV disease and good performance status may benefit from higher dose fractionation.

(b) It is important to note that routine use of concurrent chemotherapy is not recommended (Rodrigues et al., 2015b).

b) Small cell lung cancer (SCLC)

(1) SCLC accounts for 15%–18% of all diagnosed lung cancers. Approximately 80% of patients with SCLC are diagnosed at stage IV (Kahnert, Kauffmann-Guerrero, & Huber, 2016).

(2) TNM staging is recommended for SCLC; however, the Veterans Administration Lung Study Group classification dichotomy of limited stage (TNM stages I–III) and extensive stage (TNM stage IV) is often still referenced (Nicholson et al., 2016).

(3) Staging determines treatment protocols (Sun et al., 2018).

(a) In very limited (stage I) SCLC, surgery is indicated followed by adjuvant chemotherapy.

(b) With limited-stage (stage II–III) disease, concurrent chemoradiation plays an important role in preventing local recurrence.

(c) Sequential chemoradiation can be used for those unfit for concurrent therapy.

(d) Patients with extensive-stage SCLC receive palliative and supportive chemotherapy, but for those unable to tolerate systemic therapy, palliative and supportive RT is indicated.

(4) Concurrent, and if possible, accelerated hyperfractionation should be considered for limited-stage SCLC (Kahnert et al., 2016). A total dose of 45 Gy is delivered in divided 1.5 Gy fractions twice daily for three weeks (NCCN, 2020c).

(5) Decreased length of time from first day of chemotherapy to the final day of RT has shown improved survival in patients with limited-stage SCLC (Wahl & Garsa, 2018).

(6) Prophylactic cranial irradiation should be standard of care for all patients with SCLC who show response to initial chemotherapy treatment. Long-term effects, including neuropsychological toxicities, should be further evaluated, especially in very limited-stage SCLC (W. Zhang et al., 2014).

(7) Anatomic avoidance, such as hippocampal avoidance whole-brain RT, and pharmacotherapy agents, such as N-methyl-D-aspartate receptor antagonists (e.g., memantine), are being investigated to address neurocognitive toxicities associated with brain irradiation (Robin & Rusthoven, 2018).

c) Esophageal cancer

(1) The two most common types of esophageal cancer are squamous cell carcinoma, which typically occurs in the upper and middle third of the esophagus, and adenocarcinoma, which is often noted in the lower third of the esophagus near the stomach (Castro et al., 2018).

(2) Squamous cell carcinoma is the most common histologic type worldwide; however, the prevalence of adenocarcinoma has increased in the United States in recent decades (Abnet, Arnold, & Wei, 2018).

(3) Treatment of locally advanced esophageal cancer is multimodal in nature and includes neoadjuvant concurrent chemoradiation and surgical resection four to six weeks after completion of chemoradiation.

(a) Medically inoperable patients can be treated with definitive chemoradiation, and recurrent or metastatic disease can be treated with palliative and supportive RT (Shapiro et al., 2015).

(b) In the preoperative setting, a total dose of 41.4–50.4 Gy may be administered in daily 1.8–2 Gy fractions.

(c) Postoperative patients may receive a total dose of 45–50.4 Gy administered in 1.8–2 Gy daily fractions, and definitive RT total doses are 50–50.4 Gy (NCCN, 2020a).

d) Metastatic cancer

(1) In patients with oligometastatic lung disease, surgical resection is the standard of care for those who are medically operable, and RT is an alternative for those who are not (Baschnagel et al., 2013).

(2) SBRT for metastatic tumors in the lung are well tolerated with less severe toxicities. Longer disease-free interval and prolonged overall survival are seen in most oligometastatic disease, except in colorectal cancer. The reason for the exception of colorectal cancer is unclear and continues to be studied (Aoki et al., 2016).

e) Thymic malignancies

(1) Thymic malignancies are rare, but they are the most common primary tumors of the anterior mediastinum in adults (Patel, Macdonald, Nagda, Bittner, & Suntharalingam, 2012).

(a) Thymoma is the most common thymic malignancy, and it tends to have a more indolent course.

(b) Thymic carcinomas are the most aggressive form, and thymic carcinoids or neuroendocrine tumors of the thymus are extremely rare (Willmann & Rimner, 2018).

(2) The most commonly used anatomical staging system for thymic malignancies is the Masaoka-Koga system which has prognostic significance, however, the eight version of the AJCC staging system now includes both the traditional TNM staging and prognostic indicators to stage certain tumors (Willmann & Rimner, 2018).

(3) For thymoma, surgical resection is the optimal intervention (Giannopoulou, Gkiozos, Harrington, & Syrigos, 2013).

(a) Stage I disease is treated with surgery alone.

(b) For resected stage II–IV thymoma with no residual disease, RT can be considered.

(c) Resected stage II–IV thymoma with residual disease will be treated using RT alone or RT with chemotherapy.

(d) Typical dosing is 60–70 Gy (in standard 1.8–2 Gy fractions) for patients with unresectable disease and 45–60 Gy given for adjuvant RT.

f) Malignant pleural mesothelioma

(1) Mesothelioma is a rare but aggressive, and often deadly, malignancy of the pleura (Chance, Rebueno, & Gomez, 2015).

(2) Multimodal therapy remains the standard of care (Chance et al., 2015).

(3) Patients with stage I–IIIA mesothelioma are evaluated for surgery or treated with induction chemotherapy.

(a) Those receiving induction chemotherapy, who will ultimately undergo resection, may potentially get RT.

(b) The patients who have resectable disease at diagnosis and undergo extrapleural pneumonectomy will receive sequential chemotherapy and hemithoracic RT (NCCN, 2019a).

(4) High-dose adjuvant hemithoracic RT after extrapleural pneumonectomy continues to be studied. One method is known as SMART (surgery for mesothelioma after RT), in which 25 Gy are delivered in five fractions. Extrapleural pneumonectomy is performed two weeks after RT. Studies show resection at this time frame can help mitigate radiation-induced pneumonitis (de Perrot et al., 2016).

(5) Lung-sparing techniques are also the subject of large institutional studies. For example, hemithoracic intensity-modulated pleural RT (known as IMPRINT) combines chemotherapy, IMRT (50.4 Gy in 28 fractions), and pleurectomy and decortication, instead of the more aggressive extrapleural pneumonectomy (Rimner et al., 2016).

(6) Challenges exist with treatment of malignant pleural mesothelioma because of the large GTV, which can lead to serious side effects, including fatal pneumonitis (Robinson, Baas, & Kindler, 2010).

g) Immunotherapy (Chicas-Sett et al., 2019)

(1) Studies are investigating the use of immunotherapy in conjunction with RT.

(a) Trials that studied RT with immunotherapy include CHECKMATE 017 and CHECKMATE 057, which studied nivolumab; KEYNOTE-010, which studied pembrolizumab; and POPLAR, which studied atezolizumab.

(b) Limited data available from these and other studies suggest the combination of RT and immune checkpoint inhibitors may be safe, but further studies are still needed.

(2) One specific area of interest with immune checkpoint inhibitors is abscopal effects, in which local RT initiates an antitumor response that kills cancer cells, which are distant to the area being treated with RT.

(3) NSCLC has been noted to be a poorly immunogenic tumor; however, immune checkpoint inhibitors are promising in this population.

2. RT techniques
a) 3DCRT
  (1) 3DCRT uses multiple beams to match the shape of the tumor or site being treated (Behrend, 2018).
  (2) With technological advances in staging, imaging, and RT planning and delivery, 3DCRT is now used less often in thoracic RT (Ricardi et al., 2012).
b) IMRT
  (1) IMRT allows for more control and certainty, which leads to more effective sparing of healthy tissues.
  (2) This technique allows for fewer toxicities, increased efficacy, and better target coverage (Liao et al., 2010; Ling, Hess, Chen, & Daly, 2016).
  (3) IMRT may also help reduce the percentage of lung volume receiving more than 20 Gy, which may help decrease the risk of pneumonitis (Keall, Belderbos, & Kong, 2010).
  (4) With all complex RT techniques, respiratory motion management, gating, and breath hold need to be considered. Even when tumor tracking is used, motion management must be employed (Molitoris et al., 2018).
c) IGRT (Krauss, 2014)
  (1) Thoracic IGRT is complex because lung tumors are difficult to see with portal imaging; they can move significantly with respiration; and during treatment, significant changes in the internal and external anatomy may occur.
  (2) Tumor motion due to respiration must be considered, so CT images are used at coordinated phases of respiration, which allows for precision in planning and delivery of RT.
d) SBRT
  (1) SBRT is typically used in patients with early-stage NSCLC with no lymph node involvement and who are medically inoperable. It is also used in patients with pulmonary oligometastatic disease (Abreu et al., 2015).
  (2) Clinical trials have demonstrated local control rates of 90% at five years with SBRT for inoperable early-stage NSCLC (Dickhoff et al., 2018).
    (a) Peripheral tumors that are small and more than 1 cm from the chest wall can be treated with 25–34 Gy in one fraction.
    (b) If tumors are less than 1 cm from the chest wall, 40–60 Gy in three fractions are recommended.
    (c) Larger and more central tumors are treated with 48–55 Gy in 4–5 fractions, and central tumors are treated with up to 70 Gy in 8–10 fractions (NCCN, 2020b).

(3) Studies also show excellent local control without increased toxicity when using SBRT for multiple primary lung tumors and second lung cancers (Rieber et al., 2016).
(4) High dose per fraction can increase the risk of toxicities (Falkson et al., 2017).
  (a) Fistulas, pneumonitis, and hemoptysis can occur when treating centrally located tumors.
  (b) Peripheral lesions treated with SBRT can lead to increased skin toxicities, rib fractures, and brachial plexopathy.
(5) In a systematic review of SBRT in early-stage SCLC, Rathod, Koul, Bashir, Chowdhury, and Dubey (2019) cautiously noted that SBRT is a potential treatment option. They found similar outcomes without increased toxicities when compared to current regimens.
(6) Another area of study is salvage surgery after treatment with SBRT. Literature seems to show that it is technically feasible in medically operable patients; however, more research is needed in this area (Dickhoff et al., 2018).
e) Brachytherapy
  (1) Endobronchial HDR brachytherapy
    (a) Endobronchial HDR brachytherapy can be used for local control and symptom management in advanced NSCLC.
    (b) The American Brachytherapy Society consensus guidelines recommend palliative endobronchial brachytherapy for patients with central obstructing lesions. HDR is recommended over LDR brachytherapy for endobronchial treatment (Stewart et al., 2016).
    (c) It can also be used in limited cases for definitive treatment with or without RT in small tumors.
  (2) Esophageal HDR brachytherapy (Stewart et al., 2016)
    (a) Esophageal HDR brachytherapy may be used as a boost after the completion of EBRT.
    (b) It may also be used for definitive and salvage management with esophageal cancer.
    (c) It is an effective modality for palliation of dysphagia and esophageal obstruction.
  (3) LDR brachytherapy (Parashar, Arora, & Wernicke, 2013)
    (a) LDR brachytherapy can be used with surgical resection for NSCLC.
    (b) Iodine-125, cesium-131, and palladium-103 are the most commonly used isotopes.
    (c) The total delivered radiation dose to the local tissues can vary depending on the

isotope used. The depth of treatment is 0.5 cm with a 1 cm margin on both sides of the staple line.

    f) Proton beam therapy

        (1) The absence of an exit dose of protons makes proton beam therapy a reasonable choice for RT when a tumor is close to a critical structure or OAR. This is often the case with thoracic RT (Liao, Gandhi, Lin, & Bradley, 2018).

        (2) Multiple studies have shown the benefit and efficacy of proton beam therapy over photon beam therapy in early- and advanced-stage NSCLC (Higgins et al., 2017).

        (3) Despite promising outcomes, proton beam therapy is not the current standard of care. It is still associated with high cost and is not covered by many insurance companies at this time. (Higgins et al., 2017).

        (4) Toxicities and quality of life need to be further investigated when comparing proton and photon beam therapy.

3. Acute side effects

    a) Cough

        (1) Pathophysiology

            (a) According to the *Family Practice Guidelines*, acute inflammation or irritation of the respiratory tract can lead to cough (Cash & Glass, 2017).

            (b) Coughing is a medullary reflex response, but the action is also able to be somewhat controlled (Cash & Glass, 2017).

            (c) The cause is complex and controversial, but in the RT setting, cough is thought to be the result of main bronchus and large bronchiole irritation (Molassiotis, Smith, Mazzone, Blackhall, & Irwin, 2017).

        (2) Incidence and risk factors

            (a) Of all patients with cancer, 23%–37% experience cough. Of patients with lung cancer, 47%–86% experience cough (Molassiotis et al., 2017).

            (b) Continued smoking increases cough.

        (3) Assessment: Assessment of cough includes the following (Bickley, 2017).

            (a) Determination whether cough is productive or nonproductive, noting sputum color and consistency

            (b) Auscultation of breath sounds

            (c) Monitoring oxygen saturation level

            (d) Hydration and nutritional status

            (e) Association with heartburn

            (f) Examination for fever, chills, and diaphoresis

        (4) Documentation: Documentation of cough should utilize CTCAE (NCI CTEP, 2017, p. 125).

        (a) Grade 1: mild symptoms; nonprescription intervention indicated

        (b) Grade 2: moderate symptoms; medical intervention indicated; limiting instrumental ADL

        (c) Grade 3: severe symptoms; limiting self-care ADL

        (5) Collaborative management: Management of cough includes the following (Dezube, 2020; Vijayan & Groninger, 2013).

            (a) Demulcents or mucoprotective agents

            (b) Expectorants

            (c) Bronchodilators (e.g., inhalers, nebulizers)

            (d) Supplemental oxygen as needed

            (e) Chest x-ray if indicated

            (f) Antihistamines

        (6) Patient, caregiver, and family education (Memorial Sloan Kettering Cancer Center, 2018)

            (a) Clinicians should encourage smoking cessation. Continued smoking will irritate the lining of the airway and cause more coughing.

            (b) Patients can use one or two pillows to elevate their upper body while sleeping.

            (c) Instruction includes information on use of medications, including suppressants, expectorants, and bronchodilators.

            (d) Patients can use a humidifier while sleeping.

            (e) Patients should be instructed to report any signs or symptoms of infection, including fevers, change in color of secretions, shortness of breath, or dyspnea.

    b) Esophagitis

        (1) Pathophysiology (Baker & Fairchild, 2016)

            (a) Mucosal inflammation and thinning of the esophageal lining within the RT field lead to esophagitis.

            (b) The epithelium is very radiosensitive because mucosal cells have a high turnover rate. Irritation usually occurs two to three weeks after the beginning of treatment.

        (2) Incidence and risk factors (Baker & Fairchild, 2016)

            (a) In both definitive and palliative lung RT, radiation-induced esophagitis is the most common local effect.

            (b) Esophagitis is a common dose-limiting complication for thoracic RT.

            (c) Hyperfractionated RT and concurrent chemotherapy increase the risk of severe acute esophagitis.

        (3) Assessment: Assessment of esophagitis includes the following (Bickley, 2017).

            (a) Assessment for dysphagia and odynophagia

(b) Assessment for swallowing impairment

(c) Evaluation of nutritional status for impairment; close monitoring of patient weight

(d) Assessment for candidiasis (thrush)

(4) Documentation: Documentation of esophagitis focuses on the following.

    (a) Pharynx and esophagus, using CTCAE (NCI CTEP, 2017, p. 28)

        i. Grade 1: asymptomatic; clinical or diagnostic observations only; intervention not indicated

        ii. Grade 2: symptomatic, altered eating/swallowing; oral supplements indicated

        iii. Grade 3: severely altered eating/swallowing; tube feeding, [total parenteral nutrition], or hospitalization indicated

        iv. Grade 4: life-threatening consequences; urgent operative intervention indicated

        v. Grade 5: death

    (b) Pain location and intensity

    (c) Effectiveness of intervention

(5) Collaborative management: Management of esophagitis includes the following (Poirier, 2013; Sourati, Ameri, & Malekzadeh, 2017).

    (a) Consultation with RDN or RD at onset of treatment

    (b) Dietary modification and the addition of liquid nutrition supplements for inadequate intake

    (c) Pain medications, including over-the-counter medications and narcotics (oral, liquid, or transdermal); consultation for pain management if needed (see IV.C. Pain)

    (d) Acid-suppressing medications

    (e) Sitting upright for 30 minutes after eating

    (f) Antifungals for candidiasis (present or suspected)

(6) Patient, caregiver, and family education (Memorial Sloan Kettering Cancer Center, 2018)

    (a) Clinicians should discuss avoidance, or at minimum, limiting alcohol, tobacco, spicy food, caffeine, and acidic food and drinks.

    (b) Clinicians can encourage small, frequent meals and a bland and soft diet.

    (c) Patients should take pain medication prior to eating.

    (d) Patients should report any sudden increase in pain or change in ability to swallow.

    (e) Clinicians should inform patients that acute side effects may last at least three to four weeks after completion of treatment.

    (f) Clinicians should encourage smoking cessation.

c) Dyspnea

(1) Pathophysiology (Shelton et al., 2019)

    (a) Dyspnea is a subjective finding of breathlessness reported by many patients with lung cancer who receive thoracic RT.

    (b) Dyspnea can increase a patient's level of anxiety and fatigue.

(2) Incidence and risk factors

    (a) At diagnosis, 15%–55% of patients experience dyspnea (DiSalvo & Joyce, 2009).

    (b) For patients with dyspnea at baseline, 20% will have less dyspnea six months after RT (De Ruysscher et al., 2009).

    (c) Dyspnea can be exacerbated by various factors, including asthma, chronic obstructive pulmonary disease, anemia, pulmonary embolism, anxiety, and smoking.

(3) Assessment: Assessment of dyspnea should evaluate the following (Bickley, 2017).

    (a) Severity of symptoms, difference from baseline, and impact on ADLs

    (b) Heart and lung breath sounds, use of accessory muscles

    (c) Skin color

    (d) Breathing pattern and rate

    (e) Oxygen saturation level

    (f) Signs of infection, including cough, fever, or increased WBC count

    (g) Anxiety, fear, or depression

(4) Documentation: Documentation of dyspnea should utilize CTCAE (NCI CTEP, 2017, p. 125).

    (a) Grade 1: shortness of breath with moderate exertion

    (b) Grade 2: shortness of breath with minimal exertion; limiting instrumental ADL

    (c) Grade 3: shortness of breath at rest; limiting self-care ADL

    (d) Grade 4: life-threatening consequences; urgent intervention indicated

    (e) Grade 5: death

(5) Collaborative management: Management of dyspnea includes the following measures (Dudgeon, 2013).

    (a) Supplemental oxygen as needed

    (b) Chest x-ray if infection is suspected

    (c) Bronchodilators to relieve airway constriction

    (d) Corticosteroids to decrease lung irritation

    (e) Anxiolytics to decrease anxiety

    (f) Psychosocial management

(6) Patient, caregiver, and family education (Bonk, 2012)

(a) Instruction should include information on medications, including bronchodilators, steroids, pain management, and anxiolytics.

(b) Clinicians should teach patients alternative breathing techniques (e.g., pursed-lip breathing).

(c) Clinicians can provide ideas to help conserve energy.

(d) Clinicians should provide emotional support.

(e) Clinicians should encourage smoking cessation if indicated.

d) Skin reactions: Skin reactions may occur in patients receiving thoracic RT. SBRT to peripheral tumors can increase radiation skin dose (see IV.B. Skin reactions).

e) Fatigue: Patients with lung cancer frequently experience fatigue (see IV.A. Fatigue).

4. Late or delayed side effects

a) Radiation pneumonitis

(1) Pathophysiology

(a) Radiation-induced lung injury is a well-known complication of RT. Radiation pneumonitis is a subtype of radiation-induced lung injury.

(b) Cytotoxic damage to the type II pneumocytes and vascular endothelial cells leads to mitosis with cellular injury. Damage occurs in five phases (Bledsoe, Nath, & Decker, 2017).

i. Immediate phase (hours to days): Intra-alveolar edema and vascular congestion start, but patients are asymptomatic.

ii. Latent phase (days to weeks): Thick secretions accumulate; however, patients remain asymptomatic.

iii. Acute exudative phase (weeks to months): Epithelial and endothelial sloughing starts, along with clinical symptoms.

iv. Intermediate phase (months): Changes progress with increased symptoms.

v. Fibrotic phase (months to years): Injury and fibrosis develop, which diminishes lung volumes.

(2) Incidence and risk factors

(a) Exact incidence of radiation pneumonitis is difficult to quantify because it varies by primary disease and manner of diagnosis (clinical or imaging) (Bledsoe et al., 2017). Incidence of symptomatic radiation pneumonitis after SBRT can range 9%–28% (Yamashita, Takahashi, Haga, & Nakagawa, 2014).

(b) Advanced RT technology, including IMRT, IGRT, and proton therapy, has helped reduce the incidence and severity of radiation pneumonitis.

(c) There is a demonstrated relationship between dose volume and radiation pneumonitis incidence. A daily dose volume of 20 Gy or more has an increased risk of pneumonitis.

(d) Risk factors for radiation pneumonitis, beyond dose limits include fractionation schedule, chemotherapy, and hormone therapy. Immunotherapy is independently associated with pneumonitis. The impact of age, sex, tumor site, performance status, and lung disease continue to be studied (Jain & Berman, 2018).

(e) Onset of symptoms typically occurs 3–12 weeks after treatment.

(f) Angiotensin-converting enzyme inhibitor use and smoking during RT have been associated with decreased radiation pneumonitis.

(3) Assessment (Bickley, 2017)

(a) Symptom assessment includes checking for signs of dyspnea, nonproductive cough, low-grade fever, tachycardia, and pleuritic chest pain. Crackles or pleural rub may be observed.

(b) Radiation pneumonitis is a diagnosis of exclusion, so imaging such as chest x-ray and CT scan may be used to narrow the diagnosis.

i. Chest x-ray can have a variety of findings, including haziness, densities, pleural effusion, and atelectasis. It is helpful but should not be used alone to make the diagnosis.

ii. CT scans are more sensitive and can show subtle changes in the lungs; however, they are not required to make a diagnosis of radiation pneumonitis.

iii. Pulmonary function testing and bronchoscopy may also be used to rule out other causative factors.

(4) Documentation: Documentation of radiation pneumonitis should note the following.

(a) Cough, as listed previously

(b) Hemoptysis presence and characteristics

(c) Mucus color

(d) Dyspnea, as listed previously

(e) Oxygen saturation level

(5) Collaborative management (Sourati et al., 2017)

(a) Amifostine, pentoxifylline, and captopril have been reported to have preventive effects on radiation pneumonitis.

(b) Treatment of radiation pneumonitis is mainly supportive. Corticosteroids remain the treatment of choice, providing symptomatic relief, but they do not reverse or prevent fibrosis and may be contraindicated in some patients.

(c) Bronchodilators can be prescribed.

(d) Expectorants, humidifier use, increased hydration, and antitussives can also be encouraged.

(e) Supplemental oxygen can be administered.

(f) Patients can be referred for fatigue management (see also IV.A. Fatigue).

(6) Patient, care, and family education (Memorial Sloan Kettering Cancer Center, 2019)

(a) Clinicians should inform patients, caregivers, and family about interventions to manage cough and shortness of breath.

(b) Patients, caregivers, and family should know the signs and symptoms of radiation pneumonitis and which symptoms to report to the healthcare team (e.g., fever, cough, dyspnea).

(c) Clinicians should instruct patients to alternate rest and activity.

(d) Patients should avoid irritants (e.g., tobacco, pollutants).

(e) Clinicians should provide information on side effects of steroids and written steroid taper instructions to follow when appropriate.

b) Radiation fibrosis

(1) Pathophysiology (Williams, Johnston, & Finkelstein, 2010)

(a) Radiation fibrosis can develop when the cytotoxic cascade of pneumonitis progresses. The damage initiated in radiation pneumonitis can lead to tissue atrophy from cell damage and loss and fibrosis.

(b) Radiation fibrosis occurs 6–24 months after treatment and stabilizes after two years.

(2) Incidence and risk factors (Williams et al., 2010)

(a) Susceptibility to pulmonary fibrosis is seen in older adults with poor lung function, history of chronic obstructive pulmonary disease, smoking history, previous RT, use of steroids during RT, and concurrent chemoradiation.

(b) The use of some medications like amiodarone, methotrexate, and nitrofurantoin can also put patients at higher risk of developing radiation fibrosis.

(3) Assessment (Bickley, 2017)

(a) If symptoms present, they usually include dyspnea associated with progressive chronic cor pulmonale.

(b) Symptoms are proportional to the extent of lung parenchyma involved and the preexisting pulmonary reserve.

(c) CT imaging is the preferred diagnostic study.

(d) Pulmonary function studies are the most objective evaluation of the functional late effects of radiation lung toxicity. Studies may show mild deterioration as fibrosis develops.

(4) Collaborative management

(a) Anti-inflammatory treatment (corticosteroids), vascular therapy (pentoxifylline or hyperbaric oxygen), and antioxidants (superoxide dismutase, vitamin E, and pentoxifylline with vitamin E) have been recommended but with low levels of evidence (Westbury & Yarnold, 2012).

(b) Currently, no effective or proven treatment for radiation fibrosis exists.

(5) Patient, caregiver, and family education (NCI, 2016)

(a) Patient, caregivers, and family should understand signs and symptoms of radiation fibrosis.

(b) Clinicians should teach methods of avoiding further respiratory compromise, including pulmonary rehabilitation.

c) Radiation myelopathy

(1) Radiation myelopathy is white matter damage to the spinal cord that develops after RT (Kadir, Sarica, Ozgur, Cekinmez, & Nur, 2012).

(2) Incidence and risk factors

(a) Radiation myelopathy is a rare, well-described, serious complication of spinal cord irradiation. Recovery from radiation-induced motor sequelae is rare, whereas the regeneration of sensory losses is relatively frequent (Kadir et al., 2012).

(b) The dose per fraction, total dose, and absolute length of cord irradiated play an important role in determining whether radiation damage to the spinal cord occurs (Kirkpatrick, van der Kogel, & Schultheiss, 2010).

(c) When RT is given in a conventional fractionation schedule of 1.8–2 Gy per day, the incidence of radiation myelopathy is less than 1% for total doses of 50–55 Gy and less than 10% for total doses of 61 Gy (Kirkpatrick et al., 2010).

(3) Assessment (Dropcho, 2010)

(a) Lhermitte phenomenon, which is most frequently characterized by a sensation

similar to an electric shock passing down the spine in the cervicocaudal direction, is the most common symptom. The pain may be felt in the upper or lower limbs.

(b) Symptoms may develop after a latent period of 6–24 months after RT. Severity of symptoms is often progressive.

(c) Symptoms can include paresthesia or sensory deficits (unilateral or bilateral), leg weakness, clumsiness, diminished proprioception, paralysis, and bladder or sphincter dysfunction and incontinence.

(d) Examination should include the following (Bickley, 2017).

    i. Complete neurologic examination

    ii. Pain assessment

    iii. Hyperreflexia and Babinski reflex often are present.

    iv. MRI may show cord edema or hyperintensity in T2 sequences, but it may also be normal in radiation myelitis (Kadir et al., 2012).

(4) Documentation: Documentation of radiation myelopathy should note the following symptoms, using CTCAE.

(a) Peripheral motor neuropathy (NCI CTEP, 2017, p. 103)

    i. Grade 1: asymptomatic; clinical or diagnostic observations only

    ii. Grade 2: moderate symptoms; limiting instrumental ADL

    iii. Grade 3: severe symptoms; limiting self-care ADL

    iv. Grade 4: life-threatening consequences; urgent intervention indicated

    v. Grade 5: death

(b) Ataxia (NCI CTEP, 2017, p. 98)

    i. Grade 1: asymptomatic; clinical or diagnostic observations only; intervention not indicated

    ii. Grade 2: moderate symptoms, limiting instrumental ADL

    iii. Grade 3: severe symptoms; limiting self-care ADL; mechanical assistance indicated

(c) Urinary incontinence (NCI CTEP, 2017, p. 114)

    i. Grade 1: occasional (e.g., with coughing, sneezing, etc.); pads not indicated

    ii. Grade 2: spontaneous; pads indicated; limiting instrumental ADL

    iii. Grade 3: intervention indicated (e.g., clamp, collagen injections); operative intervention indicated; limiting self-care ADL

(d) Fecal incontinence (NCI CTEP, 2017, p. 28)

    i. Grade 1: occasional use of pads required

    ii. Grade 2: daily use of pads required

    iii. Grade 3: severe symptoms; elective operative intervention indicated

(5) Collaborative management: Management of radiation myelopathy involves the following (Daly & Gibbs, 2012).

(a) Careful dose calculation and administration of RT

(b) Interventions

    i. Clinicians should evaluate for other etiologies, including tumor progression, infection, or trauma.

    ii. No treatment has been shown to affect the progressive nature of myelitis; however, corticosteroids, warfarin, pentoxifylline, vitamin E, and hyperbaric oxygen have been used to palliate symptoms.

    iii. Clinicians should refer patients to rehabilitation to maximize function.

(6) Patient, caregiver, and family education (Alghamdi et al., 2018)

(a) Clinicians should educate patients, caregivers, and family on which neurologic symptoms to report.

(b) Instruction includes information on injury prevention secondary to neurologic and sensory deficits, including fall prevention.

(c) Clinicians should educate regarding corticosteroid administration, tapering, and potential side effects.

(d) Progression of symptoms depends upon the degree to which the lesion transects the spinal cord and the level of injury.

(e) Clinicians should provide psychosocial support because of the progressive nature of the symptoms.

d) Cardiac injury

(1) Pathophysiology

(a) Thoracic RT can lead to damage due to inflammation and scarring affecting vascular, structural, and myocardial tissues.

(b) Modern methods of RT delivery have decreased incidence of cardiac injury from 20% to 2.5% (Jaworski, Mariani, Wheeler, & Kaye, 2013).

(2) Incidence and risk factors

(a) Risk of cardiac damage correlates with radiation dose volume and fractionation.

(b) Late effects of RT can occur 3–29 years after treatment (Jaworski et al., 2013).

(c) Risk of radiation-induced cardiac injury can be seen in young people, those receiving high doses of RT (cumulative and fraction), concomitant anthracyclines, and pretreatment cardiac disease.

(d) Studies suggest a threefold increase in cardiac death in patients who received RT to the chest, compared to those who have not (Beggs & Pace, 2013).

(e) Of patients with esophageal cancer receiving RT, 25%–30% have been reported to have pericardial effusions (Beggs & Pace, 2013).

(3) Assessment: Assessment of cardiac injury should include the following (Bickley, 2017).

    (a) Clinical manifestations
        i. Shortness of breath
        ii. Chest pain
        iii. Fatigue
        iv. Lower extremity swelling
        v. Syncope

    (b) Physical examination
        i. Arrhythmias
        ii. Altered respiratory status
        iii. Lower extremity edema

    (c) Cardiac function studies
        i. Electrocardiogram
        ii. Resting echocardiograph and exercise echocardiography
        iii. CT or MRI

(4) Documentation: Documentation should address the following.

    (a) Fatigue (NCI CTEP, 2017, p. 41)
        i. Grade 1: fatigue relieved by rest
        ii. Grade 2: fatigue not relieved by rest; limiting instrumental ADL
        iii. Grade 3: fatigue not relieved by rest; limiting self-care ADL

    (b) Dyspnea

    (c) Chest pain, presence and characteristics

(5) Collaborative management: Management of cardiac injury includes the following (Armanious et al., 2018).

    (a) Prevention
        i. RT treatment strategies should use lower total radiation doses and minimize cardiac exposure.
        ii. Treatment should avoid concurrent cardiotoxic chemotherapy agents when possible.
        iii. Prevention involves lifestyle management and cardiovascular risk assessment and education.

    (b) Early detection (Groarke et al., 2014)
        i. Patients should be referred to cardiology for evaluation and recommendations to reduce the degree of initial cardiac injury and slow the progression of vascular, myocardial, and valvular fibrosis.
        ii. Patients should be assessed with regular electrocardiogram and echocardiograms if indicated.
        iii. Clinicians should employ aggressive treatment of cardiac risk factors, especially hyperlipidemia, at the time of cardiac therapy and during follow-up.

(6) Patient, caregiver, and family education (NCI, 2016)

    (a) Clinicians should emphasize the importance of routine follow-up with a cardiologist and cardiac rehabilitation if indicated.

    (b) Clinicians should educate on recommendations for cardiac health, including following a healthy diet, maintaining an ideal weight, and engaging in regular exercise.

    (c) Patients, caregivers, and family should know the signs and symptoms of heart disease and when to report them to a healthcare provider.

e) Esophageal injury

(1) Pathophysiology (Bandyopadhyay, Fass, Yamasaki, & Hemond, 2019)

    (a) Basal epithelial cell layer is affected, which limits the proliferation rate and causes mucosal thinning, ulceration, and an inflammatory response. This leads to congestion, edema, and erosion.

    (b) Abnormalities include impaired motility with and without mucosal edema, stricture, ulceration and pseudodiverticulum, and fistula.

(2) Incidence and risk factors

    (a) Radiation-induced esophageal injury is more frequent with concurrent chemoradiation than it is with RT alone. When concurrent chemotherapy is used, there is a 12-fold greater risk of esophagitis (Sourati et al., 2017).

    (b) Pre-RT dysphagia is associated with acute esophageal toxicity.

    (c) Accelerated twice-daily RT has also been correlated with increased esophageal toxicity (Wijsman et al., 2015).

    (d) Other contributing factors that continue to be studied include nodal involvement, mean dose to entire esophagus, female sex, and pretreatment weight loss (Z. Zhang et al., 2014).

(3) Assessment: Assessment of esophageal injury should include the following (Bickley, 2017).

    (a) Clinical manifestations
        i. Dysphagia
        ii. Hemoptysis with ulceration
        iii. Weight loss
        iv. Chest pain

    (b) Physical examination
        i. Weight loss
        ii. Difficulty swallowing solid foods

    (c) Additional studies: upper endoscopy

(4) Documentation: Documentation should address nutritional alteration.

    (a) Anorexia (NCI CTEP, 2017, p. 84)
        i. Grade 1: loss of appetite without alteration in eating habits
        ii. Grade 2: oral intake altered without significant weight loss or malnutrition; oral nutritional supplements indicated
        iii. Grade 3: associated with significant weight loss or malnutrition (e.g., inadequate oral caloric and/or fluid intake); tube feeding or [total parenteral nutrition] indicated
        iv. Grade 4: life-threatening consequences; urgent intervention indicated
        v. Grade 5: death

    (b) Nausea (NCI CTEP, 2017, p. 33)
        i. Grade 1: loss of appetite without alteration in eating habits
        ii. Grade 2: oral intake decreased without significant weight loss, dehydration, or malnutrition
        iii. Grade 3: inadequate oral caloric or fluid intake; tube feeding, [total parenteral nutrition], or hospitalization indicated

    (c) Dyspepsia (NCI CTEP, 2017, p. 26)
        i. Grade 1: mild symptoms; intervention not indicated
        ii. Grade 2: moderate symptoms; medical intervention indicated
        iii. Grade 3: severe symptoms; operative intervention indicated

(5) Collaborative management (Memorial Sloan Kettering Cancer Center, 2018)

    (a) Management depends on the specific injury.
    (b) Patients should be referred to a gastroenterologist for evaluation for potential interventions, which may include esophageal dilation, cauterization of bleeding, or placement of a stent.
    (c) Nutritional consultation should be obtained.

(6) Patient, caregiver, and family education (Memorial Sloan Kettering Cancer Center, 2018)

    (a) Clinicians should provide information on dietary suggestions and restrictions.
    (b) Clinicians should teach which signs and symptoms to report, including increased pain or difficulty swallowing.
    (c) Clinicians should provide emotional support.

References

Abnet, C.C., Arnold, M., & Wei, W.-Q. (2018). Epidemiology of esophageal squamous cell carcinoma. *Gastroenterology, 154,* 360–373. https://doi.org/10.1053/j.gastro.2017.08.023

Abreu, C.E.C.V., Ferreira, P.P.R., de Moraes, F.Y., Neves, W.F.P., Jr., Gadia, R., & Carvalho, H.A. (2015). Stereotactic body radiotherapy in lung cancer: An update. *Jornal Brasileiro de Pneumologia, 41,* 376–387. https://doi.org/10.1590/s1806-37132015000000034

Alghamdi, M., Wong, S., Medin, P., Ma, L., Lee, Y., Myrehaug, S., … Sahgal, A. (2018). Spinal cord tolerance and risk of radiation myelopathy. In E.L. Chang, P.D. Brown, S.S. Lo, A. Sahgal, & J.H. Suh (Eds.), *Adult CNS radiation oncology: Principles and practice* (pp. 533–548). Springer.

American Cancer Society. (2020). *Cancer facts and figures 2020.* https://www.cancer.org/research/cancer-facts-statistics/all-cancer-facts-figures/cancer-facts-figures-2020.html

Aoki, M., Hatayama, Y., Kawaguchi, H., Hirose, K., Sato, M., Akimoto, H., … Takai, Y. (2016). Stereotactic body radiotherapy for lung metastases as oligo-recurrence: A single institutional study. *Journal of Radiation Research, 57,* 55–61. https://doi.org/10.1093/jrr/rrv063

Armanious, M.A., Mohammadi, H., Khodor, S., Oliver, D.E., Johnstone, P.A., & Fradley, M.G. (2018). Cardiovascular effects of radiation therapy. *Current Problems in Cancer, 42,* 433–442. https://doi.org/10.1016/j.currproblcancer.2018.05.008

Baker, S., & Fairchild, A. (2016). Radiation-induced esophagitis in lung cancer. *Lung Cancer: Targets and Therapy, 7,* 119–127. https://doi.org/10.2147/lctt.s96443

Bandyopadhyay, N., Fass, R., Yamasaki, T., & Hemond, C. (2019). *Pocket handbook of esophageal disorders.* Springer. https://doi.org/10.1007/978-3-319-97331-9

Baschnagel, A.M., Mangona, V.S., Robertson, J.M., Welsh, R.J., Kestin, L.L., & Grills, I.S. (2013). Lung metastases treated with image-guided stereotactic body radiation therapy. *Clinical Oncology, 25,* 236–241. https://doi.org/10.1016/j.clon.2012.12.005

Beggs, V., & Pace, C. (2013). Radiation therapy and the heart. In A.P. Fadol (Ed.), *Cardiac complications of cancer therapy* (pp. 39–53). Oncology Nursing Society.

Behrend, S.W. (2018). Radiation treatment planning. In C. Yarbro, D. Wujcik, & B. Gobel (Eds.), *Cancer nursing: Principles and practice* (8th ed., pp. 285–332). Jones and Bartlett Learning.

Bickley, L.S. (2017). *Bates' guide to physical examination and history taking* (12th ed.). Wolters Kluwer.

Bledsoe, T.J., Nath, S.K., & Decker, R.H. (2017). Radiation pneumonitis. *Clinics in Chest Medicine, 38,* 201–208. https://doi.org/10.1016/j.ccm.2016.12.004

Bonk, A. (2012). Management of dyspnea in a patient with lung cancer. *Oncology Nursing Forum, 39,* 257–260. https://doi.org/10.1188/12.onf.257-260

Burdett, S., Rydzewska, L., Tierney, J., Fisher, D., Parmar, M.K.B., Arriagada, R., … Le Pechoux, C. (2016). Postoperative radiotherapy for non-small cell lung cancer. *Cochrane Database of Systematic Reviews, 2016*(10). https://doi.org/10.1002/14651858.cd002142.pub4

Cash, J.C., & Glass, C.A. (2017). *Family practice guidelines* (4th ed.). Springer.

Castro, C., Peleteiro, B., Morais, S., Severo, M., Bento, M.J., & Lunet, N. (2018). An explanatory and predictive model of the variation in esophageal cancer incidence on the basis of changes in the exposure to risk factors. *European Journal of Cancer Prevention, 27,* 213–220. https://doi.org/10.1097/cej.0000000000000422

Chance, W.W., Rebueno, N., & Gomez, D.R. (2015). Mesothelioma. In Y. Nishimura & R. Komaki (Eds.), *Intensity-modulated radiation therapy* (pp. 261–273). Springer. https://doi.org/10.1007/978-4-431-55486-8_13

Chicas-Sett, R., Morales-Orue, I., Castilla-Martinez, J., Zafra-Martin, J., Kannemann, A., Blanco, J., ... Lara, P.C. (2019). Stereotactic ablative radiotherapy combined with immune checkpoint inhibitors reboots the immune response assisted by immunotherapy in metastatic lung cancer: A systematic review. *International Journal of Molecular Science, 20,* 2173. https://doi.org/10.3390/ijms20092173

Daly, M.E., & Gibbs, I.C. (2012). Spinal radiosurgery: Delayed radiation-induced myelopathy. In M.A. Hayat (Ed.), *Tumors of the central nervous system: Vol. 6. Spinal tumors (part 1)* (pp. 135–140). Springer. https://doi.org/10.1007/978-94-007-2866-0_17

de Perrot, M., Feld, R., Leighl, N.B., Hope, A., Waddell, T.K., Keshavjee, S., & Cho, B.C.J. (2016). Accelerated hemithoracic radiation followed by extrapleural pneumonectomy for malignant pleural mesothelioma. *Journal of Thoracic and Cardiovascular Surgery, 151,* 468–475. https://doi.org/10.1016/j.jtcvs.2015.09.129

De Ruysscher, D., Dehing, C., Yu, S., Wanders, R., Öllers, M., Dingemans, A.-M.C., ... Lambin, P. (2009). Dyspnea evolution after high-dose radiotherapy in patients with non-small cell lung cancer. *Radiotherapy and Oncology, 91,* 353–359. https://doi.org/10.1016/j.radonc.2008.10.006

Detterbeck, F.C., Boffa, D.J., Kim, A.W., & Tanoue, L.T. (2017). The eighth edition lung cancer stage classification. *Chest, 151,* 193–203. https://doi.org/10.1016/j.chest.2016.10.010

Dezube, R. (2020). Cough in adults. In R.S. Porter (Ed.), *Merck manual: Professional version.* https://www.merckmanuals.com/professional/pulmonary-disorders/symptoms-of-pulmonary-disorders/cough-in-adults

Dickhoff, C., Rodriguez Schaap, P., Otten, R.H.J., Heymans, M.W., Heineman, D.J., & Dahele, M. (2018). Salvage surgery for local recurrence after stereotactic body radiotherapy for early stage non-small cell lung cancer: A systematic review. *Therapeutic Advances in Medical Oncology, 10,* 1758835918787989. https://doi.org/10.1177/1758835918787989

DiSalvo, W.M., & Joyce, M.M. (2009). Dyspnea. In L.H. Eaton & J.M. Tipton (Eds.), *Putting evidence into practice: Improving oncology patient outcomes* (pp. 135–148). Oncology Nursing Society.

Dropcho, E.J. (2010). Neurotoxicity of radiation therapy. *Neurologic Clinics, 28,* 217–234. https://doi.org/10.1016/j.ncl.2009.09.008

Dudgeon, D. (2013). Dyspnea in the cancer patient. In A.M. Berger, J.L. Shuster, & J.H. Von Roenn (Eds.), *Principles and practice of palliative care and supportive oncology* (4th ed., pp. 388–402). Lippincott Williams and Wilkins.

Falkson, C.B., Vella, E.T., Yu, E., El-Mallah, M., Mackenzie, R., Ellis, P.M., & Ung, Y.C. (2017). Radiotherapy with curative intent in patients with early-stage, medically inoperable, non-small-cell lung cancer: A systematic review. *Clinical Lung Cancer, 18,* 105–121.e5. https://doi.org/10.1016/j.cllc.2016.10.008

Giannopoulou, A., Gkiozos, I., Harrington, K.J., & Syrigos, K.N. (2013). Thymoma and radiation therapy: A systematic review of medical treatment. *Expert Review of Anticancer Therapy, 13,* 759–766. https://doi.org/10.1586/era.13.54

Groarke, J.D., Nguyen, P.L., Nohria, A., Ferrari, R., Cheng, S., & Moslehi, J. (2014). Cardiovascular complications of radiation therapy for thoracic malignancies: The role for non-invasive imaging for detection of cardiovascular disease. *European Heart Journal, 35,* 612–623. https://doi.org/10.1093/eurheartj/eht114

Higgins, K.A., O'Connell, K., Liu, Y., Gillespie, T.W., McDonald, M.W., Pillai, R.N., ... Behera, M. (2017). National Cancer Database analysis of proton versus photon radiation therapy in non-small cell lung cancer. *International Journal of Radiation Oncology, Biology, Physics, 97,* 128–137. https://doi.org/10.1016/j.ijrobp.2016.10.001

Jain, V., & Berman, A.T. (2018). Radiation pneumonitis: Old problem, new tricks. *Cancers, 10,* 222. https://doi.org/10.3390/cancers10070222

Jaworski, C., Mariani, J.A., Wheeler, G., & Kaye, D.M. (2013). Cardiac complications of thoracic irradiation. *Journal of the American College of Cardiology, 61,* 2319–2328. https://doi.org/10.1016/j.jacc.2013.01.090

Kadir, T., Sarica, F.B., Ozgur, K., Cekinmez, M., & Nur, A.M. (2012). Delayed radiation myelopathy: Differential diagnosis with positron emission tomography/computed tomography examination. *Asian Journal of Neurosurgery, 7,* 206–209. https://doi.org/10.4103/1793-5482.106656

Kahnert, K., Kauffmann-Guerrero, D., & Huber, R.M. (2016). SCLC—State of the art and what does the future have in store? *Clinical Lung Cancer, 17,* 325–333. https://doi.org/10.1016/j.cllc.2016.05.014

Keall, P., Belderbos, J., & Kong, F.M. (2010). Physical basis of modern radiotherapy: Dose and volume. In H.I. Pass, D.P. Carbone, D.H. Johnson, J.D. Minna, G.V. Scagliotti, & A.T. Turrisi III (Eds.), *Principles and practice of lung cancer: The official reference text of the IASCL* (4th ed., pp. 549–564). Philadelphia, PA: Lippincott Williams and Wilkins.

Kirkpatrick, J.P., van der Kogel, A.J., & Schultheiss, T.E. (2010). Radiation dose–volume effects in the spinal cord. *International Journal of Radiation Oncology, Biology, Physics, 7*(Suppl. 3), S42–S49. https://doi.org/10.1016/j.ijrobp.2009.04.095

Krauss, D.J. (2014). An overview of image-guided radiotherapy (IGRT). *OMICS Journal of Radiology, 3*(Special issue), 002. https://doi.org/10.4172/2167-7964.s1-002

Liao, Z.X., Komaki, R.R., Thames, H.D., Jr., Liu, H.H., Tucker, S.L., Mohan, R., ... Cox, J.D. (2010). Influence of technologic advances on outcomes in patients with unresectable, locally advanced non-small-cell lung cancer receiving concomitant chemoradiotherapy. *International Journal of Radiation Oncology, Biology, Physics, 76,* 775–781. https://doi.org/10.1016/j.ijrobp.2009.02.032

Liao, Z., Gandhi, S.J., Lin, S.H., & Bradley, J. (2018). Does proton therapy offer demonstrable clinical advantages for treating thoracic tumors? *Seminars in Radiation Oncology, 28,* 114–124. https://doi.org/10.1016/j.semradonc.2017.11.002

Ling, D.C., Hess, C.B., Chen, A.M., & Daly, M.E. (2016). Comparison of toxicity between intensity-modulated radiotherapy and 3-dimensional conformal radiotherapy for locally advanced non-small-cell lung cancer. *Clinical Lung Cancer, 17,* 18–23. https://doi.org/10.1016/j.cllc.2015.07.006

Memorial Sloan Kettering Cancer Center. (2018, December 12). Radiation therapy to the chest. https://www.mskcc.org/cancer-care/patient-education/radiation-therapy-chest

Memorial Sloan Kettering Cancer Center. (2019, February 4). Shortness of breath (dyspnea). https://www.mskcc.org/cancer-care/patient-education/shortness-breath-dyspnea

Moeller, B., Balagamwala, E.H., Chen, A., Creach, K.M., Giaccone, G., Koshy, M., ... Rodrigues, G. (2018). Palliative thoracic radiation therapy for non-small cell lung cancer: 2018 update of an American Society for Radiation Oncology (ASTRO) evidence-based guideline. *Practical Radiation Oncology, 8,* 245–250. https://doi.org/10.1016/j.prro.2018.02.009

Molassiotis, A., Smith, J.A., Mazzone, P., Blackhall, F., & Irwin, R.S. (2017). Symptomatic treatment of cough among adult patients with lung cancer: CHEST guideline and expert panel report. *Chest, 151,* 861–874. https://doi.org/10.1016/j.chest.2016.12.028

Molitoris, J., Diwanji, T., Snider, J.W., III, Mossahebi, S., Samanta, S., Badiyan, S.N., ... Mohindra, P. (2018). Advances in the use of motion management and image guidance in radiation therapy treatment for lung cancer. *Journal of Thoracic Disease, 10*(Suppl. 21), S2437–S2450. https://doi.org/10.21037/jtd.2018.01.155

National Cancer Institute. (2016, September 16). Late side effects of cancer treatment. https://www.cancer.gov/about-cancer/coping/survivorship/late-effects

National Cancer Institute Cancer Therapy Evaluation Program. (2017). *Common terminology criteria for adverse events* [v.5.0]. https://ctep.cancer.gov/protocolDevelopment/electronic_applications/docs/CTCAE_v5_Quick_Reference_8.5x11.pdf

National Comprehensive Cancer Network. (2019). *NCCN Clinical Practice Guidelines in Oncology (NCCN Guidelines®): Malignant pleural mesothelioma* [v.1.2020]. https://www.nccn.org/professionals/physician_gls/pdf/mpm.pdf

National Comprehensive Cancer Network. (2020a). *NCCN Clinical Practice Guidelines in Oncology (NCCN Guidelines®): Esophageal and esophagogastric junction cancers* [v.2.2020]. https://www.nccn.org/professionals/physician_gls/pdf/esophageal.pdf

National Comprehensive Cancer Network. (2020b). *NCCN Clinical Practice Guidelines in Oncology (NCCN Guidelines®): Non-small cell lung cancer* [v.4.2020]. https://www.nccn.org/professionals/physician_gls/pdf/nscl.pdf

National Comprehensive Cancer Network. (2020c). *NCCN Clinical Practice Guidelines in Oncology (NCCN Guidelines®): Small cell lung cancer* [v.3.2020]. https://www.nccn.org/professionals/physician_gls/pdf/sclc.pdf

Nicholson, A.G., Chansky, K., Crowley, J., Beyruti, R., Kubota, K., Turrisi, A., ... Rami-Porta, R. (2016). The International Association for the Study of Lung Cancer lung cancer staging project: Proposals for the revision of the clinical and pathologic staging of small cell lung cancer in the forthcoming eighth edition of the TNM classification for lung cancer. *Journal of Thoracic Oncology, 11,* 300–311. https://doi.org/10.1016/j.jtho.2015.10.008

Parashar, B., Arora, S., & Wernicke, A.G. (2013). Radiation therapy for early stage lung cancer. *Seminars in Interventional Radiology, 30,* 185–190. https://doi.org/10.1055/s-0033-1342960

Patel, S., Macdonald, O.K., Nagda, S., Bittner, N., & Suntharalingam, M. (2012). Evaluation of the role of radiation therapy in the management of malignant thymoma. *International Journal of Radiation Oncology, Biology, Physics, 82,* 1797–1801. https://doi.org/10.1016/j.ijrobp.2011.03.010

Poirier, P. (2013). Nursing-led management of side effects of radiation: Evidence-based recommendations for practice. *Nursing: Research and Reviews, 3,* 47–57. https://doi.org/10.2147/nrr.s34112

Rathod, S., Koul, R., Bashir, B., Chowdhury, A., & Dubey, A. (2019). Role of stereotactic body radiation therapy in early stage small cell lung cancer in the era of lung cancer screening: A systematic review. *American Journal of Clinical Oncology, 42,* 123–130. https://doi.org/10.1097/coc.0000000000000489

Ricardi, U., Filippi, A.R., Guarneri, A., Ragona, R., Mantovani, C., Giglioli, F., ... Scagliotti, G.V. (2012). Stereotactic body radiation therapy for lung metastases. *Lung Cancer, 75,* 77–81. https://doi.org/10.1016/j.lungcan.2011.04.021

Rieber, J., Streblow, J., Uhlmann, L., Flentje, M., Duma, M., Ernst, I., ... Guckenberger, M. (2016). Stereotactic body radiotherapy (SBRT) for medically inoperable lung metastases—A pooled analysis of the German working group "stereotactic radiotherapy." *Lung Cancer, 97,* 51–58. https://doi.org/10.1016/j.lungcan.2016.04.012

Rimner, A., Zauderer, M.G., Gomez, D.R., Adusumilli, P.S., Parhar, P.K., Wu, A.J., ... Krug, L.M. (2016). Phase II study of hemithoracic intensity-modulated pleural radiation therapy (IMPRINT) as part of lung-sparing multimodality therapy in patients with malignant pleural mesothelioma. *Journal of Clinical Oncology, 34,* 2761–2768. https://doi.org/10.1200/jco.2016.67.2675

Robin, T.P., & Rusthoven, C.G. (2018). Strategies to preserve cognition in patients with brain metastases: A review. *Frontiers in Oncology, 8,* 415. https://doi.org/10.3389/fonc.2018.00415

Robinson, B.W., Baas, P., & Kindler, H.L. (2010). Malignant mesothelioma. In H.I. Pass, D.P. Carbone, D.H. Johnson, J.D. Minna, G.V. Scagliotti, & A.T. Turrisi III (Eds.), *Principles and practice of lung cancer* (4th ed., pp. 945–960). Philadelphia, PA: Lippincott Williams and Wilkins.

Rodrigues, G., Choy, H., Bradley, J., Rosenzweig, K.E., Bogart, J., Curran, W.J, Jr., ... Videtic, G.M.M. (2015a). Definitive radiation therapy in locally advanced non-small cell lung cancer: Executive summary of an American Society for Radiation Oncology (ASTRO) evidence-based clinical practice guideline. *Practical Radiation Oncology, 5,* 141–148. https://doi.org/10.1016/j.prro.2015.02.012

Rodrigues, G., Choy, H., Bradley, J., Rosenzweig, K.E., Bogart, J., Curran, W.J., Jr., ... Videtic, G.M.M. (2015b). Adjuvant radiation therapy in locally advanced non-small cell lung cancer: Executive summary of an American

Society for Radiation Oncology (ASTRO) evidence-based clinical practice guideline. *Practical Radiation Oncology, 5,* 149–155. https://doi.org/10.1016/j.prro.2015.02.013

Shapiro, J., Van Lanschot, J.J.B., Hulshof, M.C.C.M., Van Hagen, P., Van Berge Henegouwen, M.I., Wijnhoven, B.P.L., ... Van Der Gaast, A. (2015). Neo-adjuvant chemoradiotherapy plus surgery versus surgery alone for oesophageal or junctional cancer (CROSS): Long-term results of a randomised controlled trial. *Lancet Oncology, 16,* 1090–1098. https://doi.org/10.1016/s1470-2045(15)00040-6

Shelton, B., Adames, A., Dagher, H., Dolan, E., Miller, P., Oliveira, L., ... Starr, P. (2019). Symptom interventions: Dyspnea. https://www.ons.org/pep/dyspnea?display=pepnavigator&sort_by=created&items_per_page=50

Sourati, A., Ameri, A., & Malekzadeh, M. (2017). *Acute side effects of radiation therapy: A guide to management.* Springer. https://doi.org/10.1007/978-3-319-55950-6

Stewart, A., Parashar, B., Patel, M., O'Farrell, D., Biagioli, M., Devlin, P., & Mutyala, S. (2016). American Brachytherapy Society consensus guidelines for thoracic brachytherapy for lung cancer. *Brachytherapy, 15,* 1–11. https://doi.org/10.1016/j.brachy.2015.09.006

Sun, A., Durocher-Allen, L.D., Ellis, P.M., Ung, Y.C., Goffin, J.R., Ramchandar, K., & Darling, G. (2018). Guideline for the initial management of small cell lung cancer (limited and extensive stage) and the role of thoracic radiotherapy and first-line chemotherapy. *Clinical Oncology, 30,* 658–666. https://doi.org/10.1016/j.clon.2018.06.008

Timmerman, R.D., Paulus, R., Pass, H.I., Gore, E.M., Edelman, M.J., Galvin, J., ... Choy, H. (2018). Stereotactic body radiation therapy for operable early-stage lung cancer: Findings from the NRG oncology RTOG 0618 trial. *JAMA Oncology, 4,* 1263–1266. https://doi.org/10.1001/jamaoncol.2018.1251

Videtic, G.M.M., Donington, J., Giuliani, M., Heinzerling, J., Karas, T.Z., Kelsey, C.R., ... Daly, M.E. (2017). Stereotactic body radiation therapy for early-stage non-small cell lung cancer: Executive summary of an ASTRO evidence-based guideline. *Practical Radiation Oncology, 7,* 295–301. https://doi.org/10.1016/j.prro.2017.04.014

Vijayan, J., & Groninger, J.H. (2013). Hemoptysis, airway obstruction, bronchospasm, cough, and pulmonary complications/symptoms of cancer and its treatment. In A.M. Berger, J.L. Shuster, & J.H. Von Roenn (Eds.), *Principles and practice of palliative care and supportive oncology* (4th ed., pp. 403–419). Lippincott Williams and Wilkins.

Wahl, M., & Garsa, A. (2018). Small cell lung cancer. In E.K. Hansen, & M. Roach III (Eds.), *Handbook of evidence-based radiation oncology* (3rd ed., pp. 285–291). Springer. https://doi.org/10.1007/978-3-319-62642-0_14

Westbury, C.B., & Yarnold, J.R. (2012). Radiation fibrosis—Current clinical and therapeutic perspectives. *Clinical Oncology, 24,* 657–672. https://doi.org/10.1016/j.clon.2012.04.001

Wijsman, R., Dankers, F., Troost, E.G.C., Hoffmann, A.L., van der Heijden, E.H.F.M., de Geus-Oei, L.-F., & Bussink, J. (2015). Multivariable normal-tissue complication modeling of acute esophageal toxicity in advanced stage non-small cell lung cancer patients treated with intensity-modulated (chemo-) radiotherapy. *Radiotherapy and Oncology, 117,* 49–54. https://doi.org/10.1016/j.radonc.2015.08.010

Williams, J.P., Johnston, C.J., & Finkelstein, J.N. (2010). Treatment for radiation-induced pulmonary late effects: Spoiled for choice or looking in the wrong direction? *Current Drug Targets, 11,* 1386–1394. https://doi.org/10.2174/138945011009011386

Willmann, J., & Rimner, A. (2018). The expanding role of radiation therapy for thymic malignancies. *Journal of Thoracic Disease, 10*(Suppl. 21), S2555–S2564. https://doi.org/10.21037/jtd.2018.01.154

Yamashita, H., Takahashi, W., Haga, A., & Nakagawa, K. (2014). Radiation pneumonitis after stereotactic radiation therapy for lung cancer. *World Journal of Radiology, 6,* 708–715. https://doi.org/10.4329/wjr.v6.i9.708

Zhang, W., Jiang, W., Luan, L., Wang, L., Zheng, X., & Wang, G. (2014). Prophylactic cranial irradiation for patients with small-cell lung cancer: A systematic review of the literature with meta-analysis. *BMC Cancer, 14,* 793. https://doi.org/10.1186/1471-2407-14-793

Zhang, Z., Xu, J., Zhou, T., Yi, Y., Li, H., Sun, H., ... Ying, G. (2014). Risk factors of radiation-induced acute esophagitis in non-small cell lung cancer patients treated with concomitant chemoradiotherapy. *Radiation Oncology, 9*, 54. https://doi.org/10.1186/1748-717x-9-54

E. Gastrointestinal tract and abdomen
1. Overview
   a) RT to abdominal structures may be used for treatment of certain malignancies of the gastrointestinal tract, such as distal esophageal, gastroesophageal junction, or gastric tumors; pancreatic cancers; biliary tract cancers, including those of the liver, gallbladder, bile ducts, and ampulla; and obstructive anal, colon, and colorectal tumors, or other tumors that may develop in the abdominal cavity, such as desmoid tumors or sarcomas.
   b) Incidental irradiation of the gastrointestinal tract may occur during treatment for head and neck, pelvic, thoracic, or lumbar spine malignancies (Shadad, Sullivan, Martin, & Egan, 2013).
2. Incidence (American Cancer Society, 2020)
   a) As of 2020 in the United States, gastrointestinal system cancers as a whole had an incidence of 333,680 new cases and 167,790 deaths.
   b) The highest number of new cases and deaths were in colorectal, pancreatic, and liver cancers, respectively.
3. RT techniques
   a) In certain clinical situations, advanced treatment planning techniques, such as IMRT or SBRT, have demonstrated benefit in maximizing dose to the tumor while minimizing dose to healthy tissue (Boyle, Czito, Willet, & Palta, 2015).
   b) Other modern advanced treatment planning techniques under evaluation for gastrointestinal malignancies include hypofractionated image-guided IMRT and breath holding (Stephens et al., 2018).
4. General treatment principles (Ward, Tendulkar, & Videtic, 2018)
   a) Gastric cancer: Dosing for adjuvant RT is typically 45 Gy.
   b) Hepatocellular cancer
      (1) Dosing for hepatocellular carcinoma varies but is typically 54–60 Gy.
      (2) Radiofrequency ablation can also be used for small tumors.
   c) Pancreatic cancer
      (1) RT can be given in postoperative, neoadjuvant, definitive, or palliative settings.
      (2) The dose is typically 50.4 Gy.
      (3) Palliative RT to the pancreas can help with pain control in more than half of patients.
   d) Colorectal cancer
      (1) RT can be given preoperatively or postoperatively in patients with rectal cancer.
      (2) The dose can be 25 Gy administered one week before surgery or 50.4 Gy with surgery seven to eight weeks later. If positive margins are present after surgery, the care team may consider a boost to 55–60 Gy. Both regimens are typically given with 5-fluorouracil with or without oxaliplatin.
   e) Anal cancer
      (1) Data are limited for radiation dosing for anal cancer.
      (2) Typically, RT is administered as definitive treatment, combined with chemotherapy (5-fluorouracil or mitomycin C).
      (3) IMRT can be given to help decrease toxicities, especially of the skin.
5. Treatment side effects
   a) Overview
      (1) Side effects of radiation exposure to the gastrointestinal tract may be either acute or chronic and are mediated by the total radiation dose, exposure volume, concurrent treatments (e.g., chemotherapy or immunotherapy), and other patient factors (Shadad et al., 2013).
      (2) Major dose-limiting structures in the abdomen include the small intestine, stomach, liver, kidneys, and spinal cord (Yovino et al., 2011).
      (3) Side effects tend to peak approximately one week after the completion of RT. Typically, at that time, they plateau and start to improve (Nicolini et al., 2013).
   b) Anorexia (see also IV.H. Nutritional issues)
      (1) Pathophysiology
         (a) Anorexia associated with cancer can occur as a result of the disease itself and treatments (Ezeoke & Morley, 2015).
         (b) Anorexia is affected by early satiety and distal gastrointestinal dysmotility; therefore, management of these is important in optimizing food intake (Fearon et al., 2011).
         (c) Anorexia reduces quality of life and contributes directly or indirectly to death in a large number of patients with cancer (Sadeghi et al., 2018).
      (2) Incidence
         (a) Studies have shown that unintended weight loss is the second highest predictive factor associated with colorectal, lung, pancreatic, and renal cancers and may be used as an indicator for warranting further investigation in primary care settings (Nicholson, Hamilton, O'Sullivan, Aveyard, & Hobbs, 2018).
         (b) Anorexia and weight loss occur in approximately 90% of patients undergoing intensive RT for head and neck, thoracic, abdominal, and pelvic tumors (Nicolini et al., 2013).

(c) Malnutrition is more common in gastro-intestinal cancers than other types of cancer (Nicolini et al., 2013).

(d) Patients who experience cachexia have an increased risk of reduced quality of life, overall shorter length of survival, treatment failure, and more treatment toxicities (Nicolini et al., 2013).

(e) Treatment side effects such as xerostomia, taste alterations, intense pain, esophagitis, mucositis, dysphagia, nausea, vomiting, and diarrhea contribute to anorexia and weight loss (Nicolini et al., 2013).

(3) Assessment

(a) The following factors contribute to anorexia and weight loss in patients with gastrointestinal cancer (Buduhan et al., 2018).
  i. Extent of disease
  ii. Metabolic abnormalities
  iii. Substance abuse
  iv. Socioeconomic factors
  v. Medications
  vi. Medical conditions, such as end-stage diseases, mental disorders, neurologic conditions (e.g., Parkinson disease, delirium, dementia), or chronic conditions (e.g., chronic obstructive pulmonary disease, ulcers)

(b) Loss of 10% body weight over six months with food intake less than 50% of requirements for longer than five days is considered severe or moderate malnutrition, and nutritional support is indicated (Nicolini et al., 2013).

(c) Screening tools are used as a standard of care during hospitalizations and are also recommended to be used for follow-up in other healthcare settings, such as rehabilitation facilities and clinics. Screening and assessment tools can be used along with guidelines for nutritional interventions that are appropriate for individual patients and assist in creating a plan of care (Correia et al., 2014).
  i. Malnutrition Screening Tool
  ii. Simplified Nutritional Appetite Questionnaire
  iii. Subjective Global Assessment
  iv. Mini Nutritional Assessment

(d) Dietary intake, body composition, physical activity, and predominant metabolic pattern are thought to be key variables that influence patients' overall body resource and function (Fearon et al., 2011).

(e) Physical examination findings to evaluate for signs of malnutrition include muscle protein depletion, loss of skeletal muscle, and loss of fat (Arends et al., 2017).

(f) Laboratory results may show an increase in inflammatory markers, such as C-reactive protein, and a decrease in serum albumin, prealbumin, and hemoglobin in patients with anorexia or cachexia (Letilovic & Vrhovac, 2013).

(g) Alterations in dietary intake can also affect quality of life and psychosocial factors.
  i. If patients are struggling to eat, they may feel a sense of failure, loss of independence, or that they are disappointing their family or caregivers.
  ii. Quality-of-life assessments can be helpful in this area; however, a validated tool specifically for cancer anorexia and cachexia is not yet available (Sadeghi et al., 2018).

(4) Collaborative management: Treatment of anorexia is optimized with a combination of nonpharmacologic and pharmacologic approaches (Nicolini et al., 2013).

(a) Nonpharmacologic management
  i. The goal of nutritional counseling in the cancer setting should be to supply energy, minimize weight loss, and maintain quality of life (Isenring et al., 2013).
  ii. Nutritional support can help decrease negative effects of RT on nutritional status. Nutritional counseling by an RDN or RD is considered first line (Arends et al., 2017).
  iii. The following can improve intake and nutritional status (Buduhan et al., 2018).
    • Drinking adequate fluids and high-protein and high-calorie fluids
    • Limiting fluid intake before meals and before bedtime
    • Eating small, frequent meals
    • Eating largest meal of the day when a patient feels the hungriest
    • Avoiding foods with extreme taste or smell if a patient is sensitive
    • Serving cold food and avoiding food preparation area, for patients experiencing nausea related to food odors
  iv. Additional causes of poor oral intake can be symptoms of the disease or side effects of treatment such as nausea, vomiting, constipation, reduced motility, taste changes, pain, xerostomia, mucositis, and mouth sores. Management of these symptoms is

a key method to decrease anorexia (Arends et al., 2017).

v. Patients with cancer are already at a higher risk for physical deconditioning; therefore, physical exercise is important to retain nutrients and decrease risk of muscle wasting and desensitization to anabolic factors (Arends et al., 2017).

vi. Eating food is the best way to receive nutrition; however, with certain treatments and disease patterns, this is not easy. Oral supplementation may be needed.

vii. In some cases, artificial nutrition (enteral or parenteral nutrition) may be used. Several complications can occur with these methods of giving nutrition and are reserved only for severe cases. Risks and benefits of artificial nutrition must be considered (Arends et al., 2017; Buduhan et al., 2018).

(b) Pharmacologic management

i. Progestins, such as megestrol acetate, may be prescribed to increase appetite and help patients gain weight. In a randomized trial, the addition of olanzapine to megestrol acetate resulted in improved appetite, weight gain, and increased quality of life, compared to megestrol acetate alone, in patients with advanced gastrointestinal and lung cancers (Navari & Brenner, 2010). Potential dose-related adverse effects of progestins include thromboembolic events, breakthrough bleeding, peripheral edema, hyperglycemia, hypertension, and renal suppression (Adams, Cunningham, Caruso, Norling, & Shepard, 2009).

ii. Corticosteroids, such as dexamethasone, methylprednisolone, and prednisolone, can improve treatment-related nausea and vomiting and stimulate appetite (Buduhan et al., 2018).

iii. Dronabinol acts directly on the brain to increase appetite and prevent vomiting (Badowski & Yanful, 2018). It can be given as an oral solution (5 mg/ml) or capsule. The typical dose is 2.5–5 mg (Badowski & Yanful, 2018).

(5) Documentation: Standardized sources, such as CTCAE, can be used for documentation (NCI CTEP, 2017, p. 84).

(a) Grade 1: loss of appetite without alteration in eating habits

(b) Grade 2: oral intake altered without significant weight loss or malnutrition; oral nutritional supplements indicated

(c) Grade 3: associated with significant weight loss or malnutrition (e.g., inadequate oral caloric and/or fluid intake); tube feeding or [total parenteral nutrition] indicated

(d) Grade 4: life-threatening consequences; urgent intervention indicated

(e) Grade 5: death

(6) Patient, caregiver, and family education (NCI, 2018)

(a) Education of patients, caregivers, and family includes the fundamentals of good nutrition.

(b) Nurses should emphasize the importance of healthy eating habits during and after treatment.

(c) Patients can be referred to an RDN or RD.

(d) Nurses should inform patients, caregivers, and family of symptoms from treatment affecting nutrition that should be reported.

(e) Clinicians should encourage patients, caregivers, and family to participate in development and implementation of a nutrition plan.

(f) Refer to the following websites for addition information.

i. Cancer*Care*: www.cancercare.org

ii. NCI: www.cancer.gov/cancertopics/pdq/supportivecare/nutrition/Patient

c) Nausea and vomiting

(1) Pathophysiology

(a) Knowledge on chemotherapy-induced nausea and vomiting (CINV) facilitates understanding of radiation-induced nausea and vomiting (RINV). Likewise, the approach of treatment and management for RINV is linked with treatment for CINV.

(b) The pathophysiology of RINV is not completely understood, but progress in understanding the pathophysiology and treatment of CINV has greatly influenced that of RINV (Feyer, Jahn, & Jordan, 2015).

(c) Several treatment-related factors affect RINV (Feyer et al., 2015).

i. Site of irradiation

ii. Dose of radiation and fractionation

iii. Irradiated volume

iv. RT techniques

(d) According to Von Roenn (2013), the neural pathways that mediate nausea are unknown, as most literature presents the mechanisms of vomiting rather than nausea.

(e) Both the CNS and autonomic nervous system play a role in the causation of nausea and vomiting through different mechanisms (NCI, 2020b).

(f) Nausea is a subjective symptom, most often described as feeling "queasy" or "sick in the stomach," accompanied by other autonomic symptoms, including cold sweats, pallor, diarrhea, and tachycardia. It is also referred to as "dry heaves," with unpleasant, wavelike sensations experienced in the back of the throat and the epigastric region, which can result in vomiting (NCI, 2018; Von Roenn, 2013).

(g) Vomiting is a two-phased symptom involving retching and expulsion. It is caused by a combination of complex muscular and neurophysiologic interactions (Von Roenn, 2013).

(h) Von Roenn (2013) presented the four major pathways leading to the stimulation of the vomiting center: the chemoreceptor trigger zone, vestibular system, vagal and enteric nervous system, and cerebral cortex.

    i. The chemoreceptor trigger zone is a receptor-rich area of the floor of the fourth ventricle, which has numerous dopamine, serotonin, opioid, acetylcholine, and substance P receptors.

    ii. The vagal and enteric nervous system transmits information to the brain regarding the state of the gastrointestinal system. Distention of the gut or irritation of the mucosal surface leads to activation of serotonin receptors, stimulation of vagal afferents, and an emetic response (Von Roenn, 2013). Further, the gastrointestinal tract, which is comprised of rapidly dividing cells (specifically the small intestine), are particularly sensitive to radiation damage (Urba et al., 2001).

    iii. The cerebral cortex is thought to mediate nausea and vomiting from meningeal irritation, increased intracranial pressure, psychiatric disorders, and unpleasant stimuli from the five senses (e.g., foul odor) (Von Roenn, 2013).

    iv. The vestibular system is rich in histamine and muscarinic receptors.

Its stimulation of the vomiting center mediated through labyrinthine inputs via cranial nerve VIII (vestibulocochlear nerve) plays a major role in motion sickness (Von Roenn, 2013).

(i) Serotonin, substance P, and dopamine are neurotransmitters involved in radiation-induced emesis (NCI, 2020b).

(j) Factors such as radiation or chemical factors can trigger the vomiting center and vagal nuclei (Iwamoto, Haas, & Gosselin, 2012).

(k) Vomiting is a protective reflex triggered by chemical or physical stimulation, resulting in the oral or nasal expulsion of gastric contents (Von Roenn, 2013).

(l) The key neurotransmitters involved in emesis are serotonin, dopamine, and substance P, and the main way to treat CINV is by deactivating their corresponding receptors by blocking them from binding with these neurotransmitters (Eaby-Sandy & Sherry, 2011).

(m) Gastrointestinal problems can also appear as late effects (Czito & Willett, 2011).

    i. These effects include damage to the gastric vasculature, fibrosis, and loss of mucosal and epithelial cells.

    ii. Chronic gastritis and dyspepsia can also occur.

    iii. Doses should be limited to 50 Gy when the radiation field includes a large portion of the stomach because of the risk of late gastric ulceration or perforation (Iwamoto et al., 2012).

(2) Incidence

(a) The overall cumulative incidence rate for RINV has been documented to be up to 80% (NCI, 2020b).

(b) RINV is most likely to occur if the treatment field includes the abdomen. TBI and hemibody RT to the upper body most predictably cause RINV (Stevich-Heemer, 2019).

(c) Onset may occur within the first 24 hours of treatment and within 10–15 minutes following TBI and hemibody RT (Feyer et al., 2011).

(d) Approximately 50% of people who receive conventionally fractionated RT to the abdomen have onset of symptoms within 40–90 minutes, and nausea may persist for up to 24 hours after exposure (Urba et al., 2001).

(e) Among all RT-related factors, radiation field has the most impact. Upper abdomi-

nal and craniospinal irradiation have moderate emetogenic potential, with 60%–90% risk of emesis without prophylaxis (Feyer et al., 2015).

(f) Radiation dose of 45 Gy or more can cause ulcerations in the stomach, as well as atrophy. Gastrointestinal symptoms may be noted within months and up to several years after completing RT (Iwamoto et al., 2012).

(3) Risk factors
(a) Nausea and vomiting can occur under other circumstances, such as postanesthesia nausea and vomiting (Tipton, 2014).
(b) Risk factors for RINV include gender, history of CINV and RINV, concurrent chemotherapy, alcohol consumption, and site, frequency, and dose of radiation. Individual patient and disease factors can increase the risk of developing nausea and vomiting.
(c) IV chemotherapy tends to cause more nausea than oral chemotherapy (NCCN, n.d.).
(d) Some evidence suggests that patients who have high chronic alcohol intake have less CINV than nondrinkers (Tipton, 2014).

(4) Assessment
(a) Nurses should consider all events and assess for potential factors that can lead to nausea, including constipation, intermittent bowel obstruction, electrolyte imbalances, infection, or uncontrolled cough (Tipton, 2014).
(b) Symptom assessment includes the following.
    i. Pretreatment assessment (Tipton, 2014)
       • History of cancer therapies and current chemotherapy
       • Prior experience with nausea and vomiting and current risk factors
       • Comorbidities and current disease status
       • Medications, including any previous use of an antiemetic regimen
    ii. Signs and symptoms of dehydration (Iwamoto et al., 2012)
       • Poor skin turgor
       • Electrolyte imbalance
       • Light-headedness or dizziness with postural changes
       • Nausea
       • Increased weakness or fatigue
       • Concentrated urine
       • Orthostatic hypotension
       • Oral cavity moisture

    iii. Physical examination (Iwamoto et al., 2012)
       • Height and weight
       • Vital signs, orthostatic blood pressure, and pulse
       • Skin turgor, oral cavity, bowel sounds, and abdominal tenderness or distention
       • Complete blood count to rule out associated infection and dehydration
       • Electrolytes levels to rule out dehydration and loss or imbalances
       • Oral intake over last 24 hours
    iv. Mental status
    v. Neurologic examination

(5) Collaborative management
(a) A pathophysiology-based treatment approach is generally recommended for the control of nausea and vomiting (Von Roenn, 2013).
    i. Accurate identification of the cause of nausea and vomiting can lead to effective symptom relief.
    ii. Further effective management of these symptoms is based on patient assessment, identification of source of nausea and vomiting, application of pathophysiology-based guidelines, and clinical judgment.
(b) Pharmacologic management is the mainstay for treating nausea and vomiting.
    i. Ruhlmann et al. (2017) stated, "The serotonin receptor antagonists are still the corner stone in antiemetic prophylaxis of nausea and vomiting induced by high and moderate emetic risk [RT]" (p. 309).
    ii. Preventive medications used for RINV include the following (NCI, 2020b).
       • Serotonin receptor antagonists (e.g., granisetron, ondansetron, palonosetron, dolasetron)
       • Corticosteroids (e.g., dexamethasone)
       • Dopamine receptor antagonists (e.g., metoclopramide, prochlorperazine)
    iii. Hesketh et al. (2017) noted that pharmacologic treatments are based on anatomic regions of RT and its level of emetogenicity.
    iv. Guidelines also recommended antiemetic administration schedules. Rescue therapy alone is recom-

mended for low-emetogenic RT (Hesketh et al., 2017).

v. The most effective regimens for CINV and RINV are recommended to be administered at initial treatment of symptoms (Hesketh et al., 2017).

vi. Regimens that combine a serotonin receptor antagonist (e.g., palonosetron), a neurokinin-1 receptor antagonist (e.g., netupitant), and a corticosteroid (e.g., dexamethasone) are the standard of care for managing acute and delayed CINV in patients treated with highly emetogenic chemotherapy. These medications are also effective in treating RINV (Roeland, Aapro, & Schwartzberg, 2015).

vii. Benzodiazepines can reduce the occurrence of anticipatory nausea and vomiting (Dupuis, Roscoe, Olver, Aapro, & Molassiotis, 2017).

viii. A serotonin receptor antagonist and optional short-course dexamethasone should be administered to prevent nausea and vomiting among patients receiving moderately emetic RT, including treatment to upper abdomen and craniospinal field (Ruhlmann et al., 2017).

ix. The Multinational Association of Supportive Care in Cancer (MASCC) recommends prophylactic treatment or rescue treatment utilizing serotonin receptor antagonists for patients receiving treatment to the cranium, head and neck, thorax, and pelvis (low-emetic RT) (Ruhlmann et al., 2017).

(c) Nonpharmacologic treatment can be added to an antiemetic regimen.

i. MASCC recommends behavioral therapies to prevent anticipatory nausea and vomiting. This recommendation includes progressive muscle relaxation training, systematic desensitization, and hypnosis (Dupuis et al., 2017).

ii. The following interventions can produce physiologic relaxation, which can decrease episodes of nausea and vomiting (Iwamoto et al., 2012).
• Exercise
• Hypnosis
• Music therapy
• Imagery

(d) Documentation: CTCAE should be used to standardize documentation.

i. Nausea (NCI CTEP, 2017, p. 33)
• Grade 1: loss of appetite without alteration in eating habits
• Grade 2: oral intake decreased without significant weight loss, dehydration, or malnutrition
• Grade 3: inadequate oral caloric or fluid intake; tube feeding, [total parenteral nutrition], or hospitalization indicated

ii. Vomiting (NCI CTEP, 2017, p. 39)
• Grade 1: intervention not indicated
• Grade 2: outpatient IV hydration; medical intervention indicated
• Grade 3: tube feeding, [total parenteral nutrition], or hospitalization indicated
• Grade 4: life-threatening consequences
• Grade 5: death

(e) Patient, caregiver, and family education (Iwamoto et al., 2012; NCI, 2020b; Tipton, 2014)

i. Patients must understand that nausea and vomiting are serious side effects of cancer treatment, especially chemotherapy. RT can also cause nausea and vomiting when the treatment is applied to the brain and the abdominal organs, including the liver.

ii. Clinicians should emphasize that prevention and control of nausea and vomiting is necessary to complete treatment and allow for a better quality of life. When left uncontrolled, nausea and vomiting can lead to further complications, such as chemical and mental changes in the body, loss of appetite, malnutrition, dehydration, and esophageal tear.

iii. Education includes information on when patients should see medical attention for emergent issues.
• Persistent nausea and vomiting that lasts more than one day and affects ADLs
• Blood in the vomitus
• Inability to tolerate and keep oral intake, especially fluids
• Inability to take medications, including antiemetic regimen
• Weight loss of about two pounds or more in one to two days
• Decrease in amount of urine and dark color

- Lightheadedness, dizziness, fainting, or confusion
- Fever

iv. Patients should follow up regularly with healthcare providers regarding the effectiveness of the regimen.

v. Patients should understand that nausea and vomiting can present in several ways before, during, and after treatment. It can be acute, delayed, anticipatory, breakthrough, refractory, or chronic. Patients can record episodes of nausea and vomiting in a journal.

vi. Patients should understand their risk factors for nausea and vomiting.

vii. Patients experiencing vomiting should check their weight daily.

viii. Self-care strategies can decrease nausea and vomiting (see also IV.H. Nutritional issues).
- Eating a small amount of food prior to RT
- Eating smaller, more frequent meals
- Eating bland foods, such as dry crackers, ginger ale, or chicken soup
- Not eating favorite foods when experiencing nausea
- Having someone else prepare foods; preparing meals that can be frozen and reheated
- Reducing food odors; eating foods that are room temperature or cool
- Taking antiemetic regimen as ordered or prior to meals
- Keeping the mouth clean; brushing teeth twice daily; rinsing the mouth out with water after meals
- Relaxation techniques or exercises

ix. Refer to appropriate websites for other resources.
- American Cancer Society: www.cancer.org
- ASCO: www.cancer.net
- NCCN: www.nccn.org
- NCI: www.cancer.gov

d) Diarrhea
(1) Pathophysiology
(a) Acute effects
i. RT to the abdomen or pelvis destroys the mucosal linings of the intestinal tract and can lead to radiation-induced diarrhea. Patients receiving combination therapies, such as concurrent chemotherapy, experience more severe diarrhea,

than those who receive RT alone (Muehlbauer & Lopez, 2014).

ii. Acute radiation-induced diarrhea is also classified as acute radiation enteritis when it takes place within six weeks of treatment and resolves within two to six months without specific treatment (Frazzoni et al., 2015).

iii. Damage to the intestinal mucosa leads to denuded intestinal villi, which then leads to decrease in absorption capacity of the gut. Prostaglandin is released, and bile salt malabsorption occurs, leading to increased peristaltic movement resulting in diarrhea. Ulcers also prevent proper absorption because of the decrease in the absorptive function of the mucosal linings (Frazzoni et al., 2015).

iv. Radiation affects the rapidly dividing cells of the small and large bowel. Crypt stem cells responsible for cellular replacement are affected, resulting in denudement and atrophy of villi in the small bowel and flattening of the epithelial surface in the large bowel. The loss of epithelial absorptive function results in loss of water, electrolytes, protein, and blood. Conjugated bile salts are not absorbed, enter the colon, and are compromised by bacterial flora, resulting in water retention and diarrhea (Frazzoni et al., 2015; Iwamoto et al., 2012).

v. Several other cancer treatment modalities can cause diarrhea (Muehlbauer & Lopez, 2014).
- Chemotherapy
- HSCT
- Targeted therapy and biotherapy
- Surgical resection

vi. Diarrhea can occur as a result of various mechanisms, such as osmotic, secretory, exudative, or change in motility.

vii. Either a decrease in intestinal absorption of fluids or increase in gastrointestinal secretions may cause diarrhea. The normal absorptive capacity of the intestinal tract is approximately 9–10 L of fluids (combined oral secretions and oral fluid intake). Secretory diarrhea will continue to occur despite decreased or low intake. Malabsorption disorders, infections, ileal surgery, and some medications can lead to secretory diarrhea (Muehlbauer & Lopez, 2014).

    viii. Intestinal transit time may be affected by motility disorders, leading to decreased absorption of nutrients and bile salts, thus causing an increase in bowel output. It can also lead to lactose intolerance (Iwamoto et al., 2012).

    ix. Diarrhea can significantly affect quality of life with physical and psychosocial consequences (Iwamoto et al., 2012; Lawrie et al., 2018).

(b) Chronic and late effects

    i. Radiation enteritis is a serious complication of RT, and it can occur in the small intestine, colon, and rectum. It can cause serious health issues, such as chronic ulcers, bleeding, intestinal stenosis, intestinal fistula, and perforation (Shen, Liu, & Zhu, 2018).

    ii. Chronic radiation enteritis can last for several months to years (Muehlbauer & Lopez, 2014).

    iii. Pan, Maeda, Wilson, Glynne-Jones, and Vaizey (2018) noted that late gastrointestinal toxicity after RT occurred among patients with anal cancer treated with chemotherapy and concurrent EBRT.

    iv. Several factors affect causation of radiation enteritis (NCI, 2020a).
- Total radiation dose
- Size of treatment field involving the intestines
- Size of tumor and extent of spread
- Concurrent chemotherapy
- Use of radiation implants
- Comorbidities (e.g., hypertension, diabetes, malnutrition)
- Surgery to the abdomen or pelvis

    v. Late effects may occur approximately 8–12 months after RT but can develop up to 15 years after RT secondary to vascular insufficiency caused by damaged cells in blood vessels and connective tissue in the bowel wall (Frazzoni et al., 2015; Iwamoto et al., 2012).

    vi. The small intestine is sensitive to late effects and is a dose-limiting structure in the treatment of the abdomen and pelvis. The large bowel is less radiosensitive, but radiation injury may result in colitis (Iwamoto et al., 2012).

(2) Incidence and risk factors

(a) Acute effects

    i. Diarrhea is a common toxic effect of preoperative RT for patients with rectal cancer (O'Gorman, Denieffe, & Gooney, 2014).

    ii. Diarrhea is a side effects of RT for gastric cancer and pancreatic adenocarcinoma (Ward et al., 2018).

    iii. Most patients receiving RT to the abdomen, pelvis, or rectum will show signs of acute enteritis (Iwamoto et al., 2012).

    iv. Incidence increases with higher dose fraction, larger treatment volume, concomitant chemotherapy, prior abdominal or pelvic surgery, and history of colitis, ileitis, or irritable bowel syndrome. Diarrhea usually begins to occur at 10–30 Gy (Iwamoto et al., 2012).

    v. In a patient-reported outcome study, acute gastrointestinal toxicity was highly significant in the fourth to fifth week of treatment among patients with anal cancer receiving chemoradiation, excluding rectal bleeding, which improved during treatment (Tom, Bennett, Rothenstein, Law, & Goodman, 2018).

    vi. Significant reduction in acute toxicity was noted among patients with locally advanced rectal cancer who received neoadjuvant concurrent chemoradiation utilizing IMRT (Wee et al., 2018).

    vii. When administered concurrently with chemotherapy, IMRT resulted in an acceptable acute gastrointestinal toxicity profile, with bowel cavity as the most sensitive predictor for the severity of diarrhea (Ng et al., 2018).

(b) Chronic and late effects

    i. Late gastrointestinal effects occur in 7%–64.5% of patients, and one-third present with severe side effects (Pan et al., 2018).
- Fecal incontinence (44%)
- Diarrhea (26.7%)
- Ulceration (22.6%)

    ii. Affected patients have lower quality-of-life scores (Pan et al., 2018).

    iii. IMRT appears to reduce late toxicity (Lawrie et al., 2018).

(3) Assessment

    (a) Individual risk factors: Clinicians should assess the following patient factors (Iwamoto et al., 2012).

        i. Prior abdominal surgery

        ii. History of pelvic inflammatory disease or colitis

        iii. History of lactose intolerance

        iv. History of cardiovascular disease, hypertension, or diabetes

    (b) Symptom assessment

        i. Evaluation of symptoms promptly and thoroughly allows for a better quality of life. Gastrointestinal symptoms, such as diarrhea, pain, loss of appetite, nausea, and vomiting, affect quality of life (O'Gorman, Barry, Denieffe, Sasiadek, & Gooney, 2016).

        ii. Attention to existing symptoms is required for prompt treatment, leading to improvement in the completion of planned treatments. Lawrie et al. (2018) also concluded that further study in the area of symptom management is warranted.

        iii. Symptoms of acute radiation enteritis usually resolve two to three weeks after completion of RT and include the following (Teo, Sebag-Montefiore, & Donnellan, 2015).

- Nausea and vomiting
- Abdominal cramps
- Bowel urgency
- Rectal bleeding, pain, and mucoid stool
- Watery diarrhea
- Fatigue

        iv. Symptoms of chronic radiation enteritis may begin as acute enteritis and persist after completion of RT. Symptoms may also occur several months or years after completing treatment (Teo et al., 2015).

- Colicky abdominal pain
- Bloody diarrhea
- Tenesmus
- Steatorrhea
- Weight loss
- Nausea and vomiting

    (c) Physical examination: Patient examination should include the following (NCI, 2020a).

        i. Usual pattern of elimination

        ii. The pattern of diarrhea, including onset, duration, frequency, amount, and character of stools (e.g., blood in stool)

        iii. Other symptoms, such as flatus, pain or cramping, nausea, abdominal distension, tenesmus, bleeding, and rectal excoriation

        iv. Nutritional status: weight and height, change in eating habits, and amount of residue in diet

        v. Signs of dehydration: poor skin turgor for age, serum electrolyte imbalance, increased weakness, and fatigue

        vi. Level of stress, coping patterns, and impact of symptoms on usual lifestyle

    (d) Medications: Clinicians should review medications, including over-the-counter medications and recent antibiotic history (Iwamoto et al., 2012).

    (e) Imaging: Abdominal CT, upper gastrointestinal series, and endoscopy often are required to establish the diagnosis (Iwamoto et al., 2012).

(4) Collaborative management of acute and chronic diarrhea

    (a) Dietary modification

        i. Lactose-free, low-fat, and low-fiber diets are options.

        ii. Eating small frequent meals (five to six per day) instead of three large meals is recommended (Muehlbauer & Lopez, 2014).

        iii. The following foods are also recommended.

- Foods high in soluble fiber (e.g., applesauce, oatmeal, banana, pectin-containing foods)
- Foods low in insoluble fiber or low residue (e.g., baked, broiled, or steamed skinned turkey and chicken; fish; well-cooked eggs; white toast; canned or cooked fruit without skin)
- Foods and fluids rich in electrolytes (e.g., high-potassium and high-sodium food, commercially prepared broths and soups, peach and apricot nectar, oranges, peeled potatoes)

        iv. Patients should avoid the following foods.

- Foods high in insoluble fiber (e.g., raw fruits and vegetables, whole-grain bread, nuts, popcorn, skins, seeds, legumes)
- Greasy, fried, and fatty foods; lactose products; strong spices and herbs; caffeine; alcohol; and tobacco

- Very hot or cold foods
- Hyperosmotic liquids (e.g., fruit juice, sweetened fruit drinks)

(b) Adequate fluids (Muehlbauer & Lopez, 2014)

    i. Patients should increase oral fluids to at least 8 oz per bout of diarrhea and consume at least 8–10 servings (8 oz) of fluids per day.

    ii. Room temperature liquids are also recommended.

(c) Pharmacologic management

    i. Goals of treatment are inhibition of intestinal motility, reduction in intestinal secretions, and promotion of absorption (Iwamoto et al., 2012).

    ii. Loperamide and diphenoxylate are the standard recommendation for grade 1–2 or mild diarrhea caused by RT (Muehlbauer & Lopez, 2014).

    iii. Dosing for loperamide is 4 mg at the first episode of diarrhea, followed by 2 mg after each unformed stool, with a maximum of 12–16 mg in 24 hours. This agent should be avoided in patients with suspected bowel obstruction (Iwamoto et al., 2012).

    iv. Combination diphenoxylate and atropine slows gastrointestinal transit time. Dosing is one to two tablets every four hours as needed, not to exceed eight tablets in 24 hours (Iwamoto et al., 2012).

    v. Octreotide has been found to be effective in treating radiation-induced diarrhea among patients who were refractory to loperamide. Subcutaneous doses controlled bowel symptoms in patients with rectal cancer receiving concurrent chemotherapy with pelvic RT with grade 2–3 diarrhea (Muehlbauer & Lopez, 2014).

    vi. Probiotics VSL#3® and *Lactobacillus acidophilus* have been found to decrease diarrheal symptoms in patients receiving RT. These probiotics were rated a "C" grade by the Yale Workshop on probiotics, indicating some studies have shown effectiveness, but more research is needed to establish confidence in its effectiveness (Muehlbauer & Lopez, 2014).

(d) Surgery: Surgical interventions for radiation enteritis include intestinal bypass and total intestinal resection (Huang, Guo, Yao, Li, & Li, 2016).

(e) Radiofrequency ablation: Radiofrequency ablation is an effective treatment for patients with radiation enteritis and is expected to be one of the standard treatments (Shen et al., 2018).

(5) Documentation: Documentation of grading for radiation-induced diarrhea and enteritis should adhere to CTCAE (NCI CTEP, 2017).

(6) Patient, caregiver, and family education

    (a) Nurses should teach patients about their specific type of treatment (e.g., RT, chemotherapy) before treatment begins. Patients should understand that diarrhea is an expected side effect of treatment (Gonzalez et al., 2019).

    (b) Nurses should educate patient, caregivers, and family about diarrhea management (Muehlbauer & Lopez, 2014).

        i. Patients should track and keep record of frequency, consistency, aggravating factors (e.g., foods, drinks), and symptoms (e.g., bloody stool, cramping, incontinence) (Gonzalez et al., 2019).

        ii. Nurses should teach patients preventive measures, management, treatment, and skin care in cases of incontinence.

        iii. Patients must notify the healthcare team if self-management is ineffective.

        iv. Patients must call healthcare providers immediately if any of the following symptoms occur (Gonzalez et al., 2019).

- Fever of 100.5°F (38°C)
- Blood in stool
- Severe abdominal pain and cramps
- Inability to keep oral fluids in a 12-hour period
- Dizziness, lightheadedness, weakness, increased thirst, and palpitations
- Disorientation
- Dark and concentrated urine
- Persistent diarrhea for 24 hours despite attempts to manage with loperamide

        v. Nurses should instruct on dietary modifications.

        vi. Patients require specific instructions on how to take antidiarrheal medications.

        vii. Nurses should provide recommendations for proper perineal skin care (see IV.B. Skin reactions).

    (c) Refer to the following websites.

        i. ASCO: www.cancer.net

        ii. NCI: www.cancer.gov

References

Adams, L.A., Cunningham, R.S., Caruso, R.A., Norling, M.J., & Shepard, N. (2009). ONS PEP resource: Anorexia. In L.H. Eaton & J.M. Tipton (Eds.), *Putting evidence into practice: Improving oncology patient outcomes* (pp. 31–36). Oncology Nursing Society.

American Cancer Society. (2020). *Cancer facts and figures 2020.* https://www.cancer.org/research/cancer-facts-statistics/all-cancer-facts-figures/cancer-facts-figures-2020.html

Arends, J., Bachmann, P., Baracos, V., Barthelemy, N., Bertz, H., Bozzetti, F., ... Preiser, J.-C. (2017). ESPEN guidelines on nutrition in cancer patients. *Clinical Nutrition, 36,* 11–48. https://doi.org/10.1016/j.clnu.2016.07.015

Badowski, M.E., & Yanful, P.K. (2018). Dronabinol oral solution in the management of anorexia and weight loss in AIDS and cancer. *Therapeutics and Clinical Risk Management, 14,* 643–651. https://doi.org/10.2147/tcrm.s126849

Boyle, J., Czito, B., Willett, C., & Palta, M. (2015). Adjuvant radiation therapy for pancreatic cancer: A review of the old and the new. *Journal of Gastrointestinal Oncology, 6,* 436–444. https://doi.org/10.3978/j.issn.2078-6891.2015.014

Buduhan, V., Cashman, R., Cooper, E., Levy, K., Sherriff, C., & Syme, A. (2018). *Symptom management guidelines: Anorexia and cachexia.* BC Cancer. www.bccancer.bc.ca/nursing-site/Documents/2. Anorexia and Cachexia.pdf

Correia, M.I.T.D., Hegazi, R.A., Higashiguchi, T., Michel, J.-P., Reddy, B.R., Tappenden, K.A., ... Muscaritoli, M. (2014). Evidence-based recommendations for addressing malnutrition in health care: An updated strategy from the feedM.E. global study group. *Journal of the American Medical Directors Association, 15,* 544–550. https://doi.org/10.1016/j.jamda.2014.05.011

Czito, B.G., & Willett, C.G. (2011). Stomach. In D.C. Shreve & J.S. Loeffler (Eds.), *Human radiation injury* (pp. 444–452). Lippincott Williams and Wilkins.

Dupuis, L.L., Roscoe, J.A., Olver, I., Aapro, M., & Molassiotis, A. (2017). 2016 updated MASCC/ESMO consensus recommendations: Anticipatory nausea and vomiting in children and adults receiving chemotherapy. *Supportive Care in Cancer, 25,* 317–321. https://doi.org/10.1007/s00520-016-3330-z

Eaby-Sandy, B., & Sherry, V. (2011). Updates on the understanding and management of chemotherapy-induced nausea and vomiting. *Journal of Advanced Practice Oncology, 2,* 373–380. https://doi.org/10.6004/jadpro.2011.2.6.3

Ezeoke, C.C., & Morley, J.E. (2015). Pathophysiology of anorexia in the cancer cachexia syndrome. *Journal of Cachexia, Sarcopenia and Muscle, 6,* 287–302. https://doi.org/10.1002/jcsm.12059

Fearon, K., Strasser, F., Anker, S.D., Bosaeus, I., Bruera, E., Fainsinger, R.L., ... Baracos, V.E. (2011). Definition and classification of cancer cachexia: An international consensus. *Lancet Oncology, 12,* 489–495. https://doi.org/10.1016/s1470-2045(10)70218-7

Feyer, P., Jahn, F., & Jordan, K. (2015). Prophylactic management of radiation-induced nausea and vomiting. *Biomed Research International, 2015,* 893013. https://doi.org/10.1155/2015/893013

Frazzoni, L., La Marca, M., Guido, A., Morganti, A.G., Bazzoli, F., & Fuccio, L. (2015). Pelvic radiation disease: Updates on treatment options. *World Journal of Clinical Oncology, 6,* 272–280. https://doi.org/10.5306/wjco.v6.i6.272

Gonzalez, V.J., Beckstead, J., Groer, M., McMillan, S., Ortiz, D., Marrero, S., & Saligan, L.N. (2019). Exploring the relationship between diarrhea and fatigue that can occur during cancer treatment: Using structural equation modeling. *Puerto Rico Health Sciences Journal, 38,* 81–86.

Hesketh, P.J., Kris, M.G., Basch, E., Bohlke, K., Barbour, S.Y., Clark-Snow, R.A., ... Lyman, G.H. (2017). Antiemetics: American Society of Clinical Oncology clinical practice guideline update. *Journal of Clinical Oncology, 35,* 3240–3261. https://doi.org/10.1200/jco.2017.74.4789

Huang, Y., Guo, F., Yao, D., Li, Y., & Li, J. (2016). Surgery for chronic radiation enteritis: Outcome and risk factors. *Journal of Surgical Research, 204,* 335–343. https://doi.org/10.1016/j.jss.2016.05.014

Isenring, E., Zabel, R., Bannister, M., Brown, T., Findlay, M., Kiss, N., ... Bauer, J. (2013). Updated evidence-based practice guidelines for the nutritional management of patients receiving radiation therapy and/or chemotherapy. *Nutrition and Dietetics, 70,* 312–324. https://doi.org/10.1111/1747-0080.12013

Iwamoto, R.R., Haas, M.L., & Gosselin, T.K. (Eds.). (2012). *Manual for radiation oncology nursing practice and education* (4th ed.). Oncology Nursing Society.

Lawrie, T.A., Green, J.T., Beresford, M., Wedlake, L., Burden, S., Davidson, S.E., ... Andreyev, H.J.N. (2018). Interventions to reduce acute and late adverse gastrointestinal effects of pelvic radiotherapy for primary pelvic cancers. *Cochrane Database of Systematic Reviews, 2018*(1). https://doi.org/10.1002/14651858.CD012529.pub2

Letilovic, T., & Vrhovac, R. (2013). Influence of additional criteria from a definition of cachexia on its prevalence—Good or bad thing? *European Journal of Clinical Nutrition, 67,* 797–801. https://doi.org/10.1038/ejcn.2013.121

Muehlbauer, P.M., & Lopez, R.C. (2014). Diarrhea. In C.H. Yarbro, D. Wujcik, & B.H. Gobel (Eds.), *Cancer symptom management* (4th ed., pp. 185–212). Jones and Bartlett Learning.

National Cancer Institute. (2018, March 16). Nutrition in cancer care (PDQ®) [Patient version]. https://www.cancer.gov/about-cancer/treatment/side-effects/appetite-loss/nutrition-pdq

National Cancer Institute. (2020a, April 22). Gastrointestinal complications (PDQ®) [Health professional version]. https://www.cancer.gov/about-cancer/treatment/side-effects/constipation/gi-complications-hp-pdq

National Cancer Institute. (2020b, July 23). Treatment-related nausea and vomiting (PDQ®) [Health professional version]. https://www.cancer.gov/about-cancer/treatment/side-effects/nausea/nausea-hp-pdq

National Cancer Institute Cancer Therapy Evaluation Program. (2017). *Common terminology criteria for adverse events* [v.5.0.]. https://ctep.cancer.gov/protocolDevelopment/electronic_applications/docs/CTCAE_v5_Quick_Reference_8.5x11.pdf

National Comprehensive Cancer Network. (n.d.). Nausea and vomiting. https://www.nccn.org/patients/resources/life_with_cancer/managing_symptoms/preventing_nausea.aspx

Navari, R.M., & Brenner, M.C. (2010). Treatment of cancer-related anorexia with olanzapine and megestrol acetate: A randomized trial. *Supportive Care in Cancer, 18,* 951–956. https://doi.org/10.1007/s00520-009-0739-7

Ng, M., Ho., H., Skelton, J., Guerrieri, M., Guiney, M., Chao, M., ... Melven, L. (2018). Intensity-modulated radiotherapy for anal cancer: Dose–volume relationship of acute gastrointestinal toxicity and disease outcomes. *Clinical Oncology, 30,* 634–641. https://doi.org/10.1016/j.clon.2018.07.020

Nicholson, B.D., Hamilton, W., O'Sullivan, J., Aveyard, P., & Hobbs, F.D.R. (2018). Weight loss as a predictor of cancer in primary care: A systematic review and meta-analysis. *British Journal of General Practice, 68,* e311–e322. https://doi.org/10.3399/bjgp18x695801

Nicolini, A., Ferrari, P., Masoni, M.C., Fini, M., Pagani, S., Giampietro, O., & Carpi, A. (2013). Malnutrition, anorexia and cachexia in cancer patients: A mini-review on pathogenesis and treatment. *Biomedicine and Pharmacotherapy, 67,* 807–817. https://doi.org/10.1016/j.biopha.2013.08.005

O'Gorman, C., Barry, A., Denieffe, S., Sasiadek, W., & Gooney, M. (2016). Nursing implications: Symptom presentation and quality of life in rectal cancer patients. *Journal of Clinical Nursing, 25,* 1395–1404. https://doi.org/10.1111/jocn.13234

O'Gorman, C., Denieffe, S., & Gooney, M. (2014). Literature review: Preoperative radiotherapy and rectal cancer—Impact on acute symptom presentation and quality of life. *Journal of Clinical Nursing, 23,* 333–351. https://doi.org/10.1111/jocn.12138

Pan, Y.B., Maeda, Y., Wilson, A., Glynne-Jones, A., & Vaizey, C.J. (2018). Late gastrointestinal toxicity after radiotherapy for anal cancer: A systematic literature review. *Acta Oncologica, 57,* 1427–1437. https://doi.org/10.1080/0284186X.2018.1503713

Roeland, E., Aapro, M.S., & Schwartzberg, L. (2015). Advances in the management of chemotherapy-induced nausea and vomiting: New data from recent and ongoing trials. *Clinical Advances in Hematology and Oncology, 13*(Suppl. 10), 1–14. https://www.hematologyandoncology.net/supplements/advances-in-the-management-of-chemotherapy-induced-nausea-and-vomiting-new-data-from-recent-and-ongoing-trials

Ruhlmann, C.H., Jahn, F., Jordan, K., Dennis, K., Maranzano, E., Molassiotis, A., ... Feyer, P. (2017). 2016 updated MASCC/ESMO consensus recommendations: Prevention of radiotherapy-induced nausea and vomiting. *Supportive Care in Cancer, 25,* 309–316. https://doi.org/10.1007/s00520-016-3407-8

Sadeghi, M., Keshavarz-Fathi, M., Baracos, V., Arends, J., Mahmoudi, M., & Rezaei, N. (2018). Cancer cachexia: Diagnosis, assessment, and treatment. *Critical Reviews in Oncology/Hematology, 127,* 91–104. https://doi.org/10.1016/j.critrevonc.2018.05.006

Shadad, A.K., Sullivan, F.J., Martin, J.D., & Egan, L.J. (2013). Gastrointestinal radiation injury: Symptoms, risk factors and mechanisms. *World Journal of Gastroenterology, 19,* 185–198. https://doi.org/10.3748/wjg.v19.i2.185

Shen, X.-J., Liu, L., & Zhu, Y.-J. (2018). Radiofrequency ablation in a patient with radiation enteritis: A case report. *Medicine, 97,* e13328. https://doi.org/10.1097/MD.0000000000013328

Stephens, S.J., Czito, B., Zhang, X., Duffy, E., Malicki, M., Pitcher, B., ... Palta, M. (2018). Surgical and pathologic outcomes in patients on a phase II trial of neoadjuvant chemotherapy and hypofractionated image-guided intensity modulated radiation therapy (HIGRT) in resectable and borderline resectable pancreatic cancer [Abstract]. *International Journal of Radiation Oncology, Biology, Physics, 102*(Suppl. 3), S180. https://doi.org/10.1016/j.ijrobp.2018.07.056

Stevich-Heemer, B. (2019, December 17). Management of radiation-induced nausea and vomiting. *U.S. Pharmacist, 44*(12), HS10–HS13. https://www.uspharmacist.com/article/management-of-radiationinduced-nausea-and-vomiting

Teo, M.T.W., Sebag-Montefiore, D., & Donnellan, C.F. (2015). Prevention and management of radiation-induced late gastrointestinal toxicity. *Clinical Oncology, 27,* 656–667. https://doi.org/10.1016/j.clon.2015.06.010

Tipton, J. (2014). Nausea and vomiting. In C.H. Yarbro, D. Wujcik, & B.H. Gobel (Eds.), *Cancer symptom management* (4th ed., pp. 213–240). Jones and Bartlett Learning.

Tom, A., Bennett, A.V., Rothenstein, D., Law, E., & Goodman, K.A. (2018). Prevalence of patient-reported gastrointestinal symptoms and agreement with clinician toxicity assessments in radiation therapy for anal cancer. *Quality of Life Research, 27,* 97–103. https://doi.org/10.1007/s11136-017-1700-8

Urba, S.G., Orringer, M.B., Turrisi, A., Iannettoni, M., Forastiere, A., & Strawderman, M. (2001). Randomized trial of preoperative chemoradiation versus surgery alone in patients with locoregional esophageal carcinoma. *Journal of Clinical Oncology, 19,* 305–313. https://doi.org/10.1200/JCO.2001.19.2.305

Von Roenn, J.H. (2013). Assessment and management of chronic nausea and vomiting. In A. Berger, J. Schuster, Jr., & J.H. Von Roenn (Eds.), *Principles and practice of palliative care and supportive oncology* (4th ed., pp. 163–174). Lippincott Williams and Wilkins.

Ward, M.C., Tendulkar, R.D., & Videtic, G.M.M. (Eds.). (2018). *Essentials of clinical radiation oncology.* Springer. https://doi.org/10.1891/9780826168559

Wee, C.W., Kang, H.-C., Wu, H.-G., Chie, E.K., Choi, N., Park, J.M., ... Goodman, K.A. (2018). Intensity-modulated radiotherapy versus three-dimensional conformal radiotherapy in rectal cancer treated with neoadjuvant concurrent chemoradiation: a meta-analysis and pooled-analysis of acute toxicity. *Japanese Journal of Clinical Oncology, 48,* 458–466. https://doi.org/10.1093/jjco/hyy029

Yovino, S., Poppe, M., Jabbour, S., David, V., Garofalo, M., Pandya, N., ... Regine, W.F. (2011). Intensity-modulated radiation therapy significantly improves acute gastrointestinal toxicity in pancreatic and ampullary cancers. *International Journal of Radiation Oncology, Biology, Physics, 79,* 158–162. https://doi.org/10.1016/j.ijrobp.2009.10.043

F. Bladder

1. Incidence
   a) Bladder cancer is the most common tumor of the urinary tract, with non-muscle invasive urothelial carcinoma the most frequently occurring (Jokisch, Karl, & Stief, 2015; Lotan & Choueiri, 2020; Pham, Torres, & Sharma, 2019).
   b) In the United States, bladder cancer is the sixth most common cancer, with an estimated 81,400 new cases and an estimated 17,980 deaths in 2020 (American Cancer Society, 2020; Flaig et al., 2018; Massari et al., 2017).
   c) In men, bladder cancer is the fourth most common cancer, and it is less common in women (American Cancer Society, 2020).

2. Risk factors
   a) Smoking: Approximately 50% of bladder cancers are related to smoking (American Cancer Society, 2019a; Bellmunt, Powles, & Vogelzang, 2017).
   b) Age (American Cancer Society, 2020)
      (1) Approximately 90% of people with bladder cancer are older than 55 years.
      (2) At the time of diagnosis, average age is 73 years.
   c) Sex: Bladder cancer is more common in men.
   d) Race: Bladder cancer is more prevalent in people of Caucasian descent, approximately twice as prevalent as cases in African American and Hispanic people (American Cancer Society, 2019a; Daneshmand, 2019).
   e) Family history: People with a family history of bladder cancer are more likely to develop it (American Cancer Society, 2019a).
   f) Contaminants: Arsenic in drinking water is associated with risk of bladder cancer (American Cancer Society, 2019a).
   g) Occupation (American Cancer Society, 2019a; Daneshmand, 2019; DeVita, Lawrence, & Rosenberg, 2018).
      (1) Certain jobs, such as rubber and textile workers, painters, printers, metal workers, machinists, chemical workers, and diesel truck drivers, are at higher risk of bladder cancer.
      (2) Aniline dyes and aromatic amines are two compounds that have been implicated to be related to workplace exposure.
   h) Medical history (American Cancer Society, 2019a)
      (1) Certain medical conditions, including Lynch syndrome (hereditary nonpolyposis colorectal cancer), schistosomiasis (caused by a parasite), Cowden disease (mutations in the *PTEN* gene), and chronic urinary tract infections, pose a risk of bladder cancer.
      (2) Previous treatment with pelvic irradiation also increases risk.

3. Signs and symptoms
   a) Signs of bladder cancer can include painless hematuria (65% microhematuria; up to 35% gross hema-

turia) and new onset irritative voiding symptoms, such as urinary frequency, urgency, and urinary pain (DeVita et al., 2018).

b) Generalized symptoms of decreased appetite, weight loss, fatigue, and failure to thrive can be signs of advanced or metastatic disease and signify a poorer prognosis (Daneshmand, 2019).

4. Staging

a) Depth of invasion into the bladder wall or beyond determines primary bladder cancer stage (DeVita et al., 2018).

b) Bladder cancers are classified by their stage at presentation (DeVita et al., 2018).
   (1) Non-muscle invasive bladder cancer: no invasion into the muscularis propria (true muscle of the bladder wall)
   (2) Muscle invasive bladder cancer: invasion into muscularis propria
   (3) Regional lymph node involvement
   (4) Metastatic disease

c) Bladder cancer is staged according to the TNM staging system established by the Union for International Cancer Control and AJCC (Amin et al., 2018).

d) Approximately 70%–75% of patients with bladder cancer present with non-muscle invasive disease (DeVita et al., 2018; Flaig et al., 2018; Jokisch et al., 2015).
   (1) Non-muscle invasive tumors respond well to local treatment, but despite this, 30%–85% of patients have a recurrence within two years after diagnosis (Jokisch et al., 2015).
   (2) Approximately one-half of muscle-invasive bladder cancers progress to metastatic disease despite aggressive treatment (Flaig et al., 2018).

5. Treatment options

a) The aim of all bladder cancer treatment is to achieve the best possible clinical outcome while maintaining quality of life.

b) Treatment for non-muscle invasive bladder cancer is aimed at decreasing recurrence and preventing disease progression (Flaig et al., 2018).

c) Depending on the stage and grade of disease or recurrence, bladder cancer treatment includes surgery, intravesical immunotherapy, intravesical drug therapy, chemotherapy, RT, or a combination of modalities. More recently, immune checkpoint inhibitors have become a common modality.

d) Transurethral resection of the bladder tumor is considered the standard treatment for bladder cancers and for treatment of low-grade tumors. The goal of resection is to remove all visible tumors and to obtain specimens for histopathologic inquiry (Jokisch et al., 2015).

e) In addition to resection, patients at high risk for developing recurrent disease should be considered for adjuvant intravesical drug therapy (DeVita et al., 2018).
   (1) Adjuvant intravesical drug therapy utilizes gemcitabine (preferred) or mitomycin C for low-grade Ta tumors.
   (2) For high-grade Ta tumors, intravesical immunotherapy with bacillus Calmette-Guérin (BCG) can be considered (NCCN, 2020).
   (3) For T1 tumors, repeat transurethral resection of the bladder tumor is highly recommended with consideration of cystectomy in patients with high-grade T1 disease.
   (4) If there is evidence of residual disease, adjuvant treatment with intravesical BCG or cystectomy is recommended.
   (5) If a patient has no residual disease, treatment with BCG is preferred, or intravesical drug therapy (gemcitabine or mitomycin C) can be administered (NCCN, 2020).
   (6) For any tumor in situ, adjuvant treatment with BCG is recommended (NCCN, 2020).
   (7) Ideal usage of BCG for maintenance therapy remains unclear (Jokisch et al., 2015).

f) Treatment for muscle invasive bladder cancer requires definitive local therapy (surgery or RT) with curative intent.
   (1) Systemic therapy, including neoadjuvant chemotherapy, is often used in conjunction with definitive local management (Flaig et al., 2018).
   (2) Patients need to be informed about the advantages and disadvantages of treatment options to make an informed decision.
   (3) The use of surgery and multimodal chemoradiation, along with the patient's overall health, needs to be considered before treatment decisions are made.

g) RT is considered inferior to radical cystectomy, with the overall five-year survival rate of approximately 40%, compared to approximately 50% after cystectomy (Anderson, 2018).

h) Historically, the standard of care for the management of muscle invasive bladder cancer was radical cystectomy with a bilateral pelvic lymph node dissection and the creation of a urinary diversion (DeVita et al., 2018; Smith et al., 2013).
   (1) For men, radical surgery includes removal of the prostate gland.
   (2) While providing definitive local control, radical surgery is associated with considerable morbidity, including metabolic complications, urine leak, ureteral or intestinal obstruction, stoma problems, and changes in sexual function (DeVita et al., 2018; Smith et al., 2013).
   (3) In rare instances, partial cystectomy may be an option (American Cancer Society, 2019b).

i) Approximately 30% of patients have muscle invasive bladder cancer at diagnosis. This is typically treated with neoadjuvant cisplatin followed by cystectomy with pelvic lymph node dissection and urinary diversion or with bladder-preserving trimodal therapy using maximal transurethral resection of the bladder tumor followed by radiosensitizing chemotherapy and RT (Flaig et al., 2018; Giacalone et al., 2017; Massari et al., 2017).

j) For patients with muscle invasive disease not fit to undergo cystectomy and for patients with limited disease wishing to avoid surgery, bladder-preserving therapies were developed with the goal of maintaining bladder function and form while achieving complete response (Smith et al., 2013).

    (1) Bladder-sparing EBRT for the management of muscle invasive disease involves treatment to the pelvis including the bladder, prostate, and the low external and internal iliac lymph nodes at a total dose of 40–45 Gy in 1.8–2 Gy fractions.

    (2) After repeat cystoscopy confirming complete response to treatment, the target volume is decreased to deliver an additional 15 fractions at 2–2.5 Gy per fraction to the bladder only and the primary bladder tumor (consolidation) (DeVita et al., 2018).

    (3) EBRT may not be suitable in patients who have had previous pelvic RT, a history of inflammatory bowel conditions, and previous pelvic surgery (possibility of adhesions with the bowel stuck to the bladder), as well as patients with obstruction to one or both kidneys (Anderson, 2018).

    (4) Patients receiving RT need to be instructed to empty their bladder at the time of simulation and for daily treatment to provide reproducibility of the daily treatment field and improve accuracy and adequate coverage of the bladder (DeVita et al., 2018).

    (5) Bladder brachytherapy can be used to deliver a high dose of radiation to a solitary bladder tumor within a short period of time (DeVita et al., 2018).

k) Patients with regional lymph node involvement (stages IIIA and IIIB) have a variety of treatment options available to them.

    (1) Primary treatment for stage IIIA bladder cancers include neoadjuvant cisplatin-based combination chemotherapy followed by radical cystectomy or concurrent chemotherapy and RT. For patients who are not candidates for cystectomy, concurrent chemotherapy and RT or RT alone are used (NCCN, 2020).

    (2) For stage IIIB tumors, primary treatment involves initial systemic therapy for downstaging or concurrent chemotherapy and RT with cystoscopic reassessment two to three months after treatment.

      (a) With a complete response after downstaging, consolidation cystectomy, consolidation chemotherapy and RT, or observation until disease relapse can be considered.

      (b) With a complete response after chemotherapy and RT, treatment proceeds to follow-up and surveillance until disease relapse.

      (c) With a partial response, consolidation cystectomy or chemotherapy and RT can be considered. Treatment as metastatic disease is also an option.

l) Management of advanced or metastatic disease is aimed at prolonging the quantity of life and maintaining the quality of life.

    (1) Treatment options now include immune checkpoint inhibitors (Bellmunt et al., 2017).

    (2) Bladder cancer metastasizes most commonly to the lungs, bone, liver, and brain through lymphatic and hematogenous means (DeVita et al., 2018).

    (3) Prognosis of metastatic bladder cancer is poor, with median survival of approximately 12 months (DeVita et al., 2018).

    (4) Palliative RT for invasive bladder carcinomas or metastatic disease can provide relief of bleeding and pelvic pain from the bladder cancer itself or sites of metastatic disease (Anderson, 2018).

    (5) A referral to the palliative care team is often indicated for those patients with locally advanced or metastatic disease.

6. Documentation: Documentation should utilize CTCAE for symptoms related to bladder cancer and treatment (NCI CTEP, 2017).

  a) Urinary frequency and urgency

  b) Urinary tract pain

  c) Urinary retention

  d) Urinary incontinence

  e) Dermatitis

  f) Fatigue

  g) Diarrhea

7. Collaborative management

  a) Nursing care of a patient with urothelial carcinoma will be dependent upon the type of medical treatment required.

  b) Clinicians should always assess a patient's support systems, including cultural, physical, psychological, and spiritual. Clinicians should also assess readiness to learn of patients, caregivers, and family.

  c) For patients receiving RT, early or acute urinary symptoms are a result of injury and inflammation of the epithelial layer of the bladder mucosa caused by the ionizing radiation. Inflammatory changes in the bladder mucosa can occur with exposure of subepithelial tissues to the caustic effects of urine.

d) Treatments such as RT and chemotherapy produce other symptomatic treatment sequela, including anorexia, weight loss, nausea, hemorrhagic cystitis, vomiting, diarrhea, fatigue, anxiety, and sexual dysfunction. Clinicians must be prepared to assist the patient and family in managing these symptoms (Pham et al., 2019; Vuttanon, Vichittragoonthavon, Chaisurin, & Thongchai, 2017).

8. Patient, caregiver, and family education

   a) Clinicians should instruct patients, caregivers, and family regarding lifestyle modifications.

      (1) Smoking cessation and avoidance of tobacco products

      (2) Healthy diet and regular regimen of exercise

      (3) Management of stress and anxiety

      (4) Adherence to recommended medications, treatments, and appointments

   b) Clinicians should inform patients about the possibility of bladder irritation from pelvic irradiation.

   c) Patients should decrease intake of caffeinated drinks (e.g., coffee, tea), alcohol, and carbonated beverages, as these are bladder irritants. Patients should be advised to drink 2–3 L of fluid per day (if not contraindicated) to help decrease irritation to the bladder mucosa.

   d) Clinicians should instruct patients regarding the signs and symptoms of bladder infection, such as burning on urination, increased frequency, urgency, pain in the abdomen over the bladder, low back pain, low-grade fever, foul-smelling urine, blood in urine, and painful sexual intercourse. Patients should notify the healthcare team if these symptoms occur (Barlow & Shepard, 2014).

   e) Clinicians can refer patients to the following websites for additional information.

      (1) American Cancer Society: https://www.cancer.org/cancer/bladder-cancer/treating/radiation.html

      (2) Bladder Cancer Advocacy Network: www.bcan.org

      (3) Cleveland Clinic: www.clevelandclinic.org/lp/bladder-cancer/index.html

      (4) eMedicineHealth: www.emedicinehealth.com/bladder_cancer/article_em.htm

      (5) NCI: www.cancer.gov/types/bladder/hp

      (6) U.S. National Library of Medicine: www.nlm.nih.gov/medlineplus/urinaryincontinence.html

References

American Cancer Society. (2019a). Bladder cancer risk factors. https://www.cancer.org/cancer/bladder-cancer/causes-risks-prevention/risk-factors.html

American Cancer Society. (2019b). Bladder cancer surgery. https://www.cancer.org/cancer/bladder-cancer/treating/surgery.html

American Cancer Society. (2020). Key statistics for bladder cancer. https://www.cancer.org/cancer/bladder-cancer/about/key-statistics.html

Amin, M.B., Edge, S., Greene, F., Byrd, D.R., Brookland, R.K., Washington, M.K., ... Gershenwald, J.E. (Eds.). (2018). *AJCC cancer staging manual* (8th ed.). Springer.

Anderson, B. (2018). Bladder cancer: Overview and management. Part 2: Muscle-invasive and metastatic bladder cancer. *British Journal of Nursing, 27*(18), S8–S20. https://doi.org/10.12968/bjon.2018.27.18.S8

Barlow, W., & Shepard, L.H. (2014). Care of the patient with bladder cancer. *Nursing Made Incredibly Easy, 12*(5), 40–48. https://doi.org/10.1097/01.NME.0000452685.17977.66

Bellmunt, J., Powles, T., & Vogelzang, N.J. (2017). A review on the evolution of PD-1/PD-L1 immunotherapy for bladder cancer: The future is now. *Cancer Treatment Reviews, 54*, 58–67. https://doi.org/10.1016/j.ctrv.2017.01.007

Daneshmand, S. (2019). Epidemiology and risk factors of urothelial (transitional cell) carcinoma of the bladder. In S. Shah (Ed.), *UpToDate*. Retrieved March 25, 2020, from https://www.uptodate.com/contents/epidemiology-and-risk-factors-of-urothelial-transitional-cell-carcinoma-of-the-bladder

DeVita, V.T., Jr., Lawrence, T.S., & Rosenberg, S.A. (Eds.). (2018). *DeVita, Hellman, and Rosenberg's cancer: Principles and practice of oncology* (11th ed.). Wolters Kluwer.

Flaig, T.W., Spiess, P.E., Agarwal, N., Bangs, R., Boorjian, S.A., Buyyounouski, M.K., ... Gurski, L.A. (2018). NCCN Guidelines insights: Bladder cancer, version 5.2018. *Journal of the National Comprehensive Cancer Network, 16*, 1041–1053. https://doi.org/10.6004/jnccn.2018.0072

Giacalone, N.J., Shipley, W.U., Clayman, R.H., Niemierko, A., Drumm, M., Heney, N.M., ... Efstathiou, J.A. (2017). Long-term outcomes after bladder-preserving tri-modality therapy for patients with muscle-invasive bladder cancer: An updated analysis of the Massachusetts General Hospital experience. *European Urology, 71*, 952–960. https://doi.org/10.1016/j.eururo.2016.12.020

Jokisch, J.-F., Karl, A., & Stief, C. (2015). Intravesical immunotherapy in non-muscle invasive bladder cancer. *Indian Journal of Urology, 31*, 304–311. https://doi.org/10.4103/0970-1591.166452

Lotan, Y., & Choueiri, T.K. (2020). Clinical presentation, diagnosis, and staging of bladder cancer. In S. Shah (Ed.), *UpToDate*. Retrieved March 25, 2020, from https://www.uptodate.com/contents/clinical-presentation-diagnosis-and-staging-of-bladder-cancer

Massari, F., Di Nunno, V., Cubelli, M., Santoni, M., Fiorentino, M., Montironi, R., ... Ardizzoni, A. (2018). Immune checkpoint inhibitors for metastatic bladder cancer. *Cancer Treatment Reviews, 64*, 11–20. https://doi.org/10.1016/j.ctrv.2017.12.007

National Cancer Institute Cancer Therapy Evaluation Program. (2017). *Common terminology criteria for adverse events* [v.5.0]. https://doi.org/10.1080/00140139.2010.489653

National Comprehensive Cancer Network. (2020). *NCCN Clinical Practice Guidelines in Oncology (NCCN Guidelines®): Bladder cancer* [v.5.2020]. https://www.nccn.org/professionals/physician_gls/pdf/bladder.pdf

Pham, H., Torres, H., & Sharma, P. (2019). Mental health implications in bladder cancer patients: A review. *Urologic Oncology: Seminars and Original Investigations, 37*, 97–107. https://doi.org/10.1016/j.urolonc.2018.12.006

Smith, Z.L., Christodouleas, J.P., Keefe, S.M., Malkowicz, B., & Guzzo, T.J. (2013). Bladder preservation in the treatment of muscle-invasive bladder cancer (MIBC): A review of the literature and a practical approach to therapy. *BJU International, 112*, 13–25. https://doi.org/10.1111/j.1464-410X.2012.11762.x

Vuttanon, N., Vichittragoonthavon, S., Chaisurin, P., & Thongchai, C. (2017). Symptom management for bladder cancer in Thailand. *International Journal of Urological Nursing, 11*, 82–89. https://doi.org/10.1111/ijun.12132

G. Male pelvis and prostate

1. Diagnosis

   a) According to NCCN (2020b), information needed to diagnose prostate cancer and to determine risk group includes digital rectal examination results, prostate-specific antigen (PSA) results, prostate biopsy pathology results (specifically Gleason score, TNM staging, number of positive cores, and percentage of cancerous tissue within cores), life expectancy, family history, known high-risk germline mutations, and any imaging results, if indicated.

    (1) The Gleason score is the accepted global standard for grading prostate cancer (Michalski, Pisansky, Lawton, & Potters, 2016).

        (a) This score is derived from the pathology of prostate biopsy cores.

        (b) The Gleason score is the sum of two scores: the predominant cell pattern of the biopsy specimen and the second most dominant cell pattern.

        (c) If only one cell pattern is present, both scores are given the same number.

        (d) Scores range 1–5, with 1 being entirely normal prostate tissue and 5 being the most abnormal and aggressive tissue.

    (2) Because PSA testing is commonly used to detect prostate cancer, malignancy is more often in a favorable stage when diagnosed.

        (a) Approximately 81% of newly diagnosed prostate cancer is clinically localized (T1N0M0 or T2N0M0). In these stages, it has not spread outside of the prostate, nor has it penetrated the walls of the prostate (Lardas et al., 2017).

        (b) Only 4% of prostate cancers are diagnosed with distant metastasis.

        (c) The five-year survival rate of prostate cancer is now 99% (Hussein & Cooperberg, 2016).

  b) Prostate cancer risk groups can be classified as the following (NCCN, 2020b).

    (1) Very low risk

    (2) Low risk

    (3) Favorable intermediate risk

    (4) Unfavorable intermediate risk

    (5) High risk

    (6) Very high risk

    (7) Regional (lymph node involvement)

    (8) Metastatic

2. Treatment options

  a) Multiple effective treatment options for prostate cancer are available. The following treatments can be used as a single modality or combined.

    (1) Observation

    (2) Active surveillance

    (3) EBRT

    (4) LDR brachytherapy

    (5) HDR brachytherapy

    (6) Radical prostatectomy with possible pelvic lymph node dissection if probability of lymph node metastasis is 2% or greater

    (7) Androgen deprivation therapy

    (a) According to NCCN (2020b), short-term therapy (four to six months) combined with RT is an option for treating unfavorable intermediate risk prostate cancer in patients with a life expectancy of 10 years or more.

    (b) In the high-risk and very high-risk groups, long-term therapy (one to three years) combined with RT is an option for treatment for patients with a life expectancy of more than five years.

    (c) For node-positive disease in patients with life expectancy of five years or more, androgen deprivation therapy is used in combination with abiraterone and prednisone with or without RT.

    (d) In patients with distant metastasis, androgen deprivation therapy is the treatment of choice in combination with abiraterone or docetaxel.

    (e) Androgen deprivation therapy will shrink tumor volume and lower PSA levels, which could improve local control, thus decrease metastatic disease (Walsh & Worthington, 2018).

    (f) When androgen deprivation therapy is administered prior to RT, it can reduce prostate volume. This will decrease the amount of bladder tissue that is irradiated, which has been shown to reduce the severity of urinary toxicities (Washino et al., 2018).

    (g) Androgen deprivation therapy has some harsh side effects, including loss of sexual desire and function, fatigue, hot flashes, loss of strength, weight gain, depression, and gynecomastia (Walsh & Worthington, 2018).

    (h) According to Michalski et al. (2016), EBRT is the preferred primary treatment modality for locally advanced prostate cancer, and it is often combined with androgen deprivation therapy.

       i. Neoadjuvant androgen deprivation therapy with EBRT improves outcomes, such as local tumor control and progression-free survival rates.

       ii. Adjuvant androgen deprivation therapy with EBRT also diminishes the risk for local tumor recurrence, as well as metastatic disease relapse.

       iii. Adjuvant androgen deprivation therapy may improve survival duration, particularly for patients with high-grade tumors.

    (8) Abiraterone and prednisone

    (9) Docetaxel

b) Refer to NCCN (2020b) guidelines for the accepted standard treatments that are recommended for each risk category.

c) Treatment selection depends on risk group and life expectancy.

(1) Patient choice must be taken into consideration because prostate cancer treatments have distinct effects on quality of life (e.g., bowel effects, urinary effects, sexual dysfunction).

(2) It is critical that patients are provided with pretreatment counseling about the adverse effects of treatment in order to make informed treatment decisions (O'Callaghan et al., 2017).

d) In a systematic review by Showalter, Mishra, and Bridges (2015), the most commonly presented treatment options to patients with localized prostate cancer were active surveillance, radical prostatectomy, EBRT, and brachytherapy.

(1) The best available evidence reports that no one of these treatments has better cure rates or better preserves quality of life than another option for localized prostate cancer.

(2) Having multiple comparable treatment options stresses the importance of patients taking an active role in this decision-making that is considered preference sensitive.

e) Radical prostatectomy and RT are the two primary active treatments for localized prostate cancer (Michalski et al., 2016).

(1) The choice between radical prostatectomy and RT is based on tumor characteristics, overall patient health, life expectancy, and patient choice relating to potential adverse effects to urinary, bowel, and sexual function, as well as access to therapy.

(2) Patients with preexisting comorbidities may not be selected to be treated with radical prostatectomy because of the risks involved from anesthesia and surgery.

f) Palliative RT is an option for more advanced and metastatic prostate cancer.

(1) RTOG trial 97-14 showed that 8 Gy in a single fraction is recommended most often for painful bone metastasis. It was as effective as higher doses given in multiple fractions (Howell et al., 2013).

(2) Another option for palliative RT for bone metastasis is IV radioisotopes (samarium-153 and radium-223), which can be combined with focal EBRT for improved outcome (Achary & Miyamoto, 2016).

g) Several methods of standard RT are available.

(1) Overview

(a) For almost a century, RT has been used as curative therapy for prostate cancer.

(b) The goal of RT to the prostate is to destroy malignant cells in the treated volume of tissue while minimizing damage to healthy tissues (e.g., bladder, rectum).

(c) Currently, radiation oncologists have several RT options for the management of prostate cancer.

(d) EBRT is a standard treatment modality used in patients with prostate cancer. Recent advances in EBRT include 3DCRT, IMRT, volumetric modulated arc therapy (VMAT), IGRT, SBRT, and proton beam therapy.

(e) Brachytherapy methods have also improved with advances in imaging, treatment planning software, and delivery methods.

(f) All of these techniques have helped to improve outcomes in men with prostate cancer (Michalski et al., 2016).

(g) In recent years, improvements to RT planning and real-time tracking of the target during radiation delivery have also improved outcomes by reducing acute and late urinary and bowel toxicities (Liberman, Mehus, & Elliott, 2014).

(2) EBRT (see also VIII.A. External beam radiation therapy)

(a) RT dose prescription is established by considering the relationship between the radiation dose and tumor response. The optimal dose should balance cancer control with adverse effects of radiation and effects on quality of life (Pisansky et al., 2016).

(b) NCCN (2020b) guidelines list the options for standard doses of various RT techniques (3DCRT, IMRT, image-guided IMRT, and VMAT).

(c) Regarding hypofractionation, Beckelman and Lee (2017) suggested that given conventional fractionation and hypofractionation (fewer treatments at a higher dose), which are similar in effectiveness and toxicity, the more patient-centric treatment should be chosen (see also II. Practice of Radiation Oncology).

(d) Moderate hypofractionation offers patients less-expensive medical treatment and, therefore, less out-of-pocket expenses and time away from work, as well as the convenience of a shorter treatment period that saves time and reduces travel-related costs.

(3) SBRT (see also VIII.C. Stereotactic radiosurgery)

(4) Proton beam therapy: A systematic review and meta-analysis by Di Franco et al. (2017) stated

that proton beam therapy has not been shown to be superior in prostate cancer control or toxicity profile compared to EBRT (see also VIII.G. Proton beam therapy).

(5) Brachytherapy

    (a) Overview

        i. Brachytherapy involves radioactive sources being placed directly into the prostate tissue. The radioactive sources may be left in the body permanently or temporarily.

        ii. According to NCCN (2020b), LDR or HDR brachytherapy implants are a standard option for initial treatment of prostate cancer, either used as a monotherapy for very low, low, and favorable intermediate risk groups or in combination with EBRT and androgen deprivation therapy for unfavorable intermediate, high, and very high risk groups.

        iii. Brachytherapy is not recommended for regionally advanced or metastatic disease.

        iv. There is no evidence that HDR or LDR brachytherapy is superior to the other (Walsh & Worthington, 2018).

    (b) LDR brachytherapy

        i. Before LDR brachytherapy can be administered, patients must have a prostate volume study. A prostate greater than 60 cm³ can be reduced using androgen deprivation therapy.

        ii. A follow-up volume study will determine whether the prostate is small enough to undergo LDR brachytherapy.

        iii. Transrectal ultrasound-guided LDR brachytherapy is an outpatient procedure. Patients generally recover rapidly and return to normal activity (Davis et al., 2012).

        iv. Iodine-125, palladium-103, and cesium-131 are the standard isotopes used for LDR implants.

        v. The number of seeds used depends on the size of the prostate gland—typically 70–100.

        vi. Absolute contraindications to transrectal ultrasound-guided LDR brachytherapy include the following (Davis et al., 2012).

          • Limited life expectancy
          • Unacceptable operative risk
          • Distant metastases
          • Absence of rectum

          • Large transurethral radical prostatectomy defects that preclude seed placement and acceptable radiation dosimetry
          • Ataxia telangiectasia

        vii. Relative contraindications include the following (Davis et al., 2012).

          • High International Prostate Symptom Score (typically defined as greater than 20)
          • Prior pelvic RT
          • Transurethral radical prostatectomy defects
          • Large median lobes
          • Gland size greater than 60 cm³ at time of implantation

    (c) HDR brachytherapy

        i. HDR brachytherapy can be given as a single implant or twice daily implants, both of which can be repeated if prescribed, according to NCCN (2020b) guidelines.

        ii. A single HDR implant is an outpatient procedure. While the patient is under anesthesia, the implant is placed, treatment planning occurs, and treatment is given.

        iii. HDR brachytherapy given as a twice-daily treatment is an inpatient procedure. The patient will have one implant, which will remain in place between fractions that are at least six hours apart. The patient must remain on their backs with legs lowered and very still to minimize movement of the implant. After the second fraction is delivered, the implant is removed.

        iv. HDR brachytherapy requires meticulous treatment planning and carefully executed implanting to ensure accurate delivery of radiation while avoiding excessive dose to the rectum, bladder, and urethra (Yamada et al., 2012).

        v. Iridium-192 is the most commonly used isotope for HDR brachytherapy (Yamada et al., 2012).

        vi. Absolute contraindications include preexisting rectal fistula, unacceptable operative risk, and no proof of malignancy.

        vii. Special consideration must be given to the following issues when considering HDR brachytherapy and weighed with other treatment options (Yamada et al., 2012).

- Prior rectal surgery
- Prior pelvic or prostate RT
- Inflammatory bowel disease
- Prior surgical urethral manipulation
- Large prostate volume
- Significant urinary symptoms
- High-risk prostate cancer

    viii. It should be noted that a single HDR implant takes approximately three times as long and uses more staff resources than an LDR brachytherapy procedure.

  (d) Patient, caregiver, and family education

    i. After LDR brachytherapy, patients, caregivers, and family should be educated on radiation precautions, as indicated by institutional policy.

    ii. Body wastes are not radioactive.

    iii. Sexual intercourse may be resumed with a condom two weeks after treatment. Ejaculation of a seed is uncommon.

    iv. Ejaculation may be uncomfortable at first, and the volume of ejaculate is usually reduced in the months after LDR brachytherapy (Davis et al., 2012).

    v. The ejaculate may be discolored (dark brown to black) from blood.

    vi. If a displaced seed is found, a long-handled instrument should be used to place it in a container with water. Patients should contact the RSO and oncology department as soon as possible.

    vii. After HDR brachytherapy, no radiation precautions are necessary.

h) Cryotherapy and high-intensity focused ultrasound are two nonstandard treatments.

i) Detection and treatment of cancer recurrence can involve the following (Pisansky et al., 2016; Walsh & Worthington, 2018).

  (1) Elevated PSA level is the most sensitive and earliest indicator of prostate cancer recurrence after primary treatment of prostatectomy or RT.

  (2) Elevated and rising PSA (greater than 0.2 ng/ml) after radical prostatectomy is known as *biochemical failure* or *biochemical recurrence.*

  (3) RT given after biochemical recurrence is termed *salvage RT.* When a salvage radiation dose of 66 Gy or more was used, a reduced cumulative incidence of biochemical failure was observed but not of distant metastasis.

3. Quality of life and patient-reported outcomes

  a) Ample evidence shows that a patient's choice of primary treatment for localized prostate cancer dis-tinctly affects qualify of life. Knowledge of the adverse events of different treatment options is critical for making informed treatment decisions, and it is imperative that side effects of treatment be discussed in detail with patients during pretreatment counseling (Lardas et al., 2017).

  b) Specific questionnaires or patient-reported outcome measures have been developed to evaluate adverse effects of primary prostate cancer treatments.

    (1) Available questionnaires include the Expanded Prostate Cancer Index Composite, American Urological Association Symptom Score, and International Index of Erectile Function (Lardas et al., 2017).

    (2) Patient-reported outcome measure scores are an effective way to determine improvement or worsening of adverse treatment effects.

  c) The systematic review by Lardas et al. (2017) compared the effects on quality of life for up to six years after treatment for patients with localized prostate cancer treated with radical prostatectomy, EBRT, and active surveillance.

    (1) Results showed that patient-reported quality-of-life scores after active surveillance indicated high levels, compared to radical prostatectomy and EBRT.

    (2) Patient scores indicated that radical prostatectomy has a greater negative impact on sexual and urinary function, compared to EBRT and active surveillance.

    (3) Patient scores indicated that EBRT has a greater negative impact on bowel function.

  d) A systematic review by Ávila et al. (2018) revealed the patient-reported outcomes for standard curative treatments (radical prostatectomy, EBRT, and brachytherapy) for localized prostate cancer.

    (1) EBRT techniques cause moderate sexual dysfunction, mild incontinence, and bowel dysfunction and bother.

    (2) Overall, this systematic review suggested no major patient-reported outcome differences between the standard curative therapies.

4. Treatment side effects

  a) Genitourinary side effects

    (1) Overview

      (a) Acute genitourinary side effects include frequency, urgency, nocturia, intermittency (stopping and starting of flow), hesitancy (difficulty initiating stream), dysuria, weak stream, incomplete emptying, hematuria, and retention.

      (b) Late genitourinary side effects could also include incontinence, severe frequency or dysuria, frequent (micro- or macroscopic) hematuria, reduction in bladder capacity, hemorrhagic cystitis, and necrosis.

(c) Late urinary side effects can begin long after RT is complete (Liberman et al., 2014).

(2) Pathophysiology

(a) Ionizing radiation causes irritation of the bladder detrusor or urothelial inflammation, and edema can reduce the size of the bladder, resulting in urinary symptoms of frequency, urgency, nocturia, dysuria, and cystitis (Michalski et al., 2016).

(b) Prior transurethral radical prostatectomy, larger prostate size, and more pronounced pretreatment urinary dysfunction are associated with higher rates of urinary toxicity (Liberman et al., 2014).

(c) Comparing urinary adverse effects after different types of RT for prostate cancer is difficult, but several patient factors have been shown to increase adverse urinary effects after RT (Liberman et al., 2014).

   i. More pronounced pretreatment urinary symptoms

   ii. Larger prostate volume

   iii. Prior transurethral radical prostatectomy

   iv. Worse comorbidities

(3) Incidence

(a) Incidence rates of genitourinary toxicity are dependent on specific treatment planning and modality. IMRT and 3DCRT direct radiation beams conform to targeted tissue and minimize radiation exposure to nontargeted tissue, such as the rectum and bladder (Michalski et al., 2016).

(b) A review of literature by Liberman et al. (2014) found that after EBRT, RTOG grades for adverse effects for prostate cancer are found to be 20%–43% for grade 1 and 7%–19% for grade 2, with follow-up of 10 years.

   i. Within 42 months after EBRT, mild symptoms resolve spontaneously or with treatment.

   ii. Patients had a 28%–30% three-year cumulative risk for grade 2 or greater genitourinary side effects.

   iii. Grade 3 genitourinary side effects occurred at a rate of 5%–13%. The most common grade 3 side effect seen after EBRT was radiation cystitis with gross macroscopic hematuria.

(c) Urethral strictures occur after EBRT in an estimated 1.7% of patients (Salami & Kavoussi, 2016).

(d) Patients treated with brachytherapy have a greater risk of irritating voiding symptoms, which are exacerbated in patients with a larger prostate volume and those treated with androgen deprivation therapy after brachytherapy.

   i. After brachytherapy, 4%–6% of patients have urinary incontinence one to two years after treatment, and 18% of patients have moderate or severe distress levels from overall urinary side effects (Liberman et al., 2014).

   ii. Urinary function may eventually return to baseline or close to baseline (Salami & Kavoussi, 2016).

(e) After brachytherapy for prostate cancer, incidence of genitourinary adverse effects based on RTOG grade are as follows (Liberman et al., 2014).

   i. Grade 1: 36%

   ii. Grade 2: 24%

   iii. Grade 3: 6.2%

   iv. Grade 4: 0.1%

(f) Genitourinary side effects are some of the most reported adverse effects after brachytherapy for localized prostate cancer and can range from acute edema to radiation urethritis to late chronic stricture. Acute effects improve in most patients once edema subsides (Liberman et al., 2014).

   i. Irritative genitourinary side effects were seen in approximately 50% of patients, and early (within 12 months) urinary retention was seen in 7%–25%.

   ii. Incidence of late urinary retention (after 12 months) was approximately 1%. Peak International Prostate Symptom Scores of 7–12 points greater than baseline scores were seen at 2–10 weeks after implantation.

   iii. Side effects resolved in more than 75% of patients within one year after treatment.

(4) Assessment

(a) Assessment for acute radiation-induced genitourinary side effects should note frequency, urgency, nocturia, intermittency, hesitancy, dysuria, weakened urinary stream, incomplete emptying, urge or stress incontinence, hematuria, and retention.

(b) Assessment for late radiation-induced genitourinary side effects should note incontinence, chronic severe frequency or dysuria, frequent (micro- or macroscopic) hematuria, reduction in bladder capacity, and hemorrhagic cystitis.

(c) Standard patient questionnaires are available to assess bladder function. These questionnaires are completed by patients periodically and scored to quantify bladder function and bother over time after prostate cancer treatment.

    i. American Urological Association Symptom Score and Quality of Life (also known as the International Prostate Symptom Score)

    ii. Expanded Prostate Cancer Index Composite–Bladder Domain (Michigan Medicine Department of Urology, n.d.)

(5) Documentation

(a) CTCAE should be used for documenting levels of urinary frequency, urinary incontinence, urinary retention, dysuria, and urinary urgency (NCI CTEP, 2017).

(b) Late urinary adverse effects are usually graded using the RTOG grading system.

(6) Collaborative management

(a) Patients should maintain hydration throughout daytime while decreasing fluid intake in the evening to reduce the incidence of nocturia.

(b) Patients should avoid caffeinated products.

(c) Ibuprofen can be prescribed at 400–800 mg three to four times daily orally. Ibuprofen relieves pain by inhibiting prostaglandin synthesis. It may be contraindicated if hematuria is present (IBM, n.d.).

(d) Oxybutynin chloride can be prescribed at 5 mg orally, two to three times daily (not to exceed 20 mg daily) (IBM, n.d.).

    i. Oxybutynin chloride helps overactive and neurogenic bladder and causes relaxation of the bladder smooth muscle by reducing the muscarinic effect of acetylcholine on smooth muscle.

    ii. In patients with involuntary bladder contractions, oxybutynin chloride increases bladder capacity, reduces the frequency of uninhibited contractions of the detrusor muscle, and slows the initial desire to void, leading to a decrease in urgency and frequency of incontinent episodes and voluntary urination.

(e) Phenazopyridine can be prescribed at 200 mg orally up to three times daily after meals (IBM, n.d.).

    i. Phenazopyridine hydrochloride helps with dysuria and is a urinary tract analgesic.

    ii. The precise mode of action is unknown, but when excreted in the urine, it promotes topical analgesia on the mucosa of the urinary tract, thus relieving pain, burning, urgency, and frequency.

    iii. Urine will turn a reddish-orange color.

(f) Tamsulosin hydrochloride can be prescribed at 0.4 mg once daily orally (taken 30 minutes after a meal); it can be increased to 0.8 mg daily if ineffective (IBM, n.d.).

    i. Tamsulosin hydrochloride is an alpha-1A adrenoceptor antagonist. It selectively blocks sympathetic nervous stimulation of the receptor, resulting in relaxation of the smooth muscles of the prostate, prostatic urethra, and bladder neck for improvement in urine flow rate and a reduction in symptoms of benign prostatic hyperplasia.

    ii. This medication may cause dizziness.

(g) Terazosin hydrochloride can be prescribed at 1 mg orally at bedtime; it may be increased incrementally to 2 mg, 5 mg, and then 10 mg until the desired flow rate and symptom improvement (IBM, n.d.).

    i. Terazosin hydrochloride is an alpha-1 selective adrenoceptor blocker that produces relaxation of smooth muscles in the neck of the bladder and prostate gland.

    ii. There are few alpha-1 adrenoceptors in the bladder body, which allows for lowering of bladder outlet obstruction without affecting the contractility of the organ. It also causes vasodilation, resulting in orthostatic hypotension.

(h) Doxazosin mesylate can be prescribed at 1 mg orally once daily; it can be titrated at one- or two-week intervals to a maximum dose of 8 mg (IBM, n.d.).

    i. Doxazosin mesylate, a quinazoline compound, selectively inhibits the alpha-1 adrenoceptor.

    ii. Alpha-1 receptor blockade decreases urethral resistance and may relieve symptoms of benign prostatic hyperplasia and increase urine flow.

(i) Tolterodine tartrate can be prescribed at 2 mg orally twice daily; a dose of 1 mg twice daily may be prescribed depending on tolerability and response (IBM, n.d.).

i. Tolterodine tartrate treats overactive bladder muscle with urinary frequency, urgency, or urge incontinence.

ii. Tolterodine tartrate is a competitive muscarinic receptor antagonist and increases the residual urine and decreases pressure in the detrusor muscle.

(j) Temporary suspension of RT can be considered.

(k) Patients should be referred to a urologist for evaluation and possible cystoscopy if symptoms persist.

(l) After LDR brachytherapy, an indwelling catheter may be required until acute postoperative swelling of smooth muscle decreases and urinary obstructive symptoms subside.

(7) Patient, caregiver, and family education

(a) Education includes information about the side effects of medications prescribed to alleviate urinary symptoms.

(b) For EBRT, SBRT, and brachytherapy, patients, caregivers, and family should understand acute and late urinary side effects of RT to the prostate, such as signs and symptoms of urinary tract infections and radiation-induced cystitis.

(c) Clinicians must promote adequate hydration.

(d) Clinicians should reassure patients regarding the availability of medications if symptoms become problematic.

(e) Thoroughly review side effect profiles and possible drug interactions with the patient as appropriate.

b) Gastrointestinal side effects (see also V.E. Gastrointestinal tract and abdomen)

(1) Overview

(a) The occurrence and severity of radiation-induced gastrointestinal toxicity are dependent on radiation dose and fractioning, concurrent chemotherapy, and patient-related factors, such as body mass index, smoking, history of abdominal surgery, and comorbidities (e.g., diabetes, inflammatory bowel disease, collagen vascular disease) (Frazzoni et al., 2015).

(b) Acute toxicities occur during RT or within three months. Chronic toxicities extend past three months or develop after a longer period of time.

(c) Among the most frequently reported symptoms are diarrhea, rectal urgency, rectal bleeding, and fecal incontinence (Frazzoni et al., 2015).

(d) Other acute gastrointestinal side effects include increased gas and bloating, increased stool frequency in the daytime or nighttime, softer stool or diarrhea, feeling of incomplete bowel evacuation, irritation and inflammation of existing hemorrhoids, painful defecation, cramps, tenesmus, rectal irritation and ulceration, rectal discharge, and skin ulceration in the gluteal folds.

(e) Late gastrointestinal side effects include proctitis, rectal bleeding, narrowing of the rectum, chronic diarrhea, or development of an ulcer in the rectum.

(2) Pathophysiology (Frazzoni et al., 2015)

(a) The pathogenesis of acute and chronic gastrointestinal toxicities is different.

(b) Although acute pelvic radiation-induced disease is caused by an acute inflammatory response, late-onset chronic disease is mainly caused by vascular sclerosis and fibrosis. These causes are not independent of each other.

(c) When severe acute toxicity is present, late-onset chronic toxicity is more likely to develop.

(3) Incidence

(a) Incidence rates of gastrointestinal toxicity are dependent on specific treatment planning and modality.

(b) EBRT, SBRT, and brachytherapy can cause worsened and bothersome bowel function after treatment, with eventual return to baseline function. Use of image-guided IMRT delivers a lower radiation dose to the rectum, but bowel side effects still appear in up to 11% of patients and can persist for two years after treatment (Salami & Kavoussi, 2016).

(c) Rectal morbidity, such as proctitis and ulceration, is less likely when less than 25% of the rectum receives doses less than 70 Gy (Di Franco et al., 2017).

(d) Radiation-induced diarrhea is seen most often with radiation to abdominal and pelvic areas (Thorpe et al., 2017).

(e) Acute radiation-induced enteritis can be seen in up to 70% of patients, depending on treatment and patient predisposing factors.

(4) Assessment: The Expanded Prostate Cancer Index Composite–Bowel Domain is a standard patient questionnaire to assess bowel function in patients with prostate cancer (Michigan Medicine Department of Urology, n.d.).

(5) Documentation: Documentation should adhere to CTCAE for diarrhea and proctitis (NCI CTEP, 2017).

(6) Collaborative management
    (a) Radiation-induced diarrhea
        i. Taking probiotics, such as lactobacilli and bifidobacteria strains, can help to maintain or restore the gut microflora during and after RT, lessening the chance of radiation-induced diarrhea (Frazzoni et al., 2015).
        ii. Diphenoxylate is an opioid agonist used in the treatment of radiation-induced diarrhea and prolongs transit time by slowing intestinal contractions and peristalsis. It allows the intestines to draw moisture from stool to prevent loose or liquid stools (IBM, n.d.).
        iii. Loperamide prolongs the transit time of the intestinal contents (IBM, n.d.).
        iv. Psyllium is a form of soluble fiber and has been used to treat diarrhea because of its ability to absorb fluid and increase the bulk of stools (Thorpe et al., 2017).
        v. Hydrocortisone acetate suppositories have an anti-inflammatory effect to relieve radiation proctitis and painful bowel movements (IBM, n.d.).
        vi. Clinicians should consult an RDN or RD at the onset of diarrhea or at start of treatment for diarrhea interventions.
        vii. The goal of fluid and nutrient balance is adequate intake to prevent dehydration, electrolyte imbalance, and weight loss. Refer to NCCN (2020a) guidelines for palliative care.
        viii. Clinicians should consult a proctologist or gastroenterologist if severe diarrhea is unresolved by pharmacologic interventions.
        ix. Treatment breaks may be considered during RT.
    (b) Skin alteration from diarrhea (see also IV.B. Skin reactions)
        i. If appropriate, clinicians can suggest the use of sanitary pads or adult incontinence briefs for rectal discharge or stool incontinence.
        ii. Patients should maintain good anal and personal hygiene using mild soap and tepid water to gently wash skin.
        iii. Patients can use plain, unscented, lanolin-free hydrophilic cream if skin is intact.
        iv. Patients can use over-the-counter medications (e.g., Preparation H®) as instructed by a healthcare provider.

    (c) Rectal bleeding
        i. Patients with clinically significant rectal bleeding (i.e., causing chronic anemia) should first be considered for medical management. Evidence supports the following treatments (Frazzoni et al., 2015).
            • Sucralfate twice-daily enema (two 1 g sucralfate tablets mixed with 4.5 ml of water)
            • Metronidazole 400 mg three times daily for up to 12 weeks
            • Hyperbaric oxygen of at least 30 sessions (up to 100) for chronic rectal bleeding not responding to pharmacologic treatment
        ii. Clinicians should consult a proctologist or gastroenterologist if rectal bleeding is unresolved by pharmacologic interventions.
        iii. If medical management has failed or a patient is having acute rectal bleeding that requires transfusion, then argon plasma coagulation or formalin should be used (Frazzoni et al., 2015).
        iv. Argon plasma coagulation is the treatment of choice when a patient has clinically significant rectal bleeding.
        v. Formalin is an alternative and has been proposed as a treatment for refractory severe rectal bleeding. When applied to radiation-damaged tissues, it effectively cauterizes the fragile vessels.
        vi. Treatment breaks may be considered during RT.
(7) Patient, caregiver, and family education
    (a) Patients should be informed that diarrhea and rectal bleeding are possible side effects of RT to the pelvic area.
    (b) Nurses should instruct on dietary modifications and refer patients to an RDN or RD as needed.
    (c) Instruction should include information on comfort measures (e.g., sitz baths, tepid water, cotton cloth soaks).
    (d) Nurses should explain protocols for perianal hygiene (mild soap, pat dry).
    (e) Nurses should instruct patients, caregivers, and family regarding signs and symptoms of dehydration.
    (f) Patients should record the number and consistency of bowel movements per day.
    (g) Clinicians should inform patients, caregivers, and family of medications avail-

able to alleviate treatment-related side effects.

(h) For late effects, nurses should instruct on reporting symptoms (e.g., changes in stools, rectal bleeding, pain) and when to notify a physician.

c) Sexual side effects (see IV.E. Sexual function and dysfunction)

(1) Overview

(a) Erectile dysfunction is the most commonly reported sexual dysfunction after prostate cancer treatments.

(b) Other sexual dysfunctions include absence of ejaculation, changes in orgasm, decreased libido, sexual incontinence, and loss of penile length (Jenkins & Mulhall, 2016).

(c) A literature review by Showalter et al. (2015) evaluated long-term impact of prostate cancer treatments and reported a significant negative effect on sexual relationships, which worsened during the first year after cancer treatment.

(d) Post-treatment quality of life significantly affects patients as well as sexual partners (Salami & Kavoussi, 2016).

(2) Pathophysiology

(a) Damage to blood vessels and nerves after RT can result in decreased erectile function over time (Jenkins & Mulhall, 2016).

i. Post-RT erectile dysfunction is not completely understood, but it is most likely the result of multiple factors including dose-dependent damage to neurovascular bundles, the crura, and penile bulb.

ii. The cause of impotence can be arteriogenic because of cavernosal veno-occlusive dysfunction, neurogenic dysfunction, or a combination of these.

iii. Endothelial cells that line the penile arteries and sinusoids of the corpora cavernosa are damaged in a time- and dose-dependent manner.

iv. Capillaries and sinusoids are especially sensitive, and damage to epithelial cells leads to luminal stenosis and arterial insufficiency, having a gradual progression over time.

v. The net effect of this endothelial damage is ischemia.

(b) The late progression of erectile dysfunction after RT is related to radiation damage to arteries that provide blood to the penis (Walsh & Worthington, 2018).

i. Some recent evidence points to damage to the neurovascular bundles as well, especially after brachytherapy.

ii. Radiation may also cause venous leakage.

(c) Acute changes in sexual function following LDR brachytherapy include pain with ejaculation and hematospermia (Michalski et al., 2016).

i. These symptoms generally dissipate over time and correlate with the acute prostatitis that the patient experiences.

ii. Erectile dysfunction following brachytherapy may be multifactorial, as a result of changes to a patient's neurologic, vascular, or psychological makeup.

iii. Other confounding factors include comorbidities, such as diabetes, hypertension, and smoking.

(3) Incidence

(a) The exact incidence of erectile dysfunction as a treatment-related side effect is difficult to determine because a uniform definition is not established and because older men may experience erectile dysfunction as a result of medical conditions or medications (Jenkins & Mulhall, 2016).

(b) RT has a more gradual effect on erectile function than the immediate effect of surgery (Walsh & Worthington, 2018).

i. Although sexual function may be normal shortly after completion of RT, erectile dysfunction could develop one to two years later.

ii. Radiation-induced erectile dysfunction affects 10%–70% of patients. This range is large because dysfunction depends on many factors, including the definition of erectile function, the presence of comorbidities, type of RT, and whether hormone therapy was used.

(c) The prevalence of erectile dysfunction after RT has been reported as 36%–59% after EBRT and 24%–50% after brachytherapy (Jenkins & Mulhall, 2016).

(d) When androgen deprivation therapy is combined with RT, erectile dysfunction rates are much higher. Erectile dysfunction rates do not appear to be affected in the long term by short-term (4–6 months) hormone therapy; however, long-term (18–36 months) hormone therapy does negatively affect long-term rates of erectile dysfunction.

    (e) Decreased sexual function after brachytherapy may not return to baseline function. Recovery of sexual function is worse for patients receiving androgen deprivation therapy and RT, as opposed to radiation alone (Salami & Kavoussi, 2016).

    (f) LDR brachytherapy had fewer detriments in the sexual domain than EBRT and radical prostatectomy (Michalski et al., 2016).

(4) Assessment

    (a) Assessment of sexual function after EBRT is complex and may be fraught with difficulty.

        i. Potency typically begins to diminish one to two years after RT and appears similar to the natural aging process.

        ii. Some patients have compromised potency as a result of concurrent illnesses, such as diabetes or arteriosclerosis, or as a result of medications taken for comorbid conditions.

        iii. According to single-institution reports and a meta-analysis, it appears that 50%–60% of patients remain potent after EBRT (Michalski et al., 2016).

    (b) Assessment should evaluate the following.

        i. Baseline dysfunction prior to initiation of treatment

        ii. Baseline sexual activity level

        iii. Baseline satisfaction and dissatisfaction with intercourse

        iv. Medications and comorbid conditions (e.g., hypertension, diabetes, peripheral vascular disease, neuropathy)

        v. Decreased ability to achieve erection

        vi. Decreased sensation during intercourse

        vii. Decreased ability to achieve orgasm

        viii. Therapies or medications being used to improve erections

    (c) Patient-reported outcome measures can be used.

        i. International Index of Erectile Function

        ii. Expanded Prostate Cancer Index Composite–Sexual Domain (Michigan Medicine Department of Urology, n.d.)

(5) Documentation: CTCAE should be used for documenting levels of erectile dysfunction and ejaculation disorder (NCI CTEP, 2017).

(6) Collaborative management

    (a) Factors such as stress and impaired coping may contribute to acute onset of impotence and may be helped by professional counseling.

    (b) Patients and spouses may need to be referred for professional counseling regarding the physical and psychological effects of sexual dysfunction.

    (c) Refer patient to urologist to discuss therapies described below for sexual dysfunction.

    (d) PDE5 inhibitors (e.g., sildenafil citrate, tadalafil, vardenafil, avanafil) are the first-line therapy for erectile dysfunction.

        i. These medications enable relaxation and vasodilation of vascular smooth muscle in the corpus cavernosum, allowing the inflowing of blood and resulting in erection.

        ii. Because sexual stimulation is required to initiate this chemical process, PED5 inhibitors have no effect in the absence of sexual stimulation.

        iii. Patients should seek medical help if an erection persists longer than four hours (IBM, n.d.).

        iv. Patients with a history of heart attack or irregular heartbeat in the previous six months, low or high blood pressure, congestive heart failure, chest pain, or retinitis pigmentosa, as well as those taking any nitrates (e.g., nitroglycerin), should not take PDE5 inhibitors (Walsh & Worthington, 2018).

    (e) If PDE5 inhibitors are ineffective, other nonsurgical therapies are available.

        i. Intracavernosal injection

        ii. Vacuum erection device

        iii. Intraurethral suppository

    (f) Surgical intervention, such as penile prosthesis, is also an option if other therapies fail.

(7) Patient, caregiver, and family education

    (a) The patient should verbalize understanding of importance of communication between both partners regarding concerns or issues of sexual dysfunction.

    (b) The patient should verbalize understanding of side effects of RT, radical prostatectomy, and androgen deprivation therapy as it relates to sexual dysfunction.

    (c) Clinicians should inform patients and partners about alternative medical and surgical interventions that may be available to them.

(d) Clinicians should inform patients of medications to treat some forms of sexual dysfunction. Side effect profiles and drug interactions of prescribed medications should be reviewed thoroughly.

(e) Patients and partners should be informed about resuming intercourse and sexual activity after therapy.

(f) Patients and partners should inform a nurse or physician of continued sexual dysfunction.

(g) Clinicians can use teaching tools to enhance understanding.

d) Fatigue
   (1) Fatigue is a common side effect of cancer therapies.
   (2) See IV.A Fatigue for more information.

References

Achary, M.P., & Miyamoto, C.T. (2016). Fundamentals of radiation treatment for prostate carcinoma—Techniques, radiation biology, and evidence base. In J.H. Mydlo & C.J. Godec (Eds.), *Prostate cancer: Science and clinical practice* (2nd ed., pp. 377–386). Elsevier.

Ávila, M., Patel, L., López, S., Cortés-Sanabria, L., Garin, O., Pont, A., ... Ferrer, M. (2018). Patient-reported outcomes after treatment for clinically localized prostate cancer: A systematic review and meta-analysis. *Cancer Treatment Reviews, 66*, 23–44. https://doi.org/10.1016/j.ctrv.2018.03.005

Beckelman, J.E., & Lee, W.R. (2017). Six questions to ask before we shorten radiation treatments for intact prostate cancer. *International Journal of Radiation Oncology, Biology, Physics, 97*, 718–721. https://doi.org/10.1016/j.ijrobp.2016.11.038

Davis, B.J., Horwitz, E.M., Lee, W.R., Crook, J.M., Stock, R.G., Merrick, G.S., ... Zelefsky, M.J. (2012). American Brachytherapy Society consensus guidelines for transrectal ultrasound-guided permanent prostate brachytherapy. *Brachytherapy, 11*, 6–19. https://doi.org/10.1016/j.brachy.2011.07.005

Di Franco, R., Borzillo, V., Ravo, V., Ametrano, G., Falivene, S., Cammarota, F., ... Facchini, G. (2017). Rectal/urinary toxicity after hypofractionated vs conventional radiotherapy in low/intermediate risk localized prostate cancer: Systematic review and meta analysis. *Oncotarget, 8*, 17383–17395. https://doi.org/10.18632/oncotarget.14798

Frazzoni, L., La Marca, M., Guido, A., Morganti, A.G., Bazzoli, F., & Fuccio, L. (2015). Pelvic radiation disease: Updates on treatment options. *World Journal of Clinical Oncology, 6*, 272–280. https://doi.org/10.5306/wjco.v6.i6.272

Howell, D.D., James, J.L., Hartsell, W.F., Suntharalingam, M., Machtay, M., Suh, J.H., ... Berk, L.B. (2013). Single-fraction radiotherapy versus multifraction radiotherapy for palliation of painful vertebral bone metastases—Equivalent efficacy, less toxicity, more convenient: A subset analysis of Radiation Therapy Oncology Group trial 97-14. *Cancer, 119*, 888–896. https://doi.org/10.1002/cncr.27616

Hussein, A.A., & Cooperberg, M.R. (2016). Is surgery still necessary for prostate cancer? In J.H. Mydlo & C.J. Godec (Eds.), *Prostate cancer: Science and clinical practice* (2nd ed., pp. 235–243). Elsevier

IBM. (n.d.). IBM Micromedex® [Internet application]. https://www.micromedexsolutions.com

Jenkins, L.C., & Mulhall, J.P. (2016). Impact of prostate cancer treatments on sexual health. In J.H. Mydlo & C.J. Godec (Eds.), *Prostate cancer: Science and clinical practice* (2nd ed., pp. 585–595). Elsevier.

Lardas, M., Liew, M., van den Bergh, R.C., De Santis, M., Bellmunt, J., Van den Broeck, T., ... Bourke, L. (2017). Quality of life outcomes after primary treatment for clinically localised prostate cancer: A systematic review. *European Urology, 72*, 869–885. https://doi.org/10.1016/j.eururo.2017.06.035

Liberman, D., Mehus, B., & Elliott, S.P. (2014). Urinary adverse effects of pelvic radiotherapy. *Translational Andrology and Urology, 3*, 186–195. https://doi.org/10.3978/j.issn.2223-4683.2014.04.01

Michalski, J.M., Pisansky, T.M., Lawton, C.A.F., & Potters, L. (2016). Prostate cancer. In L.L. Gunderson & J.E. Tepper (Eds.), *Clinical radiation oncology* (4th ed., pp. 1038–1095). Elsevier.

Michigan Medicine Department of Urology. (n.d.). Expanded prostate cancer index composite. https://medicine.umich.edu/dept/urology/research/epic

National Cancer Institute Cancer Therapy Evaluation Program. (2017). *Common terminology criteria for adverse events* [v.5.0]. https://ctep.cancer.gov/protocolDevelopment/electronic_applications/docs/CTCAE_v5_Quick_Reference_5x7.pdf

National Comprehensive Cancer Network. (2020a). *NCCN Clinical Practice Guidelines in Oncology (NCCN Guidelines®): Palliative care* [v.1.2020]. https://www.nccn.org/professionals/physician_gls/pdf/palliative.pdf

National Comprehensive Cancer Network. (2020b). *NCCN Clinical Practice Guidelines in Oncology (NCCN Guidelines®): Prostate cancer* [v.2.2020]. https://www.nccn.org/professionals/physician_gls/pdf/prostate.pdf

O'Callaghan, M.E., Raymond, E., Campbell, J.M., Vincent, A.D., Beckmann, K., Roder, D., ... Moretti, K. (2017). Patient-reported outcomes after radiation therapy in men with prostate cancer: A systematic review of prognostic tool accuracy and validity. *International Journal of Radiation Oncology, Biology, Physics, 98*, 318–337. https://doi.org/10.1016/j.ijrobp.2017.02.024

Pisansky, T.M., Agrawal, S., Hamstra, D.A., Koontz, B.F., Liauw, S.L., Efstathiou, J.A., ... Tendulkar, R.D. (2016). Salvage radiation therapy dose response for biochemical failure of prostate cancer after prostatectomy—A multi-institutional observational study. *International Journal of Radiation Oncology, Biology, Physics, 96*, 1046–1053. https://doi.org/10.1016/j.ijrobp.2016.08.043

Salami, S.S., & Kavoussi, L.R. (2016). Quality of life: Impact of prostate cancer and its treatment. In J.H. Mydlo & C.J. Godec (Eds.), *Prostate cancer: Science and clinical practice* (2nd ed., pp. 579–584). Elsevier.

Showalter, T.N., Mishra, M.V., & Bridges, J.F.P. (2015). Factors that influence patient preferences for prostate cancer management options: A systematic review. *Patient Preference and Adherence, 9*, 899–911. https://doi.org/10.2147/PPA.S83333

Thorpe, D.M., Byar, K.L., Conley, S., Drapek, L., Held-Warmkessel, J., Ramsdell, M.J., ... Wolles, B. (2017). Symptom interventions: Radiation-induced diarrhea. https://www.ons.org/pep/radiation-induced-diarrhea

Walsh, P.C., & Worthington, J.F. (2018). *Dr. Patrick Walsh's guide to surviving prostate cancer* (4th ed.). Grand Central Life and Style.

Washino, S., Hirai, M., Saito, K., Kobayashi, Y., Arai, Y., & Miyagawa, T. (2018). Impact of androgen deprivation therapy on volume reduction and lower urinary tract symptoms in patients with prostate cancer. *Lower Urinary Tract Symptoms, 10*, 57–63. https://doi.org/10.1111/luts.12142

Yamada, Y., Rogers, L., Demanes, D.J., Morton, G., Prestidge, B.R., Pouliot, J., ... Hsu, I.-C. (2012). American Brachytherapy Society consensus guidelines for high-dose-rate prostate brachytherapy. *Brachytherapy, 11*, 20–32. https://doi.org/10.1016/j.brachy.2011.09.008

H. Female pelvis

1. Overview
   a) RT plays an important role in the therapeutic management of pelvic malignancies (Viswanathan et al., 2014).
   b) Most common female malignancies that originate in the pelvic area are gynecologic cancers (cervical, endometrial, ovarian, vaginal, and vulvar), colorectal cancer, and bladder cancer (Nicholas et al., 2017).

2. Indications
   a) Cervical cancer
      (1) In the United States, an estimated 13,800 women will be diagnosed in 2020, and in Canada, an estimated 1,350 women will be diagnosed in 2020 (American Cancer Society, 2020; Brenner et al., 2020).
      (2) The International Federation of Gynecology and Obstetrics staging system is widely used to determine the treatment protocols for cervical cancer.
      (3) Cervical cancer is staged I–IV, with further categories within each stage based on disease and tumor factors.
   b) Vulvar cancer (NCCN, 2020c)
      (1) In the United States, an estimated 6,120 new cases of vulvar cancer will be diagnosed in 2020 (American Cancer Society, 2020).
      (2) Vulvar cancer is staged using the International Federation of Gynecology and Obstetrics staging system and TNM system.
   c) Endometrial cancer (NCCN, 2020b)
      (1) In the United States, an estimated 65,620 women will be diagnosed in 2020, and in Canada, an estimated 7,400 women will be diagnosed in 2020 (American Cancer Society, 2020; Brenner et al., 2020).
      (2) Endometrial cancer is staged most commonly using the International Federation of Gynecology and Obstetrics staging system.
   d) Vaginal cancer (Adams & Cuello, 2018)
      (1) In the United States, an estimated 6,230 cases of vaginal cancer will be diagnosed in 2020 (American Cancer Society, 2020).
      (2) Vaginal cancer is staged most commonly using the International Federation of Gynecology and Obstetrics staging system (stage 0 and I–IV).
      (3) Primary vaginal cancer is very rare, its treatment complex and patient specific, and there are many similarities between the management of primary vaginal cancer and cervical cancer due to comparable etiology and anatomical location.
   e) Rectal cancer: In the United States, an estimated 43,340 individuals will be newly diagnosed with rectal cancer in 2020, and in Canada, an estimated 26,900 new diagnoses of rectal cancer, with approximately 12,000 of them in women, in 2020 (American Cancer Society, 2020; Brenner et al., 2020; O'Sullivan et al., 2015).
3. Treatment techniques
   a) EBRT
      (1) 3DCRT (O'Sullivan et al., 2015)
         (a) CT images are used to perform a three-dimensional assessment of the tumor location and extent of disease.
         (b) The goal of this approach is to design a treatment that conforms to the target area.
      (2) IMRT (O'Sullivan et al., 2015)
         (a) IMRT is a high-precision technique in which intensity-modulated beams from multiple directions create highly conformal dose distributions in the target volumes.
         (b) IMRT allows for higher and more targeted radiation doses to be administered. It is especially beneficial with complex-shaped target volumes.
      (3) VMAT (Knapp et al., 2019)
         (a) VMAT, similar to IMRT, involves the machine rotating around the patient in an arc shape, allowing for the treatment field to be continually reshaped and providing variance of the intensity of the radiation throughout treatment.
         (b) VMAT is considered to have higher accuracy, especially when treatment areas involve complex tumors and anatomical structures, such as in gynecologic malignancies.
   b) Brachytherapy
      (1) Radioactive sources are placed into an organ (intracavity), in close proximity to the tumor, or into the tumor (interstitial) in protective capsules or applicators.
      (2) Radiation is delivered to a local area and minimal healthy tissue is exposed to radiation (O'Sullivan et al., 2015).
      (3) Brachytherapy is an essential component in cervical, endometrial, and recurrent vaginal cancer treatments.
      (4) HDR brachytherapy utilizes a high dose of radiation delivered in a short period of time (5–10 minutes) in two to five fractions. HDR is the standard of treatment in many clinical settings, rather than pulsed dose rate and LDR brachytherapy (Reed & Sadozye, 2017).
      (5) Pulsed dose-rate brachytherapy involves a series (pulses) of radiation delivered over 24 hours (Reed & Sadozye, 2017).
      (6) LDR brachytherapy, historically, was used to deliver radiation at a very low rate for four to five days. This is no longer the standard approach in gynecologic cancer treatments (Reed & Sadozye, 2017).
      (7) Image-guided brachytherapy utilizes CT or MRI to assess applicator placement and OARs surrounding tumor so that radiation is administered to the local cancerous area, which limits exposure of healthy tissue (Reed & Sadozye, 2017).

4. Treatment options
   a) Cervical cancer (NCCN, 2020a)
      (1) NCCN guidelines detail the best treatment recommendations for each stage of disease.
      (2) Premenopausal women with early-stage disease have the option of fertility-sparing and nonfertility-sparing treatments.
      (3) For early-stage cervical cancer, primary treatment can be surgery or RT. Surgery is generally the choice for fertility preservation and small lesions.
      (4) For women who are not surgical candidates and for advanced stages (IB and higher), concurrent chemoradiation is the treatment of choice.
      (5) For patients with advanced-stage cervical cancer or those being treated with definitive RT, NCCN guidelines recommend concurrent platinum-based chemotherapy and EBRT, followed by brachytherapy.
      (6) The standard dose for EBRT is 45 Gy for 25 fractions, followed by three to four fractions of HDR brachytherapy with 75–80 Gy total dose.
   b) Vulvar cancer (NCCN, 2020c)
      (1) RT is part of the primary treatment plan for locally advanced vulvar cancer and is given as adjuvant therapy after surgery.
      (2) For recurrent and metastatic disease, RT is used in the context of secondary therapy or palliation.
      (3) IMRT is a critical component of treatment, and appropriate planning is required to account for healthy tissue tolerance of the rectum, bladder, and small bowel.
      (4) For adjuvant therapy, doses can be 45–50.4 Gy in 25–28 fractions (1.8 Gy per fraction).
      (5) For unresectable diseases, doses can be 59.4–64.8 Gy in 33–36 fractions (1.8 Gy per fraction).
   c) Endometrial cancer (NCCN, 2020b)
      (1) For stage I endometrial cancer, surgery is the primary treatment with or without adjuvant RT.
      (2) EBRT and brachytherapy are the primary treatment approaches for inoperable disease.
      (3) Brachytherapy can be given preoperatively or as definitive treatment with an intact uterus.
      (4) In the context of neoadjuvant EBRT, generally accepted total doses are 45–50 Gy.
      (5) Regimens for postoperative HDR vaginal brachytherapy may include 6 Gy per fraction for five fractions, 5.5 Gy per fraction for four fractions, or 7 Gy per fraction for three fractions.
   d) Vaginal cancer (Adams & Cuello, 2018)
      (1) Histology, size of the tumor, lesion location, and patient factors (including fertility potential) all affect treatment decisions.
      (2) Surgery is limited to stage I or very early-stage disease because of the anatomic location of the lesion and proximity to the bladder, urethra, and rectum.
      (3) With advanced disease, a combination of EBRT and brachytherapy is the primary treatment of choice. Concurrent chemotherapy (platinum-based agents or 5-fluorouracil) may be included in the treatment plan.
      (4) The recommended optimal dose is 70 Gy, as higher doses have been associated with significant side effects.
   e) Rectal cancer (O'Sullivan et al., 2015)
      (1) With local recurrent disease, RT is delivered to improve local control of disease.
      (2) With surgery, RT can be neoadjuvant or adjuvant in rectal cancer management, with evidence demonstrating better outcomes with neoadjuvant radiation.
5. Treatment side effects
   a) Acute skin reactions (see also IV.B. Skin reactions)
      (1) Pathophysiology
         (a) Radiation-induced skin reactions are some of the most common side effects of RT (Bolderston et al., 2018).
         (b) Radiation-induced skin reactions result from the disruption of the continuous renewal process of the skin. Normal cell production at the basal layer and cell death at the skin surface are interrupted, leading to skin reactions (Seité, Bensadoun, & Mazer, 2017).
         (c) With pelvic irradiation, areas such as the perineum are at higher risk, as the skin is part of the treatment area (Seité et al., 2017).
         (d) Acute skin reactions typically arise in the first two to three weeks after the start of RT (Seité et al., 2017).
         (e) Severe skin reactions may lead to treatment delays and potentially compromise disease treatment outcome (Bolderston et al., 2018).
      (2) Incidence
         (a) Incidence of radiation-induced skin reactions is 50%–90% among women treated with RT for gynecologic cancers (Nicholas et al., 2017).
         (b) With some gynecologic cancers, such as vulvar cancer, in which the intended treatment area is the skin and superficial tissues, radiation-induced skin reactions cannot be prevented (Wong et al., 2013).
      (3) Risk factors
         (a) Treatment-related and patient-related factors significantly affect the onset, duration,

and severity of skin reactions (Viswanathan et al., 2014).

(b) Treatment-related factors include RT technique (i.e., use of IMRT reduces the severity of skin reactions), radiation field size, type of energy used, and length of treatment (Azria, Betz, Bourgier, Jeanneret Sozzi, & Ozshin, 2012; Nicholas et al., 2017).

(c) Patient-related factors include the following.
   i. Anatomical site (e.g., areas where the epidermis is thin, such as the perineum)
   ii. Previous surgery or other factors that may affect integrity of skin: For gynecologic cancers, such as vulvar cancer, in which RT is delivered postoperatively, women are at much higher risk for reactions (Seité et al., 2017).
   iii. Concurrent cancer treatment (e.g., chemotherapy for locally advanced cervical cancer)
   iv. Comorbidities affecting skin healing (e.g., diabetes)
   v. Older age
   vi. Inadequate nutritional intake
   vii. Smoking

(4) Clinical manifestations: See IV.B. Skin reactions for more information.

(5) Collaborative management (Bolderston et al., 2018; McQuestion, 2011)
   (a) Preservation of skin integrity is essential.
   (b) Adequate pain management and comfort is also key.
   (c) With severe skin reactions, the treatment goals may include management of wound odor and exudate, with promotion of wound healing.
   (d) Maintaining normal hygienic routine, especially in the perineal area, is recommend for physical and psychological well-being.
      i. Cleansing with mild soap and lukewarm water is recommended routine care.
      ii. Evidence shows that regular hygiene supports significant reduction in itching, erythema, and desquamation (Wong et al., 2013).
   (e) Sitz baths are recommended as a comfort measure for many women after RT for gynecologic cancers (Viswanathan et al., 2014).
   (f) Severe skin reactions (grade 3 or greater) should be evaluated, and a treatment break may be warranted (Nicholas et al., 2017).

(g) For dry desquamation, unscented water-based moisturizing cream is recommended. Saline soaks are recommended for soothing and cooling effect (Bolderston et al., 2018; McQuestion, 2011).

(h) Moist desquamation management involves the following (Bolderston et al., 2018; McQuestion, 2011; Niazi et al., 2012).
   i. Dressings promote a moist wound healing environment.
   ii. Some evidence supports the use of antibacterial dressings with patients receiving RT for anal canal or gynecologic cancers (Niazi et al., 2012).

(i) IMRT and VMAT, which allow for greater precision of target area, have significantly improved the incidence and severity of radiation-induced skin reactions (Viswanathan et al., 2014).

(6) Patient, caregiver, and family education: See IV.B. Skin reactions.

b) Acute gastrointestinal side effects
(1) Pathophysiology
   (a) RT to the pelvic region can cause injury to the healthy tissues of the gastrointestinal tract that are in close proximity to the primary tumor and are in the radiation field (Hogan, Kerin, & Joyce, 2013).
   (b) Damage of healthy tissues in the radiation field may result in disruption of the normal physiologic functions of the bowel, leading to various gastrointestinal symptoms (K.A.L. Morris & Haboubi, 2015).
   (c) The type of RT, dose, and technique all affect the extent of injury to the gastrointestinal tract (K.A.L. Morris & Haboubi, 2015).
   (d) Acute gastrointestinal side effects occur within the first three months of treatment initiation as a result of inflammatory response (K.A.L. Morris & Haboubi, 2015).

(2) Incidence: RT is commonly used in the treatment of pelvic tumors, with 60% to 70% experiencing acute gastrointestinal side effects (K.A.L. Morris & Haboubi, 2015).

(3) Risk factors (K.A.L. Morris & Haboubi, 2015; Nicholas et al., 2017; Viswanathan et al., 2014)
   (a) Treatment-related factors, such as high radiation dose, large treatment fields, and close proximity of the pelvic tumor to the bowels, contribute to development of gastrointestinal side effects.
   (b) Studies show that women treated for gynecologic malignancies who received

70 Gy or more were at significantly higher risk for acute and chronic side effects.

 (c) Technological advances with 3DCRT and IMRT have minimized the field size, thus limiting the exposure of healthy tissue to radiation.

 (d) IMRT has been proven to significantly decrease the incidence of radiation-induced gastrointestinal side effects (Viswanathan et al., 2014).

 (e) With gynecologic cancers, image-guided and HDR brachytherapy have reduced the incidence of long-term complications from 22.7% to 2.6% (Charra-Brunaud et al., 2012; Georg et al., 2012).

 (f) A multimodal approach to cancer treatment is a risk factor for developing gastrointestinal side effects.

 (g) In treatment plans using postoperative RT, such as in cases with rectal cancer, cervical cancer, and vaginal cancer, women are at higher risk because pelvic surgeries lead to the formation of adhesions surrounding the lower gastrointestinal tract, which may limit its movement and force it into the treatment area.

 (h) Women with a history of previous abdominal or pelvic surgery may be at higher risk, as discussed in the previous item.

 (i) Concurrent chemotherapy and immunotherapy can increase risk of gastrointestinal side effects.

 (j) Comorbidities such as diabetes, atherosclerosis, and inflammatory bowel disease increase risk of gastrointestinal side effects.

(4) Clinical manifestations (Gee, Andreyev, & Muls, 2018; NCI CTEP, 2017; Nicholas et al., 2017; Ní Laoire, Fettes, & Murtagh, 2017; Viswanathan et al., 2014)

 (a) Diarrhea

 (b) Urgency: sudden, immediate need to have a bowel movement

 (c) Hemorrhoids: dilated veins in the rectal area that may cause significant pain and some bleeding

 (d) Rectal bleeding

 (e) Abdominal cramping and pain

 (f) Tenesmus: persistent and sometimes painful sensation of incomplete evacuation of bowel or rectal fullness and the need to defecate frequently

(5) Collaborative management (Gee et al., 2018; Hogan et al., 2013; K.A.L. Morris & Haboubi, 2015; Viswanathan et al., 2014)

 (a) An interprofessional team includes oncologists, gastroenterologists, nutritionists, clinical nurse specialists, and specialized oncology nurses.

 (b) Comprehensive patient assessment should be completed, including the following information.

  i. Baseline bowel habits and stool consistency

  ii. Other abdominal symptoms such as pain, gas, cramping, and bloating

  iii. Physical assessment for signs and symptoms of dehydration

 (c) Diarrhea can be managed with the following options.

  i. Use of fiber products, such as psyllium and probiotics

  ii. Antidiarrheal medications (prophylactic use and increased dose with acute diarrhea)

  iii. Regular monitoring of hydration status and electrolyte imbalances in patients with significant diarrhea and possible inadequate nutritional status and dehydration

  iv. IV hydration for severe dehydration or patients unable to tolerate oral intake

  v. Replacement of electrolytes

 (d) If acute proctitis does not cause significant symptoms, treatment may not be necessary.

 (e) For hemorrhoids, comfort measures with topical and oral pain medications may be recommended.

(6) Patient, caregiver, and family education (BC Cancer, 2019)

 (a) Patients should be encouraged to keep track of the number of loose bowel movements and update the healthcare team at regular appointments.

 (b) Clinicians should encourage adequate nutritional and fluid intake with the support of the interprofessional team.

 (c) Patients should eat small, frequent meals and snacks.

 (d) Patients should avoid foods that are high in fiber, fatty, and spicy, as well as caffeinated drinks.

 (e) Patients should limit food that may cause gas, such as beans, broccoli, green leafy vegetables, prunes, chickpeas, and lentils.

 (f) Sitz baths can be used for comfort and cleansing the perianal area.

 (g) Patients can protect skin around the rectal area by regularly cleansing with mild soap and water. Moisture-retentive protective barrier ointments are recommended.

c) Chronic gastrointestinal side effects
  (1) Pathophysiology: Symptoms generally occur six months to three years after treatment (K.A.L. Morris & Haboubi, 2015).
  (2) Incidence: Receiving 70 Gy or more significantly increases the risk of developing chronic toxicity (Nicholas et al., 2017).
  (3) Clinical manifestations (K.A.L. Morris & Haboubi, 2015)
      (a) Malabsorption: Pelvic radiation can damage intestinal villi and affect production of enzymes, leading to malabsorption.
      (b) Rectal bleeding related to chronic proctitis
      (c) Urgency related to chronic proctitis
      (d) Tenesmus related to chronic proctitis
      (e) Fecal incontinence
          i. Incontinence is a major concern for patients with rectal cancer treated with RT.
          ii. The rectum and anus have tremendous nerve supplies, and damaged pelvic nerves may lead to chronic fecal incontinence.
  (4) Collaborative management
      (a) Malabsorption management will require dietary modification to a low-fat and low-residue diet with adequate caloric and fluid intake. Interprofessional management with an RDN or RD is recommended.
      (b) With chronic proctitis, leading to rectal bleeding, hyperbaric oxygen has been used to manage severe symptoms (Nicholas et al., 2017).
      (c) Steroid enemas or suppositories may be an option for symptom management of rectal bleeding, tenesmus, and urgency (K.A.L. Morris & Haboubi, 2015).
d) Acute genitourinary side effects
  (1) Pathophysiology: Pelvic irradiation may lead to upper and lower tract genitourinary complications (Viswanathan et al., 2014).
  (2) Incidence (Donovan et al., 2016; Viswanathan et al., 2014)
      (a) Acute low-grade genitourinary complications are common with EBRT, with some studies reporting incidence at 17%–40%.
      (b) Severe side effects are rare during treatment (2%–5%), and significant improvement of symptoms is generally seen by 12 months after treatment.
  (3) Risk factors (Goucher, Saad, Lukka, & Kapoor, 2019; Pascoe et al., 2019; Viswanathan et al., 2014)
      (a) Cumulative radiation dose: Total dose greater than 70 Gy increases the risk of urinary side effects.
      (b) Treatment volume
      (c) RT technique
      (d) Concurrent chemotherapy
      (e) Prior pelvic surgery
      (f) Radical hysterectomy
      (g) Smoking
  (4) Clinical manifestations (NCI CTEP, 2017)
      (a) Dysuria
      (b) Urgency
      (c) Frequency
      (d) Nocturia
      (e) Urinary incontinence
  (5) Collaborative management (Nicholas et al., 2017; Viswanathan et al., 2014)
      (a) With acute symptoms, such as dysuria, urgency, or frequency, urinalysis is recommended to rule out a urinary tract infection.
      (b) For dysuria, symptoms can be managed with NSAIDs, such as ibuprofen, or analgesics, such as phenazopyridine.
      (c) Anticholinergics are an effective pharmacologic approach to manage urinary urgency.
  (6) Patient, caregiver, and family education (NCI, 2020)
      (a) Patients must inform the healthcare team if they experience any of the following signs and symptoms of genitourinary complications.
          i. Burning or pain when urinating
          ii. Blood in urine
          iii. Difficulty initiating urination or emptying bladder completely
          iv. Feeling the need to immediately urinate or frequent need to urinate
          v. Urine leaking when pressure is applied to the pelvic area (e.g., sneezing or coughing heavily)
          vi. Fever
      (b) Clinicians should encourage patients to maintain adequate hydration with a minimum of 8 cups (2 L) of water and ensure that urine is light yellow or clear.
      (c) Patients should avoid caffeinated drinks, alcohol, spicy foods, and tobacco products, which may contribute to bladder irritation.
e) Chronic genitourinary side effects: hemorrhagic cystitis and urinary fistula
  (1) Pathophysiology
      (a) Hemorrhagic cystitis is a complication caused by damage to the mucosal lining

of the bladder. It is a collection of symptoms such as hematuria, urinary tract pain, and inflammation (Goucher et al., 2019).

 (b) Onset of cystitis can range from months to years from the start of treatment.

 (c) Early signs of hemorrhagic cystitis have been reported to occur at 3–12 months from the start of pelvic RT.

 (d) Urinary fistula is an abnormal connection between the urinary system and another anatomical site (NCI CTEP, 2017).

(2) Incidence

 (a) Incidence rates of hemorrhagic cystitis depend on multiple factors, with some studies reporting 3%–6.7% in cervical cancer and 2%–47% in bladder cancer (Goucher et al., 2019).

 (b) Major urologic complications after completion of treatment can range 1.3%–14.5% at three years (Viswanathan et al., 2014).

(3) Risk factors

 (a) Women receiving combined RT (EBRT and brachytherapy) are at high risk for chronic genitourinary complications, with some studies reporting the mean onset of hemorrhagic cystitis at three years (Viswanathan et al., 2014).

 (b) Techniques such as IMRT have significantly decreased RT-related genitourinary side effects in recent years.

(4) Clinical manifestations (Goucher et al., 2019; Viswanathan et al., 2014)

 (a) Hemorrhagic cystitis: hematuria, pain, and cystoscopic findings of urothelial damages

 (b) Urinary fistula: urinary discharge, urinary incontinence, and urethral edema

(5) Collaborative management

 (a) Hemorrhagic cystitis (Goucher et al., 2019; Nicholas et al., 2017; Viswanathan et al., 2014)

  i. Patients presenting with hematuria after RT must be carefully evaluated to rule out recurrent pathology.

  ii. For mild complications, treatment may include hydration and bladder irrigation.

  iii. Cystoscopy can be used to diagnose and treat hemorrhagic cystitis. Fulguration of vascular lesions can prevent and control hematuria.

  iv. Hyperbaric oxygen therapy is the most studied option for management of this complication. It has been demonstrated as a safe and effective approach in managing radiation-induced hemorrhagic cystitis for individuals who did not respond to cystoscopy and fulguration. Studies have shown that partial or complete treatment response was noted in 84% of patients (Goucher et al., 2019).

  v. In very rare cases, aggressive management, such as embolization, cystectomy, and urinary diversion, may be considered if all conservative approaches have been exhausted.

 (b) Urinary fistula: Surgical repair or ileal conduit may be considered in management of urinary fistula (Nicholas et al., 2017).

f) Acute gynecologic side effects (Bakker et al., 2014; Viswanathan et al., 2014)

(1) Pathophysiology

 (a) Gynecologic side effects are an expected complication with RT in the pelvic region because reproductive structures are in close proximity to the treatment area (Nicholas et al., 2017).

 (b) Acute RT gynecologic side effects are defined as those occurring during or up to six months after treatment (L. Morris, Do, Chard, & Brand, 2017).

 (c) EBRT and brachytherapy may cause acute mucosal injury, leading to side effects that occur during treatment.

 (d) The basal progenitor cells of the epithelium of the vaginal canal are sensitive to radiation, resulting in mucosal injury.

(2) Risk factors (Nicholas et al., 2017; Viswanathan et al., 2014)

 (a) Extent of vaginal mucosal involvement in the treatment field

 (b) Higher vaginal radiation dose or longer duration of treatment resulting in high cumulative dose

 (c) Combined RT modalities (e.g., EBRT in combination with brachytherapy for endometrial cancers) (Reed & Sadozye, 2017)

 (d) Concurrent chemotherapy: EBRT with concurrent cisplatin, followed by brachytherapy, is the standard curative treatment for locally advanced cervical cancer and imposes higher risk (Reed & Sadozye, 2017).

(3) Clinical manifestations

 (a) Symptoms of vaginal mucositis may include vaginal pain and mild bleeding.

 (b) Vaginal infections may manifest as changes in vaginal discharge (e.g., color, smell, increased amount), new persistent pain, vagina itchiness, cramping, and fever.

(4) Collaborative management (Nicholas et al., 2017)

    (a) Mild vaginal mucositis is generally asymptomatic and resolves when treatment is completed.

    (b) Infections related to vaginal mucosal injury and changes in vaginal pH can be managed with antifungal treatments or antibiotics.

    (c) Severe vaginal mucosal injury leading to necrosis may be managed with hydrogen peroxide douching with 1:10 saline ratio.

g) Chronic gynecologic side effects: vaginal stenosis

(1) Pathophysiology (L. Morris et al., 2017)

    (a) Delayed gynecologic side effects are defined as occurring three months after treatment completion.

    (b) RT damages the vaginal mucosa, causing atrophy and adhesion. This leads to loss of elasticity and narrowing of the vaginal canal.

(2) Incidence

    (a) Incidence rate is highly variable and is dependent on multiple factors.

    (b) Literature suggests the incidence can range 1.25%–88%, based on type of cancer, treatment protocol, RT technique, and patient-specific factors (L. Morris et al., 2017).

    (c) A study that evaluated outcomes of women with cervical cancer treated with EBRT, brachytherapy, or both found the incidence of RT-induced vaginal stenosis at 38% (Brand, Bull, & Cakir, 2006).

    (d) The highest incidence is noted to be in women who were treated with RT and brachytherapy for cervical cancer with curative intent (Kirchheiner et al., 2016).

    (e) RT-induced vaginal stenosis is not a significant concern for women who had pelvic RT for endometrial cancer (L. Morris et al., 2017).

    (f) Vaginal stenosis may result after pelvic RT for anal and rectal cancer, with one study reporting up to 66% of women experiencing some degree of stenosis (Son et al., 2015).

    (g) Up to 37.1% of women who were treated with definitive chemoradiation for anal cancer experienced vaginal stenosis (Mirabeau-Beale et al., 2015).

(3) Risk factors

    (a) Women older than 50 years are at higher risk for the development of vaginal stenosis (Nicholas et al., 2017).

    (b) Combination of EBRT and brachytherapy in a treatment protocol increases the risk of developing vaginal stenosis.

    (c) Studies suggest that an EBRT dose higher than 45 Gy in 25 fractions for cervical cancer is a definitive risk factor (Mirabeau-Beale et al., 2015).

    (d) The dose of RT and volume of vaginal tissue exposed to RT was identified as a risk factor among women treated with pelvic RT for anal and rectal cancers (Son et al., 2015).

    (e) Cigarette smoking has been identified as a risk factor (L. Morris et al., 2017).

(4) Clinical manifestations

    (a) Shortening and narrowing of the vagina due to fibrosis is the main manifestation (L. Morris et al., 2017).

    (b) Grades (NCI CTEP, 2017)

        i. Grade 1 symptoms of narrowing and shortening may be negligible and have no effect to regular sexual functioning.

        ii. Grade 2 symptoms are vaginal narrowing and shortening that does not interfere with physical examination.

        iii. Grade 3 stenosis limits vaginal examinations, use of tampons, and sexual activities, such as intercourse.

    (c) Dyspareunia (bleeding with intercourse) generally occurs in the first year of RT, but symptoms may manifest up to five years after completion of treatment (Nicholas et al., 2017).

    (d) Vaginal dryness and decreased lubrication can occur.

(5) Collaborative management

    (a) Management techniques are not supported by high-level evidence, but literature supports comprehensive patient education and psychological support for vaginal dilation after treatment (L. Morris et al., 2017).

    (b) Vaginal dilation stretches the vaginal canal, breaks down any adhesions, and promotes vaginal patency.

    (c) No single recommendation or approach to using vaginal dilators has been internationally recognized, but many guidelines recommend its usage to prevent stenosis (L. Morris et al., 2017).

(6) Patient, caregiver, and family education (Canadian Association of Nurses in Oncology, 2017)

    (a) Clinicians can recommend starting dilation two weeks after completion of RT.

(b) If the vagina or vulva is swollen, tender, or painful to touch, patients should wait until symptoms resolve to initiate dilation.

(c) Comfort is an important factor; therefore, dilation is to be started as soon as a patient is physically comfortable doing so.

(d) It is essential that vaginal dilation be started within a few weeks of completion of treatment.

(e) If additional support is needed, patients are to seek support from their healthcare team.

(f) Clinicians can instruct patients on the dilation process.

    i. Patients should initiate the dilation with the smallest dilator available. If it can be inserted easily without pain, the next size should be used.

    ii. Patients should find a quiet, comfortable place and be in a comfortable position (e.g., on back with knees bent).

    iii. A generous amount of lubricant should be used.

    iv. The dilator should be gently inserted as far as possible. It should be gently rotated side to side and moved up and down. The dilator should be kept in the vagina for 3–10 minutes at a time if possible.

    v. With the dilator insertion, stretching and pressure should be felt. Very mild discomfort may be felt, but this should improve over time.

(g) Clinicians should instruct on the duration of dilation.

    i. For the first six months, dilation should be performed three times a week.

    ii. From six months to one year, dilation should be performed once a week. If it becomes more difficult, frequency should increase to two to three times a week.

    iii. After one year, dilation should be performed once a month.

    iv. Some women may need to continue regular dilation for up to five years after treatment.

(h) The frequency of dilation can be reduced if women are having regular intercourse or other vaginal penetration. If penetration becomes difficult over time, dilation should resume as recommended.

(i) Clinicians should inform patients on when to seek medical help.

    i. Although it is common to have a small amount of bleeding with vaginal dilation, any new bleeding that requires the use of a sanitary napkin is an indication to seek immediate medical help.

    ii. If signs and symptoms of vaginal infection, such as new persistent vaginal pain, vaginal itchiness, cramping, or fever, are noted, patients should seek medical help.

(j) Clinicians can educate patients and their partners about vaginal lubricants.

    i. Lubricant is a gel-like liquid that can be used to moisten the vagina.

    ii. Lubricants can be water based, oil based, and silicone based.

    iii. Patients should avoid lubricants that contain perfume, paraben, spermicide, coloring, or flavoring, as well as lubricants with warming or tingling properties. These usually have more chemicals that can irritate the lining of the vagina.

    iv. Petroleum jelly is not recommended.

(k) Ovarian failure leading to infertility is a significant concern for premenopausal women (see also IV.F. Fertility).

References

Adams, T.S., & Cuello, M.A. (2018). FIGO cancer report 2018: Cancer of the vagina. *International Journal of Gynecology and Obstetrics, 143*(Suppl. 2), 14–21. https://doi.org/10.1002/ijgo.12610

American Cancer Society. (2020). *Cancer facts and figures 2020.* https://www.cancer.org/research/cancer-facts-statistics/all-cancer-facts-figures/cancer-facts-figures-2020.html

Azria, D., Betz, M., Bourgier, C., Jeanneret Sozzi, W., & Ozshin, M. (2012). Identifying patients at risk for late radiation-induced side effects. *Critical Reviews in Oncology/Hematology, 84*(Suppl. 1), e35–e41. https://doi.org/10.1016/j.critrevonc.2010.08.003

Bakker, R.M., ter Kuile, M.M., Vermeer, W.M., Nout, R.A., Mens, J.W.M., van Doorn, L.C., ... Creutzberg, C.L. (2014). Sexual rehabilitation after pelvic radiotherapy and vaginal dilator use consensus using the Delphi method. *International Journal of Gynecological Cancer, 24*, 1499–1506. https://doi.org/10.1097/IGC.0000000000000253

BC Cancer. (2019). *Care of radiation therapy side effects: Skin care* [Brochure]. http://www.bccancer.bc.ca/patient-and-public-info-site/Documents/BCCancer_CareOfRadiationTherapySideEffectsSkinCare_FactSheet.pdf

Bolderston, A., Cashell, A., McQuestion, M., Cardoso, M., Summers, C., & Harris, R. (2018). A Canadian survey of the management of radiation-induced skin reactions. *Journal of Medical Imaging and Radiation Sciences, 49*, 164–172. https://doi.org/10.1016/j.jmir.2018.01.003

Brand, A.H., Bull, C.A., & Cakir, B. (2006). Vaginal stenosis in patients treated with radiotherapy for carcinoma of the cervix. *International Journal of Gynecologic Cancer, 16*, 288–293.

Brenner, D.R., Weir, H.K., Demers, A.A., Ellison, L.F., Louzado, C., Shaw, A., ... Smith, L.M. (2020). Projected estimates of cancer in Canada in

2020. *Canadian Medical Association Journal, 192,* E199–E205. https://doi.org/10.1503/cmaj.191292

Canadian Association of Nurses in Oncology. (2017). *Care for women after radiation to the pelvis.* https://www.cano-acio.ca/page/radiation_pelvis

Charra-Brunaud, C., Harter, V., Delannes, M., Haie-Meder, C., Quetin, P., Kerr, C., ... Peiffert, D. (2012). Impact of 3D image-based PDR brachytherapy on outcome of patients treated for cervix carcinoma in France: results of the French STIC prospective study. *Radiation Therapy and Oncology, 103*(3), 305–310. https://doi.org/10.1016/j.radonc.2012.04.007

Donovan, J.L., Hamdy, F.C., Lane, J.A., Mason, M., Metcalfe, C., Walsh, E., ... Neal, D.E. (2016). Patient-reported outcomes after monitoring, surgery, or radiotherapy for prostate cancer. *New England Journal of Medicine, 375,* 1425–1437. https://doi.org/10.1056/NEJMoa1606221

Gee, C., Andreyev, J., & Muls, A. (2018). Developing advanced clinical practice skills in gastrointestinal consequences of cancer treatment. *British Journal of Nursing, 27,* 237–247. https://doi.org/10.12968/bjon.2018.27.5.237

Georg, P., Pötter, R., Georg, D., Lang, S., Dimopoulos, J.C.A., Sturdza, A.E., ... Dörr, W. (2012). Dose effect relationship for late side effects of the rectum and urinary bladder in magnetic resonance image-guided adaptive cervix cancer brachytherapy. *International Journal of Radiation Oncology, Biology, Physics, 82,* 653–657. https://doi.org/10.1016/j.ijrobp.2010.12.029

Goucher, G., Saad, F., Lukka, H., & Kapoor, A. (2019). Canadian Urological Association best practice report: Diagnosis and management of radiation-induced hemorrhagic cystitis. *Canadian Urological Association Journal, 13,* 15–23. https://doi.org/10.5489/cuaj.5788

Hogan, N.M., Kerin, M.J., & Joyce, M.R. (2013). Gastrointestinal complications of pelvic radiotherapy: Medical and surgical management strategies. *Current Problems in Surgery, 50,* 395–407. https://doi.org/10.1067/j.cpsurg.2013.04.004

Kirchheiner, K., Nout, R.A., Lindegaard, J.C., Haie-Meder, C., Mahantshetty, U., Segedin, B., ... Tanderup, K. (2016). *Radiotherapy and Oncology, 118,* 160–166. https://doi.org/10.1016/j.radonc.2015.12.025

Knapp, P., Eva, B., Reseigh, G., Gibbs, A., Sim, L., Daly, T., ... Bernard, A. (2019). The role of volumetric modulated arc therapy (VMAT) in gynaecological radiation therapy: A dosimetric comparison of intensity modulated radiation therapy versus VMAT. *Journal of Medical Radiation Sciences, 66,* 44–53. https://doi.org/10.1002/jmrs.311

McQuestion, M. (2011). Evidence-based skin care management in radiation therapy: Clinical update. *Seminars in Oncology Nursing, 27,* e1–e17. https://doi.org/10.1016/j.soncn.2011.02.009

Mirabeau-Beale, K., Hong, T.S., Niemierko, A., Ancukiewicz, M., Blaszkowsky, L.S., Crowley, E.M., ... Wo, J.Y. (2015). Clinical and treatment factors associated with vaginal stenosis after definitive chemoradiation for anal canal cancer. *Practical Radiation Oncology, 5,* E113–E118. https://doi.org/10.1016/j.prro.2014.09.003

Morris, K.A.L., & Haboubi, N.Y. (2015). Pelvic radiation therapy: Between delight and disaster. *World Journal of Gastrointestinal Surgery, 7,* 279–288. https://doi.org/10.4240/wjgs.v7.i11.279

Morris, L., Do, V., Chard, J., & Brand, A.H. (2017). Radiation-induced vaginal stenosis: Current perspectives. *International Journal of Women's Health, 9,* 273–279.

National Cancer Institute. (2020). Urinary and bladder problems. https://www.cancer.gov/about-cancer/treatment/side-effects/urination-changes

National Cancer Institute Cancer Therapy Evaluation Program. (2017). *Common terminology criteria for adverse events* [v.5.0]. https://ctep.cancer.gov/protocolDevelopment/electronic_applications/docs/CTCAE_v5_Quick_Reference_8.5x11.pdf

273–279. https://doi.org/10.2147/IJWH.S106796

National Comprehensive Cancer Network. (2020a). *NCCN Clinical Practice Guidelines in Oncology (NCCN Guidelines®): Cervical cancer* [v.1.2020]. https://www.nccn.org/professionals/physician_gls/pdf/cervical.pdf

National Comprehensive Cancer Network. (2020b). *NCCN Clinical Practice Guidelines in Oncology (NCCN Guidelines®): Uterine neoplasms* [v.1.2020]. https://www.nccn.org/professionals/physician_gls/pdf/uterine.pdf

National Comprehensive Cancer Network. (2020c). *NCCN Clinical Practice Guidelines in Oncology (NCCN Guidelines®): Vulvar cancer (squamous cell carcinoma)* [v.1.2020]. https://www.nccn.org/professionals/physician_gls/pdf/vulvar.pdf

Niazi, T.M., Vuong, T., Azoulay, L., Marjnen, C., Bujko, K., Nasr, E., ... Cummings, B. (2012). Silver clear nylon dressing is effective in preventing radiation-induced dermatitis in patients with lower gastrointestinal cancer: Results from a phase III study. *International Journal of Radiation Oncology, Biology, Physics, 84,* e305–e310. https://doi.org/10.1016/j.ijrobp.2012.03.062

Nicholas, S., Chen, L., Choflet, A., Fader, A., Guss, Z., Hazell, S., ... Viswanathan, A.N. (2017). Pelvic radiation and normal tissue toxicity. *Seminars in Radiation Oncology, 27,* 358–369. https://doi.org/10.1016/j.semradonc.2017.04.010

Ní Laoire, Á., Fettes, L., & Murtagh, F.E.M. (2017). A systematic review of the effectiveness of palliative interventions to treat rectal tenesmus in cancer. *Palliative Medicine, 31,* 975–981. https://doi.org/10.1177/0269216317697897

O'Sullivan, B., Brierley, J.D., D'Cruz, A.K., Fey, M.F., Pollock, R., Vermorken, J.B., & Huang, S.H. (Eds.). (2015). *UICC manual of clinical oncology* (9th ed.). John Wiley and Sons. https://doi.org/10.1002/9781119013143

Pascoe, C., Duncan, C., Lamb, B.W., Davis, N.F., Lynch, T.H., Murphy, D.G., & Lawrentschuk, N. (2019). Current management of radiation cystitis: A review and practical guide to clinical management. *British Journal of Urology International, 123,* 585–594. https://doi.org/10.1111/bju.14516

Reed, N.S., & Sadozye, A.H. (2017). Update on radiotherapy in gynaecological malignancies. *Obstetrician and Gynaecologist, 19,* 29–36. https://doi.org/10.1111/tog.12342

Seité, S., Bensadoun, R.J., & Mazer, J.M. (2017). Prevention and treatment of acute and chronic radiodermatitis. *Breast Cancer: Targets and Therapy, 9,* 551–557. https://doi.org/10.2147/BCTT.S149752

Son, C.H., Law, E., Oh, J.H., Apte, A.P., Yang, T.J., Riedel, E., ... Goodman, K.A. (2015). Dosimetric predictors of radiation-induced vaginal stenosis after pelvic radiation therapy for rectal and anal cancer. *International Journal of Radiation Oncology, Biology, Physics, 92,* 548–554. https://doi.org/10.1016/j.ijrobp.2015.02.029

Viswanathan, A.N., Lee, L.J., Eswara, J.R., Horowitz, N.S., Konstantinopoulos, P.A., Mirabeau-Beale, K.L., ... Wo, J.Y. (2014). Complications of pelvic radiation in patients treated for gynecologic malignancies. *Cancer, 120,* 3870–3883. https://doi.org/10.1002/cncr.28849

Wong, R.K.S., Bensadoun, R.-J., Boers-Doets, C.B., Bryce, J., Chan, A., Epstein, J.B., ... Lacouture, M.E. (2013). Clinical practice guidelines for the prevention and treatment of acute and late radiation reactions from the MASCC Skin Toxicity Study Group. *Supportive Care in Cancer, 21,* 2933–2948. https://doi.org/10.1007/s00520-013-1896-2

VI. Disease-Specific Management

A. Sarcomas

1. Overview: Sarcomas are rare malignant tumors named according to tissue origin and categorized as either soft tissue or bone.

   a) Soft tissue sarcomas

      (1) Soft tissue sarcomas are rare malignant tumors generating from various soft tissues, including fibrous connective tissue, fat, smooth or striated muscle, vascular tissue, peripheral neural tissue, and visceral tissue.

      (2) More than 50 histological types of soft tissue sarcoma have been identified (Amin et al., 2018).

      (3) Most commonly, sarcomas arise from connective tissue, developing in the extremities (43%); thorax (10%); viscera (19%); head and neck (9%); retroperitoneal, intra-abdominal, and gastrointestinal areas (15%); and other locations (4%) (Pisters, Weiss, Maki, & Raut, 2016; Potter, Jones, & Barrott, 2018).

      (4) Soft tissue sarcomas are classified in three histologic categories.

         (a) Malignant round cell tumors

         (b) Lipomatous tumors

         (c) Other sarcomas

   b) Bone sarcomas

      (1) Bone sarcomas commonly arise from bone material (Ferguson & Turner, 2018).

      (2) Histologic origin determines the identification of primary bone sarcoma.

         (a) Chondrosarcoma originates in cartilage.

         (b) Osteosarcomas arise from bone.

         (c) Fibrosarcoma develops in fibrogenic tissue.

      (3) Unknown histologic origin is an entire class of primary bone tumors.

      (4) Franchi (2012) found the most common subtypes are chondrosarcoma (30% in men; 29% in women), osteosarcoma (16% in men; 17% in women), Ewing sarcoma (14% in men and women), and chordoma (8% in men; 5% in women).

2. Incidence

   a) Soft tissue sarcoma is rare, accounting for only 0.8% of all new cancer diagnoses in the United States. Of these new cancer diagnoses, soft tissue sarcoma accounts for 15% of all pediatric malignancies and 1% of adult malignancies (NCI, n.d.-b).

      (1) The most common soft tissue sarcoma in the pediatric population is rhabdomyosarcoma (Alaggio & Coffin, 2015).

      (2) In 2018, approximately 13,040 patients were diagnosed with soft tissue sarcoma. Soft tissue sarcoma accounted for approximately 5,150 deaths in 2018 (NCI, n.d.-b).

   b) According to SEER data, primary malignant bone tumors (bone sarcomas) in the skeletal system are extremely rare, accounting for only 0.2% of all malignancies (NCI, n.d.-a).

      (1) The extremely rare malignant fibrous histiocytoma, fibrosarcoma, chordoma, and giant cell tumor of the bone (benign and malignant) make up approximately 1%–5% of all primary malignant bone tumors.

      (2) Age and gender play a role in primary bone sarcoma diagnoses.

         (a) Chondrosarcoma is typically diagnosed in middle-aged and older adults.

         (b) Osteosarcoma and Ewing sarcoma are typically seen in children and young adults.

         (c) Chordoma is commonly diagnosed in the fifth and sixth decades of life, with the largest demographic being men.

      (3) Because of age variations at time of diagnosis, bone sarcoma has a bimodal distribution, with the first incidence peak occurring in people younger than 20 years, and the second peak occurring in those older than 60 years (Franchi, 2012).

3. Histology and staging

   a) Staging for soft tissue sarcoma and bone tumors are performed using the AJCC TNM system.

   b) Histologic grade is an important prognostic indicator and determined using the AJCC grading system based on the French Federation of Cancer Centers Sarcoma Group guidelines.

   c) This grading system is based on tumor cell differentiation, mitotic activity, and extent of tumor necrosis, each classified on a three-point scale (Amin et al., 2018).

      (1) Tumor cell differentiation is scored on a scale of 1–3. Cancer cells appearing similar to healthy cells are classified as 1, and atypical cancer cells are classified as 3.

      (2) Mitotic activity is a scale of 1–3 based on tumor cell replication. Lower scores indicate less cell division.

      (3) Tumor necrosis defines dying tissue, scored 0–2. Lower scores indicate less tissue necrosis.

4. Prognostic factors

   a) Soft tissue sarcomas (Amin et al., 2018)

      (1) Stage and histopathology each play a role in determining overall prognosis (Amin et al., 2018).

         (a) According to SEER data for soft tissue sarcoma, the overall five-year survival rate is 64.5% (NCI, n.d.-b).

         (b) When the sarcoma is in a localized stage at diagnosis, overall survival is 80.8%.

(c) Overall survival with regional spread to lymph nodes is 58% and with distant metastasis is 16.4%.

(d) For unknown soft tissue stages at time of diagnosis, overall survival is 53.1% (see Figure 19).

(2) A correct diagnosis is a challenge in soft tissue sarcoma.

(a) A European study in 2016 found that pathologists gave different histologic grades or subtyping in approximately 35% of cases and disagreed on the sarcoma diagnosis in 8% of cases (Dei Tos, Bonvalot, & Haas, 2018).

(b) The complexity of categorizing sarcoma diagnoses is evident in this high degree of variation among pathology professionals.

(3) In light of diagnosis variation, molecular markers and genetic abnormalities are extensively being researched to encourage accurate diagnosis and therapy initiation. The clinical hope is that with further immunohistochemistry and molecular genetic assessments, customized chemotherapy and immunotherapy clinical trials can target these genetic mutations (Dei Tos et al., 2018).

b) Primary malignant bone tumors

(1) Correctly determining if a lesion is primary or secondary and central or peripheral, as well as histologic grade, size, and proximity to anatomic structures, influences primary bone tumor prognosis.

(a) The degree of surgical resection also greatly influences overall survival.

(b) Curative approaches are based on surgical resection of primary and metastatic disease (Whelan & Davis, 2018).

i. Anatomic positioning is also an influential prognostic factor. Decreased overall survival is seen with axial tumor sites when compared to cranial or appendicular positions.

ii. Justification for this variance is based on the different clinical behaviors of cranial and appendicular locations, resulting in increased overall survival for younger patients (Schneiderman, Kliethermes, & Nystrom, 2017).

iii. All these variations influence prognosis, accumulating in an overall five-year survival of 66.9% according to SEER data (NCI, n.d.-a).

(2) Molecular markers and genetic abnormalities assessments are also important prognostic factors for bone cancer (Amin et al., 2018).

(a) Customized multiagent chemotherapy is used to target specific abnormalities and provide customized care.

(b) For example, patients with personal or family history of Li-Fraumeni syndrome (*TP53* germline mutation) and familial retinoblastoma (*RB1* mutation) are at higher risk for osteosarcoma and require customized chemotherapy and RT.

5. Etiology and risk factors

a) Soft tissue sarcoma: The etiology of soft tissue sarcoma is often unknown. Known causes of soft tissue sarcoma are linked to the following (Kumar, 2017).

(1) Chemical carcinogens used in agricultural or forestry work (e.g., phenoxyacetic herbicides, chlorophenols, dioxin)

(2) Previous radiation exposure

(3) Viral infections (e.g., human herpesvirus 8)

(4) Immunodeficiency (e.g., Epstein-Barr virus)

(5) Predisposing genetic mutations (e.g., Li-Fraumeni syndrome, neurofibromatosis, hereditary retinoblastoma)

b) Bone sarcomas: Most primary bone tumors grow with no known etiology. Observed predisposing factors for bone tumors include the following (Kumar, 2017).

(1) History of Paget disease

(2) Previous radiation exposure

(3) Bone infarction or chronic osteomyelitis

(4) Preexisting benign tumors

(5) Implanted metallic hardware, joint prosthesis, and bone grafts

(6) Embryonic notochord remnants in the skull base (chordoma formation in older adults)

(7) Predisposing genetic mutations directly linked to osteosarcoma (e.g., hereditary retinoblastoma, Li-Fraumeni syndrome, Rothmund-Thomson syndrome)

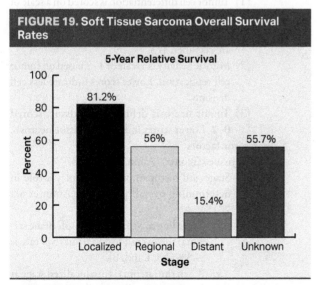

FIGURE 19. Soft Tissue Sarcoma Overall Survival Rates

5-Year Relative Survival

Note. Based on information from National Cancer Institute, n.d.-b.

(8) Ollier disease, Maffucci syndrome, and multiple osteochondromatosis (higher prevalence of chondrosarcoma)

6. Diagnostic workup and stages of treatment
   a) Both soft tissue sarcoma and bone sarcoma require biopsy for diagnosis. Wide coring needle biopsy or open incision biopsy can be used.
      (1) Coring needle biopsy is superior to fine needle aspiration due to the large tumor volume extracted for grading and subtyping.
      (2) Incision biopsies are rarely performed due to cosmetic concerns and high complication rates (Kumar, 2017).
   b) After the biopsy and diagnosis, a maximally safe surgical gross total resection should be pursued.
      (1) According to NCCN (2019) guidelines, the surgical goal should be histologically negative surgical margins to optimize tumor control and prevent recurrence.
      (2) Optimized surgery shows highest rates of overall survival particularly for patients with bone sarcoma, such as chordoma.
      (3) According to a meta-analysis of skull base chordomas by Di Maio, Temkin, Ramanathan, and Sekhar (2011), incomplete resections resulted in 3.83 times higher likelihood of recurrence at five years than complete resection.
   c) Chemotherapy and immunotherapy
      (1) Soft tissue sarcomas
         (a) Various regimens of single-agent chemotherapy and immunotherapy are used for all subtypes and nonspecific histology of soft tissue sarcoma.
         (b) Chemotherapy is often incorporated for advanced-stage disease, palliative situations, disseminated metastasis, and resected tumors with adverse functional outcomes or unresectable primary disease.
         (c) New treatment indications for regimens are being discovered regularly.
      (2) Bone sarcomas have a limited but growing list of chemotherapy and immunotherapy options for systemic therapy.
         (a) Methotrexate, doxorubicin, and cisplatin (MAP regimen) are useful in osteosarcoma treatment.
            i. New therapies are currently being studied.
            ii. A recent randomized controlled trial with methotrexate, doxorubicin, and cisplatin, with the addition of maintenance pegylated interferon alfa-2b, showed good response for resectable high-grade osteosarcoma (Bielack et al., 2015).
         (b) Chemotherapy in bone sarcoma subtypes, such as chondrosarcoma and chordoma, shows variance in improving overall survival and presents challenges with clinical replication.
         (c) Further research regarding the role of systemic chemotherapy and immunotherapy options is needed (Whelan & Davis, 2018).

7. RT options
   a) Overview
      (1) RT continues to be the gold standard of care in the treatment of soft tissue and bone sarcomas.
      (2) Previously, extremity soft tissue sarcoma treatment focused on surgical amputation.
      (3) Curative treatment in extremity sarcomas now emphasizes limb-sparing surgery and function-sparing RT.
   b) Treatment timing
      (1) For soft tissue sarcoma, RT can be used at several different stages of care, including primary, preoperative, or postoperative treatment. RT cumulative dose is always determined by tissue tolerance and anatomic location (Pisters et al., 2016).
      (2) Preoperative RT is theorized to reduce seeding during surgical manipulation and tumor resection.
         (a) Tumors may regress during preoperative RT, resulting in a smaller tumor volume.
         (b) Even if the tumor volume remains stable, the outer pseudocapsule can thicken and conform to an inert acellular form.
         (c) Regression and outer pseudocapsule thickening ease resection and decrease rates of recurrence (Dagan et al., 2011).
         (d) Preoperative RT can lead to increased wound healing complications when compared to the postoperative RT population (Albertsmeier et al., 2018).
         (e) After preoperative RT, a period of three to six weeks before surgery is recommended to allow for acute radiation reactions to resolve and decrease the risk of impaired surgical wound healing (Griffin et al., 2015).
      (3) Postoperative RT is ideal for local control in patients with positive surgical margins.
         (a) Postoperative RT boosts do not demonstrate local recurrence prevention for patients with low-grade sarcoma or surgically planned positive margins because of close proximity to anatomically fixed critical structures (Al Yami et al., 2010).
         (b) A retrospective cohort study by Alamanda, Song, Shinohara, Schwartz, and

Holt (2014) found that patients with extremity soft tissue sarcoma have no additional benefit from a postoperative boost to prevent local recurrence, distant metastasis, and mortality.

(c) Intervals between surgical resection and postoperative RT are not recommended beyond 12 weeks because of the risk of site fibrosis and malignant cell proliferation (Casabianca et al., 2017).

(4) When considering preoperative versus postoperative RT in extremity soft tissue sarcoma, several factors are considered.

(a) Late toxicities from RT, such as fibrosis, bone fracture, edema, and joint stiffness, are decreased with preoperative RT compared to postoperative.

(b) Postoperative radiation fields are typically larger because of blood, fluid, and edema filling the surgical space, thus increasing radiation surface area, leading to more significant toxicities.

(c) Preoperative RT uses targeted delineation and imaging guidance to decrease radiation dose to surrounding tissue and joint areas. Additionally, preoperative RT administers a lower total radiation dose and offers a shorter length of treatment, which is ideal in cases of large anticipated postsurgical treatment areas (El-Bared, Wong, & Wang, 2015).

(d) A recent systematic literature review and meta-analysis evaluated the role of preoperative and postoperative EBRT versus no EBRT in local recurrence and overall survival rates for soft tissue sarcomas. A total of 3,958 patients from 16 studies were analyzed, and the conclusion supported the use of preoperative EBRT because of lower local recurrence rates (Albertsmeier et al., 2018).

(e) Based on clinical data, preoperative RT shows decreased long-term side effects and beneficial rates of local control and overall survival. When considering the role of postoperative RT, the risk of local recurrence versus toxicity of postoperative RT should be individualized based on extent of tumor resection, age of patient, stage and size of tumor, and soft tissue location (El-Bared et al., 2015).

c) Brachytherapy

(1) Brachytherapy is used as a postsurgical RT technique, directly applying radioactive seeds into the tumor bed through catheters placed during surgery (NCCN, 2020).

(2) This type of RT is common for soft tissue sarcomas located in the extremities, trunk, and head and neck.

(3) Several options of brachytherapy are available: LDR, fractionated HDR, or intraoperative.

(4) LDR and HDR brachytherapy have similar rates of local disease control.

d) Intraoperative RT

(1) Intraoperative RT is a single fraction administered during surgical resection (Roeder & Krempien, 2017).

(2) Use of EBRT can be limited because of close proximity of organs with low radiation dose tolerance.

(a) Intraoperative RT can overcome these limitations and reduce toxicity.

(b) Administering a single dose of radiation during surgery enhances local control of the tumor without affecting wound healing.

(3) Recent retrospective studies at the Mayo Clinic reviewed treatment outcomes among patients with upper extremity soft tissue sarcoma (N = 61) who received intraoperative RT (Call, Stafford, Petersen, & Haddock, 2014).

(a) Local control at 5 and 10 years was 91% and 88%, respectively.

(b) This study showed excellent local control, limb preservation, and overall survival despite positive margins after resection.

e) IMRT

(1) IMRT is highly advantageous for tight radiation contours and increased control of the radiation beam.

(2) IMRT minimizes the dose of radiation to surrounding healthy tissues, resulting in less toxicity.

(3) With the addition of new image-guided techniques, such as pretreatment MRI and CT used for planning, patients experience fewer side effects and less long-term tissue toxicity from more precisely administered doses (Wang et al., 2015).

(4) IMRT reduces doses to critical structures, such as the heart, bone, gastrointestinal tract, kidneys, and blood vessels, while maintaining tumor target coverage.

(5) Recent studies showed that smaller IMRT treatment volumes reduced toxicity without increasing recurrence rates in RT margins (Shah et al., 2016).

(6) A study by O'Sullivan et al. (2013) found that long-term complications of RT, such as edema and joint stiffness, were improved with IMRT compared to conventional RT.

(7) Preoperative IMRT resulted in lower rates of wound complications for patients with

high-grade lesions when compared to conventional EBRT (O'Sullivan et al., 2013).

(8) For bone sarcomas, NCCN (2019) guidelines strongly encourage pursuing RT in combination with surgical treatments.

    (a) Various methods of specialized RT techniques, such as IMRT, particle beam RT (protons and carbon and heavy ions), SRS, or fractionated stereotactic RT, should be considered.

    (b) Maximizing dose of RT while allowing for optimal normal tissue sparing is the goal in treatment of bone sarcomas.

    (c) Each bone sarcoma diagnosis has varying goals of RT depending upon surgical resection results and timing of RT.

    (d) Providers should always review the latest NCCN guidelines for treatment algorithms because treatment pathways are rapidly developing.

f) Surgical resection and RT for bone sarcoma

    (1) A gross total surgical resection should be pursued for curative treatment intent prior to RT.

    (2) Challenging anatomical tumor locations and abutting essential vasculature can prevent a complete tumor removal.

    (3) In these cases, primary RT should be considered for borderline resected and unresectable tumors.

    (4) In a retrospective study by Goda et al. (2011), patients with extracranial high-risk chondrosarcoma received preoperative or postoperative RT. The results showed excellent and durable local tumor control, even if a complete surgical resection was not performed.

g) Proton beam therapy for bone sarcoma

    (1) Proton beam therapy is another recommended treatment for bone sarcoma.

    (a) Proton beam therapy implemented as primary therapy or in combination with photon therapy (EBRT or IMRT) is associated with excellent tumor control and long-term survival for low-grade skull base and cervical spine chordomas and chondrosarcomas according to recent research by Sahgal et al. (2015).

    (b) Proton beam therapy is excellent at sparing healthy tissue because the total radiation dose is delivered directly to the tumor bed without radiation extending beyond the tumor. Treatment results in decreased acute side effects and long-term complications (Pompos, Durante, & Choy, 2016).

    (2) Heavy carbon ion particle RT is a new form of therapy that has shown promise in the clinical radiation setting.

    (a) Carbon ions are heavier particles with higher mass than particles used in traditional RT and proton beam therapy. This results in limited scatter dose radiation effect and optimized dose effect at the tumor target.

    (b) When the carbon ion reaches the tumor volume, significant DNA damage occurs, decreasing the cancer's ability to repair the DNA damage and continue replicating (Pompos et al., 2016).

    (c) In recent research with carbon ion therapy, Uhl et al. (2014) found that it was effective for bone sarcoma in 3-year (95.9%), 5-year (88%), and 10-year (88%) local control rates and improved neurologic symptoms from baseline.

h) Palliative RT

    (1) Palliative RT can also be useful for symptom relief and improved quality of life for patients with bone and soft tissue sarcoma.

    (2) Palliative RT is an essential tool when managing unresectable and high-grade sarcoma tumors when cure is not attainable (NCCN, 2020).

8. Genetic disorders

a) Hereditary genetic disorders, such as Li-Fraumeni syndrome, show evidence of higher rates of sarcomas. Patients with Li-Fraumeni syndrome are commonly diagnosed with rhabdomyosarcoma and osteosarcoma (Ripperger et al., 2017).

b) Schneider, Zelley, Nichols, and Garber (2019) noted increased risk of second primary tumors developing from RT in patients with Li-Fraumeni syndrome.

    (1) Caution should be used to limit radiation exposure in patients with this genetic anomaly.

    (2) However, experts recommend that treatment optimization should be prioritized above concerns for late second primary malignancy.

c) A study by Archer et al. (2016) found that children with pleomorphic and embryonal rhabdomyosarcoma develop second primary malignancies independent of radiation exposure. This discovery suggests that rhabdomyosarcoma subtypes are prone to second primary malignancy formation regardless of RT.

d) Using RT to treat patients with genetic mutations is not contraindicated; however, long-term disease surveillance monitoring for second primary malignancies in these populations is essential.

9. RT side effects

a) Acute toxicities

    (1) Delayed wound healing is a common acute side effect of RT and is most common in limb and trunk sarcoma sites when RT is completed following surgery (El-Bared et al., 2015).

(2) A prospective study by Pixberg et al. (2016) found that irradiated children experienced immunosuppression when bone structures, such as the pelvis or spine, are involved in the radiation field.

    (a) Immunosuppression symptoms include anemia, oral mucositis, and increased bleeding and infection risk.

    (b) Risk of immunosuppression is higher when concurrent chemotherapy or immunotherapy is utilized during RT.

    (c) Frequent laboratory monitoring with transfusion support is recommended.

(3) Radiation-induced dermatitis and moist desquamation are common acute skin toxicities (see IV.B. Skin reactions).

(4) Patients receiving abdominal radiation can develop diarrhea, anorexia, nausea, and vomiting (El-Bared et al., 2015; see V.E. Gastrointestinal tract and abdomen).

b) Chronic toxicities

(1) Chronic radiation recall skin reactions can occur weeks to years after RT is completed (Leventhal & Young, 2017).

    (a) Triggers such as ultraviolet light, immunotherapy, chemotherapy, and various medications can cause an erythema or darkening at a previous RT site.

    (b) Using a topical corticosteroid or stopping the provoking medication will improve symptoms.

    (c) Late dermal effects, such as skin atrophy, fibrosis, and telangiectasias, can also occur after completion of RT.

(2) Chronic toxicities such as fibrosis, joint stiffness and decreased range of motion, edema, and lymphedema are common after extremity RT.

    (a) Decreasing direct radiation dose to joint areas decreases these long-term impairments.

    (b) Tumors in the lower extremities receiving greater than 63 Gy had the highest risk of moderate to severe edema and decreased range of motion (Shah et al., 2016).

    (c) These toxicities are associated with higher degrees of physical disability and impairment.

    (d) Early engagement and continued interventions with physical and occupational therapy during and after RT decreases risk of impairment.

(3) Bone stunting and fractures are serious complications in patients treated with limb-sparing surgery and RT.

    (a) Children who receive limb-sparing surgery require repeated bone-lengthening surgeries to ensure bilateral symmetry.

    (b) Repeated surgical interventions increase risk of fracture in the long term. Fractures may require multiple surgeries, prosthesis replacement, or amputation to treat (El-Bared et al., 2015; Szalontay & Shad, 2017).

    (c) Decreasing radiation dose to limb growth plates and surgically intervening only when clinically indicated can alleviate these risks.

(4) Infertility and gonadal damage can occur for patients receiving RT (see IV.F. Fertility).

(5) Renal toxicities, such as radiation nephropathy, can occur when the primary tumor is near the kidney (Szalontay & Shad, 2017).

    (a) Radiation nephritis presents after a latent period, occurring 3–12 months after completion of RT.

    (b) Radiation doses greater than 20 Gy increase risk of radiation-induced nephropathy.

    (c) Symptoms include hypertension, proteinuria, renal insufficiency, and anemia.

    (d) Measuring a comprehensive metabolic panel and urinalysis at follow-up appointments can detect renal toxicities early.

(6) Peripheral neuropathy is a common chronic side effect for patients with abdominal sarcomas requiring large volumes of intraoperative RT covering the sacral nerve plexus (El-Bared et al., 2015).

    (a) Sensory and motor neuropathy in lower extremities cause intermittent pain and varying degrees of motor weakness.

    (b) Post-RT pain symptoms are short term and resolve within six months of RT completion.

    (c) Motor weakness is a chronic impairment.

    (d) Limiting or avoiding treatment to the sacral nerve plexus decreases or removes this chronic risk.

(7) Second primary malignancies cause treatment-related mortality in long-term cancer survivors (Szalontay & Shad, 2017).

    (a) Analysis of Childhood Cancer Survivorship Study data by Friedman et al. (2010) showed 20.5% cumulative risk for patients who received RT, after 30 years of survivorship.

    (b) Second primary malignancies occur in the radiation field, and incidence increases over time with no plateau.

    (c) Common second neoplasms are soft tissue and bone sarcoma, bone cancer, and nonmelanoma skin cancer.

    (d) Underlying genetic susceptibility, such as Li-Fraumeni syndrome or familial retinoblastoma (*RB1* mutation), will also increase risk of second malignancies in survivorship settings.

   (e) In an effort to diminish the risk of long-term second primary malignancies, the clinical team should minimize doses to healthy tissues and decrease the total radiation dose when possible.

10. Follow-up and survivorship

   a) Long-term follow-up for annual screening and survivorship planning is recommended in sarcoma patients and can be completed by a primary oncology care team or specialized long-term survivorship follow-up clinics.

   b) Screening for post-traumatic stress disorder (PTSD) is important for psychological well-being and emotional health (Szalontay & Shad, 2017).

      (1) Women and children with previously diagnosed mental disorders are the most vulnerable.

      (2) Many pediatric sarcoma survivors show increased signs of resiliency and post-traumatic growth.

      (3) Overall, survivors of childhood cancers have positive concepts of identity, relationships, and life philosophy.

   c) Assessing employment and healthcare behaviors at follow-up appointments can aid in continuing support for long-term cancer survivors (Szalontay & Shad, 2017).

      (1) Childhood sarcoma cancer survivors are twice as likely to be unemployed in adulthood because of physical limitations.

      (2) Childhood cancer survivors show significant lack of knowledge and misperceptions regarding cancer diagnosis, treatment, and cancer-related health risks after completing therapy.

      (3) Continuing to educate about disease surveillance and healthy lifestyle modifications to prevent chronic conditions will positively affect the physical and psychological well-being of cancer survivors.

   d) The Children's Oncology Group (2018) and NCCN (2020) recommend long-term follow-up for patients with sarcoma receiving RT.

11. Patient, caregiver, and family education

   a) Nurses should assess patient, caregiver, and family understanding of the disease process and treatment plan, as well as overall ability and readiness to learn (Rose & Yates, 2015).

   b) Nurses should assess the need for support groups, financial assistance, and resources for emotional and spiritual coping. Patients can be referred to social workers, mental health counselors, spiritual care providers, and the palliative medicine team as indicated (Lee, Vanderwater, & Wong, 2017).

   c) Nurses should review the RT treatment procedures (e.g., intraoperative RT, brachytherapy, EBRT) with patients. Nurses should explain that an immobilization device may be fabricated for consistent positioning during RT (Rose & Yates, 2015).

   d) Nurses should review the treatment schedule and give patients a treatment calendar if they are undergoing several types of treatments (e.g., intraoperative RT plus IMRT for retroperitoneal sarcoma) (Rose & Yates, 2015).

   e) Nurses should provide instruction regarding skin care during RT (Rose & Yates, 2015).

   f) Expected acute and chronic side effects and their management should be reviewed. Nurses should reassure patients, caregivers, and family that the interprofessional medical team will be present to continually monitor and manage these acute and chronic side effects (Lee et al., 2017; Rose & Yates, 2015).

References

Alaggio, R., & Coffin, C.M. (2015). The evolution of pediatric soft tissue sarcoma classifications in the last 50 years. *Pediatric and Developmental Pathology, 18,* 481–494. https://doi.org/10.2350/15-07-1666-misc.1

Alamanda, V.K., Song, Y., Shinohara, E., Schwartz, H.S., & Holt, G.E. (2014). Postoperative radiation boost does not improve local recurrence rates in extremity soft tissue sarcomas. *Journal of Medical Imaging and Radiation Oncology, 58,* 633–640. https://doi.org/10.1111/1754-9485.12184

Albertsmeier, M., Rauch, A., Roeder, F., Hasenhütl, S., Pratschke, S., Kirschneck, M., ... Angele, M.K. (2018). External beam radiation therapy for resectable soft tissue sarcoma: A systematic review and meta-analysis. *Annals of Surgical Oncology, 25,* 754–767. https://doi.org/10.1245/s10434-017-6081-2

Al Yami, A., Griffin, A.M., Ferguson, P.C., Catton, C.N., Chung, P.W.M., Bell, R.S., ... O'Sullivan, B. (2010). Positive surgical margins in soft tissue sarcoma treated with preoperative radiation: Is a postoperative boost necessary? *International Journal of Radiation Oncology, Biology, Physics, 77,* 1191–1197. https://doi.org/10.1016/j.ijrobp.2009.06.074

Amin, M.B., Edge, S., Greene, F., Byrd, D.R., Brookland, R.K., Washington, M.K., ... Meyer, L.R. (Eds.). (2018). *AJCC cancer staging manual* (8th ed.). Springer.

Archer, N.M., Amorim, R.P., Naves, R., Hettmer, S., Diller, L.R., Ribeiro, K.B., & Rodriguez-Galindo, C. (2016). An increased risk of second malignant neoplasms after rhabdomyosarcoma: Population-based evidence for a cancer predisposition syndrome? *Pediatric Blood and Cancer, 63,* 196–201. https://doi.org/10.1002/pbc.25678

Bielack, S.S., Smeland, S., Whelan, J.S., Marina, N., Jovic, G., Hook, J.M., ... Bernstein, M. (2015). Methotrexate, doxorubicin, and cisplatin (MAP) plus maintenance pegylated interferon alfa-2b versus MAP alone in patients with resectable high-grade osteosarcoma and good histologic response to preoperative MAP: First results of the EuRAMOS-1 good response randomized controlled trial. *Journal of Clinical Oncology, 33,* 2279–2287. https://doi.org/10.1200/JCO.2014.60.0734

Call, J.A., Stafford, S.L., Petersen, I.A., & Haddock, M.G. (2014). Use of intraoperative radiotherapy for upper-extremity soft-tissue sarcomas: Analysis of disease outcomes and toxicity. *American Journal of Clinical Oncology, 37,* 81–85. https://doi.org/10.1097/COC.0b013e31826b9b3d

Casabianca, L., Kreps, S., Helfre, S., Housset, M., Anract, P., & Biau, D.J. (2017). Optimal post-operative radiation after soft-tissue sarcoma resection is achieved in less than two thirds of cases. *International Orthopaedics, 41,* 2401–2405. https://doi.org/10.1007/s00264-017-3609-9

Children's Oncology Group. (2018). *Long-term follow-up guidelines for survivors of childhood, adolescent, and young adult cancer* [Version 5.0]. http://www.survivorshipguidelines.org/pdf/2018/COG_LTFU_Guidelines_v5.pdf

Dagan, R., Indelicato, D.J., McGee, L., Morris, C.G., Kirwan, J.M., Knapik, J., ... Zlotecki, R.A. (2011). The significance of a marginal excision after preoperative radiation therapy for soft tissue sarcoma of the extremity. *Cancer, 118*, 3199–3207. https://doi.org/10.1002/cncr.26489

Dei Tos, A.P., Bonvalot, S., & Haas, R. (2018). The key role of pathology, surgery and radiotherapy in the initial management of soft tissue sarcoma. *Future Oncology, 14*(Suppl. 10), 15–23. https://doi.org/10.2217/fon-2018-0075

Di Maio, S., Temkin, N., Ramanathan, D., & Sekhar, L.N. (2011). Current comprehensive management of cranial base chordomas: 10-year meta-analysis of observational studies. *Journal of Neurosurgery, 115*, 1094–1105. https://doi.org/10.3171/2011.7.jns11355

El-Bared, N., Wong, P., & Wang, D. (2015). Soft tissue sarcoma and radiation therapy advances, impact on toxicity. *Current Treatment Options in Oncology, 16*, 19. https://doi.org/10.1007/s11864-015-0335-7

Ferguson, J.L., & Turner, S.P. (2018). Bone cancer: Diagnosis and treatment principles. *American Family Physician, 98*, 205–213. https://www.aafp.org/afp/2018/0815/p205.html

Franchi, A. (2012). Epidemiology and classification of bone tumors. *Clinical Cases in Mineral and Bone Metabolism, 9*, 92–95. https://www.ncbi.nlm.nih.gov/pmc/articles/PMC3476517

Friedman, D.L., Whitton, J., Leisenring, W., Mertens, A.C., Hammond, S., Stovall, M., ... Neglia, J.P. (2010). Subsequent neoplasms in 5-year survivors of childhood cancer: The Childhood Cancer Survivor Study. *Journal of the National Cancer Institute, 102*, 1083–1095. https://doi.org/10.1093/jnci/djq238

Goda, J.S., Ferguson, P.C., O'Sullivan, B., Catton, C.N., Griffin, A.M., Wunder, J.S., ... Chung, P.W. (2011). High-risk extracranial chondrosarcoma. *Cancer, 117*, 2513–2519. https://doi.org/10.1002/cncr.25806

Griffin, A.M., Dickie, C.I., Catton, C.N., Chung, P.W.M., Ferguson, P.C., Wunder, J.S., & O'Sullivan, B. (2015). The influence of time interval between preoperative radiation and surgical resection on the development of wound healing complications in extremity soft tissue sarcoma. *Annals of Surgical Oncology, 22*, 2824–2830. https://doi.org/10.1245/s10434-015-4631-z

Kumar, D. (2017). Pathology of bone and soft tissue sarcomas. In R. Henshaw (Ed.), *Sarcoma: A multidisciplinary approach to treatment* (pp. 23–41). Springer.

Lee, C.T., Vanderwater, C., & Wong, J. (2017). Exploring the role of collaborative patient-provider relationships in self-management during radiation therapy [Abstract]. *International Journal of Integrated Care, 17*, A50. https://doi.org/10.5334/ijic.3351

Leventhal, J., & Young, M.R. (2017). Radiation dermatitis: Recognition, prevention and management. *Oncology, 31*, 885–887, 894–899.

National Cancer Institute. (n.d.-a). Cancer stat facts: Bone and joint cancer. https://seer.cancer.gov/statfacts/html/bones.html

National Cancer Institute. (n.d.-b). Cancer stat facts: Soft tissue including heart cancer. https://seer.cancer.gov/statfacts/html/soft.html

National Comprehensive Cancer Network. (2019). *NCCN Clinical Practice Guidelines in Oncology (NCCN Guidelines®): Bone cancer* [v.1.2020]. https://www.nccn.org/professionals/physician_gls/PDF/bone.pdf

National Comprehensive Cancer Network. (2020). *NCCN Clinical Practice Guidelines in Oncology (NCCN Guidelines®): Soft tissue sarcoma* [v.6.2019]. http://www.nccn.org/professionals/physician_gls/PDF/sarcoma.pdf

O'Sullivan, B., Griffin, A.M., Dickie, C.I., Sharpe, M.B., Chung, P.W.M., Catton, C.N., ... Bell, R.S. (2013). Phase 2 study of preoperative image-guided intensity-modulated radiation therapy to reduce wound and combined modality morbidities in lower extremity soft tissue sarcoma. *Cancer, 119*, 1878–1884. https://doi.org/10.1002/cncr.27951

Pisters, P.W.T., Weiss, M., Maki, R., & Raut, C.P. (2016, June 2). Soft-tissue sarcomas. *CancerNetwork*. https://www.cancernetwork.com/cancer-management/soft-tissue-sarcomas

Pixberg, C., Koch, R., Eich, H.T., Martinsson, U., Kristensen, I., Matuschek, C., ... Steinmann, D. (2016). Acute toxicity grade 3 and 4 after irradiation in children and adolescents: Results from the IPPARCA Collaboration. *International Journal of Radiation Oncology, Biology, Physics, 94*, 792–799. https://doi.org/10.1016/j.ijrobp.2015.12.353

Pompos, A., Durante, M., & Choy, H. (2016). Heavy ions in cancer therapy. *JAMA Oncology, 2*, 1539–1540. https://doi.org/10.1001/jamaoncol.2016.2646

Potter, J.W., Jones, K.B., & Barrott, J.J. (2018). Sarcoma—The standard-bearer in cancer discovery. *Critical Reviews in Oncology/Hematology, 126*, 1–5. https://doi.org/10.1016/j.critrevonc.2018.03.007

Ripperger, T., Bielack, S.S., Borkhardt, A., Brecht, I.B., Burkhardt, B., Calaminus, G., ... Kratz, C.P. (2017). Childhood cancer predisposition syndromes—A concise review and recommendations by the Cancer Predisposition Working Group of the Society for Pediatric Oncology and Hematology. *American Journal of Medical Genetics Part A, 173*, 1017–1037. https://doi.org/10.1002/ajmg.a.38142

Roeder, F., & Krempien, R. (2017). Intraoperative radiation therapy (IORT) in soft-tissue sarcoma. *Radiation Oncology, 12*, 20. https://doi.org/10.1186/s13014-016-0751-2

Rose, P., & Yates, P. (2015). Patients' outcomes related to person-centered nursing care in radiation oncology: A case study. *European Journal of Oncology Nursing, 19*, 731–739. https://doi.org/10.1016/j.ejon.2015.05.008

Sahgal, A., Chan, M.W., Atenafu, E.G., Masson-Cote, L., Bahl, G., Yu, E., ... Laperriere, N.J. (2015). Image-guided, intensity-modulated radiation therapy (IG-IMRT) for skull base chordoma and chondrosarcoma: Preliminary outcomes. *Neuro-Oncology, 17*, 889–894. https://doi.org/10.1093/neuonc/nou347

Schneider, K., Zelley, K., Nichols, K.E., & Garber, J. (2019, November 21). Li-Fraumeni syndrome. *GeneReviews*. https://www.ncbi.nlm.nih.gov/books/NBK1311

Schneiderman, B.A., Kliethermes, S.A., & Nystrom, L.M. (2017). Survival in mesenchymal chondrosarcoma varies based on age and tumor location: A survival analysis of the SEER database. *Clinical Orthopedics and Related Research, 475*, 799–805. https://doi.org/10.1007/s11999-016-4779-2

Shah, C., Verma, V., Takiar, R., Vajapey, R., Amarnath, S., Murphy, E., ... Budd, T. (2016). Radiation therapy in the management of soft tissue sarcoma: A clinician's guide to timing, techniques, and targets. *American Journal of Clinical Oncology, 39*, 630–635. https://doi.org/10.1097/coc.0000000000000319

Szalontay, L., & Shad, A. (2017). Treatment effects and long-term management of sarcoma patients and survivors. In R.M. Henshaw (Ed.), *Sarcoma: A multidisciplinary approach to treatment* (pp. 383–411). Springer.

Uhl, M., Mattke, M., Welzel, T., Oelmann, J., Habl, G., Jensen, A.D., ... Debus, J. (2014). High control rate in patients with chondrosarcoma of the skull base after carbon ion therapy: First report of long-term results. *Cancer, 120*, 1579–1585. https://doi.org/10.1002/cncr.28606

Wang, D., Zhang, Q., Eisenberg, B.L., Kane, J.M., Li, X.A., Lucas, D., ... Kirsch, D.G. (2015). Significant reduction of late toxicities in patients with extremity sarcoma treated with image-guided radiation therapy to a reduced target volume: Results of Radiation Therapy Oncology Group RTOG-0630 trial. *Journal of Clinical Oncology, 33*, 2231–2238. https://doi.org/10.1200/jco.2014.58.5828

Whelan, J.S., & Davis, L.E. (2018). Osteosarcoma, chondrosarcoma, and chordoma. *Journal of Clinical Oncology, 36*, 188–193. https://doi.org/10.1200/jco.2017.75.1743

B. Lymphomas

1. Overview

    a) Lymphomas are a heterogeneous group of cancers that arise from the proliferation of malignant lymphocytes at varying stages of development and differentiation.

    b) Malignant cells accumulate in the lymph nodes and other extranodal sites, producing tumor masses and eventual organ dysfunction.

    c) Lymphomas develop from B lymphocytes, T lymphocytes, and natural killer cells and are categorized as either Hodgkin lymphoma or non-Hodgkin lymphoma.

d) More than 60 subtypes of lymphoma have been identified, and each subtype has distinct features in etiology, pathology, clinical presentation, and prognosis, with varying treatment trajectories (Swerdlow et al., 2016).

e) Only the most common and clinically relevant subtypes for the nurse practicing in radiation oncology will be reviewed in this section.

2. Incidence and etiology
   a) Lymphomas made up 3.5% of all cancers diagnosed internationally in 2018 (Bray et al., 2018).
   b) Although the etiology for lymphoma is largely unknown, a number of predisposing conditions increase disease risk (Tsang & Crump, 2015).
      (1) Autoimmune diseases, such as Sjögren syndrome or rheumatoid arthritis
      (2) Immunosuppression, such as with HIV infection or for organ transplantation
      (3) Viral agents, such as Epstein-Barr virus or human T-cell lymphotropic virus
      (4) Bacterial infections, such as *Helicobacter pylori*
      (5) Drugs, such as alkylating chemotherapy agents

3. Clinical presentation
   a) Lymphomas often present with lymphadenopathy in peripheral areas, such as the neck, axilla, or groin, or enlarged lymph nodes within the mediastinum or intra-abdominal regions.
   b) Classic B symptoms (systemic symptoms) include weight loss greater than 10% of body mass over six months, fevers, or night sweats (Cheson et al., 2014).
   c) Pain or other symptoms can occur in areas where lymph node enlargement is compromising organs, tissues, or vessels.

4. Diagnosis
   a) To make a diagnosis of lymphoma, an incisional or excisional lymph node biopsy, which often requires a surgical procedure, is necessary to obtain tissue for architectural and histologic evaluation by an experienced hematopathologist. Image-guided core biopsies can be considered when an incisional or excisional biopsy is not possible (Cheson et al., 2014).
   b) Further investigations at initial diagnosis include the following.
      (1) CT of the head and neck, chest, abdomen, and pelvis
      (2) Fluorodeoxyglucose PET
      (3) Blood work (Tsang & Crump, 2015)
         (a) Complete blood count
         (b) Liver function tests
         (c) Creatinine
         (d) Protein
         (e) Lactate dehydrogenase
         (f) Erythrocyte sedimentation rate (Hodgkin lymphoma)

(g) HIV serology
(h) Hepatitis screening
      (4) Bone marrow biopsy

5. Staging
   a) Staging is based on the Ann Arbor classification system.
   b) Classification as limited (stage I–II) or advanced (stage III–IV) disease is based anatomically on the number of involved lymph node sites, whether disease is present on one or both sides of the diaphragm, and the absence or presence of extranodal disease (Cheson et al., 2014).
   c) Extranodal disease includes the presence of lymphoma in the skin, lung, gastrointestinal tract, liver, bone, bone marrow, or CNS (Cheson et al., 2014).
   d) Lymphoma staging is further characterized by the absence (A) or presence (B) of B symptoms (Cheson et al., 2014).

6. Prognostic factors
   a) In addition to the Ann Arbor staging classification, various prognostic factors are used to determine the type and extent of treatment needed for Hodgkin and non-Hodgkin lymphoma.
   b) Limited-stage Hodgkin lymphoma is stratified into favorable or unfavorable risk disease. Unfavorable risk disease is defined as the presence of one or more of the following risk factors (Bröckelmann, Angelopoulou, & Vassilakopoulos, 2016).
      (1) Three or more nodal sites
      (2) Presence of extranodal disease
      (3) Bulky mediastinal mass
      (4) Erythrocyte sedimentation rate of 50 mm/hour or greater with no B symptoms
      (5) Erythrocyte sedimentation rate of 30 mm/hour or greater with B symptoms
   c) For advanced-stage Hodgkin lymphoma, the International Prognostic Score is used to determine disease risk (Bröckelmann et al., 2016).
      (1) The following risk factors are taken into account.
         (a) Male gender
         (b) Age older than 45 years
         (c) Ann Arbor stage IV disease
         (d) Hemoglobin level less than 10.5 g/dl
         (e) Albumin level less than 4 g/dl
         (f) Leukocyte count greater than 15,000/mm^3
         (g) Lymphocyte count less than 600/mm^3
      (2) Presence of risk factors are scored 0–7, with more intensive treatment approaches considered in higher scores (Bröckelmann et al., 2016).
   d) For non-Hodgkin lymphoma, the International Prognostic Index is a validated tool used to stratify disease risk and determine prognosis (Tsang & Crump, 2015).

(1) The index accounts for the following risk factors.
  (a) Age older than 60 years
  (b) Lactate dehydrogenase greater than upper limit of normal
  (c) Ann Arbor stage III or IV
  (d) Eastern Cooperative Oncology Group performance status 2–4
  (e) Extranodal involvement
(2) Presence of risk factors are scored 0–5 to predict prognosis; four to five risk factors indicate high risk.

7. Types of lymphoma (see Table 13)
  a) Hodgkin lymphoma
    (1) Hodgkin lymphoma is classically associated with Reed-Sternberg cells (Gopas et al., 2016).
    (2) Cure rates are high, but 10%–15% of limited-stage and 20%–30% of advanced-stage disease will relapse, with eventual death in half of relapses (Gopas et al., 2016).
  b) Indolent non-Hodgkin lymphoma
    (1) Indolent non-Hodgkin lymphomas are associated with very few symptoms and occasional waxing and waning (spontaneous regression) of lymphadenopathy (Tsang & Crump, 2015).
    (2) Indolent lymphomas are not curable but are associated with long-term survival attributed to advances in treatment.
    (3) Goals of therapy are to maintain quality of life with treatment indicated in early stages or those who develop symptomatic disease.
    (4) A watch-and-wait approach is reasonable in the majority of asymptomatic patients (Ardeshna et al., 2014).
    (5) Transformation to an aggressive lymphoma can occur in a small subset of patients being followed for many years (Tsang & Crump, 2015).
  c) Aggressive non-Hodgkin lymphoma
    (1) Aggressive non-Hodgkin lymphomas are associated with rapidly growing masses in nodal regions, frequent extranodal involvement (e.g., gastrointestinal tract, liver, head and neck), and symptomatic disease (Tsang & Crump, 2015).
    (2) Unlike indolent lymphomas, aggressive non-Hodgkin lymphomas are treated with curative intent.
    (3) Goals of therapy are to manage any urgent complications at presentation, establish a definitive diagnosis in a timely manner, and initiate treatment.
    (4) Prognosis will vary among subtype, staging, and additional risk factors.

8. RT options
  a) Combined modality treatment
    (1) A combined modality—chemotherapy followed by RT—is the optimal approach with curative intent for most limited-stage Hodgkin lymphomas and early-stage, aggressive non-Hodgkin lymphomas (Tsang & Crump, 2015).
    (2) The role of RT in combined modality treatment is to provide local and regional control of disease, as well as to prevent recurrence.
    (3) The recent use of fluorodeoxyglucose PET for interim response assessment has helped to limit RT in combined modality treatment for Hodgkin lymphoma. This approach carefully balances survival benefits with decreasing the risk for RT late effects (Engert et al., 2012; Radford et al., 2015).
  b) RT as a single modality
    (1) Although combined modality treatment is frequently applied for treatment of stage I and II lymphomas, RT as a single modality continues to play an important role in ensuring local control of disease.
    (2) RT alone is given to treat early-stage nodular lymphocyte-predominant Hodgkin lymphoma, early-stage indolent non-Hodgkin lymphoma, urgent complications at diagnosis (e.g., mediastinal mass compressing the trachea), or relapsed or refractory disease (symptomatic relief of bulky disease) (Tsang & Crump, 2015).
    (3) Historically, RT for the treatment of lymphoma consisted of extended field and involved field techniques, which targeted larger nodal regions and contributed to significant morbidity and mortality (Specht et al., 2014).
    (4) Modern three-dimensional planning techniques have changed the way RT is delivered to minimize exposure to surrounding healthy tissues, thus reducing acute and late effects (Specht et al., 2014).
    (5) Involved-site RT is the current standard approach. This technique uses three-dimensional planning with CT and fluorodeoxyglucose PET, as well as MRI when appropriate, to target tumor areas more accurately, avoiding healthy tissue (Specht et al., 2014).
    (6) Involved-node RT provides even more restricted coverage than involved-site RT, with treatment given only to the grossly affected lymph nodes. However, given the risk for lack of radiation exposure to potential microscopic disease, this technique is used only in limited scenarios, such as combined modality treatment for Hodgkin lymphoma (Specht et al., 2014).

9. Side effects of RT
  a) Acute effects
    (1) Acute effects associated with RT for lymphoma are related to involved nodal or extranodal radi-

TABLE 13. Types of Lymphoma and Approach to Treatment

Type of Lymphoma[a]	Description	Treatment Approach
Aggressive Non-Hodgkin Lymphoma		
Anaplastic large-cell lymphoma[b]	Separated into ALK-positive and ALK-negative Superior prognosis in ALK-positive disease	Stage I–II: combined modality Stage III–IV: chemotherapy
Angioimmunoblastic T-cell lymphoma[b]	Stage IV in 90% of cases	Stage I–II: combined modality Stage III–IV: chemotherapy
DLBCL	Most common aggressive lymphoma	Stage I–II: combined modality Stage III–IV: chemotherapy
• Primary CNS lymphoma	Subtype of DLBCL presenting in brain, cerebrospinal fluid, and eyes	Chemotherapy or combined modality
• Primary mediastinal B-cell lymphoma	Subtype of DLBCL presenting in mediastinum	Combined modality
Extranodal natural killer cell/T-cell lymphoma, nasal type[b]	Prevalent in Asia, Mexico, and South America Presents in nasal cavity and Waldeyer ring	Stage I–II: concurrent chemoradiation followed by chemotherapy Stage III–IV: chemotherapy
Mantle cell lymphoma	Considered aggressive Indolent form of disease seen in many cases	Stage I–II: combined modality Stage III–IV: chemotherapy
Peripheral T-cell lymphoma, not otherwise specified[b]	Most common T-cell lymphoma Stage III–IV in the majority of cases	Stage I–II: combined modality Stage III–IV: chemotherapy
Plasmablastic lymphoma	Often associated with immunodeficiency (e.g., HIV)	Chemotherapy or combined modality
Hodgkin Lymphoma		
Classical Hodgkin lymphoma	Stage I–II in most cases	Combined modality or chemotherapy
Nodular lymphocyte predominant Hodgkin lymphoma	5%–10% of all Hodgkin lymphomas Often stage I at presentation	RT or combined modality
Indolent Non-Hodgkin Lymphoma		
Chronic lymphocytic leukemia/small lymphocytic lymphoma	Chronic lymphocytic leukemia defined as disease in blood (lymphocyte count ≥ 5,000/mm³) and bone marrow Small lymphocytic lymphoma defined as disease in lymph nodes, spleen, or other organs without blood involvement	Chemotherapy
Follicular lymphoma	Most common indolent non-Hodgkin lymphoma	Stage I–II: RT Stage III–IV: chemotherapy
Marginal zone lymphoma	Found in extranodal sites (e.g., stomach, orbit, thyroid, skin) Stomach often associated with *Helicobacter pylori* infection	Stage I–II: RT Stage III–IV: chemotherapy
Mycosis fungoides and Sezary syndrome	Progression from skin patches to plaques, then tumors over many years	Localized: RT Advanced: topical or light therapy, chemotherapy
Primary cutaneous follicle center lymphoma	Presents as nodules or plaque-like lesions in skin	Surgical excision or RT

ALK—anaplastic lymphoma kinase; CNS—central nervous system; DLBCL—diffuse large B-cell lymphoma; RT—radiation therapy

[a] All subtypes are of B-lymphocyte origin unless otherwise indicated.

[b] T-lymphocyte origin

Note. Based on information from Grommes & DeAngelis, 2017; Tsang & Crump, 2015.

ation site and surrounding tissues. More detailed descriptions of localized acute effects can be found in V. Site-Specific Management.

(2) Radiation pneumonitis, a noninfectious inflammatory process, can occur one to six months following RT delivered to lung regions. It is associated with dry cough, dyspnea, low-grade fever, or pleuritic chest pain (Pinnix et al., 2015).

(a) Exposure to bleomycin, which is used in the treatment of Hodgkin lymphoma and known to cause pulmonary toxicity, increases risk of radiation pneumonitis.

(b) Mild cases are self-limiting; however, more severe symptoms can require corticosteroid and oxygen therapy.

(3) RT delivered to pelvic or mediastinal regions that includes bone marrow in the radiation field may cause anemia, thrombocytopenia, or neutropenia and can be exacerbated by chemotherapy in combined modality treatment (see IV.I. Neutropenia).

b) Late effects

(1) Late effects associated with RT for lymphoma are related to involved nodal or extranodal radiation site and surrounding tissues.

(2) Lymphoma survivors have significantly higher risk of developing second primary malignancies in comparison to the general population (Schaapveld et al., 2015).

(a) Breast cancer (Schaapveld et al., 2015)

    i. Breast cancer is the most common site, representing 41% of second cancers in lymphoma survivors.

    ii. Absolute excess risk for female breast cancer is 54.3 per 10,000 people per year.

    iii. Previous extended-field RT to the mantle region (axilla, mediastinal, cervical, supraclavicular, and infraclavicular areas) was associated with a 2–20 times increased risk of breast cancer, depending on patient age.

    iv. With modern three-dimensional planning techniques, more accurate targeting of tumor areas, and avoidance of axilla and infraclavicular regions, breast cancer risk has declined by 63%.

    v. It is recommended that female patients who have received RT to the mantle region before age 35–40 undergo breast screening using mammogram and MRI at age 25 years or approximately 8–10 years after treatment, whichever comes first (Hodgson, 2011).

(b) Lung cancer (Schaapveld et al., 2015)

    i. Lung cancer represents 20% of second cancers in lymphoma survivors.

    ii. Absolute excess risk is 24.6 per 10,000 people per year in comparison to the general population.

    iii. Risk is increased among those with a smoking history and who received RT above the diaphragm.

(c) Acute or chronic leukemia (Schaapveld et al., 2015)

    i. Leukemias represent 5% of second cancers in lymphoma survivors.

    ii. Absolute excess risk is 6.1 per 10,000 people per year in comparison to the general population.

(d) Various other solid tumor malignancies have absolute excess risk in comparison to the general population, including the following (Schaapveld et al., 2015).

    i. Esophageal cancer (5.6 per 10,000 people per year)

    ii. Stomach cancer (5.6 per 10,000 people per year)

    iii. Colon cancer (4.6 per 10,000 people per year)

    iv. Melanoma (3.6 per 10,000 people per year)

    v. Thyroid cancer (3.5 per 10,000 people per year)

    vi. Soft tissue sarcoma (3.3 per 10,000 people per year)

(3) Cardiac disease represents a significant late effect associated with RT to the mediastinum and neck (see also IV.K. Cardiac toxicity and cardiac implantable electronic devices).

(a) Coronary artery disease accounts for 40%–50% of complications, and valvular disease and carotid artery narrowing are less common (Hodgson, 2011).

(b) If combined modality therapy includes cardiotoxic anthracycline chemotherapy, the risk for cardiac late effects is further increased, often contributing to congestive heart failure (Hodgson, 2011).

(c) With modern three-dimensional planning techniques and more accurate targeting of disease, morbidity associated with valvular disease has improved; however, risk reduction in coronary artery disease is less clear (Hodgson, 2011).

(d) It is recommended that patients who have received RT to the mediastinal region undergo monitoring for cardiac risk factors (e.g., blood pressure, serum lipids) with appropriate treatment, if necessary (Hodgson, 2011).

(4) Lhermitte sign is associated with RT delivered to the cervical or thoracic spinal cord (Youssef et al., 2015).

(a) Lhermitte sign presents with transient electric shock sensations that radiate from the neck and down the spine to the extremities.

(b) It usually occurs within several months of completing RT and can develop spontaneously or be triggered by movement.

(c) Symptoms tend to resolve over weeks to months.

(5) Radiation myelitis is an irreversible consequence of spinal cord RT that can progress to permanent spinal cord injury. Steroids may provide some symptom relief in this late effect (Youssef et al., 2015).

10. Special circumstances: pregnancy (see also IV.G. Treatment of patients who are pregnant)

a) Pregnancy presents a significant challenge in lymphoma treatment because of concerns regarding effects of imaging tests on the fetus, level of disease aggressiveness, and potential for life-threatening organ complications if the malignancy is left untreated.

b) Recent studies suggested that delaying chemotherapy until after the first trimester may be a reasonable option if maternal safety is not compromised (Pinnix, Andraos, Milgrom, & Fanale, 2017).

c) Several studies have shown that RT can be given in pregnancy with modern shielding techniques; however, long-term fetal effects are unknown, and use of this modality should be deferred until after delivery (Pinnix et al., 2017).

References

Ardeshna, K.M., Qian, W., Smith, P., Braganca, N., Lowry, L., Patrick, P., ... Linch, D.C. (2014). Rituximab versus a watch-and-wait approach in patients with advanced-stage, asymptomatic, non-bulky follicular lymphoma: An open-label randomised phase 3 trial. *Lancet Oncology, 15,* 424–435. https://doi.org/10.1016/s1470-2045(14)70027-0

Bray, F., Ferlay, J., Soerjomataram, I., Siegel, R.L., Torre, L.A., & Jemal, A. (2018). Global cancer statistics 2018: GLOBOCAN estimates of incidence and mortality worldwide for 36 cancers in 185 countries. *CA: A Cancer Journal for Clinicians, 68,* 394–424. https://doi.org/10.3322/caac.21492

Bröckelmann, P., Angelopoulou, M., & Vassilakopoulos, T. (2016). Prognostic factors in Hodgkin lymphoma. *Seminars in Hematology, 53,* 155–164. https://doi.org/10.1053/j.seminhematol.2016.05.003

Cheson, B.D., Fisher, R.I., Barrington, S.F., Cavalli, F., Schwartz, L.H., Zucca, E., & Lister, T.A. (2014). Recommendations for initial evaluation, staging, and response assessment of Hodgkin and non-Hodgkin lymphoma: The Lugano classification. *Journal of Clinical Oncology, 32,* 3059–3067. https://doi.org/10.1200/jco.2013.54.8800

Engert, A., Haverkamp, H., Kobe, C., Markova, J., Renner, C., Ho, A., ... Diehl, V. (2012). Reduced-intensity chemotherapy and PET-guided radiotherapy in patients with advanced stage Hodgkin's lymphoma (HD15 trial): A randomised, open-label, phase 3 non-inferiority trial. *Lancet, 379,* 1791–1799. https://doi.org/10.1016/s0140-6736(11)61940-5

Gopas, J., Stern, E., Zurgil, U., Ozer, J., Ben-Ari, A., Shubinsky, G., ... Livneh, E. (2016). Reed-Sternberg cells in Hodgkin's lymphoma present features of cellular senescence. *Cell Death and Disease, 7,* e2457. https://doi.org/10.1038/cddis.2016.185

Grommes, C., & DeAngelis, L.M. (2017). Primary CNS lymphoma. *Journal of Clinical Oncology, 35,* 2410–2418. https://doi.org/10.1200/jco.2017.72.7602

Hodgson, D.C. (2011). Late effects in the era of modern therapy for Hodgkin lymphoma. *American Society of Hematology Education Program Book, 2011,* 323–329. https://doi.org/10.1182/asheducation-2011.1.323

Pinnix, C.C., Andraos, T.Y., Milgrom, S., & Fanale, M.A. (2017). The management of lymphoma in the setting of pregnancy. *Current Hematologic Malignancy Reports, 12,* 251–256. https://doi.org/10.1007/s11899-017-0386-x

Pinnix, C.C., Smith, G.L., Milgrom, S., Osborne, E.M., Reddy, J.P., Akhtari, M., ... Dabaja, B. (2015). Predictors of radiation pneumonitis in patients receiving intensity modulated radiation therapy for Hodgkin and non-Hodgkin lymphoma. *International Journal of Radiation Oncology, Biology, Physics, 92,* 175–182. https://doi.org/10.1016/j.ijrobp.2015.02.010

Radford, J., Illidge, T., Counsell, N., Hancock, B., Pettengell, R., Johnson, P., ... Barrington, S. (2015). Results of a trial of PET-directed therapy for early-stage Hodgkin's lymphoma. *New England Journal of Medicine, 372,* 1598–1607. https://doi.org/10.1056/nejmoa1408648

Schaapveld, M., Aleman, B.M.P., van Eggermond, A.M., Janus, C.P.M., Krol, A.D.G., van der Maazen, R.W.M., ... van Leeuwen, F.E. (2015). Second cancer risk up to 40 years after treatment for Hodgkin's lymphoma. *New England Journal of Medicine, 373,* 2499–2511. https://doi.org/10.1056/nejmoa1505949

Specht, L., Yahalom, J., Illidge, T., Berthelsen, A., Constine, L.S., Eich, H.T., ... Ng, A. (2014). Modern radiation therapy for Hodgkin lymphoma: Field and dose guidelines from the International Lymphoma Radiation Oncology Group (ILROG). *International Journal of Radiation Oncology, Biology, Physics, 89,* 854–862. https://doi.org/10.1016/j.ijrobp.2013.05.005

Swerdlow, S.H., Campo, E., Pileri, S.A., Harris, N.L., Stein, H., Siebert, R., ... Jaffe, E.S. (2016). The 2016 revision of the World Health Organization classification of lymphoid neoplasms. *Blood, 127,* 2375–2390. https://doi.org/10.1182/blood-2016-01-643569

Tsang, R.W.C., & Crump, M. (2015). Lymphoma. In B. O'Sullivan, J.D. Brierley, A.K. D'Cruz, M.F. Fey, R. Pollock, J.B. Vermorken, & S.H. Huang (Eds.), *UICC manual of clinical oncology* (9th ed., pp. 392–414). John Wiley and Sons.

Youssef, B., Shank, J., Reddy, J.P., Pinnix, C.C., Farha, G., Akhtari, M., ... Dabaja, B. (2015). Incidence and predictors of Lhermitte's sign among patients receiving mediastinal radiation for lymphoma. *Radiation Oncology, 10,* 206. https://doi.org/10.1186/s13014-015-0504-7

C. Benign conditions and benign tumors

1. Overview

a) RT is primarily a cancer treatment modality; however, utilizing RT for the treatment of benign conditions is sometimes indicated.

(1) It is important for professional oncology nurses to understand, embrace, and recognize the use of RT to treat benign entities.

(2) Although goals of RT delivery are commonly focused on treating malignant conditions, long-standing clinical experience has recognized the efficacy and unique radiobiologic principles of RT in treating a host of benign diagnoses.

b) Benign conditions that are considered appropriate for RT intervention may be categorized as non-neoplastic, benign neoplastic, inflammatory, and proliferative. An extensive literature review has revealed the diminished use of RT in this setting, perhaps as a result of promulgated concerns surrounding the development of radiation-induced malignancies (Taylor, Hatfield, McKeown, Prestwich, & Shaffer, 2015).

c) Use of RT for benign conditions must adhere to administration and technical guidelines.

(1) Clinical goals are to target benign disease to achieve clinical remission or cure, as well as to

minimize healthy tissue exposure to decrease risk of RT-induced cancers.

(2) Contemporary RT immobilization coupled with virtual simulation techniques enable expert dosimetry and therapeutic plans.

(3) IGRT and IMRT enhance target conformity.

(4) Quality of RT, total dose, shielding, and depth of dose must be considered.

(5) Long-term risk and benefit profiles and assessment of treatment consequences are vital.

(6) Natural history of benign diagnoses must be considered.

(7) Efficacy of other available treatment modalities must be considered.

(8) Patients must provide informed consent specific to clinical implications and short- and long-term outcomes.

(9) Proton beam therapy is an emerging option for tailored dose distribution that spares healthy tissues.

2. Tissue response

a) Tissue response is a significant predictor of both side effect and therapeutic response of benign targets.

b) Lower RT doses impose less risk in the benign setting.

c) Age, comorbidities, previous RT, and history of radiosensitivity are considered.

d) Benign diagnoses can be treated with both EBRT and brachytherapy.

e) Benign diseases are treated with a low to intermediate dose range (2–40 Gy).

f) Benign tumors are treated with standard RT dose ranges (10–50 Gy).

g) Side effect profiles vary depending on dose and duration.

h) RT field size affects side effect profile.

i) In a benign setting, conformal RT plans are indicated.

j) RT dose, quality, field size, and exposed tissues will affect response.

k) Lower dose lessens the risk and minimizes critical structures.

l) Age and comorbidities must be accounted for when predicting therapeutic response.

3. Overall effects of RT for benign conditions

a) RT will cause a degree of cellular and molecular changes.

b) Effect is related to age, field size, dose per fraction, total dose, and comorbidities.

c) Older patients commonly receive treatment to limbs, causing fewer treatment-related sequelae.

d) If radiosensitive organs are within the RT field, caution must be exercised in patients younger than 40 years old to avoid risk for development of RT-induced malignancies (Taylor et al., 2015).

4. Clinical application

a) Ocular: Graves orbitopathy (thyroid eye disease)

(1) Clinical manifestation

(a) Graves orbitopathy is an inflammatory autoimmune disease characterized by inflammation and edema of orbital tissues and extraocular muscles.

(b) Patients typically present with distorted appearances, reports of "sand" or "granules" in the eyes, excessive tearing, and diplopia.

(c) Eye examinations reveal edema of conjunctiva, retracted eyelids, and proptosis.

(d) A clinical diagnosis is made if the presence of thyroid autoantibodies is detected. Additionally, CT and MRI may be used to assess involvement of extraocular structures.

(e) If the presentation is atypical, biopsy should be considered to rule out lymphoma and other orbital malignancies (Shah, 2018).

(2) Incidence

(a) Graves orbitopathy is a rare clinical finding (3–16 cases per 100,000 people annually).

(b) It is more prevalent in women, with a 5:1 ratio (Kotwal & Stan, 2018).

(c) Graves orbitopathy is commonly associated with hyperthyroidism. It also occurs in the setting of euthyroid or hypothyroidism.

(d) Approximately 10%–15% of cases of Graves orbitopathy are associated with hypothyroidism (Hashimoto thyroiditis), which has an autoimmune association.

(e) Smoking is a risk factor, and smokers experience more severe disease.

(f) Symptoms often begin in childhood; however, it is most commonly diagnosed during middle to late adulthood.

(3) Histologic features

(a) The autoimmune histologic features of Graves orbitopathy may be the result of a phenomenon of shared autoantigens (Godfrey & Kazim, 2018).

(b) Graves orbitopathy is characterized by interstitial edema and T cell–predominant lymphocytic infiltration of the following.

i. Orbital tissues
ii. Periorbital fat
iii. Extraocular muscles
iv. Eyelids
v. Anterior orbital tissues

(c) This inflammatory cascade leads to venous engorgement, diminished drainage of interstitial fluid, periorbital edema, proptosis, and, uncommonly, compression of the optic nerve.

(d) If compression of the optic nerve occurs, irreversible neuronal death and diminished nerve function could result, leading to decreased visual acuity and papillary dysfunction with concomitant constriction of visual fields (Godfrey & Kazim, 2018).

(e) The initial clinical presentation can last a few months followed by slow decline, with symptom improvement up to two years from initial diagnosis.

(f) Avoidance of permanent fibrosis and scarring is the goal of treatment (Shah, 2018).

(4) Clinical management

(a) An interprofessional approach is required and includes medical interventions, surgery, and RT.

(b) Treatment regimens are prescribed according to severity, so not all patients will require every phase of treatment.

(5) Medical management

(a) The initial focus is treatment of underlying hyperthyroidism or hypothyroidism.

(b) Antithyroid drug therapies can be used safely.

(c) Patients should be referred to smoking cessation programs, as smoking may impair intervention.

(d) Mild Graves orbitopathy may be treated with eye lubricants and prisms to control diplopia (Kotwal & Stan, 2018).

(e) Systemic glucocorticoid therapy is the first-line medical treatment for moderate or severe Graves orbitopathy.

(6) Surgical management: If disease is resistant to steroid therapy, then orbital decompression to relieve proptosis and optic neuropathy may be indicated.

(7) RT management

(a) RT is reserved for patients who are symptomatic following a course of high-dose steroids and for those whom steroids are contraindicated.

(b) RT is effective either alone or in combination with other therapies.

i. Underlying thyroid disorders must be treated systemically in addition to locoregional treatment with EBRT (Nicosia et al., 2019).

ii. The goal of RT is to improve orbit mobility, but unfortunately control of exophthalmos is limited.

iii. RT is considered second-line treatment for mild Graves orbitopathy if response to steroids is suboptimal.

iv. Moderate to severe Graves orbitopathy is treated with IV steroids and RT if limited ocular mobility or diplopia is assessed.

(c) RT treatment plans include a CTV encompassing the extraocular muscles and bilateral retro-orbital tissue. The anterior field edge is placed posterior to the lens.

(d) Aquaplast RT™ masks are used for immobilization.

(e) Blocking focuses on sparing the contralateral lens (Kotwal & Stan, 2018).

(f) RT dose is 20 Gy in 10 fractions using small, opposed lateral fields with split beam or five-degree posterior angulation to avoid RT megavoltage dose to the lens.

(g) Data indicate that a lower dose of 10 Gy in 10 fractions over two weeks is equally effective, compared to 20 Gy in 10 fractions over two weeks. RT targeting ocular orbits is generally well tolerated (Nicosia et al., 2019).

(h) Steroids are given concurrently with RT to minimize locoregional side effects.

(i) Studies have documented the risk of radiation-induced malignancy and found no difference in mortality and an absence of intracranial tumors (Nicosia et al., 2019).

(j) Because of the possibility of secondary carcinogenesis, RT should be avoided in treating Graves orbitopathy in patients younger than 35 years (Nicosia et al., 2019).

(k) Contraindications to RT include diabetes mellitus, diabetic retinopathy, and hypertension.

(8) Nursing management

(a) Patient education should focus on the following potential side effects.

i. Cataracts

ii. Radiation retinopathy

iii. Radiation optic neuropathy, either as an acute effect (days to weeks following RT) or late effect (six months to years following completion of RT)

(b) Nurses should reassure patients regarding the precision of contemporary RT planning, fractionation, and administration, which minimizes or eliminates side effects.

b) Skin: keloids

(1) Clinical manifestation

(a) Keloids are benign fibrous growths caused by connective tissue proliferation in response to the following.

i. Surgery

ii. Burns

iii. Trauma

iv. Inflammation

v. Spontaneous occurrence

(b) Keloids are benign, cosmetically disfiguring masses of fibrous tissue that extend beyond wounds and do not regress naturally.

    i. They can present as pruritic and be painful.

    ii. Anatomic regions include areas of increased skin tension, such as the following.
- Sternum
- Back
- Posterior neck
- Ears
- Deltoids
- Anterior chest

(2) Clinical management

(a) Treatment of keloids depends on size, location, and depth of lesion.

(b) Management of keloids has been documented; however, studies often have limitations that compromise clinical outcomes (Nestor et al., 2019).

    i. Intralesional steroid injections inhibit collagen formation.

    ii. Surgical excision to reduce width is recommended only with multimodal therapy because recurrence rates are high (up to 80% in five years) if surgery is used alone.

    iii. Additional adjuvant treatments after surgery (all with limited data regarding control and or recurrence rates) include the following.
- Intralesional interferon
- Cryotherapy
- Ultraviolet irradiation
- Photodynamic therapy
- Laser therapy

(c) RT is used postoperatively with recurrence rates of 7% at 2 years, 16% at 5 years, and 27% at 10 years (Renz et al., 2018).

(d) RT is given with superficial orthovoltage x-rays or with electrons early in postoperative setting (within the first 24 hours).

(e) Single-fraction doses are 5–12 Gy, and fractionated doses are 10–15 Gy in three to five fractions (Sruthi, Chelakkot, Madhavan, Nair, & Dinesh, 2018).

(f) Conformal treatment fields are planned using custom cutouts and low-energy electrons with bolus.

(g) Local control has been reported between 70%–90% and is dose dependent.

(3) RT risks: Minor risk (0.007%) could be linked to development of skin cancer following recommended total dose range of 10–15 Gy (Flickinger, 2011).

(4) Nursing management

(a) Nurses should provide a structured approach for interprofessional team care, including disciplines from RT, PCPs, dermatology, surgery, and other fields.

(b) Dedicated nurse-led keloid clinics can focus on clinical scar management, cosmetic techniques of skin cosmesis, and techniques of skin camouflage.

(c) Patient education can focus on the use of occlusive silicone dressings to reduce scar elevation, erythema, and pruritus.

c) Soft tissue: gynecomastia

(1) Clinical manifestation

(a) Gynecomastia presents as either a unilateral or bilateral benign proliferation of glandular subareolar tissue of the male breast.

(b) It is caused by an imbalance between the stimulatory effect of estrogen and the inhibitory effect of androgen (Baumgarten & Dabaja, 2018).

(c) The most common cause is the use of antiandrogens for prostate cancer.

(d) Gynecomastia causes breasts to be tender and painful.

(e) Approximately 15% of patients receiving luteinizing hormone-releasing agonists may experience gynecomastia (Baumgarten & Dabaja, 2018).

(2) Clinical management

(a) Low-dose RT is effective in preventing and treating gynecomastia.

(b) RT should be administered either prophylactically or if symptoms occur.

(c) Optimal administration is prior to antiandrogens (Aksnessæther et al., 2018).

(d) Electrons are used for shallow depth of dose to the entire breast.

(e) Critical anatomic structures (lungs, heart, and spinal cord) are shielded.

(f) RT is administered as 10–12 Gy in a single fraction, 8–15 Gy in two fractions, or 20 Gy in five fractions.

(g) Tamoxifen can be given with RT and is effective compared to placebo. Tamoxifen alone may be more effective than RT; however, treatment is of long duration and is contraindicated with history of thromboembolic events (Viani, Bernardes da Silva, & Stefano, 2012).

(h) RT side effect profile is minimal (mild acute skin erythema).

(i) The risk of RT-induced skin or breast cancer is low (Aksnessæther et al., 2018).

(3) Nursing management

    (a) Nurses must prepare patients for comprehensive confirming diagnosis including the following.

        i. Assessment: physical examination

        ii. Laboratory tests: testosterone, luteinizing hormone, thyroid-stimulating hormone

        iii. Diagnostic studies: mammography to rule out breast cancer, testicular ultrasonography to rule out testicular cancer, CT to confirm benign gynecomastia

    (b) Patients should be educated regarding the multifaceted plan of care, which may include the following.

        i. Watchful waiting, medical or surgical intervention, and pharmacologic agents (tamoxifen)

        ii. Preparatory education during preassessment of RT immobilization, simulation, target verification, dose calculation, verification, and administration

        iii. Side effect management focused on skin care (erythema)

        iv. Psychosocial support for body image dissatisfaction, reduced self-esteem, and associated anxiety and depression

d) CNS

    (1) Cerebral AVM

    (a) Clinical manifestation (Wilke & Chung, 2020)

        i. Cerebral AVM is a congenital cerebral vascular lesion characterized by abnormal blood vessel formation.

        ii. It commonly presents as intracranial hemorrhage and neurologic deficit.

        iii. Average risk of intracranial hemorrhage is 2%–4%.

        iv. It can also manifest as seizure, headache, or sudden death.

        v. It can be detected incidentally on routine MRI screening.

        vi. Incidence of cerebral AVM is approximately 1 per 100,000.

    (b) Clinical management (Joshi et al., 2016)

        i. Options for management of cerebral AVM include observation, surgical resection, SRS, and endovascular embolization.

        ii. The focus of clinical intervention is to treat the abnormal formation of blood vessels (nidus) that forms the AVM.

        iii. Observation minimizes morbidity and mortality associated with intervention; however, risk of hemorrhage remains.

        iv. Surgical resection of the AVM carries variable risks and is dependent upon size and location.

        v. Surgery is definitive for diminishing associated risk of cerebral bleeding.

        vi. SRS is considered for small deformities that are not surgically accessible.

        vii. SRS may be used alone if patient-associated morbidities preclude surgery; however, risk of bleeding remains.

        viii. Embolization is used in conjunction with other modalities. Presurgical embolization reduces the risk of postoperative bleeding.

        ix. Management requires an interprofessional team: neurology, neurosurgery, interventional radiology, and medical and radiation oncology.

        x. Prior to choosing treatment options, patients must be assessed by age, performance status, comorbidities, and anatomic location of the AVM.

    (c) SRS management

        i. The goal of SRS is to deliver a single fraction of high-dose RT to a stereotactically defined small volume to sclerose the AVM and prevent hemorrhage.

        ii. The target must include all feeder vessels.

        iii. SRS can be delivered using proton or photon beams, with a linear accelerator, Gamma Knife®, or CyberKnife®.

        iv. SRS is more effective with smaller AVMs (less than 3 cm).

        v. Conventional RT is inferior to SRS.

        vi. Complications are rare and depend on treated target volume.

        vii. Radiation dose is 15–30 Gy in a single fraction.

        viii. The dose must correlate with best chance of obliterating the nidus.

        ix. Dose is tailored to the target size; doses greater than 16 Gy are considered therapeutic (Chen et al., 2019).

        x. Obliteration rates vary (60%–90%). Risk of hemorrhage prevails after SRS.

xi. Patients require long-term RT and neurosurgical follow-up (Ding et al., 2019).

(d) Nursing management

    i. Nurses should educate patients about the trajectory of SRS, as well as rationale, immobilization, and virtual planning.

    ii. Patients should understand side effects, such as abscopal effect of RT, fatigue, and scalp dermatitis, as well as steroid side effects.

    iii. Nurses should stress the importance of interprofessional follow-up.

    iv. End-of-treatment instructions should include follow-up appointments and reporting of symptoms such as headaches, visual changes, fatigue, light-headedness, and ataxia.

(2) Acoustic neuroma (vestibular schwannoma)

(a) Clinical manifestation

    i. Acoustic neuromas are benign intracranial brain tumors arising from Schwann cells of vestibule-cochlear nerve cells of cranial nerve VIII of the inner ear canal.

    ii. Clinical symptoms include hearing loss, headache, tinnitus, and ataxia.

    iii. Brain stem encroachment can occur with impingement on cranial nerves V and VII.

    iv. Hydrocephalus can occur as a late complication (Kittel & Suh, 2018).

    v. Incidence is approximately 1 per 100,000 (Babu et al., 2013).

    vi. Average age at diagnosis is 40 years.

    vii. MRI will yield diagnosis; therefore, biopsy is not necessary.

    viii. As a tumor enlarges, it occupies a portion of the cerebellopontine angle with possible extension into the extracanalicular spaces (DeLong, Kaylie, Kranz, & Adamson, 2011).

(b) Clinical management

    i. Acoustic neuromas display varied growth patterns. Tumors within the auditory canal typically grow slowly, and those near the cerebellopontine angle grow more quickly and may result in more rapid and permanent hearing loss.

    ii. Microsurgical removal of the acoustic neuroma with curative intent is the most effective intervention to preserve hearing and control associated symptoms.

    iii. Watchful waiting is possible if the tumor is small and indolent.

    iv. Small- to medium-sized tumors are assessed with MRI and audiology examinations.

    v. Indications for treatment include brain stem compression.

    vi. Local control can be achieved by surgery or RT.

    vii. Patients require long-term follow-up to assess regrowth.

(c) SRS management

    i. Single-fraction SRS is an established modality to treat acoustic neuroma.

    ii. A standard dose of 12 Gy provides local control rates of greater than 90% at 10 years, with low involvement of facial or trigeminal nerve side effects (Przybylowski et al., 2019).

    iii. SRS contours the target volume of the acoustic neuroma, along with adjacent healthy structures (eyes, optic nerves, and brain stem).

    iv. Fusion of CT and MRI is used to optimize a single-fraction treatment plan of 12–14 Gy (minimum dose range for acoustic neuroma).

    v. Higher doses of 16–20 Gy may provide greater long-term control; however, morbidity associated with facial nerve damage is more prevalent (Tucker et al., 2019).

    vi. Patients may experience mild facial edema with resolution after treatment.

    vii. Fractionated RT (45–56 Gy in 1.8–2 Gy fractions) has the potential advantage of improved hearing and brain stem preservation when treating larger tumors (Kharod, Herman, Amdur, & Mendenhall, 2018).

(d) Nursing management

    i. Nurses assess extent of hearing deficit.

    ii. Developmental age and concomitant comorbidities must be considered.

    iii. Tumor size should be considered because larger tumors may impinge on critical structures and cause increased side effects, hence more monitoring.

    iv. Nurses should consider patient ability to self-manage and report untoward effects or related treatment.

    v. Nurses must consider patient access to available treatment options.

(e) Long-term side effects

    i. RT imposes the possibility of malignant transformation adjacent to the brain.

    ii. Risks must be balanced against permanent surgical and RT complications.

(3) Meningiomas

  (a) Clinical manifestation (Pan, Yeboa, & Sulman, 2020)

    i. Meningiomas are well-defined and slow growing (unless anaplastic). They arise from mesodermal arachnoid cells.

    ii. World Health Organization estimates that 90% of meningiomas are grade I; 5% are grade II; and 3% are grade III.

    iii. Meningiomas account for 20%–30% of primary brain tumors.

    iv. Incidence increases with age, and women are more commonly diagnosed.

  (b) Risk factors: The following increase risk of meningiomas (Ostrom et al., 2015).

    i. RT during childhood with long latency

    ii. Genetic risk factors associated with neurofibromatosis

    iii. Hormonal vulnerability detected during reproductive years in women, with markers for progesterone, androgen, and estrogen receptors

  (c) Management of grade I meningiomas

    i. Watchful waiting is conducted with MRI surveillance.

    ii. Surgery is the favored option if a patient is symptomatic.

    iii. The goals of surgery are complete resection and a low level of morbidity.

    iv. Location predicts success rates of full resection.

    v. Meningiomas arising in the base of the skull may not be resectable. RT is initiated as an alternative or in the adjuvant setting (Rogers et al., 2015).

    vi. EBRT can be given postoperatively for newly diagnosed totally resected grade 2 or recurrent grade 1 meningioma irrespective of resection extent, with significant tumor control and minimum toxicity. Dose range is 50–55 Gy (1.8–2 Gy per fraction). (Rogers et al., 2018).

    vii. CT simulation is used with 3DCRT and IMRT.

    viii. Contouring is challenging and depends on immobilization and position verification.

    ix. SRS is recommended for small grade 1 meningiomas (less than 3–4 cm).

    x. SRS can be used as adjuvant treatment for unresectable meningiomas and for low-volume postoperative recurrence.

    xi. SRS dose range is 14–15 Gy for long-term control with diminished toxicity (Wegner et al., 2019).

    xii. No trials have compared efficacy of fractionated EBRT with SRS.

    xiii. Conformal EBRT yields superb tumor control with larger meningiomas (Islim et al., 2019).

  (d) Management of grade 2–3 meningiomas

    i. Grade 2–3 meningiomas are atypical malignant meningiomas with rare presentations.

    ii. Randomized trials comparing efficacy of surgery, EBRT, and stereotactic RT have not been conducted.

    iii. Tumor characteristics, location, and patient performance status are key factors in developing a therapeutic interprofessional approach to achieve tumor control and avoid long-term sequelae.

  (e) Nursing management

    i. Long-term side effects of EBRT (dose range 50–60 Gy) include radiation-induced cancer (malignant meningioma), and this risk increases with dose and volume.

    ii. RT to the head imposes a small risk of skin cancer to the scalp (commonly benign basal cell).

    iii. Patient education to address these possible but rare risks must be prioritized during patient trajectory of care.

e) Orthopedic and musculoskeletal: heterotopic ossification

  (1) Clinical manifestation

    (a) Heterotopic ossification is a benign complication of proliferation of mature bone in extraskeletal soft tissues following skeletal trauma, such as total hip replacement, bone fracture, and CNS injury.

    (b) The exact physiologic process is unknown. It is hypothesized that new bone formation may arise from the differentiation of bone cells into osteoblastic stem cells. This process causes soft tissues surrounding joints to ossify and transform into mature bone.

(c) Heterotopic ossification is a rare complication following hip arthroplasty. It occurs around the femoral neck adjacent to the greater trochanter (Amar, Sharfman, & Rath, 2015).

(d) It can present in a variety of joints following soft tissue trauma; medullary or brain lesions; or hip, knee, elbow, and shoulder fractures, as well as during postsurgical revisions.

(e) Prevention is important for those predisposed with history of hypertrophic osteoarthritis or high-risk skeletal disease.

(f) Clinical signs include the following.
   i. Cardinal signs: joint stiffness and pain
   ii. Advanced disease: inflammation, fever, erythema, swelling, warmth, tenderness, and impaired range of motion
   iii. Wound or prosthetic joint infection

(g) Diagnosis of hip heterotopic ossification is by an anteroposterior radiograph of the pelvis and hip.

(h) The Brooker classification of heterotopic ossification at the hip joint defines classes 1–4. This is a clinical paradigm for characterizing subjective radiographic findings (Hug, Alton, & Gee, 2015).

(2) Clinical management

(a) Surgical revision is the treatment of choice, but high recurrence rates are limiting.

(b) Providing time after trauma permits bone maturation and decreased inflammation.

(c) High-risk patients must be identified preoperatively.

(d) Prevention must be initiated within 24–48 hours postoperatively.

(e) Patients at risk for heterotopic ossification must be treated with an interprofessional team approach involving orthopedics, primary care, radiation oncology, and rheumatology.

(3) RT management

(a) RT is used in conjunction with NSAIDs to manage pain and recurrence.
   i. NSAIDs inhibit inflammatory response.
   ii. Indomethacin is currently standard treatment in this setting. Side effects include gastric irritation, bleeding, and renal and hepatic enzyme elevation (Adams, 2014).
   iii. Ibuprofen and cyclooxygenase-2 inhibitors are also prescribed; however, bleeding and cardiac toxicities

must be considered (Lavernia, Contreras, Villa, & Rossi, 2014).
   iv. RT with NSAIDs is indicated to prevent heterotopic ossification in those at risk following total hip replacement.
   v. Clinical outcomes with NSAIDs without concurrent RT are inferior.

(b) The plan of choice is single dose of 7–8 Gy targeted through anteroposterior and posteroanterior fields with inclusion of the soft tissue surrounding the hip joint.

(c) Lower total doses of RT (7–8 Gy) given within three to four days after surgery is effective. A single fraction of 7 Gy is superior to increased doses and more fractions (Shah, 2018).

(d) The radiobiologic principle that guides the use of RT is to reduce the formation of ectopic bone by targeting osteoprogenitor cells and inhibiting bone protein signal pathways.

(e) RT is indicated for patients older than 50 years.

(f) RT timing is either four hours preoperatively or 72 hours postoperatively.
   i. In a trial comparing preoperative RT of 7 Gy in a single fraction administered within four hours of surgery to a postoperative dose of 17.5 Gy in five fractions within 72 hours of surgery, researchers found that the postoperative RT was more effective (Kumar & Wilke, 2020).
   ii. Timing of postoperative RT administration is challenging because of positional variance requirements of prosthetic hip joint pain control.

(g) RT can be offered to treat heterotopic ossification of other joints; however, data on efficacy are limited.

(4) Nursing management

(a) Radiation oncology nurses interface with the interprofessional team to navigate patients and support a multipronged approach for management.

(b) Radiation oncology nurses coordinate with patients throughout the entire course of care and with each subspecialty.

(c) Patients with heterotopic ossification are treated with a short course of RT. Therefore, it is vital that comprehensive care occurs to ensure a patient's short- and long-term follow-up.

(d) Patient education focusing on interventions to control heterotopic ossification must be offered.

References

Adams, L. (2014). Heterotopic ossification. *Radiation Therapist, 23*(1), 27–48.

Aksnessæther, B.Y., Solberg, A., Klepp, O.H., Mykelbust, T.Å., Skovlund, E., Hoff, S.R., ... Lund, J.-Å. (2018). Does prophylactic radiation therapy to avoid gynecomastia in patients with prostate cancer increase the risk of breast cancer? *International Journal of Radiation Oncology, Biology, Physics, 101,* 211–216. https://doi.org/10.1016/j.ijrobp.2018.01.096

Amar, E., Sharfman, Z.T., & Rath, E. (2015). Heterotopic ossification after hip arthroscopy. *Journal of Hip Preservation Surgery, 2,* 355–363. https://doi.org/10.1093/jhps/hnv052

Babu, R., Sharma, R., Bagley, J.H., Hatef, J., Friedman, A.H., & Adamson, C. (2013). Vestibular schwannomas in the modern era: Epidemiology, treatment trends, and disparities in managment. *Journal of Neurosurgery, 119,* 121–130. https://doi.org/10.3171/2013.1.jns121370

Baumgarten, L., & Dabaja, A.A. (2018). Diagnosis and management of gynecomastia for urologists. *Current Urology Reports, 19,* 46. https://doi.org/10.1007/s11934-018-0796-x

Chen, C.-J., Kearns, K.N., Ding, D., Kano, H., Mathieu, D., Kondziolka, D., ... Sheehan, J.P. (2019). Stereotactic radiosurgery for arteriovenous malformations of the basal ganglia and thalamus: An international multicenter study. *Journal of Neurosurgery, 132,* 122–131. https://doi.org/10.3171/2018.8.jns182106

DeLong, M., Kaylie, D., Kranz, P.G., & Adamson, D.C. (2011). Vestibular schwannomas: Lessons for the neurosurgeon: Part I: Diagnosis, neuroimaging, and audiology. *Contemporary Neurosurgery, 33,* 1–5. https://doi.org/10.1097/01.cne.0000408560.95604.48

Ding, D., Chen, C.-J., Starke, R.M., Kano, H., Lee, J.Y.K., Mathieu, D., ... Sheehan, J.P. (2019). Risk of brain arteriovenous malformation hemorrhage before and after stereotactic radiosurgery: A multicenter study. *Stroke, 50,* 1384–1391. https://doi.org/10.1161/strokeaha.118.024230

Flickinger, J.C. (2011). A radiobiological analysis of multicenter data for postoperative keloid radiotherapy. *International Journal Radiation Oncology, Biology, Physics, 79,* 1164–1170. https://doi.org/10.1016/j.ijrobp.2009.12.019

Godfrey, K.J., & Kazim, M. (2018). Radiotherapy for active thyroid eye disease. *Ophthalmic Plastic and Reconstructive Surgery, 34*(Suppl. 1), S98–S104. https://doi.org/10.1097/iop.0000000000001074

Hug, K.T., Alton, T.B., & Gee, A.O. (2015). Brooker classification of heterotopic ossification after total hip arthroplasty. *Clinical Orthopaedics and Related Research, 473,* 2154–2157. https://doi.org/10.1007/s11999-014-4076-x

Islim, A.I., Mohan, M., Moon, R.D.C., Srikandarajah, N., Mills, S.J., Brodbelt, A.R., & Jenkinson, M.D. (2019). Incidental intracranial meningiomas: A systematic review and meta-analysis of prognostic factors and outcomes. *Journal of Neuro-Oncology, 142,* 211–221. https://doi.org/10.1007/s11060-019-03104-3

Joshi, N.P., Shah, C., Kotecha, R., Murphy, E.S., Chao, S.T., Rasmussen, P.A., & Suh, J.H. (2016). Contemporary management of large-volume arteriovenous malformations: A clinician's review. *Journal of Radiation Oncology, 5,* 239–248. https://doi.org/10.1007/s13566-016-0261-8

Kharod, S.M., Herman, M.P., Amdur, R.J., & Mendenhall, W.M. (2018). Fractionated radiation therapy for benign nonacoustic schwannomas. *American Journal of Clinical Oncology, 41,* 13–17. https://doi.org/10.1097/COC.0000000000000219

Kittel, J., & Suh, J. (2018). Vestibular schwannoma. In M.C. Ward, R.D. Tendulkar, & G.M.M. Videtic (Eds.), *Essentials of clinical radiation oncology* (pp. 50–57). Springer.

Kotwal, A., & Stan, M. (2018). Current and future treatments for Graves' disease and Graves' ophthalmopathy. *Hormone and Metabolic Research, 50,* 871–886. https://doi.org/10.1055/a-0739-8134

Kumar, R., & Wilke, C. (2020). Heterotopic ossification. In C. Tang & A. Farooqi (Eds.), *Pocket radiation oncology* (pp. 13–14). Wolters Kluwer.

Lavernia, C.J., Contreras, J.S., Villa, J.M., & Rossi, M.D. (2014). Celecoxib and heterotopic bone formation after total hip arthroplasty. *Journal of Arthroplasty, 29,* 390–392. https://doi.org/10.1016/j.arth.2013.06.039

Nestor, M.S., Berman, B., Goldberg, D., Cognetta, A.B., Jr., Gold, M., Roth, W., ... Glick, B. (2019). Consensus guidelines on the use of superficial radiation therapy for treating nonmelanoma skin cancers and keloids. *Journal of Clinical and Aesthetic Dermatology, 12*(2), 12–18.

Nicosia, L., Reverberi, C., Agolli, L., Marinelli, L., De Sanctis, V., Minniti, G., ... Osti, M.F. (2019). Orbital radiotherapy plus concomitant steroids in moderate-to-severe Graves' ophthalmopathy: Good results after long-term follow-up. *International Journal of Endocrinology and Metabolism, 17,* e84427. https://doi.org/10.5812/ijem.84427

Ostrom, Q., Gittleman, H., Fulop, J., Liu, M., Blanda, R., Kromer, C., ... Barnholtz-Sloan, J.S. (2015). CBTRUS statistical report: Primary brain and central nervous system tumors diagnosed in the United States in 2008–2012. *Neuro-Oncology, 17*(Suppl. 4), iv1–iv62. https://doi.org/10.1093/neuonc/nov189

Pan, H.Y., Yeboa, D.N., & Sulman, E.P. (2020). Meningioma. In C. Tang & A. Farooqi (Eds.), *Pocket radiation oncology: The MD Anderson Cancer Center handbook of radiation oncology* (e-book). Wolters Kluwer.

Przybylowski, C.J., Baranoski, J.F., Paisan, G.M., Chapple, K.M., Meeusen, A.J., Sorenson, S., ... Porter, R.W. (2019). Cyberknife radiosurgery for acoustic neuromas: Tumor control and clinical outcomes. *Journal of Clinical Neuroscience, 63,* 72–76. https://doi.org/10.1016/j.jocn.2019.01.046

Renz, P., Hasan, S., Gresswell, S., Hajjar, R.T., Trombetta, M., & Fontanesi, J. (2018). Dose effect in adjuvant radiation therapy for the treatment of resected keloids. *International Journal of Radiation Oncology, Biology, Physics, 102,* 149–154. https://doi.org/10.1016/j.ijrobp.2018.05.027

Rogers, L., Barani, I., Chamberlain, M., Kaley, T.J., McDermott, M., Raizer, J., ... Vogelbaum, M.A. (2015). Meningiomas: Knowledge base, treatment outcomes, and uncertainties. A RANO review. *Journal of Neurosurgery, 122,* 4–23. https://doi.org/10.3171/2014.7.jns131644

Rogers, L., Zhang, P., Vogelbaum, M.A., Perry, A., Ashby, L.S., Modi, J.M., ... Mehta, M.P. (2018). Intermediate-risk meningioma: Initial outcomes from NRG Oncology RTOG 0539. *Journal of Neurosurgery, 129,* 35–47. https://doi.org/10.3171/2016.11.jns161170

Shah, C. (2018). Radiation therapy for benign disease. In M.C. Ward, R.D. Tendulkar, & G.M.M. Videtic (Eds.), *Essentials of clinical radiation oncology* (pp. 614–618). Springer. https://doi.org/10.1891/9780826168559

Sruthi, K., Chelakkot, P.G., Madhavan, R., Nair, R.R., & Dinesh, M. (2018). Single-fraction radiation: A promising adjuvant therapy to prevent keloid recurrence. *Journal of Cancer Research and Therapeutics, 14,* 1251–1255. https://doi.org/10.4103/jcrt.jcrt_20_17

Taylor, R., Hatfield, P., McKeown, S., Prestwich, R., & Shaffer, R. (2015). *A review of the use of radiotherapy in the UK for the treatment of benign clinical conditions and benign tumours.* Royal College of Radiologists. https://www.rcr.ac.uk/system/files/publication/field_publication_files/BFCO%2815%291_RTBenigndisease_web.pdf

Tucker, D.W., Gogia, A.S., Donoho, D.A., Yim, B., Yu, C., Fredrickson, V.L., ... Giannotta, S.L. (2019). Long-term tumor control rates following Gamma Knife radiosurgery for acoustic neuroma. *World Neurosurgery, 122,* 366–371. https://doi.org/10.1016/j.wneu.2018.11.009

Viani, G., Bernardes da Silva, L., & Stefano, E. (2012). Prevention of gynecomastia and breast pain caused by androgen deprivation therapy in prostate cancer: Tamoxifen or radiotherapy? *International Journal of Radiation Oncology, Biology, Physics, 83,* e519–e524. https://doi.org/10.1016/j.ijrobp.2012.01.036

Wegner, R.E., Hasan, S., Abel, S., Anderson, S., Fuhrer, R., Williamson, R.W., & Karlovits, S.M. (2019). Linear accelerator-based stereotactic radiotherapy for low-grade meningiomas: Improved local control with hypofractionation. *Journal of Central Nervous System Disease, 11,* 1179573519843880. https://doi.org/10.1177/1179573519843880

Wilke, C., & Chung, C. (2020). Benign CNS. In C. Tang & A. Farooqi (Eds.), *Pocket radiation oncology* (pp. 3–14). Wolters Kluwer.

VII. Oncologic Emergencies: Spinal Cord Compression and Superior Vena Cava Syndrome

A. Overview

1. A number of conditions are considered oncologic emergencies, including febrile neutropenia, hypercalcemia, cardiac tamponade, tumor lysis syndrome, syndrome of inappropriate antidiuretic hormone, and pericardial effusions, among others.
2. RT only has a role in treating spinal cord compression and SVCS.

B. Spinal cord compression

1. Introduction
   a) Spinal cord compression associated with malignancy is a grave oncologic emergency that requires prompt recognition and intervention to preserve a patient's functional independence and quality of life and prevent permanent neurologic deficits and paralysis.
   b) The most common cause of cord compression is metastatic disease that extends into the epidural space and impinges on the spinal cord or cauda equina. This is known as epidural spinal cord compression (ESCC) (Gucalp & Dutcher, 2018; Laufer, Schiff, Kelly, & Bilsky, 2019).
   c) ESCC typically occurs in patients with advanced cancer, but in approximately 20% of cases, it is the initial manifestation of malignancy (Kaplan, 2018; Lawton et al., 2019; Rucker, 2018).
   d) Prevalence of ESCC is expected to increase as advances in cancer therapies extend life expectancies and increase the potential for metastatic disease recurrence.
   e) The median length of survival after a diagnosis of ESCC is approximately six months (Laufer, Bilsky, Schiff, & Brown, 2019).
   f) Acute-onset back pain in patients with a history of cancer is highly suspicious for ESCC (New, 2019; Viets-Upchurch, 2016).
   g) Without treatment, symptoms follow a progression from back pain to motor weakness, sensory deficits, impairment of bowel and bladder function, loss of reflexes, and, ultimately, irreversible paralysis (Kaplan, 2018).
   h) RT techniques play a key role in treating this potentially life-threatening complication.
2. Incidence
   a) ESCC occurs in 5%–14% of patients with cancer during the course of their disease (Rucker, 2018).
   b) The annual incidence of symptomatic ESCC requiring patient hospitalization is approximately 3%–5% of patients with terminal cancer (Laufer, Schiff, et al., 2019).
   c) Malignancies most frequently associated with risk of ESCC are solid tumors that often metastasize to bone, such as cancers of the breast, lung, and prostate, which together account for 60% of all ESCC cases (Brock, Toale, & Tummala, 2016; Kaplan, 2018).
      (1) Multiple myeloma accounts for 10%–15% of cases (Weinstein, 2013).
      (2) Other cancers associated with increased risk are kidney cancer, lymphomas, and cancers of unknown origin.
      (3) Figure 20 presents a list of cancers most often associated with ESCC.
   d) In the pediatric population, sarcomas, especially Ewing sarcoma, and neuroblastomas are the most frequent causes of ESCC, followed by germ cell neoplasms and Hodgkin lymphoma (Laufer, Schiff, et al., 2019).
3. Pathophysiology
   a) Three pathologic mechanisms involving the spinal column are associated with development of ESCC.
      (1) The most common mechanism (responsible for 85%–90% of cases) is the presence of metastatic disease in vertebral bone that expands into the epidural space and compresses the spinal cord and its blood supply, leading to vasogenic edema and progressive destruction in the spinal cord (Gucalp & Dutcher, 2018; Kaplan, 2018).
      (2) Less frequently (10%–15% of cases), a malignant tumor erodes vertebral bone and causes bone fragments to collapse into the epidural space, resulting in mechanical compression of the spinal cord and its blood supply. This mechanism is most commonly associated with ESCC occurring in patients with multiple myeloma (Weinstein, 2013).
      (3) The least common mechanism associated with development of ESCC is compression of the spinal cord by direct extension of tumor or a paraspinal lymph node through openings between vertebrae into the epidural space. This may occur in patients with lung cancer, lymphoma, or retroperitoneal sarcoma (Gucalp & Dutcher, 2018).
   b) Hematogenous spread of tumor cells from the primary tumor to vertebral bone marrow through the

---

FIGURE 20. Cancers Associated With Increased Risk for Epidural Spinal Cord Compression

- Breast cancer
- Hodgkin lymphoma
- Lung cancer
- Multiple myeloma
- Non-Hodgkin lymphoma
- Prostate cancer
- Renal carcinoma
- Unknown primary

Note. Based on information from Kaplan, 2018; Lawton et al., 2019; Weinstein, 2013.

Batson low-pressure venous plexus is the most common route of metastasis to the spinal column (Borke, 2019; New, 2019).

    c) The volume of bone in each area of the spine influences the distribution of cord compression. The thoracic spine, which contains the greatest amount of vertebral bone, is most frequently involved with ESCC, accounting for 70% of cases, followed by the lumbar spine (20%), and the cervical spine (10%) (Gucalp & Dutcher, 2018; Laufer, Schiff, et al., 2019).

    d) At initial diagnosis, more than one level of the spinal cord compression is present in approximately 30% of patients with ESCC (Borke, 2019). This is seen most frequently in patients with breast or prostate cancer (Gucalp & Dutcher, 2018).

4. Clinical presentation and symptoms

    a) Presenting signs and symptoms of ESCC vary with the location and severity of the compression but generally follow a similar sequence in all patients that begins with acute back pain.

    b) Back pain is the presenting symptom in 90% of patients with ESCC (Borke, 2019; Gucalp & Dutcher, 2018; Laufer, Schiff, et al., 2019).

        (1) Pain localized over the area of the cord compression is the most common initial symptom.

            (a) It is described as a constant dull ache.

            (b) Pain intensity is greatest upon awakening and in the supine position.

            (c) Until proven otherwise, this type of pain should be considered to be caused by malignancy.

        (2) Radicular pain that radiates into the extremities or across the chest or abdomen is less common. This type of pain may be described as a dull ache, a burning and shooting pain, or a tight band across the chest or abdomen.

        (3) Local and radicular pain are exacerbated by actions that increase the intra-abdominal or intrathoracic pressure, such as coughing, sneezing, and straining at stool (Valsalva maneuver).

        (4) Referred pain is difficult to localize because it involves multiple dermatomes and is experienced at an area distant from the site of cord compression (see Figure 21).

    c) Motor weakness is the second most common symptom at presentation. It is present in 85% of patients at time of diagnosis and follows pain by weeks to months (Al-Qurainy & Collis, 2016; Viets-Upchurch, 2016).

        (1) The association of motor weakness with ESCC may be missed because weakness is common in patients with advanced cancer.

        (2) Weakness generally begins in the legs regardless of the level of cord compression.

            (a) Weakness may be described as leg stiffness or heaviness.

            (b) Difficulty climbing stairs or rising from the toilet may be reported.

    d) Sensory loss follows motor weakness and is present in 50%–60% of patients at diagnosis, and manifestations depend on the level and degree of cord compression (Weinstein, 2013).

        (1) Loss of sensation of touch, pinprick, temperature, and vibration, as well as position sense, may occur early (Borke, 2019).

        (2) Numbness may be present in the toes bilaterally, ascending upward in a stocking-like fashion over time (Al-Qurainy & Collis, 2016; Weinstein, 2013).

        (3) Loss of sensation in the "saddle" area (buttocks and perineal region) reflects compression of the cauda equina and is known as *saddle anesthesia* (Dawodu et al., 2018).

        (4) Rapid onset of sensory and motor symptoms in combination is highly suspicious for ESCC (Al-Qurainy & Collis, 2016).

FIGURE 21. Types of Pain Associated With Epidural Spinal Cord Compression

Local Pain
- Definition: pain perceived within one to two spinal segments of the cord compression
- Location: back pain is localized near the midline near the site of the cord compression
- Quality: constant dull ache; may be worse in the morning; increases in intensity over time
- Exacerbating factors: reclining position; actions that increase intra-abdominal and intrathoracic pressures (e.g., coughing sneezing, straining at stool, Valsalva maneuver)
- Relieving factors: sitting or standing positions; sleeping upright

Radicular Pain
- Definition: radiating pain triggered by compression of spinal nerve roots or the cauda equina
- Location: pain radiates in a band-like pattern from back to front across the chest or abdomen, or down an extremity along dermatomes supplied by the affected nerve roots
- Quality: varies; may be constant dull ache that is difficult to localize or an easy-to-localize sharp shooting pain provoked by movement of the spine
- Exacerbating factors: movement, coughing, sneezing, Valsalva maneuver, reclining position
- Relieving factors: sitting or standing positions

Referred Pain
- Definition: pain that is perceived in an area distant from the site of spinal cord compression
- Location: pain is poorly localized due to involvement of multiple dermatomes
- Examples: Compression at first lumbar vertebra: pain may be experienced in the iliac crests, hips, or sacroiliac region. Compression at seventh cervical vertebra: pain may be referred to the area between the scapulae

Note. From "Back Pain: Is It Spinal Cord Compression?" by M. Kaplan, 2009, *Clinical Journal of Oncology Nursing, 13,* p. 594 (https://doi.org/10.1188/09 .CJON.592-595). Copyright 2009 by Oncology Nursing Society. Reprinted with permission.

e) Autonomic dysfunction is a common late finding in patients with ESCC and is associated with a poor prognosis (Gucalp & Dutcher, 2018).

(1) Bladder dysfunction, with urinary retention and incontinence, occurs most commonly.

 (a) It may be present in more than 50% of patients at diagnosis (Weinstein, 2013).

 (b) In older adults, urinary retention is a more reliable indicator of autonomic dysfunction than urinary incontinence, which can occur with increasing age (Kaplan, 2018).

(2) Bowel dysfunction results from loss of anal sphincter control and perineal sensation. Difficulty expelling stool may progress to constipation and fecal incontinence (Rucker, 2018).

(3) Newly onset impotence may be reported in men (Dawodu et al., 2018).

(4) Horner syndrome (drooping eyelid, constricted pupil, and decreased sweating on the affected side of the face) may occur with spinal cord injury at the junction of the cervical and thoracic spines (Kaplan, 2018).

(5) Autonomic hyperreflexia may occur when the spinal cord injury is located at or above the level of the sixth or seventh thoracic vertebrae.

 (a) Autonomic hyperreflexia is a medical emergency.

 (b) The following symptoms present above the level of cord compression and can be triggered by a distended bladder or bowel (Lin & Avila, 2017; Stephenson & Berliner, 2020).

 i. Pounding headache
 ii. Bradycardia
 iii. Extreme hypertension
 iv. Nasal congestion
 v. Profuse sweating
 vi. Facial flushing
 vii. Pilomotor erection (goose bumps)

5. Prognostic factors for functional and survival outcomes

a) Early diagnosis and intervention are crucial to maximizing patient outcomes because a longer time that ESCC goes untreated correlates to lower chances of neurologic recovery.

b) Patients with ESCC caused by radiosensitive tumors (myeloma, lymphoma, breast, prostate) have a better prognosis than those with radioresistant tumors (lung, renal, colon, sarcoma, bladder) (Kaplan, 2018).

c) Ability to walk at presentation is the single most important predictor of functional outcome and survival. Without timely treatment, difficulty walking can rapidly progress to irreversible paralysis (New, 2019; Weinstein, 2013).

d) After completing RT, 80% of patients who are ambulatory at presentation remain able to walk. Less than

50% of those who are nonambulatory at diagnosis will regain ambulation, and few will be alive at one year (New, 2019; Weinstein, 2013).

6. Diagnosis

a) Patient history

(1) History should comprise detailed information about known cancer history and cancer risk factors, as well as description of newly onset back pain and preexisting pain conditions.

(2) Independent predictors of risk for ESCC have been reported, including the following (Lu, Gonzalez, Jolesz, Wen, & Talcott, 2005).

 (a) Pain in the middle or upper back
 (b) Known vertebral metastases
 (c) Presence of metastatic disease at initial presentation

b) Physical examination

(1) Examination focuses on a detailed neurologic and pain evaluation.

(2) Pain induced by straight leg raising, neck flexion, or vertebral percussion may help to determine the level of cord compression (Gucalp & Dutcher, 2018).

c) Imaging studies (Brock et al., 2016; Laufer, Schiff, et al., 2019; New, 2019)

(1) MRI is the gold standard for detecting ESCC. It has a 93% sensitivity and 97% specificity ratio, as well as a 95% accuracy rate in distinguishing between benign and malignant causes of vertebral body collapse.

(2) MRI is performed without delay on anyone with suspected ESCC. The entire spine is imaged to detect all levels of compression and to provide treatment planning information for radiation oncologists and surgeons.

(3) CT myelography is reserved for patients who are unable to have an MRI (e.g., those with metallic implants, severe claustrophobia, or who cannot lie still for prolonged periods). CT myelography can also be used in treatment planning for radiosurgery.

(4) Plain film radiography of the spine has no role in the diagnosis of ESCC. It has a low sensitivity and specificity and is associated with false-negative results that can delay diagnosis.

7. Treatment decisions

a) The overall treatment goal, considering a patient's disease prognosis, is to optimize quality of life through the following (Kaplan, 2018).

(1) Relieving pain
(2) Palliating symptoms
(3) Preventing permanent disability
(4) Preserving or recovering motor and sphincter function
(5) Providing local tumor control
(6) Extending the active portion of remaining life

b) Optimal management of ESCC is an interprofessional effort. Consultation with radiation oncology and neurosurgery should occur within 24 hours of ESCC diagnosis (Lawton et al., 2019).

c) Treatment approaches are divided into initial supportive therapies (using corticosteroids and pain medications), followed by definitive therapies (RT or surgery, alone or in combination, and possibly chemotherapy) to decompress the spine and restore spinal stability (Kaplan, 2018).

d) The NOMS framework (neurologic, oncologic, mechanical stability, and systemic disease) is an individualized clinical decision-making framework for selecting appropriate primary treatment approaches that incorporates the four categories of patient factors. This framework allows for standardized assessment of metastatic spine tumors and for the incorporation of evidence-based interventions (Barzilai et al., 2017; Laufer et al., 2013).

   (1) The neurologic component evaluates the degree of spinal cord compression and the presence of functional deficits, based on clinical symptoms and MRI results.

   (2) The oncologic component assesses the radiosensitivity of tumors. Breast, prostate, ovarian, and neuroendocrine cancers are commonly radiosensitive, and renal cancer, thyroid cancer, colon cancer, NSCLC, sarcoma, and melanoma are radioresistant. The neurologic and oncologic assessments are combined to determine the optimal radiation strategy to achieve tumor control and the need for a surgical intervention.

   (3) The mechanical stability component evaluates presence of spinal instability and need for stabilization with bone cement or surgical intervention.

   (4) The systemic disease component incorporates disease prognosis, estimated life expectancy, and likelihood of tolerating the treatment.

8. Collaborative management

  a) Corticosteroids

   (1) Steroids are administered immediately to all patients with neurologic symptoms or pain, even before imaging confirmation of ESCC. Patients without neurologic deficits do not receive steroids (Brock et al., 2016; Kumar et al., 2017; Lin & Avila, 2017).

   (2) Steroids relieve pain and delay progression of neurologic symptoms by reducing inflammation and vasogenic edema in the spinal cord (Lawton et al., 2019).

   (3) Steroid use should be held in patients suspected of having ESCC caused by lymphomas until definitive diagnosis is confirmed. Steroids rapidly shrink lymphomas and can make ESCC

diagnosis difficult (Brock et al., 2016; Weinstein, 2013).

   (4) Although dexamethasone is the drug standard, optimal dosing in patients with ESCC is not known; recommendations have been to tailor the dose to the severity of a patient's neurologic symptoms (Loblaw, Mitera, Ford, & Laperriere, 2012).

     (a) For minimal symptoms, the low-dose regimen consists of an IV bolus of 10 mg dexamethasone, followed by 16 mg daily orally in divided doses. The dose is gradually tapered over weeks once definitive treatment is underway.

     (b) For severe symptoms, the high-dose regimen consists of an IV bolus of 100 mg of dexamethasone, followed by maintenance doses of up to 96 mg per day orally with taper over weeks.

     (c) A systematic review of the efficacy of steroid therapy and optimal dosing for treating ESCC revealed the need for further research (Kumar et al., 2017).

       i. The low-dose steroid regimen was found to produce fewer complications than the high-dose regimen. Proton pump inhibitors can decrease the risk of gastric complications.

       ii. Weaning from steroid therapy should occur as soon as possible after definitive treatment is initiated.

  b) Sequence of therapy

   (1) The optimal sequence of first-line therapy for ESCC (RT or surgery) depends on individual patient factors.

   (2) See Figure 22 for a comparison of indications.

  c) RT options

   (1) EBRT

     (a) Conventional EBRT is recommended as the primary therapy for patients with certain disease characteristics (George, Sundararaj, Govindaraj, Chacko, & Tharyan, 2015; Laufer, Bilsky, et al., 2019; Loblaw et al., 2012; Lutz et al., 2017; New, 2019).

       i. Radiosensitive tumors (lymphoma, multiple myeloma, SCLC, and cancers of the breast, prostate, and ovary)

       ii. Short life expectancies (less than six months)

       iii. Not surgical candidates

       iv. Total neurologic deficit below the level of cord compression for more than 24–48 hours

     (b) EBRT used alone in these patients can effectively palliate pain, improve ambulation, and provide local tumor control.

FIGURE 22. Indications for Surgery Versus Radiation Therapy as First-Line Therapy for Epidural Spinal Cord Compression

Indications for Surgery as First-Line Intervention[a]	Indications for Radiation Therapy Alone
• Vertebral bone fragments compressing cord • Intractable pain • Single vertebral level affected • Circumferential epidural tumor • Spinal instability requiring correction • Duration of loss of ambulation < 48 hours • Radioresistant tumors • Radiosensitive tumors (followed by postoperative radiation therapy) • Prior radiation therapy • Biopsy for unknown histology • Life expectancy > 3–4 months • Minimal comorbidity	• Unable to tolerate surgery • Life expectancy < 3 months • Radiosensitive tumor • Multiple vertebral levels affected • Spinal stabilization not needed • Duration of loss of ambulation > 48 hours • Inoperable tumors • Poor performance status

[a] May be followed by postoperative radiation therapy

Note. Based on information from Al-Qurainy & Collis, 2016; Laufer et al., 2019; Lawton et al., 2019; Loblaw et al., 2012.

From "Spinal Cord Compression," by M. Kaplan, in M. Kaplan (Ed.), *Understanding and Managing Oncologic Emergencies: A Resource for Nurses* (3rd ed., p. 543), 2018, Oncology Nursing Society. Copyright 2018 by Oncology Nursing Society. Adapted with permission.

(c) Although recommendations vary regarding the optimal EBRT dose and fractionation schedule, the regimen chosen is generally based on individual patient characteristics, such as radiosensitivity of tumor, disease prognosis, performance status, and life expectancy (George et al., 2015; Laufer, Bilsky, et al., 2019; Loblaw et al., 2012).

    i. Poor prognosis: single fraction of 8 Gy for those with an estimated life expectancy of three to six months

    ii. Good prognosis: 30 Gy in 10 fractions for those with an estimated life expectancy beyond six months or those receiving RT after surgical decompression

(d) The EBRT treatment field is centered on the spine, encompasses the width of the involved vertebral body and any tumor extension, and typically extends one vertebral body above and one below the area of ESCC (Laufer, Bilsky, et al., 2019).

(e) EBRT doses greater than 45–50 Gy to the spinal cord in conventional fractions increase risk of radiation myelopathy (Lawton et al., 2019).

(2) SBRT

    (a) SBRT is a highly conformal technique coupled with image-guided technology and allows delivery of high doses of radiation to precisely targeted areas of compressed spinal cord while sparing normal cord tissue (Laufer, Bilsky, et al., 2019; Osborn, Lee, & Yamada, 2018).

    (b) SBRT provides excellent pain relief and local tumor control.

    (c) Selected patients may be candidates for SBRT.

       i. Those with radioresistant tumors (e.g., melanoma, renal cell cancer) or those requiring reirradiation for recurrent ESCC after prior EBRT therapy

       ii. Those treated with surgical decompression as an alternative to EBRT for local tumor control

    (d) Postoperative SBRT is particularly useful for tumor types that are relatively radioresistant and for reirradiating recurrent ESCC.

    (e) Typical doses of SBRT delivered to the spine are 16–24 Gy given in a single fraction or 24–30 Gy in two or three fractions (Barzilai et al., 2017; Osborn et al., 2018).

    (f) Single-fraction treatment of 24 Gy is often used for patients with early-stage disease who either have radioresistant histology and/or favorable prognosis (Osborn et al., 2018).

    (g) Potential complications of SBRT depend on the area of the cord treated (Osborn et al., 2018).

       i. Acute toxicities can include nausea, fatigue, dermatitis, esophagitis, and myelitis.

       ii. Late toxicities are more significant and can include esophageal stenosis, fistula, ulcer formation, vertebral compression fracture, and radiation myelopathy.

    (h) Vertebral compression fracture is the most common risk associated with SBRT. It is more likely to occur with use of single doses greater than 20 Gy (Osborn et al., 2018).

d) Surgery (George et al., 2015; Laufer, Bilsky, et al., 2019; Lawton et al., 2019)

    (1) Spinal stability considerations

       (a) Patients with unstable spines or cord compression caused by fragments of vertebral bone require initial surgical stabilization of the spinal column (regardless of tumor radiosensitivity) in order to achieve the following.

    i. Restore mechanical stability

    ii. Provide relief of movement-induced pain

    iii. Improve neurologic function

(b) For patients with stable spines, surgery is the preferred initial treatment approach to decompress the spinal cord, and it is typically used to treat patients with the following characteristics.

    i. Good prognosis (life expectancy of at least three months and medically operable)

    ii. Single area of cord compression

    iii. Radioresistant tumors (e.g., melanoma, renal cell cancer, sarcoma, NSCLC, colon cancer)

    iv. Circumferential epidural tumor

    v. Recurrent ESCC after initial EBRT

(2) Separation surgery and postoperative SBRT (Laufer, Bilsky, et al., 2019)

(a) The goal of treatment is to remove only a sufficient volume of epidural tumor to decompress the spinal cord circumferentially and create adequate separation (3 mm or greater gap) between the remaining tumor and the cord.

(b) High-dose SBRT can then be delivered to the entire residual tumor volume to provide local tumor control while sparing the adjacent spinal cord from excessive radiation exposure.

(c) Posterior surgical approaches to the vertebral column, such as laminectomy, employ fixation devices (e.g., screw rods) to reconstruct and stabilize the spine.

(d) Anterior surgical approaches reconstruct and stabilize the spine by using bone cement to fill vertebral bone defects and placing metallic fixation devices (rods, pins, and plates).

(3) Maximal surgical excision and EBRT (Laufer, Bilsky, et al., 2019)

(a) This approach is appropriate for patients with radioresistant tumors and severe cord compression or unstable spines who do not have access to SBRT.

(b) The cord is decompressed by removing as much tumor as possible, followed within 14 days by EBRT (30 Gy in 10 days) to reduce risk of recurrence.

(4) Vertebroplasty and kyphoplasty (Kaplan, 2018; Laufer, Bilsky, et al., 2019)

(a) Vertebroplasty and kyphoplasty are minimally invasive surgical techniques that may be used for patients with short life expectancies who have painfully collapsed vertebrae without neurologic symptoms and cannot tolerate surgery.

(b) In both techniques, image-guided percutaneous injection of acrylic bone filler cement into pathologically collapsed vertebrae stabilizes and supports the spine and provides immediate pain relief.

(c) These surgeries can be done as outpatient procedures.

e) Systemic therapy (Al-Qurainy & Collis, 2016; Laufer, Bilsky, et al., 2019)

(1) Chemotherapy

(a) Chemotherapy may be useful as an adjunct to EBRT and surgery in treating ESCC caused by chemosensitive tumors (e.g., lymphomas, myeloma, breast cancer, SCLC, germ cell tumors).

(b) Used alone, chemotherapy may be sufficient to treat ESCC caused by non-Hodgkin lymphoma, which is highly chemosensitive.

(c) Chemotherapy may be used to treat recurrent ESCC at a site of previous irradiation in patients who cannot tolerate surgery.

(2) Hormone therapy: Hormone therapy may be used as adjunct therapy to EBRT or surgery for patients with ESCC caused by breast cancer who have not received antihormone therapies (tamoxifen or aromatase inhibitors), or those with prostate cancer who have not been exposed to antiandrogens.

9. Nursing implications (Kaplan, 2018; Rucker, 2018)

a) Nurses have an essential role to provide individualized care for patients being treated for ESCC, based on each patient's neurologic status, spinal stability, and type of treatment.

b) Nursing care focuses on the following issues.

(1) Pain relief

(2) Safety measures

(3) Skin integrity

(4) Sensory and motor functions

(5) Bladder and bowel management

(6) Treatment side effect assessment and management

(7) Mobilization or weight-bearing activities (as appropriate)

(8) Education about treatment modalities and rehabilitation goals

(9) Emotional support in coping with functional limitations and end-of-life issues

10. Rehabilitation and palliative care (Lawton et al., 2019; New, 2019)

a) Rehabilitation goals are individualized for each patient to prevent permanent disability, improve impaired function, and maximize quality of life. When possible, goals include the following.

    (1) Improving ambulation

    (2) Achieving weight-bearing and transfer ability

    (3) Restoring bladder and bowel function

    (4) Protecting the skin

  b) Palliative care goals for patients with brief life expectancy focus on the following.

    (1) Providing pain relief and comfort measures

    (2) Managing bladder and bowel elimination

    (3) Preventing pressure ulcers

    (4) Supporting patients and caregivers in coping with end-of-life issues as disease progresses

C. Superior vena cava syndrome

1. Introduction

  a) SVCS is an array of signs and symptoms that occur when blood flow in the superior vena cava (SVC) becomes obstructed, impeding venous return from the head, neck, and upper extremities to the right side of the heart (Shelton, 2018).

  b) Malignancy within the mediastinum, particularly lung cancer, is the most frequent cause of SVC obstruction (Drews & Rabkin, 2019; Kaplan, 2017).

  c) Nonmalignant causes of SVCS are increasing in incidence as the use of indwelling intravascular devices becomes widespread and increases the risk of thrombosis within the SVC (Friedman, Quencer, Kishore, Winokur, & Madoff, 2017; Gucalp & Dutcher, 2018).

  d) SVCS is generally not a life-threatening condition but can become a true oncologic emergency when complete obstruction of the SVC occurs suddenly and results in the following (Drews & Rabkin, 2019; Gucalp & Dutcher, 2018).

    (1) Inadequate venous blood return to the heart to support adequate cardiac output sufficient to meet the needs of the body

    (2) Respiratory compromise due to edema of the larynx and pharynx that obstructs the upper airway

    (3) Cerebral edema that leads to increased intracranial pressure and coma

2. Incidence

  a) SVCS is an uncommon oncologic complication, occurring in 3%–4% of patients who have tumors within the chest (Drews & Rabkin, 2019).

  b) Malignancy located in the thorax is responsible for 60%–85% of cases and is especially prevalent in patients with the following features (Nickloes, Kallab, & Dunlap, 2020; Shelton, 2018).

    (1) Right-sided lung cancers, especially NSCLC, but also SCLC (most cases)

    (2) Enlarged mediastinal lymph nodes associated with non-Hodgkin lymphoma

  c) Less often, metastatic disease within the mediastinum leads to SVCS. This is especially true of breast cancer, but also it occurs with thyroid cancer and melanoma (Friedman et al., 2017).

  d) SVCS may be the presenting symptom of an undiagnosed cancer in up to 60% of cases (Friedman et al., 2017).

  e) The median life expectancy of patients with malignant SVC obstruction is six months and depends on the prognosis of the underlying malignancy (Friedman et al., 2017; Straka et al., 2016).

  f) Nonmalignant causes of SVCS have increased in incidence over the years and account for 20%–40% of cases (Drews & Rabkin, 2019; Gucalp & Dutcher, 2018).

    (1) These cases are mostly related to the increased use of intravascular devices (e.g., permanent central venous access catheters, pacemaker and defibrillator leads), which can lead to thrombosis or stenosis of the SVC.

    (2) Nonmalignant causes are less often related to disease conditions in the mediastinum, such as radiation fibrosis, fibrosing mediastinitis associated with infections (e.g., histoplasmosis, tuberculosis), pericarditis, and aortic aneurysm.

3. Pathophysiology (Drews & Rabkin, 2019; Kaplan, 2017; Shelton, 2018)

  a) The SVC is a thin-walled, low-pressure blood vessel (less than 5 mm Hg) and is the major pathway for return of deoxygenated venous blood from the upper body (head, neck, arms, and upper thorax) to the right atrium of the heart.

  b) The SVC is located in the middle mediastinum, tightly surrounded by several structures: sternum, trachea, right bronchus, aorta, pulmonary artery, and lymph node chains.

  c) SVC obstruction occurs when a space-occupying tumor compresses the vessel externally or invades through the vessel wall.

  d) The presence of an intravascular device can lead to internal thrombosis or stenosis of the SVC.

  e) SVC obstruction that is partial or develops slowly allows time for the development of collateral venous pathways that return blood from the upper body to the right atrium. Collateral blood vessels become dilated and venous pressure increases in the head, neck, upper extremities, and upper thorax, resulting in the characteristic signs and symptoms of SVCS.

  f) Sudden, complete SVC obstruction often results from a combination of external tumor and internal thrombus because collateral venous pathways have not had time to develop, resulting in a life-threatening event.

4. Clinical manifestations

  a) Symptom severity depends on how rapidly and completely the SVC becomes obstructed and whether collateral blood vessels have developed. Figures 23 and 24 list early and late manifestations of SVCS.

FIGURE 23. Early Manifestations of Superior Vena Cava Syndrome

- Breast swelling in women
- Cyanosis of face and arms
- Dilated veins in neck and upper chest
- Dyspnea
- Face and periorbital area edema
- Feeling of fullness in head that is worse on awakening
- Nasal congestion
- Neck and upper extremity edema
- Nonproductive cough
- Plethora (ruddy facial complexion)
- Shirt collar and rings on fingers become tight

Note. Based on information from Kaplan, 2017; McNally, 2018; Shelton, 2018.

b) Partial SVC obstruction may be asymptomatic or produce subtle signs and symptoms that are not life threatening.

c) The characteristic symptoms of SVCS reflect venous engorgement and edema in the upper body (Friedman et al., 2017; Shelton, 2018).

   (1) Dyspnea (most common)
   (2) Nonproductive cough
   (3) Hoarseness
   (4) Nasal congestion
   (5) Shirt collars and rings feeling tight
   (6) Sense of "fullness" in the head, which may be exacerbated by lying down, bending forward, or coughing
   (7) Symptoms worsening in the morning after lying supine overnight
   (8) Symptom improvement during the day as a patient remains upright
   (9) Increased comfort with sleeping in an upright position

d) Symptoms often progress gradually over a period of weeks and may subside as collateral circulation develops.

e) SVCS that develops rapidly can produce life-threatening effects on the respiratory system, cardiac system, and CNS (Kaplan, 2017; Shelton, 2018; Straka et al., 2016).

   (1) Cardiac symptoms may include tachycardia, hypotension, and congestive heart failure.
   (2) Respiratory distress may be manifested by stridor, tachypnea, and pleural effusion.
   (3) Cerebral edema can lead to stupor, convulsions, coma, and death.

5. Prognosis (Drews & Rabkin, 2019; Gucalp & Dutcher, 2018; Nickloes et al., 2020)

   a) Survival following malignancy-associated SVCS depends on the tumor type. Death is the result of the underlying disease rather than the complication.
   b) The presence of respiratory compromise (laryngeal edema) or mental status changes (cerebral edema) is associated with a poorer prognosis.
   c) Patients with untreated malignancy-associated SVCS survive approximately 30 days.
   d) Of patients with SVCS associated with lung cancer who are treated with RT, 10% survive at least 30 months, as do 45% of patients with lymphoma and SVCS who are treated with RT.

6. Diagnosis (Friedman et al., 2017; McNally, 2018; Shelton, 2018)

   a) Clinicians should take comprehensive patient history to identify the underlying cause.
      (1) Status of known cancer and presence of metastasis
      (2) Risk factors for undiagnosed cancer
      (3) Presence of central venous catheters or pacemakers
      (4) Prior RT or infection in the thorax
   b) Clinicians should conduct a symptom review.
   c) In a physical examination, classic signs and symptoms of SVCS are usually sufficient to make the diagnosis.
      (1) Edema of the face, periorbital area, neck and chest wall, and upper extremities
      (2) Facial plethora (ruddy complexion) and cyanosis of the arms
      (3) Distended veins in the neck, chest, and upper extremities

FIGURE 24. Late Manifestations of Superior Vena Cava Syndrome

Cardiac System	Central Nervous System (related to cerebral edema)	Respiratory System (related to laryngeal or pharyngeal edema)
• Congestive heart failure • Hemodynamic compromise causing dizziness, renal insufficiency • Hypotension, syncope • Hypoxia • Tachycardia	• Horner syndrome due to pressure on cervical sympathetic nerves • Irritability • Mental status changes reflecting increased intracranial pressure: lethargy, confusion, obtundation, seizures, coma, death • Severe headache • Visual disturbances, papilledema	• Aspiration due to paralysis of the true vocal cord secondary to pressure on cranial nerve X (recurrent laryngeal nerve) • Dysphagia • Pleural effusion (mainly right-sided) • Respiratory distress (dyspnea, orthopnea, hoarseness, stridor) • Tachypnea

Note. Based on information from Drews & Rabkin, 2019; Friedman et al., 2017; McNally, 2018; Shelton, 2018; Straka et al., 2016.

From "Superior Vena Cava Syndrome," by M. Kaplan, in K. Kuebler (Ed.), *Integration of Palliative Care in Chronic Conditions: An Interdisciplinary Approach* (p. 356), 2017, Oncology Nursing Society. Copyright 2017 by Oncology Nursing Society. Adapted with permission.

d) Imaging tests can reveal the extent of SVCS (Drews & Rabkin, 2019; Nickloes et al., 2020).

  (1) Chest x-ray may reveal a tumor mass, widened mediastinum, and pleural effusion; however, it cannot image thrombosis within the SVC.

  (2) Contrast-enhanced chest CT venography is the most useful imaging test because of the following capabilities.

    (a) It provides details about the site and extent of SVC obstruction.

    (b) It determines whether an obstruction is the result of external compression or internal thrombosis.

    (c) It visualizes collateral venous circulation.

    (d) It guides biopsy procedures (e.g., mediastinoscopy, bronchoscopy, percutaneous fine-needle aspiration) when needed to attain tissue samples for a definitive cancer diagnosis.

  (3) Magnetic resonance venography allows for direct visualization of blood flow. It may be used for patients who are allergic to contrast agents, have renal failure, or will undergo SVC stenting.

  (4) Duplex ultrasound is useful for excluding thrombosis in the subclavian, axillary, and brachiocephalic veins. It is the initial imaging study for patients with mild symptoms who have an indwelling device or a malignancy at low risk for causing SVCS.

e) Histologic confirmation of cancer is required before initiation of SVCS treatment unless it is an emergency. The least invasive method possible is used to retrieve tumor cells (Drews & Rabkin, 2019; Nickloes et al., 2020).

  (1) Sputum cytology

  (2) Pleural fluid cytology

  (3) Biopsy of a palpable supraclavicular node

  (4) Bronchoscopy

  (5) Mediastinoscopy

  (6) Video-assisted thoracoscopy

  (7) Thoracotomy

7. Treatment decisions (Drews & Rabkin, 2019; Gucalp & Dutcher, 2018)

  a) Symptom relief and treatment of the underlying condition precipitating SVCS are the main goals of therapy.

  b) Treatment choice is based on the etiology of SVC obstruction (malignant tumor or thrombosis), symptom severity and treatment urgency, type and stage of cancer, disease prognosis, patient performance status, and treatment intent (palliative or curative).

8. Collaborative management (Drews & Rabkin, 2019; Kaplan, 2016, 2017; Nickloes et al., 2020; Shelton, 2018; Straka et al., 2016)

  a) Endovascular stent placement (Drews & Rabkin, 2019; Kaplan, 2016; Straka et al., 2016)

  (1) Stent placement is recommended as emergency treatment for patients with life-threatening SVCS symptoms to rapidly restore venous return.

  (2) It rapidly palliates symptoms in patients with tumors that do not respond well to chemotherapy or RT.

  (3) It is indicated for patients with recurrent SVCS previously treated with systemic therapy or RT.

  b) RT

  (1) In the past, patients with life-threatening symptoms received RT immediately; however, stent placement has supplanted RT because it rapidly relieves symptoms within 72 hours (Straka et al., 2016).

  (2) RT is the standard treatment for SVCS caused by NSCLC, and other types of radiosensitive malignancies (e.g., lymphoma) (Drews & Rabkin, 2019; McNally, 2018).

  (3) RT dose and delivery schedule have not been standardized. They are determined by the following.

    (a) Tumor radiosensitivity

    (b) Tumor size

    (c) History of prior thoracic RT

    (d) Performance status and disease prognosis

  (4) Radiation fields generally include a 2 cm margin around the tumor, as well as lymph node chains in the mediastinum, hilum, and supraclavicular areas (Drews & Rabkin, 2019).

  (5) Dose fractionation options include the following (Drews & Rabkin, 2019; Shelton, 2018; Straka et al., 2016).

    (a) 30 Gy in 10 fractions (3 Gy per day) to 50 Gy in 25 fractions (2 Gy per day)

    (b) 3–4 Gy for two to four treatments, then 1.8–2 Gy daily

    (c) Hypofractionated RT or SBRT for selected patients

  (6) Symptom relief generally begins within three to seven days of the start of RT as SVC blood flow improves (Shelton, 2018).

  c) Chemotherapy

  (1) Chemotherapy is the initial treatment of choice for chemosensitive malignancies (e.g., SCLC, non-Hodgkin lymphoma, germ cell tumors) that have not produced life-threatening symptoms (Shelton, 2018).

  (2) Symptoms usually improve within one to two weeks of treatment initiation (Straka et al., 2016).

  (3) Chemotherapy may be used concomitantly with RT to provide maximal tumor response (Friedman et al., 2017; Shelton, 2018).

    (a) Combination therapy increases the severity of side effects.

    (b) Patients require close monitoring.

d) Surgical venous bypass (Drews & Rabkin, 2019)

   (1) Surgical resection of malignant tumor and SVC bypass reconstruction is rarely used because of associated morbidity and poor survival prognoses.

   (2) Surgical venous bypass may be an option in selected patients with malignant thymoma and thymic cancer, which are resistant to both chemotherapy and RT.

e) Supportive medical therapies

   (1) Corticosteroids may be useful in selected cases.

     (a) Steroids are given in conjunction with emergency RT for patients with upper airway edema or cerebral edema who cannot be stented (Drews & Rabkin, 2019).

     (b) Steroids are used for patients with SVC obstruction caused by steroid-sensitive tumors (e.g., lymphoma, thymoma) but only after histologic confirmation of tumor type to avoid obscuring the diagnosis of these cancers (Shelton, 2018).

   (2) Loop diuretics may be used to reduce edema. However, it is important to avoid dehydration and hypovolemia, which can further reduce venous return to the heart (Shelton, 2018).

   (3) Oxygen supplementation and elevation of head of the bed provides relief of dyspnea (Shelton, 2018).

   (4) Analgesics and tranquilizers are used to relieve chest pain and allay anxiety associated with respiratory distress (Shelton, 2018).

f) Thrombolytic therapy (Kaplan, 2017; McNally, 2018)

   (1) Thrombolytic therapy is used to treat thrombosis related to the presence of intravascular devices.

   (2) It is contraindicated in patients with increased bleeding risk.

9. Nursing implications (Kaplan, 2017; McNally, 2018; Shelton, 2018)

a) Nurses can promote oxygenation by elevating head of bed or sitting patient upright, restricting activities, and providing supplemental oxygen.

b) Nurses must maintain a patient's fluid balance to avoid dehydration or fluid overload.

c) Nurses can provide analgesics and tranquilizers to relieve any chest pain and allay anxiety associated with respiratory distress.

d) Nurses should institute a bowel regimen so that a patient avoids straining at stool (i.e., Valsalva maneuver, which increases venous pressure).

e) Nurses should administer IV infusions, perform blood draws, and measure blood pressure in lower extremities when edema and elevated venous pressure are present in arms.

f) Nurses provide education to patients and caregivers regarding the cause and management of symptoms due to SVCS.

g) Nurses provide emotional support to patients and caregivers who may be concerned and frightened about the symptoms of SVCS.

h) Nurses should support the decision to decline aggressive cancer therapies, as appropriate.

References

Al-Qurainy, R., & Collis, E. (2016). Metastatic spinal cord compression: Diagnosis and management. *BMJ, 353,* i2539. https://doi.org/10.1136/bmj.i2539

Barzilai, O., Laufer, I., Yamada, Y., Higginson, D.S., Schmitt, A.M., Lis, E., & Bilsky, M.H. (2017). Integrating evidence-based medicine for treatment of spinal metastases into a decision framework: Neurologic, oncologic, mechanicals stability, and systemic disease. *Journal of Clinical Oncology, 35,* 2419–2427. https://doi.org/10.1200/jco.2017.72.7362

Borke, J. (2019, July 17). Spinal cord neoplasms. https://emedicine.medscape.com/article/779872-overview

Brock, P., Toale, K.M., & Tummala, S. (2016). Neurologic emergencies. In E.F. Manzullo, C.E. Gonzalez, C.P. Escalante, & S.-C.J. Yeung (Eds.), *Oncologic emergencies* (pp. 1–19). Springer. https://doi.org/10.1007/978-1-4939-3188-0_1

Dawodu, S.T., Bechtel, K.A., Beeson, M.S., Hodges, S.D., Humphreys, S.C., & Kellam, J.F. (2018, June 14). Cauda equina and conus medullaris syndromes. http://emedicine.medscape.com/article/1148690-overview

Drews, R.E., & Rabkin, D.J. (2019, June 27). Malignancy-related superior vena cava syndrome. In D.M.F. Savarese & K.A. Collins (Eds.), *UpToDate.* Retrieved May 14, 2020, from https://www.uptodate.com/contents/malignancy-related-superior-vena-cava-syndrome

Friedman, T., Quencer, K.B., Kishore, S.A., Winokur, R.S., & Madoff, D.C. (2017). Malignant venous obstruction: Superior vena cava syndrome and beyond. *Seminars in Interventional Radiology, 34,* 398–408. https://doi.org/10.1055/s-0037-1608863

George, R., Sundararaj, J.J., Govindaraj, R., Chacko, A.G., & Tharyan, P. (2015). Interventions for the treatment of metastatic extradural spinal cord compression in adults. *Cochrane Database of Systematic Reviews, 2015*(9). https://doi.org/10.1002/14651858.cd006716.pub3

Gucalp, R., & Dutcher, J.P. (2018). Oncologic emergencies. In J.L. Jameson, A.S. Fauci, D.L. Kasper, S.L. Hauser, D.L. Longo, & J. Loscalzo (Eds.), *Harrison's principles of internal medicine* (20th ed., e-book). McGraw-Hill Education.

Kaplan, M. (2016). Structural oncologic emergencies. In B.H. Gobel, S. Triest-Robertson, & W.H. Vogel (Eds.), *Advanced oncology nursing certification review and resource manual* (2nd ed., pp. 693–736). Oncology Nursing Society.

Kaplan, M. (2017). Superior vena cava syndrome. In K. Kuebler (Ed.), *Integration of palliative care in chronic conditions: An interdisciplinary approach* (pp. 353–361). Oncology Nursing Society.

Kaplan, M. (2018). Spinal cord compression. In M. Kaplan (Ed.), *Understanding and managing oncologic emergencies: A resource for nurses* (3rd ed., pp. 509–560). Oncology Nursing Society.

Kumar, A., Weber, M.H., Gokaslan, Z., Wolinsky, J.-P., Schmidt, M., Rhines, L., ... Fisher, C.G. (2017). Metastatic spinal cord compression and steroid treatment: A systematic review. *Clinical Spine Surgery, 30,* 156–163. https://doi.org/10.1097/bsd.0000000000000528

Laufer, I., Bilsky, M., Schiff, D., & Brown, P. (2019, December 9). Treatment and prognosis of neoplastic epidural spinal cord compression. In A.F. Eichler & D.M.F. Savarese (Eds.), *UpToDate.* Retrieved May 14, 2020, from https://www.uptodate.com/contents/treatment-and-prognosis-of-neoplastic-epidural-spinal-cord-compression

Laufer, I., Rubin, D.G., Lis, E., Cox, B.W., Stubblefield, M.D., Yamada, Y., & Bilsky, M.H. (2013). The NOMS framework: Approach to the treatment of spinal metastatic tumors. *Oncologist, 18,* 744–751. https://doi.org/10.1634/theoncologist.2012-0293

Laufer, I., Schiff, D., Kelly, H.R., & Bilsky, M. (2019, April 29). Clinical features and diagnosis of neoplastic epidural spinal cord compression. In R.E. Drews & P.Y. Wen (Eds.), *UpToDate*. Retrieved May 14, 2020, from https://www.uptodate.com/contents/clinical-features-and-diagnosis-of-neoplastic-epidural-spinal-cord-compression

Lawton, A.J., Lee, K.A., Cheville, A.L., Ferrone, M.L., Rades, D., Balboni, T.A., & Abrahm, J.L. (2019). Assessment and management of patients with metastatic spinal cord compression: A multidisciplinary review. *Journal of Clinical Oncology, 37*, 61–77. https://doi.org/10.1200/jco.2018.78.1211

Lin, A.L., & Avila, E.K. (2017). Neurologic emergencies in the patients with cancer: Diagnosis and management. *Journal of Intensive Care Medicine, 32*, 99–115. https://doi.org/10.1177/0885066615619582

Loblaw, D.A., Mitera, G., Ford, M., & Laperriere, N.J. (2012). A 2011 updated systematic review and clinical practice guideline for the management of malignant extradural spinal cord compression. *International Journal of Radiation Oncology, Biology, Physics, 84*, 312–317. https://doi.org/10.1016/j.ijrobp.2012.01.014

Lu, C., Gonzalez, R.G., Jolesz, F.A., Wen, P.Y., & Talcott, J. (2005). Suspected spinal cord compression in cancer patients: A multidisciplinary risk assessment. *Journal of Supportive Oncology, 3*, 305–312.

Lutz, S., Balboni, T., Jones, J., Lo, S., Petit, J., Rich, S.E., ... Hahn, C. (2017). Palliative radiation therapy for bone metastases: Update of an ASTRO evidence-based guideline. *Practical Radiation Oncology, 7*, 4–12. https://doi.org/10.1016/j.prro.2016.08.001

McNally, G.A. (2018). Superior vena cava syndrome. In C.H. Yarbro, D. Wujcik, & B.H. Gobel (Eds.), *Cancer nursing: Principles and practice* (8th ed., pp. 1187–1196). Jones and Bartlett Learning.

New, P.W. (2019). Rehabilitation in patients with spinal cord dysfunction. In M.D. Stubblefield (Ed.), *Cancer rehabilitation: Principles and practice* (2nd ed., pp. 601–623). Springer.

Nickloes, T.A., Kallab, A.M., & Dunlap, A.B. (2020, March 27). Superior vena cava syndrome. https://emedicine.medscape.com/article/460865-overview

Osborn, V.W., Lee, A., & Yamada, Y. (2018). Stereotactic body radiation therapy for spinal malignancies. *Technology in Cancer Research and Treatment, 17*. https://doi.org/10.1177/1533033818802304

Rucker, Y. (2018). Spinal cord compression. In C.H. Yarbro, D. Wujcik, & B.H. Gobel (Eds.), *Cancer nursing: Principles and practice* (8th ed., pp. 1153–1167). Jones and Bartlett Learning.

Shelton, B.K. (2018). Superior vena cava syndrome. In M. Kaplan (Ed.), *Understanding and managing oncologic emergencies: A resource for nurses* (2nd ed., pp. 561–587). Oncology Nursing Society.

Stephenson, R.O., & Berliner, J. (2020, March 2). Autonomic dysreflexia in spinal cord injury. http://emedicine.medscape.com/article/322809-overview

Straka, C., Ying, J., Kong, F.-M., Willey, C.D., Kaminski, J., & Kim, D.W.N. (2016). Review of evolving etiologies, implications and treatment strategies for the superior vena cava syndrome. *SpringerPlus, 5*, 229. https://doi.org/10.1186/s40064-016-1900-7

Viets-Upchurch, J.M. (2016). Malignant spinal cord compression. In K.H. Todd & C.R. Thomas, Jr. (Eds.), *Oncologic emergency medicine: Principles and practice* (pp. 161–167). Springer.

Weinstein, S.M. (2013). Management of spinal cord and cauda equina compression. In A.M. Berger, J.L. Shuster, & J.H. Von Roenn (Eds.), *Principles and practice of palliative care and supportive oncology* (4th ed., pp. 514–528). Wolters Kluwer Health/Lippincott Williams and Wilkins.

VIII. Modality-Specific Management

A. External beam radiation therapy (teletherapy)
  1. History of EBRT (Alfred & Leaver, 2016; Khan, 2020)
     a) In November 1895, Wilhelm Conrad Röntgen discovered invisible rays, which he later named x-rays.
     b) The first therapeutic application of x-rays was delivered on January 29, 1896, to a patient with carcinoma of the breast.
     c) Marie Curie and Pierre Curie discovered polonium and radium in 1898.
     d) Basal cell epitheliomas became the first cancer to be cured by radiation in 1899.
     e) In the early 1900s, Bergonié and Tribondeau discovered that tissues with higher metabolic and proliferative activity are more sensitive to radiation.
     f) In early treatments, severe tissue damage occurred after single high-dose RT treatments because radiation was focused on eradicating the tumor.
        (1) Tumor recurrences and adverse effects following RT dimmed the excitement of its usefulness in curing cancers.
        (2) However, in the 1930s, Claudius Regaud and Henri Coutard found that administering fractionated doses of radiation could achieve the same tumor response with decreased tissue injury.
     g) Surgeons and dermatologists were the first physicians to administer RT in the early 1900s, and they determined the proper length of treatment based on the amount of skin redness (erythema) present.
     h) The roentgen (or röntgen) was recognized as a unit of measurement of exposure to x-rays and gamma rays in 1928. ICRU recommended the rad as the measurement for radiation-absorbed dose in tissues in 1953. The rad was later replaced by the gray, and sometimes cGy is used.
     i) The first use of a megavoltage RT machine that produced x-rays greater than one million volts occurred in 1937 at St. Bartholomew's Hospital in London.
        (1) The high energy used deposited its maximum energy below the skin surface (skin-sparing effect) and allowed radiation to be delivered to deep-seated tumors without causing significant skin erythema.
        (2) Other megavoltage machines were eventually developed.
           (a) Betatron in 1941
           (b) Cobalt-60 machine in 1951
           (c) Linear accelerator in 1952
     j) In 1954, the first patient was treated with protons for a pituitary tumor at the Lawrence Berkley National Laboratory of the University of California.
        (1) In 1961, clinical treatment with protons began at the Harvard Cyclotron Laboratory.
        (2) Robert R. Wilson first recognized the therapeutic use of protons in 1946 (Hu, Jiang, Cui, Zhang, & Yu, 2018; Mukherji, 2018).
     k) In the 1970s and 1980s, linear accelerators were further developed to produce high-energy photon and electron beams.
        (1) Two-dimensional RT (2DRT) involved treatment with one to four radiation beams, using anatomical boundaries that resulted in homogenous dose distributions to a volume of tissue where the beams overlapped.
        (2) In 2DRT, a larger volume of normal tissue was treated rather than a conformal plan, which was developed later with advancements in imaging and physics.
     l) The practice of 3DCRT was developed to provide careful dose planning, along with beam-shaping ability that allowed for more sparing of healthy tissue.
        (1) The 1990s saw the development of multileaf collimators and IMRT.
        (2) The development of improved immobilization devices allowed SBRT to be utilized for the treatment of brain, spine, lung, and liver lesions.
     m) VMAT is an advanced form of IMRT that carefully changes the shape and intensity of the beams while the treatment unit is rotating around a patient delivering the radiation dose (Teoh, Clark, Wood, Whitaker, & Nisbet, 2011).
     n) Cone beam CT is an imaging technique that can be used prior to each treatment fraction to determine if a patient is in the same position each day and to adjust RT when needed.
        (1) Cone beam CT allows for more precise treatment and ultimately a lower dose to the surrounding healthy tissues.
        (2) It also allows visualization of any changes that may occur during treatment and provides the opportunity to implement adaptive strategies based on tumor changes.
        (3) MRI is now also being used in the same way to achieve the same goal (Srinivasan, Mohammad, & Shepherd, 2014).
  2. Commonly used types of ionizing radiation
     a) X-rays (Khan, 2020)
        (1) X-rays are delivered using high-energy (4–18 MV) linear accelerators.
           (a) Penetration is dependent upon the energy.
           (b) With higher energy levels, the x-ray penetrates more deeply, and more skin sparing is achieved.
        (2) Lower energy orthovoltage or superficial units (70–200 kV) are used to treat lesions closer to the skin surface and skin cancers.
     b) Gamma rays (Khan, 2020)
        (1) Cobalt-60 is the most commonly used source of gamma rays.

(2) Average energy of gamma rays is 1.25 MV.

(3) Penetration depth is lower than that of modern linear accelerators.

(4) The skin-sparing effect is less than the higher energy linear accelerators.

(5) Cobalt-60 teletherapy machines are now rarely used currently in high-resource countries (see VIII.H. Cobalt therapy).

(6) Cobalt-60 machines have limitations on beam shaping and require the radioactive source to be changed periodically.

(7) Cobalt-60 is also used in Gamma Knife machines used for SRS and fractionated treatment.

3. Particulate radiation

a) Electrons

(1) Electrons penetrate only a few centimeters (less than 5 cm) below the skin surface, so they can be used to deliver maximum dose to skin surfaces (Perez-Andujar & Klein, 2019).

(2) Electrons are used to treat skin or lip cancers, chest wall recurrence, and lymph nodes in patients with head and neck cancer, as well as to boost the dose to lymph nodes (Perez-Andujar & Klein, 2019).

b) Protons

(1) Protons are positively charged particles.

(2) The mass of a proton is 2,000 times the mass of an electron, so therapy requires expensive and complicated equipment such as a cyclotron to accelerate the particles.

(3) Protons can be produced by a deuterium-tritium generator or cyclotron (Khan, 2020).

(4) The radiation dose range of proton beam therapy is 70–250 MeV (Mukherji, 2018).

(a) Precise dose delivery is achieved via passive scattering or pencil beam scanning.

(b) High doses are delivered to the tumor while limiting the dose to healthy tissues.

  i. This is achieved by a very rapid fall-off of the dose deposited in the tissues beyond the target.

  ii. The Bragg peak describes the rapid decrease in energy of protons as they travel through tissue.

(5) Proton beam therapy has shown benefits in pediatric and reirradiation settings, as well as for tumors that are very close to critical structures (e.g., brain stem, optic chiasm) (Hu et al., 2018; Tsang & Patel, 2019).

(a) Proton beam therapy is used in several cancer sites, including neurologic and eye tumors, head and neck cancer, NSCLC, breast cancer, esophageal cancer, liver cancer, and prostate cancers

(b) More research is needed to understand these benefits.

(6) A narrow Bragg peak can be a limitation in proton beam therapy.

(a) If the beam is not carefully planned, the target can be missed.

(b) Other limitations include planning challenges, facility space requirements, and cost.

(c) Currently, very few proton facilities are available in North America and Europe (27 in the United States).

4. Beam delivery methods (Behrend, 2018)

a) Two-dimensional conformal beams

(1) All beams are usually aimed at a single point, often referred to as the *isocenter*.

(2) It is often used for emergency and palliative cases.

b) 3DCRT

(1) Treatments are based on three-dimensional anatomic information.

(2) This technique benefits patients with irregularly shaped tumors or tumors near complex anatomy or sensitive structures.

(3) 3DCRT can be used for most treatment sites.

c) IMRT (Gregoire, Grau, Haustermans, Muren, & Stewart, 2015)

(1) IMRT is a more focused delivery of RT dose.

(2) IMRT uses beamlets (smaller beams) of varying intensity to provide better conformality to the tumor shape while avoiding healthy tissue.

(3) Multileaf collimators are used in addition to primary and secondary collimators to shape the beam.

(a) In static IMRT, multileaf collimators do not move while the beams are active.

(b) In dynamic IMRT, leaves of the collimators move while the beam is active.

(4) IMRT has become a standard technique for most clinical sites where the technology is available.

(5) VMAT is a technique whereby treatment is delivered with the machine rotating in an arc around a patient while the beam's intensity and shape are changing.

d) IGRT (Srinivasan et al., 2014)

(1) Use of IGRT is based on the knowledge that tumor and healthy tissues may move from day to day and change over time.

(2) Movement of tissues can be categorized in the following ways.

(a) Predictable: respiratory motion

(b) Unpredictable: bowel peristalsis, gas, bladder movement

(c) Permanent: tumor shrinkage

(3) Attempts are made to image, track, and manage motion for more precise RT treatments, such as SBRT. Images are acquired using a device attached to the treatment machine.

e) SBRT and SRS (Gaya & Mahadevan, 2015)

(1) SRS is a single treatment to a small area of the brain using high-dose, carefully shaped beams. It can also use multiple fractions, using lower daily doses.

(a) Multiple radioactive sources in the machine can pinpoint a very small area, such as a single brain metastasis.

(b) SRS is most commonly used for tumors (benign and malignant) in the brain and ears.

(2) SBRT is based on the same principles as SRS. It is used to treat tumors in the body rather than the brain.

(3) SBRT and SRS allow for treatment of a small area with a low number of fractions (one to five) with a high dose per fraction.

(4) These techniques allow for precise delivery of the RT dose.

(5) The dose that can be delivered is often limited by the healthy tissue included in or near the PTV. In SBRT, the PTV is the lesion plus a margin of healthy tissue, which is smaller than that used in conventional treatments.

(6) Indications include the following.

(a) NSCLC

(b) Primary liver tumors

(c) Lung metastases

(d) Liver metastases

(e) Primary spinal tumors

(f) Vertebral metastases

(g) Pancreatic cancer

(h) Renal cancer

5. Indications for RT

a) RT is used to treat almost all cancers. An estimated 50% of patients will receive some type of RT during the course of their cancer treatment (Baskar, Lee, Yeo, & Yeoh, 2012).

b) RT administered with a curative intent has several functions (Dest, 2018).

(1) Definitive: primary RT with or without chemotherapy or immunotherapy

(2) Neoadjuvant: given before primary treatment

(3) Adjuvant: given after primary treatment to increase disease-free survival

(4) Prophylactic: given for asymptomatic patients at high risk for occurrence

c) RT administered with palliative intent has the following functions (Gosselin, 2018).

(1) RT is administered to control symptoms such as bleeding, pain, airway obstruction, neuro-logic compromise, and other structural emergencies (e.g., painful bone metastasis, increased intracranial pressure, SVCS, dyspnea).

(2) RT can also be given as anticipatory palliation for the treatment of lesions that may become symptomatic (e.g., pending spinal cord compression, airway compromise).

6. Treatment preparation

a) Simulation (Uricchio, Givens, & Keskemety, 2016)

(1) Accurate positioning is imperative to replicate daily treatment fields.

(2) Simulation usually involves a CT scan in the treatment position.

(a) If CT is not available, then fluoroscopy can be used.

(b) MRI or PET scans may be obtained and can be fused with the CT scans to provide more information about the tumor and healthy tissue location.

(3) Radiopaque markers (e.g., lead, copper, solder wire) may be used to mark specific points on a patient to assist in calculations or mark critical structures for the treatment planning phase.

(4) Contrast media may be used to enhance anatomic structures that would normally be difficult to see on CT.

(a) Barium sulfate is sometimes used in the gastrointestinal tract and is administered orally or rectally to visualize the esophagus, stomach, small bowel, or colon.

(b) Iodinated contrast helps identify vessels and organs (e.g., kidneys, bladder, gastrointestinal tract) and is administered intravenously, orally, or through catheters to enhance images.

(5) Immobilization devices are selected (Alfred & Leaver, 2016).

(a) Simple (e.g., tape, plastic or cloth straps; arm pulls; rubber bands; bite block to hold the jaw in place)

(b) Complex (e.g., plaster of paris, vacuum-formed molds, thermoplastic masks)

(6) Adjunctive motion management methods may be used (Mukherji, 2018).

(a) Deep inspiration breath hold is a technique that patients actively participate in; they will be required to breathe in deeply multiple times during each treatment, and the treatment will only be delivered during this period of breath hold.

(b) An active breathing coordinator device is a snorkel-like device used to stop a patient's breathing during the specified phase. Treatment is delivered during a defined portion of the respiratory cycle.

(c) Respiratory gating is the use of fluoroscopy or CT that is synchronized with the breathing cycle. Treatment is delivered during a specified phase.

(d) Four-dimensional CT shows the changes in the target volume during the respiratory cycle and is used at simulation to prepare for treatment planning.

7. Treatment planning (Coleman, 2016)

  a) Patient positioning
  (1) Immobilization devices help to reproduce treatment positions daily.
  (2) A radiation therapist locates landmarks (e.g., fiducials, tattoos, anatomic location).
  (3) A three-point positioning technique is common and allows the radiation therapist to align the treatment plane with the isocenter of the machine and the beams.
  (4) A patient's position is then refined more with lasers and treatment field lights.

  b) Localization
  (1) Landmarks are used to set up a patient for treatment and can be placed in a particular location (e.g., tattoos on the skin) or can already exist anatomically (e.g., umbilicus).
  (2) Planning includes the following treatment volumes.
    (a) GTV, which includes macroscopic disease
    (b) CTV, which includes the GTV and any microscopic disease
    (c) PTV, which includes the CTV plus a margin to allow for motion and treatment setup variations (see II. Practice of Radiation Oncology)

  c) Beam shaping
  (1) Blocks are used to shape photon beams.
  (2) Standardized lead blocks are rarely used, but customized blocks generally consist of Wood's metal (Cerrobend®), an alloy of bismuth, lead, tin, and cadmium.
  (3) Multileaf collimators are more commonly used than blocks.

  d) Multileaf collimators
  (1) Multileaf collimators are used in addition to primary and secondary collimators in the machine.
  (2) The field shape and size can be customized using "jaws" that have opposing leaves to form leaf pairs.
  (3) Each leaf moves independently and can produce multiple shapes and sizes.

  e) Verification imaging on the treatment unit
  (1) Verification imaging is also known as *portal imaging* and *cone beam CT*.
  (2) Images can be taken at the beginning of treatment, daily, or at intervals during the treatment

to ensure appropriate placement of the radiation beams.
  (3) The daily images and previous CT or fluoroscopic simulation images are compared, and adjustments are made if necessary.

  f) Beam-modifying devices: bolus
  (1) Bolus is material that mimics tissue.
  (2) A bolus is laid on the skin surface so that it changes the distribution of the dose. A higher dose is then delivered at the skin surface.
  (3) Common materials used include paraffin wax, petrolatum gauze, wet gauze, and water bags.
  (4) Several commercially available products, such as Superflab®, may be used.
  (5) A bolus may be used over scars, superficial nodes, variations in surface contours, or where a gap in tissue exists on a patient's body.

  g) Electron beam shields (Mukherji, 2018)
  (1) Cutouts are used to shape the beam and protect critical structures.
  (2) Shields are often made of Wood's metal—an alloy of bismuth, lead, tin, and cadmium—and inserted into the path of the beam.

8. Delivery (Mukherji, 2018)
  a) Length of treatment course depends on the type and stage of cancer.
  b) Most treatments are daily (Monday through Friday) for one to eight weeks. Some treatments are twice daily with six hours between doses (hyperfractionated RT).
  c) The rationale for hyperfractionated treatments is to reduce the probability of tumor regeneration.
  (1) It may be used for patients with advanced disease and comorbidities, as well as those who cannot receive or tolerate combined treatment modalities (e.g., chemotherapy).
  (2) Palliative courses or specific modalities, such as SBRT, require shorter treatment courses (Saunders, 1999).
  d) Before the first treatment, cone beam CT or portal images are taken to confirm that setup is accurate. These may be repeated daily, weekly, or as needed.
  e) A patient must be able to lie still on the radiation treatment couch during the treatment to decrease or eliminate movement of the treatment target. Immobilization devices may be needed, and sometimes medication can be ordered to enable patients to lie still and remain calm during the treatment.
  f) A patient lies on the table for approximately 15 minutes or longer, depending on the complexity of the setup, but the beam is on for a few minutes of that time.

9. Side effects (Dest, 2018)
  a) Tissue and organ response to radiation
  (1) Response is dependent on total dose, as well as the daily dose and fractionation schedule, and volume treated.

(2) Cells and structures in the direct path of the radiation beam are subject to damage, but tissues outside of the target area will receive a lower dose based on the treatment plan developed.

(3) Cells are most sensitive to radiation in the G_2 and M phases of the cell cycle.

(4) Tissue and organs have variable tolerances to radiation.

(5) Concurrent treatment with chemotherapy alters tissue and organ tolerance, thereby resulting in greater toxicities than would occur with radiation alone.

(6) Toxicities may be acute (occur within hours to days of RT), subacute (occur within months after RT), or late (occur within months to years after RT).

b) Implications for patient care: It is important for clinicians to know the treatment schedule and to assess the symptoms based on treatment area and the progression of the treatment course.

10. Patient, caregiver, and family education

a) Sensory information (Obinata, Yamada, & Sasai, 2019)

(1) The treatment is not painful.

(2) The machine will not touch a patient, but it will make noises as it operates and the gantry moves.

(3) A treated patient is not radioactive.

(4) The radiation beam cannot be seen or felt, but some patients who receive RT to the brain experience changes to their sense of smell.

b) Procedural information (Coleman, 2016)

(1) Nurses should provide an overview of the treatment plan.

(2) Nurses should discuss the simulation procedure.

(3) Tattoos or small marks may be made on the skin and are important, as they align the radiation beams the same way each day.

(4) A body or mask mold may be needed to help keep patients still and to ensure proper dose delivery.

(5) Additional techniques, such as use of deep inspiration breath hold, may be used to reduce the effects of breathing motion when needed.

(6) Patients should be informed that while they are alone in the treatment room, radiation therapists can see them via camera and can hear and speak to them via a speaker and microphone.

(7) Patients should not look directly at laser lights.

(8) Patients may need to change into a gown for treatment.

(9) Patients should plan on staying longer than usual at least once a week for an on-treatment visit with a physician or nurse.

c) Expected outcomes: Clinicians should explain expected outcomes and goals (e.g., cure, control, palliation).

d) Additional information: Clinicians should address any myths and misconceptions associated with RT.

References

Alfred, L., & Leaver, D.T. (2016). Treatment delivery equipment. In C.M. Washington & D.T. Leaver (Eds.), *Principles and practice of radiation therapy* (4th ed., pp. 132–155). Elsevier Mosby.

Baskar, R., Lee, K.A., Yeo, R., & Yeoh, K.-W. (2012). Cancer and radiation therapy: Current advances and future directions. *International Journal of Medical Sciences, 9*(3), 193–199. https://doi.org/10.7150/ijms.3635

Behrend, S.W. (2018). Radiation treatment planning. In C.H. Yarbro, D. Wujcik, & B.H. Gobel (Eds.), *Cancer nursing: Principles and practice* (8th ed., pp. 285–332). Jones and Bartlett Learning.

Coleman, A.M. (2016). Treatment procedures. In C.M. Washington & D.T. Leaver (Eds.), *Principles and practice of radiation therapy* (4th ed., pp. 156–177). Elsevier Mosby.

Dest, V.M. (2018). Radiation therapy: Toxicities and management. In C.H. Yarbro, D. Wujcik, & B.H. Gobel (Eds.), *Cancer nursing: Principles and practice* (8th ed., pp. 333–374). Jones and Bartlett Learning.

Gaya, A., & Mahadevan, A. (Eds.). (2015). *Stereotactic body radiotherapy: A practical guide.* Springer-Verlag.

Gosselin, T.K. (2018). Principles of radiation therapy. In C.H. Yarbro, D. Wujcik, & B.H. Gobel (Eds.), *Cancer nursing: Principles and practice* (8th ed., pp. 267–284). Jones and Bartlett Learning.

Gregoire, V., Grau, C., Haustermans, K., Muren, L.P., & Stewart, F. (2015). Principles of radiotherapy. In B. O'Sullivan, J.D. Brierley, A.K. D'Cruz, M.F. Fey, R. Pollock, J.B. Vermorken, & S.H. Huang (Eds.), *UICC manual of clinical oncology* (9th ed., pp. 108–124). Wiley-Blackwell.

Hu, M., Jiang, L., Cui, X., Zhang, J., & Yu, J. (2018). Proton beam therapy for cancer in the era of precision medicine. *Journal of Hematology and Oncology, 11,* 136. https://doi.org/10.1186/s13045-018-0683-4

Khan, F.M. (2020). *Khan's the physics of radiation therapy* (6th ed.). Wolters Kluwer Health.

Mukherji, A. (2018). *Basics of planning and management of patients during radiation therapy: A guide for students and practitioners.* Springer.

Obinata, M., Yamada, K., & Sasai, K. (2019). Unusual olfactory perception during radiation sessions for primary brain tumors: A retrospective study. *Journal of Radiation Research, 60,* 812–817. https://doi.org/10.1093/jrr/rrz060

Perez-Andujar, A., & Klein, E.E. (2019). Electron beam therapy dosimetry and treatment planning. In E.C. Halperin, D.E. Wazer, C.A. Perez, & L.W. Brady (Eds.), *Perez and Brady's principles and practice of radiation oncology* (7th ed., pp. 205–229). Wolters Kluwer.

Saunders, M.I. (1999). Head and neck cancer: Altered fractionation schedules. *Oncologist, 4*(1), 11–16.

Srinivasan, K., Mohammad, M., & Shepherd, J. (2014). Applications of linac-mounted kilovoltage cone-beam computed tomography in modern radiation therapy: A review. *Polish Journal of Radiology, 79,* 181–193. https://doi.org/10.12659/PJR.890745

Teoh, M., Clark, C.H., Wood, K., Whitaker, S., & Nisbet, A. (2011). Volumetric modulated arc therapy: A review of current literature and clinical use in practice. *British Journal of Radiology, 84*(1007), 967–996. https://doi.org/10.1259/bjr/22373346

Tsang, D.S., & Patel, S. (2019). Proton beam therapy for cancer. *Canadian Medical Association Journal, 191*(24), E664–E666. https://doi.org/10.1503/cmaj.190008

Uricchio, N., Givens, J., & Keskemety, J. (2016). Computed tomography simulation procedures. In C.M. Washington & D.T. Leaver (Eds.), *Principles and practice of radiation therapy* (4th ed., pp. 451–479). Elsevier Mosby.

B. Low-dose-rate and high-dose-rate brachytherapy
1. Overview
   a) Brachytherapy is an internal RT approach that involves placement of a radioactive source within a cavity (intracavitary) or very near (interstitial) the area of the tumor (Skowronek, 2017).
   b) Brachytherapy has been used since the early 20th century, following discovery of radium by Marie Curie (Aronowitz, 2015; Holschneider et al., 2019).
   c) Brachytherapy has been used clinically for more than 100 years (Aronowitz, 2015; Holschneider et al., 2019; Tanderup et al., 2017).
   d) The first use of afterloading occurred in 1905 (Skowronek, 2017).
      (1) Afterloaders are applicators that are placed inside the area where the brachytherapy source will be inserted.
      (2) The current brachytherapy process continues to involve the use of afterloaders (Fisher, 2019).
      (3) The afterloading process allows radiation oncologists to accurately perform implants without significant concern of exposure (Aronowitz, 2015).
   e) The use of brachytherapy declined in the 1960s and 1970s with the development of linear accelerators.
      (1) Linear accelerators limited radiation exposure to clinicians, who became wary of the risk that radium posed when used in operating rooms.
      (2) Treatments involving isotopes began to fall out of favor because of personal risks (Aronowitz, 2015).
   f) In the 1980s, interest was renewed after a 1975 Stanford University study of patients with head and neck cancer noted a decrease in cancer control rates with use of linear accelerators alone (Orio & Viswanathan, 2019).
   g) Brachytherapy can be used alone or in combination with other therapies, such as EBRT or chemotherapy.
   h) Brachytherapy delivers the radiation dose to a specified tumor volume with a rapid dose falloff to adjacent healthy tissue (Lukens, Gamez, Hu, & Harrison, 2014; Romano, Pugh, Trifiletti, Libby, & Showalter, 2017; Tanderup et al., 2017).
      (1) Brachytherapy allows for a highly focused radiation dose, which can be achieved in limited size volumes in a short treatment time.
      (2) With brachytherapy, better delineation and coverage of the tumor, more accurate treatment planning, and greater dosimetric optimization can be achieved.
      (3) This can lead to excellent local control with limited severe side effects (Banerjee & Kamrava, 2014; Lukens et al., 2014; Tanderup et al., 2017; Youroukou et al., 2017).
      (4) Local control and limited side effects can be more readily achieved thanks to increased utilization of real-time image-based treatment planning, such as CT, MRI, or ultrasound, which evaluate the position of the applicator. Compared to conventional planning, this technique is more precise and better protects OARs (Cho & Chun, 2018; Holschneider et al., 2019; Karlsson, Dreifaldt, Mordhorst, & Sorbe, 2017; Lukens et al., 2014; Romano et al., 2017; Tanderup et al., 2017; Ward, Tendulkar, & Videtic, 2018).
   i) Currently, most brachytherapy is performed with reactor-produced radionuclides (Aronowitz, 2015; Ward et al., 2018).
      (1) Cesium-137
      (2) Iridium-192
      (3) Gold-198
      (4) Radium-226
      (5) Tantalum-182
   j) Principles of radiobiology inform the use of brachytherapy (Gosselin, 2018; Lukens et al., 2014).
      (1) Alpha, beta, and gamma rays transfer energy to living matter.
      (2) Cellular reproduction process is altered. DNA is damaged.
      (3) Irradiated cells are affected directly and indirectly.
      (4) Irradiated cells die instantly or are unable to divide.
      (5) The extent of cell injury is related to the capabilities of the isotope and the amount of time the isotope is in place.
   k) Care of patients with radioactive implants is complex. Brachytherapy requires the expertise of a team of trained personnel (e.g., physician, physicist, dosimetrist, radiation therapist, radiation nurse, RSO) to implement the individualized treatment plan designed by a radiation oncologist (Orio & Viswanathan, 2019).
2. Brachytherapy procedure
   a) General principles
      (1) Brachytherapy is performed by placing a temporary or permanent sealed radioactive source into a body cavity (intracavitary), into tissue (interstitial), or on the surface of the body (e.g., plaque, custom bolus) (University of Alabama at Birmingham Medicine, n.d.).
      (2) Brachytherapy can also involve placement of catheters into the airway, gastrointestinal tract, or a blood vessel (intraluminal or intravascular) (Tanderup et al., 2017).
      (3) Brachytherapy is used as a single modality or as an adjunctive treatment in combination with EBRT to increase the total dose to a specified target (Lukens et al., 2014; Romano et al., 2017; Tanderup et al., 2017; Ward et al., 2018; Wierzbicka et al., 2016).

(4) Brachytherapy allows for the delivery of a high radiation dose that is tailored to the highest-risk area of disease while sparing the surrounding healthy tissues (Lukens et al., 2014; Youroukou et al., 2017).

(5) With temporary sealed sources, a patient is not radioactive; only the source is. Brachytherapy also allows for decreased risk of applicator movement during therapy, and no special precautions need to be taken with a patient upon removal of the implant (Mayo Clinic, n.d.; Romano et al., 2017; Youroukou et al., 2017).

b) LDR brachytherapy

(1) LDR brachytherapy enhances radiation effect by taking advantage of repair, redistribution, and repopulation principles, even in poorly oxygenated tissue (Gosselin, 2018).

(2) With LDR brachytherapy in the context of gynecologic cancers, approximately 0.4–2 Gy is given in an hour in one to two treatments, totaling 24–144 hours (Banerjee & Kamrava, 2014; Holschneider et al., 2019).

(3) Conventional LDR brachytherapy involves an operative procedure with anesthesia or sedation for placement of a hollow applicator device or catheter into body tissues or cavities.

(4) Radioactive sources are manually afterloaded into the applicators when a patient has returned to the designated hospital room (Behrend, 2018).

 (a) Hospitalization, bed rest, and specialized nursing care are required while the implant remains in place, which may be for one to several days (Banerjee & Kamrava, 2014; Mayo Clinic, n.d.).

 (b) LDR brachytherapy can be performed using remote afterloading techniques.

 (c) Strict room confinement is required for all inpatient brachytherapy (see III. Radiation Protection and Safety).

 (d) Invasive brachytherapy procedures to specific body sites, such as the pelvis and lung, carry risks of complications, such as perforation, infection, and bleeding.

c) HDR brachytherapy

(1) HDR allows for a shorter treatment time and quicker dose delivery, resulting in improved patient comfort and convenience, more reliable positioning of the source, less radiation exposure to caregivers and ancillary personnel, and performance of the procedure on an outpatient basis (elimination of hospitalization) (Aronowitz, 2015; Lukens et al., 2014; Romano et al., 2017; Youroukou et al., 2017).

(2) With HDR brachytherapy in the context of gynecologic cancers, a dose rate of approximately 0.2 Gy is delivered per minute (12 Gy per hour), over the course of four to six treatments, with each session lasting just a few minutes (Banerjee & Kamrava, 2014; Holschneider et al., 2019; Lukens et al., 2014).

(3) HDR brachytherapy involves the use of an automated remote afterloading device for the placement of the radioactive source (most often iridium-192) into the applicators, which have been placed in the tumor or cavity. Sources are remotely loaded from a storage safe in the afterloader and are delivered via source guide tubes or catheters that connect the afterloader to the applicator in the tumor or body cavity (Aronowitz, 2015; Behrend, 2018; Lukens et al., 2014).

(4) HDR brachytherapy reduces the risk of applicator displacement during treatment, decreases the uncertainty associated with applying a single treatment plan, and allows for reduced radiation exposure to medical and nursing staff (Aronowitz, 2015; Holschneider et al., 2019; Lukens et al., 2014; Romano et al., 2017; Xu-Welliver & Lin, 2013).

(5) The use of HDR brachytherapy is possible in practically all sites that can be treated by conventional LDR brachytherapy and by intracavitary, interstitial, intravascular, mold, percutaneous, or intraoperative techniques.

(6) HDR has several advantages over LDR for patients and healthcare providers.

 (a) The precise positioning of the source, lower risk of applicator displacement, infinitely variable dwell times, and custom dose planning are definite advantages.

 (b) Shorter treatment times (minutes versus days), the protection of medical personnel from radiation exposure, and cost-effectiveness are important considerations (Banerjee & Kamrava, 2014; Harkenrider, Block, Siddiqui, & Small, 2015; Romano et al., 2017; Tanderup et al., 2017).

 (c) Similarly, HDR treatments appear to be well tolerated and as effective as LDR treatments. Overall clinical outcomes and toxicities are similar (Banerjee & Kamrava, 2014; Xu-Welliver & Lin, 2013).

 (d) Because of these advantages, adoption and utilization of HDR brachytherapy has increased since the early 2000s (Banerjee & Kamrava, 2014).

(7) Anesthesia or sedation may be required depending on the site, applicator, and age or comprehension of the patient. These procedures are generally performed on an outpatient basis with or without sedation or anes-

thesia (Waring & Gosselin, 2010; Xu-Welliver & Lin, 2013).

    (8) Treatment times are shorter, but more treatments may be needed (Banerjee & Kamrava, 2014; Tanderup et al., 2017).

    (9) Caregivers and visitors are not subject to radiation exposure after the patient is discharged (Mayo Clinic, n.d.; Waring & Gosselin, 2010).

d) Equipment: The following summarizes the types of brachytherapy equipment used for various cancer diagnoses.

    (1) Gynecologic cancers (Weiner & Schwarz, 2015)

        (a) Vaginal cylinder or stump

        (b) Tandem and ovoids or tandem and ring

        (c) Interstitial needles

        (d) Template (e.g., Syed template)

    (2) Head and neck cancers (Lukens et al., 2014; NCCN, 2020c; Wierzbicka et al., 2016)

        (a) Intracavitary catheters

        (b) Interstitial catheters

    (3) NSCLC (NCCN, 2020d; Youroukou et al., 2017)

        (a) Endobronchial catheters

        (b) Interstitial catheters

    (4) Breast cancer (Deng et al., 2017; Lukens et al., 2014; NCCN, 2020a; C. Shah et al., 2018; Tanderup et al., 2017; Ward et al., 2018; see V.C. Breast)

        (a) Interstitial catheters (multicatheter interstitial brachytherapy)

        (b) Applicators

        (c) Multichannel applicators

        (d) Inflatable catheters

        (e) Intracavitary brachytherapy (MammoSite®, Xoft Axxent®, ClearPath™)

    (5) Prostate cancer (Behrend, 2018; Lukens et al., 2014; NCCN, 2020e; Tanderup et al., 2017; see V.G. Male pelvis and prostate)

        (a) Permanent interstitial radioactive seed implant (LDR)

        (b) Temporary interstitial radioactive seed implant (HDR)

3. Indications

a) The following diseases are commonly treated with LDR and HDR brachytherapy (Aronowitz, 2015; Barbarite et al., 2017; Deng et al., 2017; Lukens et al., 2014; NCCN, 2020a, 2020b, 2020c, 2020d, 2020e, 2020f, 2020g; Schefler & Kim, 2018; Tanderup et al., 2017; Ward et al., 2018; Wierzbicka et al., 2016; Youroukou et al., 2017).

    (1) Gynecologic cancers

    (2) Breast cancer

    (3) Soft tissue sarcoma

    (4) Bronchogenic cancers

    (5) Esophageal cancer

    (6) Oropharyngeal cancers

    (7) Nonmelanoma skin cancers

    (8) Head and neck cancers

    (9) Brain cancers

    (10) Meningiomas

    (11) Prostate cancer

    (12) Ocular malignancies (e.g., intraocular melanoma, retinoblastoma)

b) For the setting of cervical cancer, Banerjee and Kamrava (2014) concluded that "brachytherapy is the only demonstrated method of providing the high dose required to control cervical cancer without causing undue side effects" (p. 555).

c) LDR and HDR brachytherapy may be used as a local boost in conjunction with EBRT (Banerjee & Kamrava, 2014; Cho & Chun, 2018; Karlsson et al., 2017; Romano et al., 2017; Tanderup et al., 2017; Ward et al., 2018; Wierzbicka et al., 2016).

d) Brachytherapy is used to treat recurrent or inoperable cancers.

    (1) Lung cancer (bronchogenic)

    (2) Esophageal cancer

e) Brachytherapy is used to control disease in previously irradiated sites.

    (1) Recurrent gynecologic cancers

    (2) Head and neck cancers

    (3) Gastrointestinal cancers

4. Potential risks

a) Acute and late effects of brachytherapy are those caused by effects of ionizing radiation (Banerjee & Kamrava, 2014; Nicholas et al., 2017; Ward et al., 2018).

    (1) Complications of invasive brachytherapy procedures include perforation, infection, or bleeding (A.P. Shah, Strauss, Gielda, & Zusag, 2010).

    (2) Complications associated with bed rest, prolonged patient immobilization, and catheterization, especially for LDR brachytherapy, include thrombophlebitis, pulmonary embolus, urinary sepsis, and displacement of the applicator during treatment (Harkenrider et al., 2015; Romano et al., 2017).

b) See IV. Symptom Management and V. Site-Specific Management for information on side effect assessment and management (see site-specific assessment and management for each implant site).

5. Collaborative management

a) Gynecologic implants (LDR)

    (1) Applicators include intracavitary tandem and ovoids, vaginal cylinders, and transperineal interstitial vaginal template and needles (advanced gynecologic malignancies).

    (2) Patients should follow the pretreatment bowel preparation regimen, per institutional policy.

    (3) Clinicians should refer to institutional radiation safety guidelines for exposure limits for

staff, family, and other visitors (see also III. Radiation Protection and Safety). Portable radiation shields at a patient's bedside should be used according to institutional guidelines.

(4) Strict bed rest is mandatory to prevent dislodgment of applicators.

   (a) A Foley catheter is inserted prior to the procedure to allow a patient to remain on strict bed rest for the duration of treatment.

   (b) Moistened vaginal gauze packing or vaginal balloon-based packing are often used to secure the position of the applicators and to keep the applicator away from the bladder and rectum.

   (c) The applicator may be held in place with radiation briefs or by suturing.

   (d) Bowel management with antidiarrheal medication is given, and a low-residue diet for nutrition is provided.

   (e) The head of the bed should be raised no higher than 30°.

   (f) Clinicians should check the position of the implant every shift, modify bathing and linen change as necessary, and instruct patients on care guidelines and rationale while on bed rest (Banerjee & Kamrava, 2014).

   (g) If the applicator or radioactive source appears to be dislodged, staff must contact the RSO or designee who routinely inspects patient bed linens and surroundings for dislodged radioactive sources, as well as the radiation oncologist.

(5) Clinicians can prevent complications of immobility with use of compression stockings, postoperative deep breathing and coughing exercises, isometric exercises, and anticoagulants, if ordered.

(6) Analgesics (e.g., oral, IV, patient-controlled analgesia, transdermal, epidural) can promote patient comfort and decrease procedure-related pain (Xu-Welliver & Lin, 2013).

   (a) Pain control should be evaluated each shift or more frequently if needed.

   (b) Analgesia is required 30 minutes prior to removal of applicators, especially with interstitial needles and templates, which could cause more pain during removal than other applicators.

(7) Clinicians should reduce social isolation of patients. Frequently used items (call bell, oral hydration, tissues) should be kept within reach. Clinicians should answer calls promptly and check on patients often, as well as educate patients on the rationale of isolation.

(8) Clinicians should address issues of long-term effects of vaginal stenosis, including dyspareunia and postcoital bleeding (Harkenrider et al., 2017; Jakobsson, Ekman, & Ahlberg, 2015; Morris, Do, Chard, & Brand, 2017; see IV.E. Sexual function and dysfunction).

(9) Discharge instructions should be provided and include what symptoms to report (Gosselin, 2018).

   (a) Excessive bleeding from the bladder, vagina, or rectum

   (b) Excessive pain

   (c) Foul odor of urine or vaginal drainage

   (d) Temperature higher than 101°F (38.3°C)

   (e) Increased urinary frequency or dysuria

   (f) Inability to void after four hours

   (g) Diarrhea not controlled with diet or antidiarrheal medications

b) Gynecologic implants (HDR)

   (1) For gynecologic cancers, HDR brachytherapy applicators include tandem and ovoids, tandem and ring, interstitial needles, or vaginal cylinders or stumps.

   (2) Clinicians must teach patients, caregivers, and family what to expect during the treatment.

      (a) Treatment context, symptomatology, and passage of time are important to address during and after brachytherapy (Banerjee & Kamrava, 2014).

      (b) Clinicians should provide special instructions, such as the following.

         i. Nothing to eat or drink after midnight prior for cases requiring anesthesia (tandem and ovoid)

         ii. Light breakfast in the case of a vaginal stump or cylinder

         iii. Regular medications, per the anesthesiologist's instructions

         iv. Antidiarrheal medication, if necessary

   (3) Brachytherapy applicators need to be stabilized or anchored in place to ensure accuracy of source placement.

      (a) As with LDR application insertion, the rectum and bladder should be displaced from the applicator as much as possible (Banerjee & Kamrava, 2014; Xu-Welliver & Lin, 2013).

      (b) The applicators may be stabilized with balloon or gauze packing to minimize movement while transporting a patient.

      (c) After packing is complete, the device may be further stabilized by suturing the labia or using a less invasive approach, such as a tubular elastic mesh dressing retainer.

(d) With a vaginal cylinder applicator, a non-invasive securement device may be used for stabilization of the applicator during treatment.

(4) Patients must be assessed and prepared on arrival to the clinic.

   (a) A Foley catheter may be inserted prior to the placement of applicator for a tandem and ovoid, tandem and ring, or interstitial needles.

   (b) Oral pain medication and antianxiety medication can be administered, as necessary.

(5) Patient vital signs and pain level should be assessed throughout preparation, procedure, and recovery.

(6) Bleeding should be monitored throughout the procedure.

(7) Analgesia should be given 30 minutes prior to removal of applicators for cases that require anesthesia or sedation for implantation, especially with interstitial needles, which could cause more pain during removal than other applicators.

(8) Clinicians must provide patients with discharge instructions, including to report the following (Gosselin & Waring, 2001).

   (a) Excessive bleeding from the bladder, vagina, or rectum

   (b) Excessive pain

   (c) Foul odor of urine or vaginal drainage

   (d) Temperature higher than 101°F (38.3°C)

   (e) Increased urinary frequency or dysuria

   (f) Inability to void after four hours

   (g) Diarrhea not controlled with diet or antidiarrheal medications

(9) Patients should be educated on pelvic site-specific issues, such as vaginal stenosis and sexuality issues (see IV.E. Sexual function and dysfunction).

c) Head and neck implants (LDR)

(1) Plastic catheters are afterloaded with iridium seeds.

(2) An interstitial implant can be used alone or in combination with EBRT for treatment of oral tongue, floor of mouth, or buccal mucosa.

(3) Surface mold brachytherapy can be used for select superficial (less than 1 cm depth) initial or recurrent superficial lesions of the hard palate, lower gingiva, and floor of mouth. An impression is made of the surface to be irradiated with HDR catheters inserted into predrilled holes or grooves in the mold and sealed with dental plaster (Ward et al., 2018).

(4) Clinicians should encourage routine postoperative exercises (e.g., deep breathing, chang-

ing position in bed, ambulating inside room) if appropriate in order to prevent respiratory or cardiovascular complications.

(5) Prior to implantation, the patient should follow an aggressive bowel regimen to decrease the risk of dislodging radioactive sources while straining during bowel movement (Devine & Doyle, 2001).

(6) Prior to implantation, a patient's ability to read and write should be assessed (Devine & Doyle, 2001).

   (a) Staff should provide tools for communication if needed (e.g., pen and paper, whiteboard with marker).

   (b) If a patient is illiterate, staff must provide alternative communication strategies (e.g., cards with commonly needed items or nursing care procedures pictured).

   (c) Comprehensive patient, caregiver, and family education can reduce stress surrounding the procedure.

(7) Tracheostomy may be performed for airway obstruction resulting from edema (Devine & Doyle, 2001).

   (a) A tracheostomy set, respiratory suctioning equipment, and oxygen must be available.

   (b) Prior to implantation, clinicians should teach patients techniques for self-suctioning, oral hygiene, and tracheostomy care if indicated.

(8) While the implant is in place, nutrition and fluids can be provided via a soft or liquid diet, nasogastric tube, or IV hydration. Although some patients with head and neck implants can sip a liquid formula through a straw, most require feeding through a nasogastric tube (Otter, Holloway, Devlin, & Stewart, 2019).

(9) NSAIDs or narcotic analgesics as needed can promote patient comfort. Clinicians should be cautious to avoid overmedication, which can result in suppression of cough reflex or respirations.

(10) The implant site should be inspected for intactness at every shift.

   (a) Clinicians must discourage patients from touching the site.

   (b) Exact placement of the applicator is crucial for treatment efficacy.

(11) Patients should be informed that bleeding may occur during removal of catheters.

d) Lung implants (HDR or LDR)

(1) In the setting of lung cancer, endobronchial catheters are placed during fiber-optic bronchoscopy, and iridium-125 seed ribbons are temporarily applied (Behrend, 2018; Youroukou et al., 2017).

(a) Permanent brachytherapy is also utilized.

(b) A radioactive Vicryl® mesh (an absorbable material) with iridium-125 is placed intraoperatively in the tumor bed (Youroukou et al., 2017).

(2) Endobronchial brachytherapy can be an efficient and safe treatment option for patients with inoperable endobronchial carcinoma, and Vicryl mesh brachytherapy following sublobar resection is a feasible intraoperative procedure for patients with stage IA and IB NSCLC and a poor cardiopulmonary reserve (Youroukou et al., 2017).

(3) Placement of HDR implants is an outpatient procedure.

(a) Patients should have nothing by mouth for 8–12 hours before the procedure.

(b) Before the procedure, vital signs and oxygen saturation are monitored, and an IV is started.

(c) A nurse prepares the patient for bronchoscopy, which is used to guide a catheter to the tumor area.

(d) IV sedation, local anesthetics, and additional medications may be administered to provide comfort and to minimize gag reflex.

(e) The patient should be discharged per institutional policy.

(4) Placement of LDR implants is an inpatient procedure.

(a) Patients receiving LDR brachytherapy require hospitalization for two to seven days, depending on the radioactive source strength (Behrend, 2018).

(b) After bronchoscopy and placement of the catheter, the patient is moved to a radiation safety–approved room where the radioactive source is loaded (see also III. Radiation Protection and Safety).

(c) A nurse monitors for complications, such as bleeding, infection, and respiratory compromise.

(d) The patient is discharged after the radioactive source and catheter are removed and the patient has recovered from the procedure. A follow-up appointment is scheduled for the next day with the radiation oncologist and pulmonologist.

e) Eye plaques

(1) Eye plaques can be used to treat retinoblastoma, which is most common in pediatric patients and young adults, as well as uveal, ocular, and choroidal melanoma, which is most common in adults (Schefler & Kim, 2018).

(2) Although advanced cases of retinoblastoma are preferentially treated with systemic or intra-arterial chemotherapy, radioactive plaque brachytherapy (plaque RT) is effective as salvage therapy in cases that otherwise would have been managed with enucleation (Schefler & Kim, 2018).

(3) Plaque RT is LDR, and placement is performed in an operating room by an ophthalmologic surgeon while the patient is under anesthesia (Reiman, 2019).

(a) A radiation physicist is also present.

(b) Equipment for iodine-125 ocular plaque construction and placement includes the following (Schefler & Kim, 2018).

　i. Dummy plaque to aid in the placement of the necessary retention sutures

　ii. Gold backing with lug holes for sutures

　iii. Plastic insert to hold the radioactive iodine-125 seeds

(c) A lead eye shield is placed over the plaque in the operating room (Reiman, 2019).

(d) Each plaque is custom made to provide individualized treatment for each tumor (Duke Radiation Oncology, n.d.).

(e) Other types of plaques using various isotopes are available.

(4) Special care for adult and pediatric patients is required to protect the affected eye from trauma (e.g., creative, occlusive bandaging for pediatric patients).

(5) Acute effects are pain and operative infection.

(6) Long-term effects are cataracts, radiation retinopathy, radiation optic neuropathy, and vision loss (Schefler & Kim, 2018).

(7) Patient recovery occurs in an inpatient setting (Duke Radiation Oncology, n.d.).

(a) The plaque emits radiation for five days.

(b) After that period, it is removed.

(8) Radiation exposure from the shielded eye plaque is extremely low and does not present a significant hazard to staff or visitors (Reiman, 2019).

6. Brachytherapy for benign disease: pterygium

a) Pterygium is a growth of wedge-shaped membrane from the conjunctiva to the cornea, arising from the fissure between the eyelids. It is caused by repeated irritation to the eyes (e.g., welding, woodwork, sun, sand) (University of Alabama at Birmingham Medicine, n.d.).

b) Treatment uses a beta-emitting applicator. Treatment dose is one single fraction of 20 Gy or multiple-fraction regimens of 8–10 Gy given immediately postoperatively followed by two more treatments at seven-day intervals (University of Alabama at Birmingham Medicine, n.d.).

   c) Primary treatment for pterygium is surgery; however, rate of regrowth with surgery is high (20%–30%) (University of Alabama at Birmingham Medicine, n.d.). Brachytherapy decreases recurrence rates to 20% or less (Tripuraneni, 2009).

7. Patient, caregiver, and family education

   a) Clinicians should educate patients, caregivers, and family on the type of implant, rationale, procedure, preparation, sensory information, availability of pain medication, and care during treatment specific to the implant used.

   b) Comprehensive patient, caregiver, and family education about the brachytherapy procedure, necessary visitation restrictions, and the anticipation of potential patient problems is instrumental in preventing complications.

   c) Patients receiving HDR brachytherapy experience side effects similar to those caused by external RT, with fatigue being the most often reported symptom (Jakobsson et al., 2015).

   d) Clinicians should discuss the rationale and methods for radiation protection, such as self-care while the implant is in place and limitations on staff and visitor time in room (see also III. Radiation Protection and Safety).

   e) Clinicians must provide verbal and written discharge instructions with guidelines for activity, bathing, skin or wound care, diet, smoking restrictions (with bronchoscopy), alcohol restrictions, medication guidelines, and symptoms to report to a physician or nurse.

   f) Clinicians should instruct patients on the early and late side effects, address specific questions and concerns, and provide follow-up appointment information.

8. Related websites

   a) American Brachytherapy Society: www.american brachytherapy.org

   b) ASTRO: www.astro.org

   c) ONS: www.ons.org

References

Aronowitz, J.N. (2015). Afterloading: The technique that rescued brachytherapy. *International Journal of Radiation Oncology, Biology, Physics, 92,* 479–487. https://doi.org/10.1016/j.ijrobp.2015.02.014

Banerjee, R., & Kamrava, M. (2014). Brachytherapy in the treatment of cervical cancer: A review. *International Journal of Women's Health, 6,* 555–564. https://doi.org/10.2147/IJWH.S46247

Barbarite, E., Sick, J.T., Berchmans, E., Bregy, A., Shah, A.H., Elsayyad, N., & Komotar, R.J. (2017). The role of brachytherapy in the treatment of glioblastoma multiforme. *Neurosurgical Review, 40,* 195–211. https://doi.org/10.1007/s10143-016-0727-6

Behrend, S.W. (2018). Radiation treatment planning. In C.H. Yarbro, D. Wujcik, & B.H. Gobel (Eds.), *Cancer nursing: Principles and practice* (8th ed., pp. 285–332). Jones and Bartlett Learning.

Cho, O., & Chun, M. (2018). Management for locally advanced cervical cancer: New trends and controversial issues. *Radiation Oncology Journal, 36,* 254–264. https://doi.org/10.3857/roj.2018.00500

Deng, X., Wu, H., Gao, F., Su, Y., Li, Q., Liu, S., & Cai, J. (2017). Brachytherapy in the treatment of breast cancer. *International Journal of Clinical Oncology, 22,* 641–650. https://doi.org/10.1007/s10147-017-1155-5

Devine, P., & Doyle, T. (2001). Brachytherapy for head and neck cancer: A case study. *Clinical Journal of Oncology Nursing, 5,* 55–57.

Duke Radiation Oncology. (n.d.). Cancer care. https://radonc.duke.edu/patient-care/cancer-care

Fisher, C. (2019). Recent advances in brachytherapy. *Astronews, 22,* 18. https://www.astro.org/ASTRO/media/ASTRO/News%20and%20Publications/ASTROnews/PDFs/2019_Spring_ASTROnews.pdf

Gosselin, T.K. (2018). Principles of radiation therapy. In C.H. Yarbro, D. Wujcik, & B.H. Gobel (Eds.), *Cancer nursing: Principles and practice* (8th ed., pp. 267–284). Jones and Bartlett Learning.

Gosselin, T.K., & Waring, J.S. (2001). Nursing management of patients receiving brachytherapy for gynecologic malignancies. *Clinical Journal of Oncology Nursing, 5,* 59–63.

Harkenrider, M.M., Block, A.M., Alektiar, K.M., Gaffney, D.K., Jones, E., Klopp, A., ... Small, W., Jr. (2017). *Brachytherapy, 16,* 95–108. https://doi.org/10.1016/j.brachy.2016.04.005

Harkenrider, M.M., Block, A.M., Siddiqui, Z.A., & Small, W., Jr. (2015). The role of vaginal cuff brachytherapy in endometrial cancer. *Gynecological Oncology, 136,* 365–372. https://doi.org/10.1016/j.ygyno.2014.12.036

Holschneider, C.H., Petereit, D.G., Chu, C., Hsu, I.-C., Ioffe, Y.J., Klopp, A.H., ... Yashar, C. (2019). Brachytherapy: A critical component of primary radiation therapy for cervical cancer: From the Society of Gynecological Oncology (SGO) and the American Brachytherapy Society (ABS). *Brachytherapy, 18,* 123–132. https://doi.org/10.1016/j.brachy.2018.11.009

Jakobsson, S., Ekman, T., & Ahlberg, K. (2015). Living through pelvic radiotherapy: A mixed method study of self-care activities and distressful symptoms. *European Journal of Oncology Nursing, 19,* 301–309. https://doi.org/10.1016/j.ejon.2014.10.014

Karlsson, J., Dreifaldt, A.-C., Mordhorst, L.B., & Sorbe, B. (2017). Differences in outcome for cervical cancer patients treated with or without brachytherapy. *Brachytherapy, 16,* 133–140. https://doi.org/10.1016/j.brachy.2016.09.011

Lukens, J.N., Gamez, M., Hu, K., & Harrison, L.B. (2014). Modern brachytherapy. *Seminars in Oncology, 41,* 831–847. https://doi.org/10.1053/j.seminoncol.2014.09.015

Mayo Clinic. (n.d.). Brachytherapy. https://www.mayoclinic.org/tests-procedures/brachytherapy/about/pac-20385159

Morris, L., Do, V., Chard, J., & Brand, A.H. (2017). Radiation-induced vaginal stenosis: Current perspectives. *International Journal of Women's Health, 9,* 273–279. https://doi.org/10.2147/IJWH.S106796

National Comprehensive Cancer Network. (2020a). *NCCN Clinical Practice Guidelines in Oncology (NCCN Guidelines®): Breast cancer* [v.4.2020]. https://www.nccn.org/professionals/physician_gls/pdf/breast.pdf

National Comprehensive Cancer Network. (2020b). *NCCN Clinical Practice Guidelines in Oncology (NCCN Guidelines®): Cervical cancer* [v.1.2020]. https://www.nccn.org/professionals/physician_gls/pdf/cervical.pdf

National Comprehensive Cancer Network. (2020c). *NCCN Clinical Practice Guidelines in Oncology (NCCN Guidelines®): Head and neck cancers* [v.1.2020]. https://www.nccn.org/professionals/physician_gls/pdf/head-and-neck.pdf

National Comprehensive Cancer Network. (2020d). *NCCN Clinical Practice Guidelines in Oncology (NCCN Guidelines®): Non-small cell lung cancer* [v.6.2020]. https://www.nccn.org/professionals/physician_gls/pdf/nscl.pdf

National Comprehensive Cancer Network. (2020e). *NCCN Clinical Practice Guidelines in Oncology (NCCN Guidelines®): Prostate cancer* [v.1.2020]. https://www.nccn.org/professionals/physician_gls/pdf/prostate.pdf

National Comprehensive Cancer Network. (2020f). *NCCN Clinical Practice Guidelines in Oncology (NCCN Guidelines®): Soft tissue sarcoma* [v.1.2020]. https://www.nccn.org/professionals/physician_gls/pdf/sarcoma.pdf

National Comprehensive Cancer Network. (2020g). *NCCN Clinical Practice Guidelines in Oncology (NCCN Guidelines®): Uveal melanoma* [v.1.2020]. https://www.nccn.org/professionals/physician_gls/PDF/uveal.pdf

Nicholas, S., Chen, L., Choflet, A., Fader, A., Guss, Z., Hazell, S., ... Viswanathan, A.N. (2017). Pelvic radiation and normal tissue toxicity. *Seminars in Radiation Oncology, 27,* 358–369. https://doi.org/10.1016/j.semradonc.2017.04.010

Orio, P.F., & Viswanathan, A.N. (2019). Sustaining the art and outcomes of brachytherapy. *Astronews, 22,* 10–12. https://www.astro.org/ASTRO/media/ASTRO/News%20and%20Publications/ASTROnews/PDFs/2019_Spring_ASTROnews.pdf

Otter, S.J., Holloway, C., Devlin, P.M., & Stewart, A.J. (2019). Clinical applications of brachytherapy: Low dose rate and pulsed dose rate. In E.C. Halperin, D.E. Wazer, C.A. Perez, & L.W. Brady (Eds.), *Perez and Brady's principles and practice of radiation oncology* (7th ed., pp. 582–606). Wolters Kluwer.

Reiman, R. (2019). Radiation protection aspects of eye plaque therapy for ocular cancer. https://vmw-oesoapps.duhs.duke.edu/radsafety/nurses/eyeplaque/eyeplaque.pdf

Romano, K.D., Pugh, K.J., Trifiletti, D.M., Libby, B., & Showalter, T.N. (2017). Transition from LDR to HDR brachytherapy for cervical cancer: Evaluation of tumor control, survival, and toxicity. *Brachytherapy, 16,* 378–386. https://doi.org/10.1016/j.brachy.2016.12.005

Schefler, A.C., & Kim, R.S. (2018). Recent advancements in the management of retinoblastoma and uveal melanoma. *F1000Research, 7,* 476. https://doi.org/10.12688/f1000research.11941.1

Shah, A.P., Strauss, J.B., Gielda, B.T., & Zusag, T.W. (2010). Toxicity associated with bowel or bladder puncture during gynecologic interstitial brachytherapy. *International Journal of Radiation Oncology, Biology, Physics, 77,* 171–179. https://doi.org/10.1016/j.ijrobp.2009.04.077

Shah, C., Vicini, F., Shaitelman, S.F., Hepel, J., Keisch, M., Arthur, D., ... Wazer, D.E. (2018). The American Brachytherapy Society consensus statement for accelerated partial-breast irradiation. *Brachytherapy, 17,* 154–170. https://doi.org/10.1016/j.brachy.2017.09.004

Skowronek, J. (2017). Current status of brachytherapy in cancer treatment— Short overview. *Journal of Contemporary Brachytherapy, 9,* 581–589. https://doi.org/10.5114/jcb.2017.72607

Tanderup, K., Ménard, C., Polgar, C., Lindegaard, J.C., Kirisits, C., & Pötter, R. (2017). Advancements in brachytherapy. *Advanced Drug Delivery Reviews, 109,* 15–25. https://doi.org/10.1016/j.addr.2016.09.002

Tripuraneni, P. (2009). Benign diseases. In B.G. Haffty & L.D. Wilson (Eds.), *Handbook of radiation oncology: Basic principles and clinical protocols* (pp. 755–761). Jones and Bartlett Learning.

University of Alabama at Birmingham Medicine. (n.d.). Brachytherapy. https://www.uabmedicine.org/patient-care/treatments/brachytherapy/-/asset_publisher/3iFTIipRYIFQ/content/brain-tumors-malignant

Ward, M.C., Tendulkar, R.D., & Videtic, G.M.M. (Eds.). (2018). *Essentials of clinical radiation oncology.* Springer. https://doi.org/10.1891/9780826

Waring, J., & Gosselin, T. (2010). Developing a high-dose-rate prostate brachytherapy program. *Clinical Journal of Oncology Nursing, 14,* 199–205. https://doi.org/10.1188/10.CJON.199-205

Weiner, A.A., & Schwarz, J.K. (2015). Intracavitary brachytherapy for gynecologic malignancies: Applications and innovations. *Missouri Medicine, 112*(5), 366–372.

Wierzbicka, M., Bartochowska, A., Strnad, V., Strojan, P., Mendenhall, W.M., Harrison, L.B., ... Ferlito, A. (2016). The role of brachytherapy in the treatment of squamous cell carcinoma of the head and neck. *European Archives of Oto-Rhino-Laryngology, 273,* 269–276. https://doi.org/10.1007/s00405-014-3332-8

Xu-Welliver, M., & Lin, L.L. (2013). Evaluation of a balloon-based vaginal packing system and patient-controlled analgesia for patients with cervical cancer undergoing high-dose-rate intracavitary brachytherapy. *Practical Radiation Oncology, 3,* 263–268. https://doi.org/10.1016/j.prro.2012.11.004

Youroukou, A., Gkiozos, I., Kalaitzi, Z., Tsalafoutas, I., Papalla, K., Charpidou, A., & Kouloulias, V. (2017). The potential role of brachytherapy in the irradiation of patients with lung cancer: A systematic review. *Clinical and Translational Oncology, 19,* 945–950. https://doi.org/10.1007/s12094-017-1635-0Stereotactic radiosurgery

C. Stereotactic radiosurgery

1. Procedure

   a) Definition

   (1) SRS is a technique to deliver precisely directed, high-dose ionizing radiation to a target with the purpose of destroying tumor cells while minimizing the radiation dose to the surrounding normal tissue (Seung et al., 2013).

   (2) The term *stereotactic* describes using three-dimensional guidance to precisely perform a procedure.

   (3) The term *radiosurgery* describes the delivery of the stereotactically guided radiation treatment to the defined target volume in a single session (Belcher, Liu, Chmura, Yenice, & Wiersma, 2017; Halasz & Rockhill, 2013).

   (4) The evolution of SRS has included delivery of this high-dose, precise radiation in more than one session. In 2006, members of the American Association of Neurological Surgeons/Congress of Neurological Surgeons Washington Committee Stereotactic Radiosurgery Task Force, in conjunction with ASTRO, approved a contemporary definition of SRS to include delivery of the intended dose in one to five sessions (Seung et al., 2013; Sheehan et al., 2018).

   b) History: In 1951, Lars Leksell, a Swedish neurosurgeon, was the first to describe the concept of using single-fraction irradiation of intracranial targets to replace surgery in selected patients (Ma, Wang, Tseng, & Sahgal, 2017).

   c) Radiobiologic advantages

   (1) SRS allows for delivery of high-dose ionizing radiation to the intended target while exposing surrounding healthy tissues to a much lower dose (Song et al., 2019).

   (2) The biologically effective dose of single-fraction SRS appears to be more clinically efficacious than predicted using the linear-quadratic model. The linear-quadratic model is the most widely accepted mathematical model for describing the damaging effects of conventionally fractionated ionizing radiation on healthy and neoplastic tissue (Kondziolka, Shin, Brunswick, Kim, & Silverman, 2015; Song et al., 2019).

   (3) High-dose-per-fraction ionizing radiation causes direct cytotoxic damage related to DNA damage, as is seen in conventional low-dose fractionation. Additionally, it causes damage to supporting tissues of the neoplasm, such as microvasculature tissue and stromal tissue, which is specific to high doses (Song et al., 2019).

   (4) SRS may be more effective against radioresistant tumor stem cells, thus enhancing tumor eradication (Song et al., 2019; Thiagarajan & Yamada, 2017).

d) Optimal requirements for the use of SRS
  (1) Small target and treatment volume allow for improved tolerance of surrounding healthy tissues (Balik, Chao, & Neyman, 2018).
  (2) A sharply defined target allows irradiation with a minimal margin of surrounding healthy tissue without underdosing the target (marginal miss) (Tuleasca et al., 2019).
  (3) Accurate radiation delivery requires minimal potential for setup error, which would require a margin of healthy tissue to prevent underdosing of the target (Tuleasca et al., 2019).
  (4) High conformity can be achieved if the delivered treatment volume can be matched to the PTV (Balik et al., 2018).
  (5) Sensitive structures are excluded from the target. Radiation dose-limiting structures (e.g., optic chiasm, spinal cord) can be excluded from the PTV to limit the risk of radiation injury (Milano et al., 2018).

2. Indications
  a) Intracranial metastases
    (1) SRS plus whole-brain RT: The RTOG 95-08 trial demonstrated significant survival advantage in patients with a solitary lesion treated with combination therapy; patients with two to three lesions had significantly improved local control without survival advantage (Hatiboglu, Tuzgen, Akdur, & Chang, 2016; Kraft, Zindler, Minniti, Guckenberger, & Andratschke, 2019; Thiagarajan & Yamada, 2017).
    (2) SRS as monotherapy
      (a) Currently, SRS is an appropriate treatment for patients with 1–10 lesions, with none larger than 4 cm in diameter.
      (b) Advantages over surgical management are that SRS can treat lesions in deep or eloquent regions of the brain; it is a noninvasive outpatient procedure without anesthesia risk; and it has a short recovery time and allows for rapid initiation of systemic therapies (Hatiboglu et al., 2016; Kalash et al., 2017).
      (c) SRS as monotherapy is a reasonable treatment option but carries a higher risk of developing distant brain recurrence; thus, it requires careful, active surveillance to ensure early identification of intracranial recurrence and initiation of salvage therapy (Hatiboglu et al., 2016).
  b) Primary malignant brain tumors
    (1) SRS with a median dose of 15–24 Gy, dependent on the tumor size, has been used as salvage therapy for locally recurrent glioblastoma multiforme after standard fractionated RT and as consolidation therapy following conventional RT (Bir, Connor, Ambekar, Wilden, & Nanda, 2015; Redmond & Mehta, 2015).
    (2) The efficacy of SRS as a boost in the initial treatment of malignant gliomas has been increasing in clinical practice and has become standard of care for newly diagnosed glioblastoma multiforme (Alghamdi et al., 2018; Brehmer et al., 2018). However, Imber et al. (2017) highlighted that a retrospective report found conflicting results regarding the efficacy of adding SRS to conventional RT and that randomized trials have found no clear benefit to dose escalation or boosts.
    (3) Several prospective and retrospective studies have determined that SRS in patients with malignant gliomas may prolong survival in this setting, either alone or in combination with chemotherapy (Alghamdi et al., 2018; Redmond & Mehta, 2015).
  c) Benign tumors
    (1) Acoustic neuroma (vestibular schwannoma)
      (a) Acoustic neuromas arise from the vestibular portion of cranial nerve VIII (Lo et al., 2018).
      (b) Multiple studies have demonstrated comparable tumor control rates compared to surgical resection for small to medium lesions (Lefranc et al., 2018).
      (c) Advantages of SRS over microsurgery include a higher rate of hearing preservation; decreased incidence of facial neuropathy, brain stem dysfunction, and trigeminal neuropathy; and fewer postoperative complications (Lefranc et al., 2018).
    (2) Meningioma
      (a) Multiple studies have demonstrated a five-year local control rate of 88%–100% (Lesueur et al., 2019).
      (b) SRS is appropriate for incompletely resected or inoperable meningiomas 3 cm or smaller (Lesueur et al., 2019).
      (c) Meningiomas in the cavernous sinus and at the base of the skull have high surgical morbidity, including vascular and cranial nerve morbidity. SRS is a much less morbid option for treatment for lesions smaller than 3 cm (Leroy, Tuleasca, Reyns, & Levivier, 2018).
      (d) Research shows that 10%–20% of cavernous brain malformations are positioned in the deep brain areas, such as tumors involving the brain stem or optic apparatus, those substantially compressing the brain stem, or those that are large where surgical intervention poses a greater risk. The role of SRS for these high-risk tumors

has remained controversial (Jacobs et al., 2019).

(3) Pituitary adenoma: SRS has a 95.2% overall response rate (volume reduction) for patients with nonsecretory adenomas, 54% hormonal normalization rate in acromegaly and Cushing disease, and 44.3% remission rate for prolactinomas (Krengli, Apicella, Deantonio, Paolini, & Masini, 2015; Naeem, Darbar, & Shamim, 2018).

(4) Glomus jugulare tumors

    (a) Glomus jugulare tumors are a common site of paraganglioma involving the jugular bulb that causes lower cranial nerve symptoms, including hearing loss, tinnitus, hoarseness, vertigo, and facial weakness and numbness (Hafez, Morgan, Fahmy, & Hassan, 2018).

    (b) Research data show that SRS is an excellent treatment modality, with tumor control rates of 63%–100% (Lo et al., 2018).

    (c) SRS achieved excellent tumor control with low risk of morbidity, and 92.5% of patients reported improvement in one or more of their presenting symptoms. Actuarial tumor size control rate after Gamma Knife surgery was 97.5% at three years (Hafez et al., 2018).

d) AVM

(1) SRS has been widely used to treat AVM over the past two decades.

(2) Angiographic evidence of cure (obliteration) is seen in 80%–90% of patients after a latency period of three to five years (Song et al., 2019).

(3) The risk of hemorrhage from AVM decreases significantly during the latency period (after SRS and before angiographic obliteration) and further decreases after obliteration. The risk reduction appears greatest in patients presenting with hemorrhage (Chen et al., 2019).

(4) The risks of developing permanent symptomatic sequelae (necrosis) from SRS for AVM are significantly correlated with intracranial location and the volume of brain tissue receiving 12 Gy. The following locations are ordered from highest to lowest risk of necrosis (Lo et al., 2018).

    (a) Pons and midbrain

    (b) Basal ganglia

    (c) Thalamus

    (d) Medulla

    (e) Occipital lobe

    (f) Corpus callosum

    (g) Cerebellum

    (h) Parietal lobe

    (i) Intraventricular, temporal, and frontal lobes

(5) Management of large AVMs may include the addition of pre-SRS embolization and staged SRS in which the lesion is treated in two to three sessions separated by several months (Strauss et al., 2017; Sun, Li, Xiong, Yu, & Lv, 2019; Todnem et al., 2019).

(6) A recent study concluded that SRS was effective in improving AVM headaches but not in improving the performance status of treated patients as measured by Modified Rankin Scale. The Modified Rankin Scale is a widely accepted six-point measure of functional outcome after stroke and reflects limitations in activity and changes in lifestyle (Todnem et al., 2019).

e) Trigeminal neuralgia

(1) SRS is used for typical trigeminal neuralgia refractory to medical therapy.

(2) The maximum dose is 70–90 Gy to a 4–6 mm target area, along with the trigeminal root entry zone in the pons (Berti et al., 2018).

(3) The initial response rate is high (72%–86%) but deteriorates over time. Residual excellent and good results measured by the Barrow Neurologic Institute scale were seen in only 44%–50% five years after treatment (Berti et al., 2018; Pokhrel et al., 2017).

(4) Retreatment may need to be considered, including repeat SRS, microvascular decompression, or rhizotomy (Berti et al., 2018).

f) Spinal metastasis: Meleis et al. (2019) conducted a large, single-institution chart review of all patients treated with SRS for spinal metastases.

(1) Patients had various histologic pathologies.

(2) Patients received 12–16 Gy in a single fraction or multiple fractions (18 Gy in three fractions, 24 Gy in three fractions, 24 Gy in four fractions, and 30 Gy in five fractions).

(3) The review reported that 68.4% of patients had improvement in pain.

(4) Of those with pretreatment neurologic deficits, 55% noted improvement without a single case of radiation myelitis.

g) Extracranial sites: SBRT

(1) Lung

    (a) Medically inoperable early-stage NSCLC

        i. A recent large, multicenter, prospective trial demonstrated a survival rate of approximately 77% at two years with a 59% rate of tumor control in patients treated with standard RT (Harrison, 2019).

        ii. The dose delivered was 18 Gy for three fractions (54 Gy total) over 1.5–2 weeks, and tumors less than

2 cm from the chest wall received 12 Gy in four fractions (48 Gy total) (Harrison, 2019).

  (b) Lung metastasis: Safety and efficacy of SBRT for treatment of one to three lesions have been shown with two-year local control of 96% and a low incidence of grade 3 toxicity (Wegner et al., 2018).

(2) Liver

  (a) Primary hepatocellular carcinoma

    i. A retrospective study showed that SBRT is highly effective with doses of 45–60 Gy given in three fractions (Lee et al., 2018).

    ii. Studies of SBRT for hepatocellular carcinoma have shown encouraging outcomes, with local control rates of 66%–100% and overall survival of 52%–100% at two or three years without severe toxicities (Lee et al., 2018).

    iii. SBRT is an effective treatment for small hepatocellular carcinoma (smaller than 3 cm), with high local control rates of 96%–100% and overall survival rates of 56%–76% (Lee et al., 2018).

    iv. SBRT can be combined with transarterial chemoembolization for advanced hepatocellular carcinoma with portal vein tumor thrombosis, with minimal side effects and a response rate comparable to invasive local therapies (Murray & Dawson, 2017).

  (b) Liver metastasis

    i. In sequential phase 1 and 2 studies, SBRT was given as 22.7–62.1 Gy in six fractions. It was well tolerated as noninvasive therapy. The control rate was 49.8% at one year and 26.2% at four years (McPartlin et al., 2017).

    ii. Long-term survivors of unresected liver metastasis treated with SBRT (25–45 Gy in two to five fractions) have remained disease free (McPartlin et al., 2017).

(3) Pancreas

  (a) SBRT has been used to treat locally advanced unresectable and recurrent pancreatic adenocarcinoma.

  (b) Myrehaug et al. (2016) demonstrated that SBRT to the pancreas could be delivered effectively (greater than 70% local tumor control rate) with significant risk of late toxicity (5%–11%). However, most patients in this study died of distant disease progression.

  (c) Despite advances in surgery, systemic therapy, and RT, prognosis for pancreatic cancer remains poor (Myrehaug et al., 2016).

(4) Prostate

  (a) Typically a slowly proliferating cancer, prostate cancer is thought to be more sensitive to hypofractionated RT (Syed, Patel-Yadav, Rivers, & Singh, 2017).

  (b) Lukka et al. (2018) reported outcomes from the RTOG 0938 trial.

    i. Ultrahypofractionated SBRT was used to treat 127 patients in 5 fractions and 128 patients in 12 fractions, for clinically localized prostate cancer.

    ii. Two patients in the five-fraction arm experienced grade 3 acute treatment-related toxicity (diarrhea and urinary retention).

    iii. Two patients in the five-fraction arm experienced late grade 3 bladder or bowel toxicity; one patient experienced proctitis; and one patient experienced noninfective cystitis, urinary incontinence, and urinary tract obstruction.

    iv. No participants experienced grade 4 or 5 acute or late urinary or bowel toxicities in the five-fraction arm.

    v. In the 12-fraction arm, two patients had grade 3 acute toxicity (both proctitis).

    vi. In the 12-fraction arm, two patients experienced late grade 3 toxicities (proctitis, urinary retention, and colonic fistula). One of these patients developed a colonic fistula, which was considered a grade 3 late toxicity.

    vii. No participants developed grade 4 or 5 treatment-related urinary or bowel toxicity in the 12-fraction arm.

    viii. At two-year median follow-up, no patients had a biochemical failure in either arm.

(5) Kidney (Funayama et al., 2019)

  (a) Renal cell carcinoma is traditionally thought to be radioresistant to conventionally fractionated RT.

  (b) Multiple studies have investigated SBRT for primary and metastatic renal cell carcinoma with early evidence of efficacy for pain relief and local control.

  (c) Research studies reported positive outcomes of SBRT for a primary renal cell carcinoma lesion. It has not been determined how tumor size and renal function changes over time in a long-term follow-up.

(d) Funayama et al. (2019) highlighted the efficacy and safety of SBRT for primary renal cell carcinoma. They stated that the local progression-free rate for three years is 92.3%, and the efficacy rate was previously 84%–100%.

(e) Furthermore, Funayama et al. (2019) also found that after SBRT, all renal tumors decreased in size slowly but continuously for years. Therefore, renal cancer can be treated radically with SBRT as a radiosensitive tumor.

(6) Immunogenic effects

(a) SBRT has emerged as a platform to exploit the immunogenic effects of ionizing radiation, given its unique properties from a technical, radiobiologic, and immunologic standpoint.

(b) SBRT in combination with immunotherapy has been a logical next step in a future trial (Marciscano et al., 2019).

(c) Chajon, Castelli, Marsiglia, & De Crevoisier (2017) illuminated that the synergistic effect of RT and immunotherapy represents a plausible opportunity to improve the therapeutic ratio and to prolong tumor response.

3. SRS delivery systems

a) Gamma Knife (Berti et al., 2018; Elekta, n.d.)

(1) In 1968, Leksell and Börje Larsson installed the first prototype of Gamma Knife, which used a hemispherical array of 201 fixed cobalt-60 beams to create spherical treatment volumes of various diameter.

(2) Multiple upgrades have produced the ability to treat a broader range of lesion sizes and reduced treatment time.

b) CyberKnife: CyberKnife combines a miniaturized linear accelerator mounted on a robotic arm with continual image guidance to track target motion throughout the multiple-beam treatment (Accuray, n.d.; Nalichowski et al., 2017; Romagna et al., 2018).

c) Linear accelerator–based systems (Babic et al., 2018)

(1) Modification of a linear accelerator designed for conventional RT to be used for SRS involves hardware and software advances for improved beam shaping with circular secondary and micromultileaf collimators, stereotactic guidance systems, increased conformity dose planning, and improved immobilization and position verification.

(2) Commercially available systems include Novalis Tx™ and the XKnife™.

d) Proton beam therapy

(1) Proton beam therapy has a distinct advantage of the beam's ability to stop at a depth related to the beam's energy; hence, it lacks an exit dose. Increased ionization at the distal aspect of the beam causes increased radiobiologic effect (cell kill). The highest energy deposition occurs in the target volume (Bragg peak) (Johnson, 2018; Lesueur et al., 2019; Scaringi, Agolli, & Minniti, 2018).

(2) In the United States, a limited number of centers offer proton beam therapy. Patients may need to travel long distances, possibly out of state, to access this modality. Less than 1% of patients worldwide are treated with proton beam therapy (Mohan & Grosshans, 2017).

(3) The equipment and maintenance are much more expensive compared to conventional RT machines.

4. Immobilization (Ballangrud et al., 2018; Ma et al., 2017)

a) SRS delivery systems have specialized immobilization devices that coordinate with each system's treatment device and planning software to define the target and ensure precise patient positioning during treatment.

b) Cranial systems may have a head frame that attaches to the skull with screws (e.g., Gamma Knife, XKnife) or a frameless system using a custom-fitted thermoplastic face mask (e.g., Novalis Tx, CyberKnife).

c) Frameless techniques provide a noninvasive alternative for immobilization and patient repositioning and provide more time for planning, which increases safety and flexibility (Bennion et al., 2016).

d) Clinicians should consider patient body position and the amount of time required for fashioning the immobilization device. Pain or antianxiety medication may be required (Ballangrud et al., 2018; Lo et al., 2018; Owusu-Agyemang et al., 2016).

e) SBRT immobilization devices include custom-fitted, foam-based body molds (e.g., Alpha Cradle®) and customized external vacuum-shaped body molds (e.g., Vac-Lok™, BodyFIX®).

f) The CyberKnife system uses a custom-designed vest worn by the patient.

5. Planning

a) SRS delivery systems have complex, integrated software planning systems that coordinate all SRS treatment steps (Duan, Giles, Kirkpatrick, & Yin, 2019; Levivier, Carrillo, Charrier, Martin, & Thiran, 2018; Myrehaug et al., 2016).

(1) Imaging for target definition

(2) Development of a treatment plan using many radiation beams

(3) Successful delivery of the planned treatment with precise accuracy

b) SRS treatment planning systems integrate diagnostic imaging, such as CT, MRI, and angiogram, to define target volumes.

c) SRS and SBRT require intensive medical physics support and collaboration with multiple disciplines.

(1) Generally, for cranial SRS, neurosurgery is involved in helping define the target volume, assess the dose to critical structures, and approve the final treatment plan.

(2) For SBRT, a surgical procedure or endoscopy may be needed for placement of small metallic internal (fiducial) markers, which assist with defining and tracking the treatment target (e.g., lung tumors, liver tumors). Hence, the treatment planning period may be days or longer depending on individual institution policies and procedures. For example, if fiducial markers are needed for CyberKnife treatment, at least a week is recommended before treatment to ensure the stability of placement (Accuray, n.d.).

6. Localization: IGRT

a) A variety of technologies are used to localize and track the target, as well as to ensure reproducibility of the treatment plan, during delivery of the actual treatment (Franzone et al., 2016; Ma et al., 2017; Scaringi et al., 2018).

(1) CT scan during therapy (cone beam CT)

(2) Kilovoltage imaging

(3) Fluoroscopy

(4) Infrared imaging with skin markers

b) For SBRT, multiple methods are used to track target movement from respiratory motion, including four-dimensional CT scan. The result is the ability to match a respiratory phase and target position when the treatment beam is active (respiratory gating). This technique is used to control breathing or free breathing (Dieterich, Green, & Booth, 2018; Yoon et al., 2018).

7. Side effects

a) Acute effects

(1) Cranial SRS effects are generally minimal and include nausea, vomiting, and headache (Lo et al., 2018).

(a) Vertigo and seizures are less frequent; consequently, some patients may develop seizures within the first 24–72 hours after SRS for supratentorial lesions (Lo et al., 2018).

(b) In a large, retrospective study, Soike et al. (2019) reported that 35% of patients experienced acute sequelae, and 91% of those were mild to moderate in severity.

(c) The following symptoms were also reported, ordered by most to least frequent (Chao et al., 2012; Lo et al., 2018).

i. Headache

ii. Seizures

iii. Fluid retention and other steroid effects

iv. Neurologic changes

(2) For invasive frame-based SRS, effects include possible discomfort, bleeding, or infection at the insertion site of fixation pins (Belcher et al., 2017).

b) Late effects

(1) With cranial SRS, principal concerns are radiation necrosis and cognitive deterioration. The risk of complications increases with the volume of the target (cm³). Toxicity rapidly increases once the volume of the brain exposed to more than 12 Gy is larger than 5–10 cm³ (Pinkham, Whitfield, & Brada, 2015).

(2) For SRS to the brain stem, a maximum dose of 12 Gy is associated with less than 5% risk, an acceptable risk of toxicity, although the risk increases with lesions larger than 1 cm³. Higher doses of 13–18 Gy have been used in patients with poor prognosis with a low reported incidence of complications (Pinkham et al., 2015).

(3) SRS to the optic nerves and chiasm has a risk of RION—a painless, rapid visual loss likely caused by vasculature injury. Incidence is unlikely in a dose range of 8–12 Gy but becomes greater than 10% in doses of 12–15 Gy (Lo et al., 2018; Milano et al., 2018).

(4) Radiation dose to the cochlea should be limited to 12–14 Gy, such as when treating an acoustic neuroma to minimize the risk of SNHL (Woods, Lee, Kaprealian, Yang, & Sheng, 2018).

(5) In treatment of the spine, radiation-induced myelopathy is rare (less than 1%) with doses of 13 Gy or less in one fraction or 20 Gy or less in three fractions to the full-thickness spinal cord. Long-term data are insufficient to calculate the risk of myelopathy for partial cord radiation exposure in a hypofractionated regimen (Bennett et al., 2017; Purvis, Goodwin, Lubelski, Laufer, & Sciubba, 2017; Tseng et al., 2017).

c) Lung and thoracic toxicities

(1) Radiation pneumonitis is the most common side effect of SBRT and occurs in 9%–28% of patients. Symptoms include shortness of breath, cough, pleuritic pain, and decline in functional tests (pulmonary function test, six-minute walk, exercise capacity) (Huang & Palma, 2015; Parker, Siochi, Wen, & Mattes, 2019; Yamashita, Takahashi, & Nakagawa, 2014).

(2) Bronchial injury or stenosis has been associated with SBRT of perihilar and central tumors. To minimize this risk, the recommended SBRT

dose limit to central airways is 80 Gy (De Rose et al., 2017).

 (3) Chest wall toxicity causing severe pain or rib fracture is strongly correlated with the volume of chest wall receiving 30 Gy in three to five fractions (30% risk for chest wall volume of 35 cm³). It is recommended that the volume of chest wall receiving 30 Gy be limited to 30 cm³ (Chipko et al., 2019).

 d) Liver toxicities

  (1) Radiation-induced liver disease involves anicteric hepatomegaly, ascites, and elevated liver transaminases or alkaline phosphatase (Barry et al., 2017; Scorsetti, Clerici, & Comito, 2014).

  (2) Pathology involves occlusion and injury to central hepatocyte lobules, retrograde congestion, and secondary hepatocyte necrosis (Barry et al., 2017; Velec et al., 2017).

  (3) To reduce the risk of radiation-induced liver disease to less than 5%, broad guidelines for SBRT recommend the following doses (Michel et al., 2017).

   (a) For primary liver cancer, less than 13 Gy in three fractions and less than 18 Gy in six fractions

   (b) For liver metastases, less than 15 Gy in three fractions and less than 20 Gy in six fractions

8. Patient, caregiver, and family education

 a) Nurses should review with patients the multiple procedures required for treatment planning and delivery given the complex nature of RT (Sulé-Suso et al., 2015).

 b) Patients should be informed on the type of diagnostic imaging required for treatment planning, which may include CT, MRI, PET, angiography, or surgical or interventional radiologic placement of fiducial markers (Halasz & Rockhill, 2013; Rosenberg et al., 2019).

 c) Patients should be informed on the type of immobilization device required.

  (1) A fixed head frame is placed on the same day of SRS treatment and is invasive. A local anesthetic is used for pin placement (Lo et al., 2018).

  (2) Frameless devices, such as foam or vacuum molds, are fashioned days before SRS treatment (Ezzell, 2017).

 d) Nurses must assess for any barriers to completing treatment, including physical, cognitive, emotional, and psychological barriers (Forshaw, Hall, Boyes, Carey, & Martin, 2017).

 e) Patients should understand that treatment time is highly variable and depends on the number of targets to be treated (e.g., multiple brain metastases), complexity of the tracking, and position verification techniques required, as well as which treatment delivery system is used. Overall, the complexity of SRS generally results in a longer treatment time compared to standard RT because a traditional linear accelerator–based device utilizes one isocenter for each lesion for patients with multiple brain metastases (Ballangrud et al., 2018).

9. Follow-up and survivorship

 a) Nurses should review potential acute and late effects with patients, caregivers, and family. Possible symptoms will depend on the area of healthy tissue treated (Huang & Palma, 2015).

 b) Clinicians should ensure that patients, caregivers, and family understand when and how to contact appropriate healthcare personnel for reporting of symptoms, questions, or concerns. Clinicians should consider that much less time is required in the radiation department for delivery of SRS or SBRT compared to conventional RT because SRS utilizes a large single fraction, and SBRT delivers five or fewer daily hypofractionated sessions. In contrast, conventional fractionated RT delivers multifractionated small daily sessions over several weeks (Halvorsen et al., 2017; Newman, Sherry, Byrne, & Osmundson, 2019).

 c) The follow-up required for monitoring disease response to therapy and management of potential treatment sequelae is dependent on the disease and site treated.

References

Accuray. (n.d.). Lung SBRT with the CyberKnife® system. https://www.accuray.com/lung-sbrt-cyberknife

Alghamdi, M., Hasan, Y., Ruschin, M., Atenafu, E.G., Myrehaug, S., Tseng, C.-L., ... Soliman, H. (2018). Stereotactic radiosurgery for resected brain metastasis: Cavity dynamics and factors affecting its evolution. *Journal of Radiosurgery and SBRT, 5,* 191–200.

Babic, S., Lee, Y., Ruschin, M., Lochray, F., Lightstone, A., Atenafu, E., ... Sahgal, A. (2018). To frame or not to frame? Cone-beam CT-based analysis of head immobilization devices specific to linac-based stereotactic radiosurgery and radiotherapy. *Journal of Applied Clinical Medical Physics, 19,* 111–120. https://doi.org/10.1002/acm2.12251

Balik, S., Chao, S., & Neyman, G. (2018). Gamma knife and volumetric modulated arc therapy stereotactic radiotherapy plan quality and OAR sparing comparison for pituitary adenomas and vestibular schwannomas. *Journal of Radiosurgery and SBRT, 5,* 237–247.

Ballangrud, A., Kuo, L.C., Happersett, L., Lim, S.B., Beal, K., Yamada, Y., ... Mechalakos, J. (2018). Institutional experience with SRS VMAT planning for multiple cranial metastases. *Journal of Applied Clinical Medical Physics, 19,* 176–183. https://doi.org/10.1002/acm2.12284

Barry, A., McPartlin, A., Lindsay, P., Wang, L., Brierley, J., Kim, J., ... Dawson, L.A. (2017). Dosimetric analysis of liver toxicity after liver metastasis stereotactic body radiation therapy. *Practical Radiation Oncology, 7,* e331–e337. https://doi.org/10.1016/j.prro.2017.03.004

Belcher, A.H., Liu, X., Chmura, S., Yenice, K., & Wiersma, R.D. (2017). Toward frameless maskless SRS through real-time 6DoF robotic motion compensation. *Physics in Medicine and Biology, 62,* 9054–9066. https://doi.org/10.1088/1361-6560/aa93d2

Bennett, E.E., Berriochoa, C., Habboub, G., Brigeman, S., Chao, S.T., & Angelov, L. (2017). Rapid and complete radiological resolution of an intradural cervical cord lung cancer metastasis treated with spinal stereotactic radiosurgery: Case report. *Neurosurgical Focus, 42,* e10. https://doi.org/10.3171/2016.9.FOCUS16254

Bennion, N.R., Malouff, T., Verma, V., Denniston, K., Bhirud, A., Zhen, W., ... Lin, C. (2016). A comparison of clinical and radiologic outcomes between frame-based and frameless stereotactic radiosurgery for brain metastases. *Practical Radiation Oncology, 6,* e283–e290. https://doi.org/10.1016/j.prro.2016.05.001

Berti, A., Ibars, G., Wu, X., Sabo, A., Granville, M., Suarez, G., ... Jacobson, R.E. (2018). Evaluation of CyberKnife radiosurgery for recurrent trigeminal neuralgia. *Cureus, 10,* e2598. https://doi.org/10.7759/cureus.2598

Bir, S.C., Connor, D.E., Jr., Ambekar, S., Wilden, J.A., & Nanda, A. (2015). Factors predictive of improved overall survival following stereotactic radiosurgery for recurrent glioblastoma. *Neurosurgical Review, 38,* 705–713. https://doi.org/10.1007/s10143-015-0632-4

Brehmer, S., Grimm, M.A., Förster, A., Seiz-Rosenhagen, M., Welzel, G., Stieler, F., ... Giordano, F.A. (2019). Study protocol: Early stereotactic gamma knife radiosurgery to residual tumor after surgery of newly diagnosed glioblastoma (gamma-GBM). *Neurosurgery, 84,* 1133–1137. https://doi.org/10.1093/neuros/nyy156

Chajon, E., Castelli, J., Marsiglia, H., & De Crevoisier, R. (2017). The synergistic effect of radiotherapy and immunotherapy: A promising but not simple partnership. *Critical Reviews in Oncology/Hematology, 111,* 124–132. https://doi.org/10.1016/j.critrevonc.2017.01.017

Chao, S.T., Thakkar, V.V., Barnett, G.H., Vogelbaum, M.A., Angelov, L., Weil, R.J., ... Suh, J.H. (2012). Prospective study of the short-term adverse effects of gamma knife radiosurgery. *Technology in Cancer Research and Treatment, 11,* 117–122. https://doi.org/10.7785/tcrt.2012.500240

Chen, C.-J., Shabo, L.M., Ding, D., Ironside, N., Kano, H., Mathieu, D., ... Sheehan, J.P. (2019). Seizure presentation in patients with brain arteriovenous malformations treated with stereotactic radiosurgery: A multicenter study. *World Neurosurgery, 126,* e634–e640. https://doi.org/10.1016/j.wneu.2019.02.104

Chipko, C., Ojwang, J., Gharai, L.R., Deng, X., Mukhopadhyay, N., & Weiss, E. (2019). Characterization of chest wall toxicity during long-term follow up after thoracic stereotactic body radiation therapy. *Practical Radiation Oncology, 9,* e338–e346. https://doi.org/10.1016/j.prro.2019.01.012

De Rose, F., Franceschini, D., Reggiori, G., Stravato, A., Navarria, P., Ascolese, A.M., ... Scorsetti, M. (2017). Organs at risk in lung SBRT. *Physica Medica, 44,* 131–138. https://doi.org/10.1016/j.ejmp.2017.04.010

Dieterich, S., Green, O., & Booth, J. (2018). SBRT targets that move with respiration. *Physica Medica, 56,* 19–24. https://doi.org/10.1016/j.ejmp.2018.10.021

Duan, X., Giles, W., Kirkpatrick, J.P., & Yin, F.-F. (2019). The effect of setup uncertainty on optimal dosimetric margin in LINAC-based stereotactic radiosurgery with dynamic conformal arc technique. *Journal of Radiosurgery and SBRT, 6,* 55–65.

Elekta. (n.d.). Legacy of leadership. https://gammaknife.com/legacy-of-leadership

Ezzell, G.A. (2017). The spatial accuracy of two frameless, linear accelerator-based systems for single-isocenter, multitarget cranial radiotherapy. *Journal of Applied Clinical Medical Physics, 18,* 37–43. https://doi.org/10.1002/acm2.12044

Forshaw, K., Hall, A.E., Boyes, A.W., Carey, M.L., & Martin, J. (2017). Patients' experiences of preparation for radiation therapy: A qualitative study [Online exclusive]. *Oncology Nursing Forum, 44,* e1–e9. https://doi.org/10.1188/17.ONF.e1-e9

Franzone, P., Fiorentino, A., Barra, S., Cante, D., Masini, L., Cazzulo, E., ... Corvò, R. (2016). Image-guided radiation therapy (IGRT): Practical recommendations of Italian Association of Radiation Oncology (AIRO). *La radiologia Medica, 121,* 958–965. https://doi.org/10.1007/s11547-016-0674-x

Funayama, S., Onishi, H., Kuriyama, K., Komiyama, T., Marino, K., Araya, M., ... Takeda, M. (2019). Renal cancer is not radioresistant: Slowly but continuing shrinkage of the tumor after stereotactic body radiation therapy. *Technology in Cancer Research and Treatment, 18,* 1–8. https://doi.org/10.1177/1533033818822329

Hafez, R.F., Morgan, M.S., Fahmy, O.M., & Hassan, H.T. (2018). Long-term effectiveness and safety of stereotactic gamma knife surgery as a primary sole treatment in the management of glomus jagulare tumor. *Clinical Neurology and Neurosurgery, 168,* 34–37. https://doi.org/10.1016/j.clineuro.2018.02.037

Halasz, L.M., & Rockhill, J.K. (2013). Stereotactic radiosurgery and stereotactic radiotherapy for brain metastases. *Surgical Neurology International, 4*(Suppl. 4), S185–S191. https://doi.org/10.4103/2152-7806.111295

Halvorsen, P.R., Cirino, E., Das, I.J., Garrett, J.A., Yang, J., Yin, F.-F., & Fairobent, L.A. (2017). AAPM-RSS Medical Physics Practice Guideline 9.a. for SRS-SBRT. *Journal of Applied Clinical Medical Physics, 18*(5), 10–21. https://doi.org/10.1002/acm2.12146

Harrison, P. (2019, February 19). SBRT nearly doubles survival for early, inoperable lung cancer—Establishes evidence for peripherally located stage I NSCLC. https://www.medpagetoday.com/radiology/therapeuticradiology/78110

Hatiboglu, M.A., Tuzgen, S., Akdur, K., & Chang, E.L. (2016). Treatment of high numbers of brain metastases with gamma knife radiosurgery: A review. *Acta Neurochirurgica, 156,* 625–634. https://doi.org/10.1007/s00701-016-2707-6

Huang, K., & Palma, D.A. (2015). Follow-up of patients after stereotactic radiation for lung cancer: A primer for the nonradiation oncologist. *Journal of Thoracic Oncology, 10,* 412–419. https://doi.org/10.1097/JTO.0000000000000435

Imber, B.S., Kanungo, I., Braunstein, S., Barani, I.J., Fogh, S.E., Nakamura, J.L., ... Aghi, M.K. (2017). Indications and efficacy of gamma knife stereotactic radiosurgery for recurrent glioblastoma: 2 decades of institutional experience. *Neurosurgery, 80,* 129–139. https://doi.org/10.1227/NEU.0000000000001344

Jacobs, R., Kano, H., Gross, B.A., Niranjan, A., Monaco, E.A., & Lunsford, L.D. (2019). Defining long-term clinical outcomes and risk of stereotactic radiosurgery for brainstem cavernous malformations. *World Neurosurgery, 124,* e58–e64. https://doi.org/10.1016/j.wneu.2018.11.226

Johnson, R.P. (2018). Review of medical radiography and tomography with proton beams. *Reports on Progress in Physics, 81,* 016701. https://doi.org/10.1088/1361-6633/aa8b1d

Kalash, R., Pifer, P.M., Beriwal, S., Glaser, S.M., Vargo, J.A., & Heron, D.E. (2017). Exceptional eight-year response to stereotactic radiosurgery monotherapy for multiple brain metastases. *Cureus, 9,* e2001. https://doi.org/10.7759/cureus.2001

Kondziolka, D., Shin, S.M., Brunswick, A., Kim, I., & Silverman, J.S. (2015). The biology of radiosurgery and its clinical applications for brain tumors. *Neuro-Oncology, 17,* 29–44. https://doi.org/10.1093/neuonc/nou284

Kraft, J., Zindler, J., Minniti, G., Guckenberger, M., & Andratschke, N. (2019). Stereotactic radiosurgery for multiple brain metastases. *Current Treatment Options in Neurology, 21,* 6. https://doi.org/10.1007/s11940-019-0548-3

Krengli, M., Apicella, G., Deantonio, L., Paolini, M., & Masini, L. (2015). Stereotactic radiation therapy for skull base recurrences: Is a salvage approach still possible? *Report of Practical Oncology and Radiotherapy, 20,* 430–439. https://doi.org/10.1016/j.rpor.2014.10.007

Lee, K.H., Yu, J.L., Park, H.C., Park, S.Y., Shin, J.S., Shin, E.H., ... Lim, D.H. (2018). Is higher dose always the right answer in stereotactic body radiation therapy for small hepatocellular carcinoma? *Radiation Oncology Journal, 36,* 129–138. https://doi.org/10.3857/roj.2017.00598

Lefranc, M., Da Roz, L.M., Balossier, A., Thomassin, J.M., Roche, P.H., & Regis, J. (2018). Place of gamma knife stereotactic radiosurgery in grade 4 vestibular schwannoma based on case series of 86 patients with long-term follow-up. *World Neurosurgery, 114,* e1192–e1198. https://doi.org/10.1016/j.wneu.2018.03.175

Leroy, H.-A., Tuleasca, C., Reyns, N., & Levivier, M. (2018). Radiosurgery and fractionated radiotherapy for cavernous sinus meningioma: Systematic review and meta-analysis. *Acta Neurochirurgica, 160,* 2367–2378. https://doi.org/10.1007/s00701-018-3711-9

Lesueur, P., Calugaru, V., Nauraye, C., Stefan, D., Cao, K., Emery, E., ... Thariat, J. (2019). Proton therapy for treatment of intracranial benign tumors in adults: A systematic review. *Cancer Treatment Reviews, 72,* 56–64. https://doi.org/10.1016/j.ctrv.2018.11.004

Levivier, M., Carrillo, R.E., Charrier, R., Martin, A., & Thiran, J.-P. (2018). A real-time optimal inverse planning for gamma knife radiosurgery by convex optimization: Description of the system and first dosimetry data. *Journal of Neurosurgery, 129*(Suppl. 1), 111–117. https://doi.org/10.3171/2018.7.GKS181572

Lo, S.S., Sloan, A.E., Colussi, V.C., Sohn, J.W., Wessels, B.W., Miller, J.P., ... Machtay, M. (2018, December 19). Stereotactic radiosurgery. https://emedicine.medscape.com/article/1423298-print

Lukka, H.R., Pugh, S.L., Bruner, D.W., Bahary, J.-P., Lawton, C.A.F., Efstathiou, J.A., ... Kachnic, L.A. (2018). Patient-reported outcomes in NRG oncology RTOG 0938, evaluating two ultrahypofractionated regimens for prostate cancer. *International Journal of Radiation Oncology, Biology, Physics, 102,* 287–295. https://doi.org/10.1016/j.ijrobp.2018.06.008

Ma, L., Wang, L., Tseng, C.-L., & Sahgal, A. (2017). Emerging technologies in stereotactic body radiotherapy. *Chinese Clinical Oncology, 6*(Suppl. 2), S12. https://doi.org/10.21037/cco.2017.06.19

Marciscano, A.E., Haimovitz-Friedman, A., Lee, P., Tran, P.T., Tomé, W.A., Guha, C., ... DeWeese, T.L. (2019). Immunomodulatory effects of stereotactic body radiation therapy: Preclinical insights and clinical opportunities. *International Journal of Radiation Oncology, Biology, Physics.* Advanced online publication. https://doi.org/10.1016/j.ijrobp.2019.02.046

McPartlin, A., Swaminath, A., Wang, R., Pintilie, M., Brierley, J., Kim, J., ... Dawson, L.A. (2017). Long-term outcomes of phase 1 and phase 2 studies of SBRT for hepatic colorectal metastases. *International Journal of Radiation Oncology, Biology, Physics, 99,* 388–395. https://doi.org/10.1016/j.ijrobp.2017.04.010

Meleis, A., Jhawar, S.R., Weiner, J.P., Majmundar, N., Mahtabfar, A., Lin, Y., ... Goyal, S. (2019). Stereotactic body radiation therapy in non-surgical patients with metastatic spinal disease and epidural compression: A retrospective review. *World Neurosurgery, 122,* e198–e205. https://doi.org/10.1016/j.wneu.2018.09.210

Michel, R., Françoise, I., Laure, P., Anouchka, M., Guillaume, P., & Sylvain, K. (2017). Dose to organ at risk and dose prescription in liver SBRT. *Reports of Practical Oncology and Radiotherapy, 22,* 96–102. https://doi.org/10.1016/j.rpor.2017.03.001

Milano, M.T., Grimm, J., Soltys, S.G., Yorke, E., Moiseenko, V., Tomé, W.A., ... Naqa, I.E. (2018). Single- and multi-fraction stereotactic radiosurgery dose tolerances of the optic pathways. *International Journal of Radiation Oncology, Biology, Physics, 2018,* S0360-3016(18)30125-1. https://doi.org/10.1016/j.ijrobp.2018.01.053

Mohan, R., & Grosshans, D. (2017). Proton therapy—Present and future. *Advanced Drug Delivery Reviews, 109,* 26–44. https://doi.org/10.1016/j.addr.2016.11.006

Murray, L.J., & Dawson, L.A. (2017). Advances in stereotactic body radiation therapy for hepatocellular carcinoma. *Seminars in Radiation Oncology, 27,* 247–255. https://doi.org/10.1016/j.semradonc.2017.02.002

Myrehaug, S., Sahgal, A., Russo, S.M., Lo, S.S., Rosati, L.M., Mayr, N.A., ... Herman, J.M. (2016). Stereotactic body radiotherapy for pancreatic cancer: Recent progress and future directions. *Expert Review of Anticancer Therapy, 16,* 523–530. https://doi.org/10.1586/14737140.2016.1168698

Naeem, K., Darbar, A., & Shamim, M.S. (2018). Role of stereotactic radiosurgery in the treatment of acromegaly. *Journal of Pakistan Medical Association, 68,* 1843–1845.

Nalichowski, A., Kaufman, I., Gallo, J., Bossenberger, T., Solberg, T., Ramirez, E., ... Burmeister, J. (2017). Single fraction radiosurgery/stereotactic body radiation therapy (SBRT) for spine metastasis: A dosimetric comparison of multiple delivery platforms. *Journal of Applied Clinical Medical Physics, 18,* 164–169. https://doi.org/10.1002/acm2.12022

Newman, N.B., Sherry, A.D., Byrne, D.W., & Osmundson, E.C. (2019). Stereotactic body radiotherapy versus conventional radiotherapy for early-stage small cell lung cancer. *Journal of Radiation Oncology, 8,* 239–248. http://doi.org/10.1007/s13566-019-00395-x

Owusu-Agyemang, P., Popovich, S.M., Zavala, A.M., Grosshans, D.R., Van Meter, A., Williams, U.U., ... Mahajan, A. (2016). A multi-institutional pilot survey of anesthesia practices during proton radiation therapy. *Practical Radiation Oncology, 6,* 155–159. https://doi.org/10.1016/j.prro.2015.10.020

Parker, S.M., Siochi, R.A., Wen, S., & Mattes, M.D. (2019). Impact of tumor size on local control and pneumonitis after stereotactic body radiation ther-apy for lung tumors. *Practical Radiation Oncology, 9,* e90–e97. https://doi.org/10.1016/j.prro.2018.09.003

Pinkham, M.B., Whitfield, G.A., & Brada, M. (2015). New developments in intracranial stereotactic radiotherapy for metastases. *Clinical Oncology, 27,* 316–323. https://doi.org/10.1016/j.clon.2015.01.007

Pokhrel, D., Sood, S., McClinton, C., Saleh, H., Badkul, R., Jiang, H., ... Wang, F. (2017). Linac-based stereotactic radiosurgery (SRS) in the treatment of refractory trigeminal neuralgia: Detailed description of SRS procedure and reported clinical outcomes. *Journal of Applied Clinical Medical Physics, 18,* 136–143. https://doi.org/10.1002/acm2.12057

Purvis, T.E., Goodwin, C.R., Lubelski, D., Laufer, I., & Sciubba, D.M. (2017). Review of stereotactic radiosurgery for intradural spine tumors. *CNS Oncology, 6,* 131–138. https://doi.org/10.2217/cns-2016-0039

Redmond, K.J., & Mehta, M.P. (2015). Stereotactic radiosurgery for glioblastoma. *Cureus, 7,* e413. https://doi.org/10.7759/cureus.413

Romagna, A., Schwartz, C., Ladisich, B., Hitzl, W., Heidorn, S.-C., Winkler, P.A., & Muacevic, A. (2018). CyberKnife radiosurgery in recurrent brain metastases: Do the benefits outweigh the risks? *Cureus, 10,* e3741. https://doi.org/10.7759/cureus.3741

Rosenberg, S.A., Henke, L.E., Shaverdian, N., Mittauer, K., Wojcieszynski, A.P., Hulett, C.R., ... Bassetti, M. (2019). A multi-institutional experience MR-guided liver stereotactic body radiation therapy. *Advances in Radiation Oncology, 4,* 142–149. https://doi.org/10.1016/j.adro.2018.08.005

Scaringi, C., Agolli, L., & Minniti, G. (2018). Technical advances in radiation therapy for brain tumors. *Anticancer Research, 38,* 6041–6045. https://doi.org/10.21873/anticanres.12954

Scorsetti, M., Clerici, E., & Comito, T. (2014). Stereotactic body radiation therapy for liver metastases. *Journal of Gastrointestinal Oncology, 5,* 190–197. https://doi.org/10.3978/j.issn.2078-6891.2014.039

Seung, S.K., Larson, D.A., Galvin, J.M., Mehta, M.P., Potters, L., Schultz, C.J., ... Rosenthal, S.A. (2013). American College of Radiology (ACR) and American Society for Radiation Oncology (ASTRO) practice guideline for the performance of stereotactic radiosurgery (SRS). *American Journal of Clinical Oncology, 36,* 310–315. https://doi.org/10.1097/COC.0b013e31826e053d

Sheehan, J., Suh, J.H., Kavanagh, B., Xu, Z., Ren, L., Sheehan, K., & Lunsford, L.D. (2018). Training neurosurgery and radiation oncology residents in stereotactic radiosurgery: Assessment gathered from participants in AANS and ASTRO training course. *World Neurosurgery, 109,* e669–e675. https://doi.org/10.1016/j.wneu.2017.10.053

Soike, M.H., Hughes, R.T., Farris, M., McTyre, E.R., Cramer, C.K., Bourland, J.D., & Chan, M.D. (2019). Does stereotactic radiosurgery have a role in the management of patients presenting with 4 or more brain metastases? *Neurosurgery, 84,* 558–566. https://doi.org/10.1093/neuros/nyy216

Song, C.W., Glatstein, E., Marks, L.B., Emami, B., Grimm, J., Sperduto, P.W., ... Cho, L.C. (2019). Biological principles of stereotactic body radiation therapy (SBRT) and stereotactic radiation surgery (SRS): Indirect cell death. *International Journal of Radiation Oncology, Biology, Physics, 2019,* S0360-3016(19)30291-3. https://doi.org/10.1016/j.ijrobp.2019.02.047

Strauss, I., Haim, O., Umansky, D., Corn, B.W., Frolov, V., Shtraus, N., ... Kanner, A.A. (2017). Impact of onyx embolization on radiosurgical management of cerebral arteriovenous malformations: Treatment and outcomes. *World Neurosurgery, 108,* 656–661. https://doi.org/10.1016/j.wneu.2017.08.188

Sulé-Suso, J., Finney, S., Bisson, J., Hammersley, S., Jassel, S., Knight, R., ... Moloney, A. (2015). Pilot study on virtual imaging for patient information on radiotherapy planning and delivery. *Radiography, 21,* 273–277. https://doi.org/10.1016/j.radi.2015.02.002

Sun, Y., Li, X., Xiong, J., Yu, J., & Lv, X. (2019). Transarterial onyx embolization of residual arteriovenous malformation after surgical resection. *World Neurosurgery, 126,* e1242–e1245. https://doi.org/10.1016/j.wneu.2019.03.073

Syed, Y.A., Patel-Yadav, A.K., Rivers, C., & Singh, A.K. (2017). Stereotactic radiotherapy for prostate cancer: A review and future directions. *World Journal of Clinical Oncology, 8,* 389–397. https://doi.org/10.5306/wjco.v8.i5.389

Thiagarajan, A., & Yamada, Y. (2017). Radiobiology and radiotherapy of brain metastases. *Clinical and Experimental Metastasis, 34,* 411–419. https://doi.org/10.1007/s10585-017-9865-7

Todnem, N., Ward, A., Nahhas, M., Vender, J.R., Alleyne, C.H., & Rahimi, S.Y. (2019). A retrospective cohort analysis of hemorrhagic arteriovenous malformations treated with combined endovascular embolization and gamma knife stereotactic radiosurgery. *World Neurosurgery, 122,* e713–e722. https://doi.org/10.1016/j.wneu.2018.10.125

Tseng, C.-L., Eppinga, W., Charest-Morin, R., Soliman, H., Myrehaug, S., Maralani, P.J., ... Sahgal, A. (2017). Spine stereotactic body radiotherapy: Indications, outcomes, and points of caution. *Global Spine Journal, 7,* 179–197. https://doi.org/10.1177/2192568217694016

Tuleasca, C., Zeverino, M., Patin, D., Marguet, M., Ruiz Lopes, N., Vallet, V., ... Levivier, M. (2019). Lausanne checklist for safe stereotactic radiosurgery. *Acta Neurochirurgica, 161,* 721–727. https://doi.org/10.1007/s00701-019-03843-2

Velec, M., Haddad, C.R., Craig, T., Wang, L., Lindsay, P., Brierley, J., ... Dawson, L.A. (2017). Predictors of liver toxicity following stereotactic body radiation therapy for hepatocellular carcinoma. *International Journal of Radiation Oncology, Biology, Physics, 97,* 939–946. https://doi.org/10.1016/j.ijrobp.2017.01.221

Wegner, R.E., Ahmed, N., Hasan, S., McCormick, J., Kirichenko, A.V., & Colonias, A. (2018). Stereotactic body radiotherapy for lung metastases from colorectal cancer: A single institution experience. *Colorectal Cancer, 7.* https://doi.org/10.2217/crc-2018-0005

Woods, K., Lee, P., Kaprealian, T., Yang, I., & Sheng, K. (2018). Cochlea-sparing acoustic neuroma treatment with 4π radiation therapy. *Advances in Radiation Oncology, 3,* 100–107. https://doi.org/10.1016/j.adro.2018.01.004

Yamashita, H., Takahashi, W., & Nakagawa, K. (2014). Radiation pneumonitis after stereotactic radiation therapy for lung cancer. *World Journal of Radiology, 6,* 708–715. https://doi.org/10.4329/wjr.v6.i9.708

Yoon, K.J., Jeong, C., Kim, S.-W., Cho, B., Kwak, J., Kim, S.S., ... Lee, S.-W. (2018). Dosimetric evaluation of respiratory gated volumetric modulated arc therapy for lung stereotactic body radiation therapy using 3D printing technology. *PLOS ONE, 13,* 1–14. https://doi.org/10.1371/journal.pone.0208685

D. Total body irradiation and hematopoietic stem cell transplantation

1. Overview
   a) TBI is an RT technique that may be used as a component of preparative regimens for HSCT (ACR & ASTRO, 2017).
   b) TBI, usually in conjunction with chemotherapy agents, has proven useful for eradicating residual malignant or genetically disordered cells, for ablating hematopoietic stem cells, and for immunosuppression to reduce the risk of graft rejection (ACR & ASTRO, 2017).
   c) Unlike chemotherapy, RT does not depend on a blood supply and is not influenced by drug absorption, metabolism, biodistribution, or clearance kinetics (Wong, Filippi, Dabaja, Yahalom, & Specht, 2018).
   d) RT can reach sanctuary sites, such as the testes and brain, which can be boosted with additional radiation in conjunction with TBI (Wong et al., 2018).
2. Hematopoietic stem cells
   a) Each hematopoietic stem cell is pluripotent and able to self-replicate, proliferate, and develop along the myeloid pathway (red blood cells, platelets, neutrophils, and macrophages) or lymphoid pathway (T and B lymphocytes) (AABB et al., 2018).
   b) Myeloid progenitor cells mature into the following (Lassiter, 2016).
      (1) Megakaryocytes, which produce platelets
      (2) Erythrocytes
      (3) Mast cells
      (4) Myeloblasts
   c) Lymphoid progenitor cells mature into the following (Lassiter, 2016).
      (1) Small lymphocytes, which differentiate into bone marrow–derived cells, B cells, and T cells
      (2) Natural killer cells
3. Treatment options
   a) Low-dose TBI (2 Gy) is used in nonmyeloablative HSCT, and may be used for patients who may not be able to tolerate myeloablation because of age older than 60 years, poor performance, and comorbid conditions (Wong et al., 2018).
   b) The most common TBI schedules include the following (Wong et al., 2018).
      (1) Twice daily 2 Gy fractions given for three days (12 Gy total)
      (2) Twice daily 1.5 Gy fractions given for four to four and a half days (12–13.5 Gy total)
      (3) Three times daily 1.2 Gy fractions given for four days (12–13.2 Gy total)
      (4) Once daily 3 Gy fractions given for four days (12 Gy total)
   c) Dosing and fractionation are based on institutional and treatment protocols.
   d) Organs such as the kidneys and lungs can be shielded.
   e) Lungs are a critical OAR from TBI, and a radiation dose less than 9.4 Gy reduces the risk of developing pneumonitis, which is a major complication of HSCT (Nalichowski, Eagle, & Burmeister, 2016).
   f) Some institutions are performing total marrow irradiation as an alternative conditioning to TBI, thus reducing the radiation dose to OARs (Wong et al., 2018).
   g) Patients typically stand on a platform designed for TBI delivery, lie on a gurney or a specially designed table at floor level, or sit in a specially designed chair (Wong et al., 2018).
   h) Treatment times vary depending on treatment delivery method and can be 30 minutes or longer.
   i) Infants and young children may require anesthesia for treatment.
4. Multifaceted team approach
   a) Medical and radiation oncologists, physicists, dosimetrists, radiation therapists, and nurses are all involved in coordinating care for a successful TBI treatment.
   b) The initial patient evaluation should involve a detailed history, including a review of issues that may affect treatment tolerance; physical examination with review of systems and any pertinent diagnostic and

laboratory tests; review of previous RT treatments; and review of implanted battery-operated medical devices (ACR & ASTRO, 2017).

c) Prior to simulation and treatment, informed consent must be obtained and should include a detailed discussion of the benefits and potential tissue-specific acute and late toxicities of TBI by the radiation oncologist (ACR & ASTRO, 2017).

d) Treatment planning measurements are performed by radiation therapists according to the treatment protocol and prescription.

e) A dosimetrist calculates the dose to determine beam-on time necessary to achieve the prescribed dose homogeneity and any other relevant dose points. These dose calculations must be verified by a medical physicist (ACR & ASTRO, 2017).

f) Nurses educate patients and caregivers regarding simulation, treatment, and acute and late side effects. Nurses provide supportive care.

g) In some instances, nurse practitioners and physician assistants may also provide patient care with oncologists.

h) TBI treatments are delivered by a radiation therapist according to the written prescription.

5. Indications: In the past 30 years, HSCT has become an increasingly standard treatment for various malignant and nonmalignant diseases (Lassiter, 2016).

a) Select leukemias
b) Breast cancer
c) Ovarian cancer
d) Myelodysplastic syndromes
e) Multiple myeloma
f) Hodgkin and non-Hodgkin lymphomas
g) Germ cell tumors
h) Aplastic anemia
i) Fanconi anemia
j) Thalassemia major
k) Sickle cell anemia
l) Severe combined immunodeficiency
m) Neuroblastoma
n) Sarcoma
o) Amyloidosis

6. Sources of stem cells (Gregory, 2017)

a) Peripheral blood stem cells
   (1) Peripheral blood stem cells have become the most common source of stem cells.
   (2) The use of granulocyte–colony-stimulating factor and plerixafor increases the production of stem cells.
   (3) Stem cells are mobilized out of the bone marrow space and into the peripheral circulation and collected through apheresis.

b) Bone marrow: Stem cells are collected from the bone marrow by multiple needle aspirations from the posterior or anterior iliac crest while a donor is under anesthesia.

c) Umbilical cord blood
   (1) The cells in umbilical cord blood are used when a true human leukocyte antigen match cannot be found.
   (2) The stem cells in umbilical cord blood have not reached immunologic maturity, allowing for a less-stringent match.

7. Types of HSCT (Bashey et al., 2013; Gregory, 2017)

a) Autologous HSCT is performed using a patient's own previously collected stem cells.

b) Allogeneic HSCT is performed with the cells of a donor. It can be performed using a number of different donor sources.

c) Syngeneic HSCT is performed with stem cells donated from an identical twin who is human leukocyte antigen identical.

d) Haploidentical allogeneic HSCT uses stem cells or bone marrow from siblings, parents, or children.

8. Side effects: Many short- and long-term side effects and toxicities are associated with TBI, conditioning chemotherapy, and other previous treatment regimens.

a) Mucositis
   (1) Mucositis is an inflammatory process that affects the mucous membranes of the oral cavity and gastrointestinal tract and affects as much as 80% of patients undergoing HSCT (Cawley, 2017).
   (2) Symptoms of mouth and throat pain typically develop within 7 to 10 days after initiation of conditioning (Antin & Raley, 2013).
   (3) Healing generally corresponds with engraftment and count recovery (Antin & Raley, 2013).
   (4) Dental evaluation should occur before initiation of treatment and throughout (Cawley, 2017).
   (5) Good dental and oral hygiene should be encouraged several times a day, including brushing with a soft toothbrush and using fluoride toothpaste (Cawley, 2017).
   (6) Sodium bicarbonate mouthwashes offer deodorizing and buffering properties, and can effectively neutralize the production of acid in the mouth, while also acting as an antiseptic to help prevent infections from occurring (Majdaeen, Babaei, & Rahimi, 2015).
   (7) The use of ice chips has been found to significantly minimize the incidence and severity of oral mucositis and decrease secondary oral mucositis complications such as pain (Tayyem, 2014).

b) Nausea and vomiting
   (1) Up to 90% of patients undergoing RT will experience RINV (NCCN, 2020a).
   (2) The likelihood of developing nausea and vomiting is dependent on the anatomic site of RT, radiation dose, and size of the radiation field (Roila et al., 2016).

(3) RT to various sites presents different risk of RINV (Roila et al., 2016).

    (a) TBI presents the highest risk of developing nausea and vomiting.

    (b) RT to the upper abdomen and craniospinal area present moderate risk.

    (c) RT to the cranium, head and neck, thorax, and pelvis present low risk.

    (d) RT to the extremities and breast present minimal risk.

(4) Prior to TBI treatment, patients may be premedicated with a serotonin receptor antagonist antiemetic, such as ondansetron or granisetron, with or without dexamethasone (NCCN, 2020a).

(5) Clinicians should monitor fluid and electrolytes.

(6) Clinicians should assess food tolerances.

c) Diarrhea

(1) Radiation-induced diarrhea typically occurs within two weeks of beginning RT (Muehlbauer & Lopez, 2014).

(2) The incidence and severity of radiation-induced diarrhea are dependent on the site of RT, size of the radiation field, and dose per fraction (Muehlbauer & Lopez, 2014).

(3) The highest incidence of radiation-induced diarrhea occurs in patients receiving abdominal and pelvic irradiation (Thorpe et al., 2017).

(4) Stool testing for infection (e.g., *Clostridium difficile*), ova and parasites, fecal blood, and fecal leukocytes should be performed for newly onset diarrhea to rule out infectious etiology (Prechtel Dunphy & Walker, 2017).

(5) Four types of medications are used to treat chemotherapy-induced diarrhea (Prechtel Dunphy & Walker, 2017).

    (a) Intestinal transport inhibitors

    (b) Intraluminal agents

    (c) Proabsorptive agents

    (d) Antisecretory agents

(6) Clinicians should monitor fluid and electrolytes and administer replacement as needed.

d) Fatigue (see IV.A. Fatigue)

e) Radiation-induced skin reactions (radiation dermatitis) (see IV.B. Skin reactions)

f) Parotitis (Shaftic, 2017; Wu & Leung, 2019)

(1) Parotitis is inflammation of the parotid glands and is one of the most common radiation-induced toxicities after TBI.

(2) Parotitis can cause difficulty in mastication and swallowing and increases the risk of dental problems.

(3) Clinicians should encourage hydration (frequent sips of water) throughout the day and use of a humidifier at night.

(4) Use of artificial saliva may be helpful.

g) Alopecia (Lawenda et al., 2004)

(1) Doses as low as 2 Gy in a single fraction have been shown to cause temporary alopecia.

(2) Radiation doses greater than 40 Gy may cause permanent hair loss in the radiation treatment field.

(3) Clinicians should educate patients regarding hair loss.

(4) Clinicians should provide resources for wigs and other cosmetic interventions.

h) Pancytopenia (see also IV.I. Neutropenia)

(1) Chemotherapy and RT cause myelosuppression and, in particular, decrease the number of neutrophils, resulting in neutropenia (Rosselet, 2013).

(2) The duration of neutropenia depends on several factors, including a patient's history of chemotherapy and RT, preparative regimen, stem cell source, use of growth factors following transplantation, and post-transplant complications (Rosselet, 2013).

(3) Thrombocytopenia is a frequent consequence of myelosuppressive cancer therapy, as platelet production can be impaired with bone marrow suppression (Adams, 2017).

(4) Bone marrow aplasia may be caused by a number of conditions, in addition to cancer therapy (Arnold & Cuker, 2020).

    (a) Hematologic disease

    (b) Viral infections

    (c) Vitamin B_{12} and folate deficiencies

    (d) Direct alcohol toxicity, which also may lead to thrombocytopenia

(5) Patients undergoing aggressive active therapy may receive several units of platelets over the course of treatment. If the platelet count decreases to less than 10,000–20,000/mm³, a transfusion may be ordered; however, it may depend on whether a patient is bleeding (Camp-Sorrell, 2018).

(6) Anemia in transplant recipients has several causative factors (Rosselet, 2013).

    (a) Hemolysis

    (b) Malignancy type

    (c) Bleeding

    (d) Bone marrow suppression due to antineoplastic agents and RT

    (e) Nutritional deficiency

    (f) Hemolytic uremic syndrome

    (g) Thrombotic microangiopathy

    (h) Kidney failure due to antineoplastic agents and other drugs.

(7) Generally, when hemoglobin is less than 8 g/dl and signs or symptoms of anemia are present, transfusion is required (National Cancer Institute CTEP, 2017).

(8) Clinicians must follow institutional guidelines for transfusion criteria to prevent transfusion errors.

i) Graft-versus-host disease (GVHD)

(1) Overview

(a) GVHD is one of the classic complications of allogeneic HSCT (Antin & Raley, 2013).

(b) GVHD occurs when immunologically competent donor-derived T lymphocytes (graft) recognize the antigens and cells in the transplant recipient (host) as foreign and mount an immunologic attack.

(c) The attack of these donor-derived T lymphocytes causes damage of varying degrees of severity to host tissues (Mitchell, 2013).

(d) GVHD is classified as acute or chronic, each with two subcategories (Antin & Raley, 2013).

(2) Acute GVHD

(a) Acute GVHD predominantly affects the skin, gastrointestinal tract, and liver. Symptoms include an erythematous maculopapular rash, diarrhea, abdominal cramping, and increases in direct bilirubin, alkaline phosphatase, and aminotransferase (Shapiro, 2017).

(b) Classic acute GVHD occurs 100 days or less after HSCT. Acute GVHD features are present (Antin & Raley, 2013).

(c) Late-onset acute GVHD occurs more than 100 days after HSCT. Acute GVHD features are present (Antin & Raley, 2013).

(d) Acute GVHD is usually graded according to the modified Glucksberg scale, in which the affected organ is staged individually, and an overall grade is assigned on the basis of the severity of each organ system (Antin & Raley, 2013).

(e) Primary therapy includes steroids and calcineurin inhibitors and is effective 30%–60% of the time (Antin & Raley, 2013).

(3) Chronic GVHD

(a) Clinical manifestations of chronic GVHD are commonly observed in the skin, liver, eyes, oral cavity, lungs, gastrointestinal system, neuromuscular system, and other body systems.

(b) Symptoms include dyspigmentation, xerosis, scleroderma, lichenification, xerostomia, keratoconjunctivitis sicca, jaundice, nausea, anorexia, diarrhea, weight loss, vaginal atrophy, recurrent infections, contractures, muscle cramps, and debility (Shapiro, 2017).

(c) Classic chronic GVHD can occur early after HSCT and presents without features of acute GVHD (Antin & Raley, 2013).

(d) Overlap syndrome is seen when features of both chronic and acute GVHD appear concurrently (Antin & Raley, 2013).

(e) Risk factors for chronic GVHD include previous acute GVHD, older age, and sex mismatching (i.e., female donor and male recipient). The incidence of chronic GVHD is also higher among recipients of peripheral blood stem cells than recipients of bone marrow–derived stem cells (Shapiro, 2017).

(f) Each organ is scored depending on physical manifestations, and these scores and the number of organs or sites involved are used to grade the overall severity. Symptoms may be mild, moderate, or severe (Dhir, Slatter, & Skinner, 2014; Flowers & Martin, 2015; Shapiro, 2017).

(g) Chronic GVHD is usually treated with a combination of steroids, cyclosporine, tacrolimus, rapamycin, mycophenolate mofetil, rituximab, pentostatin, hydroxychloroquine, methotrexate, and extracorpeal photopheresis (Dhir et al., 2014; Flowers & Martin, 2015; Mitchell, 2013; Shapiro, 2019).

j) Infection

(1) Throughout the course of HSCT, a patient is susceptible to infections, and most treatment regimens require prophylactic antibiotics, antifungals, and antivirals (Gregory, 2017).

(2) Handwashing continues to be the single most critical and effective procedure for preventing infection (Antin & Raley, 2013).

(3) Hospitals that perform HSCT should have rooms with more than 12 air exchanges per hour and point-of-use HEPA filtration. HEPA filters should be able to remove particles at least as small as 0.3 mcm in diameter (Antin & Raley, 2013).

(4) Fluoroquinolones (e.g., ciprofloxacin, levofloxacin) are recommended for antibacterial prophylaxis in patients during periods of neutropenia (NCCN, 2020b).

(5) Trimethoprim-sulfamethoxazole is recommended to prevent *Pneumocystis jirovecii* pneumonia in patients with cancer. Aerosolized or IV dapsone or pentamidine is recommended if a patient is trimethoprim-sulfamethoxazole intolerant (NCCN, 2020b).

(6) Posaconazole, fluconazole, and voriconazole are recommended to prevent fungal infections (NCCN, 2020b).

(7) Acyclovir and valacyclovir are recommended for antiviral prophylaxis and prevention of herpesvirus infection (NCCN, 2020b).

(8) Some centers consider the use of letermovir as primary prophylaxis for high-risk cytomegalovirus-positive allogeneic HSCT recipients (NCCN, 2020b).

(9) The risk of infection is primarily determined by the time from transplantation, degree of immune reconstitution, and presence or absence of GVHD (Chawala & Davies, 2019; McAdams & Burgunder, 2013).

(10) Most transplantation-related infections are divided into three phases (Shapiro, 2017).
   (a) Phase 1 (pre-engraftment phase)
   (b) Phase 2 (postengraftment phase)
   (c) Phase 3 (late infection phase)

(11) During phase 1 (day 0–15), prolonged neutropenia and breaks in the mucocutaneous barrier result in a substantial risk for bacteremia and fungal infections from the following sources (Koniarczyk & Ferraro, 2016; Shapiro, 2017).
   (a) Gram-negative bacteria from gastrointestinal tract or central line catheter
   (b) Gram-positive bacteria from sinuses or respiratory tract
   (c) Invasive fungal infections, such as aspergillosis or candidemia
   (d) Herpes simplex virus reactivation

(12) During phase 2 (day 15–100), infections are primarily associated with impaired cell-mediated immunity, the scope and effect of which is determined by the extent of GVHD and the immunosuppressive therapy used to control it (Shapiro, 2017).
   (a) By this time, patients have engrafted, and neutropenia and mucositis have resolved. However, immunodeficiency and central venous catheters still present risk.
   (b) The development of acute GVHD and its treatment can greatly affect the risk of infection.
   (c) Patients usually are affected by classic opportunistic infections (Koniarczyk & Ferraro, 2016).
      i. Cytomegalovirus
      ii. Adenovirus
      iii. BK virus
      iv. Respiratory viruses
      v. *P. jirovecii* pneumonia
      vi. Toxoplasmosis
      vii. Invasive aspergillosis
      viii. Mucormycosis

(13) During phase 3 (after day 100), patients with chronic GVHD and recipients of allogeneic transplants remain most at risk for infection because of delayed or prolonged immunosuppression. The following are common infections in this setting (Koniarczyk & Ferraro, 2016; Shapiro, 2017).
   (a) Encapsulated organisms (e.g., *Streptococcus pneumoniae, Haemophilus influenzae*)
   (b) Varicella zoster virus
   (c) *P. jirovecii* pneumonia
   (d) Invasive aspergillosis or mucormycosis

(14) Sites of infection include the following (Shapiro, 2017).
   (a) Oral cavity
   (b) Skin
   (c) Central venous catheters
   (d) Lungs
   (e) Gastrointestinal tract
   (f) Genitourinary tract

(15) Monitoring of the potential sites of infection and knowledge of the types of infections can help in early detection and treatment.

k) Liver dysfunction
   (1) Hepatic sinusoidal obstruction syndrome (HSOS), formerly known as hepatic veno-occlusive disease, is a clinical syndrome most commonly associated with the administration of high-dose chemotherapy and TBI (Anderson-Reitz & Clancy, 2013).

   (2) It is a process of central venular occlusion characterized by sinusoidal endothelial injury, subendothelial edema, intrahepatic obstruction of blood flow, hepatocellular necrosis, and intense fibrosis (Antin & Raley, 2013).

   (3) HSOS most commonly occurs within the first 30 days following conditioning for HSCT (Antin & Raley, 2013).

   (4) Clinical manifestations of HSOS include the following (Shapiro, 2017).
      (a) Hyperbilirubinemia
      (b) Rapid weight gain
      (c) Ascites
      (d) Right upper quadrant pain
      (e) Hepatomegaly
      (f) Splenomegaly
      (g) Jaundice
      (h) Coagulopathy
      (i) Increased platelet consumption

   (5) In mild cases of HSOS, no treatment is needed. Patients with moderate to severe HSOS require fluid volume management and avoidance of nephrotoxic or hepatotoxic medications (Gregory, 2017).

   (6) Defibrotide has shown promise in the treatment of severe HSOS and was approved by FDA in

2016 for the treatment of adults and children with HSOS with renal or pulmonary dysfunction following HSCT (U.S. FDA, 2016).

l) Pulmonary complications

(1) Pulmonary complications occur in approximately one-third of patients who undergo HSCT. They are associated with significant morbidity and mortality (Chi, Soubani, White, & Miller, 2013).

(2) All patients should have baseline pulmonary function tests before transplantation, and an aggressive diagnostic approach should be taken early after transplantation if pulmonary problems occur (Antin & Raley, 2013).

(3) Common pulmonary complications seen in the first 30 days after transplantation include pulmonary edema, bacterial or fungal pneumonia, pulmonary hemorrhage, and acute respiratory distress syndrome associated with septic shock (Shapiro, 2017).

(4) Through day 100, patients remain at high risk for these complications and for viral pneumonia, *P. jirovecii* pneumonia, and idiopathic interstitial pneumonitis due to TBI (Shapiro, 2017).

(5) Cytomegalovirus is a common nonrespiratory viral complication of transplantation, but patients often present with respiratory symptoms (Antin & Raley, 2013).

   (a) It is more common in the allogeneic transplant population, and usually occurs two to six months after HSCT (Antin & Raley, 2013).

   (b) All HSCT candidates and allogeneic donors should be screened for evidence of cytomegalovirus immunity (Antin & Raley, 2013).

   (c) Diagnosis is based on fever, cough, signs and symptoms of upper respiratory infection, nasal washing, viral swabs, or polymerase chain reaction testing (Antin & Raley, 2013).

   (d) Oral or IV letermovir, foscarnet, valganciclovir, or ganciclovir are administered for cytomegalovirus prophylaxis and treatment (NCCN, 2020b).

   (e) Patients should be screened for evidence of cytomegalovirus reactivation.

(6) Bronchiolitis obliterans syndrome is a complication that may arise primarily in allogeneic transplant recipients and is associated with poor prognosis (Gregory, 2017).

   (a) Bronchiolitis obliterans syndrome is characterized by a slow, progressive narrowing of airways, leading to obstruction and air trapping (Antin & Raley, 2013).

   (b) It often is associated with GVHD of the lungs (Antin & Raley, 2013).

   (c) It is recommended that lung evaluation with pulmonary function tests occur six months after transplant, then annually (Chi et al., 2013).

   (d) Treatment for bronchiolitis obliterans syndrome involves corticosteroids and supportive measures, such as oxygen support (Murphy & Shannon, 2017).

(7) Aspergillosis is the most common late invasive fungal infection (Norton, Garcia, & Noonan, 2016).

   (a) Aspergillosis is primarily caused by inhalation of *Aspergillus* spores (Stephens, 2013).

   (b) It occurs in 5%–15% of HSCT recipients, and the risk is associated with local environmental factors, duration of neutropenia, and corticosteroid use (Antin & Raley, 2013).

   (c) Treatment for aspergillosis can include voriconazole, posaconazole, amphotericin B liposomal, caspofungin, or micafungin (NCCN, 2020b).

(8) Complications resulting from damage to lung tissue caused by TBI include radiation pneumonitis and radiation fibrosis (Stephens, 2013).

   (a) Radiation pneumonitis is an acute inflammation of lung tissue exposed to radiation (Webster, 2017).

   (b) Radiation pneumonitis usually occurs two to nine months after radiation exposure but can develop over months to years after initial damage (Webster, 2017).

   (c) Initially, patients present with a dry cough. One to three months after RT, symptoms may include dyspnea, productive cough, fever, and night sweats (Webster, 2017).

   (d) Clinical management of radiation pneumonitis involves corticosteroids as the primary therapy. Antibiotics may be needed for a secondary infection. Bronchodilators and sedatives may be effective for relief (Webster, 2017).

   (e) Patients who experience acute radiation pneumonitis have a higher probability of developing radiation fibrosis, a condition that is refractory to treatment (Webster, 2017).

m) Ophthalmic complications

(1) Cataracts and dry eye syndrome are the two most common ophthalmic complications following HSCT (Clark, Savani, Mohty, & Savani, 2016).

(2) Cataracts are more commonly seen in HSCT recipients after TBI and with the use of steroids.

(3) Dry eye is treated with artificial tears.

(4) Patients need to report any visual acuity changes.

(5) Regular eye examinations should occur.

(6) Clinicians should encourage the use of sunglasses if patients are in the sun.

(7) Surgery to correct the cataract may be required (Kinori et al., 2015).

n) Endocrine dysfunction

(1) Thyroid disorders can occur in patients treated with TBI and patients receiving chemotherapy conditioning alone.

(2) Hypothyroidism and hyperthyroidism are common side effects after HSCT, with hypothyroidism being more prevalent (Clark et al., 2016).

(3) Hypothyroidism has an incidence of 5%–25% in the first year after transplantation (Clark et al., 2016).

(4) Hypothyroidism has been seen in up to 58% of pediatric patients (Milenković et al., 2014).

(5) Risk factors include TBI regimens, GVHD, and cytomegalovirus infection or reactivation (Clark et al., 2016).

(6) Children need to be followed for hypothyroidism, hyperthyroidism, and thyroid cancer (Vantyghem et al., 2014).

(7) Patients will need long-term monitoring of thyroid levels after HSCT.

o) Sexuality and infertility (see IV.E. Sexual function and dysfunction and IV.F. Fertility)

p) Musculoskeletal complications

(1) Musculoskeletal complications can include avascular necrosis, osteoporosis, fracture, and osteomyelitis.

(2) Risk factors include GVHD, older age, acute leukemia, TBI, and steroid use.

(3) Pediatric patients may develop osteochondromas, avascular necrosis, and diminished bone mineral density. RT can cause stunted growth (Mulcahy-Levy et al., 2013).

(4) Treatment for these skeletal complications can include analgesics, surgical interventions, and growth hormone replacement. Patients may require physical therapy (Inamoto & Lee, 2017).

(5) Bone mineral density loss in HSCT recipients is related to corticosteroid use, gonadal failure, conditioning therapy (e.g., TBI), and long-term immunosuppression. Diminished physical activity and weight bearing have been associated with decreased bone mineral density (Vantyghem et al., 2014).

(6) Bone loss occurs 6–12 months after HSCT, and recovery of bone mineral density begins from the lumbar spine, followed by a slower recovery to the femoral heads (Inamoto & Lee, 2017).

(7) Nearly 50% of patients are found to have low bone density after HSCT (Inamoto & Lee, 2017).

(8) Prevention recommendations include vitamin D 1,000 IU daily and calcium 1,200 mg daily (Inamoto & Lee, 2017).

(9) Bisphosphonates are the primary treatment for bone loss (Inamoto & Lee, 2017).

q) Cardiotoxicity

(1) Cardiomyopathy, congestive heart failure, and arrhythmias are commonly associated with HSCT (Norton et al., 2016).

(2) These diseases have been associated with the use of anthracyclines, cyclophosphamide, and RT (Norton et al., 2016).

(3) Targeted therapy cardiotoxicities, such as dysrhythmias, hypertension, hypotension, myocardial toxicity, pericardial effusion, and QT prolongation have been associated with the use of carfilzomib, nilotinib, panobinostat, ponatinib, vandetanib, and vemurafenib (Olsen, LeFebvre, & Brassil, 2019).

(4) Radionuclide therapy with monoclonal antibodies is used to treat hematologic malignancies. These therapies are associated with prolonged cytopenias and cardiotoxicity (Gharwan & Groninger, 2016; Larson, Carrasquillo, Cheung, & Press, 2015).

(5) Patients should be assessed for cardiovascular risk factors, such as obesity, smoking, hyperlipidemia, diabetes, sedentary lifestyle, and family history. A clinical workup should include electrocardiogram, echocardiogram, chest x-ray, and stress tests. Laboratory values, including lipid profile, glucose, and thyroid function, should be regularly monitored (Norton et al., 2016).

(6) Education on diet, exercise, medication adherence, maintaining a healthy weight, and smoking cessation should be discussed with patients (Norton et al., 2016).

r) Kidney dysfunction

(1) Chronic kidney disease occurs in 20%–60% of allogeneic HSCT recipients.

(2) Chronic kidney dysfunction is defined by glomerular filtration rate.

(a) Renal failure is defined as a glomerular filtration rate of 20%–25% of normal.

(b) End-stage renal disease is defined as a glomerular filtration rate of 15%–20% of normal or less.

(3) When patients reach end-stage renal disease, treatment with dialysis is commonly initiated. Patients with chronic renal failure are generally treated on an outpatient basis (Atilla, Atilla, Toprak, & Demirer, 2017).

(4) Risk factors for renal failure include older age, hypertension, poor kidney function, and acute and chronic GVHD (Atilla et al., 2017).

(5) Kidney function should be monitored with laboratory values of creatinine, glomerular filtration rate, and urine protein.

s) Second primary malignancies

(1) RT increases the risk of second primary malignancy. The risk was found to be associated with age, hormonal influences, chemotherapy use, environmental influences, genetic predisposition, infection, and immunosuppression (Kamran, Berrington de Gonzalez, Ng, Haas-Kogan, & Viswanathan, 2016).

(2) Second primary malignancies are classified into four distinct groups (Shannon, 2013).

(a) Myelodysplastic syndrome

(b) Acute myeloid leukemia

(c) Post-transplant lymphoproliferative disorders

(d) Second solid malignancies

(3) GVHD and RT are risk factors for developing solid tumors after allogeneic HSCT (Atilla et al., 2017).

(4) Patients treated with busulfan and cyclosporine and those of older age were at risk for oral, esophageal, colon, skin, and brain and CNS cancers (Atilla et al., 2017).

(5) Nonsquamous cell carcinomas are strongly linked to conditioning regimens involving RT at an early age.

(6) Other solid tumors associated with RT include melanoma and cancers of the oral cavity, salivary glands, brain, liver, uterus, cervix, thyroid, breast, bone, and connective tissue (Atilla et al., 2017).

(7) Patients should be screened on a regular basis for any signs of second malignancies and educated to report any unusual signs and symptoms that they may have.

(a) All patients should be screened on an annual basis.

(b) Colonoscopies should start at age 50 and occur every 10 years. For pediatric patients who received RT to the abdomen, colonoscopies should begin at age 35 (Carlson, 2014).

(c) Screening mammography in women starting at age 25 or eight years after radiation exposure, whichever occurs later, but no later than age 40 (Be The Match, 2019).

(d) Pap smears are recommended every one to three years, starting by age 21 or when patients become sexually active, whichever occurs first (Pinner & Tierney, 2016).

(e) Screening for Epstein-Barr virus DNA should begin within the first month after allogeneic HSCT and should continue for at least four months. Rituximab monotherapy is the treatment of choice for Epstein-Barr post-transplant lymphoproliferative disease (Styczynski et al., 2016).

9. Post-transplantation care

a) Prognosis

(1) Prognosis after allogeneic HSCT has greatly improved (Tichelli & Rovó, 2015).

(2) Patients who are disease free two to five years after HSCT have a 10-year survival rate greater than 80% (Inamoto & Lee, 2017).

b) Specialized care: It is vital for specialized care to continue after completion of therapy for patients with a history of a hematologic malignancy, in order to maximize the benefit of cancer treatment (Luskin, Banerjee, Del Percio, & Loren, 2015).

c) Long-term care

(1) Patients will require long-term care with their oncologist and PCP.

(2) The healthcare team must be able to recognize signs and symptoms of early and long-term toxicities in order to facilitate early interventions.

(3) Patients, families, and caregivers also need to be taught early recognition of these symptoms and the importance of reporting these findings.

d) Immune recovery (Inamoto & Lee, 2017).

(1) Full immune recovery may take years.

(2) If patients are able to stop immunosuppressive medications without GVHD or recurrent disease, many recover adequate immune function by one year after HSCT.

(3) Patients with chronic GVHD remain immunodeficient and are at high risk for infections.

e) Complications: Short- and long-term complications will need to be monitored (Tichelli & Rovó, 2015).

f) Short-term side effects (Gregory, 2017)

(1) Short-term side effects of HSCT can occur based on the conditioning regimen used.

(2) Possible short-term side effects include the following.

(a) Mucositis

(b) Nausea and vomiting

(c) Low blood counts leading to bleeding and infections

(d) HSOS

(e) Pulmonary complications

(f) Cardiovascular complications

(g) Renal complications

(3) Patients may experience GVHD and graft failure.

g) Late complications: HSCT recipients are at risk for the following late complications (Atilla et al., 2017).
  (1) Neuropsychological and cognitive deficits
  (2) Depression and anxiety
  (3) Cerebrovascular disease
  (4) Cataracts and microvascular retinopathy
  (5) Hypothyroidism
  (6) Diabetes
  (7) Idiopathic pneumonia syndrome, bronchiolitis obliterans syndrome, and sinopulmonary infections
  (8) Cardiomyopathy, congestive heart failure, arrhythmias, coronary artery disease, and peripheral arterial disease
  (9) GVHD
  (10) Hepatitis B and C
  (11) Chronic kidney disease
  (12) Hypertension
  (13) Myopathy
  (14) Cutaneous sclerosis
  (15) Osteoporosis
  (16) Avascular necrosis
  (17) Peripheral neuropathy
  (18) Developmental growth delay
  (19) Second primary cancers
  (20) Fatigue
  (21) Sexual dysfunction, hypogonadism, and infertility

h) Vaccine schedule
  (1) NCCN and American Society for Transplantation and Cellular Therapy have issued a vaccine schedule for post-transplant recipients (NCCN, 2020b).
  (2) The following inactivated vaccines are recommended 6–12 months following autologous or allogeneic transplantation (NCCN, 2020c; Wilson et al., 2018).
    (a) Diphtheria, tetanus, and acellular pertussis
    (b) *H. influenzae* type b
    (c) Pneumococcal
    (d) Hepatitis B virus
    (e) Meningococcal
    (f) Polio
    (g) HPV
  (3) Live vaccines for measles, mumps, and rubella, as well as varicella zoster virus, are not recommended unless it is more than two years after transplantation and a patient is seronegative and not on immunosuppression (NCCN, 2020b).

10. Patient, caregiver, and family education
  a) Education and counseling are an essential part of preparing for HSCT.

    (1) Patients, caregivers, and family members need to understand the transplantation program.
    (2) Clinicians must explain the goals of the treatment and the short- and long-term effects of the treatment in detail.
    (3) This education needs to occur at the time of consultation, throughout the transplantation process, and during recovery and follow-up care.
    (4) Education is required for informed consent.
    (5) Patients should understand the need for long-term medications and their possible side effects.

b) The transplant team is a large group that includes but is not limited to a medical oncologist, a radiation oncologist, nurses, counselors, a dietitian, pharmacists, and spiritual support, among others.

c) The psychosocial needs of the patient should also be addressed throughout treatment.
    (1) Psychological issues, including depression, anxiety, self-image and body changes, family distress, sexual changes, infertility, employment and financial changes, and an unknown future can affect a patient's physical and emotional well-being.
    (2) Assessment of the spiritual needs of the patient should also be addressed. A patient may want to have spiritual counseling during inpatient stays.

d) HSCT recipients need to be provided with resources obtained through the counselor, social worker, or nurse.

e) The following website resources can help patients, caregivers, and families.
    (1) American Cancer Society: www.cancer.org
    (2) American Society for Transplantation and Cellular Therapy: www.astct.org
    (3) Be The Match (National Marrow Donor Program): www.bethematch.org
    (4) CancerCare: www.cancercare.org
    (5) International Myeloma Foundation: www.myeloma.org
    (6) Leukemia and Lymphoma Society: www.lls.org
    (7) NCI: www.cancer.gov
    (8) OncoLink: www.oncolink.org

References

AABB, America's Blood Centers, American Red Cross, American Society for Apheresis, American Society for Blood and Marrow Transplantation, College of American Pathologists, ... World Marrow Donor Association. (2018, October). *Circular of information for the use of cellular therapy products.* http://www.aabb.org/aabbcct/coi/Documents/CT-Circular-of-Information.pdf

Adams, P.L. (2017). Hematologic issues. In J. Eggert (Ed.), *Cancer basics* (2nd ed., pp. 491–504). Oncology Nursing Society.

American College of Radiology & American Society for Radiation Oncology. (2017). *ACR–ASTRO practice guideline for the performance of total body irradiation.* https://www.astro.org/uploadedFiles/_MAIN_SITE/Patient_Care/Clinical_Practice_Statements/Content_Pieces/ACRASTROPracticeParameterTBI.pdf

Anderson-Reitz, L., & Clancy, C. (2013). Hepatorenal complications. In S.A. Ezzone (Ed.), *Hematopoietic stem cell transplantation: A manual for nursing practice* (2nd ed., pp. 191–200). Oncology Nursing Society.

Antin, J.H., & Raley, D.Y. (2013). *Manual of stem cell and bone marrow transplantation* (2nd ed.). Cambridge University Press.

Arnold, D.M., & Cuker, A. (2020). Approach to the adult with unexplained thrombocytopenia. In J.S. Tirnauer & L. Kunins (Eds.), *UpToDate*. Retrieved June 2, 2020, from https://www.uptodate.com/contents/approach-to-the-adult-with-unexplained-thrombocytopenia

Atilla, E., Atilla, P.A., Toprak, S.K., & Demirer, T. (2017). A review of late complications of allogeneic hematopoietic stem cell transplantations. *Clinical Transplantation, 31,* e13062. https://doi.org/10.1111/ctr.13062

Bashey, A., Zhang, X., Sizemore, C.A., Manion, K., Brown, S., Holland, H.K., ... Solomon, S.R. (2013). T-cell–replete HLA-haploidentical hematopoietic transplantation for hematologic malignancies using post-transplantation cyclophosphamide results in outcomes equivalent to those of contemporaneous HLA-matched related and unrelated donor transplantation. *Journal of Clinical Oncology, 31,* 1310–1360. https://doi.org/10.1200/jco.2012.44.3523

Be The Match. (2019). HCT guidelines for referral timing and post-transplant care. http://www.bethematch.org/md-guidelines

Camp-Sorrell, D. (2018). Chemotherapy toxicities and management. In C.H. Yarbro, D. Wujcik, & B.H. Gobel (Eds.), *Cancer nursing: Principles and practice* (8th ed., pp. 497–554). Jones and Bartlett Learning.

Carlson, C.A. (2014). Late effects of childhood cancer. In N.E. Kline (Ed.), *Essentials of pediatric hematology/oncology nursing: A core curriculum* (4th ed., pp. 391–458). Association of Pediatric Hematology/Oncology Nurses.

Cawley, K.A. (2017). Mucositis. In S. Newton, M. Hickey, & J.M. Brant (Eds.), *Mosby's oncology nursing advisor: A comprehensive guide to clinical practice* (2nd ed., pp. 323–324). Elsevier.

Chawala, R., & Davies, H.D. (2019, February 13). Infections after bone marrow transplantation. http://emedicine.medscape.com/article/1013470-overview#aw2aab6b6

Chi, A.K., Soubani, A.O., White, A.C., & Miller, K.B. (2013). An update on pulmonary complications of hematopoietic stem cell transplantation. *Chest, 144,* 1913–1922. https://doi.org/10.1378/chest.12-1708

Clark, C.A., Savani, M., Mohty, M., & Savani, B.N. (2016). What do we need to know about allogeneic hematopoietic stem cell transplant survivors? *Bone Marrow Transplantation, 51,* 1025–1031. https://doi.org/10.1038/bmt.2016.95

Dhir, S., Slatter, M., & Skinner, R. (2014). Recent advances in the management of graft-versus-host disease. *Archives of Diseases in Childhood, 99,* 1150–1157. https://doi.org/10.1136/archdischild-2013-304832

Flowers, M.E.D., & Martin, P.J. (2015). How we treat chronic graft-versus-host disease. *Blood, 125,* 606–615. https://doi.org/10.1182/blood-2014-08-551994

Gharwan, H., & Groninger, H. (2016). Kinase inhibitors and monoclonal antibodies in oncology: Clinical implications. *Nature Reviews Clinical Oncology, 13,* 209–227. https://doi.org/10.1038/nrclinonc.2015.213

Gregory, S. (2017). Hematopoietic stem cell transplantation. In J. Eggert (Ed.), *Cancer basics* (2nd ed., pp. 323–354). Oncology Nursing Society.

Inamoto, Y., & Lee, S.J. (2017). Late effects of blood and marrow transplantation. *Haematologica, 102,* 614–625. https://doi.org/10.3324/haematol.2016.150250

Kamran, S.C., Berrington de Gonzalez, A., Ng, A., Haas-Kogan, D., & Viswanathan, A.N. (2016). Therapeutic radiation and the potential risk of second malignancies. *Cancer, 122,* 1809–1821. https://doi.org/10.1002/cncr.29841

Kinori, M., Bielorai, B., Souroujon, D., Hutt, D., Mizrachi, I.B.-B., & Huna-Baron, R. (2015). Ocular complications in children after hematopoietic stem cell transplantation without total body irradiation. *Graefe's Archive for Clinical and Experimental Ophthalmology, 253,* 1397–1402. https://doi.org/10.1007/s00417-015-2964-8

Koniarczyk, H., & Ferraro, C. (2016). Transplant preparative regimens, cellular infusion, acute complications, and engraftment. In B. Faiman (Ed.), *BMTCN® certification review manual* (pp. 37–68). Oncology Nursing Society.

Larson, S.M., Carrasquillo, J.A., Cheung, N.-K.V., & Press, O.W. (2015). Radio-immunotherapy of human tumours. *Nature Reviews Cancer, 15,* 347–360. https://doi.org/10.1038/nrc3925

Lassiter, M. (2016). Basic concepts and indications for transplantation. In B. Faiman (Ed.), *BMTCN® certification review manual* (pp. 1–8). Oncology Nursing Society.

Lawenda, B.D., Gagne, H.M., Gierga, D.P., Niemierko, A., Wong, W.M., Tarbell, N.J., ... Loeffler, J.S. (2004). Permanent alopecia after cranial irradiation: Dose–response relationship. *International Journal of Radiation Oncology, Biology, Physics, 60,* 879–887. https://doi.org/10.1016/j.ijrobp.2004.04.031

Luskin, M.R., Banerjee, R., Del Percio, S., & Loren, A.W. (2015). A pound of cure requires an ounce (or more) of prevention: Survivorship and complications of therapy for hematologic malignancies. *Current Hematologic Malignancy Reports, 10,* 225–236. https://doi.org/10.1007/s11899-015-0274-1

Majdaeen, M., Babaei, M., & Rahimi, A. (2015). Sodium bicarbonate containing mouthwash for preventing radiotherapy-induced oral mucositis in patients with locally advanced head and neck cancer. *Reports of Radiotherapy and Oncology, 2,* e3721. https://doi.org/10.17795/rro-3721

McAdams, F.W., & Burgunder, M.R. (2013). Transplant treatment course and acute complications. In S.A. Ezzone (Ed.), *Hematopoietic stem cell transplantation: A manual for nursing practice* (2nd ed., pp. 47–66). Oncology Nursing Society.

Milenković, T., Vujić, D., Vuković, R., Zečević, Ž., Soldatović, I., Mitrović, K., & Zdravković, D. (2014). Subclinical hypothyroidism in children and adolescents after hematopoietic stem cells transplantation without irradiation. *Vojnosanitetski Pregled: Military Medical and Pharmaceutical Journal of Serbia, 71,* 1123–1127. https://doi.org/10.2298/VSP1412123M

Mitchell, S.A. (2013). Acute and chronic graft-versus-host disease. In S.A. Ezzone (Ed.), *Hematopoietic stem cell transplantation: A manual for nursing practice* (2nd ed., pp. 103–154). Oncology Nursing Society.

Muehlbauer, P.M., & Lopez, R.C. (2014). Diarrhea. In C.H. Yarbro, D. Wujcik, & B.H. Gobel (Eds.), *Cancer symptom management* (4th ed., pp. 185–212). Jones and Bartlett Learning.

Mulcahy-Levy, J.M., Tello, T., Giller, R., Wilkening, G., Quinones, R., Keating, A.K., & Liu, A.K. (2013). Late effects of total body irradiation and hematopoietic stem cell transplant in children under 3 years of age. *Pediatric Blood Cancer, 60,* 700–704.

Murphy, V.C., & Shannon, V. (2017). Pulmonary toxicities. In J. Eggert (Ed.), *Cancer basics* (2nd ed., pp. 611–632). Oncology Nursing Society.

Nalichowski, A., Eagle, D.G., & Burmeister, J. (2016). Dosimetric evaluation of total marrow irradiation using 2 different planning systems. *Medical Dosimetry, 41,* 230–235. https://doi.org/10.1016/j.meddos.2016.06.001

National Cancer Institute Cancer Therapy Evaluation Program. (2017). *Common terminology criteria for adverse events (CTCAE)* [v.5.0]. https://evs.nci.nih.gov/ftp1/CTCAE/CTCAE_4.03/CTCAE_4.03_2010-06-14_QuickReference_5x7.pdf

National Comprehensive Cancer Network. (2020a). *NCCN Clinical Practice Guidelines in Oncology (NCCN Guidelines®): Antiemesis* [v.2.2020]. https://www.nccn.org/professionals/physician_gls/pdf/antiemesis.pdf

National Comprehensive Cancer Network. (2020b). *NCCN Clinical Practice Guidelines in Oncology (NCCN Guidelines®): Prevention and treatment of cancer-related infections* [v.2.2020]. https://www.nccn.org/professionals/physician_gls/pdf/infections.pdf

National Comprehensive Cancer Network. (2020c). *NCCN Clinical Practice Guidelines in Oncology (NCCN Guidelines®): Survivorship* [v.1.2020]. https://www.nccn.org/professionals/physician_gls/pdf/survivorship.pdf

Norton, R., Garcia, I.N., & Noonan, K. (2016). Post-transplant issues. In B. Faiman (Eds.), *BMTCN® certification review manual* (pp. 125–232). Oncology Nursing Society.

Olsen, M.M., LeFebvre, K.B., & Brassil, K.J. (Eds.). (2019). *Chemotherapy and immunotherapy guidelines and recommendations for practice*. Oncology Nursing Society.

Pinner, L.A., & Tierney, D.K. (2016). Survivorship issues. In B. Faiman (Ed.), *BMTCN® certification review manual* (pp. 233–260). Oncology Nursing Society.

Prechtel Dunphy, E., & Walker, S. (2017). Gastrointestinal symptoms. In J. Eggert (Ed.), *Cancer basics* (2nd ed., pp. 431–474). Oncology Nursing Society.

Roila, F., Molassiotis, A., Herrstedt, J., Aapro, M., Gralla, R.J., Bruera, E., ... van der Wetering, M. (2016). 2016 MASCC and ESMO guideline update for the prevention of chemotherapy- and radiotherapy-induced nausea and vomiting and of nausea and vomiting in advanced cancer patients. *Annals of Oncology, 27*(Suppl. 5), v119–v133. https://doi.org/10.1093/annonc/mdw270

Rosselet, R.M. (2013). Hematologic effects. In S.A. Ezzone (Ed.), *Hematopoietic stem cell transplantation: A manual for nursing practice* (2nd ed., pp. 155–172). Oncology Nursing Society.

Shaftic, A.M. (2017). Radiation therapy. In J. Eggert (Ed.), *Cancer basics* (2nd ed., pp. 173–196). Oncology Nursing Society.

Shannon, S.P. (2013). Relapse and secondary malignancies. In S.A. Ezzone (Ed.), *Hematopoietic stem cell transplantation: A manual for nursing practice* (2nd ed., pp. 245–250). Oncology Nursing Society.

Shapiro, T.W. (2017). Hematopoietic stem cell transplantation. In S. Newton, M. Hickey, & J.M. Brant (Eds.), *Mosby's oncology nursing advisor: A comprehensive guide to clinical practice* (2nd ed., pp. 179–205). Elsevier.

Shapiro, T.W. (2019). Nursing implications of hematopoietic stem cell transplantation. In J. Brant (Eds.), *Core curriculum for oncology nursing* (6th ed., pp. 207–216). Elsevier.

Stephens, M.L. (2013). Cardiopulmonary complications. In S.A. Ezzone (Ed.), *Hematopoietic stem cell transplantation: A manual for nursing practice* (2nd ed., pp. 201–230). Oncology Nursing Society.

Styczynski, J., van der Velden, W., Fox, C.P., Engelhard, D., de la Camara, R., Cordonnier, C., & Ljungman, P. (2016). Management of Epstein-Barr virus infections and post-transplant lymphoproliferative disorders in patients after allogeneic hematopoietic stem cell transplantation: Sixth European Conference on Infections in Leukemia (ECIL-6) guidelines. *Haematologica, 101*, 803–811. https://doi.org/10.3324/haematol.2016.144428

Tayyem, A.-Q.-M. (2014). Cryotherapy effect on oral mucositis severity among recipients of bone marrow transplantation: A literature review. *Clinical Journal of Oncology Nursing, 18*, E84–E87. https://doi.org/10.1188/14.cjon.e84-e87

Thorpe, D.M., Byar, K.L., Conley, S., Drapek, L., Held-Warmkessel, J., Ramsdell, M.J., ... Wolles, B. (2017, February 27). Symptom interventions: Radiation-induced diarrhea. https://www.ons.org/pep/radiation-induced-diarrhea

Tichelli, A., & Rovó, A. (2015). Survivorship after allogeneic transplantation—Management recommendations for the primary care provider. *Current Hematologic Malignancy Reports, 10*, 35–44. https://doi.org/10.1007/s11899-014-0243-0

U.S. Food and Drug Administration. (2016, March 30). Defitelio (defibrotide sodium). https://www.fda.gov/Drugs/InformationOnDrugs/ApprovedDrugs/ucm493278.htm

Vantyghem, M.-C., Cornillon, J., Decanter, C., Defrance, F., Karrouz, W., Leroy, C., ... Yakoub-Agha, I. (2014). Management of endocrino-metabolic dysfunctions after allogeneic hematopoietic stem cell transplantation. *Orphanet Journal of Rare Diseases, 9*, 162. https://doi.org/10.1186/s13023-014-0162-0

Webster, J.S. (2017). Structural emergencies. In S. Newton, M. Hickey, & J.M. Brant (Eds.), *Mosby's oncology nursing advisor: A comprehensive guide to clinical practice* (2nd ed., pp. 355–362). Elsevier.

Wilson, B.J., Zitella, L.J., Erb, C.H., Foster, J., Peterson, M., & Wood, S.K. (2018). Prevention of infection: A systematic review of evidence-based practice interventions for management in patients with cancer. *Clinical Journal of Oncology Nursing, 22*, 157–168. https://doi.org/10.1188/18.CJON.157-168

Wong, J.Y.C., Filippi, A.R., Dabaja, B.S., Yahalom, J., & Specht, L. (2018). Total body irradiation: Guidelines from the International Lymphoma Radiation Oncology Group (ILROG). *International Journal of Radiation Oncology, Biology, Physics, 101*, 521–529. https://doi.org/10.1016/j.ijrobp.2018.04.071

Wu, V.W.C, & Leung, K.Y. (2019). A review on the assessment of radiation induced salivary gland damage after radiotherapy. *Frontiers in Oncology, 9*, 1090. https://doi.org/10.3389/fonc.2019.01090

E. Total skin irradiation

1. Definition: Total skin irradiation is a type of RT that is delivered to the entire skin surface with electrons. It is also referred to as *total skin electron beam therapy* (Chowdhary, Song, Zaorsky, & Shi, 2019).

2. Indications

   a) The role of total skin irradiation was first described in 1951. Total skin irradiation historically is considered the single most effective method in treating cutaneous T-cell lymphoma (Chowdhary et al., 2019, Park et al., 2014).

   b) Cutaneous T-cell lymphoma comprises two major subgroups (Chowdhary et al., 2019).

      (1) Mycosis fungoides affects an estimated 5.6 in one million in the United States, according to the SEER program (Lovgren & Scarisbrick, 2019). Total skin irradiation remains a sterling treatment option (Whittaker, Hoppe, & Price, 2016).

      (2) Sézary syndrome accounts for 5% of mycosis fungoides cases and is characterized by erythroderma, lymphadenopathy, and leukemic involvement at diagnosis, with a median survival of 32 weeks (Lovgren & Scarisbrick, 2019).

   c) Total skin irradiation may be a localized treatment in patients with unilateral or localized mycosis fungoides, lymphoma cutis, and Kaposi sarcoma (Lutsyk, Ben-Yosef, Bergman, Kuten, & Bar-Sela, 2018).

   d) Total skin irradiation may be part of nonmyeloablative allogeneic HSCT (Chowdhary et al., 2019; Elsayad, Susek, & Eich, 2017; Foss & Girardi, 2017).

3. Treatment

   a) Treatment is often complex; positioning and dosing vary based on institutional guidelines and protocols (Chowdhary et al., 2019).

   b) A variety of treatments for mycosis fungoides can be used alone or in combination with chemotherapy, biotherapy, RT, or photochemotherapy (Lovgren & Scarisbrick, 2019; Piotrowski, Fundowicz, & Pawlaczyk, 2018).

   c) The management of mycosis fungoides is based on stage, and the prognosis varies significantly in low-risk (stage IA), intermediate-risk (stage IB–IIA), and high-risk cases (stage IIB–IVB) (Raychaudhury, 2017).

   d) Treatment procedure has numerous considerations related to dose, positioning, and toxicity (Chowdhary et al., 2019).

(1) Treatment typically is delivered via a 6 MeV electron beam, and a patient is placed in a standing position in front of the beam (Park et al., 2014; Platoni et al., 2019).

(2) Boost treatment may be given to areas of ulceration before total skin irradiation (Chowdhary et al., 2019).

(3) A two-day, six-field treatment approach is used that encompasses the following fields (Chowdhary et al., 2019).

    (a) Day 1: straight anterior, right posterior oblique, and the left posterior oblique

    (b) Day 2: straight posterior, right anterior oblique, and left anterior oblique

(4) Treatment typically lasts 8–10 weeks and is delivered four days a week for 30–45 minutes for a total dose of 36–40 Gy to the skin and 18–20 Gy to the hands and feet to achieve a high remission rate with acceptable toxicity (Chowdhary et al., 2019; Rivers & Singh, 2019).

    (a) Most patients eventually relapse because RT toxicity is dose dependent (Chowdhary et al., 2019).

    (b) Consequently, clinical practice is moving toward low-dose total skin irradiation of 10–12 Gy because of its improved toxicity profile, capability for disease reduction, convenience for patients, and multiple applications in relapsed disease (Chowdhary et al., 2019).

(5) Patient positioning is vital in order to minimize skinfolds. Typically, this includes special care for the breasts, perineum, and panniculi of obese patients (Piotrowski et al., 2018).

(6) Patients may have their hands and feet shielded during the six-field approach and receive supplemental therapy to these sites and the scalp, if warranted (King et al., 2017).

(7) External or internal eye shields may be used to protect the cornea and lens (Chowdhary et al., 2019).

4. Side effects
   a) Acute effects
   (1) Patients will experience epithelial reactions, including pruritus, erythema, dry desquamation, and moist desquamation (see IV.B. Skin reactions).

   (2) Superficial atrophy with wrinkling, telangiectasia, xerosis, and uneven pigmentation are the most common changes (Tandberg, Craciunescu, & Kelsey, 2015).

   (3) Patients may experience pain related to skin changes (Georgakopoulos et al., 2019).

   (4) Patients will experience alopecia, which is reversible in four to six months (Tandberg et al., 2015).

   (5) Patients will experience nail loss (Kroeger, Elsayad, Moustakis, Haverkamp, & Eich, 2017).

   (6) At higher doses (greater than 25 Gy), some patients may develop transient swelling of the hands, edema of the ankles, and occasionally large blisters. These reactions necessitate local shielding or temporary discontinuation of therapy (Georgakopoulos et al., 2019; Morris et al., 2017; see IV.B. Skin reactions).

   (7) Patients may report an inability to sweat properly for the first 6–12 months following therapy (Kaźmierska, 2014; Tandberg et al., 2015).

   (8) Gynecomastia may develop. The mechanism for this is unknown (Chowdhary, Chhabra, Kharod, & Marwaha, 2016).

   b) Late effects (Kaźmierska, 2014; Tandberg et al., 2015)
   (1) Superficial atrophy with wrinkling, telangiectasia, xerosis, and uneven pigmentation are the most common changes (Chowdhary et al., 2019; Lovgren & Scarisbrick, 2019).

   (2) Although rare, higher doses may cause permanent alopecia, frankpoikiloderma (mottled skin appearance), skin fragility, and subcutaneous fibrosis (Chowdhary et al., 2019; Lovgren & Scarisbrick, 2019).

   (3) The risk of second primary malignancies, such as squamous cell and basal cell cancers of the skin, is increased after total skin irradiation and is mostly associated with patients who have received repeated treatment with multiple therapies (Chowdhary et al., 2016).

5. Patient, caregiver, and family education
   a) Patients, caregivers, and family should be educated on the treatment procedure and the time required for the treatment each day, as well as positioning used (Duffy, Jennings, & Sahu, 2019).
   b) Clinicians should advise patients and family that most of the treatment area will be exposed during the treatment and that measures will be implemented to protect patient privacy.
   c) Clinicians should teach male patients about the potential risk of infertility caused by the dose to the testes, as well as fertility options, such as sperm banking (Chiba & Fujisawa, 2014; Skaznik-Wikiel, Gilbert, Meacham, & Kondapalli, 2015).
   d) Patients should be taught to use eye rinses to minimize irritation from eye shields.
   e) Nurses should inform patients and family about the use of skin products to minimize dry pruritus and dry desquamation (see IV.B. Skin reactions).
   f) Nurses should teach patients and family about skin care if blisters or moist desquamation arises (see IV.B. Skin reactions).

g) Patients should elevate the extremity if swelling or edema arises.

h) Patients and family should know how to perform skin checks and report any new lesions or changes in lesions.

i) Nurses should emphasize the importance of follow-up care to assess for late effects (Duffy et al., 2019).

6. Follow-up care

a) Patients may be seen frequently over the first few months after treatment, then every three months for skin assessments and to determine response to treatment (Georgakopoulos et al., 2019).

b) Patients may be followed by a dermatologist in conjunction with the radiation oncologist (Buglione et al., 2018).

References

Buglione, M., Spiazzi, L., Urips, M., Baushi, L., Avitabile, R., Pasinetti, N., ... Magrini, S.M. (2018). Light and shadows of a new technique: Is photon total-skin irradiation using helical IMRT feasible, less complex and as toxic as the electrons one? *Radiation Oncology, 13,* 158. https://doi.org/10.1186/s13014-018-1100-4

Chiba, K., & Fujisawa, M. (2014). Fertility preservation in men with cancer. *Reproductive Medicine and Biology, 13,* 177–184. https://doi.org/10.1007/s12522-014-0180-6

Chowdhary, M., Chhabra, A.M., Kharod, S., & Marwaha, G. (2016). Total skin electron beam therapy in the treatment of mycosis fungoides: A review of conventional and low-dose regimens. *Clinical Lymphoma, Myeloma and Leukemia, 16,* 662–671. https://doi.org/10.1016/j.clml.2016.08.019

Chowdhary, M., Song, A., Zaorsky, N.G., & Shi, W. (2019). Total skin electron beam therapy in mycosis fungoides—A shift towards lower dose? *Chinese Clinical Oncology, 8,* 9. https://doi.org/10.21037/cco.2018.09.02

Duffy, R., Jennings, T., & Sahu, J. (2019). Gentle skin care guidelines for patients with mycosis fungoides. *Chinese Clinical Oncology, 8,* 14. https://doi.org/10.21037/cco.2018.10.04

Elsayad, K., Susek, K.H., & Eich, H.T. (2017). Total skin electron beam therapy as part of multimodal treatment strategies for primary cutaneous T-cell lymphoma. *Oncology Research and Treatment, 40,* 244–252. https://doi.org/10.1159/000475634

Foss, F.M., & Girardi, M. (2017). Mycosis fungoides and Sezary syndrome. *Hematology/Oncology Clinics of North America, 31,* 297–315. https://doi.org/10.1016/j.hoc.2016.11.008

Georgakopoulos, I., Papadavid, E., Platoni, K., Dilvoi, M., Patatoukas, G., Kypraiou, E., ... Kouloulias, V. (2019). Clinical application of total skin electron beam (TSEB) therapy for the management of T cell cutaneous lymphomas. The evolving role of low dose (12 Gy) treatment schedule. *Clinical and Translational Radiation Oncology, 15,* 26–30. https://doi.org/10.1016/j.ctro.2018.12.002

Kaźmierska, J. (2014). Clinical results of the total skin electron irradiation of the mycosis fungoides in adults. Conventional fractionation and low dose schemes. *Reports of Practical Oncology and Radiotherapy, 19,* 99–103. https://www.sciencedirect.com/science/article/pii/S1507136713010286

King, B.J., Deufel, C.L., Locher, S.E., McLemore, L.B., Brekke-Hackman, B.S., & Martenson, J.A. (2017). A method to improve dose uniformity during total skin electron beam therapy in patients with pendulous breasts. *Advances in Radiation Oncology, 2,* 288–290. https://doi.org/10.1016/j.adro.2017.05.009

Kroeger, K., Elsayad, K., Moustakis, C., Haverkamp, U., & Eich, H.T. (2017). Low-dose total skin electron beam therapy for cutaneous lymphoma: Min-

imal risk of acute toxicities. *Strahlentherapie Und Onkologie, 193,* 1024–1030. https://doi.org/10.1007/s00066-017-1188-8

Lovgren, M.-L., & Scarisbrick, J.J. (2019). Update on skin directed therapies in mycosis fungoides. *Chinese Clinical Oncology, 8,* 7. https://doi.org/10.21037/cco.2018.11.03

Lutsyk, M., Ben-Yosef, R., Bergman, R., Kuten, A., & Bar-Sela, G. (2018). Total skin electron irradiation and sequential malignancies in mycosis fungoides patients: Longitudinal study. *Clinical Oncology, 30,* 618–624. https://doi.org/10.1016/j.clon.2018.06.006

Morris, S., Scarisbrick, J., Frew, J., Irwin, C., Grieve, R., Humber, C., ... Whittaker, S. (2017). The results of low-dose total skin electron beam radiation therapy (TSEB) in patients with mycosis fungoides from the UK Cutaneous Lymphoma Group. *International Journal of Radiation Oncology, Biology, Physics, 99,* 627–633. https://doi.org/10.1016/j.ijrobp.2017.05.052

Park, S.-Y., Ahn, B.S., Park, J.M., Ye, S.-J., Kim, I.H., & Kim, J.-I. (2014). Dosimetric comparison of 4 MeV and 6 MeV electron beams for total irradiation. *Radiation Oncology, 9,* 197. https://doi.org/10.1186/1748-717x-9-197

Piotrowski, T., Fundowicz, M., & Pawlaczyk, M. (2018). Total skin electron beam therapy with rotary dual technique as a palliative treatment for mycosis fungoides. *In Vivo, 32,* 517–522. https://doi.org/10.21873/invivo.11269

Platoni, K., Diamantopoulos, S., Dilvoi, M., Delinikolas, P., Kypraiou, E., Efstathopoulos, E., & Kouloulias, V. (2018). The first application of hemibody electron beam irradiation for Kaposi sarcoma at the lower extremities. *Journal of Balkan Union of Oncology, 23*(1), 268–272. https://www.jbuon.com/archive/23-1-268.pdf

Raychaudhury, T. (2017). Management strategies for mycosis fungoides in India. *Indian Journal of Dermatology, 62,* 137–141. https://doi.org/10.4103/ijd.ijd_71_17

Rivers, C.I., & Singh, A.K. (2019). Total skin electron beam therapy for mycosis fungoides revisited with adjuvant systemic therapy. *Clinical Lymphoma, Myeloma and Leukemia, 19,* 83–88. https://doi.org/10.1016/j.clml.2018.11.015

Skaznik-Wikiel, M.E., Gilbert, S.B., Meacham, R.B., & Kondapalli, L.A. (2015). Fertility preservation options for men and women with cancer. *Reviews in Urology, 17,* 211–219. http://medreviews.com/journal/reviews-in-urology/vol/17/no/4/fertility-preservation-options-men-and-women-cancer

Tandberg, D.J., Craciunescu, O., & Kelsey, C.R. (2015). Radiation therapy for cutaneous T-cell lymphomas. *Dermatologic Clinics, 33,* 703–713. https://doi.org/10.1016/j.det.2015.05.006

Whittaker, S., Hoppe, R., & Prince, H.M. (2016). How I treat mycosis fungoides and Sézary syndrome. *Blood, 127,* 3142–3153. https://doi.org/10.1182/blood-2015-12-611830

F. Total lymphoid irradiation

1. Overview

a) Total lymphoid irradiation (TLI), or total nodal irradiation, was initially developed in the 1970s as a curative treatment for Hodgkin lymphoma (Hautmann et al., 2015).

b) TLI has been used since then for the treatment of Hodgkin lymphoma and also as an immunosuppressive therapy in organ transplantation for several decades (Hautmann et al., 2015; Sprangers, Pirenne, Mathieu, & Waer, 2019).

c) TLI is a key component of the treatment for selected patients, including those with relapsed Hodgkin lymphoma after chemotherapy (Gentzler et al., 2014).

d) TLI remains as a significant treatment regimen with less toxicity, even when the total dose of TLI is 8 Gy in the treatment of organ rejection or bronchiolitis obliterans syndrome after organ transplantation (Hautmann et al., 2015).

2. Radiation fields
   a) TLI includes treatment to all lymph nodes in the area above and below the diaphragm (supradiaphragmatic and subdiaphragmatic), including the thymus and spleen. It is delivered through two fields: the mantle field and inverted-Y field (Lee, Kim, Choi, Ryu, & Chung, 2012; Veltri et al., 2013).
   b) Mantle fields include lymph nodes of the neck, axilla, and mediastinum. These areas include the submandibular, cervical, supraclavicular, infraclavicular, axillary, mediastinal, subcarinal, and hilar lymph nodes (Sprangers et al., 2019; see Figure 25).
   c) Inverted-Y fields include aortic, iliac, and pelvic lymph nodes, as well as the spleen (Sprangers et al., 2019; see Figure 26).

3. Indications
   a) Hodgkin lymphoma
      (1) The treatment of patients with Hodgkin lymphoma with a favorable clinical presentation typically includes two to four cycles of chemotherapy with or without low-dose RT (Terezakis, Metzger, & Constine, 2016; see also VI.B. Lymphomas).
      (2) Hodgkin lymphoma treated with chemotherapy alone most frequently relapses in the initially involved lymph nodes. Involved-site RT has been used to decrease long-term toxicities and to spare healthy structures in patients who experience relapse (Terezakis et al., 2016).
      (3) RT alone can cure some refractory or relapsed Hodgkin lymphoma when administered as a standard dose TLI (18–20 Gy). This option is used in patients with disease recurrence in a limited nodal pattern after a prolonged interval from a complete initial response (Terezakis, Hudson, & Constine, 2011).
      (4) Rimner et al. (2017) reported excellent long-term outcomes with limited toxicity in patients with relapsed and refractory Hodgkin lymphoma managed by a systematic multimodal salvage approach, including salvage chemotherapy, TLI, high-dose chemotherapy, and HSCT.
         (a) From 1985 to 2008, 186 previously unirradiated patients with biopsy-proven relapsed or refractory Hodgkin lymphoma received salvage therapy under four different institutionally approved protocols.
         (b) All patients received salvage chemotherapy, accelerated involved-field RT at 18–20 Gy to the relapsed or refractory site, followed by TLI (15–18 Gy) and high-dose chemotherapy.
         (c) Five- and 10-year overall survival rates were 68% and 56%, respectively. Five- and 10-year event-free survival rates were 62% and 56%, respectively.

FIGURE 25. Total Lymphoid Irradiation Mantle Field: Anterior and Posterior Views

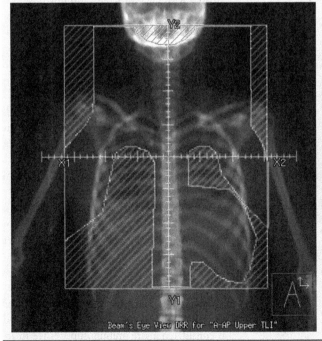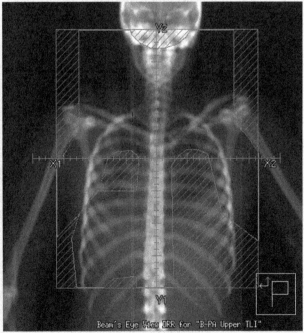

Note. Images courtesy of Susan McGovern. Used with permission.

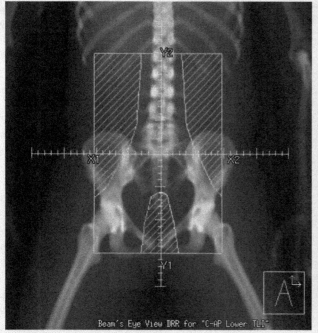 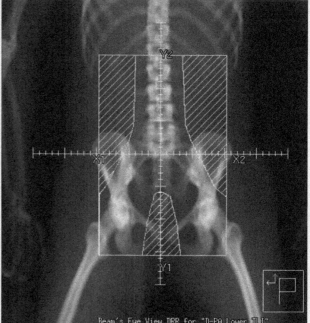

Note. Images courtesy of Susan McGovern. Used with permission.

(d) The findings also suggested that the primary refractory disease and extranodal disease were independently associated with poor disease-specific survival; eight patients experienced grade 3 or higher cardiotoxicity, accounting for three deaths (Rimner et al., 2017).

(5) In patients with relapsed or refractory classical Hodgkin lymphoma, TLI followed by high-dose chemotherapy and autologous HSCT is considered as an effective treatment strategy with low rates of treatment-related mortality and excellent long-term outcomes (Gentzler et al., 2014).

    (a) Gentzler et al. (2014) conducted a study of 51 patients with Hodgkin lymphoma (59% with primary refractory disease; 63% with active disease at autologous HSCT).

    (b) Patients were treated with TLI and autologous HSCT.

    (c) All patients received accelerated hyperfractionated TLI, administered twice daily at 1.5 Gy, five days a week for 10 days before high-dose chemotherapy (chosen by treating physician) and autologous HSCT (Gentzler et al., 2014).

    (d) In total, uninvolved nodal sites and spleen received 15 Gy, and current and previous sites received 30–34 Gy.

(e) Results showed excellent disease control and long-term survival rates.

(f) The study concluded that TLI helped to reduce relapses at the site of previous nodal involvement and eventually improved survival.

(6) Most children with Hodgkin lymphoma are treated with chemotherapy and low-dose RT. However, the RT in pediatric Hodgkin lymphoma is highly protocol dependent (Terezakis et al., 2016).

(7) RT options for unfavorable and advanced Hodgkin lymphoma are variable and protocol dependent.

    (a) In combined-modality therapy, involved-field RT and involved-site RT remain as standards, restricting RT to the areas of initial bulky disease.

    (b) Generally, RT doses are 20–36 Gy in 1.5–2 Gy fractions.

    (c) Involved-site RT fields are smaller than those of involved-field RT but larger than those of involved-node RT (Terezakis et al., 2016).

b) HSCT conditioning

(1) The literature suggests that with the advancement in RT, TLI has been increasingly used as part of conditioning regimens for HSCT and is considered a safe immunosuppressive treatment modality (Sprangers et al., 2019).

(2) Research has shown that TLI has a protectant effect against acute GVHD by increasing the percentage of natural killer cells, which helps to reduce acute GVHD (Lee et al., 2012).

(3) For patients with severe aplastic anemia, a TLI-based conditioning regimen in allogeneic HSCT provides relatively better results of engraftment and survival at long-term follow-up (Lee et al., 2012).

(a) Lee et al. (2012) reported on 20 patients with severe aplastic anemia who received TLI (7.5 Gy in a single fraction) as conditioning for HSCT, between 1995 and 2006.

(b) Patients had experienced previous graft failure or were at high risk for graft failure.

(c) These patients received TLI combined with antithymocyte globulin, followed by transplantation and GVHD prophylaxis with cyclosporine and methotrexate.

(d) Researchers found that 17 out of 20 patients (85%) had sustained engraftment at follow-up, and 12 patients (60%) showed no signs of GVHD.

(e) For all patients, overall survival was 85% at five years and 83.1% at 10 years (Lee et al., 2012).

(4) Numerous studies have shown that nonmyeloablative conditioning with TLI and antithymocyte globulin protects against acute GVHD (Veltri et al., 2013).

(a) Benjamin et al. (2014) found that TLI and antithymocyte globulin conditioning for allogeneic HSCT results in an effective graft-versus-malignancy response for control of disease.

    i. The study involved 61 patients with myelodysplastic syndromes, therapy-related myeloid neoplasms, and chronic myeloproliferative neoplasms conditioned with TLI and antithymocyte globulin for allogeneic HSCT.

    ii. The cumulative incidence of grade 2–4 acute GVHD was 14% and grade 3–4 acute GVHD was 4%.

    iii. The total incidence of nonrelapse mortality at 100 days was 0%, at 12 months was 7%, and at 36 months was 11%. At 36 months, overall survival was 41%, and progression-free survival was 35%.

    iv. A TLI and antithymocyte globulin conditioning regimen is considered safe and tolerable, as it demonstrated a low nonrelapse mortality.

(b) In a retrospective analysis of 13 patients with treatment-refractory chronic GVHD who were treated with TLI at 1 Gy, TLI represented less toxicity and sustained immunomodulatory effect (Hautmann et al., 2015).

(c) Pan et al. (2015) found that conditioning with TLI and antithymocyte globulin or TLI and regulatory T cells promoted the engraftment of embryonic stem cell allogeneic grafts.

c) Diffuse large B-cell lymphoma (DLBCL)

(1) DLBCL is a common subtype of aggressive non-Hodgkin lymphoma.

(2) Although the use of RT in this disease is controversial, international guidelines recommend chemotherapy with or without consolidative RT for the treatment of DLBCL (Sert, Kamer, Saydam, & Anacak, 2018).

(3) Sert et al. (2018) reported on 42 patients with the diagnosis of mediastinal DLBCL who received 2–10 cycles of rituximab-containing chemotherapy and involved lymphatic site RT at a total dose of 30.6–45 Gy with 1.8 Gy per fraction per day, over four to five weeks.

(a) The estimated five-year overall survival and progression-free survival rates were 84% and 77%, respectively, for all patients. For the patients without residual disease after chemotherapy, five-year overall survival and progression-free survival rates were 100% and 92%, respectively.

(b) The study showed that the response to chemotherapy is the most important factor affecting overall survival and progression-free survival.

(c) Because of a lack of phase 3 trials, the role of consolidative RT is not clear in patients treated with rituximab.

d) Acute leukemias

(1) In patients with relapsed or refractory acute leukemia undergoing HSCT with active disease, total marrow and lymphoid irradiation conditioning allows for precise delivery and more intense treatment by targeting sites of high disease burden or sites at high risk for disease involvement, while avoiding healthy tissue (Stein et al., 2017).

(2) In a phase 1 trial involving 51 patients with relapsed or refractory acute myeloid leukemia or acute lymphoblastic leukemia undergoing HSCT with active disease, all patients were treated with total marrow and lymphoid irradiation (12–20 Gy), cyclophosphamide, and etoposide. This conditioning regimen was well tolerated at a dose up to 20 Gy, with a low rate of

nonrelapse mortality at 100 days and one year and no increased risk of GVHD with higher dose of radiation (Stein et al., 2017).

e) Organ transplantation

(1) TLI has been used as an immunosuppressive therapy before transplantation of kidneys, lungs, heart, or any other organs to prevent organ rejection.

(2) In 2014, McKay, Knight, and Wright conducted a literature review to establish indications for the use of TLI. They reported that TLI may be an effective treatment for cardiac and pulmonary rejection in patients who do not respond to immunosuppressive drugs.

(3) The first clinical kidney transplants utilizing TLI were performed at the University of Minnesota and were performed on 20 patients who had previously rejected a transplant (Sprangers et al., 2019).

(a) The investigators reported an approximately 30% increase in the rate of graft survival at one year, compared to historical control data. Similar results were achieved with cyclosporine.

(b) The investigators concluded that they preferred cyclosporine over TLI because of the ease of administration.

(4) Ghadjar et al. (2010) conducted a study to assess the safety and efficacy of tailored TLI.

(a) The study consisted of seven patients who received cardiac transplants, of whom five had recalcitrant cellular cardiac allograft rejection and two had side effects of immunosuppressive drug therapy.

(b) All patients received tailored TLI to a mean dose of 6.4 Gy (range 1.6–8.8 Gy). Treatment was well tolerated.

(c) Prior to tailored TLI, the rate of rejection episode was 0.43 episodes per patient per month. After tailored TLI, this rate was 0.02 episodes per patient per month.

(d) The researchers concluded that tailored TLI is a useful and effective treatment modality for the management of recalcitrant cellular cardiac allograft rejection and in patients with significant immunosuppressive drug therapy side effects.

f) Follicular lymphoma: Guckenberger, Alexandrow, and Flentje (2012) found that TLI achieved promising overall survival and freedom from progression in stage III follicular lymphoma. They recommended that TLI be considered as a potentially curative treatment option.

4. Side effects

a) Side effects of TLI are associated with areas within the mantle and inverted-Y radiation fields (Terezakis et al., 2011).

b) Early side effects can occur shortly after the start of TLI and up to six months afterward. Early side effects may include the following (Terezakis et al., 2011).

(1) Loss of appetite

(2) Nausea and vomiting

(3) Diarrhea

(4) Reduced or sticky saliva

(5) Dry mouth

(6) Dysphagia

(7) Loss of taste

(8) Skin redness

(9) Dry skin

(10) Hair loss

(11) Fatigue

(12) Damage or inflammation to the liver, lungs, and heart

(13) Pancytopenia (increased risk of infection)

c) Late side effects can occur six months or more after TLI. Potential late side effects include the following (Guckenberger et al., 2012; Terezakis et al., 2011).

(1) Changes in normal growth and development

(2) Lung scarring leading to shortness of breath

(3) Myelitis

(4) Dental caries

(5) Testicular or ovarian damage causing sterility

(6) Second primary malignancy

d) The long-term side effects specific to TLI in children include impairment in muscle and bone development and injury to the heart, lungs, thyroid gland, and reproductive organs (Terezakis et al., 2011).

e) The following measures should be taken to manage side effects.

(1) Patients should report an elevated temperature of 100.4° F (38°C) or higher and monitor for signs of infection (Shelton, 2016).

(2) Blood counts should be monitored. Decreased counts may present in 7–10 days.

(3) Patients can maintain adequate nutrition and hydration with soft food and liquid nutrition supplements.

(4) Nurses should monitor for dysphagia, odynophagia, and diarrhea. Pain medication, dietary manipulation, and IV hydration should be administered for management (O'Leary, 2016).

5. Patient, caregiver, and family education: Patients, caregivers, and family should understand the indication, logistics, benefits, and potential short- and long-term side effects of TLI, as well as management of side effects.

References

Benjamin, J., Chhabra, S., Kohrt, H.E., Lavori, P., Laport, G.G., Arai, S., ... Lowsky, R. (2014). Total lymphoid irradiation—Antithymocyte globulin conditioning allogeneic transplantation for patients with myelodysplastic syndromes and myeloproliferative neoplasms. *Biology of Blood and Marrow Transplantation, 20,* 837–843. https://doi.org/10.1016/j.bbmt.2014.02.023

Gentzler, R.D., Evens, A.M., Rademaker, A.W., Weitner, B.B., Mittal, B.B., Dillehay, G.L., ... Winter, J.N. (2014). F-18 FDG-PET predicts outcomes for patients receiving total lymphoid irradiation and autologous blood stem-cell transplantation for relapsed and refractory Hodgkin lymphoma. *British Journal of Haematology, 165,* 793–800. https://doi.org/10.1111/bjh.12824

Ghadjar, P., Joos, D., Martinelli, M., Hullin, R., Zwahlen, M., Lössl, K., ... Mohacsi, P. (2010). Tailored total lymphoid irradiation in heart transplant patients: 10-years experience of one center. *Radiation Oncology, 5,* 3. https://doi.org/10.1186/1748-717X-5-3

Guckenberger, M., Alexandrow, N., & Flentje, M. (2012). Radiotherapy alone for stage I-III low grade follicular lymphoma: Long-term outcome and comparison of extended field and total nodal irradiation. *Radiation Oncology, 7,* 103. https://doi.org/10.1186/1748-717X-7-103

Hautmann, A.H., Wolff, D., Hilgendorf, I., Fehn, U., Edinger, M., Hoffmann, P., ... Hautmann, M.G. (2015). Total nodal irradiation in patients with severe treatment-refractory chronic graft-versus-host disease after allogeneic stem cell transplantation: Response rates and immunomodulatory effects. *Radiotherapy and Oncology, 116,* 287–293. https://doi.org/10.1016/j.radonc.2015.07.035

Lee, Y.-H., Kim, J.-Y., Choi, B.-O., Ryu, M.-R., & Chung, S.-M. (2012). Total lymphoid irradiation based conditioning for hematopoietic stem cell transplantation in severe aplastic anemia. *Radiation Oncology Journal, 30,* 165–172. https://doi.org/10.3857/roj.2012.30.4.165

McKay, C., Knight, K.A., & Wright, C. (2014). Beyond cancer treatment—A review of total lymphoid irradiation for heart and lung transplant recipients. *Journal of Medical Radiation Sciences, 61,* 202–209. https://doi.org/10.1002/jmrs.63

O'Leary, C.M. (2016). Gastrointestinal, genitourinary, and hepatic toxicities. In B.H. Gobel, S. Triest-Robertson, & W.H. Vogel (Eds.), *Advanced oncology nursing certification review and resource manual* (2nd ed., pp. 525–576). Oncology Nursing Society.

Pan, Y., Leveson-Gower, D.B., de Almeida, P.E., Pierni, A., Baker, J., Florek, M., ... Negrin, R.S. (2015). Engraftment of embryonic stem cells and differentiated progeny of host conditioning with total lymphoid irradiation and regulatory T cells. *Cell Reports, 10,* 1793–1802. https://doi.org/10.1016/j.celrep.2015.02.050

Rimner, A., Lovie, S., Hsu, M., Chelius, M., Zhang, Z., Chau, K., ... Yahalom, J. (2017). Accelerated total lymphoid irradiation-containing salvage regimen for patients with refractory and relapsed Hodgkin lymphoma: 20 years of experience. *International Journal of Radiation Oncology, Biology, Physics, 97,* 1066–1076. https://doi.org/10.1016/j.ijrobp.2017.01.222

Sert, F., Kamer, S., Saydam, G., & Anacak, Y. (2018). Role of consolidative radiation therapy for patients with mediastinal diffuse large B-cell lymphoma in the rituximab era. *Journal of Cancer Research and Therapeutics, 14,* 1397–1402. https://doi.org/10.4103/jcrt.JCRT_3_17

Shelton, B.K. (2016). Myelosuppression and second malignancies. In B.H. Gobel, S. Triest-Robertson, & W.H. Vogel (Eds.), *Advanced oncology nursing certification review and resource manual* (2nd ed., pp. 451–490). Oncology Nursing Society.

Sprangers, B., Pirenne, J., Mathieu, C., & Waer, M. (2019). Other forms of immunosuppression. In S.J. Knechtle, L. Marson, & P. Morris (Eds.), *Kidney transplantation: Principles and practice* (8th ed., pp. 313–332). Elsevier.

Stein, A., Palmer, J., Tsai, N.-C., Al Malki, M.M., Aldoss, I., Ali, H., ... Wong, J. (2017). Phase I trial of total marrow and lymphoid irradiation transplantation conditioning in patients with relapsed/refractory acute leukemia. *Biology of Blood and Marrow Transplant, 23,* 618–624. https://doi.org/10.1016/j.bbmt.2017.01.067

Terezakis, S.A., Hudson, M.M., & Constine, L.S. (2011). Hodgkin lymphoma. In E.C. Halperin, L.S. Constine, N.J. Tarbell, & L.E. Kun (Eds.), *Pediatric radiation oncology* (5th ed., pp. 137–165). Wolters Kluwer.

Terezakis, S.A., Metzger, M., & Constine, L.S. (2016). Hodgkin lymphoma. In L.S. Constine, N.J. Tarbell, & E.C. Halperin (Eds.), *Pediatric radiation oncology* (6th ed., pp. 145–174). Wolters Kluwer.

Veltri, L., Regier, M., Cumpston, A., Leadmon, S., Tse, W., Craig, M., & Hamadani, M. (2013). Incidence and pattern of graft-versus-host disease in patients undergoing allogeneic transplantation after nonmyeloablative conditioning with total lymphoid irradiation and antithymocyte globulin. *Bone Marrow Research, 2013,* 414959. https://doi.org/10.1155/2013/414959

G. Proton beam therapy

1. Overview
   a) History
      (1) Robert R. Wilson first proposed the use of protons for the treatment of cancer in 1946 (Hall, 2009).
      (2) A small number of patients were the first treated with protons in 1954 at Lawrence Berkeley National Laboratory in California (Hall, 2009).
      (3) Fractionated proton treatment for patients began at the Harvard Cyclotron Laboratory in 1970 in collaboration with physicians at Massachusetts General Hospital (Hall, 2009).
      (4) The first hospital-based proton beam therapy facility was opened in 1990 at Loma Linda University Medical Center (Smith, 2009).
   b) Protons
      (1) Protons are positively charged particles and are produced by particle accelerators.
      (2) They differ from x-rays, which are waves of energy.
      (3) In a treatment setting, protons are accelerated to therapeutic energies of 70–250 MeV with a cyclotron or a synchrotron. They are then transported to the treatment room where they enter the treatment head mounted on a rotating gantry (Mohan & Grosshans, 2017).
   c) Precision RT
      (1) Proton beam therapy is a type of precision RT.
      (2) Precision RT accurately delivers the dose to a tumor and confers little or no radiation to the surrounding healthy tissue and organs, resulting in maximum tumor control and decreasing the toxicity to the utmost extent.
2. Proton beam therapy principles
   a) The initial thin beams of protons are spread laterally and longitudinally and shaped appropriately to deliver treatments.
   b) Spreading and shaping can be achieved by electromechanical means (passively scattered proton beam therapy) or by magnetic scanning of proton beamlets (pencil beam scanning).
   c) Pencil beam scanning can be used to treat with optimized intensity-modulated proton beam therapy, the most precise proton beam therapy modality (Mohan & Grosshans, 2017).
   d) Proton beam therapy provides superior dose distributions and has a dosimetric advantage over photon beam therapy (Hu, Jiang, Cui, Zhang, & Yu, 2018).

e) When compared to photons, protons penetrate matter and decelerate continuously as a function of depth. The rate of their energy loss, or LET, increases with decreasing velocity.

    (1) Protons come to an abrupt stop when their energy is depleted, thus depositing nearly all their energy in one location.

    (2) This process of dose deposition produces a characteristic depth-dose curve (Bragg curve) for a broad beam of protons (Mohan & Grosshans, 2017).

    (3) The point of highest dose is known as the *Bragg peak* (Mohan & Grosshans, 2017).

        (a) The tissue depth where the peak occurs (i.e., range of protons) is a function of the initial energy.

        (b) Dose deposited beyond the range is negligible.

        (c) As protons traverse a medium, they also scatter laterally, but the dose outside the beam boundary falls rapidly.

f) Initially, the clinical practice and study of proton beam therapy focused on ocular tumors, skull base tumors, paraspinal tumors (chondrosarcoma and chordoma), and unresectable sarcomas, which responded poorly when treated with photon RT.

g) Proton beam therapy is now widely regarded as an ideal modality for reirradiation and pediatric cancers because it has fewer unwanted side effects as a result of lower radiation dose to healthy tissue (Hu et al., 2018).

h) During the past decade, the application of proton beam therapy has been rapidly increasing worldwide and gradually expanding for the treatment of various malignancies.

i) To date, the role of proton beam therapy in clinical settings is still controversial, and considerable challenges still exist in its application (Hu et al., 2018; Mohan & Grosshans, 2017).

j) Advantages of proton beam therapy related to precision allow it to be utilized for treatment of tumors close to critical organs, such as the eye and spinal cord.

k) Other advantages of proton beam therapy include the following (DeLaney, 2008; Durante & Loeffler, 2010; Harada et al., 2016; Mohan & Grosshans, 2017).

    (1) More accurate targeting of tumors

    (2) No exit dose

    (3) Maximum therapeutic gain

    (4) Minimal exposure to surrounding tissue

    (5) Potential to improve local control and decrease acute and long-term toxicity

    (6) Greater safety and effectiveness with combined modality therapy

3. Biologic effectiveness of protons

    a) Experimental data show clear trends in relative biologic effectiveness as a function of physical and biologic parameters (Paganetti, 2018).

    b) Other than assuming a 10% difference in required prescription doses and dose constraints, the biologic difference between proton and photon therapy is not considered quantitatively in treatment planning.

    c) Treatment planning based on variable relative biologic effectiveness values is not done clinically because of significant uncertainties, particularly for healthy tissues (Paganetti, 2018).

4. Indications

    a) Ocular tumors (uveal melanomas)

        (1) In a review of patients with ocular melanoma treated conservatively with proton beam therapy, Lane, Kim, and Gragoudas (2015) found that the cumulative melanoma-related mortality rates continued to increase up to 23 years after treatment.

        (2) Annual rates of melanoma-related death decreased considerably to less than 1% at 14 years following treatment (Lane et al., 2015).

    b) Skull base and spinal sarcomas: In a series of 77 patients, at eight years, the local control rate was 89.7%, and overall survival was 93.5% (Weber et al., 2016).

    c) Head and neck cancers

        (1) Proton beam therapy can be used to treat head and neck tumors (e.g., paranasal sinus, nasal, nasopharynx) because of their irregular configuration and proximity to critical and dose-limiting structures.

        (2) Proton beam therapy has been shown to reduce rates of feeding tube dependency in patients with head and neck cancer, when compared to conventional radiation (IMRT) (Blanchard et al., 2016).

        (3) A review of 54 patients with stage III and IV squamous cell carcinoma of the nasal cavity found that two-year and five-year actuarial local control rates were both 80%. Overall survival was 67% at two years and 47% at five years (Russo et al., 2016).

    d) Prostate cancer

        (1) For early-stage prostate cancer, protons may offer tissue-sparing advantages for the rectum and bladder and reduce treatment-related morbidities.

        (2) Takagi et al. (2017) reported on a large cohort of patients with localized prostate cancer treated with proton beam therapy, with the longest follow-up to date.

            (a) The results showed that biochemical control with proton beam therapy is favorable, particularly for high- and very high–risk

patients, with lower incidences of late genitourinary toxicity.

    (b) The study highlights the necessity of considering patient age in the treatment protocols.

   e) CNS tumors (benign and malignant)

    (1) The following CNS conditions can be treated with proton beam therapy (Shih, Chapman, Bussière, Chen, & Loeffler, 2008).

      (a) Unresectable acoustic neuromas

      (b) Unresectable or irregularly shaped meningiomas

      (c) Pituitary adenomas with treatment volumes greater than 2–3 cm or hormonally active tumors more than 5 mm from the optic chiasm

      (d) Unresectable AVMs

    (2) In a study of 20 patients with grade 2 glioma treated with proton beam therapy, Shih et al. (2015) reported the following results.

      (a) At baseline, intellectual functioning was within the normal range for the group and remained stable over time.

      (b) Visuospatial ability, attention and working memory, and executive functioning were within normal limits; however, eight patients showed baseline neurocognitive impairments in language, memory, and processing speed.

      (c) The study reported no overall decline in cognitive functioning over time.

   f) Bone and soft tissue sarcomas (DeLaney & Kirsch, 2008)

    (1) Ewing sarcoma

    (2) Retroperitoneal, pelvic, and extremity sarcomas

   g) Lung cancer

    (1) Clinical trials with dose escalation using protons for localized NSCLC are ongoing (Harada et al., 2016).

    (2) In a small study of nine patients with inoperable NSCLC, Harada et al. (2016) determined that 66 Gy (relative biologic effectiveness) is a safe dose of proton beam therapy to administer combined with chemotherapy.

   h) Breast cancer: Emerging data have shown that proton beam therapy decreases mean heart dose (Fagundes et al., 2013).

   i) Liver cancer

    (1) Proton beam therapy can significantly decrease dose to healthy liver tissue. Most of the healthy liver can be completely spared from radiation, which allows for dose escalation.

    (2) Hong et al. (2016) conducted a phase 2 multicenter clinical trial of high-dose hypofractionated proton beam therapy for localized inoperable liver cancer.

      (a) The study reported on 83 patients with hepatocellular carcinoma or intrahepatic cholangiocarcinoma.

      (b) The rates of local control at two years were 94.8% for hepatocellular carcinoma and 94.1% for intrahepatic cholangiocarcinoma.

      (c) The overall survival rates at two years were 63.2% for hepatocellular carcinoma and 46.5% for intrahepatic cholangiocarcinoma.

      (d) The most common toxicities were fatigue, rash, nausea, and anorexia.

   j) Reirradiation

    (1) Reirradiation may provide the best chance of long-term disease control and a potential cure for the patients who experience local or regional recurrence without developing distant metastasis.

    (2) The physical characteristics of proton beam therapy are particularly suited for reirradiation of head and neck, liver, and thoracic cancers (Hu et al., 2018).

   k) Pediatric cancer

    (1) In the pediatric setting, many patients require RT either for local control or to increase overall survival (Doyle-Lindrud, 2015).

    (2) Proton beam therapy offers a method to deliver a highly conformal radiation dose to a tumor while sparing sensitive, growing healthy tissue.

    (3) Proton beam therapy may significantly reduce treatment-related acute side effects related to tumor location and volume of healthy tissue in the treatment field, as well as long-term morbidities (e.g., growth disturbance, neurocognitive and neuroendocrine dysfunction, hearing loss, second malignancies) (Yock, DeLaney, Esty, & Tarbell, 2008; Yock et al., 2016).

5. Treatment setup and planning

   a) Simulation is performed in the treatment position (i.e., prone, supine, or seated) (Gottschalk, 2008).

    (1) An immobilization device is made to minimize patient motion during treatment, ensure accurate and precise daily treatment setup, and assist the patient in maintaining position.

      (a) The thickness of the device must be kept to a minimum to account for depth of the Bragg peak.

      (b) Examples include thermoplastic face masks, bite blocks, head holders, vacuum-shaped bags, and body molds.

    (2) A treatment planning CT scan is performed. Contrast may be used to help delineate normal structures or tumor volume.

    (3) CT scan data are transferred to a treatment planning system. Tumor and healthy tissue vol-

umes are contoured, or drawn, on serial CT sections throughout the treatment volume using information from clinical reports and imaging studies (CT and MRI) to accurately define the target and critical dose-limiting structures.

b) Beam application systems are used to shape and customize the beam to the target volume and minimize dose to defined healthy tissues (Gottschalk, 2008).

   (1) Passive beam shaping, most commonly used in proton beam therapy, uses a beam modulator to produce a depth-dose profile (Gottschalk, 2008).

   (2) The modulated Bragg peak, or spread-out Bragg peak, must cover the whole target homogeneously and match the distal end of the target volume. Patient-specific hardware is necessary (Mohan & Grosshans, 2017).

      (a) An aperture device customized for each treatment portal shapes the beam and eliminates protons outside the designed volume area.

      (b) A compensator accounts for differences in tissue depths within the field and the curvature of a patient's body surface. It is designed such that the distal end of the spread-out Bragg peak matches the end of the target volume.

   (3) Active beam shaping produces focused thin beams (pencil beams), allowing for three-dimensional scanning over the target field.

      (a) The dose depth for the spread-out Bragg peak is set along each pencil beam to achieve the full dose confined to the target (Gottschalk, 2008; Mohan & Grosshans, 2017).

      (b) Dose distributions can be conformed to irregular shapes without the use of patient-specific hardware, and treatment delivery is automatic via computer-controlled systems (Gottschalk, 2008; Mohan & Grosshans, 2017).

6. Treatment (Shih et al., 2008)

a) The patient is positioned using the same immobilization device used for the treatment planning CT or MRI.

b) Radiographic verification of patient position and treatment fields is obtained.

c) Treatment time varies according to the number of treatment fields and complexity of the setup.

d) Treatments are given daily (fractionated) Monday through Friday; however, single high-dose treatment is used for benign lesions (AVMs and pituitary adenomas 5 mm or more from optic nerves and chiasm).

7. Collaborative management

a) Side effects: Site-specific side effects (acute and late) are determined by the area treated and may be reduced as a result of highly conformal dose distributions and lack of exit dose, thus minimizing the dose to normal tissues (Hong et al., 2016; Shih et al., 2015; Yock et al., 2008; Yock et al., 2016).

b) Second malignancies: Proton beam therapy may reduce the risk of second malignancies, compared to photon treatment. This is especially important in pediatric patients (Durante & Loeffler, 2010; Yock et al., 2008).

c) Interprofessional collaboration

   (1) Other treatment modalities (photon radiation, chemotherapy, and surgery) may be indicated depending on the disease, stage of the disease, treatment regimen, or clinical trial. Coordination of care, patient assessment, and symptom management are essential.

   (2) Sedation is necessary for daily treatment of young children to ensure precise treatment setup and maintenance of position. Coordination and timing of these treatments are essential (see IX.B. Pediatric radiation oncology).

   (3) Patients should be referred to support services, such as nutrition services, social services, patient navigation, financial services, and chaplain, as needed.

      (a) In the United States, 15 proton beam therapy centers are operating; an estimated 70 centers are operating worldwide. Patients and families often need to travel and stay far from their home (Hu et al., 2018; Mohan & Grosshans, 2017).

      (b) Support services are especially important to ease the impact of social, emotional, and financial issues that can occur with treatment, in addition to treatment side effects.

8. Patient, caregiver, and family education

a) Nurses should teach patients, caregivers, and family members about all aspects of proton beam therapy.

b) Nurses should explain the difference between proton and photon radiation and how proton beam therapy works.

c) Nurses should provide information on the immobilization device and the importance of patient positioning and compliance.

d) Nurses should describe simulation and daily treatment. Patients should understand the treatment schedule and any special instructions necessary for daily treatment.

e) Nurses should discuss possible side effects and symptom management strategies.

f) Patients and caregivers should have information on communication with the treatment team (e.g., weekly status checks, contact information).

g) Nurses should provide information in various formats depending on patient preference and availability (e.g., written, audiovisual, verbal).

h) Nurses should confirm understanding by patients and caregivers and document this in health records.

9. Related websites

   a) Particle Therapy Co-Operative Group: www.ptcog.ch

   b) RTOG: www.rtog.org

References

Blanchard, P., Garden, A.S., Gunn, G.B., Rosenthal, D.I., Morrison, W.H., Hernandez, M., ... Frank, S.J. (2016). Intensity-modulated proton beam therapy (IMPT) versus intensity-modulated photon therapy (IMRT) for patients with oropharynx cancer—A case matched analysis. *Radiotherapy and Oncology, 120*, 48–55. https://doi.org/10.1016/j.radonc.2016.05.022

DeLaney, T.F. (2008). Clinical issues in proton radiotherapy. In T.F. DeLaney & H.M. Kooy (Eds.), *Proton and charged particle radiotherapy* (pp. 108–114). Lippincott Williams and Wilkins.

DeLaney, T.F., & Kirsch, D.G. (2008). Bone and soft tissue. In T.F. DeLaney & H.M. Kooy (Eds.), *Proton and charged particle radiotherapy* (pp. 172–185). Lippincott Williams and Wilkins.

Doyle-Lindrud, S. (2015). Proton beam therapy for pediatric malignancies. *Clinical Journal of Oncology Nursing, 19*, 521–523. https://doi.org/10.1188/15.CJON.521-523

Durante, M., & Loeffler, J.S. (2010). Charged particles in radiation oncology. *Nature Reviews Clinical Oncology, 7*, 37–43. https://doi.org/10.1038/nrclinonc.2009.183

Fagundes, M.A., Pankuch, M., Hartsell, W., Ward, C., Fang, L.C., Cahlon, O., ... Hug, E. (2013). Cardiac-sparing postmastectomy proton radiation therapy for women with stage III, loco-regional, breast cancer: A dosimetric comparison study. *International Journal of Radiation Oncology, Biology, Physics, 87*(Suppl.), S245. https://doi.org/10.1016/j.ijrobp.2013.06.637

Gottschalk, B. (2008). Treatment delivery systems: Passive beam scattering. In T.F. DeLaney & H.M. Kooy (Eds.), *Proton and charged particle radiotherapy* (pp. 33–39). Lippincott Williams and Wilkins.

Hall, E. (2009). Protons for radiotherapy: A 1946 proposal. *Lancet Oncology, 10*, 196. https://doi.org/10.1016/S1470-2045(09)70022-1

Harada, H., Fuji, H., Ono, A., Kenmotsu, H., Naito, T., Yamashita, H., ... Murayama, S. (2016). Dose escalation study of proton beam therapy with concurrent chemotherapy for stage III non-small cell lung cancer. *Cancer Science, 107*, 1018–1021. https://doi.org/10.1111/cas.12955

Hong, T.S., Wo, J.Y., Yeap, B.Y., Ben-Josef, E., McDonnell, E.I., Blaszkowsky, L.S., ... Zhu, A.X. (2016). Multi-institutional phase II study of high-dose hypofractionated proton beam therapy in patients with localized, unresectable hepatocellular carcinoma and intrahepatic cholangiocarcinoma. *Journal of Clinical Oncology, 34*, 460–468. https://doi.org/10.1200/JCO.2015.64.2710

Hu, M., Jiang, L., Cui, X., Zhang, J., & Yu, J. (2018). Proton beam therapy for cancer in the era of precision medicine. *Journal of Hematology and Oncology, 11*, 136. https://doi.org/10.1186/s13045-018-0683-4

Lane, A.M., Kim, I.K., & Gragoudas, E.S. (2015). Long-term risk of melanoma-related mortality for patients with uveal melanoma treated with proton beam therapy. *JAMA Ophthalmology, 133*, 792–796. https://doi.org/10.1001/jamaophthalmol.2015.0887

Mohan, R., & Grosshans, D. (2017). Proton therapy—Present and future. *Advanced Drug Delivery Review, 109*, 26–44. https://doi.org/10.1016/j.addr.2016.11.006

Paganetti, H. (2018). Proton relative biological effectiveness—Uncertainties and opportunities. *International Journal of Particle Therapy, 5*, 2–14. https://doi.org/10.14338/IJPT-18-00011.1

Russo, A.L., Adams, J.A., Weyman, E.A., Busse, P.M., Goldberg, S.I., Varvares, M., ... Chan, A.W. (2016). Long-term outcomes after proton beam therapy for sinonasal squamous cell carcinoma. *International Journal of Radiation Oncology, Biology, Physics, 95*, 368–376. https://doi.org/10.1016/j.ijrobp.2016.02.042

Shih, H.A., Chapman, P.H., Bussière, M.R., Chen, C.C., & Loeffler, J.S. (2008). Central nervous system. In T.F. DeLaney & H.M. Kooy (Eds.), *Proton and charged particle radiotherapy* (pp. 140–150). Lippincott Williams and Wilkins.

Shih, H.A., Sherman, J.C., Nachtigall, L.B., Colvin, M.K., Fullerton, B.C., Daartz, J., ... Yeap, B.Y. (2015). Proton therapy for low-grade gliomas: Results from a prospective trial. *Cancer, 121*, 1712–1719. https://doi.org/10.1002/cncr.29237

Smith, A.R. (2009). Vision 20/20: Proton therapy. *Medical Physics, 36*, 556–568. https://www.doi.org/10.1118/1.3058485

Takagi, M., Demizu, Y., Terashima, K., Fujii, O., Jin, D., Niwa, Y., ... Okimoto, T. (2017). Long-term outcomes in patients treated with proton therapy for localized prostate cancer. *Cancer Medicine, 6*, 2234–2243. https://doi.org/10.1002/cam4.1159

Weber, D.C., Badiyan, S., Malyapa, R., Albertini, F., Bolsi, A., Lomax, A.J, & Schneider, R. (2016). Long-term outcomes and prognostic factors of skull-base chondrosarcoma patients treated with pencil-beam scanning proton therapy at the Paul Scherrer Institute. *Neuro-Oncology, 18*, 236–243. https://doi.org/10.1093/neuonc/nov154

Yock, T.I., DeLaney, T.F., Esty, B., & Tarbell, N.J. (2008). Pediatric tumors. In T.F. DeLaney & H.M. Kooy (Eds.), *Proton and charged particle radiotherapy* (pp. 125–139). Lippincott Williams and Wilkins.

Yock, T.I., Yeap, B.Y., Ebb, D.H., Weyman, E., Eaton, B.R., & Tarbell, N.J. (2016). Long-term toxic effects of proton radiotherapy for paediatric medulloblastoma: A phase 2 single-arm study. *Lancet Oncology, 17*, 287–298. https://doi.org/10.1016/S1470-2045(15)00167-9

H. Cobalt therapy

1. Background

   a) Cobalt (Alfred & Leaver, 2016; Beyzadeoglu, Ozyigit, & Ebruli, 2010)

      (1) Cobalt is a tough, bluish-gray, stable metal.

      (2) In nonradioactive form, it can be found mixed with various natural minerals.

   b) Cobalt-60 (Alfred & Leaver, 2016)

      (1) Cobalt-60 is an unstable radioactive isotope discovered in 1930.

      (2) Cobalt-60 is commercially generated in nuclear reactors.

      (3) It produces gamma radiation through constant decay.

      (4) Cobalt-60 sources emit gamma radiation with energies of 1.17 MeV and 1.33 MeV, with an average energy of 1.25 MeV.

      (5) Machines operate at a source-to-skin distance of 80–100 cm.

      (6) Emission output decreases over time.

      (7) Cobalt-60 has a half-life of 5.26 years.

2. Cobalt-60 EBRT

   a) History of cobalt-60 EBRT units (Alfred & Leaver, 2016; Langhans et al., 2015)

      (1) The megavoltage machine was developed after World War II.

      (2) The cobalt teletherapy unit was introduced in Canada in 1951.

      (3) The original RT units could deliver a significant dose below the surface of the skin, saving the skin from the severe effects of earlier treatment forms.

(4) RT delivered via a cobalt-60 source was the most commonly used modality between 1950 and 1970.
b) External beam characteristics (Beyzadeoglu et al., 2010; Eatmon, 2016)
  (1) The radiation dose is lower than that of a linear accelerator.
  (2) Depth of penetration is less than 10 cm.
  (3) Maximum dose builds up below the skin surface (0.5 cm).
  (4) The penumbra area at the edge of the beam receives a lower dose.
  (5) Treatment time increases over time as the dose decays.
  (6) The beam source always emits radiation and requires compliance to RT safety standards for shielding.
c) Current landscape (Alfred & Leaver, 2016; Beyzadeoglu et al., 2010)
  (1) A cobalt-60 machine is mechanically simple.
  (2) Machines are highly reliable because of dependence on a radioactive isotope.
  (3) The cobalt-60 source must be replaced every five to six years.
  (4) Machines with a cobalt source constantly emit radiation, even when in the "off" position, requiring shielding of the source.
  (5) Currently, cobalt-60 machines are being replaced with newer technology.
  (6) Very few manufacturers now produce cobalt-60 RT units.
  (7) For countries that currently use cobalt-60 sources, the International Atomic Energy Agency and the World Health Organization can support source replacement, transportation, and installation if such expertise and support is needed (Page et al., 2014).
3. Cobalt-60 brachytherapy (Hajdok & Surry, 2013)
a) History of cobalt-60 HDR brachytherapy (Nandwana et al., 2015; Strohmaier & Zwierzchowski, 2011)
  (1) In the past, cobalt-60 and iridium-192 were commonly used as radioactive sources for brachytherapy.
  (2) Cobalt-60 was used in the form of pellets.
  (3) Iridium-192 began to replace cobalt-60, with the introduction of remote afterloading systems.
  (4) Cobalt-60 sources are now available in the same form as the current minute iridium-192 sources.
  (5) Cobalt-60 sources are widely used in Asian, German, and Japanese brachytherapy units.
b) Application of cobalt-60 for HDR brachytherapy
  (1) Higher levels of room shielding are required because gamma radiation is more penetrating.

(2) Because the half-life of cobalt-60 is much longer than that of iridium-192, source exchange takes place every five to six years, compared to 74 days for iridium-192. This results in 25 iridium source exchanges for every cobalt source exchange.
(3) The availability of afterloading equipment for cobalt-60 is limited.
(4) Cobalt-60 and iridium-192 have identical dose distribution.
(5) Cobalt-60 is an alternative to consider in centers with a high workload.
(6) Consideration should be given to the use of cobalt-60 for HDR brachytherapy in low-resource settings.
c) Indications for cobalt-60 brachytherapy (see also VIII.B. Low-dose-rate and high-dose-rate brachytherapy)
  (1) In the past, ocular melanoma was treated with cobalt-60 eye plaques, but now iodine-125 is more common (Echegaray, Bechrakis, Singh, Bellerive, & Singh, 2017).
  (2) Cancers of the prostate, cervix, endometrium, breast, skin, bronchus, esophagus, and head and neck, among others, can be treated with cobalt-60 brachytherapy. Cobalt is used in some centers, but other centers also use iridium, cesium, and radium (Manir et al., 2018; Strohmaier & Zwierzchowski, 2011).
4. SRS (see also VIII.C. Stereotactic radiosurgery)
a) SRS can be used to treat deep-seated tumors in the brain and benign conditions, such as AVM (Bruce & Quinn, 2007).
b) Gamma Knife, an SRS system, emits beams from cobalt-60 sources.
5. Global application
a) As of 2014, according to the Directory of Radiotherapy Centres, 2,348 cobalt RT machines are being used around the world, compared to 11,046 linear accelerators (Langhans et al., 2015).
b) Cobalt-60 RT units are widely used in Eastern Europe and in many low- and middle-income countries (Page et al., 2014; Roser, Ritchie, & Oritz-Ospina, 2019).
c) For the delivery of HDR brachytherapy, cobalt-60 can be considered as an alternative to iridium-192 for low- and middle-income countries planning RT services (Strohmaier & Zwierzchowski, 2011).
d) Cancer cases are expected to rise significantly in low- and middle-income countries, which house more than 80% of the global population and where 80% of patients currently present with advanced disease (World Health Organization, 2018).
e) Cobalt-60 RT units provide important treatment access to those who may otherwise not have access to RT.

f) In comparing cobalt-60 RT units and linear accelerators, cobalt-60 units have distinct advantages for global application (Langhans et al. 2015; Page et al., 2014).

  (1) Linear accelerators and cobalt-60 IMRT machines are cost equivalent, but linear accelerators have higher maintenance costs.

  (2) A cobalt-60 source must be replaced every five to six years. Linear accelerators require frequent quality assurance checks. The average cost to maintain a linear accelerator is $41,000, compared to $6,000 for a cobalt-60 machine (Page et al., 2014).

  (3) Linear accelerators require more highly trained staff than cobalt-60 units.

  (4) Low- and middle-income countries may be limited in their ability to provide uninterrupted power, which is important in the operation of a linear accelerator.

  (5) Cobalt-60 machines are easier to repair and are more durable.

  (6) Methods utilizing multileaf collimators and the development of tomotherapy techniques have resulted in the ability to produce flattened isodose curves for cobalt-60 machines, making them a very attractive option to deliver high-quality RT with a low-cost machine.

g) Ethical considerations (Page et al., 2014)

  (1) Cobalt-60 RT units were the most commonly used RT modality between 1950 and 1970, and millions of individuals were treated.

  (2) Currently, millions of individuals around the world do not have access to RT for treatment or palliation.

  (3) Access to treatment with a cobalt-60 RT unit could be potentially lifesaving and improve their quality of life.

  (4) Cancer centers working toward developing RT services can consider the use of cobalt-60 RT units to meet the needs of individuals who may not otherwise have treatment access.

References

Alfred, L., & Leaver, D. (2016). Treatment delivery equipment. In C.M. Washington & D. Leaver (Eds.), *Principles and practice of radiation therapy* (4th ed., pp. 132–155). Elsevier Mosby.

Beyzadeoglu, M., Ozyigit, G., & Ebruli, C. (2010). *Basic radiation oncology.* Springer.

Bruce, S.D., & Quinn, A.M. (2007). Stereotactic irradiation. In M.L. Haas, W.P. Hogle, G.J. Moore-Higgs, & T.K. Gosselin-Acomb (Eds.), *Radiation therapy: A guide to patient care* (pp. 415–430). Elsevier Mosby.

Eatmon, S. (2016). Cancer: An overview. In C.M. Washington & D. Leaver (Eds.), *Principles and practice of radiation therapy* (4th ed., pp. 1–19). Elsevier Mosby.

Echegaray, J.J., Bechrakis, N.E., Singh, N., Bellerive, C., Singh, A.D. (2017). Iodine-125 brachytherapy for uveal melanoma: A systematic review of radiation dose. *Ocular Oncology and Pathology, 3,* 193–198. https://doi.org/10.1159/000455872

Hajdok, G., & Surry, K.J.M. (2013). Image-guided brachytherapy. In J. Van Dyk (Ed.), *The modern technology of radiation oncology: A compendium for medical physicists and radiation oncologists* (Vol. 3, pp. 223–244). Medical Physics Publishing.

Langhans, M., Eshner, G., Runz, A., Baumann, M., Xu, M., Ueltzhöffer, S., ... Schlegel, W. (2015). Development, physical properties and clinical applicability of a mechanical multileaf collimator for the use in cobalt-60 radiotherapy. *Physics in Medicine and Biology, 60,* 3375–3387. https://doi.org/10.1088/0031-9155/60/8/3375

Manir, K.S., Basu, A., Choudhury, K.B., Basu, S., Ghosh, K., & Gangopadhyay, S. (2018). Interstitial brachytherapy in soft tissue sarcoma: A 5 years institutional experience with cobalt 60–based high-dose-rate brachytherapy system. *Journal of Contemporary Brachytherapy, 10,* 431–438. https://doi.org/10.5114/jcb.2018.78994

Nandwana, U., Rathore, N., Gupta, S., Shukla, A., Kumar, S., Intodia, K., ... Jain, A. (2015). Cobalt-60 is a logical, economical and comparable alternative to Ir-192: Analysis and institutional experience from western India. *Southern African Journal of Gynaecological Oncology, 7,* 60–63. https://doi.org/10.1080/20742835.2015.1083720

Page, B.R., Hudson, A.D., Brown, D.W., Shulman, A.C., Abdel-Wahab, M., Fisher, B.J., & Patel, S. (2014). Cobalt, linac, or other: What is the best solution for radiation therapy in developing countries? *International Journal of Radiation Oncology, Biology, Physics, 89,* 476–480. https://doi.org/10.1016/j.ijrobp.2013.12.022

Roser, M., Ritchie, H., & Oritz-Ospina, E. (2019). World population growth. https://ourworldindata.org/world-population-growth

Strohmaier, S., & Zwierzchowski, G. (2011). Comparison of 60Co and 192Ir sources in HDR brachytherapy. *Journal of Contemporary Brachytherapy, 3.* 199–208. https://doi.org/10.5114/jcb.2011.26471

World Health Organization. (2018). Cancer. https://www.who.int/en/news-room/fact-sheets/detail/cancer

IX. Special Populations

A. Pediatric radiation oncology

1. Incidence
   - a) In the United States in 2020, approximately 11,050 children younger than 15 years old were diagnosed with cancer (American Cancer Society, 2020).
   - b) Cancer is the leading cause of death from disease in children younger than 15 years old and is surpassed only by accidents in all causes of death in children. It was projected that approximately 1,190 children would die from cancer in 2020 (American Cancer Society, 2020).

2. Specific differences between pediatric and adult cancers
   - a) Childhood cancer is not one disease entity but a spectrum of different malignancies (American Cancer Society, 2019a).
     - (1) Pediatric cancers vary by type of histology and site of disease origin; patients vary by race, sex, and age.
     - (2) Common cancers seen in children are leukemias, brain and other CNS tumors, bone cancers, lymphomas, soft tissue sarcomas, renal cancers, and eye tumors.
     - (3) In contrast, the common cancers in adults are skin, prostate, breast, lung, and colorectal.
   - b) Childhood cancers tend to respond better to treatment with chemotherapy and RT, and children tend to tolerate treatment better than adults.
     - (1) Multimodal treatment has become the standard of care, and a significant proportion of children with cancer will receive RT as part of their clinical course.
     - (2) Patients will require follow-up for the rest of their lives, and many will need medical interventions for the long-term side effects of RT and chemotherapy.
   - c) Most children with cancer are referred to a specialized children's cancer center.
     - (1) These centers often are members of the Children's Oncology Group and associated with a university or a children's hospital.
     - (2) Treatment is coordinated by a team of experts who specialize in the diagnosis and treatment of pediatric cancers (American Cancer Society, 2019b).
     - (3) Some families may need to relocate during the time of a child's treatment.
   - d) In contrast to adults with cancer, most children with cancer will be cured of their disease (Stegmaier & Sellers, 2009).

3. Patient- and family-centered care: Patient- and family-centered care is commonly practiced in pediatric oncology settings and based on the following principles (American Academy of Pediatrics, 2012).
   - a) The child's main source of support and strength is family.
   - b) Clinical decision-making requires an understanding of the perspectives and information provided by the parents and the child or young adult.
   - c) Consideration must be given to the psychosocial and cultural needs of the family and the child throughout the course of the disease.
   - d) The goal is to help the parents develop confidence in their ability to care for their child throughout the course of the illness.

4. RT planning and treatment
   - a) Goals
     - (1) The ideal goal of RT is to increase disease-free survival while limiting normal tissue morbidity.
     - (2) If achieving disease-free survival is not possible, then the attempt is to offer a better quality of life (Stackhouse, 2013).
     - (3) RT can also palliate troublesome symptoms.
   - b) Patient evaluation: Evaluation for treatment eligibility begins at a tumor board meeting. The data reviewed includes the following (Marcus & Haas-Kogan, 2009).
     - (1) Goal of therapy: cure or palliation
     - (2) Pertinent tumor characteristics: size, location, type, and grade
     - (3) Relative volume of necrotic or poorly vascularized tissue within the treatment field, as assessed by imaging studies: tissue oxygenation and potential response of tumors to RT
     - (4) Clinical condition
     - (5) Age of the child
     - (6) Requirement of anesthesia or sedation
   - c) Target volumes: The purpose of treatment planning is to delineate target volumes and the critical anatomic structures obtained from the imaging studies (CT and MRI) in order to shape the beam to precisely match the tumor (Cotter, McBride, & Yock, 2012).
   - d) Immobilization devices
     - (1) Immobilization is necessary to achieve a more accurate radiation dose distribution at the target volume, as well as to maintain healthy tissue during RT (Yıldırım, Çelik, Bay, Pasin, & Tütüncü, 2019).
     - (2) Proper immobilization ensures the radiation is conformed directly to the shape and size of the tumor, which results in an increased radiation dose to the tumor and reduced irradiation of OARs and healthy tissues.
     - (3) The delivery of the precise treatment prescribed is possible through the use of devices such as customized masks, bite blocks, and immobilization systems or body molds. The placement of permanent skin marks or tattoos at specific locations on a child's body are also options. The following goals must be met regardless of the

device used (Cotter et al., 2012; Light & Halperin, 2011).

 (a) The child should feel comfortable and secure.

 (b) The patient setup must be reproducible.

 (c) The setup should be quick and easy.

 (d) Construction of the device should be relatively quick.

 (e) The device must not interfere with the establishment of a secure airway and monitoring devices when anesthesia is required for young children.

e) Sedation and anesthesia

 (1) The malignancies treated with RT require a specific location of the beam to spare or limit normal tissue morbidity.

 (2) Determination of the need for anesthesia often is made at the initial consultation when the child and family are seen by the anesthesiologist, the radiation oncologist, the radiation oncology nurse, social worker, child life specialist, and psychiatrist, as all play a vital role in decreasing child and family anxiety.

  (a) Several demographic, medical, child, and parental psychosocial variables are influential in making the decision.

  (b) These factors include, but are not limited to, airway management, cognitive function, fear of the environment of treatment, pain, emotional maturity, postoperative complications, and anxiety related to restraint devices (McMullen, Hanson, Bratton, & Johnstone, 2015).

   i. A behavioral program that teaches children how to cooperate with their radiation treatment without anesthesia or sedation, either through distraction or rehearsal, may be successful.

   ii. If these techniques fail to achieve the child's cooperation, anesthesia or sedation must be used (Ångström-Brännström et al., 2017).

 (3) For very young children (less than three years), anesthesia is almost always needed. Requirements for anesthesia decrease with increasing age, and typically after seven years of age, anesthesia can be omitted (Khurmi, Patel, Koushik, Daniels, & Kraus, 2018).

 (4) The following pharmaceutical and psychological measures can be employed to ensure accurate delivery of RT.

  (a) A mild sedative, such as lorazepam or diazepam, is administered one hour before treatment (Cotter et al., 2012).

  (b) Distraction therapy or behavioral rehearsal can address the separation anxiety experienced by young children. Because of the nature of RT, parents must remain outside the room, and the child is alone during treatment (Engvall et al., 2016; Woodman, 2013).

  (c) The expertise of a child life specialist is invaluable in making a child more at ease in the treatment area. With their knowledge of the various techniques of play, the child's anxiety may be reduced, and perhaps the need for sedation or anesthesia may be prevented (Scott et al., 2016).

 (5) Other deciding factors related to anesthesia and sedation include the following.

  (a) Location of malignancy: For example, retinoblastoma requires absolute immobility of the eye and prevention of disconjugate gaze during the treatment.

  (b) Length of therapy

  (c) Position required for treatment (Chalabi & Patel, 2009)

   i. Some brain tumors (e.g., medulloblastoma, germ cell tumors, CNS leukemia) require prone positioning with a flexed head for cranial and spinal irradiation.

   ii. Cranial and spinal irradiation lasts an hour, and position is difficult to maintain without anesthesia for most children younger than 11 years.

   iii. Occasionally, stabilization of the airway is required by either intubation, placement of a nasal trumpet, or laryngeal mask airway.

 (6) Anesthetic considerations

  (a) Pediatric anesthesiologists have knowledge of pediatric malignancies and appropriate anesthetic agents and can intervene in the event of complications.

  (b) Consent is obtained by the anesthesiologist at the initial consult, which will encompass all planning procedures, as well as the daily treatments.

  (c) The desired elements of pediatric anesthesia include the following (Stackhouse, 2013).

   i. Assurance of a child's immobility

   ii. Rapid onset and reliable sedation

   iii. Short duration of action

   iv. Early hospital discharge

   v. Painless administration

   vi. Assurance of patent airway despite treatment position

  (d) Anesthesia may be delivered with IV agents (e.g., ketamine, midazolam, propofol) or with inhalation agents (e.g., sevoflurane, isoflurane) (Schulman, Ferschl, Frederick, & Halperin, 2016).

    i. Propofol is the drug of choice for RT because it minimizes the rate of respiratory and cardiovascular complications in repeated RT anesthesia applications (Yıldırım et al., 2019).

    ii. Ketamine is contraindicated in children with brain tumors because it increases intracranial pressure in children with disease in the head and neck area. It causes nystagmus, which could interfere with precision of RT delivery. Recovery time is more than 20 times that of propofol.

    iii. Sevoflurane is an excellent option for children without venous access because it is delivered through inhalation. It has the advantages of quick recovery, less damage to the respiratory system, and a low distribution coefficient (Wu et al., 2019).

(e) Although adhering to fasting guidelines is important, malnutrition is a concern in the pediatric population (Brunet-Wood et al., 2016).

    i. Fasting times must balance safety with the risk of caloric deficits.

    ii. Prolonged periods of fasting can result in increased patient discomfort related to hunger and thirst, especially in younger children, as it may be difficult for them to understand the rationale behind the order.

    iii. Pediatric patients who are allowed oral intake closer to the time of anesthesia induction are likely to be better hydrated and exhibit better hemodynamic stability.

(f) Parents must be instructed on the fasting guidelines recommended by the treating institution (Williams et al., 2014).

    i. The American Society of Anesthesiologists developed evidence-based guidelines for nothing-by-mouth status prior to receiving sedation or general anesthesia for a surgical or radiologic procedure. These guidelines have been endorsed by the American Academy of Pediatrics.

    ii. These guidelines allow patients to ingest clear liquids up to two hours prior, breast milk up to four hours prior, and a regular meal up to eight hours prior to receiving sedation or anesthesia for a procedure.

(g) An RN with pediatric advanced life support certification should be available to assist the anesthesiologist, or an RN certified in CPR and airway management should be available.

(h) An emergency response policy and procedure should be in place (Schulman et al., 2016).

    i. The child must be monitored with closed-circuit television monitors clearly visible to the anesthesiologist while outside the RT room.

    ii. These monitors display electrocardiogram, pulse oximeter, blood pressure, and end-tidal carbon dioxide measurements.

    iii. All emergency equipment, including an oxygen source, suction equipment, and a pediatric code cart, must be readily available and checked daily.

(i) Continuous monitoring during the recovery period is performed until the child is fully awake and vital signs are stable.

5. Supportive care initiatives

  a) Psychosocial care of children and families

    (1) Distress

      (a) Distress is an unpleasant experience of a mental, social, spiritual, or physical quality (NCCN, 2020).

      (b) Distress can affect how an individual acts, thinks, or feels, which may make it more difficult to cope with the diagnosis of cancer, associated symptoms, or treatment.

    (2) Reaction to diagnosis

      (a) The diagnosis of cancer in a child is one of the most stressful and difficult experiences a family will ever face.

      (b) As soon as a diagnosis is known, the child's needs become the major priority, causing the family system to rapidly reorganize (Salvador, Crespo, & Barros, 2019).

      (c) Most families of a child with cancer will have the ability to successfully balance the new demands with their dynamics; however, some will struggle on a day-to-day basis.

    (3) Assessment: Clinical assessment of the child and the family should be performed at the initial visit and as clinically indicated, especially with a change in the disease state (remission, recurrence, or progression) (NCCN, 2020).

    (4) Other factors: Myriad other factors influence how patients, parents, and siblings experience the disease (Recklitis, Casey, & Zeltzer, 2009).

      (a) Status of marital relationship

      (b) Socioeconomic status

(c) Disrupted routine

(d) Fear and uncertainty

(e) Emotional state

(f) Poor relationships

(g) School performance

(h) Peer relations

(i) Self-confidence

(j) Adjustment

(5) Reaction to treatment environment

(a) How children react to the environment will have an influence on their emotions and behavior.

(b) The strongest predictor of increased anticipatory distress is the age of the child, specifically those aged two to seven years (Klosky et al., 2007).

(c) The parents' stress level has an impact on the child's stress level and behavior (Krauss & Green, 2006; Recklitis et al., 2009).

(d) Children undergoing RT frequently experience distress. Their reactions result from their fear of the unknown, the unfamiliar conditions under which the treatment will be given, the unfamiliar staff, their previous experiences with medical procedures, and the separation from their parents during the treatment (Cullen, Derrickson, & Potter, 2002; Kreitler et al., 2016).

(6) Collaborative management: The ability to help these children through their course of treatment lies in an understanding of the following.

(a) No single individual can meet all the needs of children and their families.

(b) Knowledge of the stages of child development—infancy, toddler, preschool age, school age, and adolescence—and the developmental tasks associated with each is crucial to providing the appropriate care, support, and communication to these children (Recklitis et al., 2009).

(c) Honesty can help children grow to trust that adults will not withhold information from them. Parents should be educated about the impact that withholding information has on increasing children's anxieties and fears about their illness (Recklitis et al., 2009).

(d) Children may be nonadherent at some interval during their treatment. Behavioral interventions should not be implemented until discussion with the family has occurred and they have expressed a willingness to accept and use the approach (Recklitis et al., 2009).

(7) Siblings (Fladeboe et al., 2018)

(a) The sibling relationship is affected by and affects other family dynamics and relationships within the family as a whole.

(b) Stress associated with diagnosis and treatment can affect sibling relationships because, often, one parent is the primary caregiver, while the other tends to other siblings and the home.

(c) Sibling socialization may be disrupted by long absences while the ill child receives treatment, decreasing opportunity for communication or interaction between siblings.

(d) Siblings become burdened with concern about the ill child's well-being during treatment and worry about the ill child's survival.

(e) Other feelings experienced by siblings may include isolation, loss, anger, or rivalry toward the child with cancer.

b) Nutritional status

(1) Incidence

(a) Approximately 6%–50% of pediatric patients with cancer will experience issues associated with malnutrition (Arpaci, Toruner, & Altay, 2018).

(b) Malnutrition is often seen in childhood cancers as a result of the disease itself, long-term changes in eating habits, and treatment-related factors.

(c) With so much focus being given to treating the underlying malignancy, the consequences of malnutrition (undernutrition and obesity) may be overlooked (Bhoite, 2016).

(2) Assessment

(a) Pediatric oncology nurses, along with parents, are responsible for evaluating, educating, and monitoring children at risk for nutritional problems (Arpaci et al., 2018).

(b) Nursing assessment should include a medical and surgical history, the anticipated treatments, anthropometric measurements, biochemical parameters, clinical observations, and dietary history, including the use of herbs, supplements, and other complementary and alternative therapies, use of which may require additional discussion with the radiation oncologist (Ladas et al., 2005).

(c) An RDN or RD completes the assessment and determines the nutrient requirements and relays information regarding nutritional concerns to the patient and fam-

ily at the beginning of treatment (Arpaci et al., 2018).

    (3) Intervention: The primary objectives of nutritional interventions in pediatric patients should be promotion of appropriate growth development, minimization of wasting, maintenance of body stores as close to the ideal as possible, and high quality of life (Bhoite, 2016).

    (4) RT-associated risk

      (a) Children who must fast daily for delivery of anesthesia for RT are at high risk for malnutrition.

      (b) Children could very quickly lose greater than 5% of their weight, which is the point at which nutritional interventions should be implemented (Cullen et al., 2002).

      (c) Interventions can include encouraging nutrient-dense foods and beverages, enteral tube feedings, or total parenteral nutrition.

    (5) Contributing factors: Side effects from treatment, including mouth sores, nausea and vomiting, alterations in taste, loss of appetite, diarrhea, and constipation, are all important contributing factors to malnutrition (Bhoite, 2016).

c) Radiation somnolence syndrome

    (1) Radiation somnolence syndrome is a side effect of cranial irradiation, mainly in children with leukemia receiving prophylactic cranial irradiation (Harjani, Gururajachar, & Krishnaswamy, 2016).

    (2) Symptoms include excessive sleepiness, drowsiness, fatigue, and decreased appetite that appear approximately five to six weeks after the completion of RT and may last approximately two weeks (Harjani et al., 2016).

    (3) The symptoms of this syndrome are theorized to occur because of post-RT transient demyelination (Harjani et al., 2016).

    (4) More recently, it is thought that the inflammatory response plays a primary role in development of this syndrome (Ballesteros-Zebadua, Chavarria, Celis, Paz, & Franco-Perez, 2012; Cox et al., 2015).

    (5) The most important intervention is anticipatory guidance and preparation. Failure to recognize this syndrome as a distinct RT sequela causes undue anxiety among patients and healthcare providers, and often triggers an investigation to rule out recurrence of the malignancy (Harjani et al., 2016).

d) Fatigue

    (1) NCCN defines *cancer-related fatigue* as a "distressing, persistent, subjective sense of physical, emotional, and/or cognitive tiredness or exhaustion related to cancer or cancer treatment that is not proportional to recent activity and interferes with usual functioning" (Berger et al., 2015, p. 1012).

    (2) Fatigue has been found to be one of the most distressing symptoms experienced by children receiving cancer treatment, and it is the only factor associated with poor health-related quality of life in pediatric cancer survivors (Nunes et al., 2017).

    (3) Some of the factors considered to be associated with fatigue can be divided into physical and psychosocial factors.

      (a) Tumor growth leading to competing nutrients between healthy and tumor cells

      (b) Effects from RT and chemotherapy

      (c) Inadequate nutritional intake related to nausea and vomiting from cancer therapy

      (d) Anemia

      (e) Sleep disturbances

      (f) Uncertainty about the future

      (g) Fear of death

      (h) Loss of the roles of family maintenance

e) Cerebellar mutism syndrome

    (1) Incidence and risk factors

      (a) Cerebellar mutism syndrome most frequently occurs in children after resection of a large midline cerebellar tumor (Catsman-Berrevoets, 2017).

      (b) Its incidence varies, but it has been reported to be nearly 40% (Catsman-Berrevoets, 2017).

    (2) Presentation

      (a) The syndrome typically presents 24–48 hours after resection with diminishing of speech patterns leading to mutism, emotional lability, ataxia, and hypotonia.

      (b) These symptoms may persist from weeks to months (Catsman-Berrevoets, 2017).

    (3) Sequelae

      (a) Many patients affected by cerebellar mutism syndrome will experience long-term sequelae.

      (b) Sequalae include balance difficulties, neurocognitive challenges, and speech impairments.

      (c) Functional prognosis for patients correlates with initial severity of cerebellar mutism syndrome, as well as duration of symptoms after surgery (Catsman-Berrevoets, 2017).

    (4) Prevention

      (a) It is known that surgical intervention is contributory; however, limited tumor removal is not a justifiable option unless it is known that the tumor is invading the brain stem.

(b) It is a well-supported fact that significant residual tumor is a negative prognostic indicator (Packer, MacDonald, & Vezina, 2010; Souweidane, 2010).

6. Childhood cancer survivorship
   a) Over the past 20 years, advancements in cancer treatments have increased survival rates for childhood cancer (Ljungman et al., 2014).
   b) Current overall five-year survival is 78%, compared to 28% for children diagnosed between 1966 and 1970 (Jenkins, 2013).
   c) With the high survival rate, it is important to understand the long-term and late effects of childhood cancer and treatment.
      (1) Many childhood cancer survivors are living into their second and third decades of life.
      (2) The ability to decrease the size of the RT field, thus sparing dose to healthy tissues, has provided further hopes for decreasing sequelae, which is especially crucial in children diagnosed with brain tumors (Eshelman-Kent, Gilger, & Gallagher, 2009).
   d) The healthcare team must achieve a delicate balance between effective therapy and acceptable toxicity.
      (1) A cure may be achievable at the cost of increasing morbidity.
      (2) In contrast, adhering to therapeutic regimens to minimize toxicities may increase the chance of relapse, progression, metastasis, or death (Askins & Moore, 2008).
      (3) Approximately 30% of childhood cancer survivors will develop severe, life-threatening, or disabling effects that significantly affect their health and psychosocial functioning (Jenkins, 2013). Of these complications, the most emotionally and physically devastating are second malignancies (Bhatia & Constine, 2016).
   e) The following risk factors are associated with late effects (Hutchins et al., 2019).
      (1) Age at diagnosis
      (2) Type of malignancy
      (3) Treatment modalities utilized during therapy (e.g., surgery, chemotherapy, RT, HSCT)
      (4) Presence of preexisting underlying comorbidities
   f) Long-term follow-up of pediatric cancer survivors is essential for prevention and management of treatment side effects.
      (1) The need for comprehensive, specialized follow-up care for childhood cancer survivors is growing.
      (2) Consistent follow-up with a cancer survivor clinic is an important part of a survivor's long-term health care (Cherven et al., 2014).
      (3) The Children's Oncology Group (2018) has developed a comprehensive set of guidelines to assist healthcare providers and survivors in understanding the health issues specific to the type of cancer and the treatment received.

7. Ethical considerations and clinical trials
   a) Improvements in childhood cancer survivor rates are attributed to better therapies and advances learned through clinical trials (Crane, Haase, & Hickman, 2019).
   b) Approximately 60% of pediatric patients with cancer are treated with a clinical trial protocol (Robertson et al., 2018).
   c) The decision to enroll in a clinical trial can be difficult for parents, as they can feel overwhelmed with the amount of information provided and may not fully comprehend that information.
   d) Ethical issues regarding pediatric clinical trials are more complex because of the need for parent or guardian consent and their participation in care procedures and decisions; however, ethical consideration must account for the rights of children and respect their views and wishes in relation to their developmental level and growing autonomy (Bartholdson, Lützén, Blomgren, & Pergert, 2015).
   e) The ethical considerations regarding a child's assent are difficult issues.
      (1) Questions arise regarding when it should be required and whether it is binding.
      (2) Numerous organizations, including FDA, World Health Organization, European Commission, Australian Research Council, NCI, American Academy of Pediatrics, and United Nations, have published guidance on the importance of assuring assent from pediatric patients prior to their participation in clinical trials (Lombardi et al., 2018).
      (3) Assent should be obtained from any child who is deemed mature enough to evaluate the risks and benefits of the clinical trial.
      (4) A child should understand what the clinical trial entails (goals, objectives, procedures, and risks) and any alternatives before assenting. This brings a child's maturity into question, and with that, guidance from an institutional review board is required.
      (5) The institutional review board has tremendous responsibility regarding a child's assent (Protection of Human Subjects, 2016).
         (a) An institutional review board can determine whether a child is able to provide assent, taking into consideration age, level of maturity, and psychological state.
         (b) An institutional review board may determine that assent is not a necessary condition for proceeding with the clinical trial.

(c) An institutional review board may determine that adolescents do not need parental consent if asked to participate in a low-risk study.

(d) When an institutional review board determines that a child's assent is required, it must stipulate whether and how that assent will be documented.

f) More ethical questions surface if the child or adolescent is pregnant.

g) The following principles govern the participation of children in research.

(1) Children are individuals, and their developing autonomy in decisions must be respected.

(2) A parent's wisdom in assessing what is in the best interest of a child and in guiding a child's moral development should be respected.

(3) Policies regarding assent should be amenable to the medical and psychological circumstances often seen in pediatric oncology.

h) Two questions must be asked when discussing advances in pediatric cancer therapies.

(1) What can be done next?

(2) What should be done next?

i) Good clinical trials require ethical decisions made at every level, both scientific and philosophical (Barfield & Kodish, 2009).

References

American Academy of Pediatrics. (2012). Patient- and family-centered care and the pediatrician's role. *Pediatrics, 129,* 394–404. https://doi.org/10.1542/peds.2011-3084

American Cancer Society. (2019a). Cancers that develop in children. https://www.cancer.org/cancer/cancer-in-children/types-of-childhood-cancers.html

American Cancer Society. (2019b). Treating children with cancer. https://www.cancer.org/cancer/cancer-in-children/how-are-childhood-cancers-treated.html

American Cancer Society. (2020). Key statistics for childhood cancers. https://www.cancer.org/cancer/cancer-in-children/key-statistics.html

Ångström-Brännström, C., Lindh, V., Mullaney, T., Nilsson, K., Wickart-Johansson, G., Svärd, A.M., ... Engvall, G. (2017). Parents' experiences and responses to an intervention for psychological preparation of children and families during the child's radiotherapy. *Journal of Pediatric Oncology Nursing, 35,* 132–148. https://doi.org/10.1177/1043454217741876

Arpaci, T., Toruner, E.K., & Altay, N. (2018). Assessment of nutritional problems in pediatric patients with cancer and the information needs of their parents: A parental perspective. *Asia-Pacific Journal of Oncology Nursing, 5,* 231–236. https://doi.org/10.4103/apjon.apjon_78_17

Askins, M.A., & Moore, B.D., III. (2008). Preventing neurocognitive late effects in childhood cancer survivors. *Journal of Child Neurology, 23,* 1160–1171. https://doi.org/10.1177/0883073808321065

Ballesteros-Zebadua, P., Chavarria, A., Celis, M.A., Paz, C., & Franco-Perez, J. (2012). Radiation-induced neuroinflammation and radiation somnolence syndrome. *CNS and Neurological Disorders—Drug Targets, 11,* 937–949. https://doi.org/10.2174/1871527311201070937

Barfield, R.C., & Kodish, E. (2009). Ethical considerations in pediatric oncology clinical trials. In S.H. Orkin, D.E. Fisher, A.T. Look, S.E. Lux, D. Ginsburg, & D.G. Nathan (Eds.), *Oncology of infancy and childhood* (pp. 1319–1336). Elsevier Saunders.

Bartholdson, C., Lützén, K., Blomgren, K., & Pergert, P. (2015). Experiences of ethical issues when caring for children with cancer. *Cancer Nursing, 38,* 125–132. https://doi.org/10.1097/ncc.0000000000000130

Berger, A.M., Mooney, K., Alvarez-Perez, A., Breibart, W.S., Carpenter, K.M., Cella, D., ... Smith, C. (2015). Cancer-related fatigue, version 2.2015. *Journal of the National Comprehensive Cancer Network, 13,* 1012–1039. https://doi.org/10.6004/jnccn.2015.0122

Bhatia, S., & Constine, L.S. (2016). Second primary cancers. In L.S. Constine, N.J. Tarbell, & E.C. Halperin (Eds.), *Pediatric radiation oncology* (6th ed., pp. 466–486). Wolters Kluwer Health/Lippincott Williams and Wilkins.

Bhoite, R. (2016). Importance of nutrition in pediatric oncology. *Indian Journal of Cancer, 53,* 211–212. https://doi.org/10.4103/0019-509x.197738

Brunet-Wood, K., Simons, M., Evasiuk, A., Mazurak, V., Dicken, B., Ridley, D., & Larsen, B. (2016). Surgical fasting guidelines in children: Are we putting them into practice? *Journal of Pediatric Surgery, 51,* 1298–1302. https://doi.org/10.1016/j.jpedsurg.2016.04.006

Catsman-Berrevoets, C.E. (2017). Cerebellar mutism syndrome: Cause and rehabilitation. *Current Opinion in Neurology, 30,* 133–139. https://doi.org/10.1097/wco.0000000000000426

Chalabi, J., & Patel, S. (2009). Radiation therapy in children. *International Anesthesiology Clinics, 47,* 45–53. https://doi.org/10.1097/AIA.0b013e3181a4698a

Cherven, B., Mertens, A., Meacham, L., Williamson, R., Boring, C., & Wasilewski-Masker, K. (2014). Knowledge and risk perception of late effects among childhood cancer survivors and parents before and after visiting a childhood cancer survivor clinic. *Journal of Pediatric Oncology Nursing, 31,* 339–349. https://doi.org/10.1177/1043454214532022

Children's Oncology Group. (2018). *Long-term follow-up guidelines for survivors of childhood, adolescent, and young adult cancers* [v.5.0]. http://www.survivorshipguidelines.org

Cotter, S.E., McBride, S.M., & Yock, T.I. (2012). Proton therapy for solid tumors of childhood. *Technology in Cancer Research and Treatment, 11,* 267–278. https://doi.org/10.7785/tcrt.2012.500295

Cox, M.C., Kusters, J.M., Gidding, C.E., Schieving, J.H., van Linder, E.J., Kaanders, J.H., & Janssens, G.O. (2015). Acute toxicity profile of craniospinal irradiation with intensity-modulated radiation therapy in children with medulloblastoma: A prospective analysis. *Radiation Oncology, 10,* 241. https://doi.org/10.1186/s13014-015-0547-9

Crane, S., Haase, J.E., & Hickman, S.E. (2019). Parental experiences of child participation in a phase I pediatric oncology clinical trial: "We don't have time to waste." *Qualitative Health Research, 29,* 632–644. https://doi.org/10.1177/1049732318766513

Cullen, P.M., Derrickson, J.D., & Potter, J.A. (2002). Radiation therapy. In C.R. Baggott, K.P. Kelly, D. Fochtman, & G.V. Foley (Eds.), *Nursing care of children and adolescents with cancer* (3rd ed., pp. 116–132). Saunders.

Engvall, G., Ångström-Brännström, C., Mullaney, T., Nilsson, K., Wickart-Johansson, G., Svärd, A.-M., ... Lindh, V. (2016). It is tough and tiring but it works—Children's experiences of undergoing radiotherapy. *PLOS ONE, 11,* e0153029. https://doi.org/10.1371/journal.pone.0153029

Eshelman-Kent, D., Gilger, E., & Gallagher, M. (2009). Transitioning survivors of central nervous system tumors: Challenges for patients, families, and health care providers. *Journal of Pediatric Oncology Nursing, 26,* 280–294. https://doi.org/10.1177/1043454209343209

Fladeboe, K., King, K., Kawamura, J., Gurtovenko, K., Stettler, N., Compas, B., ... Katz, L.F. (2018). Featured article: Caregiver perceptions of stress and sibling conflict during pediatric cancer treatment. *Journal of Pediatric Psychology, 43,* 588–598. https://doi.org/10.1093/jpepsy/jsy008

Harjani, R.R., Gururajachar, J.M., & Krishnaswamy, U. (2016). Comprehensive assessment of somnolence syndrome in patients undergoing radiation to the brain. *Reports of Practical Oncology and Radiotherapy, 21,* 560–566. https://doi.org/10.1016/j.rpor.2016.08.003

Hutchins, K.K., Savaşan, S., Thomas, R.L., Strathdee, L.A., Wang, Z.J., & Taub, J.W. (2019). Clinical trial enrollment is associated with improved follow-up rates among survivors of childhood cancer. *Journal of Pediatric Hematology Oncology, 41,* e18–23. https://doi.org/10.1097/mph.0000000000001169

Jenkins, A. (2013). Late effects of chemotherapy for childhood cancer. *Paediatrics and Child Health, 23,* 545–549. https://doi.org/10.1016/j.paed.2013.06.003

Khurmi, N., Patel, P., Koushik, S., Daniels, T., & Kraus, M. (2018). Anesthesia practice in pediatric radiation oncology: Mayo Clinic Arizona's experience 2014-2016. *Pediatric Drugs, 20,* 89–95. https://doi.org/10.1007/s40272-017-0259-8

Klosky, J.L., Tyc, V.L., Tong, X., Srivastava, D.K., Kronenberg, M., de Armendi, A.J., & Merchant, T.E. (2007). Predicting pediatric distress during radiation therapy procedures: The role of medical, psychosocial, and demographic factors. *Pediatrics, 119,* e1159–e1166. https://doi.org/10.1542/peds.2005-1514

Krauss, B., & Green, S.M. (2006). Procedural sedation and analgesia in children. *Lancet, 367,* 766–780. https://doi.org/10.1016/S0140-6736(06)68230-5

Kreitler, S., Ben Arush, M.W., Krivoy, E.A., Golan, H., Oren, M.Y., & Toren, A. (2016). Psychosocial aspects of radiotherapy for the child and family with cancer. In L.S. Constine, N.J. Tarbell, & E.C. Halperin (Eds.), *Pediatric radiation oncology* (6th ed., pp. 499–510). Wolters Kluwer.

Ladas, E.J., Sacks, N., Meacham, L., Henry, D., Enriquez, L., Lowry, G., ... Rogers, P. (2005). A multidisciplinary review of nutrition considerations in the pediatric oncology population: A perspective from Children's Oncology Group. *Nutrition in Clinical Practice, 20,* 377–393. https://doi.org/10.1177/0115426505020004377

Light, K.L., & Halperin, E.C. (2011). Stabilization and immobilization devices. In E.C. Halperin, L.S. Constine, N.J. Tarbell, & L.E. Kun (Eds.), *Pediatric radiation oncology* (5th ed., pp. 425–428). Lippincott Williams and Wilkins.

Ljungman, L., Cernvall, M., Grönqvist, H., Ljótsson, B., Ljungman, G., & von Essen, L. (2014). Long-term positive and negative psychological late effects for parents of childhood cancer survivors: A systematic review. *PLOS ONE, 9,* e103340. https://doi.org/10.1371/journal.pone.0103340

Lombardi, D., Squires, L., Sjostedt, P., Eichler, B., Turner, M., & Thompson, C. (2018). Industry and patient perspectives on child participation in clinical trials: The pediatric assent initiative survey report. *Therapeutic Innovation and Regulatory Science, 52,* 29–37. https://doi.org/10.1177/2168479017716490

Marcus, K.J., & Haas-Kogan, D. (2009). Pediatric radiation oncology. In S.H. Orkin, D.E. Fisher, A.T. Look, S. Lux, D. Ginsburg, & D.G. Nathan (Eds.), *Oncology of infancy and childhood* (pp. 241–256). Elsevier Saunders.

McMullen, K.P., Hanson, T., Bratton, J., & Johnstone, P.A.S. (2015). Parameters of anesthesia/sedation in children receiving radiotherapy. *Radiation Oncology, 10,* 65. https://doi.org/10.1186/s13014-015-0363-2

National Comprehensive Cancer Network. (2020). *NCCN Clinical Practice Guidelines in Oncology (NCCN Guidelines®): Distress management* [v.2.2020]. https://www.nccn.org/professionals/physician_gls/pdf/distress.pdf

Nunes, M.D.R., Jacob, E., Bomfim, E., Lopes-Junior, L.C., Garcia de Lima, R.A., Floria-Santos, M., & Nascimento, L.C. (2017). Fatigue and health related quality of life in children and adolescents with cancer. *European Journal of Oncology Nursing, 29,* 39–46. https://doi.org/10.1016/j.ejon.2017.05.001

Packer, R.J., MacDonald, T., & Vezina, G. (2010). Central nervous system tumors. *Hematology/Oncology Clinics of North America, 24,* 87–108. https://doi.org/10.1016/j.hoc.2009.11.012

Protection of human subjects, 45 C.F.R. § 46, et seq. (2016). https://www.govinfo.gov/content/pkg/CFR-2016-title45-vol1/pdf/CFR-2016-title45-vol1-part46.pdf

Recklitis, C.J., Casey, R.L., & Zeltzer, L. (2009). Psychosocial care of children and families. In S.H. Orkin, D.E. Fisher, A.T. Look, S.E. Lux, D. Ginsburg, & D.G. Nathan (Eds.), *Oncology of infancy and childhood* (pp. 1291–1318). Elsevier Saunders.

Robertson, E.G., Wakefield, C.E., Signorelli, C., Cohn, R.J., Patenaude, A., Foster, C., ... Fardell, J.E. (2018). Strategies to facilitate shared decision-making about pediatric oncology clinical trial enrollment: A systematic review. *Patient Education and Counseling, 101,* 1157–1174. https://doi.org/10.1016/j.pec.2018.02.001

Salvador, Á., Crespo, C., & Barros, L. (2019). Family management of pediatric cancer: Links with parenting satisfaction and psychological distress. *Family Process, 58,* 761–777. https://doi.org/10.1111/famp.12379

Schulman, S.R., Ferschl, M.B., Frederick, H.J., & Halperin, E.C. (2016). Anesthesia for external beam radiotherapy. In L.S. Constine, N.J. Tarbell, & E.C. Halperin (Eds.), *Pediatric radiation oncology* (6th ed., pp. 487–498). Wolters Kluwer Health/Lippincott Williams and Wilkins.

Scott, M.T., Todd, K.E., Oakley, H., Bradley, J.A., Rotondo, R.L., Morris, C.G., ... Indelicato, D.J. (2016). Reducing anesthesia and health care cost through utilization of child life specialists in pediatric radiation oncology. *International Journal of Radiation Oncology, Biology, Physics, 96,* 401–405. https://doi.org/10.1016/j.ijrobp.2016.06.001

Souweidane, M.M. (2010). Posterior fossa syndrome [Editorial]. *Journal of Neurosurgery: Pediatrics, 5,* 325–328. https://doi.org/10.3171/2009.11.PEDS09369

Stackhouse, C. (2013). The use of general anaesthesia in paediatric radiotherapy. *Radiography, 19,* 302–305. https://doi.org/10.1016/j.radi.2013.08.004

Stegmaier, K., & Sellers, W.R. (2009). Targeted approaches to drug development. In S.H. Orkin, D.E. Fisher, A.T. Look, S. Lux, D. Ginsburg, & D.G. Nathan (Eds.), *Oncology of infancy and childhood* (pp. 57–98). Elsevier Saunders.

Williams, C., Johnson, P.A., Guzzetta, C.E., Guzzetta, P.C., Cohen, I.T., Sill, A.M., ... Murray, J. (2014). Pediatric fasting times before surgical and radiologic procedures: Benchmarking institutional practices against national standards. *Journal of Pediatric Nursing, 29,* 258–267. https://doi.org/10.1016/j.pedn.2013.11.011

Woodman, H. (2013). Put yourself in their shoes ... the vulnerability of children and their families when attending for radiotherapy treatment: The role of the specialist paediatric radiotherapy radiographer. *Radiography, 19,* 311–314. https://doi.org/10.1016/j.radi.2013.08.006

Wu, X., Cao, J., Shan, C., Peng, B., Zhang, R., Cao, J., & Zhang, F. (2019). Efficacy and safety of propofol in preventing emergence agitation after sevoflurane anesthesia for children. *Experimental and Therapeutic Medicine, 17,* 3136–3140. https://doi.org/10.3892/etm.2019.7289

Yıldırım, İ., Çelik, A., Bay, S.B., Pasin, Ö., & Tütüncü, A.Ç. (2019). Propofol-based balanced anesthesia is safer in pediatric radiotherapy. *Journal of Oncology Pharmacy Practice, 25,* 1891–1896. https://doi.org/10.1177/1078155218825296

B. Adolescent and young adult radiation oncology

1. Definition
   a) NCI defines adolescent and young adult (AYA) oncology as treatment of individuals aged 15–39 years who receive a cancer diagnosis (A.W. Smith et al., 2016).
   b) The age range remains flexible.
2. Incidence: In the United States, approximately 70,000 AYAs are diagnosed with cancer annually, and cancer is one of the leading causes of death among this population (Coccia et al., 2018; Warner et al., 2016).
3. Indications: Some of the most common cancers (making up 95% of all cancers among AYAs) that may be treated with RT include the following (Coccia et al., 2018).
   a) Lymphomas
   b) Melanomas
   c) Testicular cancer and nongonadal germ cell tumors
   d) Female genital tract malignancies
   e) Thyroid cancer
   f) Bone and soft tissue sarcomas
   g) Leukemias

h) CNS cancers

i) Breast cancer

4. Customized care for AYA patients

    a) Optimizing the quality of care for AYAs involves timely detection and initiation of treatment, adherence to treatment, and access to interprofessional care delivered by healthcare professionals with expertise in this population's specific needs (Coccia et al., 2018; Gupta et al., 2016).

    b) A cancer diagnosis for AYAs is a significant interruption in their ability to move through important life milestones because, at the time of diagnosis, these patients are often completing different stages of schooling, transitioning from their childhood homes, establishing themselves in the workforce, forming intimate long-term emotional and sexual relationships, and starting a family (Ramphal et al., 2016; Warner et al., 2016).

    c) In order to optimally care for AYAs with cancer, healthcare providers, including nurses, must have a strong understanding of the unique concerns of this population (see Figure 27), provide relevant resources, and offer flexibility in approaches to clinical care (D'Agostino, Penney, & Zebrack, 2011; Mitchell, Tam, & Gupta, 2018).

5. Clinical practice guidelines

    a) NCCN publishes AYA-specific clinical practice guidelines focusing on treatment and management considerations in order to build capacity in AYA care delivery among oncology healthcare professionals (Coccia et al., 2018).

    b) Similar nursing-specific clinical practice guidelines have been established in the United Kingdom by Teenage Cancer Trust (S. Smith, Cable, Morgan, Siddall, & Chamley, 2014).

6. Assessment and intervention for AYA needs

    a) All AYAs should undergo a comprehensive assessment after a diagnosis of cancer (Coccia et al., 2018).

    b) The use of a screening tool can be an effective approach by healthcare professionals to assess and intervene on the unique care needs of the AYA population, as well as a means to approach difficult conversations (Mitchell, Tam, & Gupta, 2018).

      (1) A validated psychosocial screening tool for the AYA oncology population was developed in Australia to support healthcare professionals during the active treatment phase (Palmer, Patterson, & Thompson, 2014).

      (2) A second component of the tool focuses on screening AYA patients in the post-treatment survivorship phase.

    c) Dedicated AYA programs have been established in North America and around the world to overcome the gaps in care delivery for these patients. Although the patient age ranges and disciplines involved in these programs vary, the mission remains similar: to address the information and service needs of the defined AYA population (Mitchell, Stuart-McEwan, Panet, & Gupta, 2017; Mitchell, Tam, & Gupta, 2018; Reed, Block, & Johnson, 2014).

    d) AYA patients with cancer have unique needs; therefore, recommended clinical interventions must be tailored to those needs.

      (1) Fertility

        (a) It is well known that AYAs with cancer wish to receive information on fertility risks and preservation options (Gupta, Edelstein, Albert-Green, & D'Agostino, 2013).

        (b) Approximately 75% of AYA patients who have not had children at diagnosis express a wish for future biologic offspring (Husson, Huijgens, & van der Graaf, 2018).

        (c) See IV.F. Fertility for further information. Recommendations for addressing fertility concerns among AYAs with cancer are discussed in subsequent items.

        (d) Clinicians should discuss with patients the risks for infertility from cancer and its treatment, especially for high-risk therapies (e.g., gonadal irradiation), as well as fertility preservation options (Coccia et al., 2018).

        (e) When delivering fertility information, AYAs generally prefer to receive information directly from a healthcare pro-

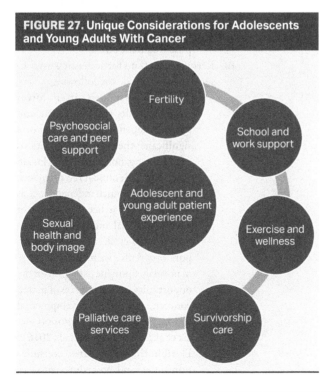

FIGURE 27. Unique Considerations for Adolescents and Young Adults With Cancer

Fertility

School and work support

Exercise and wellness

Survivorship care

Palliative care services

Sexual health and body image

Psychosocial care and peer support

Adolescent and young adult patient experience

fessional supplemented by a brochure or other written material, rather than written materials or online resources alone (Tam et al., 2018).

 (f) More in-depth discussions may be necessary for young women, given the complexities (timelines and cost) associated with oocytes and embryo cryopreservation (Mitchell, Tam, & Gupta, 2018).

 (g) Fertility should be discussed again following treatment completion, as an increasing number of survivors may have the option to undergo fertility preservation or have a fertility reassessment (Hendershot et al., 2016).

(2) Sexual function

 (a) AYA patients can experience disease- and treatment-related sexual dysfunctions.

 (b) Treatment such as RT can cause sexual side effects, including problems with erection, premature ejaculation, and early menopause (vaginal dryness, hot flashes, shrinking and loss of elasticity in vaginal tissue resulting in dyspareunia).

 (c) Sexual side effects can interfere with a younger adult's ability to engage in or enjoy sexual activity (Husson et al., 2018; Mitchell, Lewin, et al., 2018).

 (d) Recommendations for addressing sexual health problems in AYA patients with cancer include the following.

 i. At the time of diagnosis and periodically throughout treatment and survivorship follow-up, it is pertinent that healthcare professionals are holding discussions with their patients regarding sexual health and dysfunction (Carter et al., 2017; Coccia et al., 2018).

 ii. Limited evidence-based interventions for sexual changes in AYA survivors are available. An international consensus guideline was developed at the first Global Adolescents and Young Adults Cancer Congress (Mitchell, Lewin, et al., 2018).

 iii. NCCN recommends that clinicians discuss contraception with patients prior to treatment initiation (Coccia et al., 2018).

 iv. Male condoms may be safely used by male younger adults with cancer. Females have unique contraception needs, and the options are dependent on the cancer diagnosis and treatment plan (Coccia et al., 2018).

 v. Contraception is important to prevent pregnancy during treatment and sexually transmitted infections for individuals not in monogamous relationships (Mitchell, Lewin, et al., 2018).

 (e) AYAs with significant sexual side effects from treatment may benefit from a specialist referral, such as for an endocrinologist, gynecologist, pelvic floor therapist, or urologist, for a more in-depth assessment and management of symptoms (Mitchell, Lewin, et al., 2018).

(3) Psychosocial distress

 (a) The psychosocial needs of AYA patients as they relate to their unique developmental challenges and survivorship issues are well-documented in the literature (David, Williamson, & Tilsley, 2012; Husson et al., 2018; Warner et al., 2016).

 (b) Psychosocial support is critical for the continued psychological recovery and well-being of AYA patients (David et al., 2012).

 (c) Some of the common concerns of this population include the following (David et al., 2012; Husson et al., 2018; Warner et al., 2016).

 i. Isolation and relationships with peers and family

 ii. Changes in appearance and coping with body image concerns

 iii. Need for age-appropriate information

 iv. Mental health concerns (e.g., anxiety, depression, fear of cancer recurrence, post-traumatic stress)

 (d) Recommendations for addressing psychosocial needs include the following.

 i. A cancer diagnosis often forces younger adults to move home and become dependent on parents or a significant other, usually after periods of time living independently (Husson et al., 2018). Because AYAs often seek to maintain as much independence as possible, peers can become important sources of social and emotional support (David et al., 2012). Peer support programs can maintain a sense of normalcy, provide patients with the opportunity to address areas of shared concern, and reduce developmental disruption with their diagnosis (Coccia et al., 2018; Warner et al., 2016).

 ii. Flexible treatment dates, consultation times, and procedures also can reduce interruptions to normal AYA activities, allowing them to further have normalcy in their lives (Coccia et al., 2018).

(e) Physical appearance and body image are important psychosocial factors for this population.

    i. Cancer and its treatment can have a significant effect on physical appearance, body image, and self-esteem (Williamson, Harcourt, Halliwell, Frith, & Wallace, 2010).

    ii. RT can cause skin reddening and possible permanent skin pigmentation or hair loss (David et al., 2012).

    iii. It is thought that referring AYA patients to counseling services focused on self-image is most effective for addressing these specific concerns (David et al., 2012).

(f) Age-appropriate information is important for AYA patients, given that this population has significant information needs. Digital tools are important, but patients also benefit from healthcare professional guidance in navigating evidence-based online resources (David et al., 2012; Gupta et al., 2016; Mitchell, Tam, & Gupta, 2018; Warner et al., 2016).

(g) Approximately one-third of AYA patients with cancer exhibit post-traumatic distress symptoms following cancer treatment (Medlow, Patterson, & Baird, 2015). AYA patients with psychiatric symptoms (e.g., depression, anxiety) should be referred to a mental health provider for assessment and offered community-based resources that specifically provide psychosocial support to AYAs (Coccia et al., 2018).

(4) Educational, employment, and neurocognitive issues

(a) A cancer diagnosis can result in serious school and work disruptions (Husson et al., 2018).

    i. Regarding education, cancer treatment can result in absenteeism from school, inability to complete exams, and the feeling of being left behind (Husson et al., 2018).

    ii. In one study, 24% of AYAs with cancer reported unemployment because of health issues, compared to 14% of their healthy peers (Tai et al., 2012).

    iii. AYAs with cancer may be at risk for certain cognitive impairments, which have been demonstrated to increase

over time (largely associated with cranial irradiation), affecting transition back to a school or work environment. Because AYA patients experience distress related to continuing with academic, career, and personal goals in order to achieve life milestones at a similar pace as their peers, it is crucial that healthcare professionals encourage slow transitions and assist patients with establishing realistic goals (Medlow et al., 2015; Mitchell, Tam, & Gupta, 2018; Overholser, Kilbourn, & Liu, 2017).

(b) Healthcare professionals following AYAs at risk for compromised neurocognitive function should be assessing for changes in executive function, attention span, memory, and ability to process (Coccia et al., 2016; Viale, 2016).

(c) AYA patients should be referred for a formal neurocognitive assessment if they are displaying symptoms following treatment. Clinicians should provide resources on how to best manage these symptoms (Coccia et al., 2018).

(5) Medical survivorship issues

(a) RT is associated with an increased risk for the development of second malignancies, thyroid dysfunction, growth dysfunction, and cardiac dysfunction (Coccia et al., 2018).

(b) AYA survivors are at higher risk for second primary malignancy, compared to the general population or survivors of adult onset cancers (Medlow et al., 2015).

    i. Those at highest risk include survivors of non-Hodgkin and Hodgkin lymphoma, acute lymphoblastic leukemia, and acute myeloid leukemia (Chao et al., 2017).

    ii. AYA patients treated with cranial irradiation for acute lymphoblastic leukemia are at risk for CNS tumors, lymphoma, thyroid cancer, and acute myeloid leukemia (Medlow et al., 2015).

    iii. Young women (aged 10–30 years) treated with thoracic RT for Hodgkin lymphoma are shown to have a significantly elevated risk of developing breast cancer (Hodgson, Cotton, Crystal, & Nathan, 2016).

    iv. Early screening among AYA survivors at risk for second cancers should be encouraged, and the healthcare team should inform patients of these risks (Hodgson et al., 2016).

(c) Abnormalities in thyroid function resulting in hormone imbalances can occur in AYA patients who receive RT to the head and neck or CNS region.

   i. This can result in shorter stature as an adult, increased risk for obesity, and gonadal dysfunction (Coccia et al., 2018; Medlow et al., 2015).

   ii. AYA patients at risk can benefit from a consultation with an endocrinologist following treatment (Mitchell, Lewin, et al., 2018).

(d) AYA cancers demonstrate a range of cardiac complications, with a cumulative incidence of cardiac adverse outcomes that continues to increase up to 30 years after treatment.

   i. Cardiac complications include congestive heart failure, myocardial infarction, pericardial disease, and valvular abnormalities (Medlow et al., 2015).

   ii. Additional research is needed to develop AYA-specific post-treatment cardiac screening guidelines for survivors.

(6) Palliative and end-of-life care

(a) The diagnosis of advanced cancer is particularly distressing for someone young.

(b) AYA patients have less time to learn from other challenging life experiences that may help them cope with the consequences of advanced cancer (Husson et al., 2018).

(c) Little is known about specific needs of AYAs transitioning to a palliative approach to care (Donovan, Knight, & Quinn, 2015).

(d) Early palliative care involvement is encouraged. The goal of palliative care is to control symptoms, relieve emotional and physical suffering, and improve quality of life—regardless of the stage of disease or need for additional therapies (Coccia et al., 2018; Donovan et al., 2015).

(e) In order to understand the needs of AYAs with advanced cancer, Wiener et al. (2012) developed the Voicing My Choices document—a validated tool for AYA advance care planning. This tool is a guide that can support younger adults in communicating their needs to their families and healthcare providers (Wiener et al., 2012).

7. Nursing implications

a) Given the diverse needs of the AYA population, interprofessional collaboration in a team with expertise in specific AYA developmental issues (e.g., fertility, sexual health, employment, education) is vital for optimizing the care of AYA patients with cancer (Coccia et al., 2018; Mitchell, Tam, & Gupta, 2018).

b) Point-of-care nurses develop an understanding of the complex physical and psychosocial needs of their AYA patients and can offer information on resources available to these patients in hospital and community settings (A.W. Smith et al., 2016).

c) Advanced practice nurses have extensive experience and can develop an in-depth understanding of the needs of AYAs with cancer (A.W. Smith et al., 2016).

   (1) They work effectively with the interprofessional team to optimally address patient care needs.

   (2) They can further use their knowledge and expertise to educate and mentor point-of-care nursing staff.

d) Nurse leaders at the executive level are involved in strategic planning for AYA patient care at local, national, and international levels. They have advanced negotiating skills and can be influential with policy makers within an oncology institution and at a national level (A.W. Smith et al., 2016).

8. Recommended resources

a) First Descents: https://firstdescents.org

b) Living Out Loud (AYAs with advanced cancer): https://livingoutloud.life

c) NCI: www.cancer.gov/types/aya

d) Stupid Cancer: https://stupidcancer.org

e) Teen Cancer America: https://teencanceramerica.org

f) Young Adult Cancer Canada: www.youngadultcancer.ca

References

Carter, J., Lacchetti, C., Anderson, B.L., Barton, D.L., Bolte, S., Damast, S., ... Rowland, J.H. (2018). Interventions to address sexual problems in people with cancer: American Society of Clinical Oncology clinical practice guideline adaptation of Cancer Care Ontario guideline. *Journal of Clinical Oncology, 36*, 492–511. https://doi.org/10.1200/jco.2017.75.8995

Chao, C., Xu, L., Cannavale, K., Wong, F.L., Huang, P.-Y., Cooper, R., ... Armenian, S.H. (2017). Risk of subsequent malignant neoplasms in survivors of adolescent and young adult (AYA) lymphoma and leukemia. *Blood, 130*(Suppl. 1), 608. https://doi.org/10.1182/blood.V130.Suppl_1.608.608

Coccia, P.F., Pappo, A.S., Beaupin, L., Borges, V.F., Borinstein, S.C., Chugh, R., ... Shead, D.A. (2018). Adolescent and young adult oncology, version 2.2018, NCCN Clinical Practice Guidelines in Oncology. *Journal of the National Comprehensive Cancer Network, 16*, 66–97. https://doi.org/10.6004/jnccn.2018.0001

D'Agostino, N.M., Penney, A., & Zebrack, B. (2011). Providing developmentally appropriate psychosocial care to adolescent and young adult cancer survivors. *Cancer, 117*(Suppl. 10), 2329–2334. https://doi.org/10.1002/cncr.26043

David, C.L., Williamson, K., & Tilsley, D.W.O. (2012). A small scale, qualitative focus group to investigate the psychosocial support needs of teenage young adult cancer patients undergoing radiotherapy in Wales. *European*

Journal of Oncology Nursing, 16, 375–379. https://doi.org/10.1016/j.ejon.2011.08.002

Donovan, K.A., Knight, D., & Quinn, G.P. (2015). Palliative care in adolescents and young adults with cancer. *Cancer Control, 22,* 475–479. https://doi.org/10.1177/107327481502200413

Gupta, A.A., Edelstein, K., Albert-Green, A., & D'Agostino, N. (2013). Assessing information and service needs of young adults with cancer at a single institution: The importance of information on cancer diagnosis, fertility preservation, diet, and exercise. *Supportive Care in Cancer, 21,* 2477–2484. https://doi.org/10.1007/s00520-013-1809-4

Gupta, A.A., Papadakos, J.K., Jones, J.M., Amin, L., Chang, E.K., Korenblum, C., ... Giuliani, M.E. (2016). Reimagining care for adolescent and young adult cancer programs. Moving with the times. *Cancer, 122,* 1038–1046. https://doi.org/10.1002/cncr.29834

Hendershot, E., Maloncy, A.-M., Fawcett, S., Sarvanantham, S., McMahon, E., Gupta, A., & Mitchell, L. (2016). Advanced practice nurses: Improving access to fertility preservation for oncology patients. *Canadian Oncology Nursing Journal, 26,* 40–45. https://doi.org/10.5737/236880762614045

Hodgson, D., Cotton, C., Crystal, P., & Nathan, P.C. (2016). Impact of early breast cancer screening on mortality among young survivors of childhood Hodgkin's lymphoma. *Journal of the National Cancer Institute, 108,* djw010. https://doi.org/10.1093/jnci/djw010

Husson, O., Huijgens, P.C., & van der Graaf, W.T.A. (2018). Psychosocial challenges and health-related quality of life of adolescents and young adults with hematologic malignancies. *Blood, 132,* 385–392. https://doi.org/10.1182/blood-2017-11-778555

Medlow, S., Patterson, P., & Baird, H. (2015). *Exploring survivorship care for adolescent and young adult cancer survivors in Australia.* CanTeen Australia. https://www.canteen.org.au/wp-content/uploads/2016/09/Adolescent-and-Young-Adult-Cancer-Survivorship-Report.pdf

Mitchell, L., Lewin, J., Dirks, J., Wang, K., Tam, S., Katz, A., ... Gupta, A.A. (2018). Sexual health issues for the young adult with cancer: An international symposium held during the first Global Adolescents and Young Adults Cancer Congress (Edinburgh, United Kingdom). *Journal of Adolescent and Young Adult Oncology, 7,* 153–163. https://doi.org/10.1089/jayao.2017.0067

Mitchell, L., Stuart-McEwan, T., Panet, H., & Gupta, A. (2017). Adolescents and young adults: Addressing needs and optimizing care with a clinical nurse specialist. *Clinical Journal of Oncology Nursing, 21,* 123–126. https://doi.org/10.1188/17.cjon.123-126

Mitchell, L., Tam, S., & Gupta, A. (2018). Crucial conversations: Addressing informational and service needs of adolescents and young adults diagnosed with cancer. *Clinical Journal of Oncology Nursing, 22,* 483–486. https://doi.org/10.1188/18.cjon.483-486

Overholser, L., Kilbourn, K., & Liu, A. (2017). Survivorship issues in adolescent and young adult oncology. *Medical Clinics of North America, 101,* 1075–1084. https://doi.org/10.1016/j.mcna.2017.06.002

Palmer, S., Patterson, P., & Thompson, K. (2014). A national approach to improving adolescent and young adult (AYA) oncology psychosocial care: The development of AYA-specific psychosocial assessment and care tools. *Palliative and Supportive Care, 12,* 183–188. https://doi.org/10.1017/s1478951512001083

Ramphal, R., Aubin, S., Czaykowski, P., De Pauw, S., Johnson, A., McKillop, S., ... Rogers, P. (2016). Adolescent and young adult cancer: Principles of care. *Current Oncology, 23,* 204–209. https://doi.org/10.3747/co.23.3013

Reed, D., Block, R.G., & Johnson, R. (2014). Creating an adolescent and young adult cancer program: Lessons learned from pediatric and adult oncology practice bases. *Journal of the National Comprehensive Cancer Network, 12,* 1409–1415. https://doi.org/10.6004/jnccn.2014.0138

Smith, A.W., Seibel, N.L., Lewis, D.R., Albritton, K.H., Blair, D.G., Blanke, C.D., ... Zebrack, B.J. (2016). Next steps for adolescent and young adult oncology workshop: An update on progress and recommendations for the future. *Cancer, 122,* 988–999. https://doi.org/10.1002/cncr.29870

Smith, S., Cable, M., Morgan, S., Siddall, J., & Chamley, C. (2014). *Competencies: Caring for teenagers and young adults with cancer: A competence and career framework for nursing.* Teenage Cancer Trust. https://www.teenagecancertrust.org/sites/default/files/Nursing-framework.pdf

Tai, E., Buchanan, N., Townsend, J., Fairley, T., Moore, A., & Richardson, L.C. (2012). Health status of adolescent and young adult cancer survivors. *Cancer, 118,* 4884–4891. https://doi.org/10.1002/cncr.27445

Tam, S., Puri, N., Stephens, D., Mitchell, L., Giuliani, M., Papadakos, J., & Gupta, A.A. (2018). Improving access to standardized fertility preservation information for older adolescents and young adults with cancer: Using a user-centered approach with young adult patients, survivors, and partners to refine fertility knowledge transfer. *Journal of Cancer Education, 33,* 528–535. https://doi.org/10.1007/s13187-016-1108-0

Warner, E.L., Kent, E.E., Trevino, K.M., Parsons, H.M., Zebrack, B.J., & Kirchhoff, A.C. (2016). Social well-being among adolescents and young adults with cancer: A systematic review. *Cancer, 122,* 1029–1037. https://doi.org/10.1002/cncr.29866

Wiener, L., Zadeh, S., Battles, H., Baird, K., Ballard, E., Osherow, J., & Pao, M. (2012). Allowing adolescents and young adults to plan their end-of-life care. *Pediatrics, 130,* 897–905. https://doi.org/10.1542/peds.2012-0663

Williamson, H., Harcourt, D., Halliwell, E., Frith, H., & Wallace, M. (2010). Adolescents' and parents' experiences of managing the psychosocial impact of appearance change during cancer treatment. *Journal of Pediatric Oncology Nursing, 27,* 168–175. https://doi.org/10.1177/1043454209357923

Viale, P.H. (2016). Late effects: Focus on adolescent and young adult cancer survivors. *Journal of Advanced Practice Oncology, 7,* 15–16. https://doi.org/10.6004/jadpro.2016.7.1.1

C. Older adult radiation oncology

1. Incidence

   a) In developed and developing nations worldwide, cancer occurs disproportionately in older adults (Pilleron et al., 2019).

   b) Increased cancer prevalence among older patients is multifactorial and may be related to increased length of exposure to carcinogens; greater receptivity of older tissues to the effect of carcinogens; decline in immune function, which impairs processes that promote detection and destruction of neoplastic cells; and decline in endocrine function, which contributes to changes in body composition associated with common cancers (Moloney, 2014).

   c) With population aging, the number and proportion of cancers diagnosed in people aged 65 years and older is expected to increase dramatically by 2035 (Pilleron et al., 2019).

      (1) The greatest increase is expected in developing countries, with a predicted doubling of the number of new cancer cases among people aged 65 years and older.

      (2) In developed countries, including European countries, Canada, and the United States, by 2035, at least two-thirds of new cancer cases are expected to occur in those aged 65 years and older.

2. Age-associated changes

   a) Overview (World Health Organization, 2015)

      (1) Aging is characterized by changes—positive and negative—across multiple domains.

      (2) Individuals experience these changes at different times and in different ways, which can affect cancer and RT trajectory.

b) Physiologic changes

(1) Changes in cancer pathology

    (a) Some cancers are more aggressive in older adults (e.g., early-stage endometrial cancer, glioblastoma), while others become more indolent (e.g., breast, prostate), affecting the expected magnitude of locoregional control benefit of RT (G.L. Smith & Smith, 2014).

        i. A more indolent course has a lower risk of recurrence, which means the absolute benefit of RT would also be low, and therefore may not be recommended. For example, because breast cancer is more indolent in older women, less aggressive RT strategies may be used (partial breast RT, intraoperative RT), or RT may be omitted in favor of endocrine therapy alone.

        ii. Alternately, age may decrease the relative radiosensitivity of a tumor because of decreased oxygenation and proliferation of tumor cells, so RT may provide a decreased relative locoregional control benefit. In this case, treatment may be recommended, but it may be less likely to cure (Christoph & Eberhardt, 2016; G.L. Smith & Smith, 2014). For example, early-stage endometrial cancer may be more aggressive in older women, with a higher risk of locoregional recurrence, so the target volume may be greater for older as compared to younger women.

    (b) For the previously noted tumor sites, age is incorporated into risk stratification and prognostic schemes to guide decision-making for RT.

    (c) In other cancers, such as NSCLC and gastrointestinal cancers, consistent relationships between age and locoregional tumor behavior have not been identified.

(2) Decreased homeostatic reserve: Homeostatic or functional reserve refers to a person's ability to recover from stressors (i.e., physiologic or functional age) and may be indicative of a person's tolerance of RT, both in terms of treatment toxicity and completion (G.L. Smith & Smith, 2014).

(3) Changes in organ function

    (a) Age-related changes in organ function may exacerbate RT side effects associated with those organ systems (Chen & Nadalin, 2010; Haas, 2004; O'Donovan, Leech, & Gillham, 2017; see Table 14).

    (b) Changes in neurologic, cardiac, renal, and immune function may affect overall treatment tolerance and increase risk of healthy tissue damage during RT (G.L. Smith & Smith, 2014).

(4) Increased risk of chronic illness

    (a) The presence of other illnesses may affect RT tolerance, response, and outcomes.

    (b) Chronic illnesses affecting physical or cognitive functioning, such as osteoarthritis, Parkinson disease, or dementia, may prevent older adults from maintaining a position for RT that is reproducible over several days (Christoph & Eberhardt, 2016).

c) Functional changes

(1) Physiologic changes associated with aging may result in functional changes, including normal or pathologic changes in cognition, decreased mobility and increased risk of falls, and sensory changes (hearing, vision, taste, and touch).

(2) Functional changes may affect ability to access health care, communicate with healthcare professionals, follow instructions during RT, navigate the cancer care system, and engage in self-management of symptoms and side effects during the treatment course.

d) Psychosocial changes

(1) Aging is marked by positive and negative psychosocial changes, including new social roles (e.g., retirement, becoming a grandparent), the opportunity to draw on a lifetime of coping and adaptive skills, loss of close relationships that may reduce available social support, and changes in the availability of financial resources.

(2) Lack of social support and financial resources may affect ability to manage the RT trajectory, including access to transportation and ability to manage symptoms and side effects, particularly when combined with functional changes related to mobility and ADLs.

e) Existential changes

(1) Aging may be marked by heightened awareness of the nearness and inevitability of death and an increased value of time, which may lead to a shift from materialistic to more transcendent perspectives (Hannum & Rubinstein, 2016; World Health Organization, 2015).

(2) These changes may affect how an individual views the meaning of the cancer experience, as well as the goals and priorities for cancer treatment, thus shaping treatment decision-making related to RT.

3. Aging and cancer survivorship

a) Cancer survivorship affects the experience of aging (Strohschein, Fitch, & Vanderbyl, 2020).

TABLE 14. Physical Consequences of Aging and Toxicities of Radiation Treatment

Organ Site	Effects of Aging	Acute Toxicities of Radiation	Late Toxicities of Radiation
Bladder	Loss of muscle tone, leading to incomplete bladder emptying Decreased bladder capacity	Frequency Urgency Dysuria Hesitancy Hematuria	Hematuria Telangiectasia
Bone	Loss of bone density	Thrombocytopenia Neutropenia	Spinal cord myelopathy
Brain	Decrease in brain weight Loss of gray and white matter Changes in nerve cells	Cerebral edema Seizures Alopecia	Radiation necrosis Cerebral atrophy Cranial neuropathy
Breast	Less glandular tissue, more connective and fat tissue	Breast pain, swelling, tenderness Radiodermatitis Tanning/telangiectasias	Firmness Fibrosis
Colon and rectum	Slow peristalsis Decreased muscle strength in abdomen	Abdominal cramping Diarrhea	Fibrosis Diarrhea Proctitis Adhesions Stenosis
Heart	Decreased heart rate Vascular stiffness Increased platelet adhesiveness Decreased aerobic capacity	Delayed acute pericarditis Delayed pericardial effusion Diffuse myocardial fibrosis Late coronary artery disease Conduction defects	–
Lung	Reduction in glandular epithelial cells Enlargement of alveoli and alveoli ducts Reduction in respiratory muscle functioning Ossification of costal cartilage	Increasing cough, dyspnea Pain (tumor) Esophagitis Hoarseness Skin reactions (see above)	Pneumonitis Fibrosis
Oral cavity	Less production of ptyalin and amylase in saliva glands Dry mouth (medication induced) Decreased olfactory senses Decrease in mastication muscles	Mucositis/stomatitis Acute xerostomia Taste changes Pharyngitis	Osteoradionecrosis Chronic xerostomia Trismus
Prostate	Hyperplasia	Diarrhea Tenesmus Proctalgia Rectal bleeding Erectile dysfunction	Persistent bowel changes of diarrhea Fistula formation Perforation Incomplete bowel mucosa healing
Skin	Thinning of epidermis Unchanged stratum corneum, except moisture and cohesiveness Decreased melanocytes Decreased Langerhans cells Decreased fibroblasts Hypovascular endothelium Decreased mast cells	Mild to brisk erythema Dry desquamation Moist desquamation	Telangiectasias Fibrosis Necrosis
Vagina and ovaries	Atrophy of organs	Hot flashes Vagina dryness Dyspareunia	Thinning Atrophy Adhesions Shortening, narrowing

Note. Based on information from Haas, 2004, 2006.

From "Radiation Therapy," by M.L. Haas, in C.G. Varricchio, T.B. Ades, P.S. Hinds, and M. Pierces (Eds.), *A Cancer Source Book for Nurses* (8th ed., pp. 142–143), 2004, Jones and Bartlett. Copyright 2004 by Jones and Bartlett. Adapted with permission.

b) It is estimated that, by 2040, in the United States, 73% of cancer survivors will be aged 65 years or older—a 68% increase from 2016 (Bluethmann, Mariotto, & Rowland, 2016).

c) Older adult survivors include those diagnosed in older age and those diagnosed at younger ages who are aging with late effects of treatment (Strohschein et al., 2020).

d) In a cohort of cancer survivors 10 years after diagnosis, past RT was associated with low health-related quality of life (Götze, Taubenheim, Dietz, Lordick, & Mehnert, 2018).

e) Women who received RT, chemotherapy, and surgery for breast cancer have shown increased comorbidities and inflammatory changes associated with accelerated aging (Alfano et al., 2017).

f) Attention to the long-term physical and psychosocial effects of RT is important for maintaining health and quality of life among older cancer survivors (Henderson, Ness, & Cohen, 2014).
   (1) Skin protection and skin cancer screening in survivors treated with RT
   (2) Breast cancer screening in women exposed to chest irradiation at younger ages

4. Age-based disparities
   a) Age-based disparities in cancer survival and treatment suggest that healthcare providers have more to learn about appropriately addressing age-related concerns in cancer care.
   b) Improvements in cancer survival have occurred later, and to a lesser degree, in older adults, as compared to middle-aged and younger adults, suggesting that middle-aged and younger adults have experienced greater benefit from advances in screening and treatment than older adults (Liu et al., 2018; Mukhtar et al., 2018; Zeng et al., 2015).
   c) Older adults are less likely to receive guideline-concordant curative treatment than are younger adults (Fang et al., 2017).
      (1) In stage III breast cancer, older women are less likely to receive postmastectomy RT.
      (2) In stage I NSCLC, older adults are less likely to be treated with RT or surgery.
      (3) In intermediate- or high-risk prostate cancer, older men are less likely to be treated with RT or prostatectomy.
   d) Older adults are, however, more likely to receive guideline-concordant deintensified treatment (Fang et al., 2017).
      (1) In stage I–II node-negative breast cancer, older women are more likely to receive hypofractionated postlumpectomy RT.
      (2) In stage I NSCLC, older adults are more likely to be treated with SBRT instead of surgery.
   e) Treatment disparities remain despite the finding that curative RT has been shown to be well tolerated by older adults. However, poor performance status or comorbidities are predictors for decreased treatment tolerability and overall survival (Fiorica et al., 2009; Khor et al., 2015).
   f) In RT among older adults, these disparities have been associated with clinicians offering treatment less frequently, higher treatment refusal, and reluctance to travel to other centers for treatment (McAleese, Baluch, Drinkwater, Bassett, & Hanna, 2017).

5. Age-related challenges
   a) Overview
      (1) Age-based disparities are associated with important age-related challenges that affect the care of older adults with cancer.
      (2) Awareness of these challenges is central to optimizing radiation oncology nursing care for older adults.
   b) Lack of research
      (1) Large gaps in knowledge exist related to the care of older adults with cancer, particularly with respect to RT (VanderWalde, Hurria, & Jagsi, 2017).
      (2) Older adults are under-represented in clinical trials. Although people aged 65 years or older comprise more than half of the cancer population, they represent only 20%–36% of clinical trial participants (Hurria et al., 2015).
      (3) Clinicians must extrapolate from trials with younger, healthier populations to inform treatment recommendations. Recommendations may be based on chronologic age, rather than functional or physiologic age, and information concerning outcomes of importance to older adults is lacking, such as quality of life or impact on mobility, cognition, and ability to maintain independence (Hurria et al., 2015).
      (4) In radiation oncology, a need exists for better evidence concerning the tolerability, efficacy, toxicity, and relative value of various treatment options for older adults, as well as the baseline characteristics of older adults associated with positive treatment outcomes (VanderWalde, Hurria, & Jagsi, 2017).
   c) Ageism
      (1) Ageism is the "stereotypes, prejudice, or discrimination against (but also in favor of) people because of their chronological age" (Ayalon & Tesch-Römer, 2017, p. 1).
      (2) Ageism affects the quality and quantity of care that older adults with cancer receive (Wyman, Shiovitz-Ezra, & Bengel, 2018).
      (3) Radiation oncology nurses have an important role to play in addressing ageism in their own practice, in the systems within which they provide care, and in the attitudes of older patients themselves (Ayalon & Tesch-Römer, 2017;

Ben-Harush et al., 2017; Lawler, Selby, Aapro, & Duffy, 2014; Schroyen et al., 2018; Wyman et al., 2018).

  d) Heterogeneity
    (1) The best way to address ageism is to recognize the vast variation among older adults, with respect to health and functional status, life expectancy, social support and resources, and the historical experiences that they bring to their interactions with the cancer care system.
    (2) Recognizing and articulating this heterogeneity is critical in radiation oncology, as the localized nature of the treatment may mean referral of older adults deemed unfit for other treatment modalities. This variation presents important challenges in ensuring appropriate treatment (VanderWalde, Hurria, & Jagsi, 2017).
  e) Frailty
    (1) Frailty is a "complex, multidimensional, and cyclical state of diminished physiologic reserve that results in decreased resiliency and adaptive capacity and increased vulnerability to stressors" (Ethun et al., 2017, p. 364).
    (2) Understanding frailty is a valuable way of understanding the variation among older adults with cancer.
    (3) For some older adults, age-related changes may not be evident until they are exposed to stressors, such as cancer treatment (VanderWalde, Hurria, & Jagsi, 2017).
    (4) Frailty is associated with weight loss, fatigue, decreased physical activity, weakness, and impaired mobility and may occur in the absence of comorbid disease or disability in ADLs (Fried et al., 2001).
    (5) The presence of frailty in older adults with cancer is associated with increased risk of functional decline, treatment-associated complications, hospitalization, disease recurrence or progression, and death (Ethun et al., 2017).
    (6) VanderWalde, Deal, et al. (2017) identified the presence of frailty after RT in 52% of people aged 65 years and older with newly diagnosed lung or head and neck cancers who were not identified as frail at baseline, and 42% of patients who were independent in their instrumental ADLs prior to treatment were dependent in at least one instrumental ADL after treatment.
6. Treatment decision-making
  a) Age-related changes and challenges add complexity to the cancer treatment decision-making process for all those involved.
  b) Among women aged 65 years and older with breast cancer, 96% indicated that they were the primary decision maker regarding RT, with 71% indicating

doctors, family members, friends, and nurses also play an important role (Wang et al., 2017).
  c) In a qualitative study of the chemotherapy and RT treatment decision-making experiences of older adults, Sattar et al. (2018) found that most participants expressed trust in their oncologist and relied on their professional expertise, while asserting independence and autonomy in making the final decision.
  d) If patients are unable to manage the requirements and side effects of RT, they may lose trust and step away from certain aspects of care; therefore, a key element of the treatment decision-making process is an appropriate and trustworthy treatment recommendation (Strohschein, 2019).
  e) RT recommendations should be informed by a comprehensive, personalized, interprofessional risk–benefit assessment that considers locoregional tumor behavior, competing risks, functional reserve, and palliative needs (G.L. Smith & Smith, 2014).
  f) Huang and Parvathaneni (2017) presented a valuable framework and schema for developing optimal, personalized care plans for older adults, for whom RT is a potential modality for curative or palliative treatment.
    (1) According to this framework, clinicians begin by understanding patient priorities and goals of care, then they complete an initial screen for frailty to identify patients who would benefit from comprehensive geriatric assessment (CGA) and management.
    (2) If CGA is warranted, the information gained through CGA is used to determine if RT will help a patient achieve desired goals and to inform multimodal interventions that optimize treatment outcomes.
7. Patient priorities and goals of care
  a) Understanding of patients' preferences, priorities, values, and goals of care is key to optimal decision-making regarding RT for older adults with cancer (Huang & Parvathaneni, 2017; NCCN, 2020b; G.L. Smith & Smith, 2014).
  b) Assessment of priorities and goals of care involves questions that provide insight into older adults' values and preferences, such as the following.
    (1) What is important to you right now?
    (2) What are you hoping for or looking forward to?
  c) It is critical to assess if goals and values of older patients are consistent with the anticipated side effects and outcomes of treatment (NCCN, 2020b).
  d) Radiation oncology nurses have a key role to play in understanding patients' situations and enabling them to identify and communicate their values and preferences to the cancer care team (Strohschein, 2019).
8. CGA and management
  a) Overview

(1) CGA is defined as "a multidimensional, interdisciplinary diagnostic process focusing on determining an older person's medical, psychosocial, and functional capabilities to develop a coordinated and integrated plan for treatment and long-term follow-up" (Wildiers et al., 2014, p. 2595).

(2) CGA should inform the development of an optimal RT plan for older adults with cancer (Huang & Parvathaneni, 2017).

b) Screening to identify those who would benefit from CGA

(1) Limited resources often mean that CGA cannot be offered to all older adults with cancer; therefore, screening tools, such as the Vulnerable Elders Survey-13 (VES-13) and Geriatric 8 tool (G8), can be used to identify older adults who would benefit from CGA (Decoster et al., 2015; Huang & Parvathaneni, 2017).

(2) The VES-13 and G8 require minimal time for completion and can be integrated into routine practice in radiation oncology (Szumacher et al., 2018).

(3) The G8 was developed and validated for use in older adults with cancer (Bellera et al., 2012).

(a) It demonstrates good sensitivity and prognostic value in relation to other measures (Decoster et al., 2015; Soubeyran et al., 2014).

(b) It must be completed with the assistance of a healthcare professional.

(4) The VES-13 was developed for older adults living in the community and can be completed by patients themselves or a family member. It has been validated with older adults with cancer, demonstrating less sensitivity but more specificity than the G8 (Saliba et al., 2001; Soubeyran et al., 2014).

(5) In addition to the use of screening tools, clinical judgment must also be employed in identifying those in need of CGA, as clinicians may become aware of issues not flagged using these tools.

c) CGA and oncology treatment decision-making

(1) CGA provides a systematic approach to evaluating age-related concerns that may predict toxicity, adverse effects, or decrease in quality of life from cancer treatment (Hamaker, Schiphorst, ten Bokkel Huinink, Schaar, & van Munster, 2014).

(2) CGA identifies potentially reversible concerns, which are typically unnoticed in routine oncology care, enabling the use of preventive interventions that can improve treatment tolerance and adherence (Loh et al., 2018; Wildiers et al., 2014).

(3) CGA provides information that can be used to estimate life expectancy without the cancer diagnosis (Loh et al., 2018).

(4) CGA improves physician–patient communication about age-related concerns (Mohile et al., 2020).

d) Specific benefits of CGA in RT

(1) Studies suggest that CGA results are predictive of RT tolerance, showing association with treatment completion and complications (Szumacher et al., 2018).

(2) Incomplete or interrupted RT can compromise treatment efficacy and ability to deliver higher doses in the future; therefore, identification of age-related issues that may affect treatment tolerance and completion is key to treatment success (Chang, Goldstein, & Dharmarajan, 2017; NCCN, 2020b).

(3) CGA provides a baseline of health and functional status prior to RT (Haas, 2004).

(4) CGA is ideally conducted by a healthcare professional with specialization in geriatrics or a trained assessor who considers age-related concerns in four cardinal domains: physical health, functional status, psychological health, and socioenvironmental parameters (Puts & Alibhai, 2018; Rubenstein et al., 2004).

(5) In order to provide optimal care for older adults with cancer, radiation oncology nurses must be aware of age-related concerns in these domains that may affect RT toxicity and completion (O'Donovan et al., 2017; Szumacher et al., 2018).

e) Integration of CGA in nursing practice: Radiation oncology nurses have the opportunity to integrate screening and assessment of these age-related concerns into their practice during clinical interview and assessment, during telephone interactions, or in patient-report tools, to inform supportive interventions throughout the treatment trajectory (Burhenn et al., 2016). An overview of each CGA domain is provided, including recommended screening and assessment tools, as well as potential interventions that can be integrated into radiation oncology nursing practice.

(1) Comorbidities

(a) Overview

i. In 2015, 68% of Medicare-enrolled people aged 65 years or older had two or more chronic conditions (CDC, n.d.).

ii. Underlying comorbidities may worsen or accelerate toxicity associated with RT (G.L. Smith & Smith, 2014).

iii. Comorbidities are consistently associated with poorer survival among patients with cancer but are poorly considered in interprofessional decision-making (Stairmand et al., 2015; Williams et al., 2016).

    iv. Among patients undergoing palliative RT, high comorbidity is associated with major treatment interruptions but is not reflected in fractionation scheduling (Perlow et al., 2019).

  (b) Screening and assessment tools

    i. The Charlson Comorbidity Index can be used to identify comorbidities associated with an increased risk of mortality and has been shown to be an optimal measure among patients with NSCLC undergoing RT. It may be completed by chart review or questionnaire (Charlson, Pompei, Ales, & MacKenzie, 1987; DeWees, Creach, Olsen, Bradley, & Robinson, 2012; J.N. Katz, Chang, Sangha, Fossel, & Bates, 1996).

    ii. The Functional Comorbidity Index is a self-administered tool identifying the presence of comorbidities associated with functional decline (Groll, To, Bombardier, & Wright, 2005).

  (c) Potential interventions

    i. Comorbidities can be identified and accounted for in RT planning, particularly if they interfere with optimal treatment delivery or tolerance risk.

    ii. Nurses can facilitate coordination with other healthcare professionals and disciplines to ensure that appropriate baseline measures (e.g., cardiac function, pulmonary function) are collected prior to RT and that comorbidities are managed optimally during and after treatment.

(2) Polypharmacy

  (a) Overview

    i. Polypharmacy may be defined as concurrent use of five or more medications, a criterion many older adults meet prior to receiving additional medications for cancer treatment or supportive care management (Nightingale, Skonecki, & Boparai, 2017).

    ii. Nearly one-third of older adults with cancer are exposed to potentially inappropriate medications and severe drug interactions, both of which are associated with polypharmacy (Alkan et al., 2017).

    iii. In a study of people aged 70 years and older undergoing palliative RT, 72% were taking five or more daily medications (Nieder, Mannsåker, Pawinski, & Haukland, 2017).

    iv. In radiation oncology, polypharmacy is associated with increased nonadherence to medication and a greater need for assistance with medications than is recognized by healthcare professionals (Maleki et al., 2020).

  (b) Screening and assessment tools

    i. Medication review includes screening for drug interactions and medications that can be discontinued or decreased, as well as evaluating patients' ability to manage medications (Nightingale et al., 2017).

    ii. A brown bag approach (i.e., asking patients to bring in all medications) can facilitate this review (Brega et al., 2018; Mohile et al., 2018).

    iii. The Beers criteria (American Geriatrics Society 2015 Beers Criteria Update Expert Panel, 2015) and STOPP (Screening Tool of Older People's Prescriptions) and START (Screening Tool to Alert to Right Treatment) criteria (O'Mahony et al., 2010) can be used to identify potentially inappropriate medications and drug interactions (Whitman, DeGregory, Morris, & Ramsdale, 2016).

    iv. NCCN (2020b) provides a list of medications commonly used in cancer supportive care that are of concern in older adults.

  (c) Potential interventions

    i. Nurses can collaborate with interprofessional team members (physicians, pharmacists) to ensure appropriate prescribing and deprescribing as necessary (Nightingale et al., 2017).

    ii. If challenges in medication adherence are identified, use of a dosette or pharmacist-filled blister packs is recommended.

    iii. Nurses can identify people within a patient's social network or community support services able to provide medication supervision.

(3) Sensory changes

  (a) Overview

    i. Identification of sensory concerns (e.g., hearing, vision, taste, touch) is

essential to optimizing other domains, such as communication, independence in ADLs, and nutrition.
  ii. Unrecognized sensory impairment may confound assessment of other domains (e.g., cognition, mobility).
(b) Screening and assessment: Nurses can ask about the following.
  i. Hearing loss and use of hearing aids
  ii. Vision impairment, use of glasses, and cataract surgery
  iii. Peripheral neuropathy and tactile difficulty
(c) Potential interventions
  i. Nurses can ensure hearing and vision difficulty is clearly documented so that all team members optimize communication.
  ii. If sensory difficulty is noted, nurses can facilitate referral to the appropriate specialist for further assessment (e.g., audiologist, optometrist, ophthalmologist, occupational therapist).
  iii. Nurses can consider alternative ways to provide instructions and cues during RT sessions to accommodate sensory impairment, such as visual cues (lights) or auditory cues (bells) (Chang et al., 2017).
(4) Mobility and risk of falls
(a) Overview
  i. Older adults with cancer describe mobility as a key indicator of quality of life (Strohschein, 2019).
  ii. Gait speed is associated with early death, disability, falls, and hospitalization or institutionalization in older adults with cancer (Pamoukdjian et al., 2015).
  iii. Among community-dwelling older adults with cancer, difficulty with ambulation and falls are frequently experienced but rarely reported, assessed, or documented (Cheville, Beck, Petersen, Marks, & Gamble, 2009; Sattar, Alibhai, Spoelstra, & Puts, 2019).
(b) Screening and assessment tools
  i. The Short Physical Performance Battery (Guralnik et al., 1994), which includes gait speed, balance, and sit to stand, is the mobility index with the best discriminative value for six-month mortality in older adults with cancer (Pamoukdjian et al., 2020).

  ii. ASCO recommends asking, "How many falls have you had in the last 6 months (or since the last visit)?" (Mohile et al., 2018, p. 2334).
  iii. Nurses can assess for orthostatic hypotension, which may contribute to risk of falls (NCCN, 2020b).
(c) Potential interventions
  i. Patients can be referred to physiotherapy and occupational therapy for prehabilitation and for access to necessary mobility aids, fall prevention, and support in mobility and physical activity during and after RT (Mohile et al., 2018).
  ii. If orthostatic hypotension is identified, nurses can consider medication review, salt intake, hydration, and compensatory strategies (NCCN, 2020b).
  iii. Nurses can examine the RT facility for safety and ease of access, ensure space for walkers and wheelchairs in changing areas and treatment rooms, remove equipment blocking hallways and handrails, and ensure adequate assistance in positioning for treatment.
(5) ADLs
(a) Overview
  i. Approximately one-third of older adults with cancer have difficulty with basic ADLs (e.g., dressing, bathing, eating, toileting, mobilizing) (Neo, Fettes, Gao, Higginson, & Maddocks, 2017).
  ii. More than half of older adults with cancer have difficulty with instrumental ADLs (e.g., shopping, preparing meals, performing household chores, using transportation, using telephones, managing medications, managing finances), which are necessary for independent living (Neo et al., 2017).
  iii. In people aged 65 years and older with newly diagnosed lung or head and neck cancers, dependence in instrumental ADLs is predictive of decline in health-related quality of life after RT (VanderWalde, Deal, et al., 2017).
  iv. Older adults may hesitate to disclose functional challenges for fear of delaying or being deemed unfit for treatment (Cheville et al., 2009).

(b) Screening and assessment tools
   i. The Older Americans Resources and Services Program Multidimensional Functional Assessment Questionnaire includes an ADL section with straightforward questions to assess independence in basic and instrumental ADLs (Fillenbaum, 1988).
   ii. The Katz Index of Independence in ADL (S. Katz, Ford, Moskowitz, Jackson, & Jaffe, 1963) and the Lawton Instrumental ADL Scale (Lawton & Brody, 1969) are often used with older adults with cancer (Neo et al., 2017).
(c) Potential interventions
   i. Prior to treatment, nurses can identify concerns that may be exacerbated during treatment.
   ii. Patients can be referred to occupational therapy for home safety evaluation and interventions to support ADLs.
   iii. Nurses can coordinate referrals to community services and encourage patients to mobilize their social network to provide needed support.
(6) Nutrition
(a) Overview
   i. Malnutrition is associated with mortality among older adults with cancer, specifically among those undergoing RT (Szumacher et al., 2018; Zhang et al., 2019).
   ii. Among older adults undergoing RT, malnutrition or weight loss may represent an interaction between underlying disease processes; the side effects of radiation treatment, such as xerostomia, mucositis, loss of appetite, nausea, vomiting, or fatigue; and age-related concerns.
   iii. Age-related concerns affecting nutrition may include the following (Gerdes, 2017; Guigoz, Lauque, & Vellas, 2002).
      • Difficulty shopping for groceries due to mobility or cognitive issues
      • Difficulty preparing meals due to cognitive issues, vision or tactile impairment, or limited fine motor skills (osteoarthritis in hands)
      • Loss of positive sensory experiences with eating due to loss of taste or vision impairment
      • Loss of appetite due to medication-related side effects affecting saliva production or gastrointestinal functioning
      • Limited access to nutritious food or nutritional supplements due to decreased financial resources
      • Altered social patterns around meals due to loss of family members or social isolation
      • Impaired chewing ability due to dental problems
(b) Screening and assessment tools: The Mini Nutritional Assessment has been validated in older adults and is commonly used with older adults with cancer (Guigoz et al., 2002; Isenring & Elia, 2015; Vellas et al., 1999; Zhang et al., 2019).
(c) Potential interventions
   i. In addition to the standard nutritional interventions for people undergoing RT (see IV.H. Nutritional issues), it is critical to address age-related concerns.
   ii. Patients can be referred for dental care, particularly to ensure proper fit of any dentures or dental appliances.
   iii. Patients can be referred to occupational therapy or speech therapy for swallowing assessments as needed.
   iv. Patients can be referred to occupational therapy to address functional issues related to meal preparation or kitchen safety.
   v. Patients can be referred to community support services such as Meals on Wheels.
(7) Cognition (see also IX.E. Patients with cognitive changes and dementia)
(a) Overview
   i. Among older adults with cancer, cognitive impairment is associated with functional dependence, depression, and a greater risk of death (NCCN, 2020b).
   ii. Cognitive changes encompass normal cognitive changes with aging, mild cognitive impairment, dementia, and delirium (Harada, Natelson Love, & Triebel, 2013; NCCN, 2020b).
   iii. Cognitive changes may affect an older person's ability to tolerate and manage RT, thus affecting ability to understand and remember treatment instructions, verbalize discomfort during treatment sessions, report and manage treatment toxicities, navigate

the healthcare system, and maintain self-care (Chang et al., 2017; McKoy et al., 2014).

(b) Screening and assessment tools

i. The Mini-Cog is a validated, brief screening tool for dementia (Borson, Scanlan, Brush, Vitaliano, & Dokmak, 2000; Borson, Scanlan, Chen, & Ganguli, 2003) recommended for use in identifying older adults with cancer who may require further cognitive assessment (McKoy et al., 2014; NCCN, 2020b).

ii. The Mini-Mental Status Examination can be used to monitor cognitive changes over time (Folstein, Folstein, & McHugh, 1975).

iii. The Montreal Cognitive Assessment screens for mild cognitive impairment (Nasreddine et al., 2005).

iv. The Confusion Assessment Method is a validated tool to detect delirium (Inouye et al., 1990).

v. Clinicians should ensure that sensory deficits, medication side effects, or mood disorders do not confound screening and assessment of cognitive status.

(c) Potential interventions

i. Nurses can help optimize hearing and vision to ensure the best possible communication and orientation.

ii. Patients with mild cognitive impairment should be monitored for delirium, particularly during and after cancer treatment, and progressive decline (McKoy et al., 2014).

iii. As delirium is often associated with physiologic disturbances, interventions must focus on identifying and remedying the underlying cause (NCCN, 2020b).

iv. Patients with dementia may benefit from acetyl cholinesterase inhibitors, which may slow cognitive decline (McKoy et al., 2014).

v. Nurses can ensure supportive measures are in place to manage treatment and ADLs.

(8) Decision-making capacity

(a) Overview

i. Cognitive changes may affect a person's capacity to engage in decisions about treatment and care. This decision-making capacity can change over time (e.g., resolution of delir-

ium) and may depend on the situation or the decision to be made (Sessums, Zembrzuska, & Jackson, 2011).

ii. Capacity requires the ability to understand relevant information, appreciate how that information applies to one's own situation, reason about the risks and benefits of the choice, and express a choice (Appelbaum & Grisso, 1988; McFarland et al., 2020).

(b) Screening and assessment

i. Capacity is not dependent on the results of cognitive assessment tools, but should be determined with a semi-structured interview pertaining to a specific decision (McFarland et al., 2020; Sessums et al., 2011), using guidelines such as the Aid to Capacity Evaluation (Etchells et al., 1999) or the MacArthur Competence Assessment Tool (Grisso, Appelbaum, & Hill-Fotouhi, 1997).

ii. A person is always assumed to have capacity to make decisions until it is determined otherwise (Sessums et al., 2011).

(c) Potential interventions

i. Nurses can optimize capacity by ensuring optimal communication, shortening and simplifying information, providing visual aids, and addressing any reversible conditions that may affect cognition (e.g., medication adjustment, addressing causes of delirium) (Sessums et al., 2011).

ii. Nurses can facilitate engagement and support surrogate decision makers when a patient does not have the capacity to make decisions.

iii. Nurses can encourage patients and families to establish advance directives before decision-making capacity becomes a concern.

(9) Depression

(a) Overview

i. Among older adults with cancer, depression is associated with social isolation, impaired mobility, impaired cognition, poor functional status, multimorbidity, and polypharmacy, highlighting the need for screening in these at-risk groups (Canoui-Poitrine et al., 2016).

ii. Changes in mood may reflect age-related losses and side effects of treatment (Saracino, Rosenfeld, & Nelson, 2016).

   iii. Older patients with cancer are more likely to present with somatic, rather than psychological, symptoms of depression. This unique phenomenology of depression among older adults with cancer is likely to be underrecognized and untreated (Parpa, Tsilika, Gennimata, & Mystakidou, 2015; Roth, Greenstein, Weisel, & Schulberg, 2015).

(b) Screening and assessment tools

   i. The Geriatric Depression Scale is a reliable and valid tool to assess depression in older adults with or without cognitive impairment; the 15-item short form provides ease of administration (Sheikh & Yesavage, 1986).

   ii. Use of lower cutoff scores should be considered when using the Geriatric Depression Scale among older adults with cancer (Saracino, Weinberger, Roth, Hurria, & Nelson, 2017).

(c) Potential interventions

   i. Nurses can ensure optimal symptom management.

   ii. Nurses can mobilize community resources to address limitations in functional status and gaps in social support (Shahrokni, Alexander, Wildes, & Puts, 2018).

   iii. Patients can be referred to social work, psychology, or psychiatry for further assessment and support.

   iv. Nurses can collaborate with interprofessional team members in considering pharmacologic interventions.

   v. Nurses should monitor for risk of suicide (Shahrokni et al., 2018).

   vi. Nurses can provide opportunity to discuss aspects of care that may be neglected, such as psychosocial and existential concerns.

(10) Existential and spiritual concerns

(a) Overview

   i. Existential concerns or demoralization, a lack of hope or regret over the life one has lived, may face older adults with cancer near end of life (Wiesel, 2015).

   ii. A patient's spirituality may influence treatment choices (Steinhauser et al., 2006).

   iii. Among people newly diagnosed with cancer, hope decreases with age

(Duggleby, Ghosh, Cooper, & Dwernychuk, 2013).

(b) Screening and assessment

   i. The Faith, Importance, Community, Address Spiritual Assessment Tool offers an approach to identify spiritual needs (Puchalski & Romer, 2000).

   ii. A single question, such as, "Are you at peace?" can provide insight into spiritual concerns (Steinhauser et al., 2006).

(c) Potential interventions

   i. Patients can be referred to a spiritual care practitioner.

   ii. Nurses can foster hope through transitions in treatment and care, such as supporting a shift from hope for a cure to hope for comfort, peace, and maintaining relationships (Duggleby, Holtslander, Steeves, Duggleby-Wenzel, & Cunningham, 2010; Shahrokni et al., 2018).

   iii. Nurses can consider meaning-making interventions (V. Lee, 2008).

(11) Social support and resources

(a) Overview

   i. For older adults, diverse social networks are associated with decreased risk of death after cancer diagnosis (Rottenberg et al., 2014).

   ii. Nearly half of older adults with cancer report unmet support needs related to informational, medical, physical, emotional, or practical support (Williams et al., 2019).

   iii. Unmet support needs are most likely to be reported in older adults with cancer who have the following characteristics (Williams et al., 2019).
- Non-White
- Divorced
- Never married
- High symptom burden

   iv. The availability of social support may have an important impact on an older person's ability to adhere to RT regimens, such as transportation to appointments and symptom management.

   v. Caregivers experience significant emotional and physical burden (Mathew & Fulton, 2017).

   vi. Older patients may themselves be caregivers, and these caregiving responsibilities may shape their willingness and ability to manage treatment.

(b) Screening and assessment tools

    i. Nurses can ask older patients about their living situation and financial resources, as well as if they have someone to help them, if needed, during RT (NCCN, 2020b).

    ii. Nurses can create a genogram and ecomap to understand a patient's social network (Shajani & Snell, 2019).

    iii. Unmet practical and social needs can be identified with the Distress Thermometer and Problem Checklist (NCCN, 2020a).

    iv. Nurses can assess caregivers throughout the treatment trajectory for their ability to provide care and their level of distress (Given, 2015; Mathew & Fulton, 2017).

(c) Potential interventions

    i. Nurses can ensure necessary support from home care and other community resources during and after RT and follow up on effectiveness of services (Adler & Page, 2008).

    ii. Patients can be referred to social work for assistance in mobilizing necessary resources (Christ, Messner, & Behar, 2015).

    iii. Nurses can provide information and offer emotional support, coordinating biomedical and psychosocial aspects of care and following up on effectiveness of services (Adler & Page, 2008).

    iv. Caregivers experiencing health concerns can be referred to their PCP (Given, 2015).

(12) Communication

(a) Overview: Communication with older people receiving RT presents challenges because of cognitive changes, sensory deficits, functional deficits, involvement of caregivers, and ageism (Fakhreddine, Galvan, Pawlowski, & Jones, 2017; Harvey & Nelson, 2015).

(b) Assessment

    i. Assessment of sensory changes and cognition should inform communication interventions.

    ii. Nurses should remain aware of interactional dynamics when a caregiver is present, particularly if they are acting as a translator.

    iii. Nurses should recognize that patients and families may need different amounts of information (Fakhreddine et al., 2017).

(c) Interventions

    i. Nurses can ensure optimal hearing and vision (e.g., glasses, hearing aid, amplifying device) (NCCN, 2020b).

    ii. Nurses can ensure written materials (including medication labels) use large font (14 point), are written at a fourth or fifth grade level, and avoid ambiguous symbols and abbreviations (Muluneh et al., 2018; NCCN, 2020b).

    iii. In discussions, nurses should pause and ask if a patient has any questions after each item or topic. For important ideas, patients should be able to repeat the information in their own words (NCCN, 2020b).

    iv. Nurses can provide a written summary of information and instructions at the end of each visit.

f) Life expectancy

(1) The information gathered during CGA of the previously discussed domains can contribute to an estimation of life expectancy.

(2) Neither age nor comorbidities are absolute contraindications to RT unless they indicate a much shorter life expectancy than the prognosis of the cancer to be treated.

(3) Older patients themselves may consider their own life expectancy, based on their age, health, and the ages to which family members and friends lived, in their decisions about treatment (Strohschein, 2019).

(4) Evaluation of life expectancy should include consideration of chronologic age, functional status, and comorbidities.

(a) Compiled via a systematic review, ePrognosis is an online collection of prognostic indices that use information from geriatric assessment to estimate life expectancy and may be used with older adults with cancer (A. Smith et al., n.d.; NCCN, 2020b; Yourman, Lee, Schonberg, Widera, & Smith, 2012).

(b) Several CGA screening and assessment tools independently predict mortality (Mohile et al., 2018).

(5) A patient's estimated life expectancy, excluding the current cancer diagnosis, should be considered in relation to the estimated morbidity and mortality from the cancer diagnosis, considering stage of disease, likelihood of

recurrence or progression, and disease behavior (indolent versus aggressive), as well as the effectiveness and morbidity of RT (NCCN, 2020b).

    (a) This estimation can inform a risk–benefit analysis of cancer treatment and influence treatment goals and approach (i.e., curative, control, or palliative).

    (b) If the benefits of treatment outweigh the risks, clinicians should integrate interventions prior to and during RT to optimize outcomes (Huang & Parvathaneni, 2017).

    (c) If the risks outweigh the benefits, or if a patient declines treatment, clinicians must ensure ongoing access to supportive care (Huang & Parvathaneni, 2017).

9. Optimizing RT for older adults

  a) General considerations

    (1) Comorbidities and underlying age-related decline in organ function should be considered.

    (2) Considerations for older adults undergoing RT will depend on the anatomic site to be treated and the dose of radiation proposed (NCCN, 2020b).

    (3) RT can exacerbate underlying system compromise related to the intended treatment field, highlighting the importance of baseline assessments.

      (a) Pulmonary function testing prior to treating significant lung volume

      (b) Audiology examination if an ear is in the treatment field

    (4) For patients with CIEDs (e.g., pacemaker, defibrillator), clinicians must consider beam modification and post-treatment device interrogation (Zaremba, Jakobsen, Søgaard, Thøgersen, & Riahi, 2015).

  b) Technological advances in treatment approach

    (1) CT-based RT planning allows for better prediction and minimization of toxicity (Kunkler et al., 2014).

    (2) IMRT for many treatment sites allows for variation of the treatment dose across the treatment field to promote greater tissue sparing (Chang et al., 2017; Kunkler et al., 2014; O'Donovan et al., 2017).

      (a) IMRT requires more rigorous tumor and organ tracking and depends on immobilization of the patient, which may be challenging for older adults with comorbidities, such as poor respiratory function, mobility issues, or cognitive impairment.

      (b) Advancements, such as VMAT, may result in faster delivery of precisely targeted doses, which is beneficial for frail patients who may have difficulty remaining still.

      (c) IGRT facilitates precise positioning with imaging performed at each treatment session.

      (d) Techniques limiting respiratory movement (e.g., breath hold or abdominal compression) may be challenging for older adults.

      (e) 4D planning scans allow for respiratory or other predictable motion to be integrated into treatment planning.

    (3) SBRT delivers higher doses to small target volumes, reducing treatment times and revolutionizing the treatment of NSCLC in older adults, for whom preexisting frailty and comorbidities limit the use of other approaches (Kunkler et al., 2014; O'Donovan et al., 2017).

    (4) Adaptive RT uses dynamic treatment planning to account for daily variations in tumor location, healthy tissue location, biologic changes, and physical setup. These factors are important in older adults for whom treatment setup may be impacted by mobility issues and internal organ motion (Kunkler et al., 2014).

    (5) Hypofractionation of RT doses allows for shorter treatment schedules, reducing the treatment burden for patients (Chang et al., 2017).

      (a) Hypofractionation can be associated with late toxicity but may remain a valuable option for patients with limited life expectancy, for whom late effects may be less of a concern (O'Donovan et al., 2017).

      (b) In some tumor sites (e.g., breast, prostate), hypofractionated doses may offer similar rates of local control without an increase in late effects (Kunkler et al., 2014; O'Donovan et al., 2017).

      (c) Noninferiority trials exploring toxicity profiles and tumor response for hypofractionated doses that allow for shorter treatment schedules are particularly relevant to older patients managing age-related concerns (O'Donovan et al., 2017).

    (6) Kunkler et al. (2014) provided a valuable review of best practices for RT in older adults by tumor site, and VanderWalde, Hurria, and Jagsi (2017) summarized recommendations by tumor site for older adults that have been integrated into NCCN guidelines.

  c) Management of fatigue

    (1) As a common side effect of RT, fatigue may introduce important challenges for older adults, resulting from the treatment itself and the requirements of daily travel to the treatment center (O'Donovan et al., 2017).

    (2) Fatigue may contribute to increased risk of falls, which can cause treatment delays and have a detrimental effect on independence.

(3) Fatigue also may impair ability to maintain basic ADLs and instrumental ADLs, affecting ability to self-manage symptoms and side effects through treatment.

(4) Older adults may attribute fatigue to age and thus underreport the experience of fatigue to healthcare professionals.

(5) Physical activity has been shown to have benefits in reducing CRF; however, for older adults, preexisting or new mobility issues and comorbidities may make it difficult to maintain the necessary levels of physical activity to achieve these benefits (O'Donovan et al., 2017; Speck, Courneya, Masse, Duval, & Schmitz, 2010).

(6) Referrals to physical or occupational therapy may be necessary to develop an appropriate plan for physical activity before, during, and after treatment.

d) Chemoradiation
(1) Caution is advised with the use of concurrent chemotherapy and RT in older adults, and dose modification may be necessary (NCCN, 2020b).

(2) Among adults aged 66 years and older with nonmetastatic head and neck squamous cell carcinomas, VanderWalde et al. (2014) found that the addition of chemotherapy to RT did not demonstrate a survival benefit.

(3) Among adults aged 65 years or older, the use of concurrent chemotherapy and RT is significantly associated with poor tolerance of treatment in those with newly diagnosed lung or head and neck cancers, gastric tube placement in those with head and neck cancers, and increased toxicity and noncompletion of recommended treatment (Middelburg et al., 2017; VanderWalde, Deal, et al., 2017).

e) Transportation
(1) Transportation is a key factor in ensuring access to daily RT treatments and follow-up appointments.

(2) Transportation challenges may be multifactorial.
(a) Distance to treatment facility
(b) Limited access to transportation
(c) Mobility issues limiting access to public transport
(d) Fatigue or other treatment side effects that affect usual transportation options
(e) Dependence on others for transportation and desire not to be a burden
(f) Financial challenges

(3) The following interventions can address transportation issues.
(a) Volunteer or community transportation support services

(b) Temporary local housing
(c) Hospitalization during treatment
(d) Hypofractionated approach, if appropriate

f) Information provision
(1) In radiation oncology, older patients report significantly less satisfaction with the amount of information received compared to younger patients and express information needs relating to treatment benefits and side effects (Jimenez-Jimenez et al., 2018; Wang et al., 2017).

(2) Older patients should be informed not only of acute, local side effects of treatment but also of the possibility of systemic side effects, such as fatigue, depression, anorexia, nausea, sleep disturbance, headache, anemia, dermatitis, and constipation (NCCN, 2020b).

(3) Wang et al. (2017) reported that older women with breast cancer undergoing RT expressed a desire for information about what will be discussed during clinical consultations and a list of questions they should ask during the visit.

g) Coordination of care
(1) Older adults with cancer may be referred to multiple specialists for assessment prior to treatment, and they may require support from various healthcare professionals throughout the treatment trajectory in the treatment center and in the community.

(2) Communication with and among all disciplines and professionals involved in an older patient's care is essential in ensuring coordination and optimal outcomes. Patients themselves highlight the importance of care coordination (Wang et al., 2017).

(3) Nurses have an important role to play in facilitating this communication to ensure coordination of care and assist patients and family members in accessing needed services.

10. Resources
a) Guidelines: See Kunkler et al. (2014) and NCCN (2020b).
b) Handbooks and manuals
(1) Holland, J.C., Wiesel, T.W., Nelson, C.J., Roth, A.J., & Alici, Y. (Eds.). (2015). *Geriatric Psycho-Oncology: A Quick Reference on the Psychological Dimensions of Cancer Symptom Management.* Oxford University Press.

(2) Korc-Grodzicki, B., & Tew, W.P. (Eds.). (2017). *Handbook of Geriatric Oncology: Practical Guide to Caring for the Older Cancer Patient.* Demos Medical.

(3) McEvoy, L.K., & Cope, D.G. (Eds.). (2012). *Caring for the Older Adult With Cancer in the Ambulatory Setting.* Oncology Nursing Society.

c) Online education
   (1) Geriatric Oncology Nursing Education Modules (Cancer Nurses Society of Australia): www.cnsa.org.au/news/geriatric-oncology-go-nursing-education-modules
   (2) Gerontological Advanced Practice Nurses Assocation: https://library.gapna.org/gapna

d) Geriatric screening and assessment: ConsultGeri (clinical website of the Hartford Institute for Geriatric Nursing): https://consultgeri.org

e) Patient information: Sinai Health System Healthy Ageing and Geriatrics: https://sinaigeriatrics.ca/healtheducation

f) Professional association: International Society of Geriatric Oncology: www.siog.org

References

Adler, N.E., & Page, A.E.K. (Eds.). (2008). *Cancer care for the whole patient: Meeting psychosocial health needs*. National Academies Press. https://doi.org/10.17226/11993

Alfano, C.M., Peng, J., Andridge, R.R., Lindgren, M.E., Povoski, S.P., Lipari, A.M., ... Kiecolt-Glaser, J.K. (2017). Inflammatory cytokines and comorbidity development in breast cancer survivors versus noncancer controls: Evidence for accelerated aging? *Journal of Clinical Oncology, 35*, 149–156. https://doi.org/10.1200/jco.2016.67.1883

Alkan, A., Yaşar, A., Karcı, E., Köksoy, E.B., Ürün, M., Şenler, F.Ç., ... Akbulut, H. (2017). Severe drug interactions and potentially inappropriate medication usage in elderly cancer patients. *Supportive Care in Cancer, 25*, 229–236. https://doi.org/10.1007/s00520-016-3409-6

American Geriatrics Society 2015 Beers Criteria Update Expert Panel. (2015). American Geriatrics Society 2015 Updated Beers Criteria for potentially inappropriate medication use in older adults. *Journal of the American Geriatrics Society, 63*, 2227–2246. https://doi.org/10.1111/jgs.13702

Appelbaum, P.S., & Grisso, T. (1988). Assessing patients' capacities to consent to treatment. *New England Journal of Medicine, 319*, 1635–1638. https://doi.org/10.1056/NEJM198812223192504

Ayalon, L., & Tesch-Römer, C. (2017). Taking a closer look at ageism: Self- and other-directed ageist attitudes and discrimination. *European Journal of Ageing, 14*, 1–4. https://doi.org/10.1007/s10433-016-0409-9

Bellera, C.A., Rainfray, M., Mathoulin-Pélissier, S., Mertens, C., Delva, F., Fonck, M., & Soubeyran, P.L. (2012). Screening older cancer patients: First evaluation of the G-8 geriatric screening tool. *Annals of Oncology, 23*, 2166–2172. https://doi.org/10.1093/annonc/mdr587

Ben-Harush, A., Shiovitz-Ezra, S., Doron, I., Alon, S., Leibovitz, A., Golander, H., ... Ayalon, L. (2017). Ageism among physicians, nurses, and social workers: Findings from a qualitative study. *European Journal of Ageing, 14*, 39–48. https://doi.org/10.1007/s10433-016-0389-9

Bluethmann, S.M., Mariotto, A.B., & Rowland, J.H. (2016). Anticipating the "Silver Tsunami": Prevalence trajectories and comorbidity burden among older cancer survivors in the United States. *Cancer Epidemiology, Biomarkers and Prevention, 25*, 1029–1036. https://doi.org/10.1158/1055-9965.epi-16-0133

Borson, S., Scanlan, J., Brush, M., Vitaliano, P., & Dokmak, A. (2000). The Mini-Cog: A cognitive 'vital signs' measure for dementia screening in multilingual elderly. *International Journal of Geriatric Psychiatry, 15*, 1021–1027. https://doi.org/10.1002/1099-1166(200011)15:11<1021::aid-gps234>3.0.co;2-6

Borson, S., Scanlan, J.M., Chen, P., & Ganguli, M. (2003). The Mini-Cog as a screen for dementia: Validation in a population-based sample. *Journal of the American Geriatrics Society, 51*, 1451–1454. https://doi.org/10.1046/j.1532-5415.2003.51465.x

Brega, A.G., Barnard, J., Mabachi, N.M., Weiss, B.D., DeWalt, D.A., Brach, C., ... West, D.R. (2018). *AHRQ health literacy universal precautions toolkit* (2nd ed.). Agency for Healthcare Research and Quality. http://www.ahrq.gov/professionals/quality-patient-safety/quality-resources/tools/literacy-toolkit/index.html

Burhenn, P.S., McCarthy, A.L., Begue, A., Nightingale, G., Cheng, K., & Kenis, C. (2016). Geriatric assessment in daily oncology practice for nurses and allied health care professionals: Opinion paper of the Nursing and Allied Health Interest Group of the International Society of Geriatric Oncology (SIOG). *Journal of Geriatric Oncology, 7*, 315–324. https://doi.org/10.1016/j.jgo.2016.02.006

Canoui-Poitrine, F., Reinald, N., Laurent, M., Guery, E., Caillet, P., David, J.-P., ... Paillaud, E. (2016). Geriatric assessment findings independently associated with clinical depression in 1092 older patients with cancer: The ELCAPA cohort study. *Psycho-Oncology, 25*, 104–111. https://doi.org/10.1002/pon.3886

Centers for Disease Control and Prevention. (n.d.). Leading indicators for chronic diseases and risk factors. https://chronicdata.cdc.gov

Chang, S., Goldstein, N.E., & Dharmarajan, K.V. (2017). Managing an older adult with cancer: Considerations for radiation oncologists. *BioMed Research International, 2017*, 1695101. https://doi.org/10.1155/2017/1695101

Charlson, M.E., Pompei, P., Ales, K.L., & MacKenzie, C.R. (1987). A new method of classifying prognostic comorbidity in longitudinal studies: Development and validation. *Journal of Chronic Diseases, 40*, 373–383. https://doi.org/10.1016/0021-9681(87)90171-8

Chen, M.J., & Nadalin, W. (2010). Peculiarities of radiotherapy in the elderly. *Radiologia Brasileira, 43*, 324–329. https://doi.org/10.1590/S0100-39842010000500012

Cheville, A.L., Beck, L.A., Petersen, T.L., Marks, R.S., & Gamble, G.L. (2009). The detection and treatment of cancer-related functional problems in an outpatient setting. *Supportive Care in Cancer, 17*, 61–67. https://doi.org/10.1007/s00520-008-0461-x

Christ, G.H., Messner, C., & Behar, L.C. (Eds.). (2015). *Handbook of oncology social work: Psychosocial care for people with cancer*. Oxford University Press.

Christoph, D.C., & Eberhardt, W.E.E. (2016). Radiotherapy in the elderly cancer patient. In M.S. Aapro & D. Schrijvers (Eds.), *ESMO handbook of cancer in the senior patient* (2nd ed., pp. 31–38). European Society for Medical Oncology.

Decoster, L., Van Puyvelde, K., Mohile, S., Wedding, U., Basso, U., Colloca, G., ... Extermann, M. (2015). Screening tools for multidimensional health problems warranting a geriatric assessment in older cancer patients: An update on SIOG recommendations. *Annals of Oncology, 26*, 288–300. https://doi.org/10.1093/annonc/mdu210

DeWees, T.A., Creach, K.M., Olsen, J.R., Bradley, J.D., & Robinson, C.G. (2012). Defining optimal comorbidity measures for patients with medically inoperable early-stage non-small cell lung cancer (NSCLC) treated with stereotactic body radiation therapy (SBRT) [Abstract]. *International Journal of Radiation Oncology, Biology, Physics, 84*(Suppl. 3), S172. https://doi.org/10.1016/j.ijrobp.2012.07.446

Duggleby, W., Ghosh, S., Cooper, D., & Dwernychuk, L. (2013). Hope in newly diagnosed cancer patients. *Journal of Pain and Symptom Management, 46*, 661–670. https://doi.org/10.1016/j.jpainsymman.2012.12.004

Duggleby, W., Holtslander, L., Steeves, M., Duggleby-Wenzel, S., & Cunningham, S. (2010). Discursive meaning of hope for older persons with advanced cancer and their caregivers. *Canadian Journal on Aging/Revue canadienne du vieillissement, 29*, 361–367. https://doi.org/10.1017/S0714980810000322

Etchells, E., Darzins, P., Silberfeld, M., Singer, P.A., McKenny, J., Naglie, G., ... Strang, D. (1999). Assessment of patient capacity to consent to treatment. *Journal of General Internal Medicine, 14*, 27–34. https://doi.org/10.1046/j.1525-1497.1999.00277.x

Ethun, C.G., Bilen, M.A., Jani, A.B., Maithel, S.K., Ogan, K., & Master, V.A. (2017). Frailty and cancer: Implications for oncology surgery, medical oncology, and radiation oncology. *CA: A Cancer Journal for Clinicians, 67*, 362–377. https://doi.org/10.3322/caac.21406

Fakhreddine, M.H., Galvan, E., Pawlowski, J., & Jones, W.E., III. (2017). Communicating effectively with elderly cancer patients. *International Journal of*

Radiation Oncology, Biology, Physics, 98, 741–742. https://doi.org/10.1016/j.ijrobp.2017.01.213

Fang, P., He, W., Gomez, D.R., Hoffman, K.E., Smith, B.D., Giordano, S.H., ... Smith, G.L. (2017). Influence of age on guideline-concordant cancer care for elderly patients in the United States. *International Journal of Radiation Oncology, Biology, Physics, 98,* 748–757. https://doi.org/10.1016/j.ijrobp.2017.01.228

Fillenbaum, G.G. (1988). *Multidimensional functional assessment of older adults: The Duke Older Americans Resources and Services Procedures.* Lawrence Erlbaum Associates.

Fiorica, F., Cartei, F., Carau, B., Berretta, S., Spartà, D., Tirelli, U., ... Berretta, M. (2009). Adjuvant radiotherapy on older and oldest elderly rectal cancer patients. *Archives of Gerontology and Geriatrics, 49,* 54–59. https://doi.org/10.1016/j.archger.2008.05.001

Folstein, M.F., Folstein, S.E., & McHugh, P.R. (1975). "Mini-mental state": A practical method for grading the cognitive state of patients for the clinician. *Journal of Psychiatric Research, 12,* 189–198. https://doi.org/10.1016/0022-3956(75)90026-6

Fried, L.P., Tangen, C.M., Walston, J., Newman, A.B., Hirsch, C., Gottdiener, J., ... McBurnie, M.A. (2001). Frailty in older adults: Evidence for a phenotype. *Journals of Gerontology: Series A, 56,* M146–M157. https://doi.org/10.1093/gerona/56.3.M146

Gerdes, S.D. (2017). Nutrition. In B. Korc-Grodzicki & W.P. Tew (Eds.), *Handbook of geriatric oncology: Practical guide to caring for the older cancer patient* (pp. 53–61). Demos Medical.

Given, B.A. (2015). Caregiver burden. In J.C. Holland, T.W. Wiesel, C.J. Nelson, A.J. Roth, & Y. Alici (Eds.), *Geriatric psycho-oncology: A quick reference on the psychosocial dimensions of cancer symptom management.* Oxford University Press.

Götze, H., Taubenheim, S., Dietz, A., Lordick, F., & Mehnert, A. (2018). Comorbid conditions and health-related quality of life in long-term cancer survivors—Associations with demographic and medical characteristics. *Journal of Cancer Survivorship, 12,* 712–720. https://doi.org/10.1007/s11764-018-0708-6

Grisso, T., Appelbaum, P.S., & Hill-Fotouhi, C. (1997). The MacCAT-T: A clinical tool to assess patients' capacities to make treatment decisions. *Psychiatric Services, 48,* 1415–1419.

Groll, D.L., To, T., Bombardier, C., & Wright, J.G. (2005). The development of a comorbidity index with physical function as the outcome. *Journal of Clinical Epidemiology, 58,* 595–602. https://doi.org/10.1016/j.jclinepi.2004.10.018

Guigoz, Y., Lauque, S., & Vellas, B.J. (2002). Identifying the elderly at risk for malnutrition: The Mini Nutritional Assessment. *Clinics in Geriatric Medicine, 18,* 737–757. https://doi.org/10.1016/S0749-0690(02)00059-9

Guralnik, J.M., Simonsick, E.M., Ferrucci, L., Glynn, R.J., Berkman, L.F., Blazer, D.G., ... Wallace, R.B. (1994). A short physical performance battery assessing lower extremity function: Association with self-reported disability and prediction of mortality and nursing home admission. *Journal of Gerontology, 49,* 85–94. https://doi.org/10.1093/geronj/49.2.M85

Haas, M.L. (2004). Utilizing geriatric skills in radiation oncology. *Geriatric Nursing, 25,* 355–360. https://doi.org/10.1016/j.gerinurse.2004.09.001

Haas, M.L. (2006). The older adult receiving radiation therapy. In D.G. Cope & A.M. Reb (Eds.), *An evidence-based approach to the treatment and care of the older adult with cancer* (pp. 311–324). Oncology Nursing Society.

Hamaker, M.E., Schiphorst, A.H., ten Bokkel Huinink, D., Schaar, C., & van Munster, B.C. (2014). The effect of a geriatric evaluation on treatment decisions for older cancer patients—A systematic review. *Acta Oncologica, 53,* 289–296. https://doi.org/10.3109/0284186x.2013.840741

Hannum, S.M., & Rubinstein, R.L. (2016). The meaningfulness of time; Narratives of cancer among chronically ill older adults. *Journal of Aging Studies, 36,* 17–25. https://doi.org/10.1016/j.jaging.2015.12.006

Harada, C.N., Natelson Love, M.C., & Triebel, K. (2013). Normal cognitive aging. *Clinics in Geriatric Medicine, 29,* 737–752. https://doi.org/10.1016/j.cger.2013.07.002

Harvey, E., & Nelson, C.J. (2015). Communicating with older cancer patients. In J.C. Holland, T.W. Wiesel, C.J. Nelson, A.J. Roth, & Y. Alici (Eds.), *Geriatric psycho-oncology: A quick reference on the psychosocial dimensions of cancer symptom management.* Oxford University Press.

Henderson, T.O., Ness, K.K., & Cohen, H.J. (2014). Accelerated aging among cancer survivors: From pediatrics to geriatrics. *American Society of Clinical Oncology Educational Book, 34,* e423–430. https://doi.org/10.14694/edbook_am.2014.34.e423

Huang, J.C., & Parvathaneni, U. (2017). Evaluation of treatment candidacy in older adults with cancer. *International Journal of Radiation Oncology, Biology, Physics, 98,* 891–892. https://doi.org/10.1016/j.ijrobp.2016.11.024

Hurria, A., Levit, L.A., Dale, W., Mohile, S.G., Muss, H.B., Fehrenbacher, L., ... Cohen, H.J. (2015). Improving the evidence base for treating older adults with cancer: American Society of Clinical Oncology statement. *Journal of Clinical Oncology, 33,* 3826–3833. https://doi.org/10.1200/jco.2015.63.0319

Inouye, S.K., van Dyck, C.H., Alessi, C.A., Balkin, S., Siegal, A.P., & Horwitz, R.I. (1990). Clarifying confusion: The confusion assessment method. A new method for detection of delirium. *Annals of Internal Medicine, 113,* 941–948. https://doi.org/10.7326/0003-4819-113-12-941

Isenring, E., & Elia, M. (2015). Which screening method is appropriate for older cancer patients at risk for malnutrition? *Nutrition, 31,* 594–597. https://doi.org/10.1016/j.nut.2014.12.027

Jimenez-Jimenez, E., Mateos, P., Ortiz, I., Aymar, N., Vidal, M., Roncero, R., ... Sabater, S. (2018). Do patients feel well informed in a radiation oncology service? *Journal of Cancer Education, 33,* 346–351. https://doi.org/10.1007/s13187-016-1117-z

Katz, J.N., Chang, L.C., Sangha, O., Fossel, A.H., & Bates, D.W. (1996). Can comorbidity be measured by questionnaire rather than medical record review? *Medical Care, 34,* 73–84. https://doi.org/10.1097/00005650-199601000-00006

Katz, S., Ford, A.B., Moskowitz, R.W., Jackson, B.A., & Jaffe, M.W. (1963). Studies of illness in the aged: The Index of ADL: A standardized measure of biological and psychosocial function. *JAMA, 185,* 914–919. https://doi.org/10.1001/jama.1963.03060120024016

Khor, R.C., Bressel, M., Tedesco, J., Tai, K.H., Ball, D.L., Duchesne, G.M., ... Foroudi, F. (2015). Tolerability and outcomes of curative radiotherapy in patients aged 85 or more years. *Medical Journal of Australia, 202,* 153–155. https://doi.org/10.5694/mja14.00441

Kunkler, I.H., Audisio, R., Belkacemi, Y., Betz, M., Gore, E., Hoffe, S., ... Villa, S. (2014). Review of current best practice and priorities for research in radiation oncology for elderly patients with cancer: The International Society of Geriatric Oncology (SIOG) task force. *Annals of Oncology, 25,* 2134–2146. https://doi.org/10.1093/annonc/mdu104

Lawler, M., Selby, P., Aapro, M.S., & Duffy, S. (2014). Ageism in cancer care. *British Medical Journal, 348,* g1614. https://doi.org/10.1136/bmj.g1614

Lawton, M.P., & Brody, E.M. (1969). Assessment of older people: Self-maintaining and instrumental activities of daily living. *Gerontologist, 9,* 179–186.

Lee, V. (2008). The existential plight of cancer: Meaning making as a concrete approach to the intangible search for meaning. *Supportive Care in Cancer, 16,* 779–785. https://doi.org/10.1007/s00520-007-0396-7

Liu, K., Wang, P., Zhu, X., Bei, Y., Zheng, Z., & Yan, S. (2018). Disparities of age-based cancer-specific survival improvement with various clinicopathologic characteristics for kidney cancer. *Cancer Management and Research, 10,* 2259–2268. https://doi.org/10.2147/CMAR.S169192

Loh, K.P., Soto-Perez-de-Celis, E., Hsu, T., de Glas, N.A., Battisti, N.M.L., Baldini, C., ... Wildiers, H. (2018). What every oncologist should know about geriatric assessment for older patients with cancer: Young International Society of Geriatric Oncology position paper. *Journal of Oncology Practice, 14,* 85–94. https://doi.org/10.1200/JOP.2017.026435

Maleki, S., Alexander, M., Liu, C., Rischin, D., Lingaratnam, S., & Fua, T. (2020). Radiation oncology outpatient medication management needs and service gaps – A cross-sectional study of patients and clinicians. *Journal of Oncology Pharmacy Practice, 26,* 846–852. https://doi.org/10.1177/1078155219875210

Mathew, L., & Fulton, C. (2017). Social isolation and caregiver burden. In B. Korc-Grodzicki, & W.P. Tew (Eds.), *Handbook of geriatric oncology: Practical guide to caring for the older cancer patient* (pp. 99–103). Demos Medical.

McAleese, J., Baluch, S., Drinkwater, K., Bassett, P., & Hanna, G.G. (2017). The elderly are less likely to receive recommended radical radiotherapy for non-small cell lung cancer. *Clinical Oncology, 29,* 593–600. https://doi.org/10.1016/j.clon.2017.06.014

McFarland, D.C., Blackler, L., Hlubocky, F.J., Saracino, R., Masciale, J., Chin, M., ... Voigt, L. (2020). Decisional capacity determination in patients with cancer. *Oncology, 34,* 203–206. https://www.cancernetwork.com/view/decisional-capacity-determination-in-patients-with-cancer

McKoy, J.M., Burhenn, P.S., Browner, I.S., Loeser, K.L., Tulas, K.M., Oden, M.R., & Rupper, R.W. (2014). Assessing cognitive function and capacity in older adults with cancer. *Journal of the National Comprehensive Cancer Network, 12,* 138–144. https://doi.org/10.6004/jnccn.2014.0011

Middelburg, J.G., Mast, M.E., de Kroon, M., Jobsen, J.J., Rozema, T., Maas, H., ... Struikmans, H. (2017). Timed Get Up and Go test and Geriatric 8 scores and the association with (chemo-)radiation therapy noncompliance and acute toxicity in elderly cancer patients. *International Journal of Radiation Oncology, Biology, Physics, 98,* 843–849. https://doi.org/10.1016/j.ijrobp.2017.01.211

Mohile, S.G., Dale, W., Somerfield, M.R., Schonberg, M.A., Boyd, C.M., Burhenn, P.S., ... Hurria, A. (2018). Practical assessment and management of vulnerabilities in older patients receiving chemotherapy: ASCO guideline for geriatric oncology. *Journal of Clinical Oncology, 36,* 2326–2347. https://doi.org/10.1200/jco.2018.78.8687

Mohile, S.G., Epstein, R.M., Hurria, A., Heckler, C.E., Canin, B., Culakova, E., ... Dale, W. (2020). Communication with older patients with cancer using geriatric assessment: A cluster-randomized clinical trial from the National Cancer Institute Community Oncology Research Program. *JAMA Oncology, 6,* 196–204. https://doi.org/10.1001/jamaoncol.2019.4728

Moloney, E. (2014). Ageing and cancer: A complex relationship. *Cancer Forum, 38,* 235–238. https://www.cancer.org.au/content/healthprofessional/CancerForum/issues/2014-November.pdf

Mukhtar, F., Boffetta, P., Dabo, B., Park, J.Y., Tran, C.T.D., Tran, T.V., ... Luu, H.N. (2018). Disparities by race, age, and sex in the improvement of survival for lymphoma: Findings from a population-based study. *PLOS ONE, 13,* e0199745. https://doi.org/10.1371/journal.pone.0199745

Muluneh, B., Deal, A., Alexander, M.D., Keisler, M.D., Markey, J.M., Neal, J.M., ... Dressler, L.G. (2018). Patient perspectives on the barriers associated with medication adherence to oral chemotherapy. *Journal of Oncology Pharmacy Practice, 24,* 98–109. https://doi.org/10.1177/1078155216679026

Nasreddine, Z.S., Phillips, N.A., Bédirian, V., Charbonneau, S., Whitehead, V., Collin, I., ... Chertkow, H. (2005). The Montreal Cognitive Assessment, MoCA: A brief screening tool for mild cognitive impairment. *Journal of the American Geriatrics Society, 53,* 695–699. https://doi.org/10.1111/j.1532-5415.2005.53221.x

National Comprehensive Cancer Network. (2020a). *NCCN Clinical Practice Guidelines in Oncology (NCCN® Guidelines): Distress management* [v.2.2020]. https://www.nccn.org/professionals/physician_gls/pdf/distress.pdf

National Comprehensive Cancer Network. (2020b). *NCCN Clinical Practice Guidelines in Oncology (NCCN® Guidelines): Older adult oncology* [v.1.2020]. https://www.nccn.org/professionals/physician_gls/pdf/senior.pdf

Neo, J., Fettes, L., Gao, W., Higginson, I.J., & Maddocks, M. (2017). Disability in activities of daily living among adults with cancer: A systematic review and meta-analysis. *Cancer Treatment Reviews, 61,* 94–106. https://doi.org/10.1016/j.ctrv.2017.10.006

Nieder, C., Mannsåker, B., Pawinski, A., & Haukland, E. (2017). Polypharmacy in older patients ≥70 years receiving palliative radiotherapy. *Anticancer Research, 37,* 795–799. https://doi.org/10.21873/anticanres.11379

Nightingale, G., Skonecki, E., & Boparai, M.K. (2017). The impact of polypharmacy on patient outcomes in older adults with cancer. *Cancer Journal, 23,* 211–218. https://doi.org/10.1097/PPO.0000000000000277

O'Donovan, A., Leech, M., & Gillham, C. (2017). Assessment and management of radiotherapy induced toxicity in older patients. *Journal of Geriatric Oncology, 8,* 421–427. https://doi.org/10.1016/j.jgo.2017.07.001

O'Mahony, D., Gallagher, P., Ryan, C., Byrne, S., Hamilton, H., Barry, P., ... Kennedy, J. (2010). STOPP & START criteria: A new approach to detecting potentially inappropriate prescribing in old age. *European Geriatric Medicine, 1,* 45–51. https://doi.org/10.1016/j.eurger.2010.01.007

Pamoukdjian, F., Aparicio, T., Zebachi, S., Zelek, L., Paillaud, E., & Canoui-Poitrine, F. (2020). Comparison of mobility indices for predicting early death in older patients with cancer: The physical frailty in elderly cancer cohort study. *Journals of Gerontology: Series A, 75,* 189–196. https://doi.org/10.1093/gerona/glz024

Pamoukdjian, F., Paillaud, E., Zelek, L., Laurent, M., Lévy, V., Landre, T., & Sebbane, G. (2015). Measurement of gait speed in older adults to identify complications associated with frailty: A systematic review. *Journal of Geriatric Oncology, 6,* 484–496. https://doi.org/10.1016/j.jgo.2015.08.006

Parpa, E., Tsilika, E., Gennimata, V., & Mystakidou, K. (2015). Elderly cancer patients' psychopathology: A systematic review: Aging and mental health. *Archives of Gerontology and Geriatrics, 60,* 9–15. https://doi.org/10.1016/j.archger.2014.09.008

Perlow, H.K., Cassidy, V., Farnia, B., Kwon, D., Awerbuch, A.W., Ciraula, S., ... Samuels, S.E. (2019). Impact of performance status and comorbidity on palliative radiation treatment tolerance and end-of-life decision-making. *Advances in Radiation Oncology, 4,* 127–133. https://doi.org/10.1016/j.adro.2018.09.002

Pilleron, S., Sarfati, D., Janssen-Heijnen, M., Vignat, J., Ferlay, J., Bray, F., & Soerjomataram, I. (2019). Global cancer incidence in older adults, 2012 and 2035: A population-based study. *International Journal of Cancer, 144,* 49–58. https://doi.org/10.1002/ijc.31664

Puchalski, C., & Romer, A.L. (2000). Taking a spiritual history allows clinicians to understand patients more fully. *Journal of Palliative Medicine, 3,* 129–137. https://doi.org/10.1089/jpm.2000.3.129

Puts, M.T.E., & Alibhai, S.M.H. (2018). Fighting back against the dilution of the Comprehensive Geriatric Assessment. *Journal of Geriatric Oncology, 9,* 3–5. https://doi.org/10.1016/j.jgo.2017.08.009

Roth, A.J., Greenstein, M., Weisel, T.W., & Schulberg, S. (2015). Depressive spectrum disorders and grief. In J.C. Holland, T.W. Wiesel, C.J. Nelson, A.J. Roth, & Y. Alici (Eds.), *Geriatric psycho-oncology: A quick reference on the psychosocial dimensions of cancer symptom management* (pp. 59–68). Oxford University Press.

Rottenberg, Y., Litwin, H., Manor, O., Paltiel, A., Barchana, M., & Paltiel, O. (2014). Prediagnostic self-assessed health and extent of social networks predict survival in older individuals with cancer: A population based cohort study. *Journal of Geriatric Oncology, 5,* 400–407. https://doi.org/10.1016/j.jgo.2014.08.001

Rubenstein, L., Calkins, E., Andres, R., Besdine, R., Rossman, I., Jarvik, L., & Cohen, H. (2004). Comprehensive geriatric assessment: From miracle to reality. *Journal of Gerontology: Medical Sciences, 59A,* 473–477.

Saliba, D., Elliott, M., Rubenstein, L.Z., Solomon, D.H., Young, R.T., Kamberg, C.J., ... Wenger, N.S. (2001). The vulnerable elders survey: A tool for identifying vulnerable older people in the community. *Journal of the American Geriatrics Society, 49,* 1691–1699. https://doi.org/10.1046/j.1532-5415.2001.49281.x

Saracino, R.M., Rosenfeld, B., & Nelson, C.J. (2016). Towards a new conceptualization of depression in older adult cancer patients: A review of the literature. *Aging and Mental Health, 20,* 1230–1242. https://doi.org/10.1080/13607863.2015.1078278

Saracino, R.M., Weinberger, M.I., Roth, A.J., Hurria, A., & Nelson, C.J. (2017). Assessing depression in a geriatric cancer population. *Psycho-Oncology, 26,* 1484–1490. https://doi.org/10.1002/pon.4160

Sattar, S., Alibhai, S.M.H., Fitch, M., Krzyzanowska, M., Leighl, N., & Puts, M.T.E. (2018). Chemotherapy and radiation treatment decision-making experiences of older adults with cancer: A qualitative study. *Journal of Geriatric Oncology, 9,* 47–52. https://doi.org/10.1016/j.jgo.2017.07.013

Sattar, S., Alibhai, S.M.H., Spoelstra, S.L., & Puts, M.T.E. (2019). The assessment, management, and reporting of falls, and the impact of falls on cancer treatment in community-dwelling older patients receiving cancer treatment: Results from a mixed-methods study. *Journal of Geriatric Oncology, 10,* 98–104. https://doi.org/10.1016/j.jgo.2018.08.006

Schroyen, S., Adam, S., Marquet, M., Jerusalem, G., Thiel, S., Giraudet, A.-L., & Missotten, P. (2018). Communication of healthcare professionals: Is there ageism? *European Journal of Cancer Care, 27,* e12780. https://doi.org/10.1111/ecc.12780

Sessums, L.L., Zembrzuska, H., & Jackson, J.L. (2011). Does this patient have medical decision-making capacity? *JAMA, 306,* 420–427. https://doi.org/10.1001/jama.2011.1023

Shahrokni, A., Alexander, K., Wildes, T.M., & Puts, M.T.E. (2018). Preventing treatment-related functional decline: Strategies to maximize resilience. *American Society of Clinical Oncology Educational Book, 38,* 415–431. https://doi.org/10.1200/edbk_200427

Shajani, Z., & Snell, D. (2019). *Wright and Leahey's nurses and families: A guide to family assessment and intervention* (7th ed.). F.A. Davis.

Sheikh, J.I., & Yesavage, J.A. (1986). Geriatric Depression Scale (GDS): Recent evidence and development of a shorter version. *Clinical Gerontologist, 5,* 165–173. https://doi.org/10.1300/J018v05n01_09

Smith, A., Widera, E., Lee, S.J., Schonberg, M., Schoenborn, N., & Yourman, L. (n.d.). What is ePrognosis? https://eprognosis.ucsf.edu/about.php

Smith, G.L., & Smith, B.D. (2014). Radiation treatment in older patients: A framework for clinical decision making. *Journal of Clinical Oncology, 32,* 2669–2678. https://doi.org/10.1200/JCO.2014.55.1168

Soubeyran, P., Bellera, C., Goyard, J., Heitz, D., Curé, H., Rousselot, H., ... Rainfray, M. (2014). Screening for vulnerability in older cancer patients: The ONCODAGE prospective multicenter cohort study. *PLOS ONE, 9,* e115060. https://doi.org/10.1371/journal.pone.0115060

Speck, R.M., Courneya, K.S., Masse, L.C., Duval, S., & Schmitz, K.H. (2010). An update of controlled physical activity trials in cancer survivors: A systematic review and meta-analysis. *Journal of Cancer Survivorship, 4,* 87–100. https://doi.org/10.1007/s11764-009-0110-5

Stairmand, J., Signal, L., Sarfati, D., Jackson, C., Batten, L., Holdaway, M., & Cunningham, C. (2015). Consideration of comorbidity in treatment decision making in multidisciplinary cancer team meetings: A systematic review. *Annals of Oncology, 26,* 1325–1332. https://doi.org/10.1093/annonc/mdv025

Steinhauser, K.E., Voils, C.I., Clipp, E.C., Bosworth, H.B., Christakis, N.A., & Tulsky, J.A. (2006). "Are you at peace?": One item to probe spiritual concerns at the end of life. *Archives of Internal Medicine, 166,* 101–105. https://doi.org/10.1001/archinte.166.1.101

Strohschein, F.J. (2019). *Submitting to the momentum of care: Processes of treatment decision making among older people with colorectal cancer* (Doctoral thesis, McGill University, Montreal, Canada). https://escholarship.mcgill.ca/concern/theses/nz806444b

Strohschein, F.J., Fitch, M., & Vanderbyl, B. (2020). Optimizing cancer survivorship for older adults. In *Adult cancer survivorship: A self-learning resource for nurses.* Canadian Association of Nurses in Oncology.

Szumacher, E., Sattar, S., Neve, M., Do, K., Ayala, A.P., Gray, M., ... Puts, M. (2018). Use of comprehensive geriatric assessment and geriatric screening for older adults in the radiation oncology setting: A systematic review. *Clinical Oncology, 30,* 578–588. https://doi.org/10.1016/j.clon.2018.04.008

VanderWalde, N.A., Deal, A.M., Comitz, E., Stravers, L., Muss, H., Reeve, B.B., ... Chera, B. (2017). Geriatric assessment as a predictor of tolerance, quality of life, and outcomes in older patients with head and neck cancers and lung cancers receiving radiation therapy. *International Journal of Radiation Oncology, Biology, Physics, 98,* 850–857. https://doi.org/10.1016/j.ijrobp.2016.11.048

VanderWalde, N., Hurria, A., & Jagsi, R. (2017). Improving consistency and quality of care for older adults with cancer: The challenges of developing consensus guidelines for radiation therapy. *International Journal of Radiation Oncology, Biology, Physics, 98,* 721–725. https://doi.org/10.1016/j.ijrobp.2016.11.042

VanderWalde, N.A., Meyer, A.M., Deal, A.M., Layton, J.B., Liu, H., Carpenter, W.R., ... Chera, B.S. (2014). Effectiveness of chemoradiation for head and neck cancer in an older patient population. *International Journal of Radiation Oncology, Biology, Physics, 89,* 30–37. https://doi.org/10.1016/j.ijrobp.2014.01.053

Vellas, B., Guigoz, Y., Garry, P.J., Nourhashemi, F., Bennahum, D., Lauque, S., & Albarede, J.L. (1999). The Mini Nutritional Assessment (MNA) and its use in grading the nutritional state of elderly patients. *Nutrition, 15,* 116–122.

Wang, S.-Y., Kelly, G., Gross, C., Killelea, B.K., Mougalian, S., Presley, C., ... Evans, S.B. (2017). Information needs of older women with early-stage breast cancer when making radiation therapy decisions. *International Journal of Radiation Oncology, Biology, Physics, 98,* 733–740. https://doi.org/10.1016/j.ijrobp.2017.02.001

Whitman, A.M., DeGregory, K.A., Morris, A.L., & Ramsdale, E.E. (2016). A comprehensive look at polypharmacy and medication screening tools for the older cancer patient. *Oncologist, 21,* 723–730. https://doi.org/10.1634/theoncologist.2015-0492

Wiesel, T.W. (2015). Demoralization, despair, and existential concerns. In J.C. Holland, T.W. Wiesel, C.J. Nelson, A.J. Roth, & Y. Alici (Eds.), *Geriatric psycho-oncology: A quick reference on the psychosocial dimensions of cancer symptom management.* Oxford University Press.

Wildiers, H., Heeren, P., Puts, M., Topinkova, E., Janssen-Heijnen, M.L.G., Extermann, M., ... Hurria, A. (2014). International Society of Geriatric Oncology consensus on geriatric assessment in older patients with cancer. *Journal of Clinical Oncology, 32,* 2595–2603. https://doi.org/10.1200/jco.2013.54.8347

Williams, G.R., Mackenzie, A., Magnuson, A., Olin, R., Chapman, A., Mohile, S., ... Holmes, H. (2016). Comorbidity in older adults with cancer. *Journal of Geriatric Oncology, 7,* 249–257. https://doi.org/10.1016/j.jgo.2015.12.002

Williams, G.R., Pisu, M., Rocque, G.B., Williams, C.P., Taylor, R.A., Kvale, E.A. ... Kenzik, K.M. (2019). Unmet social support needs among older adults with cancer. *Cancer, 125,* 473–481. https://doi.org/10.1002/cncr.31809

World Health Organization. (2015). *World report on aging and health.* https://www.who.int/ageing/events/world-report-2015-launch/en

Wyman, M.F., Shiovitz-Ezra, S., & Bengel, J. (2018). Ageism in the health care system: Providers, patients, and systems. In L. Ayalon & C. Tesch-Römer (Eds.), *Contemporary perspectives on ageism* (pp. 193–212). Springer. https://doi.org/10.1007/978-3-319-73820-8_13

Yourman, L.C., Lee, S.J., Schonberg, M.A., Widera, E.W., & Smith, A.K. (2012). Prognostic indices for older adults: A systematic review. *JAMA, 307,* 182–192. https://doi.org/10.1001/jama.2011.1966

Zaremba, T., Jakobsen, A.R., Søgaard, M., Thøgersen, A.M., & Riahi, S., (2015). Radiotherapy in patients with pacemakers and implantable cardioverter defibrillators: A literature review. *EP Europace, 18,* 479–491. https://doi.org/10.1093/europace/euv135

Zeng, C., Wen, W., Morgans, A.K., Pao, W., Shu, X.-O., & Zheng, W. (2015). Disparities by race, age, and sex in the improvement of survival for major cancers: Results from the National Cancer Institute Surveillance, Epidemiology, and End Results (SEER) Program in the United States, 1990 to 2010. *JAMA Oncology, 1,* 88–96. https://doi.org/10.1001/jamaoncol.2014.161

Zhang, X., Tang, T., Pang, L., Sharma, S.V., Li, R., Nyitray, A.G., & Edwards, B.J. (2019). Malnutrition and overall survival in older adults with cancer: A systematic review and meta-analysis. *Journal of Geriatric Oncology, 10,* 874–883. https://doi.org/10.1016/j.jgo.2019.03.002

D. Patients with special needs

1. Definition

   a) Special needs are defined in a variety of ways, depending on the country or geographic region or the context in which special needs are addressed, such as education, health care, or government.

   b) In North America, the term is often linked to diagnostic or functional development and refers to individuals with medical, physical, and psychological or mental disabilities, including those requiring additional support beyond what is required by the general group or population.

   c) In the context of RT, *special needs* refer to comorbidities and disabilities affecting the delivery or side effects of treatment, psychosocial and functional concerns of patients undergoing RT, and special populations (e.g., pediatric, older adult) or unique concerns of populations of patients receiving RT.

2. Medical comorbidities
   a) Definition
      (1) A comorbidity is a disease that coexists with a cancer diagnosis (Sarfati, Koczwara, & Jackson, 2016).
      (2) As individuals age, comorbidities increase.
      (3) A comorbidity is present for a year or more and requires medical attention.
      (4) These can also affect an individual's ADLs.
   b) Prognosis
      (1) Medical comorbidities represent a major prognostic factor in the long-term survival of patients with cancer.
      (2) Patients diagnosed with the four cancers of highest incidence have high rates of comorbidities (NCI, 2016).
         (a) Lung: 52.9%
         (b) Colorectal: 40.7%
         (c) Breast: 32.2%
         (d) Prostate: 30.5%
      (3) Comorbidities can add complexity to cancer care and management (Pirschel, 2017b).
   c) Survival rates: According to NCI, patients aged 66 years and older with a comorbidity have an increased probability of death (NCI, 2013).
   d) Challenges
      (1) A patient, cancer diagnosis, and comorbidities should be managed holistically, not only as a single diagnosis of cancer (Sarfati et al., 2016).
      (2) The severity of comorbidities affects a patient's trajectory of care, as well as the influence of confounding medical issues, age, sex, ethnicity, and socioeconomic status.
3. Treatment side effects
   a) As a result of aging and associated limitations in organ systems that prolong plasma levels of chemotherapy, older adults are at an increased risk for treatment-related toxicity and poor outcomes (Hurria et al., 2016).
   b) Geddie, Loerzel, and Norris (2016) reported that, although cancer treatment often results in a myriad of treatment-related symptoms, the degree of symptoms may be more related to comorbid illnesses rather than cancer and its treatment.
   c) Loerzel (2018) confirmed that comorbid illness symptoms may make treatment-related symptoms worse.
   d) Presence of a comorbidity, such as diabetes mellitus, renal disease, heart disease, and lung disease, decreases the ability to tolerate treatment (Cope, Reb, Schwartz, & Simon, 2018).
   e) The presence of comorbidity can also have a myriad of nursing practice implications related to symptom management.
      (1) Assessment tools for functional status, nutritional assessment, social support availability, cognitive screening, and chemotherapy toxicity screening can be helpful in clinical practice (Goldberg, Burhenn, & Ginex, 2018).
      (2) As the population ages, more patients will be living with cancer and comorbidities.
      (3) Coordination with other specialties in managing comorbidities is essential (Goldberg et al., 2018).
         (a) Patients could be referred to a physical therapist or an occupational therapist as needed to build or maintain function.
         (b) Referral to an RDN or RD is warranted if a patient is not eating well, experiencing weight loss, or experiencing changes in appetite.
4. Physical disability
   a) Definition (World Health Organization, 2018)
      (1) The International Classification of Functioning, Disability and Health defines *disability* as a broad term for impairments, limitations in activity, and restrictions in participation.
      (2) Disability is largely related to interaction between people with health conditions and personal and environmental factors (e.g., negative attitudes, transportation, building access, social supports).
   b) Pretreatment practice implications
      (1) Clinical and RT staff (nurses and radiation therapists), nurse navigators, or social workers (if available) may need to intervene to set up transportation arrangements for daily treatment. Some patients may rely on a caregiver and family for transportation, but they may not be prepared or able to assist with appropriate equipment.
      (2) Transportation assistance may be available for patients with disabilities.
         (a) Availability of insurance-assisted transportation may be determined by income requirements.
         (b) Community RT centers may not have access to the same level of transportation assistance that may be available in urban areas.
         (c) Scheduling of appointments may be contingent on transportation schedules.
      (3) RT nurses need to educate staff and provide appropriate equipment to facilitate safe transfers.
      (4) RT staff, patients, and caregivers must anticipate increased time for treatment administration and physical examinations during visits.
   c) Treatment practice implications
      (1) The goal is to maintain a patient's functional independence or preexisting level of function during and after treatment.

(2) Staff should anticipate and reduce the occurrence of secondary conditions.

d) Post-treatment practice implications

(1) Many patients may need referral to various therapies during or after active treatment to rebuild their strength, endurance, and physical stability.

(2) Clarke, Radford, Coffey, and Stewart (2016) reviewed the official guidelines regarding rehabilitation of patients with head and neck cancer. These guidelines included pretreatment assessment of speech and swallowing, as well as ongoing exercises to aid the patient in their rehabilitation.

(3) Patients without an initial disability may develop a disability related to the treatments they have undergone, resulting in a need for referral to physical therapy, speech therapy, lymphedema therapy, and other rehabilitation specialists (American Cancer Society, 2019).

(4) Cheville et al. (2017) suggested that the need for cancer rehabilitation is increasing, but current models of rehabilitation have not been validated.

(a) Oncology rehabilitation can help a patient recover from the disease, treatment, and associated physical changes.

(b) Rehabilitation can help a patient achieve maximum recovery.

(c) Rehabilitation is an appropriate option for cancer survivors who are experiencing weakness, experiencing more fatigue than prior to cancer diagnosis, having difficulty with ADLs, or having difficulty recovering from the treatment (Livestrong, n.d.).

5. Obesity

a) Definition

(1) CDC (2020) defines obesity as a body mass index greater than 30 (i.e., more than what is healthy for the given height of an individual).

(2) Morbid obesity is a body mass index greater than 40.

(3) Obesity increases the risk of diabetes, hypertension, and cardiovascular diseases.

b) Practice implications

(1) Appropriate supplies and equipment should be accessible to facilitate patient care.

(a) Extra-large hospital gowns

(b) Scale with weight capacity of greater than 350 pounds

(c) Patient lift with appropriate weight capacity

(d) Large blood pressure cuffs

(e) Large wheelchairs for transport

(2) CT planning and the use of daily cone beam imaging may provide challenges with morbidly obese patients because of the machine's small opening (bore) and difficulty moving equipment around the patient when using cone beam imaging.

(3) Nurses provide assistance as required on and off the treatment table. Nurses must always treat patients with respect and dignity.

(4) Clinicians should evaluate for sarcopenic obesity, a medical condition in which patients have low muscle mass and strength but high fat mass (Lindsey, Astroth, & Kumar, 2016).

(a) Patients undergoing treatments with predicted weight loss as a side effect should be evaluated for sarcopenic obesity.

(b) Treatment for sarcopenic obesity is physical therapy to increase muscle mass and strength.

(c) Clinicians should provide dietary referrals as needed.

6. Visual impairment and blindness

a) Preexisting visual impairment and blindness

(1) Patients with visual impairments or blindness can encounter unique challenges that can hinder access to safe, patient-centered care.

(2) Several actions can be taken to ensure patient understanding and trust in clinicians.

(a) Read aloud what is being written in the medical record.

(b) Speak directly to the patient.

(c) Explain to the patient what will be done.

(d) Let the patient feel the equipment before treatment if possible.

(e) Always say goodbye when leaving a patient's room or treatment area.

b) Practice implications: Vision Australia (n.d.) recommended the following interventions for healthcare providers to improve the overall cancer treatment experience for patients with visual impairments or blindness.

(1) Communication

(a) All RT team members participating in a patient interaction should introduce themselves.

(b) Team members should address the patient by name so that he or she is cognizant of the conversation.

(c) Clinicians should speak to patients in a normal tone of voice.

(d) Clinicians must ensure that a patient is aware when the radiation therapist is exiting the treatment room and will be monitoring by intercom and camera.

(e) Clinicians must explain all procedures to a patient and always inform a patient prior to commencement of any physical contact.

(2) Respect

    (a) The patient must be central in all discussions about the cancer diagnosis and planned RT because visual impairment does not hinder ability to fully participate in healthcare decision-making.

    (b) Clinicians must ask the patient what assistance, if any, is required.

(3) Physical access and mobility

    (a) Clinicians should orient a patient to the examination room or radiation suite by utilizing a central point.

    (b) Clinicians should accompany the patient in new clinical areas, which will aid the patient in deciphering both spatial and sensory cues.

    (c) Guide dogs are permitted in patient areas.

      i. Guide dogs cannot be refused entry to the hospital or cancer center. This is supported through federal legislation.

      ii. Guide dogs should not be touched when they are wearing a working harness.

      iii. During the RT session, a guide dog can remain with staff outside the treatment unit.

    (d) Clinicians should invite the patient to take their arm for guiding purposes.

(4) Access to information: Whenever possible, information regarding cancer diagnosis and RT should be provided in Braille, large print, or audio format.

c) Treatment-related visual impairment

(1) Patients whose RT fields encompass critical eye structures may lose their vision immediately or over time as a result of RT (e.g., patients with brain or nasopharyngeal cancers where treatment margins are close to or involve the optic nerve or optic chiasm) (Ferguson, Huecker, Huang, McClelland, & Van Stavern, 2017).

(2) Clinicians must provide education, supportive counseling, and referral to resources for patients who will lose their vision immediately or over time as a result of RT.

7. Hearing impairment

a) Preexisting hearing impairment

(1) Patients with preexisting hearing impairment are at risk for not understanding their diagnosis or treatment options.

(2) They may use many different forms of communicating.

b) Practice implications: Interventions for hearing-impaired individuals include the following (Funk, Garcia, & Mullen, 2018; Newton & Shah, 2013).

(1) Clinicians must ask the patient about preference in communication style and make appropriate accommodations as needed, such as the usage of interpreters, emails, and faxes.

(2) Staff should ensure privacy so that a patient can ask questions without fearing others will overhear.

(3) Staff must be mindful not to speak loudly in public places when speaking with a patient because of privacy issues.

(4) Staff must provide a quiet environment for all interactions.

(5) Assessment rooms should have appropriate lighting to facilitate communication (e.g., lip reading).

(6) Clinicians should ask for permission to discuss sensitive subjects in the presence of a caregiver.

(7) Staff should always face the patient when speaking.

(8) Clinicians should speak slowly and in simple sentences.

(9) An interpreter or communication service should be employed if needed.

(10) Clinicians must always inform a patient prior to touching or physical contact.

(11) Clinicians should ask questions about treatment and care to ensure that a patient understands.

(12) Clinicians can use visual aids (pictures or drawings), if necessary, to explain.

(13) Clinicians should provide important information in writing, such as appointment times and medication instructions.

(14) Staff should ask the patient if the current communication style is effective, and if not, what measures could be employed to rectify unsatisfactory circumstances.

c) Treatment-related hearing impairment practice implications

(1) Clinicians should provide referrals for routine and follow-up hearing assessment for patients who are at risk of hearing loss as a result of RT or combined modality treatment (e.g., IMRT and cisplatin chemotherapy for head and neck cancers).

(2) Clinicians must advocate for assistance and funding of hearing aids or assistive devices.

8. Frailty (see also IX.C. Older adult radiation oncology)

a) "Frailty is defined as a disability in those of advanced age, often with comorbidities, poor nutritional status, cognitive decline, and reduced functional status" (Overcash, Cope, & Van Cleave, 2018, p. 8).

b) CGA is recommended.

c) NCCN (2020b) recommends the following measures related to collaboration in older adult oncology settings.

(1) Referral to a geriatrician to help assess patient

(2) Assessment of cognitive impairment, dementia, and delirium
(3) Assessment of life expectancy to aid in advance care planning and guardianship
(4) Assessment of functional or physical impairment, mobility issues, or disability
(5) Assessment of multimorbidity, including vision and hearing impairments
(6) Polypharmacy evaluation
(7) Assessment of weight loss (5% or greater unintentional weight loss in the previous three months) and anorexia
(8) Referral to an RDN or RD to assist with nutritional status

9. Psychosocial issues
  a) Distress and coping (see also IV.D. Distress and coping)
    (1) Definition: NCCN (2020a) defines distress in cancer as "a multifactorial unpleasant experience of a psychological (i.e., cognitive, behavioral, emotional), social, spiritual, and/or physical nature that may interfere with the ability to cope effectively with cancer, its physical symptoms, and its treatment. Distress extends along a continuum, ranging from common normal feelings of vulnerability, sadness, and fears to problems that can become disabling, such as depression, anxiety, panic, social isolation, and existential and spiritual crisis" (p. DIS-1).
    (2) Susceptible patients: NCCN (2020a) identified the following preexisting patient factors that place an individual with cancer at increased risk for emotional distress throughout the care experience.
      (a) History of depression or suicide attempt
      (b) Uncontrolled symptoms
      (c) Substance abuse
      (d) Diminished cognitive functioning
      (e) Multiple medical comorbidities
      (f) Spiritual or religious conflicts
      (g) Limited support network
      (h) Family or caregiver discord
      (i) Financial concerns
      (j) Living alone
      (k) Dependent child or children
      (l) Younger age and female sex
      (m) Communication issues (e.g., language, literacy, speech and hearing problems)
      (n) Past abuse (physical and/or sexual)
      (o) Psychiatric disorder
    (3) Pretreatment distress
      (a) The timing between initial visit and initiation of treatment can cause distress for patients.
      (b) Often, additional tests, exams, referrals for procedures, or physician visits add to the length of time between initial evaluation and the start of treatment.
      (c) It is important for RT staff to give thorough instructions about procedures, such as simulation, and answer questions about treatment options and available resources.
      (d) The establishment of trust during the first visit helps ease the fears and distress of patients, caregivers, and family (Hamilton, Kruse, Holcomb, & Freche, 2018).
    (4) Distress during treatment
      (a) Clinicians should assess distress at the beginning of treatment and at any change in condition utilizing the NCCN Distress Thermometer or a similar tool (NCCN, 2020a).
      (b) Clinicians should refer patients to support services (e.g., social services, spiritual and chaplain services, psychological and psychiatric services, palliative care) as needed (NCCN, 2020a).
    (5) Post-treatment distress
      (a) After completion of treatment, clinicians can utilize phone calls to check on patients as needed (Bunch, 2016).
      (b) Clinicians should assess patients on follow-up visits to check how they are feeling and coping.
    (6) Treatment implications and recommended interventions
      (a) Clinicians must identify clinically significant distress in patients with cancer because it can have profound implications on treatment outcomes.
      (b) Clinicians should encourage early intervention when predictors of distress have been noted.
      (c) Clinicians should continually assess distress and be aware of predictors to improve communication between nurses and patients and expedite referrals to appropriate psychosocial support services (Hamilton et al., 2018).
      (d) Clinicians can anticipate stressful situations and recognize patients who are vulnerable to experience emotional discord.
        i. Interventions for those requiring emotional support during an aspect of their oncology trajectory of care are both situational and patient dependent.
        ii. NCCN (2020a) recommends the following options to improve patients' overall emotional status.
          • Symptom management

- Psychosocial interventions
- Pharmacology options
- Complementary and integrative therapies
- Referral to mental health team
- Counseling
- Referral for spiritual care

b) Anxiety (see also IV.D. Distress and coping)
  (1) Pretreatment anxiety
    (a) The planning phase prior to the initiation of RT involves periods of waiting, multiple consultations, and various medical investigations—all of which can produce emotional suffering for a patient with cancer (NCCN, 2020a).
    (b) Different forms of patient education are available to help reduce anxiety.
    (c) Marquess et al. (2017) conducted a pilot evaluation study of a virtual reality program and its effect on reducing anxiety. They concluded that the virtual reality module was effective in reducing anxiety.
  (2) Anxiety during treatment
    (a) Clinicians should educate patients about treatment, how treatment works, and positioning.
    (b) Clinicians should answer any patient questions.
    (c) Clinicians should offer reassurance to patients regarding any issues as needed.
  (3) Post-treatment anxiety
    (a) Anxiety levels increase as a patient awaits medical follow-up or results of diagnostic tests for disease surveillance (NCCN, 2020a).
    (b) A study by Giuliani et al. (2016) of supportive care needs in 89 patients with lung cancer (median age 71 years) found that the top three unmet needs were fear of cancer progression (52%), lack of energy and tiredness (48%), and uncertainty about the future (44%).
  (4) Treatment implications and recommended interventions
    (a) Recognition of anxiety in patients with cancer receiving RT is necessary to provide patient-centered care and manage needs effectively.
    (b) Screening tools are an efficient and reliable means of identifying anxiety in this patient population (NCCN, 2020a).
    (c) The oncology team should be aware of circumstances that may heighten anxiety and offer patient-specific interventions, which may include any of the following (NCCN, 2020a).
      i. Exclusion of appropriate intervention for potential contributing factors, such as medications, medical states, and substance withdrawal
      ii. Emotional support (e.g., referral to community resources)
      iii. Education (i.e., problem solving)
      iv. Referral to psychiatry or psychology for interventions such as cognitive behavioral therapy, supportive psychotherapy, or individual, couples, or family counseling
      v. Pharmacologic interventions
      vi. Spiritual counseling when appropriate
      vii. Wellness activities (e.g., yoga, Reiki, meditation)

c) Claustrophobia
  (1) Definition: Claustrophobia (n.d.) is an extreme or irrational fear of confined spaces.
  (2) Pretreatment and active treatment
    (a) Patients should be assessed for claustrophobia as needed.
    (b) At the discretion of the radiation oncologist, medication can be prescribed.
  (3) The planning phase of RT and the treatment itself can be extremely challenging for patients with claustrophobia, particularly those who require immobilization of the body part being treated.
    (a) The panic experienced may be heightened for patients with head and neck cancer who require a hard plastic mesh mask placed over their face and shoulders to secure them to the radiation table to minimize movement (Wiant et al., 2016).
    (b) Using elevators to get to daily treatment can also pose challenges.
  (4) Practice implications
    (a) The oncology team must identify patients with claustrophobia early in the care process to enable timely referrals and prevent delays with diagnosis and treatment.
    (b) Treatment will depend on the patient and severity of the claustrophobic disorder and may include the following.
      i. Referral to psychology, psychiatry, social work, or pastoral care for cognitive behavioral therapy
      ii. Use of previously listed interventions for anxiety disorders, including sedatives (see IV.D. Distress and coping)
      iii. Provision of detailed information on the particular test or procedure to support and prepare a patient to cope with procedures and treatment

d) Depression (see also IX.F. Patients with mental illness)

(1) Patients may experience an array of emotions, such as sadness, fear, anger, and shock, with their diagnosis.

(2) In pretreatment, clinicians should assess patients for any depression prior to starting RT and make appropriate referrals.

(3) During treatment, patients should be assessed during weekly treatment visits, and clinicians should make referrals as needed.

(4) In post-treatment follow-up, clinicians should assess for depression at visits and make referrals as needed.

(5) Interventions for depression can include the following.

　(a) Appropriate referral to psychiatry or family physician for pharmacologic intervention

　(b) Psychosocial interventions
　　i. Cognitive behavioral therapy
　　ii. Supportive psychotherapy
　　iii. Individual, couples, or family counseling
　　iv. Referral to other team members, such as social work, psychology, or pastoral care

e) Cognitive impairment (see also IX.E. Patients with cognitive changes and dementia)

(1) Overview

　(a) Cognitive impairment is a symptom commonly found in patients with cancer that results in distress and debilitating effects.

　(b) Subjective complaints of cognitive impairment are voiced by many patients and their family (Von Ah, 2015).

　(c) Cognitive impairment in a patient with cancer can be the result of multiple conditions, some of which may be preexisting, including dementia, delirium, brain tumors, mental illness, developmental delays, learning disabilities, medication side effects, and medical comorbidities, among others.

(2) Treatment considerations

　(a) Patients with cognitive impairment may not be able to provide informed consent because of their inability to understand the reason for treatment or inability to understand the risk versus benefit.

　(b) The healthcare team should recognize the need for appropriate consultations such as psychiatry, neuropsychology, and patient advocacy groups.

　(c) If decision-making capacity is impeded, involvement of the substitute decision maker or medical power of attorney is required.

　(d) A patient's ability to be compliant during treatment must be considered, such as the ability to attend daily treatments and be immobilized for therapy.

　(e) Cognitive impairment can be worsened by the malignant disease process, side effects, and medications.

　(f) The effect on a patient's ability to perform ADLs must be considered.

　(g) Patients and families may benefit from support groups.

(3) Assessment

　(a) Listening to patients when they voice concerns regarding memory, organizing information related to medications and appointments, and distress about problems with functioning is essential.

　(b) Revelations of cognitive impairment during visits can guide clinicians to further evaluation, then to referrals as needed (Von Ah, Jansen, & Allen, 2014).

　(c) Clinicians should use validated screening and assessment tools.

　(d) NCCN (2020b) recommends further cognitive assessment in any of the following circumstances.
　　i. Concern that cognitive impairment would affect treatment planning or delivery
　　ii. Concern from the medical team regarding decision-making capacity
　　iii. Patient history of recent delirium or late-onset depression
　　iv. Suspicion of cognitive impairment by the healthcare team
　　v. Suggestion of cognitive impairment by the patient's family

10. Social and family issues

a) Social support and family burden of care

(1) A diagnosis of cancer and its treatment can result in disruption of an individual's and family members' lives.

(2) A patient's routine must now accommodate daily RT, new medication regimens, and numerous self-care measures.

(3) As treatment progresses and side effects worsen, a patient may find it difficult to cope with the expectations of the new schedules, especially those patients with limited support networks.

(4) Furthermore, a patient may continue to struggle during the initial periods after treatment through recovery and reestablishment of old routines.

(5) Often, family members assist patients with these functional aspects of life.

b) Practice implications

    (1) The healthcare team must make appropriate and timely referrals (e.g., social work, home care, meal delivery services).

    (2) Online resources are available for caregivers (U.S. Department of Health and Human Services, n.d.).

        (a) American Cancer Society: www.cancer.org

        (b) NCI: www.cancer.gov

        (c) National Institutes of Health: www.nih.gov

c) Financial issues

    (1) A diagnosis of cancer and its sequelae can have a devastating impact on one's financial circumstances because of the inability or reduced ability to work, lack of sick leave benefits, and overall cost of oncologic care.

        (a) Patients need to be referred to social work and to financial counselors early in the treatment process.

        (b) Patients can be referred to discuss application for disability benefits if appropriate.

        (c) Social workers and nurses need to be available to assist patients with information provision and review of available insurance or other sources of support for care and treatment.

    (2) Insurance and drug coverage

        (a) Referral to a social worker is necessary for assessment regarding qualification and, if appropriate, assistance with applications to various government or compassionate assistance plans.

        (b) Medical supplies, such as dressings, wound care supplies, or ostomy supplies, are additional expenses that often are not covered by insurance plans.

        (c) The following organizations can provide resources and assistance to patients (Pirschel, 2017a).

            i. American Cancer Society

            ii. Cancer*Care*'s financial assistance program

            iii. Cancer Financial Assistance Coalition

            iv. HealthWell Foundation

            v. Leukemia and Lymphoma Society

        (d) ONS (2017) has published a navigation toolkit for financial issues.

d) Transportation

    (1) With the majority of patients receiving RT on an outpatient basis, this requires individuals to travel to the treatment facility for their daily therapy.

    (2) The encumbrance of daily travel on patients can include the following (Pisu, Azuero, Benz, McNees, & Meneses, 2017).

        (a) Travel time

        (b) Travel expenses

        (c) Driving during hazardous weather conditions

        (d) Reliance on family or friends for rides

        (e) Fatigue or exhaustion upon arrival to the treatment facility or on return home

    (3) Transportation solutions

        (a) The oncology team may refer a patient to organizations that provide transportation through volunteers.

        (b) The use of volunteer drivers can decrease burden on a patient and family.

        (c) Such volunteer services often transport more than one patient, resulting in individuals waiting for extended periods of time for others to complete their treatments and appointments.

e) Accommodations

    (1) Patients who live far from the treating facility or find the daily travel unmanageable may opt to stay at lodgings closer to the hospital, such as a patient hotel, which typically offer accommodations and various support services for independent patients and their spouse or partner for a reasonable cost.

    (2) In larger metropolitan areas and around academic centers, hotel accommodations may be more available.

    (3) Although patient hotels tend to offer discounted fees for patients and their spouse or partner, this cost can still represent an added expense and financial burden.

    (4) Referral to social work may help with financial assistance or the waiving of patient hotel fees for those with limited household income.

    (5) Clinicians should discuss the potential of a family member or caregiver staying with the patient at the hotel during treatment.

    (6) For patients who find it difficult being away from family or friends, clinicians should recommend returning home on weekends.

f) Access to care

    (1) Urban healthcare facilities may have larger university or teaching-based oncology programs or cancer-focused hospitals connected to them. These hospital services may not be equally available to inner-city neighborhoods or urban populations (Fung et al., 2019).

    (2) A shortage of primary care physicians can result in fewer screenings, assessments, and required

diagnostics, thus making referrals to oncology specialists difficult for some populations.

    (3) Rural communities tend to have limited hospital resources per capita compared to cities.

    (4) Cultural barriers can affect access to care.

    (5) A system of private care and lack of insurance greatly limits access to care.

    (6) Some residents may be unaware of obtainable or affordable health care in their communities.

g) Treatment adherence

    (1) Definition: Adherence occurs when a patient follows recommended courses of treatment (i.e., takes full course of treatment, either radiation, chemotherapy, or immunotherapy without treatment delays).

    (2) Barriers to adherence

        (a) A patient's ability to effectively cope with symptoms from the disease and resulting side effects from RT can negatively affect not only quality of life but also capacity to tolerate further treatment.

        (b) A patient's inability to fully appreciate and comprehend the diagnosis and potential outcomes of treatment can affect adherence. This lack of understanding can be the result of multiple and often coexisting patient factors, including cultural background, education and literacy levels, socioeconomic status, age, and gender (Rangarajan & Jayaraman, 2017).

        (c) Physical barriers that can impede patient attendance to daily RT include transportation issues and distance from the treatment center.

        (d) Lack of health insurance coverage may influence adherence.

        (e) Inability to take time off from work because of financial obligations or inflexible work schedules can affect adherence.

        (f) Patients may become emotionally overwhelmed by life circumstances such that they can no longer manage the demands of daily treatment.

    (3) Practice implications and interventions

        (a) Clinicians should address medications and side effect management at each visit and ensure the patient is taking medications as prescribed.

        (b) Clinicians can utilize teach-back methods when addressing side effects related to RT and self-care measures to assess comprehension (Agency for Healthcare Research and Quality, 2015).

        (c) Clinicians must intervene with appropriate strategies to ensure that patients are able to attend all scheduled appointments because risk of cancer recurrence can increase with missing as few as two RT appointments (NCI, 2016).

h) Language

    (1) Barriers to nurse–patient communication affect nursing practice as well as patient care.

    (2) With increasing diversity, communication becomes more complex (Squires, 2018).

    (3) For precise interpretation to occur, a healthcare interpreter must be utilized.

    (4) Family and friends of the patient should not be used for translation or interpretation.

    (5) Interpretation services can include the following.

        (a) Hospital-employed interpreters

        (b) Language lines (e.g., telephone service, interpretation phone lines)

        (c) Outside agencies with interpreters

    (6) Patient education material that is culturally sensitive and in common languages should be available whenever possible.

    (7) A healthcare team member who is bilingual may act as an interpreter if other options are not available.

i) Culture and multicultural knowledge

    (1) The U.S. Census Bureau (2018) reported that the next 30 years will see significant change in demographics.

        (a) In the United States, there will be more people older than 65 years than children.

        (b) The population will grow at a slower rate and become more racially and ethnically diverse.

        (c) Immigration will play a large part in some demographic changes.

        (d) To effectively help patients, it is vital for healthcare professionals caring for patients with cancer to learn about other cultures (Dauvrin & Lorant, 2015).

    (2) Family structure and roles

        (a) The family interaction is important to recognize because many cultures differ in their interpretation of roles.

        (b) Training in cultural understanding and sensitivity is imperative.

    (3) Communication styles

        (a) Medical interpreters or language services must be used rather than family members of patients.

        (b) Healthcare professionals must focus on effective communication and expressing empathy (Weber, Sulstarova, & Singy, 2016).

    (4) Western views of medical care

        (a) With changing demographics and information more easily available to people, it is

essential for nurses to be aware of varying health practices that may affect a patient's RT and overall care.

(b) Nurses should understand CAM health practices that patients across cultures may be using or interested in exploring.

(5) Diet

(a) Diet has significance in each culture in regard to general well-being, treatment of illness, and socialization, and it can be a means to comfort the individual.

(b) It is important to discuss dietary preferences.

(c) Referral to an RDN or RD for culturally based recommendations may be required (Guerdoux-Ninot et al., 2016).

(6) Sexuality: Healthcare professionals must have knowledge of sexual concerns and be sensitive to individual and cultural norms.

j) Literacy

(1) Illiteracy: Many people who do not read or write may be reluctant to share this with clinicians, and they may compensate with statements such as, "I forgot my glasses," or use strategies to avoid a focus on their perceived limitations.

(2) Health literacy (Cartwright, Dumenci, Cassel, Thomson, & Matsuyama, 2017)

(a) Health literacy addresses the ability of patients to comprehend medical information that will affect their access to and use of healthcare systems, resources, and information.

(b) Low health literacy is associated with increased hospitalizations in patients with cancer.

(3) Guidelines for low literacy

(a) The American Cancer Society provides easily read information related to side effects of treatment and pain.

(b) The Agency for Healthcare Research and Quality (2017) suggests strategies for teaching patients.

    i. Use simple language and avoid medical terminology.
    ii. Converse at a slow pace.
    iii. Avoid information overload.
    iv. Repeat instructions.
    v. Use pictures and stories to facilitate a patient's comprehension.
    vi. Use a teach-back method rather than ask if a patient understands.
    vii. Always be courteous and sensitive to the patient.
    viii. Written patient education materials should be at a grade 4–8 reading level.
    ix. Videos and interactive computer programs may be beneficial.

k) Return to work

(1) Resources are available through the National Institutes of Health to assist patients as they prepare to return to work.

(2) A patient will need to work with the physician regarding accommodations for work and possible limitations (U.S. Department of Health and Human Services, 2019).

(3) Cognitive impairment causes distress to patients and families and has an impact on return to work. Some patients return to work but often work fewer hours, and some return to work but in a different job (Von Ah et al., 2016).

(4) The healthcare team should assist the patient in identifying accommodations required to facilitate a smooth and successful transition back to the workplace.

(a) Support should be provided to the patient in order to make appropriate arrangements and to complete necessary work-related forms.

(b) A referral to social work, occupational therapy, or neuropsychology may be required to assist the patient with returning to work.

11. Rare cancers

a) In the United States, approximately 20% of all cancers are classified as a rare cancer (DeSantis, Kramer, & Jemal, 2017).

b) Those diagnosed with rare cancers often have challenges in finding a physician with the expertise to diagnose, treat, or refer to an RT facility.

c) Although RT often can be available closer to a patient's home, referral to RT centers with more experience in the management of rare cancers, infrastructures to provide access to combined-modality treatment including clinical trials, and an interprofessional team to support a patient should be considered.

d) Patients may need to be referred to centers with specialized equipment, including IMRT or proton beam therapy machines, to manage specific cases.

12. Pediatric cancers (see also IX.B. Pediatric radiation oncology)

a) Conscious sedation for procedures

(1) Depending on the developmental age of a child, the number of RT fractions, the time required for daily treatment, the level of anxiety, and the need to be motionless during treatment, conscious or deep sedation or general anesthesia may be required.

(2) A team of well-trained personnel is required to safely manage the sedation and recovery (Chang, 2018).

b) Distress: Children younger than 12 years of age often experience procedural distress (Trentacosta et al., 2016).

c) Transition to adult centers: The age at which children transition to receiving care in an adult facility may vary depending on the center, the program, and the location of the treating and follow-up center (Psihogios et al., 2019).

d) Long-term follow-up

(1) It is important to identify high-risk patients based on the site and volume irradiated, as well as when the treatment was delivered.

(2) Young adults may develop chronic conditions after RT, so they require frequent follow-up with their physicians (Bright et al., 2019; Ramsay et al., 2018).

(3) Patients at high risk for recurrence or with large treatment volumes require close monitoring and frequent follow-up so that possible long-term side effects may be diagnosed early (Henson et al., 2016).

(4) Late effects depend on the systems within the treatment field.

(a) Cardiovascular

i. Adult survivors of pediatric cancers are at increased risk of myocardial infarction and stroke.

ii. Depending on area treated, survivors experience different effects to the heart, such as arrhythmias, autonomic dysfunction, carotid disease, and valve abnormalities.

iii. Pediatric cancer survivors should have an annual physical assessment (Henson et al., 2016).

(b) Pulmonary

i. Treatment fields involving the lungs impose an increased risk of pulmonary fibrosis.

ii. A history and physical should be performed, along with pulmonary function tests, every one to two years depending on results.

iii. A chest CT should be ordered for any abnormal pulmonary function test.

(c) Cranial irradiation: Patients who were treated with cranial irradiation should undergo cognitive screening based on age.

(d) Gastrointestinal and genitourinary

i. Gastrointestinal and genitourinary effects of RT may include asplenia with lifelong risk of sepsis, gastrointestinal obstruction secondary to fibrosis, nephropathy, and bladder damage.

ii. Routine monitoring should involve an annual history and physical.

(e) Thyroid

i. Hypothyroidism has been associated with thoracic, cranial, and neck irradiation.

ii. Thyroid levels should be checked during an annual history and physical.

(f) Gonadal impairment

i. Gonadal impairment depends on RT dose.

ii. Routine history and physical should include hormone levels.

(g) Second primary cancers: Pediatric survivors are at risk for second cancers after RT.

13. Sexual orientation and gender

a) People define themselves based on race, ethnicity, social and religious beliefs, and gender identification (Christensen, 2019).

(1) Most clinical assessment tools are heterocentric, with questions related to social support and marriage or partner relationships, and these tools often identify sex as only male or female.

(2) There is a need to address sexual orientation and gender identification to best meet the needs of patients and support them through RT and other treatments.

(3) Patients should be asked by which pronoun they prefer to be identified (e.g., he, she, they).

b) Studies addressing the needs of gay or lesbian individuals tend to be focused on traditional disease sites (breast, gynecologic, or prostate cancer). Future research should focus on other disease sites beyond the sexual organs (e.g., colon, anal, head and neck cancer) and address side effects, late effects, sexuality, and body image concerns.

c) To create a welcoming environment, staff may require training in regard to cultural competence in sensitivity to the LGBTQ population. A nondiscrimination policy should be in place, and educational materials on sexuality and gender identity should be available (Christensen, 2019).

References

Agency for Healthcare Research and Quality. (2015). Use the teach-back method: Tool 5. In *Health literacy universal precautions toolkit* (2nd ed.). https://www.ahrq.gov/professionals/quality-patient-safety/quality-resources/tools/literacy-toolkit/healthlittoolkit2-tool5.html

Agency for Healthcare Research and Quality. (2017). *Health literacy: Hidden barriers and practical strategies* [PowerPoint slides]. https://www.ahrq.gov/health-literacy/quality-resources/tools/literacy-toolkit/tool3a/index.html

American Cancer Society. (2019). *Cancer treatment and survivorship facts and figures 2019–2021.* https://www.cancer.org/content/dam/cancer-org/research/cancer-facts-and-statistics/cancer-treatment-and-survivorship-facts-and-figures/cancer-treatment-and-survivorship-facts-and-figures-2019-2021.pdf

Bright, C.J., Reulen, R.C., Winter, D.L., Stark, D.P., McCabe, M.G., Edgar, A.B., ... Hawkins, M.M. (2019). Risk of subsequent primary neoplasms in survivors of adolescent and young adult cancer (Teenage and Young Adult Cancer Survivor Study): A population-based, cohort study. *Lancet Oncology, 20,* 531–545. https://doi.org/10.1016/s1470-2045(18)30903-3

Bunch, L. (2016). The role of post discharge phone calls in the radiation therapy department. *Journal of Medical Imaging and Radiation Sciences, 47*(Suppl. 1), S2. https://doi.org/10.1016/j.jmir.2015.12.007

Cartwright, L.A., Dumenci, L., Cassel, J.B., Thomson, M.D., & Matsuyama, R.K. (2017). Health literacy is an independent predictor of cancer patients' hospitalizations. *Health Literacy Research and Practice, 1,* e153–e162. https://doi.org/10.3928/24748307-20170808-01

Centers for Disease Control and Prevention. (2020, April 3). Defining adult overweight and obesity. https://www.cdc.gov/obesity/adult/defining.html

Chang, W.-T.W. (2018). Pediatric sedation. *Medscape.* https://emedicine.medscape.com/article/804045-overview

Cheville, A.L., Mustian, K., Winter-Stone, K., Zucker, D.S., Gamble, G.L., & Alfano, C.M. (2017). Cancer rehabilitation: An overview of current need, delivery models, and levels of care. *Physical Medicine Rehabilitation Clinics of North America, 28,* 1–17. https://doi.org/10.1016/j.pmr.2016.08.001

Christensen, D. (2019, January 15). The case of the gender gaffe. *ONS Voice.* https://voice.ons.org/news-and-views/the-case-of-the-gender-gaffe

Clarke, P., Radford, K., Coffey, M., & Stewart, M. (2016). Speech and swallow rehabilitation in head and neck cancer: United Kingdom National Multidisciplinary Guidelines. *Journal of Laryngology and Otology, 130*(Suppl. 2), S176–S180. https://doi.org/10.1017/s0022215116000608

Claustrophobia. (n.d.). In *Oxford English Dictionary* (2nd ed.).

Cope, D.G., Reb, A., Schwartz, R., & Simon, J. (2018). Older adults with lung cancer: Assessment, treatment options, survivorship issues, and palliative care strategies. *Clinical Journal of Oncology Nursing, 22*(Suppl.), 26–35. https://doi.org/10.1188/18.cjon.s2.26-35

Dauvrin, M., & Lorant, V. (2015). Leadership and cultural competence of healthcare professionals: A social network analysis. *Nursing Research, 64,* 200–210. https://doi.org/10.1097/nnr.0000000000000092

DeSantis, C.E., Kramer, J.L., & Jemal, A. (2017). The burden of rare cancers in the United States. *CA: A Cancer Journal for Clinicians, 67,* 261–272. https://doi.org/10.3322/caac.21400

Ferguson, I., Huecker, J., Huang, J., McClelland, C., & Van Stavern, G. (2017). Risk factors for radiation-induced optic neuropathy: A case-control study. *Clinical and Experimental Ophthalmology, 45,* 592–597. https://doi.org/10.1111/ceo.12927

Fung, C.Y., Chen, E., Vapiwala, N., Pohar, S., Trifiletti, D., Truong, M.-T., ... Royce, T. (2019). The American Society for Radiation Oncology 2017 radiation oncologist workforce study. *International Journal of Radiation Oncology, Biology, Physics, 103,* 547–556. https://doi.org/10.1016/j.ijrobp.2018.10.020

Funk, A., Garcia, C., & Mullen, T. (2018). Understanding the hospital experience of older adults with hearing impairment. *American Journal of Nursing, 118,* 28–34. https://doi.org/10.1097/01.NAJ.0000534821.03997.7b

Geddie, P.I., Loerzel, V.W., & Norris, A.E. (2016). Family caregiver knowledge, patient illness characteristics, and unplanned hospital admissions in older adults with cancer. *Oncology Nursing Forum, 43,* 453–463. https://doi.org/10.1188/16.onf.453-463

Giuliani, M.E., Milne, R.A., Puts, M., Sampson, L.R., Kwan, J.Y., Le, L.W., ... Jones, J. (2016). The prevalence and nature of supportive care needs in lung cancer patients. *Current Oncology, 23,* 258–265. https://doi.org/10.3747/co.23.3012

Goldberg, J.I., Burhenn, P.S., & Ginex, P.K. (2018). Nursing education: Review of assessment, clinical care, and implications for practice regarding older adult patients with cancer. *Clinical Journal of Oncology Nursing, 22*(Suppl. 6), 19–25. https://doi.org/10.1188/18.cjon.s2.19-25

Guerdoux-Ninot, E., Kilgour, R.D., Janiszewski, C., Jarlier, M., Meuric, J., Poirée, B., ... Senesse, P. (2016). Meal context and food preferences in cancer patients: Results from a French self-report survey. *SpringerPlus, 5,* 810. https://doi.org/10.1186/s40064-016-2538-1

Hamilton, J., Kruse, H., Holcomb, L., & Freche, R. (2018). Distress and psychosocial needs. Demographic predictors of clinical distress after a diagnosis of cancer. *Clinical Journal of Oncology Nursing, 22,* 390–397. https://doi.org/10.1188/18.cjon.390-397

Henson, K.E., Reulen, R.C., Winter, D.L., Bright, C.J., Fidler, M.M., Frosbisher, C., ... Hawkins, M.M. (2016). Cardiac mortality among 200,000 five-year survivors of cancer diagnosed at 15 to 39 years of age: The teenage and young adult cancer survivor study. *Circulation, 134,* 1519–1531. https://doi.org/10.1161/circulationaha.116.022514

Hurria, A., Mohile, S., Gajra, A., Klepin, H., Muss, H., Chapman, A., ... Tew, W.P. (2016). Validation of a prediction tool for chemotherapy toxicity in older adults with cancer. *Journal of Clinical Oncology, 34,* 2366–2371. https://doi.org/10.1200/jco.2015.65.4327

Lindsey, S., Astroth, K.S., & Kumar, P. (2016). Improving awareness, identification, and management of sarcopenic obesity in cancer survivors: An evidence-based toolbox. *Clinical Journal of Oncology Nursing, 20,* E123–E138. https://doi.org/10.1188/16.cjon.e132-e138

Livestrong. (n.d.). Rehabilitation after cancer. https://www.livestrong.org/we-can-help/healthy-living-after-treatment/rehabilitation-after-cancer

Loerzel, V.W. (2018). Symptom self-management: Strategies used by older adults receiving treatment for cancer. *Clinical Journal of Oncology Nursing, 22,* 83–90. https://doi.org/10.1188/18.cjon.83-90

Marquess, M., Johnston, S.P., Williams, N.L., Giordano, C., Leiby, B.E., Hurwitz, M.D., ... Den, R.B. (2017). A pilot study to determine if the use of a virtual reality education module reduces anxiety and increases comprehension in patients receiving radiation therapy. *Journal of Radiation Oncology, 6,* 317–322. https://doi.org/10.1007/s13566-017-0298-3

National Cancer Institute. (2013, December 16). *Annual report to the nation on the status of cancer, 1975–2010, featuring prevalence of comorbidity and impact on survival among persons with lung, colorectal, breast or prostate cancer: Questions and answers* [Press release]. https://web.archive.org/web/20190110171657/https://www.cancer.gov/news-events/press-releases/2013/ReportNationDec2013QandA

National Cancer Institute. (2016, February 26). Missed radiation therapy sessions increase risk of cancer recurrence. https://www.cancer.gov/news-events/cancer-currents-blog/2016/missed-radiation-therapy

National Comprehensive Cancer Network. (2020a). *NCCN Clinical Practice Guidelines in Oncology (NCCN® Guidelines): Distress management* [v.2.2020]. https://www.nccn.org/professionals/physician_gls/pdf/distress.pdf

National Comprehensive Cancer Network. (2020b). *NCCN Clinical Practice Guidelines in Oncology (NCCN® Guidelines): Older adult oncology* [v.1.2020]. https://www.nccn.org/professionals/physician_gls/pdf/senior.pdf

Newton, V.E., & Shah, S.R. (2013). Improving communication with patients with a hearing impairment. *Community Eye Health, 26,* 6–7.

Oncology Nursing Society. (2017). *Oncology nurse navigator toolkit: Helping patients navigate financial issues.* https://www.ons.org/sites/default/files/ONS_ONN_Toolkit_Financial_Issues_050417.pdf

Overcash, J., Cope, D.G., & Van Cleave, J.H. (2018). Frailty in older adults: Assessment, support, and treatment implications in patients with cancer. *Clinical Journal of Oncology Nursing, 22*(Suppl. 6), 8–18. https://doi.org/10.1188/18.cjon.s2.8-18

Pirschel, C. (2017a). Financial toxicity and its burden on cancer care. *ONS Voice.* https://voice.ons.org/news-and-views/financial-toxicity-and-its-burden-on-cancer-care

Pirschel, C. (2017b). The impact of comorbidities on patient care. *ONS Voice.* https://voice.ons.org/news-and-views/comorbidities-in-cancer-patient-care

Pisu, M., Azuero, A., Benz, P., McNees, P., & Meneses, K. (2017). Out-of-pocket costs and burden among rural breast cancer survivors. *Cancer Medicine, 6,* 572–581. https://doi.org/10.1002/cam4.1017

Psihogios, A.M., Schwartz, L.A., Deatrick, J.A., Ver Hoeve, E.S., Anderson, L.M., Wartman, E.C., & Szalda, D. (2019). Preferences for cancer survivorship care among adolescents and young adults who experienced healthcare transitions and their parents. *Journal of Cancer Survivorship, 13,* 620–631. https://doi.org/10.1007/s11764-019-00781-x

Ramsay, J.M., Mann, K., Kaul, S., Zamora, E.R., Smits-Seemann, R.R., & Kirchhoff, A.C. (2018). Follow-up care provider preferences of adolescent and young adult cancer survivors. *Journal of Adolescent and Young Adult Oncology, 7,* 204–209. https://doi.org/10.1089/jayao.2017.0083

Rangarajan, R., & Jayaraman, K. (2017). Barriers affecting adherence to radiation treatment and strategies to overcome those barriers. *Indian Journal of Cancer, 54,* 458–460. https://doi.org/10.4103/ijc.ijc_260_17

Sarfati, D., Koczwara, B., & Jackson, C. (2016). The impact of comorbidity on cancer and its treatment. *CA: A Cancer Journal for Clinicians, 66,* 337–350. https://doi.org/10.3322/caac.21342

Squires, A. (2018). Strategies for overcoming language barriers in healthcare. *Nursing Management, 49,* 20–27. https://doi.org/10.1097/01.numa.0000531166.24481.15

Trentacosta, C.J., Harper, F.W., Albrecht, T.L., Taub, J.W., Phipps, S., & Penner, L.A. (2016). Pediatric cancer patients' treatment-related distress and longer-term anxiety: An individual differences perspective. *Journal of Developmental and Behavioral Pediatrics, 37,* 753–761. https://doi.org/10.1097/dbp.0000000000000327

U.S. Census Bureau. (2018, March 13). *Older people projected to outnumber children for first time in U.S. history* [Press release]. https://www.census.gov/newsroom/press-releases/2018/cb18-41-population-projections.html

U.S. Department of Health and Human Services. (n.d.). Resources for caregivers. https://www.cancer.gov/resources-for-caregivers

U.S. Department of Health and Human Services. (2019, January 24). Going back to work. https://www.cancer.gov/about-cancer/coping/day-to-day/back-to-work

Vision Australia. (n.d.). Caring for patients. https://www.visionaustralia.org/information/family-friends-carers/caring-for-patients

Von Ah, D. (2015). Cognitive changes associated with cancer and cancer treatment: State of the science. *Clinical Journal of Oncology Nursing, 19,* 47–56. https://doi.org/10.1188/15.cjon.19-01ap

Von Ah, D., Jansen, C.E., & Allen, D.H. (2014). Evidence-based interventions for cancer- and treatment-related cognitive impairment. *Clinical Journal of Oncology Nursing, 18*(Suppl.), 17–25. https://doi.org/10.1188/14.cjon.s3.17-25

Von Ah, D., Storey, S., Tallman, E., Nielsen, A., Johns, S.A., & Pressler, S.J. (2016). Cancer, cognitive impairment, and work-related outcomes: An integrative review. *Oncology Nursing Forum, 43,* 602–616. https://doi.org/10.1188/16.onf.602-616

Weber, O., Sulstarova, B., & Singy, P. (2016). Cross-cultural communication in oncology: Challenges and training interests. *Oncology Nursing Forum, 43,* E24–E33. https://doi.org/10.1188/16.onf.e24-e33

Wiant, D., Squire, S., Liu, H., Maurer, J., Lane Hayes, T., & Sintay, B. (2016). A prospective evaluation of open face masks for head and neck radiation therapy. *Practical Radiation Oncology, 6,* e259–e267. https://doi.org/10.1016/j.prro.2016.02.003

World Health Organization. (2018, January 16). Disability and health. https://www.who.int/en/news-room/fact-sheets/detail/disability-and-health

E. Patients with cognitive changes and dementia
  1. Normal changes with aging
    a) Worldwide, people are living longer; thus, the population of older adults is increasing.
    b) Aging affects all systems in the body differently, and normal changes due to the physiology of aging can affect function.
    c) Normal aging affects cognition, and changes related to aging affect individuals to varying degrees (Grayston, 2018; Harada, Natelson Love, & Triebel, 2013).
    d) Cognitive abilities can be divided into two components—fluid intelligence and crystallized intelligence—and aging affects these two components differently (Grayston, 2018; Harada et al., 2013).
      (1) *Fluid cognition* refers to the innate ability to think abstractly, process and learn new information, use logic, and solve problems (Grayston, 2018; Harada et al., 2013).
        (a) Most fluid cognitive abilities peak in the third decade of life and slowly decline.
        (b) Examples of fluid cognitive abilities include executive function, processing speed, memory, and psychomotor ability.
      (2) *Crystallized intelligence* describes the use of knowledge and skills that are learned.
        (a) Examples of crystallized abilities are vocabulary, numeracy, and general knowledge (Grayston, 2018; Harada et al., 2013).
        (b) Crystallized abilities remain stable or increase into the sixth and seventh decade of life (Harada et al., 2013; Salthouse, 2010).
        (c) As a result of learning experiences leading to an accumulation of information, older adults tend to perform as well or better at tasks that require crystallized abilities compared to younger adults (Harada et al., 2013).
  2. Executive function
    a) *Executive function* is defined as the capacities that allow a person to successfully engage in purposeful behavior (Harada et al., 2013).
      (1) Executive function includes the ability to plan, organize, reason, solve problems, and self-monitor.
      (2) Mental flexibility is also an executive function. Research has shown that types of executive function such as mental flexibility, concept formation, abstraction, and reasoning with unfamiliar information decline with aging (Fjell, McEvoy, Holland, Dale, & Walhovd, 2014; Harada et al., 2013).
    b) Other types of executive function, such as the ability to reason with familiar situations, identify similarities, and describe the meaning of proverbs, remain stable throughout life (Harada et al., 2013).
  3. Processing speed: With increasing age, processing speed declines, starting in the third decade of life, and this slowing can negatively impact other cognitive functions (Fjell et al., 2014; Harada et al., 2013).
  4. Attention
    a) The ability to concentrate and focus on a specific stimulus involving simple auditory attention span (immediate memory) declines only slightly with age (Harada et al., 2013).
    b) However, more complex tasks, such as those requiring selective attention (i.e., tasks that require focus on specific information while ignoring other information) and divided attention (i.e., activities that require focus on multiple activities at the same time), are more affected with aging (Harada et al., 2013).
    c) With increasing age, individuals may experience more difficulty performing tasks that require work-

ing memory (i.e., the ability to hold information in the memory while manipulating the information at the same time) (Harada et al., 2013).

5. Memory
   a) Age-related changes in memory are among the most common complaints in older adults.
   b) Aging affects an older adult's episodic and semantic (use of language) memory differently.
      (1) The episodic memory declines after age 50–60 years.
      (2) Semantic memory declines in late life (Fjell et al., 2014; Harada et al., 2013).
      (3) Implicit (nondeclarative) memory includes procedural memory, allowing individuals to remember how to perform a task (e.g., ride a bicycle) and does not change with increasing age.
      (4) The ability to form new information into memory (acquisition) and memory retrieval decline with aging.

6. Language
   a) Language requires both fluid and crystallized cognitive abilities.
   b) Overall language ability remains intact with aging, and vocabulary improves.
   c) Visual confrontation naming (i.e., naming common objects when one sees them) and verbal fluency (i.e., finding words within a certain category) in a set time decline with aging (Salthouse, 2010).

7. Age-related changes in the structure and function of the brain
   a) A great deal of research is dedicated to age-related changes in function and structure of the brain.
   b) With aging, gray matter volume declines, with most of the atrophy seen in the prefrontal cortex (Fjell et al., 2014; Harada et al., 2013).
   c) Death of neurons is a cause of gray matter volume loss.
   d) With age, neurons also decrease in size, and the number of connections between them also decreases (i.e., reduction in synaptic density).

8. Mild cognitive impairment
   a) Mild cognitive impairment is the clinical intermediate stage between normal aging and early dementia (Brodaty et al., 2017; Hugo & Ganguli, 2014).
   b) Although mild neurocognitive disorder increases the risk of dementia, currently, the risk of conversion from mild neurocognitive disorder to dementia is not clearly defined, as studies have used different methodology.
   c) The fifth edition of *Diagnostic and Statistical Manual of Mental Disorders* (DSM-5) now uses the term *mild neurocognitive disorder* (American Psychiatric Association [APA], 2013).
   d) A diagnosis of mild neurocognitive disorder requires the following conditions (APA, 2013).

      (1) A cognitive complaint or concern, ideally corroborated by another person
      (2) Objective evidence of cognitive impairment that is abnormal for the age (usually defined as one to two standard deviations below normal)
      (3) No effect on the ability to perform everyday activities
   e) Diagnosis of mild neurocognitive disorder is important to assess for any potentially reversible causes of cognitive impairment, to allow for counseling, and to plan care and therapeutic strategies (Petersen et al., 2018).
   f) The American Academy of Neurology practice guidelines recommend assessing patients if they have complained about their cognitive function or a close contact has voiced concern about a patient's cognitive function (Petersen et al., 2018).
      (1) Subjective cognitive complaints are not sufficient for a diagnosis, and validated assessment tools should be used.
      (2) Patients with screening results suggestive of impairment should be referred for a formal clinical assessment.
      (3) Nurses working in radiation oncology settings are in a position to administer cognitive screening tools if patients or their caregivers express concerns about cognitive function.
      (4) American Academy of Neurology guidelines recommend that in cases involving a concern for memory loss and clinicians lacking experience in managing cognitive impairment, patients be referred to a specialist with experience in cognition, such as a geriatrician, neurologist, internal medicine specialist, psychiatrist, or psychologist (Petersen et al., 2018).
      (5) The American Academy of Neurology guidelines recommend counseling patients and their families about the potential benefits of regular exercise twice weekly (Petersen et al., 2018).
   g) The difference between mild neurocognitive disorder and dementia is in impact on function (Hugo & Ganguli, 2014; Petersen et al. 2018).
      (1) A diagnosis of dementia requires evidence of impairment in function that limits the ability to perform ADLs; clinicians need to assess for the presence of functional impairments related to cognition prior to a diagnosis of dementia.
      (2) Although FDA-approved agents for mild neurocognitive disorder are available (only for the treatment of dementia), it is important to assess for changes in cognitive status over time and review medications (including medication side effects), general medical conditions, sleep, and depression, as these all can contribute to mild neurocognitive disorder.

9. Dementia
   a) Overview
      (1) DSM-5 refers to dementia as *major neurocognitive disorder*. Diagnosis requires substantial cognitive impairment in one or more cognitive domains that interferes with independence ADLs (Hugo & Ganguli, 2014).
      (2) The prevalence of dementia increases exponentially with age and doubles every five years after age 65 years (Hugo & Ganguli, 2014; Livingston et al., 2017).
         (a) The prevalence is estimated to be 5%–10% in higher income countries, such as the United States, and higher in women than in men (Hugo & Ganguli, 2014).
         (b) In the United States, higher prevalence has been reported in African American and Latino/Hispanic populations, compared to non-Hispanic White populations.
      (3) Current research is examining pathways to identify who with mild neurocognitive disorder will develop Alzheimer disease based on atrophy pattern, what amyloid-related changes in the brain represent Alzheimer disease pathology, and what is part of the normal aging process (Fjell et al., 2014).
      (4) Neuropathologic examination is the standard for diagnosis of Alzheimer disease.
      (5) With dementia, symptoms such as memory loss, word-finding difficulties, and visuospatial problems lead to functional impairment (Albert et al., 2011; Alzheimer's Association, 2019).
   b) Dementia subtypes
      (1) Alzheimer disease (Alzheimer's Association, 2019; Livingston et al., 2017)
         (a) Alzheimer disease is the most common form of neurodegenerative disease, characterized by progressive loss of synapses and neurons and an accumulation of amyloid plaques and neurofibrillary tangles.
         (b) It is most commonly diagnosed in the eighth or ninth decade of life but can be diagnosed as early as the fifth decade.
         (c) The average disease duration is four to eight years, but exceptions of more than 20 years have also been reported.
      (2) Vascular dementia (Hugo & Ganguli, 2014)
         (a) Vascular dementia includes the major and minor vascular neurocognitive disorders.
         (b) Cognitive deficits are attributed to cerebrovascular disease.
         (c) It is the second most common cause of dementia and is frequently present with Alzheimer disease; co-occurrence is known as *mixed dementia*.
         (d) The location of the vascular lesion is more important than atrophy.
         (e) The progression of the cognitive decline can occur in an acute stepwise pattern, a gradual pattern, or a rapid decline.
         (f) Cognitive decline is mostly seen in the domains of executive function and complex attention.
      (3) Lewy body dementia (Hugo & Ganguli, 2014)
         (a) Lewy body dementia is the third most common neurodegenerative dementia, characterized by alpha-synuclein misfolding and aggregation with the pathognomonic Lewy bodies.
         (b) Onset occurs between the sixth and ninth decade of life, and the survival after onset is on average five to seven years.
         (c) Lewy body dementia presents with a gradual onset and progression; the most common observed cognitive deficits are in the domain of attention, visuospatial ability, and executive function.
         (d) Additional core symptoms include fluctuating cognition, recurrent visual hallucinations, and Parkinsonism features.
         (e) The distinction between Lewy body dementia and dementia of Parkinson disease is based on the timing of the cognitive impairment—whether the cognitive function precedes the onset of Parkinsonism or vice versa.
         (f) Approximately 75% of those with Parkinson disease will develop dementia.
      (4) Frontotemporal dementia (FTD) (Kansal et al., 2016)
         (a) FTD is less common and is characterized by atrophy of the frontal and temporal lobes with a gradual onset and progression.
         (b) With the mean age of onset in the sixth decade of life, it is a common cause of early-onset dementia.
         (c) An estimated 20%–25% of those with FTD are aged 65 years and older.
         (d) There are two different subtypes.
            i. FTD-amyotrophic lateral sclerosis subtype (median survival 2.5 years)
            ii. FTD-semantic dementia subtype (median survival 12 years)
10. Cognition in older adults with cancer
   a) Incidence of cancer and neurocognitive disorders increase with age, and for older adults with cancer, a diagnosis of dementia affects treatment decision-making, as well as prognosis (Karuturi et al., 2016).

b) Individuals undergoing cancer treatment must be able to understand and process information in order to receive cancer treatment. However, because mild neurocognitive disorder and major neurocognitive disorder are underdiagnosed, it is currently unclear how many older adults with cancer have either disorder.

c) Cognitive impairment can affect the reporting of symptoms, side effects, and disease-related outcomes.

  (1) Head and neck cancer and brain cancer can cause neurocognitive impairment; however, few studies have examined the prevalence of neurocognitive impairment prior to the start of cancer treatment in patients with head and neck cancer (Piai et al., 2019).

    (a) In studies in patients with head and neck cancer, the reported prevalence of neurocognitive impairment was 21%–36%, with more than 55% of these studies using the Montreal Cognitive Assessment to diagnose the cognitive impairment (Piai et al., 2019).

    (b) In a prospective nationwide cohort study of 254 patients with head and neck cancer in the Netherlands (mean age 62 years), the prevalence of mild cognitive impairment was 12%, and prevalence of severe cognitive impairment was 26% (Piai et al., 2019).

      i. The researchers used the Trail Making Test parts A and B, Hopkins verbal learning test, and letter fluency test.

      ii. The discrepancy between studies reporting a higher prevalence of cognitive impairment and the Piai et al. (2019) study is the result of the lower sensitivity and specificity of the Montreal Cognitive Assessment compared to other tests.

  (2) Brain metastases are the most common neurologic complication of any type of cancer, affecting approximately 30%–40% of patients with cancer (Lynch, 2019).

    (a) Lung cancer, breast cancer, and melanoma are the three most common types of primary cancer that have a high likelihood of metastasizing to the brain.

    (b) Treatment of brain metastases can include surgery (for single lesions and depending on location) and RT. Patients with brain metastases can undergo whole-brain RT as a preventive, therapeutic, or palliative treatment.

    (c) Whole-brain RT can lead to serious toxicity, which occurs in three phases (initial symptoms, early-delayed/subacute, and late delayed) on a continuum (Lynch, 2019).

      i. Initial symptoms (0–6 weeks) include headache, nausea, and hypersomnia, with worsening of preexisting neurologic dysfunction.

      ii. The early-delayed/subacute phase includes somnolence syndrome—excessive drowsiness, memory loss, attention deficits, and radiologic damage.

      iii. The late-delayed phase (six months and more after early-delayed/subacute) is irreversible, can continue to worsen over time, and includes symptoms such as ataxia, urinary incontinence, and dementia.

      iv. Initial symptoms and early-delayed/subacute phases can have spontaneous resolution.

    (d) The mechanisms underlying cognitive dysfunction following whole-brain RT are not completely understood (Jacob et al., 2018; Lynch, 2019; Wilke, Grosshans, Duman, Brown, & Li, 2018).

    (e) Research demonstrates that RT to the brain can cause a significant deterioration in cognition and decreases quality of life (Wilke et al., 2018).

  (3) Primary brain tumors can also present with cognitive impairment.

    (a) Reported prevalence of radiation-induced cognitive impairment is 27%–90% of adults with brain tumors (Ali et al., 2018).

    (b) Seizures and cognitive impairment are the two dominant presenting symptoms in patients with glioma (Ali et al., 2018).

11. Cognitive testing for dementia

  a) In addition to taking a history, it is important to perform cognitive testing.

  b) Cognitive tests can be influenced by language, culture, and educational background; thus, it is important to choose the correct test for each individual patient (Budson & Solomon, 2016).

  c) Several types of cognitive testing are available.

    (1) Mini-Cog (Borson, Scanlan, Brush, Vitaliano, & Dokmak, 2000; Budson & Solomon, 2016; Cordell et al., 2013)

      (a) Two items

      (b) Score out of 5 (3 points for three-word recall and 2 points for clock drawing)

      (c) Domains assessed: executive function, short-term memory recall, visuospatial

      (d) Administration time: three minutes

(e) Benefits: developed for and validated in primary care, appropriate for those with limited language or education, culturally appropriate

(f) Limitation: not diagnostic

(2) Montreal Cognitive Assessment (Budson & Solomon, 2016; Cordell et al., 2013; Nasreddine et al., 2005)

  (a) 12 items

  (b) Score out of 30; abnormal score less than 25

  (c) One extra point for less than a high school education

  (d) Domains assessed: orientation, recall, attention, naming, repetition, verbal fluency, abstraction, visuospatial, executive function

  (e) Administration time: 5–10 minutes

  (f) Sensitivity for mild cognitive impairment: 90%; sensitivity for mild Alzheimer disease: 100%

  (g) Specificity: 87%

  (h) Benefits: sensitive test for mild cognitive impairment, available in multiple languages

  (i) Limitations: limited studies in primary care settings, education bias

(3) Rowland Universal Dementia Assessment Scale (Rowland et al., 2007)

  (a) Six items

  (b) Score out of 30; abnormal score less than 22

  (c) Domains assessed: memory, visuospatial, praxis, executive function, memory recall, language

  (d) Sensitivity: 89%

  (e) Specificity: 98%

  (f) Benefits: little education or language bias, created for multicultural population

  (g) Limitations: new test, thus limited evidence and use; validated in Australian population

(4) Folstein Mini-Mental Status Exam (Budson & Solomon, 2016; Cordell et al., 2013; Folstein, Folstein, & McHugh, 1975)

  (a) 19 items

  (b) Score out of 30; abnormal score less than 25

  (c) Domains assessed: orientation, registration, recall, attention, naming, repetition, three-step command, visuospatial, language

  (d) Administration time: 5–10 minutes

  (e) Sensitivity to mild cognitive impairment: 18%; sensitivity to mild Alzheimer disease: 78%

  (f) Specificity: 100%

  (g) Benefit: commonly used as a reference for comparative evaluations

  (h) Limitations: biased by education, language, and culture

    i. Highly educated patients will perform well even if they have impairments.

    ii. It can only be used for memory because the instrument is proprietary.

(5) St. Louis University Mental Status Exam (Budson & Solomon, 2016; Cordell et al., 2013; Saint Louis University, 2019)

  (a) 11 items

  (b) Score out of 30; abnormal score less than 27 for high school education; abnormal score less than 25 for less than high school education

  (c) Domains assessed: orientation, recall, calculation, naming, attention, executive function

  (d) Benefit: no education bias

  (e) Limitations: studied in Veterans Affairs geriatric clinic with predominantly White male patients; new test, thus limited evidence and use

12. Evaluation

  a) General: It is important to note that the diagnosis of dementia is clinical; laboratory investigations and neuroimaging are used to identify treatable causes, which are rare, and comorbid conditions (Harper, Lyons, & Potter, 2019).

  b) Laboratory tests

    (1) Routine laboratory tests include the following (American Academy of Neurology, 2004; Livingston et al., 2017).

      (a) Complete blood count

      (b) Serum electrolytes

      (c) Blood urea nitrogen

      (d) Creatinine

      (e) Fasting glucose

      (f) Thyrotropin

      (g) Vitamin B_{12}

      (h) Liver function tests (aspartate transaminase, alanine transaminase, bilirubin)

    (2) Based on clinical examination and suspicion, further testing can include the following.

      (a) Rapid plasma regain

      (b) HIV testing

      (c) Lyme disease testing

    (3) Screening for syphilis should occur only if a patient has risk factors (e.g., living in high incidence region, sexual history, immunocompromise) (American Academy of Neurology, 2004; Budson & Solomon, 2016).

c) Neuroimaging
  (1) Which types of patients should be tested with neuroimaging is a subject of debate with no clear consensus.
  (2) American Academy of Neurology guidelines stated, "structural neuroimaging with either a noncontrast CT or [MRI] scan in the routine initial evaluation of patients with dementia is appropriate" (Knopman et al., 2001, p. 1148).
  (3) In 1997, the American Association for Geriatric Psychiatry, the Alzheimer's Association, and the American Geriatrics Society published a consensus statement on the diagnosis and treatment of dementia (Small et al., 1997).
    (a) The consensus concluded that imaging studies are optional; however, they are recommended by many clinicians and experts.
    (b) Noncontrast CT of the head is adequate in most circumstances.
  (4) The Alzheimer's Association recommends neuroimaging as an additional aid in the diagnosis of dementia, especially in the case of abnormal neurologic findings from examination (Cordell et al., 2013). They also recommend considering neuroimaging if the patient has rapidly progressing dementia, is younger than 65 years old at onset, and has a history of head trauma.
  (5) The American Geriatrics Society recommends that neuroimaging may be useful in cases of dementia in the following situations (Harper et al., 2019).
    (a) Onset before 65 years old
    (b) Sudden or rapidly progressing symptoms
    (c) Abnormal neurologic examination with focal or asymmetrical signs
    (d) Concern for normal pressure hydrocephalus (gait disorder, unexplained incontinence, onset within one year)
    (e) History of recent fall or head trauma
  (6) ACR Appropriateness Criteria lean toward recommending neuroimaging (ACR, 2019).
    (a) ACR utilizes a 1–9 scale, with 1 being least appropriate and 9 being the most appropriate.
    (b) MRI without contrast is the preferred imaging study (ACR, 2019).
      i. MRI is more sensitive.
      ii. It can exclude stroke, subdural hematoma, normal pressure hydrocephalus, and mass.
      iii. It can help determine dementia subtype based on pattern of atrophy seen.
      iv. Several issues should be considered with MRI: longer duration of test, noise level, difficulty in obtaining, claustrophobia, and patients with behavioral symptoms (Budson & Solomon, 2016).
      (c) Refer to the full ACR Appropriateness Criteria (ACR, 2019) for recommendations related to other diagnostic procedures.
13. Differential diagnosis: It is important to be aware of diseases and circumstances that can mimic dementia, including the following.
  a) Delirium (Budson & Solomon, 2016)
    (1) Delirium is characterized by acute onset, fluctuations in level of consciousness, and inattention.
    (2) Delirium is a geriatric emergency and requires immediate investigation and management.
    (3) Diagnosis of dementia should not be made in the setting of delirium.
  b) Depression: Depression can be an early sign of dementia or can present as a "pseudodementia" (Feldman et al., 2008).
  c) Medication: Dementia may be caused by medications, such as anticholinergics and benzodiazepines.
  d) Normal aging memory loss: If concerned about dementia, clinicians should address previously discussed reversible causes and reassess memory.
14. Functional decline associated with cognitive impairment and assessment of ADLs
  a) Functional dependency
    (1) Being functionally dependent is defined as being unable to live independently without assistance.
    (2) A focused assessment, such as CGA, can identify areas of concern in older adults, such as deficits in basic ADLs, instrumental ADLs, and diminished cognitive capacity (Mohile et al., 2018).
    (3) Functional dependency may be the result of cognitive impairment; therefore, it is important to assess for a baseline prior to RT.
    (4) It is also important to assess instrumental ADLs in order to understand patients' functional abilities prior to RT to appreciate if they will require assistance at home and at the treatment facility.
    (5) It is important to know why a patient is unable to perform these functions (e.g., impaired cognition, physical impairment).
    (6) Clinicians should assess upper and lower mobility prior to treatment to determine if patients can transfer, get on and off of the treatment table, move their arms, and lie flat for the duration of the treatment (Cree, O'Donovan, & O'Hanlon, 2019).
    (7) Before, during, and after RT, healthcare professionals should assess patients' basic and instru-

mental ADLs, such as ability to bathe, dress, toilet, transfer, and feed themselves (Katz, 1983).

(8) If patients require assistance in one or more basic or instrumental ADLs, it is important to assess their cognition using previously discussed tools and diagnostic tests, as well as their functional status. Assessment should determine whether they will be able to function at home alone after treatment (Cree et al., 2019).

(9) The following questions can assist in assessing instrumental ADLs (Fillenbaum & Smyer, 1981).

(a) Is the patient able to use the telephone independently?

(b) Can the patient see the telephone and push the correct phone numbers?

(c) Can the patient shop independently or make meals?

(d) Can the patient do housework?

(e) Can the patient take medications without forgetting?

(f) Can the patient see a medication label well enough to read it?

(g) Is the patient able to manage finances and pay bills correctly and on time?

b) Falls

(1) Several factors may increase risk of falls in older adults.

(a) Sarcopenia (loss of skeletal mass)

i. Sarcopenia has been associated with the development of functional impairment; it increases the risk of falls and the risk of death in older adults (Williams, Rier, McDonald, & Shachar, 2019).

ii. In 2014, approximately 2.8 million older adults sought treatment in emergency departments in the United States for falls; fractures from falls are relatively common (Grossman et al., 2018; Guirguis-Blake, Michael, Perdue, Coppola, & Beil, 2018).

iii. A bone mineral density test is recommended in older adults (varies by country). Decreased bone mineral density may require medication management, such as vitamin D or calcium supplementation or antiresorptive therapy.

(b) RT

i. RT may cause bladder cystitis, leading to urgency and frequency, and this may pose concerns for patients who are cognitively impaired, especially during the night.

ii. RT may also cause diarrhea, involving frequent washroom visits, which may lead to falls.

iii. Strategies to prevent falls in these situations could include a commode at the bedside in the home or adult absorptive pads in the case of incontinence.

(c) Cognitive impairment

i. It is important to assess cognitive impairment prior to RT.

ii. Patients may require extra guidance and support to navigate the hospital setting.

iii. It is recommended to improve signage, orient the patient to the hospital prior to starting treatment, provide flexible appointment times, educate the staff, and provide the patient with identifiers (e.g., badges, bracelets) to alert others if they need assistance (Cree et al., 2019).

(d) Postural hypotension

i. Postural hypotension is common in older adults for several reasons (e.g., medications, comorbidities, weakened circulatory system, poor fluid intake).

ii. Postural hypotension may affect blood pressure, ultimately leading to more falls.

(2) Addressing fall risk for older adults is essential.

(a) Daily RT can be challenging, especially for patients with cognitive impairment who do not fully comprehend the treatment plan.

(b) The oncology team should consider a tailored RT plan for those with cognitive impairment.

(c) Prior to RT initiation, clinicians should consider referral for physiotherapy, a geriatric falls prevention program that consists of a geriatric assessment, occupational therapy in the home for a home safety assessment to prevent falls, proper footwear for each season, and gait aids if necessary.

(d) Home hazard modifications have been proven to be effective in reducing falls in the home (Grossman et al., 2018).

(e) Other strategies to help prevent falls in older adults can include assessing postural blood pressure, assessing for dizziness, and assessing lower extremities for edema, circulation, neuropathy, and pain.

c) Pain

(1) Few pain assessment tools are available for cognitively impaired older adults; nonethe-

less, pain scales, guarding, and facial grimacing have been effective tools in pain assessment (Fry, Arendts, & Chenoweth, 2017).

   (2) Clinicians should assess pain and skin of the RT site daily for those with cognitive impairment because they may not be able to verbalize their pain or effects of RT.

d) Nutrition

   (1) Cognitive impairment and malnutrition directly and indirectly decrease ability to perform ADLs in older adults living at home and receiving home nursing care (Furuta et al., 2013).

   (2) It is vital to assess nutritional intake and hydration daily with cognitively impaired patients.

   (3) Patients with cognitive impairment often forget to eat, struggle to go grocery shopping, do not remember how to perform their personal banking to purchase groceries, are unable to cook for themselves, leave kitchen appliances on, or forget how to use appliances.

   (4) To help patients and families with these difficulties, healthcare professionals can recommend a nutrition diary, an RDN or RD consult, and nutritional supplements.

   (5) If a patient has limited social supports, clinicians should recommend home nursing care or personal support service.

e) Vision and hearing

   (1) Very little is known about how RT affects vision and hearing, but vision, hearing, sensory, and cognitive changes occur as a part of normal aging.

   (2) SNHL can be an adverse event of RT to the head and neck region (Theunissen et al., 2013).

   (3) Some systemic therapies may also cause ototoxicity (Theunissen et al., 2013).

   (4) Researchers have focused on the otoprotective effect of several agents in humans (Theunissen et al., 2013).

   (5) In the United States, 75% of individuals aged 70 years or older have hearing loss (Lin et al., 2013). Lin et al. (2013) reported that older adults with hearing loss displayed a 30%–40% accelerated rate of cognitive decline compared to those with normal hearing.

   (6) It is recommended that older adults have their vision and hearing assessed regularly. Clinicians should perform a pretreatment and post-treatment audiologic evaluation with special emphasis on high frequencies (Theunissen et al., 2013).

   (7) Vision and hearing should be assessed for a baseline prior to starting RT. Assessment should occur during and after RT, if any changes are noted.

   (8) A sound amplifier, or pocket talker, is a useful tool for those with hearing issues.

   (9) Improved signage, orientation, and reduction of stimulation and clutter are recommended (Cree et al., 2019).

   (10) Music therapy has also been recommended to promote a calming environment (Cree et al., 2019).

15. Frailty associated with cognitive impairment

   a) Definition: Frailty has many definitions in the research but is generally associated with weakness, vulnerability, functional deficits, comorbidities, advanced age, polypharmacy, poor nutritional status, and cognitive decline (Rodríguez-Mañas et al., 2012).

   b) Screening tools

   (1) The VES-13 or G8 can be effective tools for healthcare professionals to identify frailty in older adults (Decoster et al., 2015).

   (2) The VES-13 and G8 assess cognition; an abnormal score on either warrants further cognitive screening and functional assessment.

   (3) The VES-13 was designed to assess those older than age 65 years living in the community with functional decline (Saliba et al., 2001).

   (a) It involves a questionnaire that can be administered by the patient, family, or healthcare professional and takes four to five minutes to complete.

   (b) The VES-13 focuses on functional status, ADLs, and age; it also has a self-rated health question.

   (4) In a study of older patients with cancer, Rowbottom et al. (2019) reported that those who scored positive (vulnerable) on the VES-13 had higher cognitive impairment and worse physical outcomes compared to those who were VES-13 negative.

   (5) The G8 is a quick screening tool that was developed for those aged 70 years and older who are undergoing first-line chemotherapy. The G8 includes a self-rated health question and measures health, function, cognition, and nutrition (Soubeyran et al., 2014).

   (6) CGA may be warranted when assessing frailty in those with suspected cognitive impairment undergoing RT; it can be used to refine diagnosis and treatment.

   (7) A reduced RT plan may be necessary for patients if cure is not the goal, if reduced RT will not compromise survival, or if a patient has dementia (Alibhai et al., 2018).

   c) Quality of life

   (1) Radiation-induced cognitive impairment may have significant effects on quality of life for older adults.

(2) To date, very little research has focused on long-term side effects of radiation-induced cognitive impairment, as well as proven treatments or preventive strategies.

(3) Medications should be assessed at the beginning of RT to identify inappropriate medications that may induce cognitive impairment in older adults. The Beers criteria and the STOPP criteria may be helpful (O'Mahony et al., 2015).

16. Treatment decision-making and RT tolerance in older adults with cognitive issues

a) Older patients can experience treatment-related toxicities that affect quality of life, treatment compliance and effectiveness, and treatment-related mortality (Chang, Goldstein, & Dharmarajan, 2017).

b) RT-related burdens can be significant and include intensive schedules, travel demands, costs, and temporary or permanent loss of functional independence (Chang et al., 2017).

(1) For this reason, it is suggested that patients may benefit from hypofractionated treatment schedules, aimed to deliver the same total doses of conventional RT schedules but in fewer treatment sessions (Chang et al., 2017).

(2) Reduction of treatment volumes has also been utilized in a number of tumor sites, including lymphoma and breast cancer (Cree et al., 2019).

(3) SRS and SBRT have been used to treat brain metastasis and early-stage lung cancer, respectively. These treatments are beneficial to older patients because of reduced toxicity compared to standard RT (Cree et al., 2019).

c) Research demonstrates that performing a CGA prior to treatment can modify up to 30%–40% of initial treatment plans in older adults with cancer (Hamaker, Schiphorst, ten Bokkel Huinink, Schaar, & van Munster, 2014; Puts et al., 2014).

(1) In RT, the use of CGA prior to treatment has demonstrated the potential to predict side effects and tolerability (Chang et al., 2017; Szumacher et al., 2018).

(2) Low vitamin D levels and slow gait speeds detected in a CGA were found to be associated with post-RT esophagitis and emesis, respectively (Ulger et al., 2015).

(3) Determining RT risks in older adults can maximize the benefits and minimize the risks of treatment in each unique individual, within the following framework (Chang et al., 2017).

(a) Clinicians must recognize individuals who can benefit from standard treatment and those for whom the therapeutic risks would outweigh the benefits, resulting in loss of function and independence (Chang et al., 2017).

(b) Implementation of personalized medical and psychosocial interventions may improve the tolerance to cancer therapy (Chang et al., 2017).

(c) CGA and validated prediction tools assist in the development of CGA-based interventions and recommendations to the cancer treatment plan. These tools inform discussion of treatment risks and benefits, identify goals of care, and assist in modifying toxicity risk (Chang et al., 2017; Mohile et al., 2018).

(d) Risk prediction tools in both surgical and medical oncology have demonstrated reduced toxicity in older adults who have undergone these treatment routes, but evidence to reduce RT toxicity in this population is sparse (Hurria et al., 2011; Mohanty et al., 2016; Szumacher et al., 2018).

17. Life expectancy

a) Dementia affects prognosis (Todd, Barr, Roberts, & Passmore, 2013).

b) Research has demonstrated the effectiveness of using ePrognosis (see https://eprognosis.ucsf.edu) to assist oncologists, patients, families, and caregivers in discussions of treatment decision-making, quality of life, and patient priorities by providing an estimation of life expectancy independent of cancer diagnosis.

(1) Created from a systematic review, ePrognosis is an online tool that can calculate mortality risk, independent of the cancer diagnosis, based on markers of frailty, medical conditions, age, and sex, among others. It was designed for older adults who do not have a dominant terminal illness (Yourman, Lee, Schonberg, Widera, & Smith, 2012).

(2) It is important to note that validated prognostic indices used in ePrognosis cannot predict with absolute certainty how long an older adult will live; however, these indices may improve the accuracy of prognostic assumptions that affect clinical decisions (Yourman et al., 2012).

(3) ASCO Clinical Practice Guidelines also recommend the use ePrognosis to estimate life expectancy (excluding the diagnosis of cancer) to aid in treatment decision-making with patients and their families considering chemotherapy (Mohile et al., 2018).

(4) Mohile et al. (2018) recommended the Schonberg Index (Schonberg, Li, Marcantonio, Davis, & McCarthy, 2017) or Lee Index (Lee, Lindquist, Segal, & Covinsky, 2006) for older adults (see https://eprognosis.ucsf.edu/calculators.php).

(5) Mohile et al. (2018) highlighted that the quality of evidence to support these tools to

predict mortality is high, but the evidence that using these tools improves outcomes or decision-making is insufficient.

18. Improving RT tolerance in older adults
    a) Telephone nursing support in cancer care has demonstrated a reduction in social isolation, caregiver burden, cancer symptoms, toxicity to treatment, emotional distress, and improvement in symptom self-management and health-related quality of life (Chen & Schulz, 2016; Chi & Demiris, 2015; Craven, Hughes, Burton, Saunders, & Molassiotis, 2013; Suh & Lee, 2017).
    b) Close follow-up of CGA-based interventions is key to successfully optimizing the health of older adults, which can result in improved tolerance of cancer treatment (Burhenn et al., 2016; Mohile et al., 2018).
    c) The effectiveness of the CGA-process lies with a well-established follow-up plan, guided by a goal-directed care plan established with the patient and family or caregiver (Mohile et al., 2018).
    d) Much of the follow-up and monitoring of the interventions from CGA can be done by nursing through proactive monitoring and integration, as well as collaboration with the circle of care (Burhenn et al., 2016).

19. Nursing approaches to patient and caregiver support
    a) Addressing needs of older patients
        (1) Addressing the interaction between aging and cancer can be further complicated for nurses by unique individual and family needs, geriatric syndromes, frailty, communication challenges, and limitations in health literacy (Bridges, Wengström, & Bailey, 2016; Fields, Rodakowski, James, & Beach, 2018; Kelley et al., 2012; Morgan & Tarbi, 2016).
        (2) The following measures can be implemented to address geriatric challenges (Korc-Grodzicki & Tew, 2017).
            (a) Enhancing communication techniques to work with cognitively impaired older adults, such as providing written information in large font to help recall what was discussed
            (b) Increasing signage and proper orientation to facilities prior to treatment
            (c) Taking breaks in discussions and allowing a patient to paraphrase information provided
            (d) Nurses acting as advocates for a patient with aggressive family
        (3) Nurses must include the collateral information from caregivers, family, and community care providers to clarify the symptoms and unmet needs of older adults with cognitive impairment (Burhenn et al., 2016).

        (4) Nurses need to assess for presence and adequacy of a caregiver, living conditions, level of income, and access to transportation prior to, during, and after RT to uncover unmet needs (Burhenn et al., 2016).
    b) Health education
        (1) Providing education and support to the caregiver is imperative to the health outcomes of the care recipient (Fields et al., 2018).
        (2) Twenty percent of caregivers demonstrated low health literacy, which dramatically increases the odds of encountering difficulty with healthcare communication and system navigation (Fields et al., 2018).
        (3) Poor health literacy results in higher levels of caregiver burden and correlates to decline in physical and mental health outcomes secondary to the unmet care needs of the care recipient (Bobay, Jerofke, Weiss, & Yakusheva, 2010).
    c) Navigation and care coordination
        (1) Care facilitation, integration, and system navigation are important roles of nurses in supporting the cancer care of older adults (Gorin et al., 2017; Korc-Grodzicki & Tew, 2017; Manderson, McMurray, Piraino, & Stolee, 2012).
        (2) Integration of care with the broader care team (e.g., PCP, visiting nurse, physiotherapy, pharmacy) can help manage symptoms and preserve function and independence in this population (Korc-Grodzicki & Tew, 2017).
        (3) Nurses can facilitate reminder calls to patients and identify and assist navigation needs before and during clinic visits, especially for those with cognitive, mobility, and functional impairments. Support with navigating the healthcare system is shown to reduce barriers to care in older adults with chronic illness (Manderson et al., 2012).
    d) Social support
        (1) Evidence shows lack of social connections increases the risk for premature mortality in adults of all age groups (Holt-Lunstad, Smith, Baker, Harris, & Stephenson, 2015).
            (a) Older adults are thought to be particularly vulnerable to social isolation as a result of being widowed, living alone, having multiple health conditions, and having functional impairments (Holt-Lunstad et al., 2015).
            (b) Social isolation often goes undetected and unaddressed by oncology teams (Rosario et al., 2019).
        (2) Social isolation and marginalization are considered independent predictors of mortality in older adults with cancer, as sufficient social

support enhances resilience against the stress inherent in having cancer (Holt-Lunstad et al., 2015).

(3) Functional status greatly affects the ability to socialize. Functional status is a strong predictor of morbidity and mortality (Hurria et al., 2011).

(4) Adequate social support is pivotal for several aspects of RT, including transportation, access to care to manage treatment toxicities, and emotional and physical support to the patient during treatment (Chang et al., 2017).

(5) Emotional loneliness is associated with mortality among older adults in nursing homes with or without cognitive impairment (Drageset, Eide, Kirkevold, & Ranhoff, 2013).

   (a) Nurses should be attuned to signs of emotional loneliness in older adults and inquire about the presence of a confidant or supportive people in a patient's day-to-day life who provide emotional support (Drageset et al., 2013).

   (b) It is important for nurses to be aware that depression in older adults often goes unrecognized and untreated and that detection of depression in adults with dementia is challenging because of the lack of a validated, brief screening tool (Brown, Raue, & Halpert, 2015).

(6) Referrals to a social worker or relevant community supports should be initiated by a nurse to meet these needs (Burhenn et al., 2016).

e) Transportation

(1) Transportation barriers limit access to timely health care for older adults, and strategies to improve access to transportation services for oncology visits can improve health outcomes and facilitate cancer treatment adherence (Syed, Gerber, & Sharp, 2013).

(2) It is thought that older adults are particularly limited by transportation barriers because of illness, functional limitations, and multiple medical visits, yet there is a lack of research to support this because of poor representation of this population (Syed et al., 2013).

(3) Nurses need to assess this often unmet need and provide the following assessments and interventions.

   (a) Ask how patients get to medical appointments.

   (b) Identify barriers in accessing transportation services.

   (c) Connect patients to community services and volunteer drivers.

f) Home care

(1) Building adequate home care through community support programs to assist in symptom management with enhanced collaboration and communication with the broader care team will assist in improving access to care for this population (Burhenn et al., 2016).

(2) Families and caregivers require support and education from nurses to provide support and management to their loved ones. Effective caregivers are able to coordinate a patient's treatment with the following actions (Korc-Grodzicki & Tew, 2017).

   (a) Timely recognition of treatment complications

   (b) Arrangement of transportation for medical visits

   (c) Bridging communication gaps between a patient, family, and practitioners

   (d) Facilitating problem solving and adherence to care plans

(3) It is also important to note that an older adult with cancer may also be a caregiver to another person. This situation will require the facilitation of community supports for the other person to enable the patient to attend scheduled treatments.

g) Caregiver burden

(1) Caregiver burden of family caregivers is an important consideration when engaging the health of older adults.

(2) Caregivers of patients with dementia experience a higher physical and mental burden than caregivers of relatives without dementia (Cheng, 2017; Kim, Chang, Rose, & Kim, 2012).

(3) A study examining family caregivers of patients undergoing RT concluded that caregivers experience sleep disturbance, anxiety, perceived poor family support, and high levels of patient fatigue, which put caregivers at highest risk for prolonged fatigue. These issues require assessment from the healthcare team (Fletcher et al., 2009).

(4) Better assessment and support for caregivers may improve their well-being before and after bereavement, as well as improve quality of care for patients and reduce hospital admissions (De Korte-Verhoef et al., 2015).

(5) Many caregiver burden screening tools have been validated in those caring for older adults with cognitive impairment; however, none are specific to older adults with cognitive impairment and cancer undergoing RT (Applebaum, 2019).

h) Elder abuse

(1) Elder abuse is an essential consideration for oncology nurses caring for older adults with cognitive impairment.

(2) Several tools are available to screen for elder abuse (Gallione et al., 2017).

(3) Nurses need to be aware of the types of elder abuse (Pillemer, Burnes, Riffin, & Lachs, 2016).
  (a) Physical
  (b) Psychological
  (c) Sexual assault
  (d) Material and financial exploitation
  (e) Neglect
(4) Strong risk factors for elder abuse specific to older adult patients include the following (Pillemer et al., 2016).
  (a) Functional dependence and disability
  (b) Poor physical health
  (c) Cognitive impairment
  (d) Poor mental health
  (e) Low socioeconomic status
(5) The U.S. Preventive Services Task Force has a recommendation statement and guidelines for healthcare professionals on its website (see www.uspreventiveservicestaskforce.org).

References

Albert, M.S., DeKosky, S.T., Dickson, D., Dubois, B., Feldman, H.H., Fox, N.C., ... Phelps, C.H. (2011). The diagnosis of mild cognitive impairment due to Alzheimer's disease: Recommendations from the National Institute on Aging-Alzheimer's Association workgroups on diagnostic guidelines for Alzheimer's disease. *Alzheimer's and Dementia, 7,* 270–279. https://doi.org/10.1016/j.jalz.2011.03.008

Ali, F.S., Hussain, M.R., Gutiérrez, C., Demireva, P., Ballester, L.Y., Zhu, J.-J., ... Esquenazi, Y. (2018). Cognitive disability in adult patients with brain tumors. *Cancer Treatment Reviews, 65,* 33–40. https://doi.org/10.1016/j.ctrv.2018.02.007

Alibhai, S.M.H., Jin, R., Loucks, A., Yokom, D.W., Watt, S., Puts, M., ... Berger, A. (2018). Beyond the black box of geriatric assessment: Understanding enhancements to care by the geriatric oncology clinic. *Journal of Geriatric Oncology, 9,* 679–682. https://doi.org/10.1016/j.jgo.2018.03.012

Alzheimer's Association. (2019). *2019 Alzheimer's disease facts and figures.* https://www.alz.org/media/Documents/alzheimers-facts-and-figures-2019-r.pdf

American Academy of Neurology. (2004). *AAN guideline summary for clinicians: Detection, diagnosis and management of dementia.* https://www.aan.com/Guidelines/home/GuidelineDetail/42

American College of Radiology. (2019). *ACR Appropriateness Criteria®: Dementia.* https://acsearch.acr.org/docs/3111292/Narrative

American Pyschiatric Association. (2013). *Diagnostic and statistical manual of mental disorders* (5th ed.). Author.

Applebaum, A.J. (Ed.). (2019). *Cancer caregivers.* Oxford University Press.

Bobay, K.L., Jerofke, T.A., Weiss, M.E., & Yakusheva, O. (2010). Age-related differences in perception of quality of discharge teaching and readiness for hospital discharge. *Geriatric Nursing, 31,* 178–187. https://doi.org/10.1016/j.gerinurse.2010.03.005

Borson, S., Scanlan, J., Brush, M., Vitaliano, P., & Dokmak, A. (2000). The Mini-Cog: A cognitive 'vital signs' measure for dementia screening in multilingual elderly. *International Journal of Geriatric Psychiatry, 15,* 1021–1027. https://doi.org/10.1002/1099-1166(200011)15:11<1021::aid-gps234>3.0.co;2-6

Bridges, J., Wengström, Y., & Bailey, D.E., Jr. (2016). Educational preparation of nurses caring for older people with cancer: An international perspective. *Seminars in Oncology Nursing, 32,* 16–23. https://doi.org/10.1016/j.soncn.2015.11.003

Brodaty, H., Aerts, L., Crawford, J.D., Heffernan, M., Kochan, N.A., Reppermund, S., ... Sachdev, P.S. (2017). Operationalizing the diagnostic criteria for mild cognitive impairment: The salience of objective measures in predicting incident dementia. *American Journal of Geriatric Psychiatry, 25,* 485–497. https://doi.org/10.1016/j.jagp.2016.12.012

Brown, E.L., Raue, P.J., & Halpert, K. (2015). Evidence-based practice guideline: Depression detection in older adults with dementia. *Journal of Gerontologic Nursing, 41*(11), 15–21. https://doi.org/10.3928/00989134-20151015-03

Budson, A.E., & Solomon, P.R. (2016). *Memory loss, Alzheimer's disease and dementia: A practical guide for clinicians.* Elsevier.

Burhenn, P.S., McCarthy, A.L., Begue, A., Nightingale, G., Cheng, K., & Kenis, C. (2016). Geriatric assessment in daily oncology practice for nurses and allied health care professionals: Opinion paper of the Nursing and Allied Health Interest Group of the International Society of Geriatric Oncology (SIOG). *Journal of Geriatric Oncology, 7,* 315–324. https://doi.org/10.1016/j.jgo.2016.02.006

Chang, S., Goldstein, N.E., & Dharmarajan, K.V. (2017). Managing an older adult with cancer: Considerations for radiation oncologists. *BioMed Research International, 2017,* 1695101. https://doi.org/10.1155/2017/1695101

Chen, Y.-R., & Schulz, P.J. (2016). The effect of information communication technology interventions on reducing social isolation in the elderly: A systematic review. *Journal of Medical Internet Research, 18,* e18. https://doi.org/10.2196/jmir.4596

Cheng, S.-T. (2017). Dementia caregiver burden: A research update and critical analysis. *Current Psychiatry Reports, 19,* 64. https://doi.org/10.1007/s11920-017-0818-2

Chi, N.-C., & Demiris, G. (2015). A systematic review of telehealth tools and interventions to support family caregivers. *Journal of Telemedicine and Telecare, 21,* 37–44. https://doi.org/10.1177/1357633x14562734

Cordell, C.B., Borson, S., Boustani, M., Chodosh, J., Reuben, D., Verghese, J., ... Fried, L.B. (2013). Alzheimer's Association recommendations for operationalizing the detection of cognitive impairment during the Medicare annual wellness visit in a primary care setting. *Alzheimer's and Dementia, 9,* 141–150. https://doi.org/10.1016/j.jalz.2012.09.011

Craven, O., Hughes, C.A., Burton, A., Saunders, M.P., & Molassiotis, A. (2013). Is a nurse-led telephone intervention a viable alternative to nurse-led home care and standard care for patients receiving oral capecitabine? Results from a large prospective audit in patients with colorectal cancer. *European Journal of Cancer Care, 22,* 413–419. https://doi.org/10.1111/ecc.12047

Cree, A., O'Donovan, A., & O'Hanlon, S. (2019). New horizons in radiotherapy for older people. *Age and Ageing, 48,* 605–612. https://doi.org/10.1093/ageing/afz089

Decoster, L., Van Puyvelde, K., Mohile, S., Wedding, U., Basso, U., Colloca, G., ... Extermann, M. (2015). Screening tools for multidimensional health problems warranting a geriatric assessment in older cancer patients: An update on SIOG recommendations. *Annals of Oncology, 26,* 288–300. https://doi.org/10.1093/annonc/mdu210

De Korte-Verhoef, M.C., Pasman, H.R., Schweitzer, B.P.M., Francke, A.L., Onwuteaka-Philipsen, B.D., & Deliens, L. (2015). How could hospitalisations at the end of life have been avoided? A qualitative retrospective study of the perspectives of general practitioners, nurses and family carers. *PLOS ONE, 10,* e0118971. https://doi.org/10.1371/journal.pone.0118971

Drageset, J., Eide, G.E., Kirkevold, M., & Ranhoff, A.H. (2013). Emotional loneliness is associated with mortality among mentally intact nursing home residents with and without cancer: A five-year follow-up study. *Journal of Clinical Nursing, 22,* 106–114. https://doi.org/10.1111/j.1365-2702.2012.04209.x

Feldman, H.H., Jacova, C., Robillard, A., Garcia, A., Chow, T., Borrie, M., ... Chertkow, H. (2008). Diagnosis and treatment of dementia: 2. Diagnosis. *Canadian Medical Association Journal, 178,* 825–836. https://doi.org/10.1503/cmaj.070798

Fields, B., Rodakowski, J., James, A.E., & Beach, S. (2018). Caregiver health literacy predicting healthcare communication and system navigation difficulty. *Families, Systems, and Health, 36,* 482–492. https://doi.org/10.1037/fsh0000368

Fillenbaum, G.G., & Smyer, M.A. (1981). The development, validity, and reliability of the OARS multidimensional functional assessment questionnaire. *Journal of Gerontology, 36,* 428–434. https://doi.org/10.1093/geronj/36.4.428

Fjell, A.M., McEvoy, L., Holland, D., Dale, A.M., & Walhovd, K.B. (2014). What is normal in normal aging? Effects of aging, amyloid and Alzheimer's disease on the cerebral cortex and the hippocampus. *Progress in Neurobiology, 117,* 20–40. https://doi.org/10.1016/j.pneurobio.2014.02.004

Fletcher, B.A.S., Schumacher, K.L., Dodd, M., Paul, S.M., Cooper, B.A., Lee, K., ... Miaskowski, C. (2009). Trajectories of fatigue in family caregivers of patients undergoing radiation therapy for prostate cancer. *Research in Nursing and Health, 32,* 125–139. https://doi.org/10.1002/nur.20312

Folstein, M.F., Folstein, S.E., & McHugh, P.R. (1975). "Mini-mental state": A practical method for grading the cognitive state of patients for the clinician. *Journal of Psychiatric Research, 12,* 189–198. https://doi.org/10.1016/0022-3956(75)90026-6

Fry, M., Arendts, G., & Chenoweth, L. (2017). Emergency nurses' evaluation of observational pain assessment tools for older people with cognitive impairment. *Journal of Clinical Nursing, 26,* 1281–1290. https://doi.org/10.1111/jocn.13591

Furuta, M., Komiya-Nonaka, M., Akifusa, S., Shimazaki, Y., Adachi, M., Kinoshita, T., ... Yamashita, Y. (2013). Interrelationship of oral health status, swallowing function, nutritional status, and cognitive ability with activities of daily living in Japanese elderly people receiving home care services due to physical disabilities. *Community Dentistry and Oral Epidemiology, 41,* 173–181. https://doi.org/10.1111/cdoe.12000

Gallione, C., Dal Molin, A., Cristina, F.V.B., Ferns, H., Mattioli, M., & Suardi, B. (2017). Screening tools for identification of elder abuse: A systematic review. *Journal of Clinical Nursing, 26,* 2154–2176. https://doi.org/10.1111/jocn.13721

Gorin, S.S., Haggstrom, D., Han, P.K.J., Fairfield, K.M., Krebs, P., & Clauser, S.B. (2017). Cancer care coordination: A systematic review and meta-analysis of over 30 years of empirical studies. *Annals of Behavioral Medicine, 51,* 532–546. https://doi.org/10.1007/s12160-017-9876-2

Grayston, F. (2018). Normal changes of ageing. *InnovAiT, 11,* 627–633. https://doi.org/10.1177/1755738018793446

Grossman, D.C., Curry, S.J., Owens, D.K., Barry, M.J., Caughey, A.B., Davidson, K.W., ... Tseng, C.-W. (2018). Interventions to prevent falls in community-dwelling older adults: US Preventive Services Task Force recommendation statement. *JAMA, 319,* 1696–1704. https://doi.org/10.1001/jama.2018.3097

Guirguis-Blake, J.M., Michael, Y.L., Perdue, L.A., Coppola, E.L., & Beil, T.L. (2018). Interventions to prevent falls in older adults: Updated evidence report and systematic review for the US Preventive Services Task Force. *JAMA, 319,* 1705–1716. https://doi.org/10.1001/jama.2017.21962

Hamaker, M.E., Schiphorst, A.H., ten Bokkel Huinink, D., Schaar, C., & van Munster, B.C. (2014). The effect of a geriatric evaluation on treatment decisions for older cancer patients—A systematic review. *Acta Oncologica, 53,* 289–296. https://doi.org/10.3109/0284186x.2013.840741

Harada, C.N., Natelson Love, M.C., & Triebel, K.L. (2013). Normal cognitive aging. *Clinics in Geriatric Medicine, 29,* 737–752. https://doi.org/10.1016/j.cger.2013.07.002

Harper, G.M., Lyons, W.L., & Potter, J.F. (Eds.). (2019). *Geriatric review syllabus: A core curriculum in geriatric medicine.* American Geriatrics Society.

Holt-Lunstad, J., Smith, T.B., Baker, M., Harris, T., & Stephenson, D. (2015). Loneliness and social isolation as risk factors for mortality: A meta-analytic review. *Perspectives on Psychological Science, 10,* 227–237. https://doi.org/10.1177/1745691614568352

Hugo, J., & Ganguli, M. (2014). Dementia and cognitive impairment: Epidemiology, diagnosis, and treatment. *Clinics in Geriatric Medicine, 30,* 421–442. https://doi.org/10.1016/j.cger.2014.04.001

Hurria, A., Togawa, K., Mohile, S.G., Owusu, C., Klepin, H.D., Gross, C.P., ... Tew, W.P. (2011). Predicting chemotherapy toxicity in older adults with cancer: A prospective multicenter study. *Journal of Clinical Oncology, 29,* 3457–3465. https://doi.org/10.1200/jco.2011.34.7625

Jacob, J., Durand, T., Feuvret, L., Mazeron, J.-J., Delattre, J.-Y., Hoang-Xuan, K., ... Maingon, P. (2018). Cognitive impairment and morphological changes after radiation therapy in brain tumors: A review. *Radiotherapy and Oncology, 128,* 221–228. https://doi.org/10.1016/j.radonc.2018.05.027

Kansal, K., Mareddy, M., Sloane, K.L., Minc, A.A., Rabins, P.V., McGready, J.B., & Onyike, C.U. (2016). Survival in frontotemporal dementia phenotypes: A meta-analysis. *Dementia and Geriatric Cognitive Disorders, 41,* 109–122. https://doi.org/10.1159/000443205

Karuturi, M., Wong, M.L., Hsu, T., Kimmick, G.G., Lichtman, S.M., Holmes, H.M., ... Mohile, S. (2016). Understanding cognition in older patients with cancer. *Journal of Geriatric Oncology, 7,* 258–269. https://doi.org/10.1016/j.jgo.2016.04.004

Katz, S. (1983). Assessing self-maintenance: Activities of daily living, mobility, and instrumental activities of daily living. *Journal of the American Geriatrics Society, 31,* 721–727. https://doi.org/10.1111/j.1532-5415.1983.tb03391.x

Kelley, A.S., Back, A.L., Arnold, R.M., Goldberg, G.R., Lim, B.B., Litrivis, E., ... O'Neill, L.B. (2012). Geritalk: Communication skills training for geriatric and palliative medicine fellows. *Journal of the American Geriatrics Society, 60,* 332–337. https://doi.org/10.1111/j.1532-5415.2011.03787.x

Kim, H., Chang, M., Rose, K., & Kim, S. (2012). Predictors of caregiver burden in caregivers of individuals with dementia. *Journal of Advanced Nursing, 68,* 846–855. https://doi.org/10.1111/j.1365-2648.2011.05787.x

Knopman, D.S., DeKosky, S.T., Cumming, J.L., Chui, H., Corey-Bloom, J., Relkin, N., ... Stevens, J.C. (2001). Practice parameter: Diagnosis of dementia (an evidence-based review): Report of the Quality Standards Subcommittee of the American Academy of Neurology. *Neurology, 56,* 1143–1153. https://doi.org/10.1212/WNL.56.9.1143

Korc-Grodzicki, B., & Tew, W. (Eds.). (2017). *Handbook of geriatric oncology: Practical guide to caring for the older cancer patient.* Demos Medical.

Lee, S.J., Lindquist, K., Segal, M.R., & Covinsky, K.E. (2006). Development and validation of a prognostic index for 4-year mortality in older adults. *JAMA, 295,* 801–808. https://doi.org/10.1001/jama.295.7.801

Lin, F.R., Yaffe, K., Xia, J., Xue, Q.-L., Harris, T.B., Purchase-Helzner, E., ... Simonsick, E.M. (2013). Hearing loss and cognitive decline in older adults. *JAMA Internal Medicine, 173,* 293–299. https://doi.org/10.1001/jamainternmed.2013.1868

Livingston, G., Sommerlad, A., Orgeta, V., Costafreda, S.G., Huntley, J., Ames, D. ... Mukadam, N. (2017). Dementia prevention, intervention, and care. *Lancet, 390,* 2673–2734. https://doi.org/10.1016/s0140-6736(17)31363-6

Lynch, M. (2019). Preservation of cognitive function following whole brain radiotherapy in patients with brain metastases: Complications, treatments, and the emerging role of memantine. *Journal of Oncology Pharmacy Practice, 25,* 657–662. https://doi.org/10.1177/1078155218798176

Manderson, B., McMurray, J., Piraino, E., & Stolee, P. (2012). Navigation roles support chronically ill older adults through healthcare transitions: A systematic review of the literature. *Health and Social Care in the Community, 20,* 113–127. https://doi.org/10.1111/j.1365-2524.2011.01032.x

Mohanty, S., Rosenthal, R.A., Russell, M.M., Neuman, M.D., Ko, C.Y., & Esnaola, N.F. (2016). Optimal perioperative management of the geriatric patient: A best practices guideline from the American College of Surgeons NSQIP and the American Geriatrics Society. *Journal of the American College of Surgeons, 222,* 930–947. https://doi.org/10.1016/j.jamcollsurg.2015.12.026

Mohile, S.G., Dale, W., Somerfield, M.R., Schonberg, M.A., Boyd, C.M., Burhenn, P.S., ... Hurria, A. (2018). Practical assessment and management of vulnerabilities in older patients receiving chemotherapy: ASCO guideline for geriatric oncology. *Journal of Clinical Oncology, 36,* 2326–2347. https://doi.org/10.1200/jco.2018.78.8687

Morgan, B., & Tarbi, E. (2016). The role of the advanced practice nurse in geriatric oncology care. *Seminars in Oncology Nursing, 32,* 33–43. https://doi.org/10.1016/j.soncn.2015.11.005

Nasreddine, Z.S., Phillips, N.A., Bédirian, V., Charbonneau, S., Whitehead, V., Collin, I., ... Chertkow, H. (2005). The Montreal Cognitive Assessment, MoCA: A brief screening tool for mild cognitive impairment. *Journal of the American Geriatrics Society, 53,* 695–699. https://doi.org/10.1111/j.1532-5415.2005.53221.x

O'Mahony, D., O'Sullivan, D., Byrne, S., O'Connor, M.N., Ryan, C., & Gallagher, P. (2015). STOPP/START criteria for potentially inappropriate prescribing in older people: Version 2. *Age and Ageing, 44,* 213–218. https://doi.org/10.1093/ageing/afu145

Petersen, R.C., Lopez, O., Armstrong, M.J., Getchius, T.S.D., Ganguli, M., Gloss, D., ... Rae-Grant, A. (2018). Practice guideline update: Mild cognitive impairment; Report of the Guideline Development, Dissemination, and Implementation Subcommittee of the American Academy of Neurology. *Neurology, 90,* 126–135. https://doi.org/10.1212/wnl.0000000000004826

Piai, V., Prins, J.B., Verdonck-de Leeuw, I.M., Leemans, C.R., Terhaard, C.H.J., Langendijk, J.A., ... Kessels, R.P.C. (2019). Assessment of neurocognitive impairment and speech functioning before head and neck cancer treatment. *JAMA Otolaryngology—Head and Neck Surgery, 145,* 251–257. https://doi.org/10.1001/jamaoto.2018.3981

Pillemer, K., Burnes, D., Riffin, C., & Lachs, M.S. (2016). Elder abuse: Global situation, risk factors, and prevention strategies. *Gerontologist, 56*(Suppl. 2), S194–S205. https://doi.org/10.1093/geront/gnw004

Puts, M.T.E., Santos, B., Hardt, J., Monette, J., Girre, V., Atenafu, E.G., ... Alibhai, S.M.H. (2014). An update on a systematic review of the use of geriatric assessment for older adults in oncology. *Annals of Oncology, 25,* 307–315. https://doi.org/10.1093/annonc/mdt386

Rodríguez-Mañas, L., Féart, C., Mann, G., Viña, J., Chatterji, S., Chodzko-Zajko, W., ... Vega, E. (2012). Searching for an operational definition of frailty: A Delphi method based consensus statement. The Frailty Operative Definition-Consensus Conference Project. *Journals of Gerontology: Series A, 68,* 62–67. https://doi.org/10.1093/gerona/gls119

Rosario, C.O., Puts, M., Jang, R., Bezjak, A., Yokom, D., & Alibhai, S.M.H. (2019). Exploring the geriatric needs of oncology inpatients at an academic cancer centre. *Journal of Geriatric Oncology, 10,* 824–828. https://doi.org/10.1016/j.jgo.2018.12.001

Rowbottom, L., Loucks, A., Jin, R., Breunis, H., Syed, A.T., Watt, S., ... Alibhai, S.M.H. (2019). Performance of the vulnerable elders survey 13 screening tool in identifying cancer treatment modification after geriatric assessment in pre-treatment patients: A retrospective analysis. *Journal of Geriatric Oncology, 10,* 229–234. https://doi.org/10.1016/j.jgo.2018.10.018

Rowland, J., Conforti, D., Basic, D., Vrantsidis, F., LoGiudice, D., Russel, M., ... Lucero, K. (2007). A study to evaluate the Rowland Universal Dementia Assessment Scale (RUDAS) in two populations outside of the Sydney South West Area Health Service. Australian Government Department of Health and Ageing. https://www.dementia.org.au/sites/default/files/20110303-Nat-CALD-RUDASvalidation2007.pdf

Saint Louis University. (2019). Saint Louis University mental status exam. https://www.slu.edu/medicine/internal-medicine/geriatric-medicine/aging-successfully/assessment-tools/mental-status-exam.php

Saliba, D., Elliott, M., Rubenstein, L.Z., Solomon, D.H., Young, R.T., Kamberg, C.J., ... Wenger, N.S. (2001). The vulnerable elders survey: A tool for identifying vulnerable older people in the community. *Journal of the American Geriatrics Society, 49,* 1691–1699. https://doi.org/10.1046/j.1532-5415.2001.49281.x

Salthouse, T.A. (2010). The paradox of cognitive change. *Journal of Clinical and Experimental Neuropsychology, 32,* 622–629. https://doi.org/10.1080/13803390903401310

Schonberg, M.A., Li, V., Marcantonio, E.R., Davis, R.B., & McCarthy, E.P. (2017). Predicting mortality up to 14 years among community-dwelling adults aged 65 and older. *Journal of the American Geriatrics Society, 65,* 1310–1315. https://doi.org/10.1111/jgs.14805

Small, G.W., Rabins, P.V., Barry, P.P., Buckholtz, N.S., DeKosky, S.T., Ferris, S.H., ... Tune, L. (1997). Diagnosis and treatment of Alzheimer disease and related disorders. Consensus statement of the American Association for Geriatric Psychiatry, the Alzheimer's Association, and the American Geriatrics Society. *JAMA, 278,* 1363–1371. https://doi.org/10.1001/jama.1997.03550160083043

Soubeyran, P., Bellera, C., Goyard, J., Heitz, D., Curé, H., Rousselot, H., ... Rainfray, M. (2014). Screening for vulnerability in older cancer patients: The ONCODAGE prospective multicenter cohort study. *PLOS ONE, 9,* e115060. https://doi.org/10.1371/journal.pone.0115060

Suh, S.-R., & Lee, M.K. (2017). Effects of nurse-led telephone-based supportive interventions for patients with cancer: A meta-analysis. *Oncology Nursing Forum, 44,* E168–E184. https://doi.org/10.1188/17.onf.e168-e184

Syed, S.T., Gerber, B.S., & Sharp, L.K. (2013). Traveling towards disease: Transportation barriers to health care access. *Journal of Community Health, 38,* 976–993. https://doi.org/10.1007/s10900-013-9681-1

Szumacher, E., Sattar, S., Neve, M., Do, K., Ayala, A.P., Gray, M., ... Puts, M. (2018). Use of comprehensive geriatric assessment and geriatric screening for older adults in the radiation oncology setting: A systematic review. *Clinical Oncology, 30,* 578–588. https://doi.org/10.1016/j.clon.2018.04.008

Theunissen, E.A.R., Bosma, S.C.J., Zuur, C.L., Spijker, R., van der Baan, S., Dreschler, W.A., ... Rasch, C.R.N. (2013). Sensorineural hearing loss in patients with head and neck cancer after chemoradiotherapy and radiotherapy: A systematic review of the literature. *Journal of the Sciences and Specialties of the Head and Neck, 37,* 281–292. https://doi.org/10.1002/hed.23551

Todd, S., Barr, S., Roberts, M., & Passmore, A.P. (2013). Survival in dementia and predictors of mortality: A review. *International Journal of Geriatric Psychiatry, 28,* 1109–1124. https://doi.org/10.1002/gps.3946

Ulger, S., Kizilarslanoglu, M.C., Kilic, M.K., Kilic, D., Cetin, B.E., Ulger, Z., & Karahacioglu, E. (2015). Estimating radiation therapy toxicity and tolerability with comprehensive assessment parameters in geriatric cancer patients. *Asian Pacific Journal of Cancer Prevention, 16,* 1965–1969. https://doi.org/10.7314/apjcp.2015.16.5.1965

Wilke, C., Grosshans, D., Duman, J., Brown, P., & Li, J. (2018). Radiation-induced cognitive toxicity: Pathophysiology and interventions to reduce toxicity in adults. *Neuro-Oncology, 20,* 597–607. https://doi.org/10.1093/neuonc/nox195

Williams, G.R., Rier, H.N., McDonald, A., & Shachar, S.S. (2019). Sarcopenia and aging in cancer. *Journal of Geriatric Oncology, 10,* 374–377. https://doi.org/10.1016/j.jgo.2018.10.009

Yourman, L.C., Lee, S.J., Schonberg, M.A., Widera, E.W., & Smith, A.K. (2012). Prognostic indices for older adults: A systematic review. *JAMA, 307,* 182–192. https://doi.org/10.1001/jama.2011.1966

F. Patients with mental illness

1. Psychological distress
   a) Overview
      (1) Psychological distress in patients with cancer occurs along a continuum from the expected levels of sadness and anxiety in the context of health crisis to symptoms of greater severity, duration, or associated dysfunction that meet criteria for a psychiatric disorder, such as adjustment disorder or major depressive disorder (Howell et al., 2015; Riba et al., 2019).
      (2) Psychological distress can arise at multiple points along the disease trajectory (Howell et al., 2015).
         (a) Cancer screening
         (b) Diagnostic workup
         (c) Time of diagnosis
         (d) Start of active treatment
         (e) Development of new cancer symptoms
         (f) Completion of treatment (survivorship)
         (g) Relapse or recurrence
      (3) In the RT population, changes in appearance and treatment-induced side effects, including pain, nausea, and inanition (mental fatigue related to malnutrition) can lead to significant disability and resulting distress (Yuppa & Braun, 2015).

(4) Psychological distress is associated with poor cancer outcomes, including nonadherence to oncology management and decreased quality of life (Riba et al., 2019).

b) Relationship between cancer and psychological distress

(1) The healthcare community and lay public alike have long been interested in the connection between psychological distress and cancer incidence, advancement, and mortality.

(2) To the extent beliefs about the connection between psychological states and cancer are held, patients may feel the need to maintain positivity and disavow negative affect in order to prevent disease progression.

(3) At present, research evidence is inconsistent in this area, with some findings suggesting that psychological distress in patients with cancer is associated with decreased survival, others showing no relationship, and others showing an inverse relationship (Brower, 2014).

(4) Theoretical mechanisms for the possible link between distress and cancer include diminishment of natural killer cell function or dysregulation of the HPA axis (Batty, Russ, MacBeath, Stamatakis, & Kivimäki, 2017; Kiecolt-Glaser, McGuire, Robles, & Glaser, 2002).

(5) It is also possible that distress and cancer are linked through other mechanisms, such as unhealthy behaviors or social determinants of health, such as poverty (Kissane, 2009).

(6) Causality may be reversed, in that cancer and the associated physiologic changes cause psychiatric symptoms.

(7) Regardless, patients and families may benefit from reassurance that they are not to blame for their cancer and that cancers are a heterogenous group of diseases with multiple causes that are still being researched and have yet to be fully understood.

(8) Although some psychological distress in the cancer population is to be expected, significant distress that affects functioning and may lead to a psychiatric diagnosis, such as major depressive disorder, can be seen as a comorbidity that may complicate cancer treatment, therefore demanding clinical attention of the oncology team as a whole.

c) Risk factors

(1) Determinants of psychological distress in cancer populations include the following (Riba et al., 2019).

(a) Communication barriers
(b) History of psychiatric disorders
(c) History of trauma
(d) Cognitive impairment
(e) Uncontrolled symptoms of cancer
(f) Severe comorbid medical illness
(g) Conflicts with caregivers or family
(h) Living alone
(i) Financial or other practical problems
(j) Younger age
(k) Spiritual/religious concerns

(2) Attachment style

(a) Attachment theory is an evidence-based explanatory framework that can aid healthcare providers in understanding the patient experience of the crisis of cancer and the differences among patients in how they express distress and access support from others.

(b) There are two main dimensions of attachment: anxious (or preoccupied) attachment, which refers to a tendency to express distress and uncertainty about caregiver availability, and avoidant (or dismissive) attachment, which refers to a tendency to avoid expressions of distress and reliance on others (Hunter & Maunder, 2017).

i. Anxiously attached patients are often those in need of more support and guidance. These patients benefit from more frequent and regular clinical care, reassurance, and information.

ii. Avoidantly attached patients are those who benefit from maximizing their sense of control and autonomy while receiving nonintrusive supports.

(c) Patients who have both high attachment anxiety and avoidance are often those who are most problematic for healthcare teams to support, as these patients may appear to be both seeking help and avoiding or rejecting help.

i. This attachment style often overlaps with a significant trauma history and borderline personality disorder diagnosis.

ii. These patients often require a cohesive and organized treatment team that can be supportive, understanding, and tolerant of expressions of distress and the higher complexity of care.

d) Distress screening

(1) Psychological distress screening is recommended for all patients with cancer to ensure appropriate selection for diagnosis and treatment. Screening is recommended when the initial diagnosis of cancer is made and periodically thereafter, as clinically indicated at treatment

transitions or disease progression (Andersen et al., 2014; Howell et al., 2015; Riba et al., 2019).

(2) The Distress Thermometer is a validated self-administered Likert scale to screen level of distress in patients with cancer (Donovan, Grassi, McGinty, & Jacobsen, 2014).

    (a) This scale has been translated into more than 20 languages (Donovan et al., 2014).

    (b) A prospective study of 462 patients with various cancer diagnoses found that the Distress Thermometer had a sensitivity of 87% to detect emotional distress with a cutoff score of greater than 4 (Thalén-Lindström, Larsson, Hellbom, Glimelius, & Johansson, 2013).

(3) Alternative screening tools have been used to detect the full range of self-report distress and include thresholds for detection of depressive or anxiety disorders (Andersen et al., 2014).

    (a) Nine-item Personal Health Questionnaire (PHQ-9) and two-item PHQ (PHQ-2) for depressive symptoms

    (b) Generalized Anxiety Disorder (GAD-7) scale for anxiety symptoms

(4) A 2016 U.S. feasibility study that assessed screening tools for depression in patients with cancer receiving RT found that the PHQ-2 and PHQ-9 were superior to the Distress Thermometer in detecting depression (Wagner et al., 2017).

(5) Integrated care models may include screening of patients receiving RT by nurses and referral to specialized psychosocial care (Holtzman, Pereira, & Yeung, 2018).

(6) Despite improvements in distress screening within oncology, a proportion of patients may underreport symptoms on screening measures; therefore, screening tools cannot replace the clinician assessment.

e) Management

(1) Initial efforts to mandate distress screening as part of cancer care did not improve outcomes, and it is widely acknowledged that although screening may help to detect those needing clinical attention, there needs to be an assessment and management protocol beyond the screening process to affect outcomes (Li, Macedo, et al., 2016; McCarter, Britton, et al., 2018).

(2) The majority of psychological distress is initially assessed and managed by clinicians at the point of care, including nurses in radiation oncology.

(3) Initial assessment and management by clinicians should include exploration of the nature, intensity, and duration of distress; effect on functioning; and possible contributing factors and causes.

    (a) In cases of low to moderate distress, patients may benefit from supportive techniques.

        i. Normalization

        ii. Validation

        iii. Assistance with problem solving

        iv. Encouragement of adaptive coping strategies (e.g., seeking social support, sleep, exercise)

        v. Information about psychosocial oncology resources available in the hospital, community, or online

    (b) In cases of moderate to high distress or if safety is a concern, patients may require referral for formal psychiatric assessment and management.

(4) A proportion of patients, despite symptom reporting, may not wish to receive support or referrals for specialized psychosocial care.

    (a) This may be the result of stigma surrounding mental health issues or discomfort with vulnerability and expression of emotional distress (avoidant attachment style).

    (b) This is a challenging subgroup to help, and they may benefit from a nonintrusive approach emphasizing strengths and adaptive coping strategies, psychoeducation about distress as a common symptom in cancer care that can affect cancer management and outcomes, and information about the range of supports available.

2. Incidence of psychiatric disorder in cancer care

  a) It is well known that levels of psychiatric disorders, particularly mood and anxiety disorders, are higher in cancer populations than in the general population.

  b) A U.S. registry study compared the incidence of mental disorders (adjustment disorder, depressive disorder, anxiety disorder, somatic symptom disorder, and substance use disorders) among individuals with and without cancer (Lu et al., 2016).

    (1) After age, sex, and education were matched in the two groups, the incidence of mental disorders was elevated in the cancer population at almost seven times compared to the noncancer group (hazard ratio 6.7; 95% confidence interval, 6.1–7.4).

    (2) The rate decreased over time but remained elevated 10 years after diagnosis (hazard ratio 1.1; 95% confidence interval, 1.1–1.2).

  c) Studies outside of North America have shown that approximately one-third of individuals with cancer have psychiatric comorbidities. A meta-analysis of 1,448 individuals with cancer assessed with validated instruments revealed at least one mental disorder (adjustment, depressive, anxiety, post-traumatic stress, somatic symptom, or substance use disorders) was present in 32% (Singer, Das-Munshi, & Brähler, 2010).

d) A cross-sectional German study of 2,141 individuals found that 32% of participants with cancer had at least one mental disorder (adjustment, depressive, anxiety, somatic symptom, or substance use disorders) (Mehnert et al., 2014).

3. Psychiatric disorders within radiation oncology

a) Risk

(1) Patients undergoing RT are at high risk for mental health disorders, such as anxiety and depression.

(a) A Spanish study of 103 patients undergoing RT reported that 46% were diagnosed with a depressive, anxiety, or adjustment disorder during treatment (Blázquez & Cruzado, 2016).

(b) A German study of 87 patient undergoing RT found 51% prevalence of any mental health disorder in patients undergoing RT (Fritzsche, Liptai, & Henke, 2004).

(2) Early detection of psychiatric disorders by radiation-specific nursing staff was shown to be feasible with implementation of screening (Holtzman et al., 2018).

b) Adjustment disorder

(1) Diagnosis

(a) Adjustment disorders are diagnosed if significant psychological distress and/or behavioral symptoms are present in response to a stressor, such as cancer. These symptoms exceed what would be expected in severity and impair social, occupational, or other areas of functioning.

(b) This diagnosis is applied when a patient does not meet criteria for another disorder (e.g., major depression, generalized anxiety disorder) (APA, 2013).

(c) Clinical utility of this diagnostic syndrome has been controversial because of its lack of clarity and the subjective determination of diagnostic threshold (Semprini, Fava, & Sonino, 2010).

(d) In settings that require a psychiatric diagnosis to qualify for mental health supports or employment benefits, this may be a useful category.

(2) Incidence: The point prevalence of adjustment disorders in patients with cancer is approximately 10%–20% (Howell et al., 2015).

(3) Management

(a) Psychosocial approaches

i. Psychological approaches are first-line treatments for adjustment disorder (Yuppa & Braun, 2015).

ii. General management strategies include psychoeducation, relaxation, and individual and family therapies (Yuppa & Braun, 2015).

iii. Some evidence supports interventions targeting quality of life and adjustment, including yoga, specifically for the RT population (Tolia et al., 2018).

(b) Pharmacologic approaches

i. Medications may be beneficial in patients with adjustment disorder, especially those who do not benefit from supportive or psychotherapeutic approaches (Strain & Diefenbacher, 2008).

ii. As with most pharmacotherapy, selection should be based on consideration of potential drug interactions, side effects, and benefit for physical symptoms (see Table 15).

c) Depressive disorders

(1) Diagnosis

(a) A major depressive episode can be diagnosed when a minimum of five out of nine symptoms are present for at least two weeks. At least one symptom must include depressed mood or loss of interest or pleasure (APA, 2013).

(b) The other symptoms include changes in appetite, changes in sleep, psychomotor agitation or retardation, decreased energy, feelings of worthlessness or guilt, concentration difficulties, and suicidal ideation (APA, 2013).

(c) In patients with cancer, diagnosis of depression can be confounded by the cancer or its treatment, which may cause changes in appetite, weight, sleep, energy, and cognitive effects.

(d) Some cancer treatments and supportive care therapies (e.g., interferon, high-dose steroids) can be associated with depressive symptoms. In these cases, depression may be diagnosed as a substance-induced depressive disorder.

(2) Incidence

(a) The point prevalence of major depressive disorder in patients with active cancer is approximately 5%–20% (Krebber et al., 2013; Walker et al., 2014).

(b) The increased rate of diagnosis of depression is highest in the first week after diagnosis of cancer and decreases thereafter (Lu et al., 2016).

(3) Risk factors (Burgess et al., 2005; Hill et al., 2011; Suppli et al., 2014; Walker et al., 2014; Zhao et al., 2014)

   (a) Prior history of major depression

   (b) Social deprivation (e.g., low income, limited education)

   (c) Living alone, being unmarried, and having poor social support

   (d) General medical comorbidity

   (e) Pain

   (f) Metastases or advanced disease

   (g) Impairment of functioning (e.g., self-care, work)

(4) Screening: Ongoing screening is supported by oncology practice guidelines (tools listed previously) to guide the best approach along the continuum of psychosocial care.

(5) Management

   (a) Overview (Li, Kennedy, et al., 2016)

      i. Treatment of depressive symptoms in patients with cancer includes pharmacologic and psychosocial interventions, depending on clinical severity, patient preference, and available resources.

      ii. These factors should be assessed by a stepped-care model, with each line of treatment to progress from psychosocial approaches to pharmacologic and neurostimulation modalities.

      iii. Initial goals include psychoeducation, destigmatization, empathic communication, and understanding patient treatment preferences.

   (b) Psychosocial approaches

      i. A wide variety of psychotherapeutic or counseling modalities have demonstrated benefit in management of depressive disorders in the cancer setting.

      ii. The symptom severity, stage of illness, and individual patient factors guide choice of treatment.

      iii. Psychoeducation, structured physical activity programs, peer support, cognitive behavioral therapy, behavioral activation, and problem-solving approaches have been recommended by Cancer Care Ontario and ONS guidelines (Cope et al., 2019b; Li, Kennedy, et al., 2016).

      iv. In a Scottish randomized controlled trial, nurse-delivered complex intervention improved the symptoms of depression, compared to usual care alone, for patients with a variety of cancers and major depressive disorder at three months for up to 12 months (Strong et al., 2008).

      v. Some evidence supports use of complementary interventions targeting depression in RT patients.

      vi. A U.S. study involving patients with head and neck cancer compared two meditation modalities during 12 weeks of RT. Three groups were compared: treatment as usual, meditation with a coach, and self-meditation with an audio CD. The meditation groups showed a decrease from baseline on the Hospital Anxiety and Depression Scale and Distress Thermometer at 6 and 12 weeks (Boxleitner et al., 2017).

   (c) Pharmacologic approaches

      i. Multiple psychotropic agents have been developed to treat depression.

      ii. Selection is based on side effect profile and utility for multiple symptoms (see Table 15).

   (d) Neurostimulation: Neurostimulation treatments, including electroconvulsive therapy and repetitive transcranial magnetic therapy, have been safely and efficiently evaluated for the treatment of major depression; however, there are no large trials evaluating their efficacy for patients with cancer (Milev et al., 2016).

d) Anxiety disorders and trauma- and stressor-related disorders

(1) Definition: Within the categories of anxiety disorders and trauma- and stressor-related disorders in the DSM-5, there are a number of different diagnoses (APA, 2013).

   (a) Generalized anxiety disorder is classified as excessive worry, over at least a six-month period, that is difficult to control. Worry may be related to cancer trajectory, treatment outcomes, side effects, and the future. This anxiety may interfere with communication around cancer treatment and decision-making processes.

   (b) Specific phobias are persistent fears of a situation or object, such as blood injection injury phobias during chemotherapy infusions or blood draws, or the fear of confined spaces (claustrophobia), which may limit patients from participating in necessary procedures, such as

imaging, initial RT simulation, or RT treatments.

    (c) PTSD involves reexperiencing symptoms of past psychological trauma, with features of avoidance, hyperarousal, and negative cognitions for more than one month.

    (d) Acute stress disorder (ASD) has similar criteria to PTSD, but duration of symptoms is less than one month.

    (e) Panic disorder involves recurrent panic attacks—a cascade of physical symptoms, such as tachycardia, dyspnea, sweating, chest pain, and fear of losing control or dying.

        i. Many other anxiety disorders also are associated with panic attacks.

        ii. Other medical issues can cause panic-like symptoms, and these possible etiologies should be ruled out before attributing physical symptoms to anxiety.

    (f) Anxiety disorder due to a general medical condition involves anxiety symptoms due to underlying medical pathology such as direct or indirect cancer effects (e.g., endocrine imbalances, cardiac arrhythmias, sepsis, or seizures). Substance or medication-induced anxiety disorder may be caused by cancer treatments including corticosteroids or chemotherapy (Traeger, Greer, Fernandez-Robles, Temel, & Pirl, 2012; Yuppa & Braun, 2015).

(2) Incidence

    (a) General rates of anxiety or trauma- and stressor-related disorders in oncology are approximately 10% (Mehnert et al., 2014; Mitchell et al., 2011).

    (b) A prospective German study of 166 patients with breast cancer showed that 3.6% were diagnosed with ASD or PTSD at cancer diagnosis, and 2% were diagnosed with ASD or PTSD one year later. In addition, at least one ASD symptom was present in 83% of patients at diagnosis and 57% at the one-year follow-up, highlighting that subthreshold symptoms may persist in the cancer population (Voigt et al., 2017).

    (c) A Spanish study of 103 patients undergoing RT found that 16%–18% met criteria for an anxiety disorder on a self-report tool during treatment (before, one week after, and/or one month after treatment) (Blázquez & Cruzado, 2016).

    (d) An Australian survey demonstrated that up to 49% of patients attending RT appointments experienced anxiety and distress symptoms (Holmes & Williamson, 2008).

    (e) Brachytherapy for gynecologic cancers can be distressing, particularly for some patients with trauma history.

    (f) An Austrian study of 50 patients undergoing brachytherapy for cervical cancer found that 15 of 50 patients had ASD symptoms and 20 of 49 patients had PTSD symptoms three months after treatment (Kirchheiner et al., 2014).

    (g) An Australian study of 100 patients with head and neck cancer undergoing mask fitting for RT found that the prevalence of anxiety symptoms was 26%, using a modified Distress Thermometer screening tool (Nixon et al., 2018).

(3) Risk factors (Traeger et al., 2012)

    (a) Comorbid medical or psychiatric illnesses

    (b) Cancer-related factors (e.g., metastases, hypercalcemia, hypoxia, paraneoplastic syndromes, thromboembolic disease)

    (c) Treatment-related factors (e.g., glucocorticoid steroids)

(4) Management

    (a) Treatment of anxiety in patients with cancer includes pharmacologic and psychosocial interventions, depending on clinical severity, patient preference, and available resources.

    (b) Evidence-based psychosocial interventions include education, cognitive behavioral therapy, mindfulness approaches, supportive-expressive therapy, supportive counseling, and creative art therapies (Cope et al., 2019a; Yuppa & Braun, 2015).

    (c) An Australian systematic review of radiation therapist–led psychosocial interventions found that increased communication, psychoeducation, and screening were feasible to provide and reduced patient anxiety (Elsner, Naehrig, Halkett, & Dhillon, 2017).

    (d) An Australian multisite radiation therapist–led intervention (psychoeducation, assessment of psychosocial needs, and coaching) involving 190 patients produced lower psychological distress and lower Hospital Anxiety and Depression Scale scores compared to usual care (Halkett et al., 2018).

    (e) A U.S. randomized controlled trial of 78 patients showed that a protocolized music therapy intervention had benefits in

TABLE 15. Psychotropic Medications Commonly Used in Cancer Care

Class/Drug	Cancer Care Considerations
Antipsychotics	–
• Aripiprazole	Can be activating Shows efficacy in mood stabilization, psychosis, and delirium Side effects: metabolic syndrome, akathisia
• Haloperidol	Shows efficacy in mood stabilization, psychosis, and delirium Side effects: extrapyramidal side effects
• Olanzapine	Shows efficacy in mood stabilization, psychosis, and delirium Side effects: metabolic syndrome, sedation, orthostasis, QT prolongation, weight gain
• Quetiapine	Exhibits less extrapyramidal side effects Shows efficacy in mood stabilization, psychosis, and delirium Side effects: metabolic syndrome, sedation, orthostasis, cataracts, QT prolongation, weight gain
• Risperidone	Shows efficacy in mood stabilization, psychosis, and delirium Side effects: metabolic syndrome, sedation, orthostasis, cataracts, QT prolongation, weight gain, blood dyscrasias, elevated prolactin levels, extrapyramidal side effects
Atypical antidepressants	First-line agents for depression and anxiety
• Agomelatine	Shows benefits for insomnia Requires liver function test monitoring Side effects: nausea, dizziness, somnolence, insomnia, headache
• Bupropion	Activating Has seizure risk at high doses Side effects: insomnia, dizziness, sweating, tachycardia, appetite suppression, minimal sexual dysfunction
• Mirtazapine	Shows benefits for nausea, low appetite, and insomnia Side effects: sedation, appetite stimulation, weight gain, dry mouth, constipation, minimal sexual dysfunction
• Trazodone	Used primarily as a sleep aid Side effects: sedation, orthostasis, anticholinergic effects, priapism
Benzodiazepines	Tolerance and dependence potential Used in anxiety disorders May have antinausea function Side effects: sedation, confusion, ataxia, cognitive impairment
• Alprazolam	Rebound anxiety from short half-life Has addiction potential with high potency and short half-life
• Clonazepam	Used in seizure disorders and sleep disorders
• Diazepam	Used in seizure disorders and alcohol withdrawal Side effect: respiratory depression
• Lorazepam	Used in seizure disorders, alcohol withdrawal, and patients with liver disease Side effect: respiratory depression
Mood stabilizers	–
• Gabapentin	Mood stabilizer, anticonvulsant, analgesic in neuropathic pain, antiemetic properties Side effects: somnolence, dizziness, peripheral edema, ataxia
• Lamotrigine	Mood stabilizer, anticonvulsant Side effects: rash that may progress to Stevens-Johnson syndrome or toxic epidermal necrolysis, photosensitivity, headache, gastrointestinal upset, ataxia
• Pregabalin	Mood stabilizer, anticonvulsant, analgesic in neuropathic pain Shows efficacy in generalized anxiety and social anxiety disorders Side effects: somnolence, dizziness, peripheral edema, ataxia

(Continued on next page)

TABLE 15. Psychotropic Medications Commonly Used in Cancer Care *(Continued)*

Class/Drug	Cancer Care Considerations
Mood stabilizers *(cont.)*	–
• Valproic acid/divalproex sodium	Mood stabilizer, anticonvulsant Requires blood monitoring Side effects: somnolence, dizziness, gastrointestinal upset, ataxia, hepatitis, blood dyscrasias, alopecia, weight gain
Selective serotonin reuptake inhibitors	First-line agents for depression and anxiety Side effects: nausea, diarrhea, dyspepsia, sweating, headache, anxiety, insomnia, sexual dysfunction
• Acetabularia	Risk of cardiac arrhythmias at high doses Few drug interactions
• Citalopram	Risk of cardiac arrhythmias at high doses Few drug interactions
• Fluoxetine	Longest half-life Stronger drug interactions with hepatic enzymes
• Paroxetine	More anticholinergic than other drugs in this class May be sedating Stronger drug interactions with hepatic enzymes Shortest half-life (risk of withdrawal symptoms)
• Sertraline	Few drug interactions
Serotonin norepinephrine reuptake inhibitors	First-line agents for depression and anxiety Side effects: nausea, constipation, dyspepsia, sweating, headache, anxiety, insomnia, sexual dysfunction
• Desvenlafaxine	Shows benefits for hot flashes Renal metabolism
• Duloxetine	Should be avoided with liver impairment Shows benefits for neuropathic pain
• Venlafaxine	Increases blood pressure at high doses Few drug interactions Discontinuation symptoms common Shows benefits for hot flashes and neuropathic pain

Note. Based on information from Fitzgerald et al., 2014; Fitzgerald et al., 2015; Procyshyn et al., 2019. Yuppa & Braun, 2015.

reducing Distress Thermometer scores and State-Trait Anxiety Inventory scores during RT simulation (Rossetti et al., 2017).

(f) See Table 15 for common evidence-based pharmacologic treatments for anxiety symptoms.

e) Serious and persistent mental illness (SPMI)
   (1) Overview
      (a) SPMIs include psychiatric diagnoses that lead to significant impairment of functioning and are longstanding in nature, such as schizophrenia, schizoaffective disorder, bipolar disorder, or persistent depressive disorder.
      (b) Unlike adjustment, mood, or anxiety disorders, which may be longstanding diagnoses or newly diagnosed in the context of cancer treatment, SPMIs usually predate the cancer diagnosis, and patients often have received mental health care before they present for cancer care, highlighting the need for effective communication and a liaising between oncology and mental health teams.
      (c) Challenges during RT for those with SPMI can include exacerbation of psychiatric symptoms and inability to adhere to treatment regimen or schedule.
   (2) Barriers to care and mortality risk
      (a) Research suggests that patients with a psychiatric disorder have a 30% higher fatality rate from cancer, even when the incidence is no greater than the general population. This disparity has been attributed

to more advanced stage of disease at diagnosis and to less specialized interventions (Kisely, Crowe, & Lawrence, 2013).

(b) Individuals with significant preexisting mental illness may be diagnosed at a more advanced stage of disease for several reasons.

    i. Examples include care avoidance and lack of primary health care, other medical comorbidities, and socioeconomic factors, such as homelessness and unemployment.

    ii. Many individuals with a preexisting mental illness are less likely to access and use preventive healthcare services and may experience disparities in health education and health literacy (Muirhead, 2014).

    iii. In addition, some of these patients may have difficulty coping with the diagnosis and treatment of cancer and, as a result, may ignore symptoms, resulting in delayed access to care (Inagaki et al., 2006).

(c) Health service factors also influence care in this patient population, with access to primary care having been identified as an unmet need for people with mental illnesses.

(d) Stigma associated with mental illness has also been identified as a barrier to health care in people with mental illness (Canadian Mental Health Association, 2008).

    i. Stigma can occur from the perspective of the patient, creating fear of seeking health care.

    ii. It can also occur from the perspective of the healthcare provider and includes the phenomenon of diagnostic overshadowing, whereby physical complaints are misdiagnosed as being psychiatric.

(3) Incidence

(a) North American research suggests that approximately 4% of the adult population have a serious mental illness (Weinstein et al., 2016).

(b) Evidence from epidemiological studies has been conflicting with some reports that cancer rates in those with SPMI are higher, lower, or equal to rates in the general population (Weinstein et al., 2016).

(c) Much of this variability may depend on whether socioeconomic factors, environmental factors, and behavioral factors are controlled for in the research.

(4) Management

(a) Common evidence-based approaches to treatment of SPMIs usually involve multiple dimensions of care.

    i. Monitoring

    ii. Attending to social needs (e.g., housing, education, employment)

    iii. Psychotherapeutic supports (e.g., psychoeducation, supportive techniques, structured psychotherapeutic modalities)

    iv. Pharmacotherapy targeting psychiatric symptoms (see Table 15)

(b) Given the challenges of cancer care for those with a significant psychiatric comorbidity, it is important to consider interventions at the individual, interpersonal, community, organizational, and health system level (Weinstein et al., 2016).

(c) Collaboration between the oncology team, mental health team, and informal supports is essential to help these patients throughout cancer care.

(d) Patients may need specialized support of medical psychiatry teams during their care, optimization of psychiatric treatment before cancer care, consistency of and familiarity with the cancer care team ahead of time, and adjustments or simplifications to the care plan, such as consolidation of appointments or brief hospitalizations for chemotherapy or RT to ensure adherence (Irwin, Henderson, Knight, & Pirl, 2014).

(e) For those at the point of care, collaboration with formal or informal mental health supports may help in understanding a patient's baseline symptoms and how these may affect care, as well as provide suggestions about how to tailor communication (e.g., simplifying language for those with cognitive deficits or concrete thinking) (Irwin et al., 2014).

(f) Homelessness is common in those with SPMIs and is itself associated with higher rates of cancer and complications to treatment adherence. Patients with housing issues need integrated and flexible care and may require hospitalization for care that is typically outpatient (Bauer, Baggett, Stern, O'Connell, & Shtasel, 2013; O'Connell et al., 2010).

(g) Healthcare professionals may fear patients becoming violent if they are disorganized, agitated, or psychotic (Friedman, 2006).

    i. The absolute risk of violence in those with major mental illness is low, although mildly increased, compared to the general population.

    ii. Risk is higher in those with history of assault, victimization by violence, comorbid substance use, or uncontrolled psychiatric symptoms.

    iii. Screening for risk factors and treating psychosis and substance use may help to decrease risk and aid in safe management.

4. Substance use disorders
   a) Overview
     (1) Substance use disorders are defined as a problematic pattern of use leading to clinically significant impairment or distress (APA, 2013).
     (2) The problematic pattern of use may include the following (APA, 2013).
       (a) Use of greater amounts or for greater duration than intended
       (b) A great deal of time spent to obtain, use, or recover from substance effects
       (c) Cravings
       (d) Desire or unsuccessful attempts to control use
       (e) Recurrent impacts on social and occupational obligations
       (f) Continued use despite knowledge of negative impacts
       (g) Physical hazards secondary to use
       (h) Tolerance and withdrawal symptoms
   b) Challenges in cancer care
     (1) Substance use disorders are associated with high rates of psychiatric comorbidities, including anxiety, mood, and co-occurring substance use disorders (Kessler, Chiu, Demler, & Walters, 2005).
     (2) Cancer care in those with substance use disorders may also be complicated because of the higher prevalence of other medical comorbidities (e.g., cardiovascular events, respiratory complications, neurologic complications) (National Institute on Drug Abuse, 2017).
     (3) Substance use can come with many challenges that can impact health outcomes through nonadherence to treatment, stigmatization, and bidirectional mistrust between patients and healthcare teams.
     (4) Within the cancer setting, the effects of substances on patient mental status may be altered if a change in route of administration occurs (e.g., oral to gastrostomy tube) or if health status worsens due to malnutrition or cancer-related sedation and fatigue.
     (5) Some in the field of addictions in cancer have emphasized that substance use behaviors exist on a spectrum from what may be considered normal use to more problematic use. Healthcare providers need to be mindful of differing cultural or social norms and how these contribute to stigma and mistrust (Yuppa & Braun, 2015).
   c) Incidence
     (1) A 2017 national survey showed that approximately 7.2% of individuals in the United States over age 12 had a substance use disorder in the past year, including approximately 5.3% with an alcohol use disorder (Substance Abuse and Mental Health Services Administration, 2018b).
     (2) Tobacco and alcohol are also significant risk factors for cancer; therefore, the representation of substance use disorders will be prevalent in the oncology setting. Tobacco use has been identified to negatively impact overall survival by diminishing effects of cancer treatment including RT, increase complications of wound healing and infections, and can be associated with at least 30% of all cancer-related deaths (Warren, Kasza, Reid, Cummings, & Marshall, 2013).
     (3) According to a national U.S. study, the overall prevalence of active smoking among cancer survivors is approximately 23% during the first year after diagnosis (Bellizzi, Rowland, Jeffery, & McNeel, 2005).
     (4) In a British study of patients with cancer, the prevalence of active alcohol use was reported to be 18% (Webber & Davies, 2012).
     (5) A U.S. study of 280 patients with head and neck cancer reported that 45% continued to consume alcohol 12 months after diagnosis (Potash, Karnell, Christensen, Vander Weg, & Funk, 2010).
     (6) An Australian cross-sectional study of more than 300 patients with head and neck cancer undergoing RT found that 21% had two or more co-occurring problems, including current smoking, hazardous alcohol use, and positive screens for a major depressive episode (McCarter, Baker, et al., 2018).
   d) Screening and monitoring
     (1) Multiple screening tools have been validated to assess substance use disorders in conjunction with clinical assessment for different populations.
       (a) For alcohol use, the Alcohol Use Disorders Identification Test (or AUDIT) has been validated in the primary care setting (Saunders, Aasland, Babor, de la Fuente, & Grant, 1993).
       (b) However, because of the length of the AUDIT questionnaire, the CAGE tool

(acronym for *cutting* down use, *annoyance* from inquiry, *guilt* from use, and *eye-opener* consumption) is another clinical tool that can guide further inquiry (Maisto & Saitz, 2003).

 (c) The Opioid Risk Tool and the Screener and Opioid Assessment for Patients with Pain can be used prior to initiating opioid therapy to assess risk for aberrant drug-related behavior (Butler, Budman, Fernandez, & Jamison, 2004; Webster & Webster, 2005).

 (d) The Fagerstrom test has been used for assessing nicotine dependence (Prokhorov, Pallonen, Fava, Ding, & Niaura, 1996).

(2) An assessment by a mental healthcare specialist is recommended to assess potential comorbidities, such as depression and anxiety.

(3) Given the medical complexity of some patients, assessment for potential intoxication or withdrawal should be considered.

 (a) In alcohol intoxication, symptoms include slurred speech, unsteady gait, nystagmus, impaired cognition and sedation, and depressed mental status (APA, 2013).

 (b) Common signs of opioid intoxication include decreased breathing rate, sedation and depressed mental status, slurred speech, impaired attention or memory, and constricted pupils (APA, 2013; Substance Abuse and Mental Health Services Administration, 2018a; Taha, 2018).

 (c) The Clinical Institute Withdrawal Assessment for Alcohol scale is a validated, symptom-triggered tool for monitoring and managing acute alcohol withdrawal (Sullivan, Sykora, Schneiderman, Naranjo, & Sellers, 1989).

 (d) The Clinical Opiate Withdrawal scale has been used to assess symptoms of opioid withdrawal (Taha, 2018).

e) Management

(1) An interprofessional team approach involving nursing staff, radiation therapists, oncologists, and mental health specialists is recommended for individuals with substance use disorders.

(2) A collaborative approach and shared treatment goals are necessary, with a range of possible goals, from abstinence to harm reduction to relapse prevention.

(3) Best practice guidelines recommend a stepped-care model, with the least invasive level to be the first-line approach, including education on substance use and effects, ongoing assessment, and consideration of the continuum of care, depending on needs of the individual. This approach includes supporting harm reduction, abstinence, relapse prevention, and referrals to appropriate community supports (Taha, 2018).

(4) Trust can be facilitated when healthcare providers take an empathic, nonjudgmental approach to gathering history and using screening tools. A focus on patient comfort, by preventing withdrawal or compounding adverse effects from treatment interactions, can further aid in the therapeutic alliance and equity of treatment (Substance Abuse and Mental Health Services Administration, 2018a; Taha, 2018; Yuppa & Braun, 2015).

(5) Psychosocial approaches to substance use disorders include supportive counseling to patients and family members.

 (a) Optimizing coping strategies and stress management via mindfulness and social supports can be helpful during any stage of substance use.

 (b) Motivational interviewing and contingency management have shown positive outcomes in treatment engagement in alcohol and opioid use disorders (APA, 2013; Substance Abuse and Mental Health Services Administration, 2018a; Taha, 2018).

 (c) Community programs, such as 12-step programs, can provide further benefits (Kaskutas, Subbaraman, Witbrodt, & Zemore, 2009).

(6) Pharmacologic approaches may include medications that can support harm reduction, withdrawal management, and abstinence.

 (a) For alcohol use disorders, benzodiazepines, under appropriate supervision, have been used to manage symptoms and adverse side effects (e.g., seizures, delirium) (APA, 2018).

 (b) Pharmacotherapy for reducing cravings and preventing relapse for alcohol use disorders include naltrexone, acamprosate, and disulfiram (APA, 2018).

 (c) In opioid use disorders, U.S. and Canadian evidence-based guidelines support the use of methadone, naloxone, and clonidine (Bruneau et al., 2018; Substance Abuse and Mental Health Services Administration, 2018a; Taha, 2018).

 (d) Opioid agonists such as methadone and buprenorphine have been used to diminish cravings and reduce relapse (Bruneau et al., 2018).

 (e) Naloxone kits are recommended for harm reduction for the reversal of acute opioid intoxication (Taha, 2018).

(f) Medications should be prescribed under the guidance of health specialists (Bruneau et al., 2018; Substance Abuse and Mental Health Services Administration, 2018a; Taha, 2018).

5. Suicidality
   a) Identification: Suicidal ideation in patients with cancer can have multiple meanings and may refer to a current and active plan and intent to take one's own life, a request for medical assistance in dying, desire for hastened death, a wish to stop active cancer treatment, an expression of more general distress or despair, or acceptance of impending death in those with advanced disease (Spoletini et al., 2011).
   b) Incidence
      (1) Studies using direct assessment of nonpsychiatric oncology populations have found the prevalence of suicidal ideation to be 8%–17.7%, compared to reported prevalence of 1.1%–19.8% in the general population (Robson, Scrutton, Wilkinson, & MacLeod, 2010).
      (2) Reported incidence of completed suicide in patients with cancer ranges as a standardized mortality ratio of 1–11 (ratio of observed to expected deaths), with variability related to study methodology and setting (Robson et al., 2010).
      (3) The majority of studies have found that suicide risk is highest in the acute phase following diagnosis (Robson et al., 2010).
   c) Risk factors
      (1) Risk factors for suicide in the general population include the following (Robson et al., 2010).
         (a) Previous self-harm or suicide attempts
         (b) Psychiatric diagnosis
         (c) Male sex
         (d) Older age
         (e) Significant physical health problems
         (f) Social isolation
         (g) Substance use
      (2) Additional risk factors for suicidality in patients with cancer include the following (Anguiano, Mayer, Piven, & Rosenstein, 2012).
         (a) Poorly controlled pain
         (b) Poorer prognosis or advanced stage
         (c) Physical impairment
         (d) Hopelessness
         (e) Certain cancer types (lung, bronchus, stomach, head and neck, prostate, pancreas)
      (3) It is widely acknowledged that, despite understanding risk factors, clinical ability to accurately predict suicidal behavior among those expressing suicidal ideation is poor.

      (4) Suicidal ideation can fluctuate, and suicidal behavior in some cases is impulsive and inherently unpredictable. Despite this, oncology clinicians should be able to identify high-risk patients and work to address risk factors such as distress, depression, and pain.
   d) Management: Within oncology clinics, including radiation clinics, staff need to be able to do the following (Anguiano et al., 2012).
      (1) Respond to suicidal ideation when expressed.
      (2) Understand the different potential meanings of this ideation (e.g., intent to end life, passive wish to die, wish to stop treatment).
      (3) Identify risk factors and attend to possible contributory factors (e.g., pain, depression, anxiety, other stressors).
      (4) Provide initial support.
      (5) Communicate hope in the alleviation of suffering.
      (6) Facilitate referral for further psychiatric assessment and care if needed.

6. Safety in radiation oncology
   a) Workplace violence is defined as any act in which a person is abused, threatened, intimidated, or assaulted during their employment.
   b) A Canadian study found that 59 out of 78 radiation technicians experienced at least one verbal abuse event in their career. In addition, 18 respondents reported a threatening action toward them and five experienced physical assault in the cancer setting (Sperduti et al., 2018).
   c) Early intervention by staff may help to de-escalate distressed patients and prevent aggression and safety incidents.
   d) Consensus guidelines created for verbal de-escalation of psychiatric patients in emergency settings focus on the importance of ensuring the safety of the patient, staff, and others in the area; helping the patient manage emotions and distress and maintain agency of behaviors; and avoiding coercive interventions and restraints when possible (Richmond et al., 2012).
      (1) Ten principles to de-escalation are emphasized (Richmond et al., 2012).
         (a) Respect personal space.
         (b) Do not be provocative.
         (c) Establish verbal contact.
         (d) Communicate concisely.
         (e) Listen intently to what the patient is saying.
         (f) Identify wants and feelings.
         (g) Agree or agree to disagree.
         (h) Clarify boundaries.
         (i) Offer choices and optimism.
         (j) Follow up to debrief the patient and staff.
      (2) The focus on collaborative approaches with less coercive interventions may result in bene-

fits to reduce progressive distress leading into agitation.

(3) Empowering the patient to stay in control while building trust with the healthcare team supports confidence in patients to seek help proactively in the future, which, in turn, avoids subsequent episodes of agitation (Richmond et al., 2012).

References

American Psychiatric Association. (2013). *Diagnostic and statistical manual of mental disorders* (5th ed.). Author.

American Psychiatric Association. (2018). *The American Psychiatric Association practice guideline for the pharmacological treatment of patients with alcohol use disorder*. Author. https://doi.org/10.1176/appi.books.9781615371969

Andersen, B.L., DeRubeis, R.J., Berman, B.S., Gruman, J., Champion, V.L., Massie, M.J., ... Rowland, J.H. (2014). Screening, assessment, and care of anxiety and depressive symptoms in adults with cancer: An American Society of Clinical Oncology guideline adaptation. *Journal of Clinical Oncology, 32,* 1605–1619. https://doi.org/10.1200/jco.2013.52.4611

Anguiano, L., Mayer, D.K., Piven, M.L., & Rosenstein, D. (2012). A literature review of suicide in cancer patients. *Cancer Nursing, 35,* E14–E26. https://doi.org/10.1097/ncc.0b013e31822fc76c

Batty, G.D., Russ, T.C., MacBeath, M., Stamatakis, E., & Kivimäki, M. (2017). Psychological distress in relation to site specific cancer mortality: Pooling of unpublished data from 16 prospective cohort studies. *BMJ, 356,* j108. https://doi.org/10.1136/bmj.j108

Bauer, L.K., Baggett, T.P., Stern, T.A., O'Connell, J.J., & Shtasel, D. (2013). Caring for homeless persons with serious mental illness in general hospitals. *Psychosomatics, 54,* 14–21. https://doi.org/10.1016/j.psym.2012.10.004

Bellizzi, K.M., Rowland, J.H., Jeffery, D.D., & McNeel, T. (2005). Health behaviors of cancer survivors: Examining opportunities for cancer control intervention. *Journal of Clinical Oncology, 23,* 8884–8893. https://doi.org/10.1200/jco.2005.02.2343

Blázquez, M.H., & Cruzado, J.A. (2016). A longitudinal study on anxiety, depressive and adjustment disorder, suicide ideation and symptoms of emotional distress in patients with cancer undergoing radiotherapy. *Journal of Psychosomatic Research, 87,* 14–21. https://doi.org/10.1016/j.jpsychores.2016.05.010

Boxleitner, G., Jolie, S., Shaffer, D., Pasacreta, N., Bai, M., & McCorkle, R. (2017). Comparison of two types of meditation on patients' psychosocial responses during radiation therapy for head and neck cancer. *Journal of Alternative and Complementary Medicine, 23,* 355–361. https://doi.org/10.1089/acm.2016.0214

Brower, V. (2014). Evidence accumulating that depression may hinder survival. *Journal of the National Cancer Institute, 106,* djt446. https://doi.org/10.1093/jnci/djt446

Bruneau, J., Ahamad, K., Goyer, M.-E., Poulin, G., Selby, P., Fischer, B., ... Wood, E. (2018). Management of opioid use disorders: A national clinical practice guideline. *Canadian Medical Association Journal, 190,* E247–E257. https://doi.org/10.1503/cmaj.170958

Burgess, C., Cornelius, V., Love, S., Graham, J., Richards, M., & Ramirez, A. (2005). Depression and anxiety in women with early breast cancer: Five year observational cohort study. *BMJ, 330,* 702. https://doi.org/10.1136/bmj.38343.670868.d3

Butler, S.F., Budman, S.H., Fernandez, K., & Jamison, R.N. (2004). Validation of a screener and opioid assessment measure for patients with chronic pain. *Pain, 112,* 65–75. https://doi.org/10.1016/j.pain.2004.07.026

Canadian Mental Health Association. (2008, December). The relationship between mental health, mental illness and chronic physical conditions. https://ontario.cmha.ca/documents/the-relationship-between-mental-health-mental-illness-and-chronic-physical-conditions

Cope, D.G., Coignet, H., Conley, S., Doherty, A., Drapek, L., Feldenzer, K., ... Walker, D.K. (2019a). Anxiety. https://www.ons.org/pep/anxiety

Cope, D.G., Coignet, H., Conley, S., Doherty, A., Drapek, L., Feldenzer, K., ... Walker, D.K. (2019b). Depression. https://www.ons.org/pep/depression

Donovan, K.A., Grassi, L., McGinty, H.L., & Jacobsen, P.B. (2014). Validation of the Distress Thermometer worldwide: State of the science. *Psycho-Oncology, 23,* 241–250. https://doi.org/10.1002/pon.3430

Elsner, K., Naehrig, D., Halkett, G.K.B., & Dhillon, H.M. (2017). Reduced patient anxiety as a result of radiation therapist–led psychosocial support: A systematic review. *Journal of Medical Radiation Sciences, 64,* 220–231. https://doi.org/10.1002/jmrs.208

Fitzgerald, P., Li, M., Grassi, L., & Rodin, G. (2014). Pharmacotherapy of depression in cancer patients. In L. Grassi & M. Riba (Eds.), *Psychopharmacology in oncology and palliative care: A practical manual* (pp. 145–161). Springer. https://doi.org/10.1007/978-3-642-40134-3_9

Fitzgerald, P., Miller, K., Li, M., & Rodin, G. (2015). Depressive disorders. In J.C. Holland, W.S. Breitbart, P.N. Butow, P.B. Jacobsen, M.J. Loscalzo, & R. McCorkle (Eds.), *Psycho-oncology* (3rd ed., pp. 281–288). Oxford University Press.

Friedman, R.A. (2006). Violence and mental illness—How strong is the link? *New England Journal of Medicine, 355,* 2064–2066. https://doi.org/10.1056/nejmp068229

Fritzsche, K., Liptai, C., & Henke, M. (2004). Psychosocial distress and need for psychotherapeutic treatment in cancer patients undergoing radiotherapy. *Radiotherapy and Oncology, 72,* 183–189. https://doi.org/10.1016/j.radonc.2004.03.015

Halkett, G., O'Connor, M., Jefford, M., Aranda, S., Merchant, S., Spry, N., ... Schofield, P. (2018). RT prepare: A radiation therapist–delivered intervention reduces psychological distress in women with breast cancer referred for radiotherapy. *BJC, 118,* 1549–1558. https://doi.org/10.1038/s41416-018-0112-z

Hill, J., Holcombe, C., Clark, L., Boothby, M.R.K., Hincks, A., Fisher, J., ... Salmon, P. (2011). Predictors of onset of depression and anxiety in the year after diagnosis of breast cancer. *Psychological Medicine, 41,* 1429–1436. https://doi.org/10.1017/s0033291710001868

Holmes, N., & Williamson, K. (2008). A survey of cancer patients undergoing a radical course of radiotherapy, to establish levels of anxiety and depression. *Journal of Radiotherapy in Practice, 7,* 89–98. https://doi.org/10.1017/s1460396908006304

Holtzman, A.L., Pereira, D.B., & Yeung, A.R. (2018). Implementation of depression and anxiety screening in patients undergoing radiotherapy. *BMJ Open Quality, 7,* e000034. https://doi.org/10.1136/bmjoq-2017-000034

Howell, D., Keshavarz, H., Esplen, M.J., Hack, T., Hamel, M., Howes, J., ... Ali, M. (2015). Pan-Canadian practice guideline: Screening, assessment and management of psychosocial distress, depression and anxiety in adults with cancer. *Supportive Care in Cancer, 21,* 2695–2706. https://www.capo.ca/resources/Documents/Guidelines/3APAN-~1.PDF

Hunter, J., & Maunder, R. (Eds.). (2017). *Improving patient treatment with attachment theory: A guide for primary care practitioners and specialists.* Springer. https://doi.org/10.1007/978-3-319-23300-0

Inagaki, T., Yasukawa, R., Okazaki, S., Yasuda, H., Kawamukai, T., Utani, E., ... Horiguchi, J. (2006). Factors disturbing treatment for cancer in patients with schizophrenia. *Psychiatry and Clinical Neurosciences, 60,* 327–331. https://doi.org/10.1111/j.1440-1819.2006.01509.x

Irwin, K.E., Henderson, D.C., Knight, H.P., & Pirl, W.F. (2014). Cancer care for individuals with schizophrenia. *Cancer, 120,* 323–334. https://doi.org/10.1002/cncr.28431

Kaskutas, L.A., Subbaraman, M.S., Witbrodt, J., & Zemore, S.E. (2009). Effectiveness of making Alcoholics Anonymous easier: A group format 12-step facilitation approach. *Journal of Substance Abuse Treatment, 37,* 228–239. https://doi.org/10.1016/j.jsat.2009.01.004

Kessler, R.C., Chiu, W.T., Demler, O., & Walters, E.E. (2005). Prevalence, severity, and comorbidity of 12-month DSM-IV disorders in the National Comorbidity Survey Replication. *Archives of General Psychiatry, 62,* 617–627. https://doi.org/10.1001/archpsyc.62.6.617

Kiecolt-Glaser, J.K., McGuire, L., Robles, T.F., & Glaser, R. (2002). Psychoneuroimmunology: Psychological influences on immune function and health.

Journal of Consulting and Clinical Psychology, 70, 537–547. https://doi.org/10.1037//0022-006x.70.3.537

Kirchheiner, K., Czajka-Pepl, A., Ponocny-Seliger, E., Scharbert, G., Wetzel, L., Nout, R.A., ... Pötter, R. (2014). Posttraumatic stress disorder after high-dose-rate brachytherapy for cervical cancer with 2 fractions in 1 application under spinal/epidural anesthesia: Incidence and risk factors. *International Journal of Radiation Oncology, Biology, Physics, 89,* 260–267. https://doi.org/10.1016/j.ijrobp.2014.02.018

Kisely, S., Crowe, E., & Lawrence, D. (2013). Cancer-related mortality in people with mental illness. *JAMA Psychiatry, 70,* 209–217. https://doi.org/10.1001/jamapsychiatry.2013.278

Kissane, D. (2009). Beyond the psychotherapy and survival debate: The challenge of social disparity, depression and treatment adherence in psychosocial cancer care. *Psycho-Oncology, 18,* 1–5. https://doi.org/10.1002/pon.1493

Krebber, A.M.H., Buffart, L.M., Kleijn, G., Riepma, I.C., de Bree, R., Leemans, C.R., ... Verdonck-de Leeuw, I.M. (2013). Prevalence of depression in cancer patients: A meta-analysis of diagnostic interviews and self-report instruments. *Psycho-Oncology, 23,* 121–130. https://doi.org/10.1002/pon.3409

Li, M., Kennedy, E.B., Byrne, N., Gérin-Lajoie, C., Katz, M.R., Keshavarz, H., ... Green, E. (2016). Management of depression in patients with cancer: A clinical practice guideline. *Journal of Oncology Practice, 12,* 747–756. https://doi.org/10.1200/jop.2016.011072

Li, M., Macedo, A., Crawford, S., Bagha, S., Leung, Y.W., Zimmermann, C., ... Rodin, G. (2016). Easier said than done: Keys to successful implementation of the distress assessment and response tool (DART) program. *Journal of Oncology Practice, 12,* e513–e526. https://doi.org/10.1200/jop.2015.010066

Lu, D., Andersson, T.M.L., Fall, K., Hultman, C.M., Czene, K., Valdimarsdóttir, U., & Fang, F. (2016). Clinical diagnosis of mental disorders immediately before and after cancer diagnosis. *JAMA Oncology, 2,* 1188–1196. https://doi.org/10.1001/jamaoncol.2016.0483

Maisto, S.A., & Saitz, R. (2003). Alcohol use disorders: Screening and diagnosis. *American Journal on Addictions, 12*(Suppl. 1), s12–s25. https://doi.org/10.1111/j.1521-0391.2003.tb00493.x

McCarter, K., Baker, A.L., Britton, B., Wolfenden, L., Wratten, C., Bauer, J., ... Oldmeadow, C. (2018). Smoking, drinking, and depression: Comorbidity in head and neck cancer patients undergoing radiotherapy. *Cancer Medicine, 7,* 2382–2390. https://doi.org/10.1002/cam4.1497

McCarter, K., Britton, B., Baker, A.L., Halpin, S.A., Beck, A.K., Carter, G., ... Wolfenden, L. (2018). Interventions to improve screening and appropriate referral of patients with cancer for psychosocial distress: Systematic review. *BMJ Open, 8,* e017959. https://doi.org/10.1136/bmjopen-2017-017959

Mehnert, A., Brähler, E., Faller, H., Härter, M., Keller, M., Schulz, H., ... Koch, U. (2014). Four-week prevalence of mental disorders in patients with cancer across major tumor entities. *Journal of Clinical Oncology, 32,* 3540–3546. https://doi.org/10.1200/JCO.2014.56.0086

Milev, R.V., Giacobbe, P., Kennedy, S.H., Blumberger, D.M., Daskalakis, Z.J., Downar, J., ... Ravindran, A.V. (2016). Canadian Network for Mood and Anxiety Treatments (CANMAT) 2016 clinical guidelines for the management of adults with major depressive disorder: Section 4. Neurostimulation treatments. *Canadian Journal of Psychiatry, 61,* 561–575. https://doi.org/10.1177/0706743716660033

Mitchell, A.J., Chan, M., Bhatti, H., Halton, M., Grassi, L., Johansen, C., & Meader, N. (2011). Prevalence of depression, anxiety, and adjustment disorder in oncological, haematological, and palliative-care settings: A meta-analysis of 94 interview-based studies. *Lancet Oncology, 12,* 160–174. https://doi.org/10.1016/s1470-2045(11)70002-x

Muirhead, L. (2014). Cancer risk factors among adults with serious mental illness. *American Journal of Preventive Medicine, 46*(Suppl. 1), S98–S103. https://doi.org/10.1016/j.amepre.2013.10.028

National Institute on Drug Abuse. (2017, March). Health consequences of drug misuse. https://www.drugabuse.gov/related-topics/health-consequences-drug-misuse

Nixon, J.L., Cartmill, B., Turner, J., Pigott, A.E., Brown, E., Wall, L.R., ... Porceddu, S.V. (2018). Exploring the prevalence and experience of mask anxiety for the person with head and neck cancer undergoing radiotherapy.

Journal of Medical Radiation Sciences, 65, 282–290. https://doi.org/10.1002/jmrs.308

O'Connell, J.J., Oppenheimer, S.C., Judge, C.M., Taube, R.L., Blanchfield, B.B., Swain, S.E., & Koh, H.K. (2010). The Boston Health Care for the Homeless Program: A public health framework. *American Journal of Public Health, 100,* 1400–1408. https://doi.org/10.2105/AJPH.2009.173609

Potash, A.E., Karnell, L.H., Christensen, A.J., Vander Weg, M.W., & Funk, G.F. (2010). Continued alcohol use in patients with head and neck cancer. *Head and Neck, 32,* 905–912. https://doi.org/10.1002/hed.21281

Procyshyn, R.M., Bezchlibnyk-Butler, K.Z., & Jeffries, J.J. (2019). *Clinical handbook of psychotropic drugs* (23rd ed.). Hogrefe.

Prokhorov, A.V., Pallonen, U.E., Fava, J.L., Ding, L., & Niaura, R. (1996). Measuring nicotine dependence among high-risk adolescent smokers. *Addictive Behaviors, 21,* 117–127. https://doi.org/10.1016/0306-4603(96)00048-2

Riba, M.B., Donovan, K.A., Andersen, B., Braun, I., Breitbart, W.S., Brewer, B.W., ... Darlow, S. D. (2019). Distress management, version 3.2019, NCCN clinical practice guidelines in oncology. *Journal of the National Comprehensive Cancer Network, 17,* 1229–1249. https://doi.org/10.6004/jnccn.2019.0048

Richmond, J.S., Berlin, J.S., Fishkind, A.B., Holloman, G.H., Zeller, S.L., Wilson, M.P., ... Ng, A.T. (2012). Verbal de-escalation of the agitated patient: Consensus statement of the American Association for Emergency Psychiatry Project BETA De-Escalation Workgroup. *Western Journal of Emergency Medicine, 13,* 17–25. https://doi.org/10.5811/westjem.2011.9.6864

Robson, A., Scrutton, F., Wilkinson, L., & MacLeod, F. (2010). The risk of suicide in cancer patients: A review of the literature. *Psycho-Oncology, 19,* 1250–1258. https://doi.org/10.1002/pon.1717

Rossetti, A., Chadha, M., Torres, B.N., Lee, J.K., Hylton, D., Loewy, J.V., & Harrison, L.B. (2017). The impact of music therapy on anxiety in cancer patients undergoing simulation for radiation therapy. *International Journal of Radiation Oncology, Biology, Physics, 99,* 103–110. https://doi.org/10.1016/j.ijrobp.2017.05.003

Saunders, J.B., Aasland, O.G., Babor, T.F., de la Fuente, J.R., & Grant, M. (1993). Development of the Alcohol Use Disorders Identification Test (AUDIT): WHO collaborative project on early detection of persons with harmful alcohol consumption-II. *Addiction, 88,* 791–804. https://doi.org/10.1111/j.1360-0443.1993.tb02093.x

Semprini, F., Fava, G.A., & Sonino, N. (2010). The spectrum of adjustment disorders: Too broad to be clinically helpful. *CNS Spectrums, 15,* 382–388. https://doi.org/10.1017/s1092852900029254

Singer, S., Das-Munshi, J., & Brähler, E. (2010). Prevalence of mental health conditions in cancer patients in acute care—A meta-analysis. *Annals of Oncology, 21,* 925–930. https://doi.org/10.1093/annonc/mdp515

Sperduti, A., Hindle, D., Shessel, A., Pidgeon, B., Akmal, H., Chaulk, G., ... Rosewall, T. (2018). Treating too lightly? Radiation therapists' experiences of workplace violence when providing care to cancer patients and their families. *Journal of Medical Imaging and Radiation Sciences, 49,* 56–61. https://doi.org/10.1016/j.jmir.2017.11.001

Spoletini, I., Gianni, W., Caltagirone, C., Madaio, R., Repetto, L., & Spalletta, G. (2011). Suicide and cancer: Where do we go from here? *Critical Reviews in Oncology/Hematology, 78,* 206–219. https://doi.org/10.1016/j.critrevonc.2010.05.005

Strain, J.J., & Diefenbacher, A. (2008). The adjustment disorders: The conundrums of the diagnoses. *Comprehensive Psychiatry, 49,* 121–130. https://doi.org/10.1016/j.comppsych.2007.10.002

Strong, V., Waters, R., Hibberd, C., Murray, G., Wall, L., Walker, J., ... Sharpe, M. (2008). Management of depression for people with cancer (SMaRT oncology 1): A randomised trial. *Lancet, 372,* 40–48. https://doi.org/10.1016/s0140-6736(08)60991-5

Substance Abuse and Mental Health Services Administration. (2018a). Medications for opioid use disorder for healthcare and addiction professionals, policymakers, patients, and families. https://medicine.yale.edu/edbup/quickstart/TIP_63_338482_42801_v1.pdf

Substance Abuse and Mental Health Services Administration. (2018b). *Results from the 2017 national survey on drug use and health: Detailed tables.*

https://www.samhsa.gov/data/sites/default/files/cbhsq-reports/NSDUH DetailedTabs2017/NSDUHDetailedTabs2017.pdf

Sullivan, J.T., Sykora, K., Schneiderman, J., Naranjo, C.A., & Sellers, E.M. (1989). Assessment of alcohol withdrawal: The revised Clinical Institute Withdrawal Assessment for Alcohol scale (CIWA-Ar). *British Journal of Addiction, 84,* 1353–1357. https://doi.org/10.1111/j.1360-0443.1989 .tb00737.x

Suppli, N.P., Johansen, C., Christensen, J., Kessing, L.V., Kroman, N., & Dalton, S.O. (2014). Increased risk for depression after breast cancer: A nationwide population-based cohort study of associated factors in Denmark, 1998–2011. *Journal of Clinical Oncology, 32,* 3831–3839. https://doi.org/10.1200 /jco.2013.54.0419

Taha, S. (2018, August). *Best practices across the continuum of care for the treatment of opioid use disorder.* https://www.ccsa.ca/sites/default/files/2019-04 /CCSA-Best-Practices-Treatment-Opioid-Use-Disorder-2018-en.pdf

Thalén-Lindström, A., Larsson, G., Hellbom, M., Glimelius, B., & Johansson, B. (2013). Validation of the Distress Thermometer in a Swedish population of oncology patients; Accuracy of changes during six months. *European Journal of Oncology Nursing, 17,* 625–631. https://doi.org/10.1016/j.ejon.2012 .12.005

Tolia, M., Tsoukalas, N., Nikolaou, M., Mosa, E., Nazos, I., Poultsidi, A., ... Kyrgias, G. (2018). Utilizing yoga in oncologic patients treated with radiotherapy: Review. *Indian Journal of Palliative Care, 24,* 355–358.

Traeger, L., Greer, J.A., Fernandez-Robles, C., Temel, J.S., & Pirl, W.F. (2012). Evidence-based treatment of anxiety in patients with cancer. *Journal of Clinical Oncology, 30,* 1197–1205. https://doi.org/10.1200/jco.2011.39.5632

Voigt, V., Neufeld, F., Kaste, J., Bühner, M., Sckopke, P., Wuerstlein, R., ... Hermelink, K. (2017). Clinically assessed posttraumatic stress in patients with breast cancer during the first year after diagnosis in the prospective, longitudinal, controlled COGNICARES study. *Psycho-Oncology, 26,* 74–80. https://doi.org/10.1002/pon.4102

Wagner, L.I., Pugh, S.L., Small, W., Jr., Kirshner, J., Sidhu, K., Bury, M.J., ... Bruner, D.W. (2017). Screening for depression in cancer patients receiving radiotherapy: Feasibility and identification of effective tools in the NRG Oncology RTOG 0841 trial. *Cancer, 123,* 485–493. https://doi.org/10 .1002/cncr.29969

Walker, J., Hansen, C.H., Martin, P., Symeonides, S., Ramessur, R., Murray, G., & Sharpe, M. (2014). Prevalence, associations, and adequacy of treatment of major depression in patients with cancer: A cross-sectional analysis of routinely collected clinical data. *Lancet Psychiatry, 1,* 343–350. https://doi.org /10.1016/s2215-0366(14)70313-x

Warren, G.W., Kasza, K.A., Reid, M.E., Cummings, K.M., & Marshall, J.R. (2013). Smoking at diagnosis and survival in cancer patients. *International Journal of Cancer, 132,* 401–410. https://doi.org/10.1002/ijc.27617

Webber, K., & Davies, A.N. (2012). An observational study to determine the prevalence of alcohol use disorders in advanced cancer patients. *Palliative Medicine, 26,* 360–367. https://doi.org/10.1177/0269216311409474

Webster, L.R., & Webster, R.M. (2005). Predicting aberrant behaviors in opioid-treated patients: Preliminary validation of the Opioid Risk Tool. *Pain Medicine, 6,* 432–442. https://doi.org/10.1111/j.1526-4637.2005.00072.x

Weinstein, L.C., Stefancic, A., Cunningham, A.T., Hurley, K.E., Cabassa, L.J., & Wender, R.C. (2016). Cancer screening, prevention, and treatment in people with mental illness. *CA: A Cancer Journal for Clinicians, 66,* 133–151. https://doi.org/10.3322/caac.21334

Yuppa, D.P., & Braun, I.M. (2015). Psychotropic medications in cancer care. In J.C. Holland, W.S. Breitbart, P.N. Butow, P.B. Jacobsen, M.J. Loscalzo, & R. McCorkle (Eds.), *Psycho-oncology* (3rd ed., pp. 419–428). Oxford University Press.

Zhao, L., Li, X., Zhang, Z., Song, C., Guo, C., Zhang, Y., ... Han, L. (2014). Prevalence, correlates and recognition of depression in Chinese inpatients with cancer. *General Hospital Psychiatry, 36,* 477–482. https://doi.org/10 .1016/j.genhosppsych.2014.05.005

X. Chemical Modifiers of Treatment

A. Radiosensitizers and concurrent chemotherapy and biotherapy

  1. Combined modality therapy

    a) Combined modality therapy is the use of RT, chemotherapy, and surgery in sequence or concurrently in a variety of combinations and has improved cancer outcomes compared to RT alone for many cancers.

    b) The past few decades have seen an increase in the combination of therapeutic modalities to improve organ preservation, cosmesis, overall survival, and local-regional control (Willey, Yang, & Bonner, 2016).

    c) RT can be given as definitive, neoadjuvant, adjuvant, prophylactic, or palliative treatment, as well as concurrent with other therapeutic modalities (see VIII. Modality-Specific Management for more information).

    d) Many challenges exist in finding a concise list of chemotherapy agents used in combination with RT, as research has led to frequent changes. Many combined chemotherapy regimens are not endorsed by NCCN.

    e) Minimal evidence regarding the interactions of chemotherapy with protons is available. Photons and electrons appear to have similar interactions with medications (Lehnert, 2015).

    f) Many combined chemotherapy agents are excreted in body fluids like urine and feces, sometimes for days after a patient has received a dose. Radiation oncology nurses should follow relevant body fluid and chemotherapy safety precautions.

  2. Radiosensitizers

    a) Definition

      (1) Radiosensitizers are chemical agents administered in conjunction with RT for the enhancement of antitumor efficacy (Mowery, Yoo, & Brizel, 2019).

      (2) The decision to use a medication in combination with RT is based on safety and demonstrated benefit to the patient.

    b) Rationale

      (1) Radiosensitizers are utilized to enhance damage to tumor cells while minimizing toxicity in healthy tissue (Morgan, Parsels, Maybaum, & Lawrence, 2014).

      (2) The utility of a radiosensitizer is determined by the therapeutic ratio.

        (a) Therapeutic ratio (also known as *therapeutic index* or *therapeutic margin*) is a ratio of the tumor control probability (likelihood of killing cancer cells) in relation to the normal tissue complication probability (likelihood of damaging healthy tissue) (Mowery et al., 2019).

        (b) An agent's ability to improve the efficacy of treatment and the degree to which it adds to morbidity together determine its overall usefulness (Mowery et al., 2019).

    c) Types of radiosensitizers

      (1) Augmented oxygenation of tumor cells

        (a) Ionizing radiation creates oxygen free radicals, which, in turn, lead to cell death.

        (b) Well-oxygenated cells are approximately 2.5 times more sensitive to a given dose of ionizing radiation than hypoxic cells (Mowery et al., 2019).

        (c) Severely hypoxic cells require double to triple the dosage of radiation to sustain damage compared to well-oxygenated cells (Mowery et al., 2019).

      (2) Targeting tumor vasculature

        (a) Blood supply to a tumor can be modified or normalized to reduce tumor hypoxia, thereby improving tumor radiosensitization.

        (b) Bevacizumab is a monoclonal antibody that binds to and neutralizes VEGF (Lehnert, 2015).

          i. This antiangiogenesis agent targets the growth of new blood vessels.

          ii. Use of this agent has been controversial because of the theoretical risk of decreasing blood flow to a tumor and causing hypoxia, decreasing radiosensitivity.

        (c) Tyrosine kinase inhibitors act by preventing growth factor receptor activation. Some tyrosine kinase inhibitors affect angiogenesis and thus face the same theoretical risk.

      (3) Agents targeting hypoxic cells: Mitomycin C is an alkylating agent that is preferentially cytotoxic to hypoxic cells and metabolized in regions of low oxygen concentration.

      (4) Biotherapy agents

        (a) Biotherapy agents are given concurrently with RT with the goal of improving control of locoregional disease and improving survival versus RT alone. This benefit is weighed against toxicities (Milenic, Baidoo, Kim, & Brechbiel, 2015).

        (b) Some molecular-targeted therapy agents have radiosensitizing potential in addition to their primary clinical application.

        (c) These agents have their own toxicities and challenges for management.

        (d) Cetuximab is a monoclonal antibody directed against epidermal growth factor receptor. Inhibition of the epidermal

growth factor receptor pathway enhances the response to RT (Bonner et al., 2006).

    i. Cetuximab is a biotherapy that has been tested concurrently with RT and multiple chemotherapy agents (Lehnert, 2015).

    ii. Cetuximab can cause myelosuppression. Leukopenia occurs in approximately 25% of patients, and anemia occurs in 16% of patients. Complete blood count and differential should be monitored during therapy (Wilkes & Barton-Burke, 2020).

    iii. Hypomagnesemia occurs in 55% of patients, and the time to onset and severity can be highly variable (Wilkes & Barton-Burke, 2020).

    iv. Nausea, vomiting, diarrhea, anorexia, constipation, and mucositis are considered mild to moderate. However, for treatment of head and neck cancers, mucositis can exacerbate the expected RT side effects.

    v. Cetuximab is associated with a rash, and a more severe rash appears to be associated with a stronger beneficial reaction to treatment (Chu & DeVita, 2021).

    vi. Rashes occur in 76%–88% of patients (Wilkes & Barton-Burke, 2020).

    vii. The incidence and severity of radiation dermatitis can be compounded by the addition of cetuximab (Langendijk & Oosting, 2011).

3. Agents used in concurrent chemotherapy

  a) 5-Fluorouracil (Chu & DeVita, 2021; Willey et al., 2016)

    (1) 5-Fluorouracil has been used with RT since the 1950s. It has been combined with RT to treat several forms of gastrointestinal cancers.

    (2) 5-Fluorouracil is thought to target radioresistant cells in the S phase.

  b) Leucovorin calcium folate (Wilkes & Barton-Burke, 2020)

    (1) Leucovorin is often given intravenously in conjunction with 5-fluorouracil to potentiate the antitumor activity.

    (2) It also enhances the toxicity of 5-fluorouracil.

      (a) Myelosuppression is dose limiting. Complete blood count should be monitored during treatment.

      (b) Anorexia is common in patients with gastric and pancreatic cancer receiving 5-fluorouracil.

      (c) Nausea and vomiting occur in 30%–50% of patients and is dose dependent.

      i. This same symptom may also be caused by the RT itself depending on the treatment field.

      ii. Altered nutrition and fluid and electrolyte abnormalities should be regularly assessed.

    (d) Diarrhea is a dose-limiting toxicity and can be severe. Patients should be monitored for fluid and electrolyte imbalances.

    (e) Mucositis can lead to pain, poor nutritional status, reduced fluid intake, and increased risk for dehydration, as well as increase risk of infection.

      i. Symptomatic treatment may be required.

      ii. Anal and oral mucositis can occur with 5-fluorouracil.

    (f) Palmar-plantar erythrodysesthesia (hand-foot syndrome) can be dose limiting and is most often observed with continuous infusion therapy (characterized by tingling, numbness, pain, erythema, dryness, rash, swelling, increased pigmentation, nail changes, pruritus of the hands and feet, and desquamation).

    (g) Neurotoxicity is rare, but it is characterized by somnolence, confusion, seizures, cerebellar ataxia, and possible encephalopathy. Therapy must be discontinued immediately if encephalopathy is suspected.

  c) Capecitabine

    (1) Capecitabine is an oral form of 5-fluorouracil that has proven to have an equivalent survival rate to continuous IV 5-fluorouracil (Chionh, Lau, Yeung, Price, & Tebbutt, 2017).

    (2) In several randomized trials, capecitabine demonstrated at least equivalent outcomes to 5-fluorouracil and leucovorin. Capecitabine is now commonly used as an alternative to IV 5-fluorouracil in several regimens (Lehnert, 2015).

    (3) Capecitabine should be taken by mouth with a glass of water within 30 minutes after a meal.

    (4) Patients may have questions related to when they should start capecitabine in relation to RT, as well as how to take capecitabine (Wilkes & Barton-Burke, 2020).

    (5) Capecitabine has the potential for multiple toxicities (Wilkes & Barton-Burke, 2020).

      (a) Myelosuppression is less common with capecitabine than with IV 5-fluorouracil.

      (b) Nausea and vomiting occur in 50% of patients. Clinicians should screen for altered nutrition and fluid and electrolyte abnormalities as part of regular assessment.

(c) Anorexia is common in patients with gastric and pancreatic cancer.

(d) Diarrhea occurs in 55% of patients, is dose limiting, and can be severe enough to require symptomatic management.

(e) Mucositis can lead to pain, poor nutritional status, reduced fluid intake, and increased risk for dehydration, as well as increased risk of infection. Symptomatic treatment may be required.

(f) Electrolyte imbalances and dehydration related to nausea, vomiting, mucositis, and diarrhea should be monitored and corrected as necessary.

(g) Severe hand-foot syndrome occurs in up to 20% of patients and is similar in presentation to continuous IV 5-fluorouracil.

(h) Capecitabine has multiple food and drug interactions.

d) Cisplatin

(1) Cisplatin is a platinum-based agent that acts similarly to alkylating agents, and it has been a known radiosensitizer since the 1970s (Willey et al., 2016).

(2) Cisplatin has an extensive toxicity profile that can be challenging to manage (Wilkes & Barton-Burke, 2020).

(a) Complete blood count and differential should be monitored during treatment.

(b) Cisplatin is highly emetogenic and causes acute and delayed nausea and vomiting. Antiemetic regimens are scheduled and can be more complex.

(c) Cisplatin causes magnesium and potassium wasting, which can manifest days after the drug administration.

  i. Potassium and magnesium levels should be monitored, and supplementation may be required.

  ii. This can manifest as heart rhythm changes.

(d) Ototoxicity manifests as high-frequency hearing loss and tinnitus. Hearing loss is reversible if addressed early, but it can become permanent if not addressed.

(e) Cisplatin causes cumulative, dose-limiting nephrotoxicity, and renal function can be altered permanently if not addressed in a timely manner.

(f) Dysgeusia and anorexia are common side effects.

(g) Peripheral neuropathy can be severe and can become irreversible.

e) Gemcitabine

(1) Gemcitabine is a fluorine-substituted deoxycytidine analog.

(2) As a radiosensitizer, gemcitabine has been studied with NSCLC, head and neck cancer, gastrointestinal cancer, cervical cancer, breast cancer, bladder cancer, and glioblastoma (Lehnert, 2015).

(3) The following toxicities can occur with gemcitabine (Wilkes & Barton-Burke, 2020).

(a) Myelosuppression is dose limiting.

  i. Of patients treated with gemcitabine, 73% develop anemia, 63% develop leukopenia, and 36% develop thrombocytopenia.

  ii. Complete blood count with differential should be monitored during treatment.

(b) Nausea and vomiting occur in 69% of patients; of that group, 15% experience severe nausea and vomiting. Nausea and vomiting should be monitored, along with associated electrolyte imbalances and altered nutritional status.

(c) Flu-like symptoms occur in one-fifth of patients, and 41% of patients experience transient febrile episodes.

(d) Erythematous, pruritic, and/or maculopapular rash to the face and trunk occurs in 30% of patients.

(e) Liver and renal function should be monitored during treatment.

(f) Up to 30% will experience edema, which is usually peripheral but can involve the face or pulmonary system.

(4) Toxicities have been clinically unacceptable with higher dose gemcitabine in many disease sites, but it is currently used with pancreatic cancers.

f) Temozolomide

(1) Temozolomide combined with RT has become the standard of care in glioblastoma treatment (Karachi, Dastmalchi, Mitchell, & Rahman, 2018; Ward, Tendulkar, & Videtic, 2018).

(2) The combination of temozolomide and RT has shown significant improvements in median survival and overall survival (Willey et al., 2016).

(3) Temozolomide is an oral medication.

(a) Absorption is optimized on an empty stomach; the rate and extent the drug is absorbed is affected by food (Chu & DeVita, 2021).

(b) Patients may have questions regarding the coordination of medication and RT.

(4) The following toxicities can occur with temozolomide treatment (Wilkes & Barton-Burke, 2020).

(a) Myelosuppression is a well-known toxicity of temozolomide.

      i. Leukopenia and thrombocytopenia occur in 40% of patients.

      ii. Myelosuppression is dose limiting.

      iii. Monitoring complete blood count during treatment is essential, and patients may need to be placed on precautions related to risk for bleeding or risk for infection.

(b) Nausea and vomiting occurs in 75% of patients and is usually mild. It can be difficult to differentiate temozolomide-induced nausea and vomiting from nausea and vomiting related to increased intracranial pressure due to inflammation caused by RT.

(c) Lethargy, ataxia, headache, dizziness, and fatigue were noted in 40% of patients with malignant glioma, but it is unclear if this was the result of malignancy or treatment.

(d) Stomatitis can occur in up to 20% of patients.

(e) Diarrhea, constipation, and anorexia affect up to 40% of patients.

g) Mitomycin C

(1) Mitomycin C is a hypoxic cell sensitizer with cytotoxic effects that has greatly affected anal cancer treatment.

(2) In anal cancer treatment, the addition of mitomycin C to 5-fluorouracil and RT improved local control, overall survival, and colostomy-free survival when compared to 5-fluorouracil and RT without mitomycin C (Chin, Hong, & Ryan, 2012).

(3) Mitomycin C can cause the following toxicities (Wilkes & Barton-Burke, 2020).

(a) Myelosuppression is a dose-limiting toxicity, and thrombocytopenia and leukopenia are common. Complete blood count and differential should be monitored during treatment.

(b) Anorexia is a common side effect.

(c) Nausea and vomiting are usually mild to moderate and readily controllable with antiemetics.

(d) Mitomycin C can cause increased creatinine level.

(4) Toxicities are more severe with the addition of mitomycin C to 5-fluorouracil chemotherapy.

(5) Mitomycin C is not used as single-agent primary therapy (Wilkes & Barton-Burke, 2020).

h) Etoposide

(1) Etoposide is a plant alkaloid derived from the mandrake plant and is used concurrently with cisplatin and RT in the treatment of stage III or higher lung cancer (Liang et al., 2017).

(2) Etoposide can cause the following toxicities (Wilkes & Barton-Burke, 2020).

(a) Myelosuppression is a dose-limiting toxicity. Complete blood count should be monitored during RT.

(b) Liver and renal function may be affected, so these should be monitored during therapy.

(c) Nausea and vomiting occur in 30%–40% of patients. Symptoms are generally mild to moderate, and anorexia is possible (Chu & DeVita, 2021).

(d) Etoposide is known to cause radiation recall reactions.

(e) Alopecia is dose dependent.

i) Carboplatin

(1) Carboplatin is an alkylating platinum agent.

(2) Carboplatin can cause the following toxicities (Wilkes & Barton-Burke, 2020).

(a) Myelosuppression is possible. Complete blood count and differential should be monitored during therapy.

(b) Carboplatin is considered less emetogenic than high-dose cisplatin, and incidence of delayed-onset nausea and vomiting is lower (Chu & DeVita, 2021).

(c) Renal function and electrolyte levels should be monitored, particularly magnesium and potassium (Chu & DeVita, 2021).

(d) Less than 10% of patients develop peripheral neuropathy (Chu & DeVita, 2021).

(e) Liver enzymes increase mildly during therapy, but this is reversible (Chu & DeVita, 2021).

j) Oxaliplatin

(1) Oxaliplatin is an IV platinum compound.

(2) This medication has been used concurrently with RT when combined with 5-fluorouracil for esophageal and colon cancers (Ward et al., 2018).

(3) Oxaliplatin may cause the following toxicities (Wilkes & Barton-Burke, 2020).

(a) Myelosuppression may occur. Complete blood count and differential should be monitored during therapy.

(b) Renal function may be affected and should be monitored during therapy.

(c) Acute neurotoxicity may occur, and clinicians should monitor for this.

(d) Cold hypersensitivity occurs in 56% of patients and can require diet and lifestyle modifications.

(e) Peripheral sensory neuropathy is usually transient, and exposure to cold can worsen or precipitate the neuropathy.

k) Paclitaxel
  (1) Paclitaxel is a taxane used in combination with RT and carboplatin. It has been tested in a variety of regimens.
  (2) Paclitaxel can cause the following toxicities (Wilkes & Barton-Burke, 2020).
    (a) Myelosuppression may occur. Complete blood count and differential should be monitored during treatment.
    (b) Sensory neuropathy occurs in 60% of patients and should be assessed and monitored for paresthesias.
    (c) Nausea and vomiting occur in 52% of patients (Wilkes & Barton-Burke, 2020).
    (d) Mild diarrhea occurs in 38% of patients.
    (e) Stomatitis is less common with infusions shorter than 24 hours.
l) Irinotecan
  (1) Irinotecan is a cell cycle–nonspecific agent with activity throughout the cell cycle (Wilkes & Barton-Burke, 2020).
  (2) Irinotecan may cause the following toxicities.
    (a) Myelosuppression is a dose-limiting toxicity. Complete blood count and differential should be monitored during treatment.
    (b) Early diarrhea is significant with irinotecan and can occur during the infusion and for the next 24 hours due to a cholinergic response accompanied by diaphoresis and abdominal cramping (Chu & DeVita, 2021).
    (c) Late diarrhea is also possible with irinotecan and can be severe (Chu & DeVita, 2021).
    (d) Fluid and electrolyte abnormalities need to be monitored, and rehydration and supplementation should be implemented as clinically indicated.
m) Docetaxel
  (1) Docetaxel is a taxane in the same family as paclitaxel (Wilkes & Barton-Burke, 2020).
  (2) Docetaxel may cause the following toxicities (Wilkes & Barton-Burke, 2020).
    (a) Myelosuppression, leading to neutropenia, is a dose-limiting toxicity.
      i. Complete blood count and differential should be monitored during treatment.
      ii. Patients should receive myelosuppression precaution education.
    (b) Nausea and vomiting are generally mild and controllable with an antiemetic regimen. Nausea appears in up to 42% of patients, and vomiting occurs in 22%.
    (c) Diarrhea is reported to occur in up to 42% of patients.
    (d) Stomatitis occurs in 51% of patients.
    (e) Fluid and electrolyte imbalances, liver function, pain, weight loss, and nutritional status need to be monitored.
    (f) Cutaneous reactions can include edema and erythema on the extremities, as well as changes to the fingernails and toenails.
      i. Pruritic, erythematous, and maculopapular rashes can occur, usually on the extremities but also on the thorax.
      ii. Skin reactions usually resolve within a week after the final dose.
    (g) Cystoid macular edema, which causes acute vision changes, has been reported. If a patient develops vision loss while on treatment, referral to an ophthalmologist is recommended.
n) Vinblastine
  (1) Vinblastine is a vinca alkaloid derived from the periwinkle plant.
  (2) Vinblastine may cause the following toxicities (Wilkes & Barton-Burke, 2020).
    (a) Myelosuppression can be severe. Complete blood count and differential should be monitored during treatment.
    (b) Nausea and vomiting are rare.
    (c) Stomatitis can be severe, but this is not a common side effect.
    (d) Constipation should be monitored for and reported.
    (e) Peripheral neuropathy should be monitored for and reported.
o) Vincristine
  (1) Vincristine is a vinca alkaloid derived from the periwinkle plant (Wilkes & Barton-Burke, 2020).
  (2) Vincristine may cause the following toxicities (Wilkes & Barton-Burke, 2020).
    (a) Myelosuppression is generally mild.
    (b) Neurotoxicity is a dose-limiting toxicity.
    (c) Constipation is a common symptom and can progress to paralytic ileus and abdominal pain.
    (d) Nausea, vomiting, and diarrhea are rare.
    (e) Amenorrhea and azoospermia are possible.
p) Hydroxyurea
  (1) Hydroxyurea is an antimetabolite (Wilkes & Barton-Burke, 2020).
  (2) Hydroxyurea may cause the following toxicities (Wilkes & Barton-Burke, 2020).
    (a) Myelosuppression can be severe.
    (b) Nausea, vomiting, mucositis, and liver dysfunction are rare. Abnormal liver function can occur.

(c) Renal function should be monitored.

(d) Drowsiness, confusion, disorientation, headaches, and vertigo are possible side effects.

(e) This drug is associated with radiation recall.

q) Pemetrexed

(1) Pemetrexed is an antimetabolite used in conjunction with cisplatin (Senan et al., 2016; Wilkes & Barton-Burke, 2020).

(2) Pemetrexed may cause the following toxicities.

(a) Myelosuppression is a dose-limiting toxicity. Complete blood count with differential should be monitored during therapy (Chu & DeVita, 2021).

(b) Nausea, vomiting, and mucositis can interfere with fluid and electrolyte intake. Renal and liver function panel should be monitored during treatment.

(c) Bowel function can be altered, with constipation and diarrhea being possible.

(d) A rash may develop and can be ameliorated with prophylactic steroid use.

(e) NSAIDs should be avoided during therapy because of an increased risk of renal dysfunction.

r) Other agents: Currently, doxorubicin, bleomycin, and methotrexate are no longer recommended by NCCN for concurrent RT regimens.

4. Commonly approved regimens: A complete listing of all regimens and recommended supportive care, searchable by disease site and agent, is available for free at NCCN's website (see www.nccn.org/professionals/OrderTemplates/Default.aspx).

References

Bonner, J.A., Harai, P.M., Giralt, J., Azarnia, N., Shin, D.M., Cohen, R.B., ... Ang, K.K. (2006). Radiotherapy plus cetuximab for squamous-cell carcinoma of the head and neck. *New England Journal of Medicine, 354,* 567–578. https://doi.org/10.1056/nejmoa053422

Chin, J.Y., Hong, T.S., & Ryan, D.P. (2012). Mitomycin in anal cancer: Still the standard of care. *Journal of Clinical Oncology, 30,* 4297–4301. https://doi.org/10.1200/jco.2012.44.8878

Chionh, F., Lau, D., Yeung, Y., Price, T., & Tebbutt, N. (2017). Oral versus intravenous fluoropyrimidines for colorectal cancer. *Cochrane Database of Systematic Reviews, 2017*(7). https://doi.org/10.1002/14651858.CD008398.pub2

Chu, E., & DeVita, V.T., Jr. (Eds.). (2021). *Physicians' cancer chemotherapy drug manual.* Jones and Bartlett Learning.

Karachi, A., Dastmalchi, F., Mitchell, D.A., & Rahman, M. (2018). Temozolomide for immunomodulation in the treatment of glioblastoma. *Neuro-Oncology, 20,* 1566–1572. https://doi.org/10.1093/neuonc/noy072

Langendijk, J.A., & Oosting, S.F. (2011). Grading system and management guidelines for dermatitis induced by head and neck radiotherapy plus cetuximab: Clinical validation required. *Annals of Oncology, 22,* 2157–2159. https://doi.org/10.1093/annonc/mdr410

Lehnert, S. (2015). *Radiosensitizers and radiochemotherapy in the treatment of cancer.* CRC Press.

Liang, J., Bi, N., Wu, S., Chen, M., Lv, C., Zhao, L., ... Wang, L. (2017). Etoposide and cisplatin versus paclitaxel and carboplatin with concurrent thoracic radiotherapy in unresectable stage III non-small cell lung cancer: A multicenter randomized phase III trial. *Annals of Oncology, 28,* 777–783. https://doi.org/10.1093/annonc/mdx009

Milenic, D.E., Baidoo, K.E., Kim, Y.-S., & Brechbiel, M.W. (2015). Evaluation of cetuximab as a candidate for targeted α-particle radiation therapy of HER1-positive disseminated intraperitoneal disease. *mAbs, 7,* 255–264. https://doi.org/10.4161/19420862.2014.985160

Morgan, M.A., Parsels, L.A., Maybaum, J., & Lawrence, T.S. (2014). Improving the efficacy of chemoradiation with targeted agents. *Cancer Discovery, 4,* 280–291. https://doi.org/10.1158/2159-8290.CD-13-0337

Mowery, Y.M., Yoo, D.S., & Brizel, D.M. (2019). Chemical modifiers of radiation response. In E.C. Halperin, D.E. Wazer, C.A. Perez, & L.W. Brady (Eds.), *Perez and Brady's principles and practice of radiation oncology* (7th ed., pp. 715–725). Wolters Kluwer.

Senan, S., Brade, A., Wang, L.-H., Vansteenkiste, J., Dakhil, S., Biesma, B., ... Vokes, E. (2016). PROCLAIM: Randomized phase III trial of pemetrexed-cisplatin or etoposide-cisplatin plus thoracic radiation therapy followed by consolidation chemotherapy in locally advanced nonsquamous non–small-cell lung cancer. *Journal of Clinical Oncology, 34,* 953–962. https://doi.org/10.1200/jco.2015.64.8824

Ward, M.C., Tendulkar, R.D., & Videtic, G.M.M. (Eds.). (2018). *Essentials of clinical radiation oncology.* Springer. https://doi.org/10.1891.9870826168559

Wilkes, G.M., & Barton-Burke, M. (2020). *2020–2021 oncology nursing drug handbook.* Jones and Bartlett Learning.

Willey, C.D., Yang, E.S.-H., & Bonner, J.A. (2016). Interaction of chemotherapy and radiation. In L.L. Gunderson & J.E. Tepper (Eds.), *Clinical radiation oncology* (4th ed., pp. 63–79.e4). https://doi.org/10.1016/b978-0-323-24098-7.00004-6

B. Radioimmunotherapy and radiopharmaceuticals

1. Overview

a) Radioimmunotherapy is a selective internal RT using radioisotopes conjugated to tumor-directed antibodies (monoclonal antibodies) or their fragments (Sgouros, 2019).

b) Radioimmunotherapy is used for directed treatment of cancer or for palliation of tumor-related symptoms, such as pain (ACR, 2019).

c) Radioimmunotherapy allows for the delivery of high-dose therapeutic radiation to cancer cells, while minimizing the exposure of healthy cells (Jadvar, 2017).

d) Engineered monoclonal antibodies paired with radioactive materials are known as *radiopharmaceuticals* (molecules containing radioactive isotopes). These agents are generally administered intravenously, but some can also be inhaled or swallowed (Dandapani & Wong, 2016; Jadvar, 2017; Ramos et al., 2017).

(1) Radioisotopes are chosen based on half-life, energy path length, and ability to conjugate the radioisotope to the tumor target without altering the target (Dandapani & Wong, 2016).

(2) The radioisotopes emit short-range particles (often alpha, beta, and gamma) and are used for therapy because they expend all their

energy over a very short distance, thus causing significant local damage, such as cell destruction (Kunos & Capala, 2018; Kunos, Capala, Finnigan, Smith, & Ivy, 2019; Marcu, Bezak, & Allen, 2018).

    (3) The dose equivalency of an alpha-emitting therapeutic radiopharmaceutical refers to the absorbed dose received by the target. Alpha irradiation has a fivefold higher toxicity than an x-ray (Marcu et al., 2018).

2. Radiopharmaceutical terms
  a) Dosimetry
    (1) For purpose of radioimmunotherapy, *dosimetry* refers to measuring and characterizing the effects of radiation in organs, including activity and absorbed radiation dose in an organ and biologic effects after administration of a radiopharmaceutical (Kesner & Bodei, 2018; Kunos & Capala, 2018; Peştean, Veloso Jéronimo, & Hogg, 2016).

    (2) Dosimetry guides the selection of a reasonably safe therapeutic radiation administered to patients. Biodistribution estimates vary significantly for different radiopharmaceuticals and protocols, as well as among centers. Currently, standards for documenting and reporting biodistribution measurements do not exist (Kesner & Bodei, 2018).

  b) Activity: *Activity* refers to the number of transitions or decays per unit of time in a given amount of radioactive material (Menzel, 2017; U.S. FDA, 2019).

  c) Mass dose: The mass dose is the dose (mass unit) of the pharmaceutical administered per body surface area (Menzel, 2017; U.S. FDA, 2019).

  d) Radiation administered dose: Radiation administered dose is the amount of radioactivity administered to patients and expressed as the unit of activity (i.e., in units of Mbq or mCi) (Menzel, 2017; U.S. FDA, 2019).

  e) Radiation absorbed dose
    (1) Radiation absorbed dose is the ionizing radiation energy deposited per unit mass of an organ or tissue (Menzel, 2017; U.S. FDA, 2019).

    (2) See also II. Practice of Radiation Oncology.

  f) Equivalent dose
    (1) Equivalent dose is a measure of biologic effect of the radioactive dose that considers both the absorbed dose and biologic effectiveness of the radiation, and hence, the radiation type (Menzel, 2017; U.S. FDA, 2019).

    (2) The equivalent dose is dependent on the ratio of biologic effectiveness of one type of ionizing radiation to another radiation of interest (e.g., gamma rays or beta particles to alpha particles). Ratio of biologic effectiveness has no unit (Menzel, 2017; U.S. FDA, 2019).

    (3) See also II. Practice of Radiation Oncology.

  g) Half-life of radiopharmaceuticals (Menzel, 2017; Ramos et al., 2017; U.S. FDA, 2019)
    (1) Biologic half-life is the half-life of the pharmaceutical in the living system.

    (2) Physical half-life is the half-life of the radionuclide itself, not affected by surrounding conditions, independent of the living system.

    (3) Effective half-life is the half-life of radionuclide in a living system and affected by the conditions (i.e., a function of elimination due to the elimination of the ligand that carries it).

  h) Ligand: *Ligand* refers to any part of the molecule that can be divided and used to bond to the radionuclide or to deliver or target the radionuclide to the organ or tissue (U.S. FDA, 2019).

  i) Organ (Shen et al., 2018; U.S. FDA, 2019)
    (1) The source organ takes up the radiopharmaceutical and contains significant levels of radioactivity.

    (2) The target organ is where the energy is deposited from the source organ (e.g., an organ adjacent to the source organ).

    (3) All source organs are target organs.

3. Radiopharmaceutical target and penetration
  a) Mechanism (Peştean et al., 2016; Sgouros, 2019; U.S. FDA, 2019)
    (1) Radioimmunotherapy exploits the immune protein as a carrier for radioactivity, as a tracer or targeted therapeutic.

    (2) Once injected, the antibody is distributed by blood flow, diffusion, or convection to its natural target—an antigen-binding site on tumor cells.

    (3) The radiation effects are the result of energy release that occurs during radioactive decay, and the process is one of the most energy efficient known.

    (4) For example, a dose of 80 Gy or more from high-energy beta emitter yttrium-90 increased overall survival in patients with hepatocellular carcinoma, compared to a dose less than 80 Gy (Peştean et al., 2016; Vermeulen, Vandamme, Bormans, & Cleeren, 2019).

  b) Bystander effects
    (1) Cancer cells subjected to ionizing radiation may release signals that can influence nearby nonirradiated cells—termed *bystander effects* (Shen et al., 2018; Toossi, Khademi, Azimian, Mohebbi, & Soleymanifard, 2017).

    (2) The transmission of bystander effects among cancer cells involves the activation of inflammatory cytokines, death ligands, and reactive oxygen and nitrogen species (Shen et al., 2018; Toossi et al., 2017).

  c) Nontarget effects
    (1) In addition to bystander effects, two other forms of nontarget effects have been identi-

fied in RT: cohort effects and abscopal effects (Shen et al., 2018; Toossi et al., 2017).

    (2) Cohort effects represent the phenomenon in which irradiated cells can produce signals that reduce the survival of neighboring cells within an irradiated volume (Shen et al., 2018; Toossi et al., 2017).

    (3) Abscopal effects describe the nontarget effects that typically occur in nonirradiated cells distant from an irradiated target.

    (4) These effects can be mediated primarily by immune cells (T cells) (Runcie, Budman, John, & Seetharamu, 2018; Shen et al., 2018; Wang, Xu, Huang, & Lu, 2018).

  d) Radiopharmaceuticals for solid tumors

    (1) Research in radiolabeled antibodies for treatment of solid cancers has been more varied and seen limited clinical success, compared to treatment of hematologic cancers (Runcie et al., 2018).

    (2) Solid tumors, unlike hematologic tumors, have a diversity of cells in their tumor deposits (i.e., hypoxic areas), and radioimmunotherapy may not penetrate beyond a few tumor cell layers, thus leaving the burden of tumor intact (Dandapani & Wong, 2016; Runcie et al., 2018).

    (3) Bispecific and trispecific antibodies are showing promise in solid tumor therapeutics (Runcie et al., 2018).

    (4) Some of these promising target antigens are not only tumor markers but molecules found to be essential in tumor cell survival and proliferation (Li et al., 2018; Runcie et al., 2018).

4. Types of radiation and application in radiopharmaceuticals: Isotopes that emit alpha particles or beta particles are commonly used in radiopharmaceuticals, and new drugs are emerging in clinical trials (Marcu et al., 2018).

  a) Alpha emitters (Marcu et al., 2018; Vermeulen et al., 2019)

    (1) Astatine-211 has a half-life of 7.2 hours. A monoclonal antibody radiolabeled with astatine-211 is being studied in clinical trials for treatment of CNS cancer.

    (2) Radium-223 has a half-life of 11.4 days. The radiopharmaceutical radium-223 dichloride is approved for bone metastases of castration-resistant prostate cancer with only bone disease.

    (3) Actinium-225 has a half-life of 10 days. Monoclonal antibodies radiolabeled with actinium-225 are being studied for treatment of leukemia, neuroendocrine cancer, and breast cancer.

  b) Beta emitters (Marcu et al., 2018; Vermeulen et al., 2019)

    (1) Strontium-89 has a half-life of 50.6 days. It is used in combination with chemotherapy or RT for bone metastases.

    (2) Yttrium-90 has a half-life of 2.67 days, and several radiopharmaceuticals in trials contain this isotope.

      (a) Yttrium-90–radiolabeled monoclonal antibodies for lymphoma and breast cancer

      (b) Yttrium-90 peptides for neuroendocrine tumors

      (c) Yttrium-90–radiolabeled monoclonal antibody for renal cell carcinoma and ovarian cancer

    (3) Iodine-131 has a half-life of approximately eight days. Radiopharmaceutical iobenguane iodine-131 is indicated for neuroendocrine tumors. Iobenguane iodine-131 is being studied to treat neuroblastoma (Jimenez, Erwin, & Chasen, 2019; U.S. NRC, 2019).

    (4) Samarium-153 has a half-life of 1.94 days. Radiopharmaceutical samarium-153 lexidronam is indicated for bone metastases (Lantheus Medical Imaging, 2018; Vermeulen et al., 2019).

    (5) Lutetium-177 has a half-life of 6.65 days. Several radiopharmaceuticals are being studied (ACR, 2017, 2019; Hagemann et al., 2017; Vermeulen et al., 2019).

      (a) Lutetium-177 monoclonal antibody for prostate cancer (Hosono et al., 2019)

      (b) Lutetium-177 monoclonal antibodies for renal cancer and ovarian cancer (Marcu et al., 2018)

      (c) Lutetium-177 monoclonal antibodies for lymphoma (Marcu et al., 2018)

      (d) Lutetium-177 peptides for neuroendocrine tumors (Hosono et al., 2019)

5. Common radiopharmaceuticals (ACR, 2016, 2017, 2019; Peştean et al., 2016; U.S. FDA, 2019)

  a) Yttrium-90 ibritumomab tiuxetan (Acrotech Biopharma, 2019)

    (1) Yttrium-90 ibritumomab tiuxetan is indicated for transformed B-cell follicular non-Hodgkin lymphomas that are cluster of differentiation (CD) 20 positive.

    (2) See Figure 28 for exclusion criteria for treatment.

    (3) See Figure 29 for patient preparation and data.

  b) Samarium-153 (ACR, 2017, 2019; Handkiewicz-Junak et al., 2018; Lantheus Medical Imaging, 2018)

    (1) Samarium-153 accumulates in osteoblastic lesions more than in healthy bone.

FIGURE 28. Exclusion Criteria for Treatment With Yttrium-90 Ibritumomab Tiuxetan

- Pregnancy and continued breastfeeding
- Known hypersensitivity to yttrium-90 ibritumomab tiuxetan, yttrium chloride, other murine proteins, or any of their components
- Children and adolescents younger than 18 years of age
- Marked bone marrow suppression (leukocytes < 1,500/mm³; thrombocytes < 100,000/mm³)
  - The peripheral blood cell count should not be lower than these limits; however, lower blood counts do not constitute an absolute contraindication.
  - Low blood counts increase the risk of severe and prolonged bone marrow suppression and, subsequently, infection and bleeding.
- Previous external beam radiation therapy involving > 25% of active bone marrow
- Greater than 25% of bone marrow infiltration by lymphoma cells, as judged by bone marrow biopsy
- Poor bone marrow reserve or high tumor burden in the bone marrow; requires coordination with physicians trained in the safe use of radionucleotides to proceed
- Detectable human antimurine antibody, depending on titer

Note. Based on information from Acrotech Biopharma, 2019.

---

(2) Greater number of metastatic lesions correlates to more skeletal uptake of samarium-153 radioactivity.

(3) It is indicated for relief of pain in patients with confirmed osteoblastic metastatic bone lesions that enhance on radionuclide bone scan.

c) Lutetium-177 dotatate (ACR, 2017; Raedler, 2019; Runcie et al., 2018)

(1) Lutetium-177 dotatate is a radiolabeled somatostatin analog indicated for the treatment of somatostatin receptor–positive gastroenteropancreatic neuroendocrine tumors, including foregut, midgut, and hindgut tumors in adults.

(2) Long-acting octreotide should be discontinued four weeks prior to treatment initiation. Short-acting octreotide should be discontinued 24 hours prior to treatment initiation.

(3) Premedication of an antiemetic is administered.

(4) Lutetium-177 dotatate is administered with an amino acid solution (see Table 16).

(a) The IV amino acid solution contains lysine and arginine.

(b) Amino acid solution administration begins 30 minutes before beginning

---

FIGURE 29. Patient Preparation and Data

- Patient information: age, sex, height, weight, diagnoses (ICD-10)
- Indication for the therapy
- Information on the previous therapies
  - Data should include previously completed RT and/or autologous or allogeneic HSCT.
  - Previous chemotherapy, especially if recent, or EBRT involving active bone marrow can worsen radionuclide-induced leukocytopenia and thrombocytopenia.
- Bone marrow biopsy
  - A representative (>2 cm long cylinder) bone marrow biopsy from the iliac crest must not show a > 25% tumor infiltration (number of lymphoma cells as a percentage of nucleated cells).
  - The bilateral bone marrow biopsy must have been performed no earlier than the previous time at which disease progression was detected or in any case a maximum of 3 months before the scheduled therapy date.
  - The density of cells under normal hematopoiesis must be judged adequate to ensure satisfactory hematopoietic recovery after myelosuppressive therapy.
  - Bilateral cores are recommended, and the pathologist should provide the percent of cellular elements involved in the marrow.
  - Cytogenetics should include FISH for known MDS markers. A trend toward an increased risk of MDS with radioimmunotherapy has been suggested.
- Pregnancy excluded prior to radionuclide therapy; breastfeeding discontinued
- Current medications, especially those that can affect coagulation or blood cell counts
- Laboratory tests
  - Blood profile, prothrombin time (international normalized ratio), serum creatinine, and bilirubin tests should be obtained within 1 week prior to therapy.
  - There is no adequate experience with the use of yttrium-90 ibritumomab tiuxetan in patients with increased creatinine or bilirubin levels.
  - It is advised that therapy should not be performed if these values are greater than 2.5 times the upper normal limit of the local laboratory.
- Hepatitis B surface antigen and hepatitis B core antibody testing in all patients prior to therapy with rituximab
- Life expectancy
  - An estimated life expectancy > 3 months, with a Karnofsky index > 70, is recommended.
  - A patient with a life expectancy < 3–4 weeks is unlikely to benefit from treatment.
  - Patients showing rapidly progressing disease are not candidates for radioimmunotherapy because of delayed efficacy of the treatment.

EBRT—external beam radiation therapy; FISH—fluorescence in situ hybridization; HSCT—hematopoietic stem cell transplantation; ICD—International Classification of Diseases; MDS—myelodysplastic syndrome; RT—radiation therapy

Note. Based on information from Acrotech Biopharma, 2019; Handkiewicz-Junak et al., 2018; Mallol, 2015; Tennvall et al., 2007.

TABLE 16. Amino Acid Solution

Item	Specification
Arginine HCl content	18–24 g
Lysine HCl content	18–24 g
Osmolarity	< 1,050 mOsmol
Volume	1.5–2.2 L

Note. Based on information from Acrotech Biopharma, 2019; National Comprehensive Cancer Network, 2020.

lutetium-177 dotatate and continues during drug infusion and for three hours after infusion.

(c) Clinicians should use a three-way valve to administer the amino acid solution using the same venous access as lutetium-177 dotatate, or the amino acid solution can be administered through a separate venous access in the patient's other arm.

(d) The dose of the amino acid solution must not be reduced if the dose of lutetium-177 dotatate is reduced.

(5) See Table 17 for dose modifications of lutetium-177 dotatate for adverse reactions. (Advanced Accelerator Applications, 2018).

d) Iobenguane iodine-131 (Progenics Pharmaceuticals, 2018)

(1) Iobenguane iodine-131 is indicated for the treatment of adult and pediatric patients aged 12 years and older with iobenguane scan–positive, unresectable, locally advanced, or metastatic pheochromocytoma or paraganglioma who require systemic anticancer therapy.

(2) Iobenguane is taken up by the norepinephrine transporter in adrenergic nerve terminals and accumulates in adrenergically innervated tissues, such as the heart, lungs, adrenal medulla, salivary glands, liver, and spleen, as well as tumors of neural crest origin.

(3) The risks of radiation associated with iobenguane iodine-131 are greater in pediatric patients than in adult patients because of greater absorbed radiation doses and longer life expectancy. Clinical decisions must weigh the therapeutic benefit of iobenguane iodine-131 against risks prior to treatment in pediatric patients.

(4) A thyroid blockade of inorganic iodine begins at least 24 hours before and continuing for 10 days after each iobenguane iodine-131 dose.

(5) See Table 18 for recommended dose modifications of iobenguane iodine-131 for adverse reactions.

(6) See Table 19 for recommended dose or dose reduction for the second therapeutic dose of iobenguane iodine-131 for myelosuppression.

(7) See Figure 30 for iobenguane iodine-131 drug interactions.

e) Radium-223 dichloride: Radium-223 dichloride is an alpha particle–emitting agent indicated for the treatment of patients with castration-resistant prostate cancer, symptomatic bone metastases, and no known visceral metastatic disease (Bayer Healthcare Pharmaceuticals, 2019; U.S. FDA, 2019).

f) Iodine-131 tositumomab: Iodine-131 tositumomab was withdrawn permanently from the U.S. market in 2014 because of low usage ("GlaxoSmithKline LLC; Withdrawal of Approval," 2013).

6. Nursing management of radiopharmaceuticals (ACR, 2016, 2017; Kunos, Capala, Finnigan, Smith, & Ivy, 2019; U.S. FDA, 2019)

a) Administration (Hosono et al., 2019; Peştean et al., 2016)

(1) It is not necessary for a patient to be fasting before therapy, but care must be taken to ensure adequate hydration.

(2) Premedication and concomitant medications are administered per prescribing information and safety protocol with radiopharmaceuticals.

(3) The radiopharmaceutical agent must be infused via a venous catheter or an indwelling infusion device to ensure safe IV administration and prevent perivascular infiltration. Venous access should be checked before administration.

(4) Clinicians must always verify that the radiopharmaceutical will be administered with a compatible solution.

(5) Nurses must always follow radiopharmaceutical administration guidelines.

(6) The residual radiation activity in the needle, infusion kit, or catheter can be measured to calculate the precise radiation activity administered. Nurses must be aware that the most common radiopharmaceuticals (e.g., yttrium-90 ibritumomab tiuxetan) are injected. The administered radiation activity in the 10 ml syringe must be measured using a calibrator.

b) Extravasation (van der Pol, Vöö, Bucerius, & Mottaghy, 2017)

(1) Nurses must monitor patients closely for evidence of extravasation during radiopharmaceutical therapy.

(2) If extravasation is suspected, the infusion must be stopped immediately and restarted in another limb if possible.

(3) Extravasation can lead to radionecrosis.

(4) There is no specific therapy for perivenous infiltration.

TABLE 17. Recommended Dose Modification of Lutetium-177 Dotatate for Adverse Reactions

Adverse Reactions	Severity of Adverse Reaction	Dose Modification
Anemia and neutropenia	Grade 3 or 4	Withhold dose until complete or partial resolution (grade 0, 1, or 2). Resume at 3.7 Gbq (100 mCi) in patients with complete or partial resolution. If reduced dose does not result in grade 3 or 4 anemia or neutropenia, administer next dose at 7.4 Gbq (200 mCi). Permanently discontinue for grade 3 or higher anemia or neutropenia requiring a treatment delay of 16 weeks or longer. Permanently discontinue for recurrent grade 3 or 4 anemia or neutropenia.
Hepatotoxicity	Defined as one of the following: • Bilirubinemia greater than 3 times the upper limit of normal (grade 3 or 4) • Hypoalbuminemia less than 3 g/dl with a decreased prothrombin ratio less than 70%	Withhold dose until complete resolution. Resume at 3.7 Gbq (100 mCi) in patients with complete resolution. If reduced dose does not result in hepatotoxicity, administer next dose at 7.4 Gbq (200 mCi). Permanently discontinue for hepatotoxicity requiring a treatment delay of 16 weeks or longer. Permanently discontinue for recurrent hepatotoxicity.
Other nonhematologic toxicity	Grade 3 or 4	Withhold dose until complete or partial resolution (grade 0, 1, or 2). Resume at 3.7 Gbq (100 mCi) in patients with complete resolution. If reduced dose does not result in toxicity, administer next dose at 7.4 Gbq (200 mCi). Permanently discontinue for toxicity requiring a treatment delay of 16 weeks or longer. Permanently discontinue for recurrent grade 3 or 4 toxicity.
Renal toxicity	Defined as one of the following: • Creatinine clearance less than 40 ml/min, calculated using Cockcroft Gault with actual body weight • 40% increase in baseline serum creatinine • 40% decrease in baseline creatinine clearance, calculated using Cockcroft Gault with actual body weight	Withhold dose until complete resolution. Resume at 3.7 Gbq (100 mCi) in patients with complete resolution. If reduced dose does not result in renal toxicity, administer next dose at 7.4 Gbq (200 mCi). Permanently discontinue for renal toxicity requiring a treatment delay of 16 weeks or longer. Permanently discontinue for recurrent renal toxicity.
Thrombocytopenia	Grade 2, 3, or 4	Withhold dose until complete or partial resolution (grade 0 or 1). Resume at 3.7 Gbq (100 mCi) in patients with complete or partial resolution. If reduced dose does not result in grade 2, 3, or 4 thrombocytopenia, administer next dose at 7.4 Gbq (200 mCi). Permanently discontinue for grade 2 or higher thrombocytopenia requiring a treatment delay of 16 weeks or longer. Permanently discontinue for recurrent grade 2, 3, or 4 thrombocytopenia.

Note. Based on information from Advanced Accelerator Applications, 2018; National Cancer Institute, 2020; Raedler, 2019.

(5) If extravasation occurs, use of local hyperthermia, elevation of the limb, and light massage may favor lymphatic drainage and thereby reduce the local radiation dose.

(6) The radiation oncologist must evaluate the patient, and the RSO records the event in the procedure report (ACR, 2019; van der Pol et al., 2017).

(7) A patient may need to be admitted and assessed for further management (e.g., vascular surgery, reconstructive surgery).

c) Anaphylactic and other hypersensitivity reactions

(1) Anaphylactic and other hypersensitivity reactions have been reported in less than 1% of patients following the IV administration of autologous proteins (Gülsen, Wedi, & Jappe, 2020).

(2) Blood pressure and pulse should be monitored with any administration of monoclonal antibodies.

(3) An emergency kit including glucocorticoids and antihistamines should be available (Guan, Zhou, Sun, & Chen, 2015).

d) Discharge

(1) A patient cannot be discharged until radioactivity levels and exposure rates comply with federal and local regulations (ACR, 2017, 2019).

TABLE 18. Dose Modifications of Iobenguane Iodine-131 for Adverse Reactions

Adverse Reaction	Dose Modification
Myelosuppression	Do not administer the first therapeutic dose for platelet count < 80,000/mm³ or absolute neutrophil count < 1,200/mm³. Do not administer the second therapeutic dose until platelets and neutrophils return to baseline or to the normal range. Reduce the second therapeutic dose for the following: • Platelet count < 25,000/mm³ • Absolute neutrophil count < 500/mm³ • Life-threatening anemia for more than 7 days • Febrile neutropenia • Platelet count < 50,000/ mm³ with active bleeding
Pneumonitis	Do not administer the second therapeutic dose if pneumonitis is diagnosed after the first therapeutic dose.

Note. Based on information from Progenics Pharmaceuticals, 2018.

(2) Radioactivity levels are calculated using clearance activity measured in urine.

(3) Based on type of radiopharmaceutical decay, clearance activity is determined on the cumulative dose of exposure once a patient is released and calculated on the effective dose rate of 1 m from surface of the patient's body (Hosono et al., 2019).

(4) The patient is discharged after completion of the infusion and an adequate period of observation for side effects (Handkiewicz-Junak et al., 2018).

(5) The nursing staff attending hospitalized patients and caregivers dealing with patient excretions should wear rubber gloves to prevent skin contamination for contact with patient excretion based on type of radiopharmaceutical, route of elimination, and decay (Handkiewicz-Junak et al., 2018; U.S. FDA, 2019).

e) Outpatient setting: Although no radiopharmaceutical is completely risk free, social contact with other people and pets has relatively minimal risk of radiation exposure; therefore, concerns about exposure should not interfere with prompt, appropriate medical treatment if needed (Handkiewicz-Junak et al., 2018; U.S. FDA, 2019).

f) Side effects

(1) Blood counts and creatinine levels are commonly affected.

(a) Baseline complete blood count and creatinine levels should be obtained.

(b) A reduction of 30%–70% in leukocyte and platelet counts from baseline levels is possible, sometimes very rapidly (Guan et al., 2015).

(c) Nadir can occur approximately four to nine weeks after therapy (median 60 days), occurring later than with chemotherapy (Guan et al., 2015).

(d) Weekly blood tests are recommended, until a patient reaches baseline levels.

TABLE 19. Recommended Dose or Dose Reduction for Second Therapeutic Dose of Iobenguane Iodine-131 for Myelosuppression

Patient Weight	If First Therapeutic Dose was Weight Based	If First Therapeutic Dose was Reduced Based on Critical Organ Limits
Greater than 62.5 kg	Reduce the second therapeutic dose to 425 mCi.	Reduce second therapeutic dose to 85% of the first dose.
62.5 kg or less	Reduce the second therapeutic dose to 7 mCi/kg.	Reduce second therapeutic dose to 85% of the first dose.

Note. Based on information from American College of Radiology, 2016; Progenics Pharmaceuticals, 2018.

FIGURE 30. Iobenguane Iodine-131 Drug Interactions

Do not administer these drugs until at least 7 days after each iobenguane iodine-131 dose:
• Alpha-agonist or alpha/beta-agonist (e.g., pseudoephedrine, phenylephrine, ephedrine, phenylpropanolamine, naphazoline)
• Botanicals that may inhibit reuptake of norepinephrine, serotonin, or dopamine (e.g., ephedra, ma huang, St John's Wort, yohimbine)
• Central monoamine depleting drugs (e.g., reserpine)
• Central nervous system stimulants or amphetamines (e.g., cocaine, methylphenidate, dextroamphetamine)
• Monoamine oxidase inhibitors (e.g., phenelzine, linezolid)
• Nonselected beta-blockers (e.g., labetalol)
• Norepinephrine and dopamine reuptake inhibitors (e.g., phentermine)
• Norepinephrine and serotonin reuptake inhibitors (e.g., tramadol)
• Tricyclic antidepressants or norepinephrine reuptake inhibitors (e.g., amitriptyline, bupropion, duloxetine, mirtazapine, venlafaxine)

Note. Based on information from Kunos & Capala, 2018; Progenics Pharmaceuticals, 2018.

(e) If blood counts decrease more rapidly than expected, short-term controls should be instituted.

(f) If platelets decrease to less than 50,000/mm³, levels should be monitored closely, and treatment should be discontinued if levels do not recover in six to eight weeks despite supportive care (Pawson et al., 2020).

(g) Platelet transfusions and growth factors should be administered if indicated.

(h) Patients should also be informed of the increased risk of infection and bleeding (Acrotech Biopharma, 2019; Pawson et al., 2020).

(2) See Table 20 for adverse events associated with yttrium-90 ibritumomab tiuxetan (Acrotech Biopharma, 2019).

(3) Gastrointestinal side effects are common with select radiopharmaceuticals.

(4) Because of the unknown potential for additive effects on bone marrow, radiopharmaceuticals should not be given concurrently with chemotherapy or EBRT unless the clinical benefits outweigh the risks (Acrotech Biopharma, 2019).

(5) Consideration should be given to a patient's current clinical and hematologic status and bone marrow response history to treatment with myelotoxic agents (Guan et al., 2015).

(6) Metastatic prostate and other cancers can be associated with disseminated intravascular coagulation. Caution should be exercised in treating patients whose platelet counts are decreased or those who have other clinical or laboratory findings suggesting disseminated intravascular coagulation (ACR, 2019).

(7) Spinal cord compression occurs in patients with known bone metastases to the cervical, thoracic, or lumbar spine, and precautions are exercised when using radiopharmaceuticals (ACR, 2019; Lo et al., 2014).

(8) The combination of abiraterone acetate, prednisone or prednisolone, and radium-223 increases risk of bone fractures and death (Janssen Biotech, 2019).

(9) Serious infusion reactions, prolonged and severe cytopenias, and severe cutaneous and mucocutaneous reactions, including death within 24 hours of infusion, have occurred with radiopharmaceuticals combined with monoclonal antibodies (Dandapani & Wong, 2016; Guan et al., 2015).

g) Renal function

(1) Renal function should be monitored during and after treatment with radiopharmaceuticals.

TABLE 20. Adverse Events of Yttrium-90 Ibritumomab Tiuxetan

Adverse Event	Occurrence
Hematologic	
• Anemia	61% all grades; 17% grade 3–4
• Ecchymosis	7% all grades; < 1% grade 3–4
• Neutropenia	77% all grades; 60% grade 3–4
• Thrombocytopenia	95% all grades; 63% grade 3–4
Nonhematologic	
• Asthenia	35%
• Chills	21%
• Fever	13%
• Headache	9%
• Nausea	25%
• Throat irritation	9%

Note. Based on information from Acrotech Biopharma, 2019.

(2) Urinary radiopharmaceutical excretion is a concern, and patients with baseline renal impairment may be at greater risk for toxicity and treatment discontinuation with severe renal impairment (creatinine clearance less than 30 ml/min) (Dandapani & Wong, 2016; Guan et al., 2015; Handkiewicz-Junak et al., 2018).

h) Elimination (Bayer Healthcare Pharmaceuticals, 2019; NCCN, 2020)

(1) The major route of elimination for radium is through fecal excretion.

(2) For radium-223 dichloride, at 48 hours after injection, the cumulative fecal excretion was 13% (range 0%–34%), and the cumulative urine excretion was 2% (range 1%–5%) (Bayer Healthcare Pharmaceuticals, 2019).

(3) Intestinal transit rate, which is highly variable throughout the population, influences the rate of elimination of radium-223 dichloride from the gastrointestinal tract (Bayer Healthcare Pharmaceuticals, 2019).

(a) Patients with a slower intestinal transit rate could potentially receive a higher intestinal radiation exposure.

(b) It is not known whether slower intestinal transit results in increased gastrointestinal toxicity.

i) Laboratory values (Bayer Healthcare Pharmaceuticals, 2019; NCCN, 2020)

(1) Before the first administration of radium-223 dichloride, a patient should have the following laboratory values.

(a) ANC: 1,500/mm³ or greater

(b) Platelets: 100,000/mm³ or greater

(c) Hemoglobin: 10 g/dl or greater

(2) Before subsequent administrations of radium-223 dichloride, a patient should have the following laboratory values (Bayer Healthcare Pharmaceuticals, 2019).

(a) ANC: 1,000/mm³

(b) Platelets: 50,000/mm³

(3) If there is no recovery to these values within six to eight weeks after the previous administration of radium-223 dichloride, despite receiving supportive care, further treatment with radium-223 dichloride should be discontinued.

(4) Patients with evidence of compromised bone marrow reserve should be monitored closely and provided with supportive care measures when clinically indicated.

(5) Radium-223 dichloride should be discontinued in patients who experience life-threatening complications despite supportive care for bone marrow failure.

j) Late toxicities (ACR, 2017, 2019; NCI, 2020; NCCN, 2020; U.S. FDA, 2019)

(1) An assessment of late radiation toxicities is warranted when patients have a long life expectancy that could be affected by late radiation effects.

(2) After repeat exposure to radiopharmaceuticals, patients can experience ongoing watery eyes with possible conjunctivitis as acute and late toxicities.

(3) Pneumonitis may arise one to three months after radiopharmaceutical treatment.

(4) Long-term fibrosis can develop after radiopharmaceutical exposure.

(5) Bone marrow hypoplasia can occur as a late toxicity of repeated radiopharmaceutical exposure.

(6) Long-term cumulative radiation exposure is associated with increased risk of second cancers.

7. Reproductive toxicities (NCI, 2020; U.S. FDA, 2019)

a) General

(1) Radiopharmaceuticals are genotoxic and thus can affect human reproductive cells.

(2) Many radiopharmaceuticals have effective half-lives of a week or longer.

b) Contraception (NCI, 2020; NCCN, 2020; U.S. FDA, 2019)

(1) Clinicians should communicate the importance of contraception use before, during, and after treatment. This education should be documented.

(2) Female patients should be advised to use contraception during treatment and for at least a minimum of five effective half-lives after treatment completion, as well as an additional six months after the final dose of the radiopharmaceutical.

(a) The half-life of daughter cell decays also should be considered.

(b) Five effective half-lives allow elimination of approximately 97% of the radioactivity, and the additional six months ensures that damaged follicles and oocytes are released before fertilization.

(c) Medical physicists are a possible resource for questions regarding half-lives.

(d) Each radiopharmaceutical requires protocols for administration as part of institution accreditation.

(e) These protocols must be made available for all staff involved in delivering direct care to patients receiving treatment (Kesner & Bodei, 2018).

(f) Given that biodistribution estimates vary significantly and a lack of current standards in measurement exists, female patients of childbearing potential should be advised to use adequate contraception for a minimum of 12 months (ACR, 2019; Kesner & Bodei, 2018; U.S. FDA, 2019).

(3) Male patients with female partners of reproductive potential should be advised to use contraception during treatment and for a minimum of five effective half-lives after treatment completion, as well as an additional three months after the final dose of the radiopharmaceutical (ACR, 2019).

(a) The half-life of daughter cell decays also should be considered, along with varying biodistribution estimates (ACR, 2019).

(b) Five effective half-lives allow elimination of approximately 97% of the radioactivity, and the additional three months considers the duration of spermatogenesis and residence time of unejaculated sperm (ACR, 2019; Kesner & Bodei, 2018).

c) Lactation

(1) Lactating women should be advised not to breastfeed during treatment with an oncology therapeutic radiopharmaceutical and, if applicable, for a specific period of time after the final dose (ACR, 2019).

(2) If a decision is made to pump and discard breast milk, a period during which a woman should not breastfeed should be long enough to limit the radiation effective dose to the nursing child to 1 mSv or less (ACR, 2019).

(3) An actual duration for advising against breastfeeding after treatment should be proposed and should be supported by estimation of radioactivity present in the breast milk at the end of this period and an assumption of complete absorption by the nursing child (ACR, 2019).

(4) Any residual milk should be discarded before nursing resumes (ACR, 2019).

8. Radiopharmaceutical quality and safety (ACR, 2019; Mallol, 2015)

   a) Required patient preparation and data (see Figure 29).

   b) Patient information and instruction (ACR, 2016; U.S. FDA, 2019)

      (1) Prior to planning the treatment, the nuclear medicine physician or radiation physicist, who is directly responsible for the treatment and subsequent follow-up, must personally verify the safety-related suitability criteria of the patient and discuss all technical and clinical aspects of the radioimmunotherapy with the patient.

      (2) The patient should be provided with written guidelines on the radiopharmaceutical therapy, anticipated adverse events, contact telephone numbers, and the precautions that should be followed during the treatment (see Figure 31).

      (3) After informing the patient both verbally and in writing, the patient must give consent to the treatment. Legal provisions must be observed, including obtaining written informed consent.

   c) Safe administration protocols (ACR, 2019; Hosono et al., 2019)

      (1) Therapy with radiopharmaceuticals should only be performed in facilities capable of meeting the standards for treatment with unsealed radioactive sources and licensed according to national regulations.

      (2) The treatment must be performed in close collaboration with the physicians treating the patient for the underlying disease.

      (3) Administration should only occur where resuscitation measures are immediately available.

      (4) The personnel engaged in the procedures must have the required qualification and the appropriate government authorization for the use and manipulation of radionuclides.

      (5) A representative of the nuclear medicine service is responsible for synchronizing and organizing the coordination of all pretreatment and treatment steps, along with referring hematology–oncology service, the services preparing the radiopharmaceutical agent, and other participants.

      (6) Proof of training in radiochemical labeling procedures, including quality control, is required.

FIGURE 31. Generic Guidelines Describing Administration and Information Relevant to Radioimmunotherapy Regimens

Patient education
- Contact a healthcare professional for severe signs and symptoms of infusion reactions.
- See specific information describing the yttrium-90 ibritumomab tiuxetan treatment, including possible adverse events and safety precautions required during actual treatment.
- Take premedications as prescribed.
- Report any signs or symptoms of cytopenias (e.g., bleeding, easy bruising, petechiae or purpura, pallor, weakness, worsening fatigue).
- Avoid medications that interfere with platelet function, except as directed by a healthcare professional.
- Seek prompt medical evaluation for diffuse rash, bullae, or desquamation of the skin or mouth.
- Immediately report symptoms of infection (e.g., fever, pyrexia).
- Immunization with live viral vaccines is not recommended for 12 months following the yttrium-90 ibritumomab tiuxetan therapeutic regimen.
- Risk of radiation exposure to people and animals in contact with the patient is minimal.
- During treatment, patients do not need to change their routine activities, and no special precautions are required, such as separate toilet, cutlery, and dishes. Family members and caregivers should avoid exposure to a patient's body fluids (e.g., vomit, urine, stool) for 3 days (72 hours) after treatment.
- Prior treatment with chemotherapy may contribute to the low incidence of second malignancies (1.5%) observed after yttrium-90 ibritumomab tiuxetan treatment, which is in the range reported following alkylator-based chemotherapy alone (1%–8%).

Following treatment for 1 week
- Patients should use condoms if they engage in sexual activity.
- Kissing should be avoided for the first 24 hours.
- Men should urinate sitting down. Any spilled urine should be cleaned, and cleaning cloths should be disposed of in a plastic bag before being put in the waste disposal. Flushable items can be flushed down the toilet.
- All patients should wash their hands after bathroom use.

Contraceptive advice
- As with other anticancer treatments, contraception to avoid pregnancy is recommended for 1 year following treatment.
- Yttrium-90 ibritumomab tiuxetan may cause fetal harm when administered to a pregnant woman.
- Male patients may experience a temporary loss of fertility and may have a low risk of permanent sterility.
  - There are no studies validating this risk, but yttrium-90 ibritumomab tiuxetan treatment results in a radiation dose to the testes.
  - Thus, if prior therapies have not damaged sperm quality, male patients should be advised to consider semen cryopreservation.

Note. Based on information from Acrotech Biopharma, 2019; National Comprehensive Cancer Network, 2020.

(7) The radiopharmaceutical agent may be received, used, and administered only by authorized personnel (e.g., radiation oncologist, nuclear medicine physician) in designated settings. Its receipt, storage, use, transfer, and disposal are subject to national regulations.

d) Accidental exposure and spills (ACR, 2019; Hosono et al., 2019)

(1) In case of contact with skin or eyes, the affected area should be flushed immediately with water.

(2) In the event of spillage of radiopharmaceuticals, the RSO should be contacted immediately to initiate the necessary measurements and required procedures to decontaminate the area. A complexing agent, such as ethylene-diaminetetraacetic acid (EDTA) solution, is recommended to remove contamination.

e) Protective equipment (ACR, 2019; Hosono et al., 2019)

(1) Protective shields for needles and containers must be used.

(2) Clinicians must observe local regulations for procedures involving unsealed radioactive resources.

(3) Use of 1 cm thick acrylic glass or lead-loaded acrylic glass shields during labeling is required.

(4) Forceps and tongs should be used as gripping tools.

(5) Plastic gloves, disposable waterproof gowns, and acrylic glass eye protection should be used.

9. Follow-up and monitoring (ACR, 2016, 2019; Hosono et al., 2019)

a) A nuclear medicine physician or radiation oncologist must participate in the administration of radiopharmaceuticals and follow-up care of a patient as a part of the management team.

b) Advanced practice nurses are a valued part of the oncology team and should be involved in follow-up care. Because of licensing and certification requirements for administration of radiopharmaceuticals, advanced practice nurses should not directly administer radiopharmaceuticals to patients (ACR, 2016, 2019).

c) Monitoring response should be assessed after therapy using fluorodeoxyglucose PET-CT scan no earlier than six weeks.

(1) It should be emphasized that quality of response may still be improved beyond three months (Kitajima et al., 2019).

(2) An important role for radioisotopes is the ability to assess tumor burden to quantify the activity of radionuclide therapies (Zhao et al., 2018).

10. Patient, caregiver, and family education (ACR, 2016, 2019; U.S. FDA, 2019)

a) Myelosuppression

(1) Patients should contact their healthcare provider for any signs or symptoms of myelosuppression or infection (e.g., fever, chills, dizziness, shortness of breath, increased bleeding, bruising).

(2) Clinicians should instruct patients to follow up with repeat blood counts weekly for eight weeks starting one to two weeks after injection.

(3) Hematologic events are the most common adverse events and usually are reversible.

b) Precautions need to be taken for at least 12 hours after administration (Hosono et al., 2019).

c) Second primary malignancy: Patients should understand the potential for second cancers, including myelodysplastic syndrome and acute leukemia.

d) Renal toxicity: Patients must be advised to hydrate and urinate frequently during and after administration of radiopharmaceuticals.

e) Hepatotoxicity: Patients will require periodic laboratory testing to monitor for hepatotoxicity.

f) Neuroendocrine hormonal crisis: Clinicians should advise patients to contact their healthcare provider for signs or symptoms that may occur following tumor hormone release, including severe flushing, diarrhea, bronchospasm, and hypotension.

g) Pain flare (Bayer Healthcare Pharmaceuticals, 2019)

(1) Clinicians should educate patients that mild and transient flare of pain may occur within 72 hours of injection.

(2) Patients may notice pain relief one week after administration of treatment, and maximal pain relief generally occurs at three to four weeks after radiopharmaceutical injection.

h) Toileting (Hosono et al., 2019)

(1) Patients should flush the toilet at least two times after each use.

(2) Patients should use a toilet rather than a urinal.

(3) Spilled urine or blood should be immediately cleaned up with flushable toilet paper and disposed via the toilet or nonflushable paper or cloths placed in a separate bag for storage and disposal outside the home.

(4) Patients should wash hands thoroughly with soap and water after using the toilet.

i) Laundry: Soiled clothing or linens should be immediately washed separately from other items or stored in a bag for one to two weeks prior to washing to allow for radioactive decay prior to mingling.

j) Hypothyroidism: Clinicians should advise patients that treatment with several radiopharmaceuticals necessitates lifelong monitoring for hypothyroidism (Guan et al., 2015).

k) Handling body fluids (Hosono et al., 2019)

(1) Caregivers should use universal precautions for patient care, such as gloves and barrier gowns, when handling body fluids (most notably feces) to avoid contamination.

(2) Wearing gloves and handwashing will protect caregivers when handling body fluids.

11. Outlook of radiopharmaceuticals
    a) Advances in genetic engineering have allowed for development of polyspecific monoclonal antibodies, genetically engineered proteins that can simultaneously engage two or more different types of epitopes (Runcie et al., 2018).
    b) As Kunos and Capala (2018) stated, the new insights in cancer biology, radiobiology, and radiochemistry have repositioned radiopharmaceutical therapies at the leading edge of personalized medicine oncology research. The forecast is promising.
12. Recommended websites
    a) ACR: www.acr.org
    b) ASTRO: www.astro.org
    c) National Library of Medicine: www.nlm.nih.gov
    d) NCCN: www.nccn.org
    e) Society of Nuclear Medicine and Molecular Imaging: www.snmmi.org
    f) World Nuclear Association: www.world-nuclear.org
13. Side effects reporting: Patients and healthcare professionals are encouraged to report negative side effects of prescription drugs to FDA by visiting www.fda.gov/medwatch, or by calling 1-800-332-1088.

References

Acrotech Biopharma. (2019). *Zevalin® (ibritumomab tiuxetan)* [Package insert].

Advanced Accelerator Applications. (2018). *Lutathera® (lutetium Lu 177 dotatate)* [Package insert].

American College of Radiology. (2016). *ACR–SPR technical standard for diagnostic procedures using radiopharmaceuticals.* https://www.acr.org/-/media/ACR/Files/Practice-Parameters/Radiopharmaceuticals.pdf

American College of Radiology. (2017). *ACR–AAPM–SPR technical standard for therapeutic procedures using radiopharmaceuticals.* https://www.acr.org/-/media/ACR/Files/Practice-Parameters/RadioPharm.pdf

American College of Radiology. (2019). *ACR-ACNM-ASTRO-SNMMI practice parameter for the performance of therapy with unsealed radiopharmaceutical sources.* https://www.acr.org/-/media/ACR/Files/Practice-Parameters/UnsealedSources.pdf

Bayer Healthcare Pharmaceuticals. (2019). *Xofigo® (radium Ra 223 dichloride)* [Package insert].

Dandapani, S.V., & Wong, J. (2016). Radioimmunotherapy. In K. Olivier Jr. & S.A. Hurvitz (Eds.), *Antibody-drug conjugates: Fundamentals, drug development, and clinical outcomes to target cancer* (pp. 409–429). John Wiley and Sons.

GlaxoSmithKline LLC; withdrawal of approval of the indication for treatment of patients with relapsed or refractory, low grade, follicular, or transformed CD20 positive non-Hodgkin's lymphoma who have not received prior rituximab; BEXXAR, 78 Fed. Reg. 63226 (October 23, 2013). https://www.federalregister.gov/d/2013-24840

Guan, M., Zhou, Y.-P., Sun, J.-L., & Chen, S.-C. (2015). Adverse events of monoclonal antibodies used for cancer therapy. *Biomed Research International, 2015,* 428169. https://doi.org/10.1155/2015/428169

Gülsen, A., Wedi, B., & Jappe, U. (2020). Hypersensitivity reactions to biologics (part I): Allergy as an important differential diagnoses in complex immune-derived adverse events. *Allergo Journal International, 29,* 97–125. https://doi.org/10.1007/s40629-020-00126-6

Hagemann, U.B., Mihaylova, D., Uran, S.R., Borrebaek, J., Grant, D., Bjerke, R.M., ... Cuthbertson, A.S. (2017). Targeted alpha therapy using novel CD70 targeted thorium-227 conjugate in *in vitro* and *in vivo* models of renal cell carcinoma. *Oncotarget, 8,* 56311–56326. https://doi.org/10.18632/oncotarget.16910

Handkiewicz-Junak, D., Poeppel, T.D., Bodei, L., Aktolun, C., Ezziddin, S., Glammarile, F., ... Gabriel, M. (2018). EANM guidelines for radionuclide therapy of bone metastases with beta-emitting radionuclides. *European Journal of Nuclear and Molecular Imaging, 45,* 846–859. https://doi.org/10.1007/s00259-018-3947-x

Hosono, M., Ikebuchi, H., Kinuya, S., Yanagida, S., Nakamura, Y., Yamada, T., ... Hatazawa, J. (2019). Manual on the proper use of yttrium-90-labeled anti-P-cadherin antibody injection for radionuclide therapy in clinical trials. *Annals of Nuclear Medicine, 33,* 787–805. https://doi.org/10.1007/s12149-019-01409-x

Jadvar, H. (2017). Targeted radionuclide therapy: An evolution toward precision cancer treatment. *American Journal of Roentgenology, 209,* 277–288. https://doi.org/10.2214/AJR.17.18264

Janssen Biotech. (2019). *Zytiga® (abiraterone acetate)* [Package insert].

Jimenez, C., Erwin, W., & Chasen, B. (2019). Targeted radionuclide therapy for patients with metastatic pheochromocytoma and paraganglioma: From low-specific-activity to high-specific-activity iodine-131 metaiodobenzylguanidine. *Cancers, 11,* 1018. https://doi.org/10.3390/cancers11071018

Kesner, A.L., & Bodei, L. (2018). Modern radiopharmaceutical dosimetry should include robust biodistribution reporting. *Journal of Nuclear Medicine, 59,* 1507–1509. https://doi.org/10.2967/jnumed.118.208603

Kitajima, K., Okada, M., Kashiwagi, T., Yoshihara, K., Tokugawa, T., Sawada, A., ... Yamakado, K. (2019). Early evaluation of tumor response to ^{90}Y-ibritumomab radioimmunotherapy in relapsed/refractory B cell non-Hodgkin lymphoma: What is the optimal timing for FDG-PET/CT? *European Radiology, 29,* 3935–3944. https://doi.org/10.1007/s00330-019-06134-7

Kunos, C.A., & Capala, J. (2018). National Cancer Institute programmatic collaboration for investigational radiopharmaceuticals. *American Society of Clinical Oncology Educational Book, 38,* 488–494. https://doi.org/10.1200/EDBK_200199

Kunos, C.A., Capala, J., Finnigan, S., Smith, G.L., & Ivy, S.P. (2019). Radiopharmaceuticals for relapsed or refractory ovarian cancers. *Frontiers in Oncology, 9,* 180. https://doi.org/10.3389/fonc.2019.00180

Lantheus Medical Imaging. (2018). *Quadramet® (samarium Sm 153 lexidronam injection)* [Package insert].

Li, Y., Zhou, C., Li, J., Liu, J., Lin, L., Li, L., ... Wang, Z. (2018). Single domain based bispecific antibody, Muc1-Bi-1, and its humanized form, Muc1-Bi-2, induce potent cancer cell killing in muc1 positive tumor cells. *PLOS ONE, 13,* e0191024. https://doi.org/10.1371/journal.pone.0191024

Lo, S.S.-M., Ryu, S., Chang, E.L., Galanopoulos, N., Jones, J., Kim, E.Y., ... Vassil, A.D. (2014). *Metastatic epidural spinal cord compression and recurrent spinal metastasis* [ACR Appropriateness Criteria®]. American College of Radiology. https://www.acsearch.acr.org/doc/3091670/narrative

Mallol, J. (2015). Registration dossier for radiopharmaceuticals products. *Pharmaceuticals, Policy and Law, 17,* 213–220. https://doi.org/10.3233/PPL-140408

Marcu, L., Bezak, E., & Allen, B.J. (2018). Global comparison of targeted alpha vs targeted beta therapy for cancer: In vitro, in vivo and clinical trials. *Critical Reviews in Oncology/Hematology, 123,* 7–20. https://doi.org/10.1016/j.critrevonc.2018.01.001

Menzel, H.-G. (2017). International commission on radiation units and measurements. *Journal of the ICRU, 14,* 1–2. https://doi.org/10.1093/jicru/ndx006

National Cancer Institute. (2020, April 2). Late effects of treatment for childhood cancer (PDQ®) [Health professional version]. https://www.cancer.gov/types/childhood-cancers/late-effects-hp-pdq

National Comprehensive Cancer Network. (2020). *NCCN Clinical Practice Guidelines in Oncology (NCCN Guidelines®): B-cell lymphomas* [v.1.2020]. https://www.nccn.org/professionals/physician_gls/pdf/b-cell.pdf

Pawson, A., Ghumman, Z., Kuo, P.H., Jadvar, H., Bartel, T., Shayegan, B., & Kukotynski, K. (2020). A review of prostate cancer imaging, positron emission tomography, and radiopharmaceutical based therapy. *Canadian Urological Association Journal, 14,* 130–138. https://doi.org/10.5489/cuaj.6506

Peştean, C., Veloso Jéronimo, V., & Hogg, P. (Eds.). (2016). *Radionuclide metabolic therapy: Clinical aspects, dosimetry and imaging; A technologist's guide.* European Association of Nuclear Medicine. https://www.eanm.org/content-eanm/uploads/2016/11/Radionuclide_Metabolic_Therapy.pdf

Progenics Pharmaceuticals. (2018). *Azedra® (iobenguane I 131)* [Package insert].

Raedler, L.A. (2019, April 24). Lutathera (lutetium lu 177 dotatate) first radio-active drug approved for gastroenteropancreatic neuroendocrine tumors. *American Health and Drug Benefits.* http://www.ahdbonline.com/select-drug-profiles/2752-lutathera-lutetium-lu-177-dotatate-first-radioactive-drug-approved-for-gastroenteropancreatic-neuroendocrine-tumors

Ramos, S.M.O., Thomas, S., Pinheiro, M.A., Coelho, F.A.R.F.B., Albernaz, M.S., dos Santos, C.L.G., ... de Souza, S.A.L. (2017). Internal radiation dose and modeling codes in nuclear medicine: A fresh look at old problems. *International Journal of Radiology and Radiation Therapy, 4,* 439–443 https://doi.org/10.15406/ijrrt.2017.04.00111

Runcie, K., Budman, D.R., John, V., & Seetharamu, N. (2018). Bi-specific and tri-specific antibodies—the next big thing in solid tumor therapeutics. *Molecular Medicine, 24,* 50. https://doi.org/10.1186/s10020-018-0051-4

Sgouros, G. (2019). Radiopharmaceutical therapy. *Health Physics, 116,* 175–178. https://doi.org/10.1097/hp.0000000000001000

Shen, N., Qian, H.-L., & Fan, C.-F. (2018). Optimizing radiotherapy strategy: Combining radiotherapy with immunotherapy. *Journal of International Translational Medicine, 6,* 55–56. https://doi.org/10.11910/2227-6394.2018.06.02.01

Tennvall, J., Fischer, M., Delaloye, A.B., Bombardieri, E., Bodei, L., Giammarile, F., ... Brans, B. (2007). EANM procedure guideline for radioimmunotherapy for B-cell lymphoma with ^{90}Y-radiolabelled ibritumomab tiuxetan (Zevalin). *European Journal of Nuclear and Molecular Imaging, 34,* 616–622. https://doi.org/10.1007/s00259-007-0372-y

Toossi, M.T.B., Khademi, S., Azimian, H., Mohebbi, S., & Soleymanifard, S. (2017). Assessment of the dose-response relationship of radiation-induced bystander effect in two cell lines exposed to high doses of ionizing radiation (6 and 8 Gy). *Cell Journal, 19,* 434–442. https://doi.org/10.22074/cellj.2017.4343

U.S. Food and Drug Administration. (2019, October). *Oncology therapeutic radiopharmaceuticals: Nonclinical studies and labeling recommendations guidance for industry.* https://www.fda.gov/media/129547/download

U.S. Nuclear Regulatory Commission. (2018, June 21). Licensing of lutetium-177 (STC-18-042). https://www.nrc.gov/docs/ML1815/ML18156A589.pdf

U.S. Nuclear Regulatory Commission. (2019, May 28). Information for patients administered radioactive iodine (I-131). https://www.nrc.gov/materials/miau/patient-release.html

van der Pol, J., Vöö, S., Bucerius, J., & Mottaghy, F.M. (2017). Consequences of radiopharmaceutical extravasation and therapeutic intervention: A systematic review. *European Journal of Nuclear Medicine and Molecular Imaging, 44,* 1234–1243. https://doi.org/10.1007/s00259-017-3675-7

Vermeulen, K., Vandamme, M., Bormans, G., & Cleeren, F. (2019). Design and challenges of radiopharmaceuticals. *Seminars in Nuclear Medicine, 49,* 339–356. https://doi.org/10.1053/j.semnuclmed.2019.07.001

Wang, J.-C., Xu, Y., Huang, Z.-M., & Lu, X.-J. (2018). T cell exhaustion in cancer: Mechanisms and clinical implications. *Journal of Cellular Biochemistry, 119,* 4279–4286. https://doi.org/10.1002/jcb.26645

Zhao, W., Esquinas, P.L., Hou, X., Uribe, C.F., Gonzales, M., Beauregard, J.-M., ... Celler, A. (2018). Determination of gamma camera calibration factors for quantitation of therapeutic radioisotopes. *EJNMMI Physics, 5,* 8. https://doi.org/10.1186/s40658-018-0208-9

C. Immunotherapy

1. Introduction
   a) For decades, surgery, chemotherapy, and RT have stood as the main anticancer treatment strategies.
   b) Although these treatments have offered significant benefit to many patients with cancer, disease relapse remains a significant issue (Arruebo et al., 2011).
   c) The concept of utilizing the body's own immune system to attack cancer cells has become an alternative in eradicating tumor cells, and the combination of immunotherapy with RT has become an actively growing field of clinical investigation.

2. Combined RT and immunotherapy
   a) Once thought to be immunosuppressive due to large treatment fields encompassing a significant portion of bone marrow, RT had not been acknowledged as a modality that could be used in combination with immunotherapy.
      (1) Advances in radiation oncology have led to treatments that spare healthy surrounding tissue while delivering a highly focused, ablative dose to the tumor.
      (2) These new techniques, such as SRS and SBRT, along with the realization that RT has a mechanism of action extending well beyond that of DNA damage, have opened the door to numerous clinical trials investigating the mechanisms of synergy between RT and immunotherapy.
   b) Several studies have demonstrated that the immune system plays a significant role in the therapeutic effects of RT (Deng et al., 2014; Ferrara, Hodge, & Gulley, 2009; Formenti & Demaria, 2013; Rotstein, Blomgren, Petrini, Wasserman, & Baral, 1985; Wattenberg, Fahim, Ahmed, & Hodge, 2014).
      (1) As far back as 1979, Slone, Peters, and Milas demonstrated the need for lower doses of RT to control a chemically induced fibrosarcoma when they stimulated the immune system with a crude bacteria preparation, suggesting that the host immune system can influence the efficacy of RT.
      (2) When determining RT's role with immunotherapy, two important questions drive further investigation.
         (a) The first is to determine if immunotherapy added to definitive RT can improve locoregional control. Radiosensitizing chemotherapy has been used to augment RT. Thus, could there be a role for radiosensitizing immunotherapy?
         (b) The second question is the reverse. Can adding RT to immunotherapy contribute to the control of distant or systemic disease via the abscopal effect?

3. The immune system and radiation
   a) Antigen response
      (1) Studies have suggested that the immune system plays a critical role in the therapeutic effects of radiation by promoting tumor cell death within the radiation field.
      (2) How the immune system and radiation interact is unclear, but preclinical data demonstrate that RT generates tumor antigen–specific immune responses that were not present prior to the initiation of RT (Walle et al., 2018).
      (3) This release of tumor-specific antigens combined with the increase in the cell surface expression of the antigen and receptors all

influence T-cell response and subsequent trafficking of T cells, as well as antitumor activity.

b) Major histocompatibility complex (MHC) molecules

(1) MHC molecules, also known as *human leukocyte antigens*, are found on the cell surface and function by presenting foreign peptides to cytotoxic T cells crucial for the immune response.

(2) Many tumors are capable of downregulating MHC molecule expression as a means of escaping immune recognition.

(3) Several studies have shown that upregulation of MHC class I molecules occurs after RT, allowing for better recognition of tumor cells (Reits et al., 2006; Walle et al., 2018).

(4) RT also functions to upregulate several other immune responses, such as release of Fas, a cell surface molecule responsible for inducing apoptosis; chemokines; and high mobility group box 1, an abundant protein that can have a positive or negative effect on tumor development based on its location.

(5) Inside the nucleus, high mobility group box 1 functions in DNA repair, transcription, and telomere maintenance, thus serving in an antitumor capacity, while outside the nucleus it is essential to each of the six hallmarks of cancer and could act to stimulate living tumor cell proliferation.

(6) Unscheduled cell death and local changes in the stroma associated with tissue invasion generate damage-associated molecular pattern molecules that act as danger signals and activate antigen-presenting cells, attracting the attention of the immune system (see Figure 32).

c) PD-1 and PD-L1

(1) PD-1 and PDL-1 are two types of proteins found on cell surfaces whose interactions act as an "off" switch, alerting T cells to disengage and leave the area of attack. Some tumor cells express a large amount of these proteins, thus enabling them to escape immune response.

(2) Antibody therapies targeted at PD-1 and PD-L1 (immune checkpoint inhibitors) have demonstrated survival benefit in patients with metastatic NSCLC, and combining RT with this type of immunotherapy became a logical next step in clinical trials (Huang et al., 2018).

(3) The PACIFIC trial was the first to study immune checkpoint inhibitors alongside RT in a clinical setting (Antonia et al., 2018).

(a) In this study, 713 patients with unresectable stage III NSCLC were treated with a platinum-based chemotherapy and RT.

(b) If disease did not progress, they were randomized to receive durvalumab, which prevents PD-L1 from binding to PD-1, thus preventing T-cell exhaustion, versus a placebo.

(c) The primary endpoints were progression-free survival and overall survival.

(d) At 12 months, the progression-free survival rate for durvalumab was 55.9% versus 35.3% for placebo, and the improvement was maintained at 18 months with 44.2% in the durvalumab arm versus 27% in the placebo arm.

(e) This led to a new standard of care for consolidation therapy of patients with unresectable stage III NSCLC without disease progression.

(f) Safety profiles were similar, with grade 3 or 4 toxicities occurring in 30.5% of patients in the durvalumab group, compared to 26.1% in the placebo group. The most common adverse event was pneumonitis in both groups (Antonia et al., 2018).

(g) The most recently published three-year overall survival rates from this trial show continued survival benefit. Overall survival was 57% for durvalumab and 43.5% for placebo, confirming the PACIFIC regimen as the standard treatment in this patient population (Gray et al., 2020).

(4) Perhaps the most compelling evidence of the synergy of RT and checkpoint blockade comes from the retrospective analysis of patients on KEYNOTE-001. This phase 1 trial utilizing pembrolizumab in patients with metastatic NSCLC showed that patients who received RT at some point in their treatment appeared to have improved overall and progression-free survival, compared with those who never received RT (Herbst et al., 2016).

4. Abscopal effect

a) Overview (Reynders, Illidge, Siva, Chang, & De Ruysscher, 2015)

(1) RT has long been considered to have immunosuppressive effects because older RT techniques included large amounts of bone marrow and circulating blood within the treatment field.

(2) However, advances in RT delivery with more precise targeting have led to the reemergence of a phenomenon known as the *abscopal effect* (see Figure 33).

(3) First reported more than 50 years ago, the abscopal effect refers to the ability of localized RT to illicit an antitumor response in an area outside the radiation field.

(4) This rare effect has been reported in the treatment of several cancers, including melanoma, renal cell carcinoma, breast cancer, hepatocel-

FIGURE 32. Cellular and Molecular Effects of ADT and RT as They Relate to the Development of Antitumor Immunity

Effects of RT	Implication for Anti-Tumor Immune Responses	Effects of ADT
Antigen Recognition		
Releases DAMPS	Promotes immunogenic cell death	
Releases tumor antigens upon cell death	Promotes uptake of tumor antigens by DC for presentation to T cells	Releases tumor antigens upon cell death
Increases MHC I expression on tumor cells	Improves T cell recognition of tumor antigens	Mitigates tolerance to prostate antigens
Adaptive Immune Responses		
DNA and protein damage	Generates novel tumor antigens that may be immunogenic	
	Promotes development of anti-tumor immune responses	Promotes thymopoiesis, lymphocyte development, increased peripheral naive T and B cells
Tumor Infiltration		
Up-regulates adhesion molecules on immune cells	Facilitates immune cell extravasation	
Stimulates pro-inflammatory cytokine and chemokine production	Promotes immune cell infiltration, activates local innate immune cells	Promotes tumor immune cell infiltration
T cell Effector Function		
Increases Fas expression on tumor cells	Induces tumor cell apoptosis through engagement of FasL on T cells	
	Supports development of anti-tumor CTL	Promotes T$_H$1 differentiation

ADT—androgen deprivation therapy; CTL—cytotoxic T lymphocyte; DAMPs—danger-associated molecular patterns; DC—dendritic cell; FasL—Fas ligand; MHC—major histocompatibility complex; RT—radiation therapy; T$_H$1—T helper cell type 1

Note. From "Immune Modulation by Androgen Deprivation and Radiation Therapy: Implications for Prostate Cancer Immunotherapy," by J.L. Kalina, D.S. Neilson, A.P. Comber, J.M. Rauw, A.S. Alexander, J. Vergidis, and J.J. Lum, 2017, *Cancers, 9,* 13, p. 9 (https://doi.org/10.3390/cancers9020013). Copyright 2017 by the authors. Licensed under Attribution 4.0 International (CC BY 4.0; https://creativecommons.org/licenses/by/4.0).

lular carcinoma, and other metastatic solid tumors.

(5) A growing body of evidence suggests that combining RT and immunotherapy can boost the abscopal effect in patients with cancer (Demaria et al., 2004; Liu et al., 2018; Stamell, Wolchok, Gnjatic, Lee, & Brownell, 2013).

b) Mechanism of action

(1) Although a complete mechanism of action of how radiation can boost the abscopal effect is still not understood, several studies have helped to clarify why combining RT and immunotherapy could potentiate the effect (Portella & Scala, 2019).

(a) When a tumor is irradiated, the injury incurred by the cell leads to the release of tumor-specific antigens.

(b) A substantial increase in tumor-specific antigens can elicit a tumor-specific immune response (Portella & Scala, 2019).

  i. Tumor-specific antigens are engulfed by antigen-presenting cells, then presented to CD8+ T cells.

  ii. These specific T cells can then recognize and attack the primary tumor, as well as metastatic disease.

(c) Irradiated tumor cells may also release cellular danger-associated molecular patterns and cytokines that enhance trafficking of immune cells.

(d) Collectively, these events encourage tumor cell elimination by CD8+ T cells.

(e) Unfortunately, the tumor microenvironment does not allow the therapeutic effects of primed CD8+ T cells and acts to suppress their beneficial activity against the tumor.

(f) Tumors release immunosuppressive cytokines, such as transforming growth factor-beta, and surface receptors expressed on T cells, such as CTLA-4, can inhibit the function of the T cells.

(g) Several preclinical studies have consistently shown the benefit of combining RT with immunotherapy to improve abscopal response rates, compared to RT alone. Anti-CTLA-4 or anti-PD-1 therapies have shown to increase the T-cell activity directed against tumor cells.

(2) The perfect timing, dosage, and combinations of RT and immunotherapy are still yet to be determined.

(3) Many studies have reported a substantial increase in abscopal responses when administering immunotherapy after RT; however, the optimal dosing and fractionation for each cancer type requires further investigation (Formenti & Demaria, 2009).

(a) Both single-fraction and multiple-fraction RT regimens have been shown to boost the abscopal effect when combined with immunotherapy.

(b) A preclinical study combining anti-CTLA-4 treatments for breast and colon cancer models concluded that three fractions of 8 Gy was superior to five fractions of 6 Gy or a single ablative dose of 12 Gy (Van Limbergen et al., 2017).

(c) Other studies have shown synergy when using a large single fraction (Van Limbergen et al., 2017).

FIGURE 33. Abscopal Effect

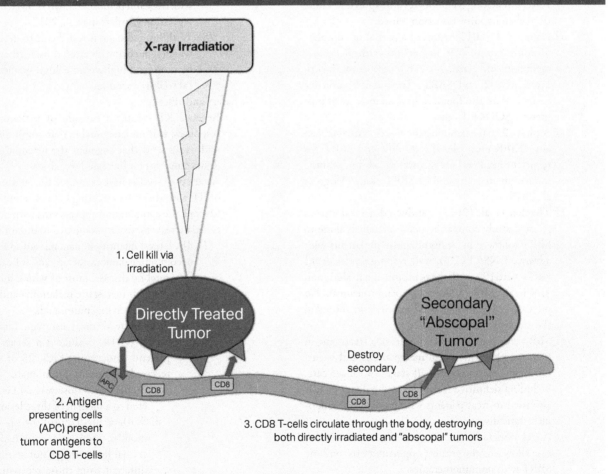

The image illustrates the mechanism of action of abscopal effect in causing DNA damage at distant sites. Radiation causes several changes during the cell-killing process that leads to an eruption of inflammatory mediators from the dying cancer cell. The mediators then stimulate an immune response against tumors elsewhere in the body.

(4) The combination of RT with PD-L1 blockade resulted in significantly delayed tumor growth in mouse models.

    (a) Dovedi et al. (2017) discovered that concurrent but not sequential administration of RT and anti-PD-L1 therapy led to tumor regression of distal nonirradiated lesions.

    (b) RT given before or concurrently with CTLA-4 blockade stunted tumor growth and increased survival in melanoma mouse models compared to anti-CTLA-4 therapy alone (Van Limbergen et al., 2017).

5. SRS and SBRT

    a) SRS has dramatically changed the treatment of various tumors, and its indications continue to expand.

    b) Compared to regimens with lower doses per fraction, higher doses of RT are considered to be more immunogenic because of increased tumor antigen release and improved antigen presentation and T-cell infiltration.

    c) Fewer circulating lymphocytes are exposed to radiation when hypofractionation is used.

    d) Seung et al. (2012) reported a partial or complete response rate of 67% in patients with metastatic melanoma or renal cell carcinoma treated with interleukin-2 and SBRT. Treatment-responsive patients were also found to have an increase of proliferating CD4+ T cells.

    e) A phase 2 trial examining the use of cetuximab, an anti-EGFR monoclonal antibody, and SBRT for recurrent head and neck cancer showed substantial improvement compared to SBRT alone (Vargo et al., 2015).

    f) Theelen et al. (2018) conducted a randomized phase 2 study comparing pembrolizumab alone to SBRT followed by pembrolizumab in patients with advanced NSCLC. Overall response rates at 12 weeks were 19% with the pembrolizumab alone and 41% in the SBRT followed by pembrolizumab. No increase in treatment-related toxicities was noted in the experimental arm.

    g) SBRT has proven to be an effective treatment in patients with widespread malignancies and is currently incorporated into all stages of cancer care, including definitive treatment and palliation. It is also used to treat patients who present with oligometastatic disease.

    h) A lack of data in the setting of oligometastatic disease allows for the greatest opportunity to combine SBRT with immunotherapies.

6. Dosage and timing

    a) Dosage

        (1) Utilizing RT to evoke antitumor immunity depends largely on the total dose and dose per fraction (Theelen et al., 2018).

        (2) Many different doses and fractions have been used when studying RT with immunotherapy; however, at the time of this publication, no significant clinical evidence exists as to what fractionation schedule is optimal with immunotherapy.

    b) Timing

        (1) Timing and sequencing of RT also play an important role in the efficacy of RT and immunotherapy.

        (2) In a study of 46 patients diagnosed with metastatic melanoma, patients who received SRS for new brain metastases during or before ipilimumab therapy had better intracranial disease control than those who received SRS after (Buchwald et al., 2018; Kiess et al., 2015).

        (3) The aforementioned PACIFIC trial noted excellent response rates with RT followed by immunotherapy (Antonia et al., 2018).

        (4) A small study of 21 patients with melanoma and brain metastases treated concurrently with SRS and pembrolizumab showed marked regression (Anderson et al., 2017).

        (5) With limited data, it is difficult to determine which sequencing is better; thus, further investigation with high-volume, high-quality clinical trials is warranted.

7. Safety and efficacy

    a) Because RT creates a cascade of inflammatory responses, it is understandable that combining RT with treatments that augment the immune system draws concerns for increased toxicities.

    b) A variety of studies have examined the combination of RT with therapies targeting CTLA-4 and PD-1. Overall, the combination appears safe, with no additional increase in toxicity compared to monotherapy.

        (1) The largest quantity of data related to toxicity of combining immunotherapy and RT exists for intracerebral disease, most of which included patients with metastatic melanoma and brain metastases receiving ipilimumab.

        (a) A study by Verma, Cushman, Tang, and Welsh (2018) evaluated a series of 58 patients undergoing SRS, 25 of whom received concurrent ipilimumab.

           i. Median SRS dose was 20 Gy delivered to a median of three lesions.

           ii. With a median follow-up of six months, seven cases (28%) had intracranial hemorrhage, not statistically different from those receiving SRS alone (30%).

           iii. No cases of treatment-related radiation necrosis were reported.

        (b) A study by Fang et al. (2017) at University of Texas MD Anderson Cancer Center specifically evaluated radiation necrosis in a series of 137 patients receiving RT and immunotherapy.

    i. Eighty percent of patients received SRS, and the remainder received whole-brain RT.

    ii. Ipilimumab was administered in 87% of patients; pembrolizumab was administered in 9%; and both were administered in 4%.

    iii. The median follow-up was 10 months from RT, and the overall crude rate of radiation necrosis was 27%.

(2) One of the biggest limiting factors in determining associations between combination RT and immune checkpoint blockade is that toxicities from both modalities can manifest months or years—in the case of RT—after treatment is completed. Thus, long-term follow-up is essential.

c) In the PACIFIC trial, the rates of any grade 3 and 4 events were 30% in the durvalumab arm and 26% in the placebo arm. Durvalumab did not appear to appreciably increase radiation pneumonitis, as the rate was 1.3% in both groups (Antonia et al., 2018).

d) Other published data at the time of this publication suggest that combined immunotherapy and RT offer encouraging safety profiles, and evidence shows that the combination does produce an overt increase in high-grade toxicities (Fuchs et al., 2018; Kiess et al., 2015; Seiwert et al., 2016).

(1) However, many studies had limitations, and further prospective experiences are greatly needed.

(2) Increased toxicities directly related to immunotherapy and RT may generally relate to larger treatment volumes and anatomically sensitive areas, as is similar to RT alone.

(3) Dosimetric parameters, as well as dose and fractionation considerations, should be exercised in the immunotherapy and RT setting.

(4) Presently, no data indicate the need to alter dosimetric objectives or dose constraints based on the receipt (prior, concomitant, or future) of immunotherapy.

8. Nursing implications

  a) Toxicity recognition

    (1) Oncology nurses caring for this unique population of patients hold the responsibility of educating patients and their caregivers on the possible risks and toxicities of combined RT and immunotherapy.

    (2) If symptoms should arise, detection and rapid management are key to preventing potentially life-threatening events.

    (3) Patients receiving concurrent therapy will be more likely to report adverse side effects to their radiation oncology team because they will be in the department daily for treatment.

    (4) Familiarity with the common side effects of rash, diarrhea, hepatotoxicity, endocrinopathy, and pneumonitis allows radiation oncology nurses to provide effective communication to the medical oncology team.

  b) Risk of toxicity (Verma et al., 2018)

    (1) Patients at greater risk for toxicities with RT and immunotherapy are the same patients at higher risk for RT toxicities.

    (2) Patients with a history of collagen vascular diseases or previous RT should be observed carefully for adverse reactions.

    (3) Patients with a history of autoimmune disease or those on multiple immunotherapies may be at greater risk for toxicity from combined therapies.

  c) Pneumonitis (Sears et al., 2019)

    (1) Risk of pneumonitis may be increased in patients undergoing RT with immunotherapy, specifically consisting of PD-1 or PD-L1 inhibitors.

    (2) Radiation oncology nurses must encourage patients receiving this course of treatment to immediately report shortness of breath or a nagging, persistent cough.

    (3) Because pneumonitis often develops months after RT is complete, it is imperative that patients understand this delayed reaction.

    (4) Radiation recall pneumonitis is a phenomenon in which patients experience pneumonitis only in the previously irradiated lung fields. It can occur in patients previously treated with RT to the chest followed by immune checkpoint inhibitors.

    (5) Because symptoms can mimic tumor progression, diagnosis may be delayed. Nurses must encourage patients to report symptoms immediately, as early initiation of corticosteroids may lead to complete resolution of symptoms.

  d) Radiation necrosis (Weingarten, Kruser, & Bloch, 2019)

    (1) Radiation necrosis is a common side effect of brain irradiation. It occurs when brain tissue around the targeted lesion becomes injured and dies.

    (2) This condition can be debilitating and causes severe headaches, nausea and vomiting, cognitive issues, and neural dysfunction. It often mimics tumor progression on MRI.

    (3) Radiation necrosis is a late side effect not seen until months or even years after completing RT and may have increased incidence in patients receiving immunotherapy.

    (4) It is important for radiation oncology nurses to encourage patients to immediately report

any changes in cognitive function or motor weakness.

 (5) Treatment for brain necrosis often consists of corticosteroids with the addition of bevacizumab and hyperbaric oxygen therapy.

e) Colitis (Thompson et al., 2019)

 (1) Patients who have received immunotherapy and abdominal irradiation may experience an exacerbation of colitis.

 (2) Grade 1 colitis can usually be managed with loperamide or diphenoxylate and atropine.

 (3) Educating patients to follow a bland diet, avoid high amounts of fiber and lactose, and hydrate consistently are important steps for successful earlier intervention.

 (4) If diarrhea persists, a stool sample should be obtained to rule out infectious etiology. If infectious causes are ruled out, then management with corticosteroids should begin immediately.

f) Interprofessional collaboration

 (1) Communication with the medical oncology team and close observation of the patient are key to successful treatment.

 (2) Interprofessional communication and collaboration are essential in this patient population.

 (3) As timing of treatments varies, patients may have discontinued immunotherapy and commenced RT; thus, late effects of immunotherapy may emerge during RT.

 (4) Conversely, patients may develop recall immune-related adverse events that are localized to a previous radiation field; thus, communication regarding prior RT treatment to the medical oncology team is essential.

g) Future directions

 (1) At the time of this publication, the combination of RT and immunotherapy is still a relatively new form of treatment.

 (2) Further research is warranted to determine both acute and late toxicities that may emerge from the combination of these two modalities, as well as appropriate medical management.

References

Anderson, E.S., Postow, M.A., Wolchok, J.D., Young, R.J., Ballangrud, Å., Chan, T.A., ... Beal, K. (2017). Melanoma brain metastases treated with stereotactic radiosurgery and concurrent pembrolizumab display marked regression; efficacy and safety of combined treatment. *Journal for ImmunoTherapy of Cancer, 5*, 76. https://doi.org/10.1186/s40425-017-0282-x

Antonia, S.J., Villegas, A., Daniel, D., Vicente, D., Murakami, S., Hui, R., ... Özgüroğlu, M. (2018). Overall survival with durvalumab after chemoradiotherapy in stage III NSCLC. *New England Journal of Medicine, 379*, 2342–2350. https://doi.org/10.1056/nejmoa1809697

Arruebo, M., Vilaboa, N., Sáez-Gutierrez, B., Lambea, J., Tres, A., Valladares, M., & González-Fernández, Á. (2011). Assessment of the evolution of cancer treatment therapies. *Cancers, 3*, 3279–3330. https://doi.org/10.3390/cancers3033279

Buchwald, Z.S., Wynne, J., Nasti, T.H., Zhu, S., Mourad, W.F., Yan, W., ... Khan, M.K. (2018). Radiation, immune checkpoint blockade and the abscopal effect: A critical review on timing, dose and fractionation. *Frontiers in Oncology, 8*, 612. https://doi.org/10.3389/fonc.2018.00612

Demaria, S., Ng, B., Devitt, M.L., Babb, J.S., Kawashima, N., Liebes, L., & Formenti, S.C. (2004). Ionizing radiation inhibition of distant untreated tumors (abscopal effect) is immune mediated. *International Journal of Radiation Oncology, Biology, Physics, 58*, 862–870. https://doi.org/10.1016/j.ijrobp.2003.09.012

Deng, L., Liang, H., Burnette, B., Beckett, M., Darga, T., Weichselbaum, R., & Fu, Y.-X. (2014). Irradiation and anti-PD-L1 treatment synergistically promote antitumor immunity in mice. *Journal of Clinical Investigation, 124*, 687–695. https://doi.org/10.1172/jci67313

Dovedi, S.J., Cheadle, E.J., Popple, A.L., Poon, E., Morrow, M., Stewart, R., ... Illidge, T.M. (2017). Fractionated radiation therapy stimulates antitumor immunity mediated by both resident and infiltrating polyclonal T-cell populations when combined with PD-1 blockade. *Clinical Cancer Research, 23*, 5514–5526. https://doi.org/10.1158/1078-0432.ccr-16-1673

Fang, P., Jiang, W., Allen, P., Glitza, I., Guha, N., Hwu, P., ... Li, J. (2017). Radiation necrosis with stereotactic radiosurgery combined with CTLA-4 blockade and PD-1 inhibition for treatment of intracranial disease in metastatic melanoma. *Journal of Neuro-Oncology, 133*, 595–602. https://doi.org/10.1007/s11060-017-2470-4

Ferrara, T.A., Hodge, J.W., & Gulley, J.L. (2009). Combining radiation and immunotherapy for synergistic antitumor therapy. *Current Opinion in Molecular Therapeutics, 11*, 37–42.

Formenti, S.C., & Demaria, S. (2009). Systemic effects of local radiotherapy. *Lancet Oncology, 10*, 718–726. https://doi.org/10.1016/s1470-2045(09)70082-8

Formenti, S.C., & Demaria, S. (2013). Combining radiotherapy and cancer immunotherapy: A paradigm shift. *Journal of the National Cancer Institute, 105*, 256–265. https://doi.org/10.1093/jnci/djs629

Fuchs, C.S., Doi, T., Jang, R.W., Muro, K., Satoh, T., Machado, M., ... Yoon, H.H. (2018). Safety and efficacy of pembrolizumab monotherapy in patients with previously treated advanced gastric and gastroesophageal junction cancer: Phase 2 clinical KEYNOTE-059 trial. *JAMA Oncology, 4*, e180013. https://doi.org/10.3410/f.732851580.793549623

Gray, J.E., Villegas, A., Daniel, D., Vicente, D., Murakami, S., Hui, R., ... Antonia, S.J. (2020). Three-year overall survival with durvalumab after chemoradiotherapy in stage III NSCLC—Update from PACIFIC. *Journal of Thoracic Oncology, 15*, 288–293. https://doi.org/10.1016/j.jtho.2019.10.002

Herbst, R.S., Bass, P., Kim, D.W., Felip, E., Pérez-Garcia, J.L., Han, J.Y., ... Garon, E.B. (2016). Pembrolizumab versus docetaxel for previously treated, PD-L1-positive, advanced non-small-cell lung cancer (KEYNOTE-010): A randomised controlled trial. *Lancet, 387*, 1540–1550. https://doi.org/10.3410/f.726044364.793539633

Huang, Q., Zhang, H., Hai, J., Socinski, M.A., Lim, E., Chen, H., & Stebbing, J. (2018). Impact of PD-L1 expression, driver mutations and clinical characteristics on survival after anti-PD-1/PD-L1 immunotherapy versus chemotherapy in non-small-cell lung cancer: A meta-analysis of randomized trials. *Oncoimmunology, 7*, e1396403. https://doi.org/10.1080/2162402X.2017.1396403

Kiess, A.P., Wolchok, J.D., Barker, C.A., Postow, M.A., Tabar, V., Huse, J.T., ... Beal, K. (2015). Stereotactic radiosurgery for melanoma brain metastases in patients receiving ipilimumab: Safety profile and efficacy of combined treatment. *International Journal of Radiation Oncology, Biology, Physics, 92*, 368–375. https://doi.org/10.1016/j.ijrobp.2015.01.004

Liu, Y., Dong, Y., Kong, L., Shi, F., Zhu, H., & Yu, J. (2018). Abscopal effect of radiotherapy combined with immune checkpoint inhibitors. *Journal of Hematology and Oncology, 11*, 104. https://doi.org/10.1186/s13045-018-0647-8

Portella, L., & Scala, S. (2019). Ionizing radiation effects on the tumor microenvironment. *Seminars in Oncology, 46*, 254–260. https://doi.org/10.1053/j.seminoncol.2019.07.003

Reits, E.A., Hodge, J.W., Herberts, C.A., Groothuis, T.A., Chakraborty, M., Wansley, E.K., ... Neefjes, J.J. (2006). Radiation modulates the peptide repertoire, enhances MHC class I expression, and induces successful antitumor immunotherapy. *Journal of Experimental Medicine, 203,* 1259–1271. https://doi.org/10.1084/jem.20052494

Reynders, K., Illidge, T., Siva, S., Chang, J.Y., & De Ruysscher, D. (2015). The abscopal effect of local radiotherapy: Using immunotherapy to make a rare event clinically relevant. *Cancer Treatment Reviews, 41,* 503–510. https://doi.org/10.1016/j.ctrv.2015.03.011

Rotstein, S., Blomgren, H., Petrini, B., Wasserman, J., & Baral, E. (1985). Long term effects on the immune system following local radiation therapy for breast cancer. I. Cellular composition of the peripheral blood lymphocyte population. *International Journal of Radiation Oncology, Biology, Physics, 11,* 921–925. https://doi.org/10.1016/0360-3016(85)90114-2

Sears, C.R., Peikert, T., Possic, J.D., Naidoo, J., Nishino, M., Patel, S.P., ... Rivera, M.P. (2019). Knowledge gaps and research priorities in immune checkpoint inhibitor-related pneumonitis. *American Journal of Respiratory and Critical Care Medicine, 200,* 31–43. https://doi.org/10.1164/rccm.201906-1202st

Seiwert, T.Y., Burtness, B., Mehra, R., Weiss, J., Berger, R., Eder, J.P., ... Chow, L.Q. (2016). Safety and clinical activity of pembrolizumab for treatment of recurrent or metastatic squamous cell carcinoma of the head and neck (KEY-NOTE-012): An open-label, multicentre, phase 1b trial. *Lancet Oncology, 17,* 956–965. https://doi.org/10.1016/s1470-2045(16)30066-3

Seung, S.K., Curti, B.D., Crittenden, M., Walker, E., Coffey, T., Siebert, J.C., ... Urba, W.J. (2012). Phase 1 study of stereotactic body radiotherapy and inter-leukin-2—tumor and immunological responses. *Science Translational Medicine, 4,* 137ra74. https://doi.org/10.1126/scitranslmed.3003649

Slone, H., Peters, L.J., & Milas, L. (1979). Effect of host immune capability on radiocurability and subsequent transplantability of a murine fibrosarcoma. *Journal of the National Cancer Institute, 63,* 1229–1235. https://doi.org/10.1093/jnci/63.5.1229

Stamell, E.F., Wolchok, J.D., Gnjatic, S., Lee, N.Y., & Brownell, I. (2013). The abscopal effect associated with a systemic anti-melanoma immune response. *International Journal of Radiation Oncology, Biology, Physics, 85,* 293–295. https://doi.org/10.1016/j.ijrobp.2012.03.017

Theelen, W., Peulen, H., Lalezari, F., de Vries, J., De Langen, J., Aerts, J., ... Baas, P. (2018). Randomized phase II study of pembrolizumab after stereotactic body radiotherapy (SBRT) versus pembrolizumab alone in patients with advanced non-small cell lung cancer: The PEMBRO-RT study. *Journal of Clinical Oncology, 36*(Suppl. 15), 9023. https://doi.org/10.1200/jco.2018.36.15_suppl.9023

Thompson, J.A., Schneider, B.J., Brahmer, J., Andrews, S., Armand, P., Bhatia, S., ... Scavone, J.L. (2019). Management of immunotherapy-related toxicities, version 1.2019, NCCN Clinical Practice Guidelines in Oncology. *Journal of the National Comprehensive Cancer Network, 17,* 255–289. https://doi.org/10.6004/jnccn.2019.0013

Van Limbergen, E.J., De Ruysscher, D.K., Olivo Pimentel, V., Marcus, D., Ber-bee, M., Hoeben, A., ... Lambin, P. (2017). Combining radiotherapy with immunotherapy: The past, the present and the future. *British Journal of Radiology, 90,* 20170157. https://doi.org/10.1259/bjr.20170157

Vargo, J.A., Ferris, R.L, Ohr, J., Clump, D.A., Davis, K.S., Duvvuri, U., ... Heron, D.E. (2015). A prospective phase 2 trial of reirradiation with stereotactic body radiation therapy plus cetuximab in patients with previously irradiated recurrent squamous cell carcinoma of the head and neck. *International Journal of Radiation Oncology, Biology, Physics, 91,* 480–488. https://doi.org/10.1016/j.ijrobp.2014.11.023

Verma, V., Cushman, T.R., Tang, C., & Welsh, J.W. (2018). Toxicity of radiation and immunotherapy combinations. *Advances in Radiation Oncology, 3,* 506–511. https://doi.org/10.1016/j.adro.2018.08.003

Walle, T., Martinez Monge, R., Cerwenka, A., Ajona, D., Melero, I., & Lecanda, F. (2018). Radiation effects on antitumor immune responses: Current per-spectives and challenges. *Therapeutic Advances in Medical Oncology, 10.* https://doi.org/10.1177/1758834017742575

Wattenberg, M., Fahim, A., Ahmed, M.M., & Hodge, J.W. (2014). Unlocking the combination: Potentiation of radiation-induced antitumor responses with immunotherapy. *Radiation Research, 182,* 126–138. https://doi.org/10.1667/RR13374.1

Weingarten, N., Kruser, T.J., & Bloch, O. (2019). Symptomatic radiation necrosis in brain metastasis patients treated with stereotactic radiosurgery and immunotherapy. *Clinical Journal of Neurology and Neurosurgery, 179,* 14–18. https://doi.org/10.1016/j.clineuro.2019.02.010

XI. General Radiation Oncology Issues

A. Survivorship

1. History
   a) Cancer survivorship has been an essential part of cancer care since the 1980s.
   b) Fitzhugh Mullan, an American physician who was diagnosed with cancer in 1975, believed that the challenges and long-term side effects from cancer treatment deserved an independent title from "cure." In 1985, Mullan introduced the concepts of "survivorship" and the "seasons of survival" (Khan, Rose, & Evans, 2012; Mullan, 1985).
   c) The National Coalition for Cancer Survivorship, founded by Mullan and others in 1986, advocated for and addressed the needs of cancer survivors (Khan et al., 2012; National Coalition for Cancer Survivorship, 2014).
   d) In 1997, the Lance Armstrong Foundation (now the Livestrong Foundation) was established to raise awareness and develop resources for survivorship care (Corcoran, Dunne, & McCabe, 2015).
   e) In 2018, Aiuppa, Hewitt, and Nass (2018) authored *Long-Term Survivorship Care After Cancer Treatment: Proceedings of a Workshop* for the Health and Medicine Division of the National Academies of Sciences, Engineering, and Medicine (formerly the Institute of Medicine).
      (1) The authors evaluated the progress of survivorship care since the 2006 report *From Cancer Patient to Cancer Survivor: Lost in Transition* (Hewitt, Greenfield, & Stovall, 2006).
      (2) The workshop also addressed the current evidence-based impact of physical, psychosocial, and socioeconomic considerations for survivors.

2. Definition
   a) Despite the term's wide use across multiple disciplines, several definitions for *cancer survivor* exist (Khan et al., 2012).
   b) The Office of Cancer Survivorship, established by NCI in 1996, defines someone as a *cancer survivor* "from the time of diagnosis, through the balance of his or her life" (NCI Office of Cancer Survivorship, n.d., para. 1).
   c) The National Coalition for Cancer Survivorship (2014) delineates a *cancer survivor* as someone "living with, through, and beyond a cancer diagnosis" (para. 1). This definition includes the family members, friends, and caregivers who are affected by the diagnosis.

3. Cancer statistics
   a) As of 2020, an estimated 16.9 million cancer survivors are living in the United States (American Cancer Society, 2020). By 2031, that number is projected to increase to 22.1 million (American Cancer Society, 2019).
   b) Improved treatment technologies and early-detection methods have contributed to the increase in cancer survivors (American Cancer Society, 2019; Corcoran et al., 2015).
   c) RT is one of three primary treatments for cancer.
      (1) Almost two-thirds of patients diagnosed with cancer will receive RT.
      (2) RT can be used for curative intent or to relieve cancer-related pain (Wang et al., 2018).
   d) From 2013 to 2017, the cancer death rate per year decreased by 1.8% and 1.4% for men and women, respectively (NCI, 2020).
   e) As of January 31, 2019, the most common cancer sites for survivors were the following (American Cancer Society, 2019).
      (1) Female breast: 3.8 million
      (2) Prostate: 3.6 million
      (3) Colorectal: 1.5 million
      (4) Gynecologic: 1.3 million
      (5) Melanoma: 1.2 million

4. Survivorship standards
   a) *Optimal Resources for Cancer Care (2020 Standards)* (ACoS CoC, 2019)
      (1) The updated standards focus on the development of a survivorship program to meet the needs of patients who are being treated with curative intent.
      (2) Survivorship care plans (SCPs) are still valuable and encouraged; however, they are no longer required for patients who are being treated with curative intent.
      (3) Each program may determine the patient population best served by an SCP.
      (4) Programs have the following requirements.
         (a) The program must have a designated leader or coordinator.
         (b) Identified teams, services, and programs should be in place to address the needs of cancer survivors.
         (c) Annual reporting must occur on patients participating in three identified services offered by the program and the required resources needed for improvement.
            i. The survivorship program team determines a list of services and programs that address the needs of cancer survivors.
            ii. A minimum of three services offered each year should be formally documented.
            iii. These services may be continued year to year, but the goal is to enhance existing services over time, along with development of new services.

(d) Survivorship programs may include SCPs and treatment summaries, as well as the following services.

    i. Screening for recurrence and new cancers

    ii. Education and seminars

    iii. Rehabilitation services

    iv. Nutrition services

    v. Psychological support and psychiatric services

    vi. Support groups and services

    vii. Formalized referrals to experts in cardiology, pulmonary services, sexual dysfunction, and fertility counseling

    viii. Financial support services

    ix. Physical activity programs

b) National Accreditation Program for Breast Centers SCPs (ACoS, 2017)

  (1) Patient eligibility criteria

    (a) Diagnosed with stage 0 (in situ), I, II, or III breast cancer; stage IV considered maintenance (not definitive treatment)

    (b) Treated with curative intent (definitive treatment); stage IV considered maintenance treatment (not definitive; no SCP required)

    (c) Considered an analytic case

    (d) Completed active therapy (i.e., chemotherapy and/or RT), though still may be receiving hormone or targeted therapy

  (2) Process requirements

    (a) An SCP should be completed 12 months from the time of diagnosis; however, this can be extended to 18 months if the patient is receiving hormonal or targeted therapy.

    (b) The SCP should be manually or electronically prepared by the healthcare providers. Eligible team members include the following.

      i. Physicians

      ii. Registered nurses

      iii. Advanced practice nurses

      iv. Nurse Practitioners

      v. Physician assistants

      vi. Credentialed clinical navigators (does not include lay navigators)

  (3) Compliance

    (a) A comprehensive process should be established to prepare and disseminate a breast cancer SCP. Eligible patients should receive a treatment summary within six months of completing active treatment and within 12 months from the date of diagnosis.

    (b) An annual compliance review should be completed by the breast program leadership committee and documented in meeting minutes.

5. SCPs

  a) An SCP is a document that summarizes the patient's treatment and includes updated guidelines for follow-up care, ongoing surveillance, and potential late or long-term side effects.

  b) SCPs are important communication tools to facilitate transition of care, promote communication, and improve quality of life (Haylock, 2015).

  c) A survivorship visit can help patients to cope with the possible mental, physical, and late or long-term side effects they can experience after treatment (Denlinger et al., 2014).

  d) NCCN guidelines for survivorship care discuss general survivorship principles, late or long-term effects on psychosocial and physical issues, and preventive health (see https://www.nccn.org/professionals/physician_gls/default.aspx).

  e) From Cancer Patient to Cancer Survivor: Lost in Transition recommends that every survivor should receive an SCP, which should include a treatment summary, surveillance plan, and post-treatment care (Aiuppa et al., 2018; Hewitt et al., 2006).

    (1) Treatment summary components include general information, diagnosis and treatment information, and the names and contact information of the care team (Huenerberg et al., 2018).

    (2) Surveillance plan components should include follow-up recommendations based on current guidelines, signs and symptoms of recurrence, secondary cancers, health maintenance, late or long-term side effects of the specific treatment (e.g., chemotherapy, immunotherapy, targeted therapy), and cancer-related resources (Denlinger et al., 2014; Huenerberg et al., 2018).

  f) Examples of treatment summaries and SCP template builders (Klemanski, Browning, & Kue, 2015)

    (1) ASCO Treatment Summary and Survivorship Care Plan (ASCO, n.d.; see Figure 34)

    (2) ASTRO survivorship template specific to radiation oncology (Chen et al., 2016)

    (3) Penn Medicine's OncoLife template builder (https://oncolife.oncolink.org)

6. Models of care

  a) A wide variety of survivorship care models exist; however, a consensus on a recommended model has left healthcare professionals with the challenge of providing national guidance on a care model that addresses survivor needs and quality of life (Halpern et al., 2015; McCabe et al., 2013; Oeffinger & McCabe, 2006).

  b) Models of survivorship care may include a variety of care providers, including oncologists, nurses, family physicians, and advanced practice providers, and may be dependent on the clinical setting. The goal of any

FIGURE 34. ASCO Treatment Summary and Survivorship Care Plan

General Information

Patient Name: _____   Patient DOB: _____

Patient phone: _____   Email: _____

Health Care Providers (Including Names, Institution) _____

Primary Care Provider: _____

Surgeon: _____

Radiation Oncologist: _____

Medical Oncologist: _____

Other Providers: _____

Treatment Summary

Diagnosis _____   Diagnosis Date (year): _____

Cancer Type/Location/Histology Subtype: _____
_____

Stage: ☐ I   ☐ II   ☐ III   ☐ Not applicable

Treatment _____

Surgery ☐ Yes ☐ No   Surgery Date(s) (year): _____

Surgical procedure/location/findings: _____
_____

Radiation ☐ Yes   ☐ No   Body area treated: _____   End Date (year): _____

Systemic Therapy (chemotherapy, hormonal therapy, other)   ☐ Yes   ☐ No

Names of Agents Used	End Dates (year)

Persistent symptoms or side effects at completion of treatment: ☐ No   ☐ Yes (enter type(s)) : _____
_____
_____

(Continued on next page)

FIGURE 34. ASCO Treatment Summary and Survivorship Care Plan *(Continued)*

Familial Cancer Risk Assessment

Genetic/hereditary risk factor(s) or predisposing conditions: _____

_____

Genetic counseling: ☐ Yes ☐ No   Genetic testing results: _____

_____

Follow-up Care Plan

Need for ongoing (adjuvant) treatment for cancer ☐ Yes ☐ No

Additional treatment name	Planned duration	Possible Side effects

Schedule of clinical visits

Coordinating Provider	When/How often

Cancer surveillance or other recommended related tests

Coordinating Provider	When/When/How often

Please continue to see your primary care provider for all general health care recommended for a (man) (woman) your age, including cancer screening tests. Any symptoms should be brought to the attention of your provider:

Anything that represents a brand new symptom;

Anything that represents a persistent symptom;

Anything you are worried about that might be related to the cancer coming back.

Possible late- and long-term effects that someone with this type of cancer and treatment may experience: _____

_____

(Continued on next page)

Follow-up Care Plan *(Continued)*

Cancer survivors may experience issues with the areas listed below. If you have any concerns in these or other areas, please speak with your doctors or nurses to find out how you can get help with them.

☐ Emotional and mental health
☐ Fatigue
☐ Weight changes
☐ Stopping smoking
☐ Physical Functioning

☐ Insurance
☐ School/Work
☐ Financial advice or assistance
☐ Memory or concentration loss

☐ Parenting
☐ Fertility
☐ Sexual functioning
☐ Other_____

A number of lifestyle/behaviors can affect your ongoing health, including the risk for the cancer coming back or developing another cancer. Discuss these recommendations with your doctor or nurse:

☐ Tobacco use/cessation
☐ Diet

☐ Alcohol use
☐ Sun screen use

☐ Weight management (loss/gain)
☐ Physical activity

Resources you may be interested in: _____

_____

Other comments:_____

_____

Prepared by: _____   Delivered on: _____

- This Survivorship Care Plan is a cancer treatment summary and follow-up plan is provided to you to keep with your health care records and to share with your primary care provider.
- This summary is a brief record of major aspects of your cancer treatment. You can share your copy with any of your doctors or nurses. However, this is not a detailed or comprehensive record of your care.

model is to increase the quality of life for the cancer survivor and provide comprehensive, coordinated, and patient-specific care (Haylock, 2015).

c) Types of models

(1) Academic models can be consultative or longitudinal and have been adopted by most academic cancer centers in the United States, Europe, Australia, and Canada (McCabe et al., 2013).

(a) In a consultative model, the survivor is seen for a one-time comprehensive visit to review the treatment summary and SCP.

i. If specialized referrals are needed, these are usually coordinated at this visit.

ii. Continued follow-up care is performed by the survivor's oncologist or PCP (McCabe et al., 2013).

(b) In a longitudinal model, the survivor is provided ongoing survivorship care for one to five years after treatment. Once the oncologist believes the risk of recurrence

is low, the survivor is transitioned back to the PCP (McCabe et al., 2013).

(2) The disease-specific model was initially developed for breast cancer survivors to address common late effects of treatment, including fatigue, lymphedema, weight gain, and psychological distress. Disease-specific models for other cancer sites have been developed using the breast cancer survivorship paradigm (Haylock, 2015).

(3) The multidisciplinary clinic model has been most commonly used in the pediatric survivor setting; however, nurse navigators have used this model to help facilitate disciplines for adult survivorship (Haylock, 2015).

(4) In an integrated care model, the patient receives the SCP from the oncology nurse practitioner, who is also a member of the healthcare team. Long-term follow-up care is provided by the oncologist and nurse practitioner (Haylock, 2015).

(5) In community practice models, the focus is on enhancing survivorship care at community hospitals. NCI provides funding through the NCI

Community Cancer Centers Program for this particular model (McCabe et al., 2013).

(6) A shared care model typically uses a risk stratification approach and facilitates coordination between the oncologist and the other providers involved in the survivor's care.

    (a) The oncology specialist will be the cancer care provider during the most crucial times when the patient is at highest risk for recurrence.

    (b) The PCP will also be involved in addressing any non–cancer-related needs of the patient.

    (c) The treatment summary and SCP will be provided to the patient and the PCP for continuity of care (Haylock, 2015; McCabe et al., 2013).

(7) The transition clinic model focuses on transitioning back to the PCP from the oncologist (Halpern et al., 2015).

(8) The personalized cancer survivorship care model is based on initiating, integrating, and safeguarding a partnership with the patient. A patient-centered focus and clinical practice guidelines are essential elements of this model (Loonen et al., 2018).

    (a) A patient-centered focus will include an informed and involved patient, a responsible and receptive healthcare professional, and a coordinated and well-integrated healthcare environment (Loonen et al., 2018).

    (b) Ideal clinical practice guidelines should help to address and treat late effects, improve patient quality of care, and reduce costs (Loonen et al., 2018).

7. Barriers to survivorship visits (Haylock, 2015)

  a) Time commitment required to prepare treatment summary and SCP

  b) Lack of reimbursement for preparation time

  c) Lack of defined role for completing and updating guidelines for SCPs

  d) Lack of communication between oncology providers and PCP

  e) Limited information documenting improved outcomes or quality of life

  f) Existing templates not being compatible with electronic health records

8. Role of advanced practice nurses in survivorship care (Corcoran et al., 2015)

  a) An estimated 3,000 oncology advanced practice nurses work in the United States. In Canada, that number shrinks to 1,000, and internationally, the number further diminishes.

  b) Advanced practice nurses have the knowledge and expertise to discuss the key components of survivorship care and provide excellent, impactful care to patients.

  c) Advanced practice nurses provide comprehensive follow-up care in a variety of settings and can work independently or in collaboration with other healthcare professionals.

9. Late and long-term side effects (see IV. J. Late effects of treatment)

  a) Late effects develop months or years after the completion of a cancer treatment (Cancer.Net, 2019).

  b) Long-term effects develop during treatment and persist after completion of a cancer treatment (e.g., fatigue, pain, cognitive impairment, sexual dysfunction) (Sjödahl, 2015).

  c) RT and multimodal treatments can increase the likelihood of second malignancies, as these methods are believed to accelerate the aging process to many organs (Kline et al., 2018).

  d) Common late and long-term effects, and their associated nursing interventions, include the following.

    (1) CRF

      (a) CRF continues to be one of the most prevalent adverse effects of cancer survivors even after treatment has completed (Mustian et al., 2017).

      (b) Exercise and psychological interventions are the first-line treatment (e.g., aerobic, anaerobic, or strength exercises).

      (c) Psychological intervention with cognitive behavioral therapy has also shown to improve CRF.

      (d) A combination of exercise and psychological intervention was shown to be the most effective treatment in the cancer survivor population.

    (2) Sleep disruption

      (a) Sleep hygiene techniques, such as avoiding napping and not drinking caffeine later in the day, have reduced sleep disruption (Howell et al., 2013).

      (b) Cognitive behavioral therapy can address issues affecting sleep and can incorporate relaxation training to promote sleep (Howell et al., 2013).

      (c) Short-term use of hypnotic medications may be considered through particularly stressful times during the cancer journey (Howell et al., 2013).

    (3) Cognitive impairment

      (a) Cognitive impairment is typically first noted with chemotherapy but can persist in many survivors as a long-term side effect. It can subjectively have a significant impact on patient quality of life (Miller et al., 2016).

      (b) Brain irradiation carries the risk for cognitive impairment as a late and/or long-term effect from cancer treatment (Scoccianti et al., 2012).

(4) Distress

    (a) More than 50% of patients diagnosed with cancer will experience distress (Mehnert et al., 2017).

    (b) Distress is defined as an emotional response to a condition that can either be physical or psychological in nature (Hammelef, Friese, Breslin, Riba, & Schneider, 2014).

    (c) ACoS CoC requires that all patients with cancer be screened for distress and appropriate referrals placed (ACoS CoC, 2019; Zebrack et al., 2015).

        i. This screening should take place at a "pivotal medical visit," as determined by the specific program.

        ii. Each year, the cancer committee implements a policy and procedure for providing and monitoring psychosocial distress screening and referral for psychosocial care.

    (d) Untreated distress can affect quality of life and inhibit adherence to treatment (Yee et al., 2017).

    (e) NCCN guidelines for distress management are available (see www.nccn.org/professionals/physician_gls/pdf/distress.pdf).

e) Late and long-term effects related to chemotherapy and immunotherapy include the following.

    (1) Potential side effects related to systemic treatment include cardiac toxicity, neuropathy, osteopenia and osteoporosis, menopausal symptoms, fatigue, cognitive impairment, and sexual issues and dysfunction (Mullen & Mistry, 2018; Wefel, Kesler, Noll, & Schagen, 2014).

    (2) Immunotherapy drugs, specifically used for treatment of lung cancer, can potentially cause toxicities related to the immune response (e.g., pneumonitis, colitis, nephritis, endocrinopathy) (Miller et al., 2016).

f) Radiation-related late and long-term effects are dependent on cancer site.

    (1) Breast cancer

        (a) Breast and arm lymphedema can be a late effect of RT. The extent of the breast surgery, as well as chronic pain, also contribute to lymphedema (Hille-Betz et al., 2015).

        (b) Compression corsets have been shown to be effective in reducing pain and treating lymphedema (Hansdorfer-Korzon, Teodorczyk, Gruszecka, Wydra, & Lass, 2016).

        (c) Fibrosis of the skin with unfavorable cosmetic outcomes can occur (Hille-Betz et al., 2015).

        (d) Telangiectasia, pneumonitis, cardiac toxicity, and brachial plexopathy with nodal irradiation are all rare late effects (Hille-Betz et al., 2015).

        (e) Second primary lung cancer and heart disease are long-term effects of breast irradiation (Taylor et al., 2017).

            i. The risk of these side effects is dependent upon the radiation dose received by the heart and lungs.

            ii. Smokers are 20 times more likely to be diagnosed with lung cancer and 4 times more likely to experience a cardiac event than nonsmokers (Taylor et al., 2017).

    (2) Colon and rectal cancer (Miller et al., 2016)

        (a) Chronic diarrhea occurs in approximately one-half of cancer survivors and can be caused by combination chemotherapy and RT.

        (b) Bowel dysfunction is a common late effect of RT and can include frequency of bowel movements, incontinence, radiation proctitis, and perianal irritation.

        (c) Urinary changes, sexual dysfunction, and body image issues can be experienced.

        (d) Second malignancy is also a risk.

    (3) Lung cancer

        (a) Radiation pneumonitis diagnosed six months after treatment is known as *radiation-induced lung fibrosis*, and symptoms include a dry and nonproductive cough, dyspnea, chest discomfort, and fatigue (Giridhar, Mallick, Rath, & Julka, 2015).

        (b) Radiation recall pneumonitis is an inflammatory response within the previously irradiated field with the administration of a pharmacology agent (i.e., taxanes and anthracyclines).

            i. Nivolumab has also been linked to radiation recall pneumonitis (Shibaki, Akamatsu, Fujimoto, Koh, & Yamamoto, 2017).

            ii. Considerations for nursing management revolve around supportive care, mobilization of airway secretions, anti-inflammatory therapy, and decreasing acute exacerbation flares (Giridhar et al., 2015).

            iii. Treatment is typically steroids (inhaled or oral), angiotensin-converting enzyme inhibitors, and consideration of pentoxifylline (Giridhar et al., 2015; Simone, 2017).

            iv. Referral to appropriate specialists can be considered.

(c) Combination chemotherapy and RT has the risk of late radiation esophagitis (usually mild) and myelosuppression (He et al., 2016).

(d) Cardiac toxicity can also be a late effect (Simone, 2017).

(4) Prostate cancer

(a) Long-term effects from RT include lower urinary tract complaints, bowel changes, and erectile dysfunction (Miller et al., 2016). The most common severe late effects are noted as urinary obstruction and urethral stricture (Matta et al., 2019).

   i. Radiation-induced urethral strictures are most commonly managed by dilation or visual internal urethrotomy.

   ii. Continued recurrence of the stricture can be common (Matta et al., 2019).

(b) Rectal and urinary bleeding are potential late effects that can be recurrent over time with treatment dependent upon the grading (severity) of the bleeding (Matta et al., 2019).

(c) The following information describes grades of radiation proctitis and interventions (Matta et al., 2019; McElvanna, Wilson, & Irwin, 2014).

   i. Grade 1 (mild): no intervention indicated

   ii. Grade 2 (moderate): sucralfate enemas self-administered twice daily for six weeks or minor cauterization

   iii. Grade 3 (severe): transfusion, radiologic endoscopic, or elective operative intervention indicated

   iv. Grade 4 (life threatening): immediate intervention. Hyperbaric oxygen has been used to promote healing of radiation proctitis (Yildiz, Ercan, & Demirer, 2016).

(d) The following information describes grades of radiation cystitis and interventions (Matta et al., 2019).

   i. Grade 1 (mild): microscopic hematuria, asymptomatic; intervention not indicated

   ii. Grade 2 (moderate): symptomatic, requiring urinary catheter or bladder irrigation

   iii. Grade 3 (severe): gross hematuria; transfusions, IV medication, or hospitalization; consideration of elective endoscopic, radiologic, or operative intervention

   iv. Grade 4 (life threatening): immediate intervention. Hyperbaric oxy-

gen has been used to promote healing through capillary angiogenesis. Hyperbaric oxygen can improve symptoms, if not completely resolve the hematuria (Hayne & Smith, 2008; Yildiz et al., 2016).

(e) Erectile dysfunction is a common side effect as the patient ages, but radiation can also play a role. Treatment should be based on the individual (Donovan et al., 2016; Gaither et al., 2017; Le, Tsambarlis, & Hellstrom, 2018).

   i. PDE5 inhibitors (generics available)

   ii. Intraurethral suppositories

   iii. Vasoactive injectable agents

(f) Increased hip fracture risk has been documented (Matta et al., 2019).

(g) Urinary or gastrointestinal fistula can be a rare late complication (Matta et al., 2019).

(5) Uterine corpus cancer

(a) Long-term effects of radiation include bladder and bowel dysfunction, atrophic vaginitis, and stenosis.

(b) Lower extremity lymphedema after radiation can be a late effect (especially after pelvic lymphadenectomy) (Miller et al., 2016).

(c) Sexual problems, anxiety, and depression are common after pelvic radiation and should be addressed (Eaton et al., 2017).

(d) Vaginal dryness can cause pain with intercourse (Boa & Grénman, 2018).

   i. Vaginal estrogen can be controversial in the setting of some gynecologic cancers; if this is the case, water-, silicone-, mineral oil–, or plant oil–based lubricants and moisturizers should be used (Edwards & Panay, 2016).

   ii. The patient should be encouraged to have regular sexual intercourse with full penetration or use a dilator, which can reduce the risk of radiation-induced vaginal stenosis (Boa & Grénman, 2018).

   iii. A step-by-step guide on dilator use and care for women after pelvic radiation is available online at www.cano-acio.ca/page/radiation_pelvis (Canadian Association of Nurses in Oncology, 2017).

   iv. Referral to a sex therapist or psychologist with special interest in sexual health should be considered for some survivors (Boa & Grénman, 2018; see www.aasect.org).

(6) Head and neck cancer
  (a) The Union for International Cancer Control TNM system (8th edition) has changed in relation to patients with head and neck cancer who are p16 positive. This is a more favorable prognostic indicator (Rasmussen et al., 2018). Patients with what would have been stage IV disease (7th edition) are now considered stage II or III with this marker. As a result, survivors who were previously diagnosed with stage IV head and neck cancer can now be included in the survivorship criteria if their p16-positive status changes.
  (b) The American Cancer Society, with modification from an ASCO expert panel, has created a cancer survivorship care guideline specific to head and neck cancer (Nekhlyudov, Lacchetti, & Siu, 2018).
  (c) Late effects can be exacerbated by receiving chemotherapy with radiation treatments (Dong et al., 2017).
  (d) Radiation-related late and long-term effects include physical appearance changes with resultant psychological impact, dysphagia, odynophagia, dysgeusia, xerostomia, thick saliva, and mucositis (Ackerman, Laszlo, Provisor, & Yu, 2018).
  (e) Radiation-associated dysphagia is difficulty swallowing as the result of tissue fibrosis, strictures, or lower cranial neuropathy from treatment (De Felice et al., 2018).
      i. The gold standard for evaluation of this condition is a videofluorographic swallowing study, which includes a modified barium swallow and esophagography to visualize the phases of swallowing (i.e., oral, pharyngeal, and esophageal) (De Felice et al., 2018).
      ii. Referral to a speech-language pathologist can assist the survivor with swallowing function and improve their quality of life.
      iii. The patient can also be taught exercises to improve coordination of structural movement during swallowing (De Felice et al., 2018).
  (f) Nutritional issues are a common late effect. Patients should be educated about the slow recovery process and realistic expectations during the post-treatment phase (Ackerman et al., 2018; McQuestion, Fitch, & Howell, 2011).
  (g) Xerostomia is dry mouth related to salivary gland dysfunction. It can also affect dentition and taste (Ringash et al., 2015).
  (h) Dental caries can be a result of changes in saliva.
      i. The fluoride is lost from the tooth enamel from xerostomia.
      ii. Survivors should have daily fluoride treatments and meticulous oral hygiene, which decreases the risk of deterioration of the teeth (Ringash et al., 2015).
  (i) Patients are also at risk for osteoradionecrosis, which affects the bones within the radiation field and can delay healing related to lack of oxygen and blood flow to the tissue. Osteoradionecrosis is rare in areas that received less than 60 Gy but is more common in survivors who have received combination chemotherapy and radiation (Ringash et al., 2015).
  (j) Radiation-induced fibrosis can decrease range of motion to the tongue and jaw, and subsequent decreased oral and pharyngeal swallowing performance can also impede swallowing (King, Dunlap, Tennant, & Pitts, 2016). Fibrosis affecting the shoulder and neck can also inhibit range of motion (Ringash et al., 2015).
10. Pediatric survivorship
  a) In 2017, an estimated 15,270 children and adolescents aged 0–19 years were diagnosed with cancer, and 1,790 died of the disease (NCI, 2020).
  b) The overall cancer death rate for children aged 0–14 years decreased an average of 1.4% per year during 2013–2017 (NCI, 2020).
  c) The type and stage of cancer determine the treatment modality (surgery, RT, chemotherapy, targeted therapy) (Miller et al., 2016).
  d) Survival rates have also improved with early detection and treatment advances. In 2005–2011, the five-year survival from birth to 14 years was 83%, as opposed to a 58% survival from 1975–1977 (Miller et al., 2016).
  e) The most commonly diagnosed cancers for children are leukemia (30%), brain and CNS tumors (26%), and soft tissue sarcomas (7%) (Miller et al., 2016).
  f) The most commonly diagnosed cancers for adolescents are brain and CNS tumors (20%), leukemia (14%), and Hodgkin lymphoma (13%) (Miller et al., 2016).
  g) Cancer survivors who had treatment during childhood are more at risk for developing a second cancer (Lewis-Patterson, Palos, Dains, & Jackson, 2016).
      (1) Approximately 30 years after initial treatment, almost 10% of childhood cancer survivors have been diagnosed with a second cancer, most commonly breast (female), thyroid, brain, and other CNS tumors (Armstrong et al., 2015).

(2) Treatment-related leukemia can develop approximately five to nine years after exposure to RT (Lewis-Patterson et al., 2016).

(3) Survivorship follow-up care is extremely important in the pediatric patient population to ensure proper surveillance and prevention screening of other cancers (Armstrong et al., 2015).

h) Pediatric long-term and late effects of treatment (see IX.A. Adolescent and young adult radiation oncology)

(1) Treatment for pediatric cancers from the 1970s through the 1980s was very aggressive, putting this patient population at an increased risk for late long-term effects, cardiomyopathies, cognitive impairments, infertility, psychosocial distress, and second malignancies.

(2) Fertility should be discussed with AYA patients prior to receiving treatments such as chemotherapy and RT, as this can impair sexual function and fertility. As the survivor ages, uncertainty over fertility can cause distress and anxiety (Nahata, Quinn, & Tishelman, 2018).

(3) Pediatric cancer survivors can develop late effects from their cancer treatment, even 10–20 years later (Oeffinger & McCabe, 2006).

(a) Long-term follow-up guidelines for pediatric survivors are available through the Children's Oncology Group (https://survivorshipguidelines.org) and the Pediatric Oncology Group of Ontario (see www.pogo.ca).

(b) Long-term follow-up programs were developed to address the ongoing needs of children and adolescents treated for cancer. Once two years off therapy, survivors should be transitioned from the oncology team to the long-term follow-up program (Oeffinger & McCabe, 2006).

(c) Annual follow-up should be based specifically on the type of treatment received and include monitoring for late effects, recurrence, and screening for secondary cancers, while promoting health maintenance (Oeffinger & McCabe, 2006).

11. Support programs and organizations

a) Livestrong Foundation is active in raising awareness of survivorship (Corcoran et al., 2015).

b) ASCO include many tools to guide survivors (Corcoran et al., 2015).

(1) Survivorship guidelines with focus on late and long-term effects

(2) Simplified treatment summaries and care plan

(3) Clinical practice guidelines with prevention and management addressing physical and psychological needs

c) The American Cancer Society established the National Cancer Survivorship Resource Center to develop survivorship guidelines for certain cancers (Corcoran et al., 2015).

d) NCCN updates clinical practice survivorship guidelines (Corcoran et al., 2015).

e) ONS has an active online community focusing on survivorship issues.

f) Canadian Association of Nurses in Oncology has a survivorship special interest group and has published a series of self-learning modules for survivorship care (see www.cano-acio.ca/page/survivorship_module).

g) The Canadian Cancer Society has resources for survivors and families (see www.cancer.ca/en/?region=on).

h) Imerman Angels is a resource for survivors interested in mentoring services (see https://imermanangels.org/about-us-2). This free service that uniquely partners people of any age, gender, or cancer type around the world for support and camaraderie.

References

Ackerman, D., Laszlo, M., Provisor, A., & Yu, A. (2018). Nutrition management for the head and neck cancer patient. In E. Maghami & A.S. Ho (Eds.), *Multidisciplinary care of the head and neck cancer patient* (pp. 187–208). https://doi.org/10.1007/978-3-319-65421-8_11

Aiuppa, L., Hewitt, M., & Nass, S.J. (2018). *Long-term survivorship care after cancer treatment: Proceedings of a workshop.* https://doi.org/10.17226/25043

American Cancer Society. (2019). *Cancer treatment and survivorship facts and figures 2019–2021.* https://www.cancer.org/content/dam/cancer-org/research/cancer-facts-and-statistics/cancer-treatment-and-survivorship-facts-and-figures/cancer-treatment-and-survivorship-facts-and-figures-2019-2021.pdf

American Cancer Society. (2020). *Cancer facts and figures 2020.* https://www.cancer.org/content/dam/cancer-org/research/cancer-facts-and-statistics/annual-cancer-facts-and-figures/2020/cancer-facts-and-figures-2020.pdf

American College of Surgeons. (2017). *National accreditation program for breast centers standards manual.* https://accreditation.facs.org/accreditationdocuments/NAPBC/Portal%20Resources/2018NAPBCStandardsManual.pdf

American College of Surgeons Commission on Cancer. (2019). *Optimal resources for cancer care (2020 standards).* https://www.facs.org/-/media/files/quality-programs/cancer/coc/optimal_resources_for_cancer_care_2020_standards.ashx

American Society of Clinical Oncology. (n.d.). *ASCO cancer treatment and survivorship care plans.* https://www.cancer.net/survivorship/follow-care-after-cancer-treatment/asco-cancer-treatment-and-survivorship-care-plans

Armstrong, G.T., Yasui, Y., Chen, Y., Leisenring, W.M., Gibson, T.M., Mertens, A., ... Robison, L.L. (2015). Reduction in late mortality among 5-year survivors of childhood cancer: A report from the Childhood Cancer Survivor Study (CCSS). *Journal of Clinical Oncology, 33*(Suppl. 15), LBA2. https://doi.org/10.1200/jco.2015.33.15_suppl.lba2

Boa, R., & Grénman, S. (2018). Psychosexual health in gynecologic cancer. *International Journal of Gynecology and Obstetrics, 143,* 147–152. https://doi.org/10.1002/ijgo.12623

Canadian Association of Nurses in Oncology. (2017, February 27). *Care for women after radiation to the pelvis.* https://cdn.ymaws.com/www.cano-acio.ca/resource/resmgr/Resources/Vaginal_Dilator_Booklet_LONG.pdf

Cancer.Net. (2019, December). Managing late effects of childhood cancer. https://www.cancer.net/navigating-cancer-care/children/managing-late-effects-childhood-cancer

Chen, R.C., Hoffman, K.E., Sher, D.J., Showalter, T.N., Morrell, R., Chen, A.B., ... Hardenbergh, P. (2016). Development of a standard survivorship care plan template for radiation oncologists. *Practical Radiation Oncology, 6,* 57–65. https://doi.org/10.1016/j.prro.2015.10.001

Corcoran, S., Dunne, M., & McCabe, M.S. (2015). The role of advanced practice nurses in cancer survivorship care. *Seminars in Oncology Nursing, 31,* 338–347. https://doi.org/10.1016/j.soncn.2015.08.009

De Felice, F., de Vincentiis, M., Luzzi, V., Magliulo, G., Tombolini, M., Ruopolo, G., & Polimeni, A. (2018). Late radiation-associated dysphagia in head and neck cancer patients: Evidence, research and management. *Oral Oncology, 77,* 125–130. https://doi.org/10.1016/j.oraloncology.2017.12.021

Denlinger, C.S., Carlson, R.W., Are, M., Baker, K.S., Davis, E., Edge, S.B., ... Freedman-Cass, D. (2014). Survivorship: Introduction and definition. Clinical practice guidelines in oncology. *Journal of the National Comprehensive Cancer Network, 12,* 34–45. https://doi.org/10.6004/jnccn.2014.0005

Dong, Y., Ridge, J.A., Li, T., Lango, M.N., Churilla, T.M., Bauman, J.R., & Galloway, T.J. (2017). Long-term toxicities in 10-year survivors of radiation treatment for head and neck cancer. *Oral Oncology, 71,* 122–128. https://doi.org/10.1016/j.oraloncology.2017.05.009

Donovan, J.L., Hamdy, F.C., Lane, J.A., Mason, M., Metcalfe, C., Walsh, E., ... Neal, D.E. (2016). Patient-reported outcomes after monitoring, surgery, or radiotherapy for prostate cancer. *New England Journal of Medicine, 375,* 1425–1437. https://doi.org/10.1056/NEJMoa1606221

Eaton, L., Kueck, A., Maksut, J., Gordon, L., Metersky, K., Miga, A., ... Bradley, A. (2017). Sexual health, mental health, and beliefs about cancer treatments among women attending a gynecologic oncology clinic. *Sexual Medicine, 5,* e175–e183. https://doi.org/10.1016/j.esxm.2017.04.002

Edwards, D., & Panay, N. (2016). Treating vulvovaginal atrophy/genitourinary syndrome of menopause: How important is vaginal lubricant and moisturizer composition? *Climacteric, 19,* 151–161. https://doi.org/10.3109/13697137.2015.1124259

Gaither, T.W., Awad, M.A., Osterberg, E.C., Murphy, G.P., Allen, I.E., Chang, A., ... Breyer, B.N. (2017). The natural history of erectile dysfunction after prostatic radiotherapy: A systematic review and meta-analysis. *Journal of Sexual Medicine, 14,* 1071–1078. https://doi.org/10.1016/j.jsxm.2017.07.010

Giridhar, P., Mallick, S., Rath, G.K., & Julka, P.K. (2015). Radiation induced lung injury: Prediction, assessment and management. *Asian Pacific Journal of Cancer Prevention, 16,* 2613–2617. https://doi.org/10.7314/apjcp.2015.16.7.2613

Halpern, M.T., Viswanathan, M., Evans, T.S., Birken, S.A., Basch, E., & Mayer, D.K. (2015). Models of cancer survivorship care: Overview and summary of current evidence. *Journal of Oncology Practice, 11,* e19–e27. https://doi.org/10.1200/jop.2014.001403

Hammelef, K.J., Friese, C.R., Breslin, T.M., Riba, M., & Schneider, S.M. (2014). Implementing distress management guidelines in ambulatory oncology. *Clinical Journal of Oncology Nursing, 18*(Suppl. 1), 31–36. https://doi.org/10.1188/14.cjon.s1.31-36

Hansdorfer-Korzon, R., Teodorczyk, J., Gruszecka, A., Wydra, J., & Lass, P. (2016). Relevance of low-pressure compression corsets in physiotherapeutic treatment of patients after mastectomy and lymphadenectomy. *Patient Preference and Adherence, 10,* 1177–1187. https://doi.org/10.2147/ppa.s108326

Haylock, P.J. (2015). Evolving nursing science and practice in cancer survivorship. *Seminars in Oncology Nursing, 31,* 3–12. https://doi.org/10.1016/j.soncn.2014.11.002

Hayne, D., & Smith, A.E. (2008). Hyperbaric oxygen treatment of chronic refractory radiation proctitis: A randomized and controlled double-blind crossover trial with long-term follow-up. *International Journal of Radiation Oncology, Biology, Physics, 72,* 1621. https://doi.org/10.1016/j.ijrobp.2008.08.027

He, J., Huang, Y., Chen, Y., Shi, S., Ye, L., Hu, Y., ... Zeng, Z. (2016). Feasibility and efficacy of helical intensity-modulated radiotherapy for stage III non-small cell lung cancer in comparison with conventionally fractionated 3D-CRT. *Journal of Thoracic Disease, 8,* 862–871. https://doi.org/10.21037/jtd.2016.03.46

Hewitt, M., Greenfield, S., & Stovall, E. (Eds.). (2006). *From cancer patient to cancer survivor: Lost in transition.* https://doi.org/10.17226/11468

Hille-Betz, U., Vaske, B., Bremer, M., Soergel, P., Kundu, S., Klapdor, R., ... Henkenberens, C. (2015). Late radiation side effects, cosmetic outcomes and pain in breast cancer patients after breast-conserving surgery and three-dimensional conformal radiotherapy. *Strahlentherapie und Onkologie, 192,* 8–16. https://doi.org/10.1007/s00066-015-0899-y

Howell, D., Oliver, T.K., Keller-Olaman, S., Davidson, J., Garland, S., Samuels, C., ... Taylor, C. (2013). A Pan-Canadian practice guideline: Prevention, screening, assessment, and treatment of sleep disturbances in adults with cancer. *Supportive Care in Cancer, 21,* 2695–2706. https://doi.org/10.1007/s00520-013-1823-6

Huenerberg, K.J., Anderson, B.M., Tevaarwerk, A.J., Neuman, H.B., Wilke, L.G., Seaborne, L.A., & Sesto, M. (2018). Integrating survivorship care planning in radiation oncology workflow. *Journal of Community and Supportive Oncology, 16,* e66–e71. https://doi.org/10.12788/jcso.0392

Khan, N.F., Rose, P.W., & Evans, J. (2012). Defining cancer survivorship: A more transparent approach is needed. *Journal of Cancer Survivorship, 6,* 33–36. https://doi.org/10.1007/s11764-011-0194-6

King, S.N., Dunlap, N.E., Tennant, P.A., & Pitts, T. (2016). Pathophysiology of radiation-induced dysphagia in head and neck cancer. *Dysphagia, 31,* 339–351. https://doi.org/10.1007/s00455-016-9710-1

Klemanski, D.L., Browning, K.K., & Kue, J. (2015). Survivorship care plan preferences of cancer survivors and health care providers: A systematic review and quality appraisal of the evidence. *Journal of Cancer Survivorship, 10,* 71–86. https://doi.org/10.1007/s11764-015-0452-0

Kline, R.M., Arora, N.K., Bradley, C.J., Brauer, E.R., Graves, D.L., Lunsford, N.B., ... Ganz, P.A. (2018). Long-term survivorship care after cancer treatment: Summary of a 2017 national cancer policy forum workshop. *Journal of the National Cancer Institute, 110,* 1300–1310. https://doi.org/10.1093/jnci/djy176

Le, T.V., Tsambarlis, P., & Hellstrom, W.J.G. (2018). Pharmacodynamics of the agents used for the treatment of erectile dysfunction. *Expert Opinion on Drug Metabolism and Toxicology, 15,* 121–131. https://doi.org/10.1080/17425255.2019.1560421

Lewis-Patterson, P., Palos, G.R., Dains, J., & Jackson, T.L. (2016). Cancer prevention in the survivorship setting. *Seminars in Oncology Nursing, 32,* 291–305. https://doi.org/10.1016/j.soncn.2016.05.009

Loonen, J.J., Blijlevens, N.M., Prins, J., Dona, D.J., Den Hartogh, J., Senden, T., ... Hermens, R.P. (2018). Cancer survivorship care: Person centered care in a multidisciplinary shared care model. *International Journal of Integrated Care, 18,* 4. https://doi.org/10.5334/ijic.3046

Matta, R., Chapple, C.R., Fisch, M., Heidenreich, A., Herschorn, S., Kodama, R.T., ... Nam, R.K. (2019). Pelvic complications after prostate cancer radiation therapy and their management: An international collaborative narrative review. *European Urology, 75,* 464–476. https://doi.org/10.1016/j.eururo.2018.12.003

McCabe, M.S., Bhatia, S., Oeffinger, K.C., Reaman, G.H., Tyne, C., Wollins, D.S., & Hudson, M.M. (2013). American Society of Clinical Oncology statement: Achieving high-quality cancer survivorship care. *Journal of Clinical Oncology, 31,* 631–640. https://doi.org/10.1200/jco.2012.46.6854

McElvanna, K., Wilson, A., & Irwin, T. (2014). Sucralfate paste enema: A new method of topical treatment for haemorrhagic radiation proctitis. *Colorectal Disease, 16,* 281–284. https://doi.org/10.1111/codi.12507

McQuestion, M., Fitch, M., & Howell, D. (2011). The changed meaning of food: Physical, social and emotional loss for patients having received radiation treatment for head and neck cancer. *European Journal of Oncology Nursing, 15,* 145–151. https://doi.org/10.1016/j.ejon.2010.07.006

Mehnert, A., Hartung, T.J., Friedrich, M., Vehling, S., Brähler, E., Härter, M., ... Faller, H. (2017). One in two cancer patients is significantly distressed: Prevalence and indicators of distress. *Psycho-Oncology, 27,* 75–82. https://doi.org/10.1002/pon.4464

Miller, K.D., Siegel, R.L., Chieh, C., Mariotto, A.B., Kramer, J.L., Rowland, J.H., ... Jemal, A. (2016). Cancer treatment and survivorship statistics, 2016. *CA: A Cancer Journal for Clinicians, 66,* 271–289. https://doi.org/10.3322/caac.21349

Mullan, F. (1985). Seasons of survival: Reflections of a physician with cancer. *New England Journal of Medicine, 313,* 270–273. https://doi.org/10.1056/nejm198507253130421

Mullen, E., & Mistry, H. (2018). Managing cancer survivorship issues. *Journal for Nurse Practitioners, 14,* 337–343. https://doi.org/10.1016/j.nurpra.2017.12.022

Mustian, K.M., Alfano, C.M., Heckler, C., Kleckner, A.S., Kleckner, I.R., Leach, C.R., ... Miller, S.M. (2017). Comparison of pharmaceutical, psychological, and exercise treatments for cancer-related fatigue. *JAMA Oncology, 3,* 961–968. https://doi.org/10.1001/jamaoncol.2016.6914

Nahata, L., Quinn, G.P., & Tishelman, A.C. (2018). Counseling in pediatric populations at risk for infertility and/or sexual function concerns. *Pediatrics, 142,* e20181435. https://doi.org/10.1542/peds.2018-1435

National Cancer Institute. (2020). Annual report to the nation 2020: Overall cancer statistics. https://seer.cancer.gov/report_to_nation/statistics.html

National Cancer Institute Office of Cancer Survivorship. (n.d.). OCS home. https://cancercontrol.cancer.gov/ocs

National Coalition for Cancer Survivorship. (2014, July 24). Defining cancer survivorship. https://www.canceradvocacy.org/news/defining-cancer-survivorship

Nekhlyudov, L., Lacchetti, C., & Siu, L.L. (2018). Head and neck cancer survivorship care guideline: American Society of Clinical Oncology clinical practice guideline endorsement summary. *Journal of Oncology Practice, 14,* 167–171. https://doi.org/10.1200/jop.2017.029041

Oeffinger, K.C., & McCabe, M.S. (2006). Models for delivering survivorship care. *Journal of Clinical Oncology, 24,* 5117–5124. https://doi.org/10.1200/jco.2006.07.0474

Rasmussen, J.H., Håkansson, K., Rasmussen, G.B., Vogelius, I.R., Friborg, J., Fischer, B.M., ... Specht, L. (2018). A clinical prognostic model compared to the newly adopted UICC staging in an independent validation cohort of P16 negative/positive head and neck cancer patients. *Oral Oncology, 81,* 52–60. https://doi.org/10.1016/j.oraloncology.2018.04.009

Ringash, J., Bernstein, L.J., Cella, D., Logemann, J., Movsas, B., Murphy, B., ... Ridge, J. (2015). Outcomes toolbox for head and neck cancer research. *Head and Neck, 37,* 425–439. https://doi.org/10.1002/hed.23561

Scoccianti, S., Detti, B., Cipressi, S., Iannalfi, A., Franzese, C., & Biti, G. (2012). Changes in neurocognitive functioning and quality of life in adult patients with brain tumors treated with radiotherapy. *Journal of Neuro-Oncology, 108,* 291–308. https://doi.org/10.1007/s11060-012-0821-8

Shibaki, R., Akamatsu, H., Fujimoto, M., Koh, Y., & Yamamoto, N. (2017). Nivolumab induced radiation recall pneumonitis after two years of radiotherapy. *Annals of Oncology, 28,* 1404–1405. https://doi.org/10.1093/annonc/mdx115

Simone, C.B., Jr. (2017). Thoracic radiation normal tissue injury. *Seminars in Radiation Oncology, 27,* 370–377. https://doi.org/10.1016/j.semradonc.2017.04.009

Sjödahl, R. (2015). Short- and long-term side effects from adjuvant and neoadjuvant treatment of rectal cancer. In G. Baatrup (Ed.), *Multidisciplinary treatment of colorectal cancer: Staging, treatment, pathology, palliation* (pp. 147–153). https://doi.org/10.1007/978-3-319-06142-9_15

Taylor, C., Correa, C., Duane, F.K., Aznar, M.C., Anderson, S.J., Bergh, J., ... McGale, P. (2017). Estimating the risks of breast cancer radiotherapy: Evidence from modern radiation doses to the lungs and heart and from previous randomized trials. *Journal of Clinical Oncology, 35,* 1641–1649. https://doi.org/10.1200/jco.2016.72.0722

Wang, Y., Deng, W., Li, N., Neri, S., Sharma, A., Jiang, W., & Lin, S.H. (2018). Combining immunotherapy and radiotherapy for cancer treatment: Current challenges and future directions. *Frontiers in Pharmacology, 9,* 185. https://doi.org/10.3389/fphar.2018.00185

Wefel, J.S., Kesler, S.R., Noll, K.R., & Schagen, S.B. (2014). Clinical characteristics, pathophysiology, and management of noncentral nervous system cancer-related cognitive impairment in adults. *CA: A Cancer Journal for Clinicians, 65,* 123–138. https://doi.org/10.3322/caac.21258

Yee, M.K., Sereika, S.M., Bender, C.M., Brufsky, A.M., Connolly, M.C., & Rosenzweig, M.Q. (2017). Symptom incidence, distress, cancer-related distress, and adherence to chemotherapy among African American women with breast cancer. *Cancer, 123,* 2061–2069. https://doi.org/10.1002/cncr.30575

Yildiz, H., Ercan, E., & Demirer, Z. (2016). Evaluation of hyperbaric oxygen therapy in the treatment of radiation-induced hemorrhagic cystitis. *Urology, 96,* 178. https://doi.org/10.1016/j.urology.2016.05.063

Zebrack, B., Kayser, K., Sundstrom, L., Savas, S.A., Henrickson, C., Acquati, C., & Tamas, R.L. (2015). Psychosocial distress screening implementation in cancer care: An analysis of adherence, responsiveness, and acceptability. *Journal of Clinical Oncology, 33,* 1165–1170. https://doi.org/10.1200/jco.2014.57.4020

B. Palliative care

1. Definition: The term *palliative care* is described as "an approach that improves the quality of life of patients and their families facing the problems associated with life-threatening illness, through the prevention and relief of suffering by means of early identification and impeccable assessment and treatment of pain and other problems, physical, psychosocial, and spiritual" (World Health Organization, n.d., para. 1).

2. Benefits
   a) Relief of symptoms related to advanced cancers (e.g., pain, dyspnea, bleeding, neurologic deficits caused by metastases arising from brain, bone, lung, or spine) results in improved quality of life (Dalal & Bruera, 2017).
   b) May et al. (2015) found that a palliative care consultation within two days of hospital admission reduced inpatient care costs by 24%.
   c) Advance care planning provides assistance in determining the best treatment based on patient factors (e.g., performance status, advanced age, comorbidities), cancer diagnosis (e.g., metastatic, locally advanced disease), and previous cancer treatments (Zhi & Smith, 2015).
   d) Palliative care can reduce burden on caregivers.
   e) Bakitas et al. (2015) provided strong evidence that early integration of palliative care improved overall survival (14 months vs. 8.5 months).

3. Barriers to care
   a) Patient and family barriers include denial of deteriorating health, fear of addiction and abuse of opioids, stoicism, and cognitive factors (Coyne, Mulvenon, & Paice, 2018).
   b) Healthcare provider barriers include inadequate assessment of pain, lack of recognition of pain, fear of addiction and diversion, and lack of skill in prescribing opioids (Coyne et al., 2018).
   c) Healthcare system barriers include cost prohibition, restrictive formularies limiting access to opioids, lack of insurance coverage, lack of pain management specialists, and lack of resources and education for challenging pain cases (Coyne et al., 2018).

4. Key recommendations
   a) ASCO clinical practice guidelines indicate that patients with advanced cancer, whether inpatient or outpatient, "should receive dedicated palliative care services early in the disease course, concurrent with active treatment. Referring patients to interdisciplinary palliative care teams is optimal, and services may complement existing programs. Providers may refer caregivers of patients with early or advanced cancer to palliative care services" (Ferrell et al., 2017, p. 97).
5. Nursing role
   a) According to a position statement by ANA (2018), "Nurses have an ethical responsibility to provide clinically excellent care to address a patient's pain. Clinically excellent pain management considers clinical indications, mutual identification of goals for pain management, . . . interprofessional collaboration and awareness of professional standards for the assessment and management of different types of pain" (p. 6).
   b) Expectations of the nursing role (McMenamin, Ross, & Jones, 2014)
      (1) Assess knowledge of the patient's understanding of their disease (e.g., prognosis, goals of proposed treatment).
      (2) Discuss potential treatments and expected outcomes.
      (3) Monitor patients for symptoms related to their disease (e.g., pain, dyspnea, nausea).
      (4) Address interventions necessary to reduce symptoms (e.g., analgesia, oxygen, comfort strategies).
      (5) Ensure that the patient and family agree with the plan and understand that the goal is for palliation and not cure.
6. Palliative RT
   a) Goals of treatment
      (1) RT given with palliative intent is most often given to patients with advanced or metastatic cancer with the goal of rapid and durable symptom relief (McMenamin et al., 2014).
      (2) This type of RT has been used successfully in the palliative setting and is a time-efficient and cost-effective way to reduce the level of suffering in symptomatic patients.
   b) Dosing
      (1) Palliative treatment requires lower total doses, shifting focus to symptom control while minimizing treatment burden by using shorter courses of larger fraction size (Spencer, Parrish, & Barton, 2018).
      (2) The radiation dose in this context depends on patient condition (e.g., prognosis, performance status, prior treatment) and considers patient expressed wishes and goals of care.
      (3) Treatment courses may include a single fraction to 5–10 fractions depending on many factors (Fareed, Krishnan, Balboni, & Yu, 2018).

   c) Palliative care teams (Tseng et al., 2014)
      (1) Many cancer centers have developed palliative programs to help with collaboration and decision-making.
      (2) These rapid-access palliative teams have improved timely access to RT for symptom management and enhance patient, family, and team satisfaction with care.
   d) Side effects
      (1) Side effects are dictated by which tissues receive a substantial dose of radiation. For example, radiation to the thoracic spine may cause esophagitis or nausea depending on the level of spine treated (Sourati, Ameri, & Malekzadeh, 2017).
      (2) Fatigue is a common side effect and can affect quality of life and limit activity level in up to two-thirds of patients (Sourati et al., 2017).
      (3) Acute side effects of treatment usually resolve within four to six weeks after completion of treatment.
      (4) Long-term side effects are uncommon in palliative radiation management (Sourati et al., 2017).
   e) Barriers
      (1) Although rapid access teams exist to quickly assess and treat patients (even same-day treatment is often possible), there remains an underutilization of this service (Chow et al., 2017).
      (2) Livergant, Howard, and Klein (2019) identified barriers to referral in a systematic review, including lack of understanding of expected outcomes and toxicities of treatment, perceptions of patient inconvenience, and patient preferences.
      (3) A lack of understanding exists of the benefits of palliative RT among family physicians and palliative care specialists. These providers are most likely to see the patients who would most benefit from this type of symptomatic treatment, especially in the community setting (Lutz, Jones, & Chow, 2014).
   f) Palliative RT at the end of life (Park et al., 2017)
      (1) Park et al. (2017) examined symptomatic improvement and survival in a systematic review of palliative RT given in the last 30 days of life. Findings revealed that when survival is short, palliative RT may have minimal clinical benefit for patients, delay referral to hospice care, and impede access to end-of-life care delivery.
      (2) Overestimation of life expectancy may contribute to inappropriate use of longer fractionation regimens, as well as a high rate of incomplete RT; however, a good rate of pain reduction and better quality of life was seen as early as 10 days after a single fraction of radiation and is

preferred to minimize time spent on treatment and improve quality of time outside the hospital environment.

7. Site-specific palliative RT

a) Brain metastases

(1) Brain metastases are common in patients with lung cancer, breast cancer, and melanoma, as well as other primary site cancers. Based on various studies, incidence is 9%–17% for all patients (Nayak, Lee, & Wen, 2012).

(2) Options for management include whole-brain RT, stereotactic RT, surgical resection, or supportive care (Nayak et al., 2012).

(3) Stereotactic RT is typically used in patients with fewer than 10 lesions that are no more than 3–4 cm in size. Practice in this area is continually changing, and some centers are performing stereotactic RT on a higher number of lesions (Nayak et al., 2012).

(4) The typical course for whole-brain radiation is 20–30 Gy in 5–10 fractions, depending on patient factors (Nayak et al., 2012).

(5) The QUARTZ trial is the first randomized controlled trial to compare whole-brain RT with best supportive care in patients with primary NSCLC.

(a) Results showed that whole-brain treatment had little additional clinically significant survival or quality-of-life benefit.

(b) However, improved survival was shown with whole-brain RT in patients less than 60 years old.

(c) A potential survival benefit exists in patients with good performance status and controlled primary lung disease (Mulvenna et al., 2016).

(6) Major prognostic factors include age, performance status, and extent of extracranial metastatic disease (Soffietti et al., 2017).

(7) Neurosurgical opinion is suggested if substantial edema or hydrocephalus is present (Soffietti et al., 2017).

(8) Symptom/nursing management includes monitoring for seizures, elevated intracranial pressure, neurologic loss, visual deficits, and side effects of steroids (Soffietti et al., 2017).

(9) Use of steroids is important, especially if edema is on scan and/or neurologic symptoms are present. A single morning dose is ideal and may taper off after RT (Soffietti et al., 2017).

(10) Patient education includes medication management (antiepileptics and steroids), harm reduction strategies, support for finances, medication coverage, assistive devices, and referral to social work or palliative and homecare services (Soffietti et al., 2017).

b) Spinal metastases: See VII.B. Spinal cord compression for information on management.

c) Lung metastases (Bezjak, Fairchild, & Macbeth, 2018)

(1) Many of the common symptoms from intrathoracic disease are well palliated by RT and include cough, hemoptysis, and chest pain.

(a) Response rate is 50%–90%.

(b) Dyspnea has been shown to be a more challenging symptom to palliate, as it may be caused by a number of other factors (e.g., obstructive airway disease, cardiac disease, lymphangitis carcinomatoses, pleural effusion).

(2) SVC obstruction due to tumor compression may also be relieved by palliative RT when stenting is not possible.

(3) The choice of palliative dose depends on performance status, extent of intra- and extrathoracic disease, prognosis, expected volume of radiation, estimated toxicity, and availability of other systemic treatments.

(4) A summary of systematic reviews indicates that if a patient's performance status is poor (Eastern Cooperative Oncology Group score 2–4), then they should receive a shorter course of RT for effective symptom control (8–10 Gy in a single fraction or 17 Gy in two fractions).

(a) A fractionation schedule of 20 Gy in five fractions is also commonly prescribed, as it is well tolerated and has proven palliative benefit.

(b) When performance status is 0 or 1, it may be possible to obtain a more durable response and increased survival when giving a higher dose (36–39 Gy in 12 or 13 fractions).

(5) The most common side effects from palliative RT to the thorax include fatigue and esophagitis.

(a) The severity of esophagitis is dose related and resolves in a week on average.

(b) Radiation pneumonitis may occur if large fields and higher doses are used.

d) Bone metastases: See IV.L. Bone metastases for information on management.

References

American Nurses Association. (2018). *The ethical responsibility to manage pain and the suffering it causes* [Position statement]. https://www.nursingworld .org/~495e9b/globalassets/docs/ana/ethics/theethicalresponsibilitytoman agepainandthesufferingitcauses2018.pdf

Bakitas, M., Tosteson, T.D., Li, Z., Lyons, K.D., Hull, J.G., Li, Z., ... Ahles, T.A. (2015). Early versus delayed initiation of concurrent palliative oncology care: Patient outcomes in the ENABLE III randomized controlled trial. *Journal of Clinical Oncology, 33,* 1438–1445. https://doi.org/10.1200/jco.2014.58.6362

Bezjak, A., Fairchild, A., & Macbeth, F. (2018). Palliative radiotherapy for lung cancer. In H.I. Pass, D. Ball, & G.V. Scagliotti (Eds.), *IASLC thoracic oncology* (2nd ed., pp. 382–392). Elsevier.

Chow, R., Hoskin, P., Chan, S., Mesci, A., Hollenberg, D., Lam, H., ... Chow, E. (2017). Efficacy of multiple fraction conventional radiation therapy for painful uncomplicated bone metastases: A systematic review. *Radiotherapy and Oncology, 122,* 323–331. https://doi.org/10.1016/j.radonc.2016.12.031

Coyne, P., Mulvenon, C., & Paice, J.A. (2018). American Society for Pain Management Nursing and Hospice and Palliative Nurses Association position statement: Pain management at the end of life. *Pain Management Nursing, 19,* 3–7. https://doi.org/10.1016/j.pmn.2017.10.019

Dalal, S., & Bruera, E. (2017). End-of-life care matters: Palliative cancer care results in better care and lower costs. *Oncologist, 22,* 361–368. https://doi.org/10.1634/theoncologist.2016-0277

Fareed, M.M., Krishnan, M., Balboni, T.A., & Yu, H.M. (2018). SA–CME information: Indications, barriers and paths to advancement in palliative radiation oncology. *Applied Radiation Oncology.* https://cdn.agilitycms.com/applied-radiation-oncology/PDFs/issues/ARO_06-18_Fareed_web.pdf

Ferrell, B.R., Temel, J.S., Temin, S., Alesi, E.R., Balboni, T.A., Basch, E.M., ... Smith, T.J. (2017). Integration of palliative care into standard oncology care: American Society of Clinical Oncology clinical practice guideline update. *Journal of Clinical Oncology, 35,* 96–112. https://doi.org/10.1200/jco.2016.70.1474

Livergant, J., Howard, M., & Klein, J. (2019). Barriers to referral for palliative radiotherapy by physicians: A systematic review. *Clinical Oncology, 31,* e75–e84. https://doi.org/10.1016/j.clon.2018.09.009

Lutz, S.T., Jones, J., & Chow, E. (2014). Role of radiation therapy in palliative care of the patient with cancer. *Journal of Clinical Oncology, 32,* 2913–2919. https://doi.org/10.1200/jco.2014.55.1143

May, P., Garrido, M.M., Cassel, J.B., Kelley, A.S., Meier, D.E., Normand, C., ... Morrison, R.S. (2015). Prospective cohort study of hospital palliative care teams for inpatients with advanced cancer: Earlier consultation is associated with larger cost-saving effect. *Journal of Clinical Oncology, 33,* 2745–2752. https://doi.org/10.1200/JCO.2014.60.2334

McMenamin, E., Ross, N., & Jones, J. (2014). Palliative radiotherapy and oncology nursing. *Seminars in Oncology Nursing, 30,* 242–252. https://doi.org/10.1016/j.soncn.2014.08.006

Mulvenna, P., Nankivell, M., Barton, R., Faivre-Finn, C., Wilson, P., McColl, E., ... Langley, R.E. (2016). Dexamethasone and supportive care with or without whole brain radiotherapy in treating patients with non-small cell lung cancer with brain metastases unsuitable for resection or stereotactic radiotherapy (QUARTZ): Results from a phase 3, non-inferiority, randomised trial. *Lancet, 388,* 2004–2014. https://doi.org/10.1016/s0140-6736(16)30825-x

Nayak, L., Lee, E.Q., & Wen, P.Y. (2012). Epidemiology of brain metastases. *Current Oncology Reports, 14,* 48–54. https://doi.org/10.1007/s11912-011-0203-y

Park, K.R., Lee, C.G., Tseng, Y.D., Liao, J.J., Reddy, S., Bruera, E., & Yennurajalingam, S. (2017). Palliative radiation therapy in the last 30 days of life: A systematic review. *Radiotherapy and Oncology, 125,* 193–199. https://doi.org/10.1016/j.radonc.2017.09.016

Soffietti, R., Abacioglu, U., Baumert, B., Combs, S.E., Kinhult, S., Kros, J.M., ... Weller, M. (2017). Diagnosis and treatment of brain metastases from solid tumors: Guidelines from the European Association of Neuro-Oncology (EANO). *Neuro-Oncology, 19,* 162–174. https://doi.org/10.1093/neuonc/now241

Sourati, A., Ameri, A., & Malekzadeh, M. (2017). *Acute side effects of radiation therapy: A guide to management.* Springer.

Spencer, K., Parrish, R., & Barton, R. (2018). Palliative radiotherapy. *BMJ, 360,* k821. https://doi.org/10.1136/bmj.k821

Tseng, Y., Krishnan, M.S., Jones, J.A., Sullivan, A.J., Gorman, D., Taylor, A., ... Balboni, T.A. (2014). Supportive and palliative radiation oncology service: Impact of a dedicated service on palliative cancer care. *Practical Radiation Oncology, 4,* 247–253. https://doi.org/10.1016/j.prro.2013.09.005

World Health Organization. (n.d.). WHO definition of palliative care. https://www.who.int/cancer/palliative/definition/en

Zhi, W.I., & Smith, T.J. (2015). Early integration of palliative care into oncology: Evidence, challenges and barriers. *Annals of Palliative Medicine, 4,* 122–131. https://doi.org/10.3978/j.issn.2224-5820.2015.07.03

C. Cancer clinical trials

1. Benefits
   a) Clinical trials involve one or more people who voluntarily agree to be prospectively assigned to one or more interventions to evaluate the effects of the treatment on their disease (Canadian Cancer Society, n.d.; National Institutes of Health, 2017).
   b) Clinical trials help to improve the quality of life of people living with cancer not only during their treatment but also after treatment (Canadian Cancer Society, n.d.; National Institutes of Health, 2017).
   c) Clinical trials allow researchers to test new ways to prevent, detect, treat, or manage cancer through the following.
      (1) Evaluation of the safety and efficacy of novel treatments or devices
      (2) Assessment of the safety and efficacy of new combinations and indications for existing regulatory-approved treatments (e.g., FDA, Health Canada, European Medicines Agency)

2. Phases (American Cancer Society, 2017)
   a) Phase 0 trials introduce human participants and determine how a drug is processed in and effects the body. These trials have a small number of participants who are given small doses of the drug (NCCN, n.d.).
   b) Phase 1 trials determine the route, frequency, dose, and preliminary safety information for a new treatment.
   c) Phase 2 trials assess the effectiveness and continued appraisal of safety for a new treatment.
   d) Phase 3 trials evaluate the effectiveness of a new treatment or combination of treatments compared to the standard treatment.
   e) Phase 4 trials appraise a treatment after it has been FDA approved and market it to further assess effectiveness and safety over a longer period of time.
   f) Some trials are designed to combine phases (e.g., phase 1/2, phase 2/3) in a single protocol, allowing research questions to be answered more quickly or with fewer participants (Cancer Research UK, 2019).

3. Types (Canadian Cancer Society, n.d.; U.S. FDA, 2018b)
   a) Treatment trials determine the safety and effectiveness of both new and existing treatments. These trials generally involve an intervention such as a medication, medical device, or new approach to RT or surgery.
      (1) Medical devices
         (a) A medical device is a healthcare product that does not achieve its principal purpose

by chemical action or metabolization (U.S. FDA, 2019b).

    (b) In the United States, different classes of medical devices (based on level of risk) require different pre- and post-market approvals by FDA.

    (c) In Canada, manufacturers and importers must meet the requirements set out by the Food and Drugs Act in order to sell a device for the purpose of conducting investigational testing (Health Canada, 2018).

  (2) Multimodal treatments

    (a) This treatment combines more than one treatment strategy, such as surgery and RT, or RT and chemotherapy.

    (b) Multiple regulations and clinical practices may need to be taken into consideration during the design and conduct of these trials (Almquist, Mosalpuria, & Ganti, 2016).

b) Preventive clinical trials explore new ways to prevent cancer from developing or returning and focus on the general population and specific high-risk groups.

c) Trials that focus on screening appraise new methods of detecting cancer in populations of people before they have any symptoms. The goal may also be to assess an overall benefit to detecting the cancer early.

d) Diagnostic trials assess new ways to identify or stage cancer.

e) Quality-of-life or supportive care trials evaluate interventions to improve comfort and quality of life for patients with cancer and survivors.

4. Oncology clinical trial nurses (OCTNs)

a) OCTNs are highly skilled and specialized oncology nurses who are integral to the conduct and outcomes of a clinical research study.

b) Inherent to this role is the ability to integrate oncology nursing practice while adhering to stringent regulatory and protocol requirements (Klimaszewski et al., 2016; National Institutes of Health, 2019; ONS, 2016).

  (1) Role delineation of the OCTN has been reviewed in the literature and demonstrates variability in title and responsibilities (Matsumoto, Nagamura, Ogami, Yamashita, & Kamibeppu, 2011; Ness & Royce, 2017; Purdom, Petersen, & Haas, 2017).

  (2) This subspecialty of oncology nursing requires radiation clinical trial nurses to develop a myriad of competencies that integrate protocol adherence and clinical nursing care (Brinkman-Denney, 2013).

  (3) With multimodal treatment, nurse assessments are essential in the identification of adverse events for data collection, analysis, and patient care.

  (4) Although oversight remains with the principal investigator, study nurses can be delegated to identify the attribution and grading of adverse events, which uses their knowledge, skill, and judgment.

c) The ONS Clinical Trials Nurse Competencies framework identified fundamental duties of the OCTN (ONS, 2016).

  (1) Adherence to ethical standards

  (2) Protocol compliance

  (3) Informed consent

  (4) Patient recruitment and retention

  (5) Management of clinical trial patients

  (6) Documentation and document management

  (7) Data management and information technology

  (8) Financial stewardship

  (9) Leadership and professional development

d) Underpinning these fundamental duties are three principles defined as the following (ONS, 2016).

  (1) Advocacy for patient safety and protocol integrity: Nurses must understand each patient's needs and challenges and be able to identify any barriers that may impede their ability to comply with a protocol's required treatments and procedures.

  (2) Adherence to nursing standards: Trial nurses must abide by the practice standards set by their licensing bodies.

  (3) Communication: Written and verbal communication are essential elements in the conduct of clinical trials.

e) For a more in-depth description of the role and competencies of the clinical trial nurse, refer to ONS's *Manual for Clinical Trials Nursing* (Klimaszewski et al., 2016).

5. Informed consent process

a) One of the key functions delegated to the OCTN is the process of informed consent.

b) The OCTN must be knowledgeable about regulatory requirements and the process for obtaining ongoing consent.

c) Informed consent is the process of learning the key facts about a clinical trial before deciding whether to participate (NCI, 2020; U.S. FDA, 2019a).

  (1) Informed consent is a continuing process throughout a study to provide information to participants.

  (2) The basis of this process is the principle of respect for people, by which there is recognition of a participant's personal dignity and autonomy, or the right of participants to act in their best interest, as well as recognition that participants with diminished autonomy (e.g., children, older adults) require additional protection.

  (3) *The Belmont Report* guides the informed consent process in the United States (National Com-

mission for the Protection of Human Subjects of Biomedical and Behavioral Research, 1979).

(4) In Canada, the *Tri-Council Policy Statement* sets the ethical standards around the informed consent process (Canadian Institutes of Health Research, Natural Sciences and Engineering Research Council of Canada, & Social Sciences and Humanities Research Council, 2018).

(5) Elements of the informed consent process include the following (Shah, Thornton, & Hipskind, 2020).

  (a) Information

    i. Individuals, knowing that the procedure is neither necessary for their care nor perhaps fully understood, can decide whether they wish to participate in the furthering of knowledge.

    ii. Even when some direct benefit to them is anticipated, the participant should clearly understand the range of risk and the voluntary nature of participation.

    iii. The participant should receive any new information relevant to the participant's consent in a timely manner (U.S. FDA, 2018a).

  (b) Comprehension

    i. Because the participant's ability to understand is a function of intelligence, rationality, maturity, and language, it is necessary to adapt the presentation of information to the participant's capacities.

    ii. Investigators are responsible for determining whether the participant has understood the information.

    iii. Although an obligation exists to ascertain that information about risk to participants is complete and adequately comprehended, when the risks are more serious, that obligation increases.

    iv. On occasion, it may be suitable to give some oral or written tests of comprehension.

  (c) Voluntariness (Canadian Institutes of Health Research, Natural Sciences and Engineering Research Council of Canada, & Social Sciences and Humanities Research Council, 2018)

    i. An agreement to participate in research constitutes a valid consent only if it has been voluntarily given— free of coercion and undue influence.

    ii. Consent can be withdrawn at any time, and the participant can request

the withdrawal of their data or human biological materials.

    iii. Researchers should recognize and be aware of situations in which undue influence, coercion, or the offer of incentives may affect a participant's decision-making during the consent process.

6. Nurse role in the informed consent process

  a) Preparing for the consent process

  (1) Nurses should use various communication techniques, such as video, interactive computer programs, and discussions, and supplemental materials (written materials) whenever possible and appropriate (U.S. FDA, 2018a).

  (2) Nurses should assess informed consent for appropriate reading, sight, and hearing levels, as well as spoken language (Health Canada, 2014; National Institutes of Health, 2019; U.S. FDA, 2018a, 2019a).

  (3) Nurses should ensure that the content of the informed consent includes the essential elements to comply with FDA Section 50.25 (U.S. FDA, 2018a, 2019a).

  (a) What the study entails; explanation of purpose; expected duration for participation; description of procedures, including which are experimental, any foreseeable risks, benefits, side effects and alternative treatments; and name and contact information of the principle investigator

  (b) Statement around confidentiality of records, to whom it will be disclosed and for what purpose, and the expiration date for transferring protected health information

  (c) Notice that the participant's involvement is voluntary and that their refusal to participate or withdraw will not involve penalty or loss of benefits

  (d) Statement around compensation for research involving more than minimal risk explaining what treatments are available if injury occurs and how that will be facilitated

  (e) Additional elements

    i. Risk to embryo or fetus

    ii. Additional costs that the participant may need to incur while participating

    iii. Approximate number of individuals expected to participate

    iv. Current institutional review board version and date of consent form

  (4) Clinicians should assess a patient's decision-making capacity prior to the informed consent discussion and provide the participant or their

advocate with information at his or her level of understanding to allow autonomous decision-making (Klimaszewski et al, 2016; ONS, 2016; U.S. FDA, 2019a).

b) Executing the informed consent process (ONS, 2016; U.S. FDA, 2018a, 2019a)

   (1) Provide the participant with a copy of the consent form(s) to read, review, and consider their participation.

   (2) Thoroughly review the contents of the consent form(s), allowing the participant adequate time to ask questions.

   (3) Outline the progression of the protocol and what the participant can expect at each stage, as well as his or her responsibilities as a trial participant.

   (4) Clarify and expand on information given by physicians or delegate by facilitating a meaningful discussion (Farmer & Lundy, 2017).

   (5) Provide and assist the participant in gathering additional relevant sources of information or clarification.

   (6) Emphasize that participation is voluntary. A participant may choose to discontinue participation at any time without penalty or loss of benefits to which they would otherwise be entitled. Emphasize that refusal to participate will involve no penalty or loss of benefits.

   (7) Verify understanding of content on a continual basis (ANA, 2016; Cook, 2016).

   (8) Inform the participant that new information is provided throughout study, and if required, an updated informed consent document is presented to the patient for signature and date.

   (9) Provide ongoing teaching around monitoring and reporting of side effects (e.g., skin reactions, difficulty swallowing, concomitant medications).

   (10) Ensure that the consent is signed and dated and that the participant has a copy for their own reference (Health Canada, 2014; U.S. FDA, 2019a).

7. The OCTN's role in clinical trial patient management (ANA, 2016; Klimaszewski et al., 2016; ONS, 2016)

a) OCTNs should understand the barriers and facilitators to clinical trial recruitment.

b) OCTNs verify that the potential participant meets study eligibility criteria.

c) OCTNs assess the participant for adverse events and assist in the management of side effects.

d) OCTNs provide contact numbers of clinical trials team members and instructions for after-hours care.

e) OCTNs prepare ongoing education for participants regarding how and when to report changes in health status.

f) OCTNs coordinate protocol-related tests and appointments within defined time frames.

g) OCTNs perform timely identification, documentation, and communication of serious or unexpected side effects.

h) OCTNs determine whether a dose-limiting toxicity has occurred based on adverse event assessments and protocol guidelines and communicate this to the study team.

i) OCTNs ensure compliance with the protocol with the following actions (Klimaszewski et al., 2016; ONS, 2016).

   (1) Assess the participant's ability to adhere to protocol requirements (e.g., completing diaries and quality-of-life surveys, keeping the treatment schedule).

   (2) Ensure that protocol guidelines, processes, and procedures are followed.

   (3) Ensure accurate and timely completion of research data.

   (4) Prepare for monitor and auditor reviews.

j) OCTNs facilitate clinical trial–related communication with the following actions (ANA, 2016; CRN 2010 Domain of Practice Committee, 2009; Klimaszewski et al., 2016; ONS, 2016).

   (1) Act as a liaison among the patient, physician, study team, IRB, and study sponsor.

   (2) Provide clinical trial information to healthcare professionals within the organization and develop relationships with referring departments and organizations to promote accrual and improve protocol compliance.

   (3) Coordinate site initiation visits with the study sponsor and study team members.

   (4) Provide community education and outreach regarding clinical trials.

k) OCTNs ensure appropriate clinical trial–related documentation (Klimaszewski et al., 2016; ONS, 2016).

   (1) Follow protocol, institutional, and institutional review board requirements related to appropriate documentation in source data. Documentation must also comply with organizational nursing policies and licensure requirements.

   (2) Educate study team members regarding the protocol, institutional, and institutional review board requirements for documentation in source data.

   (3) Confirm that all data can be verified within source documents.

l) OCTNs ensure ethical practice in the conduct of clinical trials with the following actions (Klimaszewski et al., 2016; ONS, 2016; U.S. FDA, 2018a).

   (1) Adhere to ethical principles, including informed consent, patient autonomy, justice, and beneficence.

   (2) Identify and protect the rights of vulnerable patient populations participating in clinical trials.

(3) Report scientific misconduct according to institutional guidelines.

m) OCTNs practice financial stewardship in the conduct of clinical trials with the following actions (Klimaszewski et al., 2016; ONS, 2016).

  (1) Guide participants in verifying healthcare coverage.

  (2) Identify routine care costs versus research-related costs and the impact on the research participant.

  (3) Identify financial factors that may influence the cost of trial conduct.

n) The privacy and confidentiality of the participant's personal health information should be protected and respected in accordance with local regulatory requirements (U.S. FDA, 2018a). See the following resources for further information.

  (1) American Medical Association: www.ama-assn .org

  (2) European Union General Data Protection Regulation: https://gdpr-info.eu

  (3) Health Insurance Portability and Accountability Act: www.hhs.gov/hipaa/for-professionals/ index.html

  (4) Personal Information Protection and Electronic Documents Act (Canada): www.priv .gc.ca/en/privacy-topics/privacy-laws-in -canada/the-personal-information-protection -and-electronic-documents-act-pipeda/r_o_p

  (5) U.S. Department of Health and Human Services: www.hhs.gov/ocr/privacy

8. Additional resources

  a) ACR Imaging Network: www.acrin.org

  b) Applied Clinical Trials: www.appliedclinicaltrials online.com

  c) ClinicalTrials.gov: https://clinicaltrials.gov

  d) FDA Medical Devices: www.fda.gov/Medical -Devices

  e) NCI: www.cancer.gov

  f) NCI Center for Cancer Research: https://ccr.cancer .gov

  g) NCI Dictionary of Cancer Terms: www.cancer.gov/ dictionary

  h) ONS: www.ons.org

  i) RTOG: www.rtog.org

  j) U.S. Department of Health and Human Services Office for Human Research Protections: www.hhs.gov/ohrp

References

Almquist, D., Mosalpuria, K., & Ganti, A.K. (2016). Multimodality therapy for limited-stage small-cell lung cancer. *Journal of Oncology Practice, 12,* 111–117. https://doi.org/10.1200/JOP.2015.009068

American Cancer Society. (2017). What are the phases of clinical trials? https:// www.cancer.org/treatment/treatments-and-side-effects/clinical-trials/what -you-need-to-know/phases-of-clinical-trials.html

American Nurses Association. (2016). *Clinical research nursing: Scope and standards of practice.*

Brinkman-Denney, S. (2013). An international comparison of the clinical trials nurse role. *Nursing Management, 20,* 32–40. https://doi.org/10.7748 /nm2013.12.20.8.32.e1060

Canadian Cancer Society. (n.d.). Clinical trials. http://www.cancer.ca/en /cancer-information/diagnosis-and-treatment/clinical-trials/?region=on

Canadian Institutes of Health Research, Natural Sciences and Engineering Research Council of Canada, & Social Sciences and Humanities Research Council. (2018). *Tri-Council policy statement: Ethical conduct for research involving humans.* Secretariat on Responsible Conduct of Research. https:// ethics.gc.ca/eng/documents/tcps2-2018-en-interactive-final.pdf

Cancer Research UK. (2019, February 13). Phases of clinical trials. https:// www.cancerresearchuk.org/about-cancer/find-a-clinical-trial/what-clinical -trials-are/phases-of-clinical-trials

Cook, W. (2016). "Sign here": Nursing value and the process of informed consent. *Plastic Surgical Nursing, 36,* 182–186. https://doi.org/10.1097/PSN .0000000000000168

CRN 2010 Domain of Practice Committee. (2009). *Building the foundation for clinical research nursing: Domain of practice for the specialty of clinical research nursing.* National Institutes of Health. http://www.cc.nih.gov/nursing/crn /DOP_document.pdf

Farmer, L., & Lundy, A. (2017). Informed consent: Ethical and legal considerations for advanced practice nurses. *Journal for Nurse Practitioners, 13,* 124–130. https://doi.org/10.1016/j.nurpra.2016.08.011

Health Canada. (2014, August). *Requirements for informed consent documents.* https://www.canada.ca/content/dam/hc-sc/migration/hc-sc/sr-sr/alt _formats/pdf/advice-avis/reb-cer/consent/document-consent-document-eng.pdf

Health Canada. (2018, November 9). Applications for medical device investigational testing authorizations guidance document—Summary. https:// www.canada.ca/en/health-canada/services/drugs-health-products/medical -devices/application-information/guidance-documents/investigational -testing-authorizations-guidance.html

Klimaszewski, A.D., Bacon, M., Eggert, J.A., Ness, E., Westendorp, J.G., & Willenberg, K. (Eds.). (2016). *Manual for clinical trials nursing* (3rd ed.). Oncology Nursing Society.

Matsumoto, K., Nagamura, F., Ogami, Y., Yamashita, N., & Kamibeppu, K. (2011). Difficulties of nursing staff involved in phase 1 oncology trials in Japan. *Cancer Nursing, 34,* 369–375. https://doi.org/10.1097/NCC .0b013e31820809ad

National Cancer Institute. (2020). Informed consent. https://www.cancer.gov /about-cancer/treatment/clinical-trials/patient-safety/informed-consent

National Commission for the Protection of Human Subjects of Biomedical and Behavioral Research. (1979, April 18). *The Belmont Report: Ethical principles and guidelines for the protection of human subjects of research.* https://www .hhs.gov/ohrp/policy/belmont.html

National Comprehensive Cancer Network. (n.d.). Phases of clinical trials. https://www.nccn.org/patients/resources/clinical_trials/phases.aspx

National Institutes of Health. (2017, August 8). NIH's definition of a clinical trial. https://grants.nih.gov/policy/clinical-trials/definition.htm

National Institutes of Health. (2019, January 24). Guidelines on communicating informed consent for individuals who are deaf or hard-of-hearing and scientists. https://www.nih.gov/health-information/nih-clinical-research -trials-you/guidelines-communicating-informed-consent-individuals-who -are-deaf-or-hard-hearing-scientists

Ness, E.A., & Royce, C. (2017). Clinical trials and the role of the oncology clinical trials nurse. *Nursing Clinics of North America, 52,* 133–148. https://doi .org/10.1016/j.cnur.2016.10.005

Oncology Nursing Society. (2016). *2016 oncology clinical trials nurse competencies.* https://www.ons.org/sites/default/files/2018-10/Oncology_Clinical _Trials_Nurse_Competencies.PDF

Purdom, M.A., Petersen, S., & Haas, B.K. (2017). Results of an oncology clinical trial nurse role delineation study. *Oncology Nursing Forum, 44,* 589–595. https://doi.org/10.1188/17.ONF.589-595

Shah, P., Thornton, I., & Hipskind, J.E. (2020, March 30). *Informed consent.* https://www.ncbi.nlm.nih.gov/books/NBK430827

U.S. Food and Drug Administration. (2018a). *E6(R2) good clinical practice: Integrated addendum to ICH E6(R1)*. https://www.fda.gov/media/93884/download

U.S. Food and Drug Administration. (2018b, January 4). What are the different types of clinical research? https://www.fda.gov/forpatients/clinicaltrials/types/default.htm

U.S. Food and Drug Administration. (2019a). A guide to informed consent: Guidance for institutional review boards and clinical investigators. https://www.fda.gov/RegulatoryInformation/Guidances/ucm126431.htm#process

U.S. Food and Drug Administration. (2019b). How to determine if your product is a medical device. https://www.fda.gov/medicaldevices/deviceregulationandguidance/overview/classifyyourdevice/ucm051512.htm

XII. Patient, Caregiver, and Family Education

A. Overview

1. Patient education is a planned, systematic process that uses various techniques such as teaching, counseling, and behavior modification to help people develop and understand health-related behaviors (e.g., knowledge, skills, attitudes, values).

2. It is a sequential, logical, and scientific course of action used to foster a dynamic and interactive process between the teacher and learner, which leads to outcomes of mutually desired behavior changes (Bastable & Gonzalez, 2019).

3. Patient and caregiver education has long been an essential aspect of the role of the professional nurse.

4. Current trends in health care require patients and caregivers to be adequately prepared for self-care and have the requisite knowledge and skills to deliver care (Bastable & Gonzalez, 2019; U.S. Department of Health and Human Services, 2019).

   a) The terms *family caregiver* and *informal caregiver* refer to an unpaid family member, friend, or neighbor who provides care to an individual with an acute or chronic illness who needs assistance to manage a variety of tasks, including ADLs, medical care (e.g., wound care, tube feedings, medications), social support, and advocacy (Berry, Dalwadi, & Jacobson, 2017).

   b) Caregivers are an integral component of the education process. As more outpatient treatments increase in complexity and toxicity, so too do the educational demands on the caregiver, which may lead to caregiver strain (Berry et al., 2017; Nejad, Aghdam, Hassankhani, & Sanaat, 2016). The Family Caregiver Alliance (2019) reported that the majority of caregivers are women, the average caregiver age is 49.2 years old, the average age of a care recipient is 69.4 years old, and of family caregivers who provide complex care, 46% perform medical and nursing tasks.

   c) Caregiver preparedness is associated with lower levels of caregiver role strain. It is essential to assess caregiver readiness when structuring education (Hendrix et al., 2016; Marshall & Hale, 2017).

   d) Caregivers should be educated from a proactive approach to help them understand how to monitor the patient, anticipate issues, and intervene early (Berry et al., 2017).

5. Lack of adequate educational preparation may worsen anxiety and distress in both the patient and caregiver, significantly affecting quality of life and sense of well-being (Berry et al., 2017; Northouse et al., 2014).

6. Negative emotional status, cognitive and physical impairment, lower socioeconomic status, ethnicity, and low literacy may be significant obstacles to patient care and may impact treatment decision-making by the patient and caregivers (Sullivan et al., 2019; Wong & Szumacher, 2012). The use of written materials and decision aids may help to improve the decision-making process and should be presented in a way that is in the best interest of the patient (Sullivan et al., 2019).

B. Learning theories

1. Learning theories provide a framework for patient education (Braungart, Braungart, & Gramet, 2019; Doak, Doak, & Root, 1996).

2. Numerous theories have been proposed over the past decades and originate from various schools of thought, including communications, psychology, education, nursing, sociology, and more contemporary theory related to technology.

3. Nurses should have a familiarity with education theory to achieve optimal patient outcomes and to adjust to any changes in a patient's health or medical condition (Braungart et al., 2019; Syx, 2008).

C. Effective education

1. Components of the patient education process include assessment, planning, implementation, and evaluation (Bastable & Myers, 2019).

2. Evidence suggests that effective education and learner participation are both required and that nurses should assess and implement the appropriate environment that fosters learning through a patient-centric and empowering approach (Bastable & Gonzalez, 2019; Kelliher, 2013).

3. Patient and caregiver participation in healthcare education and decision-making helps to facilitate informed consent and to increase the satisfaction and simultaneously decrease the anxiety associated with cancer treatments (Bonin et al., 2018; Northouse et al., 2014).

D. Role of radiation oncology nurses in education

1. Historically, patient education has been a core role component of the radiation oncology nurse (Abshire & Lang, 2018).

2. Key elements of radiation oncology education include rationale for treatment, treatment modalities, complicated regimens, symptom reporting and management, complex combination therapies, radiation safety, potential late effects of treatment, patient advocacy, and survivorship (Quinn, 2010).

3. The growing complexity of radiation treatments has resulted in complicated decision-making between the provider and patient (Wong & Szumacher, 2012).

   a) The radiation nurse is an essential part of the process and is tasked with explaining treatment regimens, schedules, and possible side effects.

   b) A descriptive study by Güleser, Taşci, and Kaplan (2012) found that 83% of patients who experienced problems during RT wanted to have more information.

c) Addressing educational needs can alleviate caregiver strain, build confidence in meeting care needs, optimize health outcomes, and improve quality of life (Nejad et al., 2016).

E. Rationale for patient education

1. The Patient Care Partnership establishes a patient's right to information about diagnosis, treatment, prognosis, procedures, medical consequences, personnel, and the hospital (American Hospital Association, 2003). The ONS (2019) position statement on quality cancer care outlines a patient's right to information throughout the cancer care continuum.

2. State nurse practice acts and ANA's (2015) *Nursing: Scope and Standards of Practice* define the scope of nursing practice and designate health or patient education as an independent function of the professional nurse.

3. *Oncology Nursing: Scope and Standards of Practice* (Lubejko & Wilson, 2019) states that it is the responsibility of oncology nurses to assess, implement, and evaluate educational programs for patients, significant others/caregivers, and the public. Additionally, *Standards of Oncology Education: Patient/Significant Other and Public* upholds the nursing role of educator and endorses evidence-based practice and current practice trends to achieve quality education (Blecher, Ireland, & Watson, 2016).

4. Accreditation organizations, such as the Joint Commission, have delineated patient safety goals that include educational components (Joint Commission, 2019).

5. Interventional studies of preparatory education for patients receiving RT have measured various outcomes such as patient satisfaction, self-care behaviors, anxiety, distress, and quality of life.

   a) Studies testing various delivery methods for patient education have consistently reported increased patient satisfaction and reduced stress and anxiety with preparatory information (Hyde et al., 2018; Nathoo, 2017; Smith, Milross, & Dhillon, 2016).

   (1) Misconceptions, lack of knowledge, and inadequate communication about treatment may compound anxiety in patients, reduce their sense of control, and decrease their confidence in healthcare professionals (Williams, Blencowe, Ind, & Willis, 2017).

   (2) In a study comparing written materials from hospital radiation departments versus cancer control organizations, Smith et al. (2016) found that patients wanted to receive information on both acute and chronic/long-term side effects of RT. Resources analyzed were more likely to contain more information about short-term effects than long-term side effects (87% vs. 47%).

   b) Other studies have explored the effects that specific interventions have on self-care and the symptom experience.

   (1) Henderson et al. (2013) found that a mindfulness-based stress reduction program intervention for women with breast cancer undergoing RT appeared to facilitate psychosocial adjustment, including better quality of life with enhanced sense of emotional and social-family well-being, greater coping abilities, decreased feelings of helplessness and need for avoidance, and significantly decreased general psychological distress.

   (2) Another study by Park, Chun, Jung, Bae, and Jung (2018) examined the effects of an integrated psychoeducational program for distress management in women newly diagnosed with breast cancer. The program consisted of individual face-to-face education and telephone health coaching sessions. These interventions were effective in reducing distress, determining supportive care needs, and increasing patient quality of life.

   (3) A pilot study by Bergin et al. (2016) developed a novel psychoeducational intervention to improve psychosocial outcomes for gynecologic–oncologic patients treated with RT by combining nursing consultations with telephone peer support during pretreatment, mid-treatment, at the end of treatment, and post-treatment. The intervention was designed to provide tailored support and self-care strategies for physical, psychosocial, and psychosexual effects from RT and was found to be feasible, relevant, and acceptable to participants and clinicians.

   c) Numerous studies have addressed the use of audiovisual materials in patient education.

   (1) Audiovisual aids can be very effective instructional tools that can stimulate the visual and hearing senses and potentially improve information retention (Hainsworth & Keyes, 2019).

   (2) An extensive literature review over the past three decades by Nathoo (2017) found that educational videos have a positive impact on increasing knowledge, understanding and making informed treatment decisions, reducing stress, coping, and enhancing self-care practices that optimize psychological well-being.

   (3) A study by Koss, Bires, Cline, and Mason (2018), which evaluated an educational video aimed at addressing typical concerns about treatment regimens, reported significant value for the patient and caregiver in reducing anxiety and enhancing the ability to absorb new information and instructions.

   (4) A study by Laszewski et al. (2016) found that, when given a choice, patients preferred verbal or video instruction over written instruction.

Providing instructional options may improve overall patient satisfaction with the educational process.

    (5) Innovative, multimodal education tools and computer technology are increasingly being used in clinical settings to improve patient and caregiver understanding and engagement (Saeed, 2018).

       (a) Williams et al. (2017) employed the use of live footage video and three-dimensional visualization software to explain the process for RT.

       (b) Approximately 98% of patients found the videos useful, and 50% reported a decrease in self-reported anxiety levels.

    (6) ONS has made the use of technology for identification of symptoms and symptom management a top priority for oncology nurses (LoBiondo-Wood et al., 2014).

       (a) In a literature review by Carrasco and Symes (2018), electronic assessment of patient-reported symptoms was feasible, acceptable, and easy to use in most studies.

       (b) Symptom reporting was also found to improve symptom detection and management, quality of life, and patient satisfaction.

F. Assessment

1. Learning needs

    a) Learning needs are gaps in knowledge, skills, or attitudes (Kitchie, 2019).

    b) Most patients want to be fully informed about procedures, including risks, benefits, and alternatives, primarily so they can be active participants in their therapy. As such, patients should be provided with clear and accessible information (Bonin et al., 2018; Forshaw, Hall, Boyes, Carey, & Martin, 2017; Saeed, 2018).

    c) The increasing complexity of patient and caregiver needs in health care and nursing responsibilities requires a full understanding of what is important to the patient and caregiver as well and their motivation and readiness to learn (Inott & Kennedy, 2011).

    d) Ongoing assessment is essential, as information needs change over time and exist across the continuum of cancer care (Kitchie, 2019; Piervil, Odedina, & Young, 2019).

    e) Studies have indicated the need to improve patient education on preparation for RT, and it is essential for patients to understand treatment options (Rosenberg et al., 2017; Shabason, Mao, Frankel, & Vapiwala, 2014).

    f) Additionally, in an analysis by Rosenberg et al. (2017), information on academic radiation oncology websites was typically written at an 11th grade level or higher. This information should be targeted to a sixth-grade level for better understanding.

2. Readiness to learn (Kitchie, 2019)

    a) *Readiness* refers to the time when the patient is both receptive and willing to learn.

    b) Four realms of readiness exist: physical, emotional, experiential, and knowledge.

3. Learning style

    a) Learning style is defined as the way that the patient perceives and processes information (Savage, Arif, Smoke, & Farrell, 2017).

    b) Many learning style theories exist.

    c) One commonly used approach to describing learning style is the VARK method developed by Neil Fleming, which represents the visual (V), aural or auditory (A), reading or writing (R), and kinesthetic (K) senses for learning. This style is very conducive to patient education (Auguste, Al-Muhaiteeb, & Chan, 2018; Blevins, 2018; Savage et al., 2017).

       (1) Visual: prefers information through illustrations, pictures, and words (e.g., printed materials)

       (2) Aural or auditory: prefers information by spoken word, discussion, web chat, discussion groups (e.g., nurse verbally explains with minimal distractions that can interfere with hearing)

       (3) Reading or writing: preference for information displayed specifically as words (e.g., written text, reading and writing)

       (4) Kinesthetic: learning through actual doing or manipulation (e.g., practicing with physical aids or simulation)

4. Health literacy

    a) Health literacy is "the degree to which individuals can obtain, process, and understand the basic health information and services they need to make appropriate health decisions" (Papadakos et al., 2018, p. 4202).

    b) As technology continues to expand, having a high health literacy is important to process and handle information, explore new opportunities, and initiate change.

    c) Low literacy is a barrier to patient education and may adversely affect informed consent, self-management, treatment outcomes, and quality of life (Papadakos et al., 2018).

    d) Health literacy skills vary widely.

       (1) An essential component of literacy is the ease with which materials can be read and understood (Lambert & Keogh, 2014; Prabhu et al., 2016).

       (2) The American Medical Association and National Institutes of Health have recommended that reading materials be written

between a third- and a seventh-grade level to meet the needs of the average American (Prabhu et al., 2016).

   (3) More than 80 million American adults have limited health literacy, and the average adult has a seventh- to ninth-grade reading level (Rosenberg et al., 2017).

   e) Screening tools for health literacy
   (1) Screening tools for health literacy include the Rapid Estimate of Adult Literacy in Medicine (Dumenci, Matsuyama, Kuhn, Perera, & Siminoff, 2013) and the Test of Functional Health Literacy in Adults, which has short and long forms available (Housten et al., 2018).
   (2) The U.S. Health Literacy Scale and the Health Literacy Questionnaire are more comprehensive tools that can be used to identify individuals with limited health literacy; however, both are lengthy and may limit practical use in clinical settings (Ylitalo et al., 2018). Descriptions of these tools, including benefits and limitations of use, can be found in a review by Ylitalo et al. (2018).
   (3) The single screening questions, "How confident are you filling out medical forms by yourself?" and "How often do you have someone help you read hospital materials?" were found to be effective in identifying clinic patients with limited and marginal health literacy skills. Limitations in the studies, however, prevent generalization to other populations (Jain, Sheth, Bender, Weisbord, & Green, 2014; University of Arkansas for Medical Sciences Center for Health Literacy, 2017; Woods & Chesser, 2017).

   f) Informal, subtle cues that may indicate low literacy include lack of interest, expression of frustration, slow reading speed, desire to let someone else read first, claims of "forgotten glasses," inability to complete forms, no attempt to seek clarification, diversion of the conversation, or the false appearance of information comprehension (Smith et al., 2013).
   g) Patients aged 65 years and older typically have lower health literacy than that of younger age groups (Chesser, Woods, Smothers, & Rogers, 2016).

G. Planning

1. The patient teaching plan should be formulated with objectives that are SMART—specific, measurable, attainable, realistic, and timed (Revello, 2015).
2. Patients require sensory, procedural, and self-care information tailored to the individual and caregiver early in the course of treatment and throughout the trajectory of illness (Forshaw et al., 2017; Wright et al., 2015).
3. The patient teaching plan may include the following topics.

   a) Goal of treatment
   (1) Cure
   (2) Control
   (3) Palliation
   b) Type of treatment
   (1) EBRT (3DCRT, IMRT, IGRT, SRS, SBRT, proton beam therapy)
   (2) Brachytherapy
   (3) Systemic RT (radiopharmaceuticals, radioimmunotherapy)
   (4) Intraoperative
   (5) Hyperthermia
   (6) Photodynamic therapy
   c) Simulation
   (1) Purpose
   (2) Preparation: disrobing, use of contrast material, laxative, enema
   (3) Description of procedure: duration, staff present, bowel preparation, indwelling catheter, oral/IV contrast, positioning, immobilization devices, x-rays, CT/MRI scans, tattoos
   (4) Postsimulation care: care of markings, laxative
   d) EBRT treatment schedule
   (1) Monday through Friday: once or twice daily
   (2) Total number of fractions and days
   (3) Days to be seen for "status check" appointments with physician and nurse, called *on treatment visit* and usually every fifth treatment
   (4) Days to receive laboratory work, if necessary
   (5) Timing of concurrent chemotherapy/immunotherapy, if necessary
   e) EBRT treatment experience
   (1) Staff administering the treatment
   (2) Positioning
   (3) Video and audio monitoring system
   (4) Sensory aspects: size of machine, sounds of machine, temperature of the room
   (5) Duration
   (6) Port films
   f) Possible side effects
   (1) General and site-specific side effects
   (2) Causes of symptoms
   (3) Expected onset and duration
   (4) Use of medications
   (5) Reassurance that patient is not radioactive with EBRT
   g) Self-care activities
   (1) Preventive measures to initiate at start of treatment
   (2) Interventions to initiate as symptoms develop
   (3) Use of complementary/integrative care therapies
   (4) Activity and nutrition recommendations
   (5) Assessment of caregiver burden and self-care
   h) Physician and nurse contact information
   (1) Indications for calling

     (2) Telephone numbers to call during business hours, evenings, and weekends

   i) Resources for assistance

     (1) Support groups

     (2) Dietitian

     (3) Social worker

     (4) Spiritual care counselor

     (5) Community agencies

     (6) Caregiver support services and resources

   j) Instructions at the completion of treatment

     (1) Treatment side effects, including patterns of recovery and self-care

     (2) Possible emotional effects (e.g., anxiety, worry, distress) during the post-treatment transition related to resumption of social responsibilities, desire to regain a sense of normalcy, loss of continued contact with oncology team, persistent physical symptoms, and fears of cancer recurrence (Bergin et al., 2016; Forshaw et al., 2017; Northouse et al., 2014)

     (3) Resources for psychosocial support and counseling; survivorship programs

     (4) Indications for calling the oncology team prior to a scheduled follow-up visit

   k) Survivorship care: Instructions should be incorporated into a patient's comprehensive SCP and given during the post-treatment or follow-up phase to enhance self-management of living with cancer as a chronic illness (Denlinger et al., 2018; Hewitt, Greenfield, & Stovall, 2006).

     (1) Cancer type, stage, and treatment received

     (2) Potential late effects of treatment and self-care practices to mitigate late effects

     (3) Recommended follow-up schedule and practices, including cancer screening guidelines

     (4) Cancer prevention measures; health promotion activities related to diet, exercise, and smoking cessation; and other behaviors to enhance well-being; health goals

     (5) Community psychosocial resources

     (6) Legal protections regarding employment and access to health insurance

H. Implementation

1. Nurses must include significant others and informal caregivers in teaching.
2. Nurses must work to build a trusting relationship.
3. Nurses should use teaching strategies appropriate for the developmental stage of the learner (Bastable & Myers, 2019).

   a) Older adults are increasingly using computer technology to access information.

     (1) Processing information and recall is often diminished in this population compared to younger adults (Bol, van Weert, de Haes, Loos, & Smets, 2015).

     (2) Bol et al. (2015) found that combining audio-visual information with conversational style is the best way to present eHealth information to both younger and older adults.

   b) Children with cancer treated with RT experience distress as a reaction to confronting fear of procedures, meeting hospital staff, and being separated from parents, often requiring more creative teaching strategies, distraction interventions, and psychological preparation (Engvall et al., 2018).

4. Nurses should schedule time for patient education.
5. An effective learning environment should be private, quiet, and free from distractions.
6. Nurses should attend to a patient's comfort needs before initiating a teaching session.
7. Verbal instruction involves the following techniques.

   a) Avoid using medical or technical terminology.

   b) Divide complex information or tasks into smaller subunits of instruction.

   c) Use advanced organizers or simple category names that are meaningful to the patient.

   d) Tailor or personalize the instruction to fit patient/caregiver needs.

   e) Allow time for questions and answers.

   f) Provide contact information for staff.

8. Learning tools can reinforce verbal instructions.

   a) Print materials matched to the reading skills of the patient

   b) Videotapes

   c) Audiotapes

   d) Computer-assisted instruction

   e) Internet

   f) Flip charts

   g) Models or simulation

   h) Calendars or journals

9. Nurses can use various methods of teaching.

   a) Personal session

   b) Group instruction or class

   c) Family or caregiver conference

   d) Role-play

   e) Demonstration and teach-back

10. Nurses should provide immediate feedback to the learner to increase motivation or the desire to learn (Braungart et al., 2019). Feedback consists of positive reinforcement, such as suggestions for improvement, use of teach-back method, and appropriate readability of educational materials (Vaartio-Rajalin et al., 2015; Wittink & Oosterhaven, 2018).

11. Strategies for teaching patients with low literacy skills include the following (Bastable & Gonzalez, 2019; Wittink & Oosterhaven, 2018).

   a) Using multiple teaching methods and tools

   b) Partitioning information into smaller parts

   c) Speaking slowly and clearly

   d) Using present tense with short sentences

   e) Using vivid visuals

f) Using simple pictures or drawings

g) Encouraging interaction during the educational session

h) Offering examples or testimonials

i) Using audiovisual aids

I. Evaluation

1. Nurses should obtain verbal feedback from patients.
2. Nurses should observe return demonstration.
3. Teaching plans can be modified to enhance learning (Hinkle & Cheever, 2017).
4. Nurses should reinforce learning at subsequent patient visits.

J. Documentation

1. Assessment: In the medical record, document preparedness, identified learning needs, and any other factors that may influence a patient's learning.
2. Planning: Document learning objectives.
3. Implementation: Document who was taught and the topics and methods used.
4. Evaluation: Document the patient's response to teaching, as well as a plan for reinforcement and further evaluation.

K. Selected online resources

1. American Cancer Society: www.cancer.org
2. ASCO: www.asco.org
3. Literacy Information and Communication System: https://lincs.ed.gov
4. Medline Plus: https://medlineplus.gov
5. National Center for Complementary and Integrative Health: www.nccih.nih.gov
6. National Coalition for Cancer Survivorship: www.canceradvocacy.org
7. NCI: www.cancer.gov
8. NCI Office of Cancer Survivorship: https://cancercontrol.cancer.gov/ocs
9. ONS: www.ons.org
10. RT Answers: www.rtanswers.org

References

Abshire, D., & Lang, M.K. (2018). The evolution of radiation therapy in treating cancer. *Seminars in Oncology Nursing, 34,* 151–157. https://doi.org/10.1016/j.soncn.2018.03.006

American Hospital Association. (2003). *The patient care partnership: Understanding expectations, rights and responsibilities.* https://www.aha.org/system/files/2018-01/aha-patient-care-partnership.pdf

American Nurses Association. (2015). *Nursing: Scope and standards of practice* (3rd ed.).

Auguste, B.L., Al-Muhaiteeb, A., & Chan, C.T. (2018). The effect of learning styles on adverse events in home hemodialysis patients. *Clinical Journal of the American Society of Nephrology, 13,* 782–783. https://doi.org/10.2215/CJN.12161017

Bastable, S.B., & Gonzalez, K.M. (2019). Overview of education in health care. In S.B. Bastable (Ed.), *Nurse as educator: Principles of teaching and learning for nursing practice* (5th ed., pp. 3–34). Jones and Bartlett Learning.

Bastable, S.B., & Myers, G.M. (2019). Developmental stages of the learner. In S.B. Bastable (Ed.), *Nurse as educator: Principles of teaching and learning for nursing practice* (5th ed., pp 169–218). Jones and Bartlett Learning.

Bergin, R.J., Grogan, S.M., Bernshaw, D., Juraskova, I., Penberthy, S., Mileshkin, L.R., ... Schofield, P.E. (2016). Developing an evidence-based, nurse-led psychoeducational intervention with peer support in gynecologic oncology. *Cancer Nursing, 39,* E19–E30. https://doi.org/10.1097/NCC.0000000000000263

Berry, L.L., Dalwadi, S.M., & Jacobson, J.O. (2017). Supporting the supporters: What family caregivers need to care for a loved one with cancer. *American Society of Clinical Oncology, 13,* 35–41. https://doi.org/10.1200/JOP.2016.017913

Blecher, C.S., Ireland, A.M., & Watson, J.L. (2016). *Standards of oncology education: Patient/significant other and public* (4th ed). Oncology Nursing Society.

Blevins, S. (2018). Nurses as educators: The art of patient education. *MedSurg Nursing, 27,* 401–402.

Bol, N., van Weert, J.C.M., de Haes, H.C.J.M., Loos, E.F., & Smets, E.M.A. (2015). The effect of modality and narration style on recall of online health information: Results from a Web-based experiment. *Journal of Medical Internet Research, 17,* e104. https://doi.org/10.2196/jmir.4164

Bonin, K., McGuffin, M., Lechtman, E., Cumal, A., Harth, T., Calabrese, E., ... Szumacher, E. (2018). Evaluation of an online education resource on radiation therapy created for patients with postprostatectomy prostate cancer and their caregivers. *Journal of Medical Imaging and Radiation Sciences, 49,* 365–370. https://doi.org/10.1016/j.jmir.2018.07.007

Braungart, M.M., Braungart, R.G., & Gramet, P.R. (2019). Applying learning theories to healthcare practice. In S.B. Bastable (Ed.), *Nurse as educator: Principles of teaching and learning for nursing practice* (5th ed., pp. 69–116). Jones and Bartlett Learning.

Carrasco, S., & Symes, L. (2018). Patient use of electronic methods to self-report symptoms: An integrative literature review. *Oncology Nursing Forum, 45,* 399–416. https://doi.org/10.1188/18.ONF.399-416

Chesser, A.K., Woods, N.K., Smothers, K., & Rogers, N. (2016). Health literacy and older adults: A systematic review. *Gerontology and Geriatric Medicine, 2,* 1–13. https://doi.org/10.1177/2333721416630492

Denlinger, C.S., Sanft, T., Baker, K.S., Broderick, G., Demark-Wahnefried, W., Friedman, D.L., ... Freedman-Cass, D.A. (2018). Survivorship, version 2.2018; NCCN Clinical Practice Guidelines in Oncology. *Journal of the National Comprehensive Cancer Network, 16,* 1216–1247. https://doi.org/10.6004/jnccn.2018.0078

Doak, C.C., Doak, L.G., & Root, J.H. (1996). *Teaching patients with low literacy skills* (2nd ed.). Lippincott.

Dumenci, L., Matsuyama, R.K., Kuhn, L., Perera, R.A., & Siminoff, L.A. (2013). On the validity of the shortened Rapid Estimate of Adult Literacy in Medicine (REALM) scale as a measure of health literacy. *Communication Methods and Measures, 7,* 134–143. https://doi.org/10.1080/19312458.2013.789839

Engvall, G., Lindh, V., Mullaney, T., Nyholm, T., Lindh, J., & Ångström-Brännström, C. (2018). Children's experiences and response towards an intervention for psychological preparation for radiotherapy. *Radiation Oncology, 13,* 9. https://doi.org/10.1186/s13014-017-0942-5

Family Caregiver Alliance. (2019, April 17). Caregiver statistics: Demographics. https://www.caregiver.org/caregiver-statistics-demographics

Forshaw, K., Hall, A.E., Boyes, A.W., Carey, M.L., & Martin, J. (2017). Patients' experiences of preparation for radiation therapy: A qualitative study. *Oncology Nursing Forum, 44,* E1–E9. https://doi.org/10.1188/17.ONF.E1-E9

Güleser, G.N., Taşci, S., & Kaplan, B. (2012). The experience of symptoms and information needs of cancer patients undergoing radiotherapy. *Journal of Cancer Education, 27,* 46–53. https://doi.org/10.1007/s13187-011-0254-7

Hainsworth, D.S., & Keyes, K. (2019). Instructional materials. In S.B. Bastable (Ed.), *Nurse as educator: Principles of teaching and learning for nursing practice* (5th ed., pp. 505–548). Jones and Bartlett Learning.

Henderson, V.P., Massion, A.O., Clemow, L., Hurley, T.G., Druker, S., & Hébert, J.R. (2013). A randomized controlled trial of mindfulness-based stress reduction for women with early-stage breast cancer receiving radiotherapy. *Integrative Cancer Therapies, 12,* 404–413. https://doi.org/10.1177/1534735412473640

Hendrix, C.C., Bailey, D.E., Jr., Steinhauser, K.E., Olsen, M.K., Stechuchak, K.M., Lowman, S.G., ... Tulsky, J.A. (2016). Effects of enhanced caregiver training program on cancer caregiver's self-efficacy, preparedness, and psychological well-being. *Supportive Care in Cancer, 24,* 327–336. https://doi.org/10.1007/s00520-015-2797-3

Hewitt, M., Greenfield, S., & Stovall, E. (Eds.). (2006). *From cancer patient to cancer survivor: Lost in transition.* https://doi.org/10.17226/11468

Hinkle, J.L., & Cheever, K.H. (2017). *Brunner and Suddarth's textbook of medical-surgical nursing* (14th ed.). Wolters Kluwer Health/Lippincott Williams and Wilkins.

Housten, A.J., Lowenstein, L.M., Hoover, D.S., Leal, V.B., Kamath, G.R., & Volk, R.J. (2018). Limitations of the S-TOFHLA in measuring poor numeracy: A cross-sectional study. *BMC Public Health, 18,* 1–9. https://doi.org/10.1186/s12889-018-5333-9

Hyde, L., Mackenzie, L., Boyes, A.W., Evans, T.-J., Symonds, M., & Sanson-Fisher, R. (2018). Prevalence and correlates of patient-centered preparatory information provision to computed tomography and magnetic resonance imaging outpatients: A cross-sectional study. *Patient Education and Counseling, 101,* 1814–1822. https://doi.org/10.1016/j.pec.2018.05.025

Inott, T., & Kennedy, B.B. (2011). Assessing learning styles: Practical tips for patient education. *Nursing Clinics of North America, 46,* 313–320. https://doi.org/10.1016/j.cnur.2011.05.006

Jain, D., Sheth, H., Bender, F.H., Weisbord, S.D., & Green, J.A. (2014). Evaluation of a single-item screening question to detect limited health literacy in peritoneal dialysis patients. *Advances in Peritoneal Dialysis, 30,* 27–30.

Joint Commission. (2019). *Hospital national patient safety goals.* https://www.jointcommission.org/assets/1/6/2019_HAP_NPSGs_final2.pdf

Kelliher, F. (2013). *Nurses and patient education.* Association française pour le développement de l'éducation thérapeutique. https://www.connecting-nurses.com/-/media/Project/One-Sanofi-Web/Websites/Global/Connecting-Nurses/Home/disease-knowledge/nurse-practice-education/afdet-nurses-patient-education.pdf

Kitchie, S. (2019). Determinants of learning. In S.B. Bastable (Ed.), *Nurse as educator: Principles of teaching and learning for nursing practice* (5th ed., pp. 119–162). Jones and Bartlett Learning.

Koss, T.S., Bires, A.M., Cline, T.W., & Mason, D.L. (2018). Evaluation of an educational video: What to expect on the first day of chemotherapy. *Critical Care Nursing Quarterly, 41,* 142–160. https://doi.org/10.1097/CNQ.0000000000000194

Lambert, V., & Keogh, D. (2014). Health literacy and its importance for effective communication. Part 1. *Nursing Children and Young People, 26,* 31–37. https://doi.org/10.7748/ncyp2014.04.26.3.31.e387

Laszewski, P., Zelko, C., Andriths, L., Vera Cruz, E., Bauer, C., & Magnan, M.A. (2016). Patient preference for instructional reinforcement regarding prevention of radiation dermatitis. *Clinical Journal of Oncology Nursing, 20,* 187–191. https://doi.org/10.1188/16.CJON.187-191

LoBiondo-Wood, G., Brown, C.G., Knobf, M.T., Lyon, D., Mallory, G., Mitchell, S.A., ... Fellman, B. (2014). Priorities for oncology nursing research: The 2013 national survey. *Oncology Nursing Forum, 41,* 67–76. https://doi.org/10.1188/14.ONF.67-76

Lubejko, B.G., & Wilson, B.J. (2019). *Oncology nursing: Scope and standards of practice.* Oncology Nursing Society.

Marshall, K., & Hale, D. (2017). Caregiver education and support. *Home Healthcare Now, 36,* 341–342. https://doi.org/10.1097/NHH.0000000000000554

Nathoo, D. (2017). Video material as an effective educational tool to address informational and educational needs of cancer patients undergoing radiation therapy. *Journal of Cancer Education, 32,* 219–227. https://doi.org/10.1007/s13187-015-0933-x

Nejad, Z.K., Aghdam, M.A., Hassankhani, H., & Sanaat, Z. (2016). The effects of a patient-caregiver education and follow-up program on the Breast Cancer Caregiver Strain Index. *Iranian Red Crescent Medical Journal, 18,* 1–6. https://doi.org/10.5812/ircmj.21627

Northouse, L., Schafenacker, A., Barr, K.L., Katapodi, M., Yoon, H., Brittain, K., ... An, L. (2014). A tailored web-based psychoeducational intervention for cancer patients and their family caregivers. *Cancer Nursing, 37,* 321–330. https://doi.org/10.1097/NCC.0000000000000159

Oncology Nursing Society. (2019). *Access to quality cancer care* [Position statement]. https://www.ons.org/sites/default/files/2019-05/Access_to_Quality_Cancer_Care_2019.pdf

Papadakos, J.K., Hasan, S.M., Barnsley, J., Berta, W., Fazelzad, R., Papadakos, C.J., ... Howell, D. (2018). Health literacy and cancer self-management behaviors: A scoping review. *Cancer, 124,* 4202–4210. https://doi.org/10.1002/cncr.31733

Park, J.H., Chun, M., Jung, Y.S., Bae, S.H., & Jung, Y.M. (2018). Psychoeducational approach to distress management of newly diagnosed patients with breast cancer. *Journal of the Korean Academy of Nursing, 48,* 669–678. https://doi.org/10.4040/jkan.2018.48.6.669

Piervil, E., Odedina, F., & Young, M.E. (2019). The role and influence of prostate cancer caregivers across the care continuum. *Health Promotion Practice, 20,* 436–444. https://doi.org/10.1177/1524839918764667

Prabhu, A.V., Gupta, R., Kim, C., Kashkoush, A., Hansberry, D.R., Agarwal, N., & Koch, E. (2016). Patient education materials in dermatology: Addressing the health literacy needs of patients. *JAMA Dermatology, 152,* 946–947. https://doi.org/10.1001/jamadermatol.2016.1135

Quinn, K.L. (2010). The role of the radiation oncology nurse: Being the best that you can be. *Oncology Nurse Advisor,* 34–36. https://2k9bc93shxit2dn8sp21nwtz-wpengine.netdna-ssl.com/wp-content/uploads/sites/13/2019/01/ona_radiation0510_3274.pdf

Revello, K. (2015). An educational intervention to increase nurse adherence in eliciting patient daily goals. *Rehabilitation Nursing, 40,* 320–326. https://doi.org/10.1002/rnj.201

Rosenberg, S.A., Francis, D.M., Hullet, C.R., Morris, Z.S., Brower, J.V., Anderson, B.M., ... Kimple, R.J. (2017). Online patient information from radiation oncology departments is too complex for the general population. *Practical Radiation Oncology, 7,* 57–62. https://doi.org/10.1016/j.prro.2016.07.008

Saeed, N. (2018). Patient education in radiation oncology: Evolution and innovation. *Applied Radiation Oncology, 7,* 43–49. https://pdfs.semanticscholar.org/644d/ff3f1da7374e3dd79326149b5810a96491bc.pdf

Savage, K., Arif, S., Smoke, M., & Farrell, T. (2017). Preferences in learning styles and modes of information delivery in patients receiving first-day education for radiation therapy. *Journal of Medical Imaging and Radiation Sciences, 48,* 193–198. https://doi.org/10.1016/j.jmir.2016.10.011

Shabason, J.E., Mao, J.J., Frankel, E.S., & Vapiwala, N. (2014). Shared decision-making and patient control in radiation oncology: Implications for patient satisfaction. *Cancer, 120,* 1863–1870. https://doi.org/10.1002/cncr.28665

Smith, S.K., Milross, B.Y., & Dhillon, H.M. (2016). Radiation therapy for people with cancer: What do written information materials tell them? *European Journal of Cancer Care, 25,* 675–685. https://doi.org/10.1111/ecc.12366

Smith, S.K., Zhu, Y., Dhillon, H.M., Milross, C.G., Taylor, J., Halkett, G., & Zilliacus, E. (2013). Supporting patients with low health literacy: What role do radiation therapists play? *Supportive Care in Cancer, 21,* 3051–3061. https://doi.org/10.1007/s00520-013-1875-7

Sullivan, D.R., Eden, K.B., Dieckmann, N.F., Golden, S.E., Vranas, K.C., Nugent, S.M., & Slatore, C.G. (2019). Understanding patients' values and preferences regarding early stage lung cancer treatment decision making. *Lung Cancer, 131,* 47–57. https://doi.org/10.1016/j.lungcan.2019.03.009

Syx, R.L. (2008). The practice of patient education: The theoretical perspective. *Orthopaedic Nursing, 27,* 50–54. https://doi.org/10.1097/01.NOR.0000310614.31168.6b

University of Arkansas for Medical Sciences Center for Health Literacy. (2017, January 27). *Patient health literacy measures.* https://afmc.org/wp-content/uploads/2017/01/Literacy-Tools-UAMS-CHL-DHS-2017.pdf

U.S. Department of Health and Human Services (2019, October 23). About the Affordable Care Act. https://www.hhs.gov/healthcare/about-the-aca/index.html

Vaartio-Rajalin, H., Huumonen, T., Iire, L., Jekunen, A., Leino-Kilpi, H., Minn, H., & Paloniemi, J. (2015). Patient education process in oncologic context:

What, why, and by whom? *Nursing Research, 64,* 381–390. https://doi.org/10.1097/NNR.0000000000000114

Williams, K., Blencowe, J., Ind, M., & Willis, D. (2017). Meeting radiation therapy patients informational needs through educational videos augmented by 3D visualisation software. *Journal of Medical Radiation Sciences, 64,* 35–40. https://doi.org/10.1002/jmrs.220

Wittink, H., & Oosterhaven, J. (2018). Patient education and health literacy. *Musculoskeletal Science and Practice, 38,* 120–127. https://doi.org/10.1016/j.msksp.2018.06.004

Wong, J., & Szumacher, E. (2012). Patients' decision-making in radiation oncology. *Expert Review of Pharmacoeconomics and Outcomes Research, 12,* 95–104. https://doi.org/10.1586/erp.11.82

Woods, N.K., & Chesser, A.K. (2017). Validation of a single question health literacy screening tool for older adults. *Gerontology and Geriatric Medicine, 3,* 1–4. https://doi.org/10.1177/2333721417713095

Wright, K.M., Simpson, G.K., Koh, E.-S., Whiting, D., Gillet, L., Simpson, T., & Firth, R. (2015). Development and evaluation of information resources for patients, families, and healthcare providers addressing behavioral and cognitive sequelae among adults with a primary brain tumor. *Journal of Neuroscience Nursing, 47,* 135–145. https://doi.org/10.1097/JNN.0000000000000132

Ylitalo, K.R., Meyer, M.R.U., Lanning, B.A., During, C., Laschober, R., & Griggs, J.O. (2018). Simple screening tools to identify limited health literacy in a low-income patient population. *Medicine, 97,* e0110. https://doi.org/10.1097/MD.0000000000010110

Index

The letter *f* after a page number indicates that relevant content appears in a figure; the letter *t*, in a table.

bladder cancer, 129
  documentation of, 242
  incidence/risk factors, 240
  management of, 242–243
  patient/family education on, 243
  resources on, 242
  sexual dysfunction with, 72
  signs/symptoms of, 240–241
  staging of, 241
  treatment options for, 241–242
Bladder Cancer Advocacy Network, 243
bladder dysfunction, 129–130
bleomycin, 275
blindness, 376–377
body fluids, radioactivity of, 24, 28–29
body image, 355
body scan (relaxation technique), 42
bolus, 302
bone fractures, 135–136, 270, 326
bone marrow, 100, 321
bone metastases
  assessment of, 155
  incidence of, 154
  management of, 155–156
  pathophysiology of, 154
  patient/family education on, 157
  prognosis for, 154–155
  RT side effects, 156–157
bone sarcomas, 265
  chemotherapy/immunotherapy for, 267
  diagnosis of, 267
  incidence of, 265
  patient/family education on, 271
  prognostic factors, 265–266
  proton beam therapy for, 339
  risk factors for, 266–267
  RT options for, 267–269
  RT side effects, 269–271
  staging for, 265
  survivorship issues, 271
boost (extra RT dose), 204, 331
brachial plexopathy, 125–127, 212–213
brachytherapy, 6, 19, 20t–21t, 24, 29–31, 304
  for bladder cancer, 242
  for breast cancer, 207
  with cobalt-60, 342
  equipment for, 306
  for female pelvic cancers, 255
  for head and neck, 308
  HDR, 305–306, 309
  indications for, 306
  LDR, 305, 309
  for lung cancer, 219–220, 308–309
  management of, 306–309
  patient/family education on, 310
  potential risks of, 306
  procedure for, 304–306
  for prostate cancer, 245–247
  for pterygium, 309–310
  for soft tissue sarcomas, 268
Bragg Peak, 208
brain/CNS cancers
  acute RT side effects, 160–172
  assessment/documentation of effects, 160, 167f

cognitive changes with, 389
  incidence/epidemiology of, 159–160
  late RT side effects, 105–111, 174–178
  localized symptoms of, 166t–167t
  management of effects, 167
  palliative RT with, 454
  patient/family education on, 168
  proton beam therapy for, 339
  resources on, 168f
  RT standard of care, 160, 161t–165t
  SRS for, 312
  subacute RT side effects, 172–174
  tumor categories, 159
BRCA1/BRCA2 gene mutations, 209
breakthrough pain, 58
breast cancer
  acute RT side effects, 209–210
  brachial plexopathy with, 126–127, 212–213
  brachytherapy for, 207
  cardiac effects from RT, 143–144
  effects in survivorship, 447
  incidence of, 202
  late side effects of RT, 210–214
  with lymphoma, 276
  in men, 70
  patient/family education on, 212
  postmastectomy RT, 207
  pregnancy after, 213–214
  proton beam therapy for, 339
  RT dosages/fractionation, 204–205
  RT techniques for, 205–208
  sexual dysfunction with, 70
  staging of, 202
  targeted tissue/radiation field for, 203–204
  treatment goals for, 202–203
breast-conserving surgery, 203
bronchial injury/stenosis, after SRS, 316–317
bronchiolitis obliterans syndrome, 325
bystander effects, 421

C

cachexia, 38, 87. See also malnutrition
CAGE tool, 408–409
Canada's Food Guide, 96
Canadian Association of Nurses in Oncology
  (CANO), 1, 450
Canadian Association of Psychosocial Oncol-
  ogy, 64–65
Canadian Cancer Society, 450
Canadian Nuclear Safety Commission, 21, 32
Canadian Nutrition Screening Tool, 88
Canadian Problem Checklist, 63
Canadian Radiation Protection Bureau,
  21–22
cancer cachexia. See cachexia
Cancer Care Ontario, 2
Cancer Financial Assistance Coalition, 381
Cancer Index, 67
Cancer Support Community, 67
cancer survivorship. See survivorship
cancer-related anemia. See anemia
cancer-related fatigue (CRF). See fatigue
Cancer.Net, 43, 67

CancerCare, 67, 381
cannabis, medical, 59
capecitabine, 416–417
capsular contracture, after breast cancer RT,
  214
carboplatin, 418
carcinogenesis, 7
cardiac implantable electronic device (CIED),
  146–150, 369
cardiac injury/toxicity, 142
  in AYA patients, 356
  from combination therapy, 145–146
  from HSCT, 326
  with lymphoma, 276
  pathophysiology of, 142–146
  prevention of, 150
  risk-based monitoring plan, 148, 149f
  surveillance of, 150–151
  from thoracic RT, 124–125, 143, 213, 224–
  225
  types of, 144–145
cardio-oncology, 151–152. See also cardiac
  injury/toxicity
cardiomyopathy, 326
cardiopulmonary resuscitation (CPR), 31–32
caregiver burden, 396
caregivers, defined, 461. See also patient/
  caregiver/family education
cataracts, 17, 325–326
caution signs, 27–28, 28f
Cavilon No Sting Barrier Film, 53
cell cycle phase, radiosensitivity in, 8
cell death, radiation-induced, 7
Center for Cancer Research (NCI), 459
Centers for Disease Control and Prevention
  (CDC), 77
centigray (cGy), 6
cerebellar mutism syndrome, 349–350
cerebral AVM, 281–282
cerebrovascular accident (stroke), 120–121
certified nurse midwife, 2
certified registered nurse anesthetist, 1–2
cervical cancer, 255
  sexual dysfunction with, 71–72
  treatment for, 256
cesium-137, 19
  half-value layer of, 26
  in LDR treatment, 6
cetuximab, 415–416
Charlson comorbidity index, 363
CHECKMATE immunotherapy trials, 218
chemoreceptor trigger zone, 232
chemotherapy. See also combined/concurrent
  modality therapy
  cardiotoxicity of, 145
  with RT, 9, 415–420, 447–448
  for spinal cord compression, 292
  for SVCS, 295
child life specialist, 346
children. See pediatric patients
Children's Oncology Group, 271, 345, 350,
  450
chondrosarcoma, 265
chordoma, 265
choroid plexus tumors, 159

K

Karnofsky Performance Scale, 167f
Kegel exercises, 75
keloids, 279–280
ketamine, 347
KEYNOTE immunotherapy trials, 218, 433
kidney cancer, SBRT for, 314–315
kidney dysfunction, from HSCT, 326–328
kilovoltage x-ray imagers, 11

L

lactation
    after breast cancer RT, 213
    during radiopharmaceutical therapy, 427–429
language/culture concerns, 382–383
lanolin, 53
late effects, 105
    of brain/CNS RT, 105–111
    defined, 15
    of head and neck RT, 111–122
    of lung cancer RT, 222–226
    in pediatric populations, 384, 450
    of radiopharmaceuticals, 428
    sexual, 69
    in survivorship, 446–449
late-responding tissues, 8
learning needs, assessment of, 463
learning styles, 463
learning theories, 461
Lee Index, 394
Lesbian, gay, bisexual, transgender, queer or
    questioning (LGBTQ) patients, 70, 77,
    384
leucovorin, 416
leukemia
    with lymphoma, 276
    radiation-induced, 17
    TLI for, 335–336
Leukemia and Lymphoma Society, 328, 381
leukoencephalopathy, RT-induced, 178
Lewy body dementia, 388
Lhermitte sign, 198–199, 223–224, 276–277
Li-Fraumeni syndrome, 266, 269
licensure, 2
Life Span Study of atomic bomb survivors, 17
ligand, 421
linear accelerator-based SRS, 315
linear accelerators, 5, 5f, 11, 304
linear energy transfer (LET), 9, 17
linear no-threshold model, of effect risk, 17
Literacy Information and Communication
    System, 466
liver cancer, 314, 339
liver metastasis, 314
liver toxicities
    from HSCT, 324
    from SRS, 317
Livestrong Foundation, 85, 441, 450
Living Out Loud, 356
localization, 302, 316

long-term effects
    in pediatric populations, 450
    sexual, 69
    on skin, 55
    in survivorship, 446–449
*Long-Term Survivorship Care After Cancer
    Treatment: Proceedings of a Workshop*, 441
longitudinal model, of survivorship care,
    445
loop diuretics, 296
loperamide, 238, 251
low-dose-rate (LDR) treatment, 6, 305, 309
low-energy gamma emitters, 24
lung cancer, 216–217
    acute RT side effects, 220–222
    brachytherapy for, 308–309
    distress with, 62
    effects in survivorship, 447–448
    late RT effects, 222–226
    with lymphoma, 276
    proton beam therapy for, 339
    RT techniques, 219–220
    sexual dysfunction with, 73
lung metastases, 218, 314, 454
lutetium-177, 422–424, 424t–425t
lymphedema
    with breast cancer, 210–211, 447
    with head and neck cancers, 121–123
    with uterine cancer, 448
lymphomas, 272–273
    incidence of, 273
    pregnancy with, 277
    presentation/diagnosis of, 273
    prognostic factors, 273–274
    RT options for, 274
    RT side effects, 274–277
    staging of, 273
    types of, 274, 275t

M

MacArthur Competence Assessment Tool,
    366
major depressive episodes, 402
major histocompatibility complex (MHC)
    molecules, 433, 434f
male fertility issues, 81–84, 132. *See also* infer-
    tility
male sexual dysfunction, 69–70, 72–73,
    75–77. *See also* sexual function/
    dysfunction
malignant pleural mesothelioma, 218
malnutrition, 87–90. *See also* nutritional
    deficits/disturbances
    with abdominal RT, 230
    in older adults, 365
    in pediatric patients, 348
    screening/assessment for, 87–89
Malnutrition Screening Tool, 88, 230
Managing Cancer Side Effects, 96
Manual for Clinical Trials Nursing (ONS),
    456
Masaoka-Koga system, for thymic cancer stag-
    ing, 218

mass dose, in radioimmunotherapy, 421
MD Anderson Symptom Inventory, 63
measurement, of radiation, 6–7
medical cannabis, 59
medical device trials, 455–456, 459
medical sources, of radiation exposure,
    18–19
meditation, 42
Medline Plus, 466
megaelectron volt (McV), 5
megavoltage imagers, 5, 11
megavolts (MV), 5
megestrol acetate, 231
memory, 387
meningiomas, 159, 283, 312–313
Mepilex dressings, 54
Mepitel film dressing, 54
mesothelioma, 218
methotrexate, 267
millicuries (mCi), 7
millirem (mrem), 7
mindfulness-based stress reduction, 66, 462
Mini Nutritional Assessment, 230, 365
Mini-Cog assessment, 366, 389–390
Mini-Mental Status Exam, 366
mirtazapine, for sleep disturbance, 41
misrepair, 7
mitomycin C, 415, 418
mixed dementia, 388
mobility, in older adults, 364
moist desquamation, 46
    assessment of, 48
    management of, 55
moisturizers, 49–54
mometasone furoate, 53
monitoring devices, 26–27, 27f
monoamine oxidase (MAO) inhibitors, for
    depression management, 41
Montreal Cognitive Assessment, 366, 390
mucositis, 92–93
    documentation of, 183
    from HSCT, 321
    management of, 183
    pathophysiology of, 181–182
    patient/family education on, 183–184
    vaginal, 260–261
Multidimensional Fatigue Inventory, 40
Multidimensional Functional Assessment
    Questionnaire, 365
multidisciplinary clinic model, of survivor-
    ship care, 445
multileaf collimators, 86, 302
multimodal therapy. *See* combined/
    concurrent modality therapy
muscle metabolism, 37
music therapy, 66
mutations, 7, 209
mycosis fungoides, 330
myelopathy
    of cranial nerves, 108, 174–175
    with lung cancer RT, 223–224
myelosuppression, during radiopharmaceuti-
    cal therapy, 430
myelotoxicity, 99
myocardial disease, 144–145

ovarian transposition, 71–72, 82
oxaliplatin, 418
oxybutynin, 249
oxygen, radiosensitivity affected by, 8, 415
oxygenation, of tumor cells, 415

P

pacemakers, 146–147
PACIFIC trial, 433, 437
packed RBCs, for anemia, 40
paclitaxel, 418
pain
   assessment/screening of, 58–59
   barriers to assessment of, 58–59
   documentation of, 59
   incidence/prevalence of, 58
   management of, 40, 44, 59–60
   in older adults, 392–393
   pathophysiology of, 58
   patient/family education on, 59–60
pain flare
   during bone metastases RT, 156–157
   during radiopharmaceutical therapy, 430
palladium-103, 29
palliative care, 452
   for AYA patients, 356
   barriers to, 452–453
   nursing role in, 453
   recommendations for, 453
palliative RT, 13, 59, 62, 453–454
   for bone/soft tissue sarcomas, 269
   for breast cancer, 203
   for prostate cancer, 245
Pan-Canadian Oncology Symptom Triage and
   Remote Support, 67
pancreatic cancer, 62, 314
pancytopenia, 322–323
panic disorder, 404
parallel OARs, 10
paraspinal nerve tumors, 159
parenteral nutrition, 94–95
Parkinson disease, 388
parotitis, 322
partial-breast RT, 204–206
Particle Therapy Co-Operative Group, 341
particulate radiation, 5, 5f, 300
pathologic staging, 202
Patient Care Partnership, 462
Patient Health Questionnaire, 63
patient positioning, 302
patient- and family-centered care, for pediatric cancer, 345
Patient-Reported Outcomes CTCAE
   (PRO-CTCAE), 43, 63
Patient's Assessment of Own Functioning
   Inventory, 177
patient/caregiver/family education, 461
   assessment in, 463–464
   documentation of, 466
   evaluation of, 466
   implementation of, 465–466
   nurses' role in, 461–462
   planning of, 464–465

rationale for, 462–463
   resources on, 466
PD-1/PD-L1 proteins, 433
pediatric cancers
   differences vs. adult cancers, 345
   incidence of, 345
   proton beam therapy for, 339
   RT planning/treatment, 345–347
Pediatric Oncology Group of Ontario, 450
pediatric patients, 383–384
   in clinical trials, 350–351
   long-term follow-up of, 350, 384
   nutritional issues in, 348–349
   psychosocial support for, 347–348
   sedation/anesthesia for, 346–347, 383
   siblings of, 348
   survivorship in, 350, 384, 449–450
pembrolizumab, 433
pemetrexed, 419
penile cancer, 73
Penn Medicine, OncoLife survivorship template, 442
pentoxifylline, 193, 196
Perception of Cognition Questionnaire, 177
pericardial disease, 144
periodontitis, 187–188
peripheral blood stem cells, 321
peripheral neuropathy, 224, 270
permanent brachytherapy, 6
Personal Health Questionnaires (PHQs),
   400
Personal Information Protection and Electronic Documents Act (Canada), 459
personal monitoring devices, 26–27, 27f
personalized cancer survivorship care model,
   446
phenazopyridine, 249
phobias, 403–404
phosphodiesterase type 5 (PDE5) inhibitors,
   76, 253, 448
physical activity
   for distress management, 66
   for fatigue management, 41–42
physical disability, 375–376
physical half-life, 421
Piper Fatigue Score-12, 40
pituitary adenoma, 313
Planning Healthy Meals, 96
planning OAR volume, 10
planning target volume (PTV), 10, 10f, 11
pleural mesothelioma, 218
pneumonitis
   after SRS, 316
   after thoracic RT, 123–124, 447
   with breast cancer RT, 212
   with lung cancer RT, 222–223
   with lymphoma, 275
   with RT and immunotherapy, 437
pocket ion chamber dosimeters, 27
polypharmacy, in older adults, 363
POPLAR immunotherapy trial, 218
portal imaging, 302
positioning, of patient, 302
post-radiation fibrosis, 47, 449. See also skin
   reactions

post-traumatic stress disorder, 271, 355,
   404
potassium-40, 18
pregnancy
   after breast cancer, 213–214
   in cancer patients, 85–86
   lymphoma during, 277
   radiation exposure in, 31
   risks/protection during, 86
prescriptive authority, of nurse practitioners, 2
preventive clinical trials, 456
primary hepatocellular carcinoma, 314
Princess Margaret Cancer Foundation, 97
privacy/confidentiality, in clinical trials, 459
probiotics, 238
procedure-related pain, 58
processing speed, 386
proctitis, RT-induced, 128–129, 258, 448
professional nursing practice, 1–2
progestins, 231
progressive muscle relaxation, 42, 67
proliferative capacity, radiosensitivity in, 8
prophylactic treatment, RT as, 12–13
propofol, 347
prostate cancer
   diagnosis of, 243–244
   effects in survivorship, 448
   genitourinary side effects, 247–250
   proton beam therapy for, 338–339
   quality of life with, 247
   SBRT for, 314
   sexual dysfunction with, 72
   treatment options for, 244
prostate implants, 29–31. See also brachytherapy
prostatectomy, 245
proton beam therapy, 86, 145, 300, 315
   administration of, 340
   for bone sarcomas, 269
   for breast cancer, 208
   history of, 337
   indications for, 338–339
   for lung cancer, 220
   patient/family education on, 340–341
   planning/setup for, 339–340
   principles of, 337–338
   for prostate cancer, 245–246
   resources on, 341
protons, 5, 300, 337
pruritus, 46, 54
psychiatric disorders, 401–402. See also
   distress
psychosocial distress. See distress
psychosocial interventions
   for fatigue, 42
   for pediatric patients, 347–348
   for sexual dysfunction, 74–75
psychotropic medications, 405t–406t
psyllium, 251
pterygium, 309–310
pulmonary complications, from HSCT,
   325
pure alpha particle emitters, 23
pure beta emitters, 23, 28

skin reactions, 133–135, 222
  affecting sexual function, 69
  assessment of, 47–48, 49t
  with breast cancer, 447
  healing of, 47
  incidence/prevalence of, 47, 256
  long-term, 55
  management of, 48–55, 50t–53t
  pathophysiology of, 45–47, 45f, 256
  patient/family education on, 55
  risk factors for, 46–47, 209, 256–257
Skin Toxicity Assessment Tool, 48
sleep disorders/disturbance
  fatigue with, 38
  management of, 41
  in survivorship, 446
small cell lung cancer (SCLC), 217
SMART objectives, in patient education planning, 465
smoking
  psychological distress with, 62, 66
  RT side effects enhanced by, 15
social/family issues, 380–381
Society of Nuclear Medicine and Molecular Imaging, 431
soft tissue sarcomas, 265
  chemotherapy/immunotherapy for, 267
  diagnosis of, 267
  incidence of, 265
  patient/family education on, 271
  Prognostic factors, 265–266
  proton beam therapy for, 339
  risk factors for, 266–267
  RT options for, 267–269
  RT side effects, 269–271
  staging for, 265
  survivorship issues, 271
solid tumors
  with lymphoma, 276
  radiation-induced, 17
  radiopharmaceuticals for, 422
somnolence syndrome, 173–174, 349
source organs, in radioimmunotherapy, 421
special needs, definitions of, 374
sperm cryopreservation, 83
spills, of radiopharmaceuticals, 430
spinal cord compression, 287
  diagnosis of, 289
  incidence of, 287, 287f
  management of, 290–292, 291f
  nursing implications, 292
  pathophysiology of, 287–288
  prognostic factors, 289
  rehabilitation/palliative care, 292–293
  signs/symptoms of, 288, 288f
  treatment decisions, 289–290
Spinal Instability Neoplastic Score (SINS), 156
spinal metastases, 313, 454
spirituality, 67, 367
St. Louis University Mental Status Exam, 390
standards of care, 1, 462
Standards of Oncology Education: Patient/ Significant Other and Public, 462
START screening tool, 363
state licensure, 2

state nurse practice acts, 462
state regulatory commissions/agencies, 21, 23f
stereotactic body RT (SBRT), 12, 301, 436
  for lung cancers, 218–219, 313–314
  in older adult patients, 369
  for spinal cord compression, 291
stereotactic radiosurgery (SRS), 12, 281–282, 301, 436
  advantages of, 311
  for brain metastases, 454
  with cobalt-60, 342
  definition of, 311
  delivery systems, 315
  history of, 311
  indications for, 312–315
  patient/family education on, 317
  planning for, 315–316
  side effects of, 316–317
steroids
  for ESCC, 290–291, 291f
  for pain management, 59
  with palliative RT, 454
  topical, 53
stochastic effects, 17
STOPP screening tool, 363
stroke, 120–121
strontium-89, 28, 422
Stupid Cancer, 356
subacute side effects, defined, 172
subacutely responding tissues, 8
Subjective Global Assessment, 88, 230
substance use disorders, 408–410
suicide, incidence of, 62
suicide ideation, 410
superior vena cava obstruction, 454
superior vena cava syndrome (SVCS), 293–296, 294f
superoxide dismutase, 196
Support for People with Oral and Head and Neck Cancer (SPOHNC), 97
supportive care trials, 456
surveillance plans, in SCPs, 442
survivorship
  APN role in, 446
  in AYA patients, 355–356
  barriers to care in, 446
  definitions/statistics of, 441
  history of, 441
  models of care, 442–446
  nutrition issues in, 96–97
  in older adult patients, 358–360
  in pediatric populations, 350, 384, 449–450
  resources on, 450
  standards of, 441–442
survivorship care plans (SCPs), 441–442, 443f–445f
survivorship programs, 441–442
swallowing study, 449

T

tamulosin, 249
target organs, in radioimmunotherapy, 421
taste changes, 189–190, 449

taxanes, 145
Teen Cancer America, 356
Teenage Cancer Trust, 353
telephone peer support, 462
teletherapy, 19
temozolomide, 417–418
temporary brachytherapy, 6
terazosin, 249
Test of Functional Health Literacy in Adults, 464
testicular cancer, sexual dysfunction with, 73
testicular tissue cryopreservation, 83
therapeutic radionuclide information sheets, 28
therapeutic ratio, 415
three-dimensional conformal RT (3DCRT), 11–12, 46, 219, 299–300
thrombolytic therapy, 296
thymic malignancies, 218
thymoma, 218
time, radiation safety and, 24–25
tissue tolerance dose, 13, 13t–14t
tobacco use. *See* smoking
tocopherol, 193
toileting, during radiopharmaceutical therapy, 430
tolterodine tartrate, 249–250
topical steroids, 53
total body irradiation (TBI), 17, 73, 320
total lymphoid irradiation (TLI), 332–333
  indications for, 333–336
  patient/family education on, 336
  radiation fields for, 333, 333f–334f
  side effects of, 336
total skin irradiation, 330–332
transition clinic model, of survivorship care, 446
transportation/accommodation issues, 370, 381, 396
trastuzumab, 145
treated volume, 10, 10f
treatment adherence, 382
treatment planning, 11, 301–302
treatment simulator, 11, 301
treatment summaries, in SCPs, 442
treatment trials, 455–456
treatment volume, 10, 10f
Tri-Council Policy Statement (Canada), on informed consent, 457
tricyclic antidepressants, 41
trigeminal neuralgia, 313
trismus, 117–119, 188, 194–195
trispecific antibodies, 422
tumor board meetings, 345
tumor genetics, 209
tumor necrosis factor-alpha (TNF-α), 37
tumor node metastasis (TNM) staging system, 216, 218
tumor size, radiosensitivity affected by, 8
tumor vasculature, targeting of, 415
tumor-specific antigens, 432–433
Twist Out Cancer, 67
two-dimensional RT (2DRT), 299–300
tyrosine kinase inhibitors, 415

U

U.S. Department of Health and Human Services, 459

U.S. Food and Drug Administration (FDA), 21, 32, 459

U.S. Health Literacy Scale, 464

U.S. National Library of Medicine, 243

U.S. Nuclear Regulatory Commission (NRC), 20–21

umbilical cord blood, 321

Union for International Cancer Control, TNM system, 449

United Nations Environment Programme (UNEP), 18

unsealed radioactive sources, 19, 21*t*, 24, 29, 30*f*

urethral stricture/fibrosis, 131–132

urinary incontinence, 224

uterine cancer, effects in survivorship, 448

uveal melanomas, proton beam therapy for, 338

V

vaccines, 104, 328

vagal afferent nerve activation, fatigue from, 37

vaginal cancer, 255–256

vaginal dilation, 74–75, 77, 261–262, 448

vaginal dryness, 75, 132, 261, 448

vaginal infections, 260–261

vaginal stenosis, 71–72, 77, 132–133, 261

valvular disease, 144

Varian real-time position management system, 208

VARK model, of learning styles, 463

vascular changes
  from breast cancer RT, 213
  from head and neck RT, 197–198

vascular dementia, 388

vasculopathy, RT-induced, 109–110, 177–178

verification imaging, 86, 302

verification simulation, 11

vestibular schwannoma, 282–283

videofluorographic swallowing study, 449

vinblastine, 418

vincristine, 418

visual impairment, 376–377, 393

voice changes, with head and neck cancers, 115–116, 190–191

volume. *See* dose/volume

volumetric modulated arc therapy (VMAT), 245, 255, 299–300, 369

vomiting, 232. *See also* nausea/vomiting

Vulnerable Elders Survey-13 (VES-13), 362

vulvar cancer, 71, 255–256

W

Walking . . . A Step in the Right Direction (brochure), 43

white blood cells (WBCs), 99–100

whole-brain radiation, 389, 454

whole-breast RT, 203–204

work, return to, 355, 383

workplace safety, 410–411

World Nuclear Association, 431

wound healing, delayed after RT, 269–270

X

X-rays, 5, 5*f*, 18–19, 299

xerostomia, 93, 449
  with head and neck cancers, 112–114, 186–188

Y

Young Adult Cancer Canada, 356

yttrium-90, 28, 422, 423*f*, 427*t*

Z

Z0011 study (ACoS Oncology Group), 206